CURRENT THERAPY IN GASTROENTEROLOGY AND LIVER DISEASE

FOURTH EDITION

CURRENT THERAPY SERIES

CURRENT THERAPY IN
GASTROENTEROLOGY AND
LIVER DISEASE

FOURTH EDITION

THEODORE M. BAYLESS, M.D.
Professor of Medicine
The Johns Hopkins University School of Medicine
Clinical Director
Meyerhoff Digestive Disease-Inflammatory Bowel Disease Center
The Johns Hopkins Hospital
Baltimore, Maryland

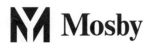

Mosby

St. Louis Baltimore Boston Chicago London Madrid Philadelphia Sydney Toronto

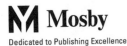
Mosby

Dedicated to Publishing Excellence

Executive Editor: Susan M. Gay
Senior Managing Editor: Lynne Gery
Project Manager: Linda Clarke
Project Supervisor: Vicki Hoenigke

FOURTH EDITION
Copyright © 1994 by Mosby–Year Book, Inc.

Previous editions copyrighted 1984, 1986, 1990

Printed in the United States of America

Mosby–Year Book, Inc.
11830 Westline Industrial Drive
St. Louis, Missouri 63146

NOTICE: The authors and publisher have made every effort to ensure that the patient care recommended herein, including choice of drugs and drug dosages, is in accord with the accepted standards and practice at the time of publication. However, since research and regulation constantly change clinical standards, the reader is urged to check the product information sheet included in the package of each drug, which includes recommended doses, warnings, and contraindications. This is particularly important with new or infrequently used drugs.

ISBN 0-8151-0421-9
94 95 96 97 GW/MY 9 8 7 6 5 4 3 2 1

CONTRIBUTORS

STEVEN A. AHRENDT, M.D.

Surgical Resident, The Johns Hopkins Medical Institutions, Baltimore, Maryland

ESTELLA M. ALONSO, M.D.

Assistant Professor of Pediatrics, University of Chicago Pritzker School of Medicine, Chicago, Illinois

DONALD A. ANTONIOLI, M.D.

Associate Professor of Pathology, Harvard Medical School; Associate Chief, Department of Pathology, Beth Israel Hospital, and Consultant in Gastrointestinal Pathology, The Children's Hospital, Boston, Massachusetts

DAVID A. APPEL, M.D.

Resident in General Surgery, Medical College of Wisconsin, Milwaukee, Wisconsin

ARTHUR H. AUFSES, Jr., M.D.

Franz W. Sichel Professor and Chairman, Department of Surgery, Mount Sinai Medical Center; Chairman, Department of Surgery, The Mount Sinai Hospital, New York, New York

JOHN BAILLIE, M.B., Ch.B., F.R.C.P. (Glasg.)

Associate Professor of Medicine, Duke University School of Medicine; Associate Director of Gastrointestinal Endoscopy, Division of Gastroenterology, Duke University Medical Center, Durham, North Carolina

JAMIE S. BARKIN, M.D., F.A.C.G., F.A.C.P.

Professor of Medicine, University of Miami School of Medicine, Miami; Chief, Division of Gastroenterology, Mt. Sinai Medical Center, Miami Beach, Florida

JOHN G. BARTLETT, M.D.

Professor of Medicine, and Chief, Infectious Disease Division, The Johns Hopkins University School of Medicine, Baltimore, Maryland

IVAN T. BECK, M.D. Ph.D., F.R.C.P.C., F.A.C.P., F.A.C.G.

Emeritus Professor of Medicine and of Physiology, Queen's University Faculty of Medicine; Consultant in Gastroenterology, Hotel Dieu Hospital and the Kingston General Hospital, Kingston, Ontario, Canada

JOHN R. BENNETT, M.D., F.R.C.P.

Consultant Physician, Hull Royal Infirmary, Hull, England

CARL L. BERG, M.D.

Instructor in Medicine, Harvard Medical School; Associate Physician, Gastroenterology Division, Brigham and Women's Hospital, Boston, Massachusetts

HENRY J. BINDER, M.D.

Professor of Medicine, Yale University School of Medicine, New Haven, Connecticut

INGVAR BJARNASON, M.D., M.Sc., M.R.C.Path.

Senior Lecturer and Honorary Consultant, Department of Clinical Biochemistry, King's College School of Medicine and Dentistry; Honorary Consultant Physician, Northwick Park Hospital, London, England

ANDRES T. BLEI, M.D.

Associate Professor of Medicine, Northwestern University School of Medicine; Attending Physician, Northwestern Memorial Hospital and Lakeside VA Medical Center, Chicago, Illinois

EDGAR C. BOEDEKER, M.D.

Professor of Medicine, Uniformed Services University School of Medicine, Bethesda, Maryland; Chief, Department of Gastroenterology, Walter Reed Army Institute of Research, Washington, D.C.

HERBERT L. BONKOVSKY, M.D.

Professor of Medicine, Biochemistry, and Molecular Biology, University of Massachusetts Medical School; Director, Center for Study of Disorders of Iron and Porphyrin Metabolism, and Director, Division of Digestive Disease and Nutrition, University of Massachusetts Medical Center, Worcester, Massachusetts

PATRICK G. BRADY, M.D.

Professor of Internal Medicine, University of South Florida College of Medicine; Chief, Section of Digestive Diseases and Nutrition, James A. Haley VA Medical Center, Tampa, Florida

DAVID W. BUCHHOLZ, M.D.

Associate Professor of Neurology, The Johns Hopkins University School of Medicine; Director, Neurological Consultation Clinic, The Johns Hopkins Outpatient Center, and Neurologic Consultant, The Johns Hopkins Swallowing Center, Baltimore, Maryland

HANS A. BÜLLER, M.D.

Co-Director, Pediatric Gastroenterology, Academisch Medisch Centrum, Amsterdam, The Netherlands

MICHAEL CAMILLERI, M.D.

Professor of Medicine, Mayo Medical School; Consultant in Gastroenterology and Physiology, Mayo Clinic, Rochester, Minnesota

PAOLO CARACENI, M.D.

Research Associate, Oklahoma Medical Research Foundation, Oklahoma City, Oklahoma

LESLIE E. CASHEL, M.D.

Associate Medical Director, Harvard Community Health Plan of New England, Providence, Rhode Island

DONALD O. CASTELL, M.D.

Kimbel Professor and Chairman, Department of Medicine, Graduate Hospital; Clinical Professor of Medicine, University of Pennsylvania, Philadelphia, Pennsylvania

RICHARD E. CHAISSON, M.D.

Associate Professor of Medicine, Epidemiology and International Health, The Johns Hopkins University School of Medicine and School of Hygiene and Public Health; Director, AIDS Services, The Johns Hopkins University School of Medicine, Baltimore, Maryland

EUGENE B. CHANG, M.D.

Professor of Medicine, University of Chicago Pritzker School of Medicine, Chicago, Illinois

LAWRENCE J. CHESKIN, M.D.

Assistant Professor of Medicine (Gastroenterology) and International Health (Human Nutrition), The Johns Hopkins University School of Medicine and School of Hygiene and Public Health; Staff Physician, Francis Scott Key Medical Center and The Johns Hopkins Hospital, Baltimore, Maryland

JUDY H. CHO, M.D.

Research and Clinical Fellow, Department of Medicine, University of Chicago Pritzker School of Medicine, Chicago, Illinois

JAMES CHONG, M.D.

Senior Fellow, Division of Gastroenterology, University of Miami School of Medicine, Miami, Florida

PAUL J. CICLITIRA, M.D., Ph.D., F.R.C.P.

Consultant Physician and Senior Lecturer, Gastroenterology Unit, St. Thomas' Hospital, London, England

ZANE COHEN, M.D., F.R.C.S.C., F.A.C.S.

Professor of Surgery, University of Toronto Faculty of Medicine; Surgeon-in-Chief, Mount Sinai Hospital, Toronto, Ontario, Canada

ROBERT E. CONDON, M.D., M.S.

Ausman Foundation Professor and Chairman, Department of Surgery, Medical College of Wisconsin; Chairman, Department of Surgery, Froedtert Memorial Lutheran Hospital, Milwaukee, Wisconsin

PETER F. CROOKES, M.D.

Assistant Unit Chief, Foregut Surgery Service, Los Angeles County-University of Southern California Medical Center, Los Angeles, California

MOUNES DAKKAK, M.D., Ph.D., M.R.C.P.

Specialist Gastroenterologist, Hull Royal Infirmary, Hull, England

BESS DAWSON-HUGHES, M.D.

Associate Professor of Medicine, Tufts University School of Medicine; Chief, Calcium and Bone Metabolism Laboratory, USDA Human Nutrition Research Center on Aging at Tufts University, Boston, Massachusetts

ARTHUR J. DeCROSS, M.D.

Senior Gastroenterology Fellow, University of Virginia, Charlottesville, Virginia

TOM R. DeMEESTER, M.D.

Professor and Chairman, Department of Surgery, University of Southern California School of Medicine, Los Angeles, California

STEPHEN F. DEUTSCH, M.D.

Attending Physician, West Suburban Hospital Medical Center, Oak Park, Illinois

ANNA MAE DIEHL, M.D.

Associate Professor of Medicine, Division of Gastroenterology, The Johns Hopkins University School of Medicine, Baltimore, Maryland

WILLIAM O. DOBBINS III, M.D.

Professor Emeritus of Internal Medicine, University of Michigan Medical School, Ann Arbor, Michigan

SUDHIR K. DUTTA, M.D.

Professor of Medicine, University of Maryland School of Medicine; Director, Division of Gastroenterology, Department of Medicine, Sinai Hospital of Baltimore, Baltimore, Maryland

STEFANO FAGIUOLI, M.D.

Senior Fellow in Transplant Medicine, Oklahoma Transplant Institute, Baptist Medical Center of Oklahoma, Oklahoma City, Oklahoma

RICHARD G. FARMER, M.D., F.A.C.P.

Clinical Professor of Medicine, Georgetown University Medical Center, Washington, D.C.

VICTOR W. FAZIO, M.D.

Chairman, Department of Colorectal Surgery, The Cleveland Clinic Foundation, Cleveland, Ohio

JEFFREY S. FEIN, M.D.

Chief Fellow, Gastroenterology, Memorial Sloan-Kettering Cancer Center, New York, New York

M. BRIAN FENNERTY, M.D.

Assistant Professor of Medicine, Assistant Chief of Medicine, and Director, Gastrointestinal Endoscopy, Arizona Health Sciences Center, Tucson, Arizona

FRANCIS D. FERDINAND, M.D.

Chief Resident in Thoracic Surgery, The University of Chicago, Chicago, Illinois

GEORGE D. FERRY, M.D.

Associate Professor of Clinical Pediatrics, Nutrition, and Gastroenterology, Baylor College of Medicine; Chief, Nutrition and Gastroenterology Clinic, Texas Children's Hospital, Houston, Texas

BARRY FINN, M.D.

Post-Doctoral Fellow in Gastroenterology, Northwestern University Medical School, Chicago, Illinois

JOSEF E. FISCHER, M.D.

Christian R. Holmes Professor and Chairman, Department of Surgery, University of Cincinnati College of Medicine; Surgeon-in-Chief, University Hospital and Christian R. Holmes Division, University of Cincinnati Medical Center, Cincinnati, Ohio

J. LAWRENCE FITZPATRICK, M.D.

Assistant Professor of Surgery, University of Maryland School of Medicine, Baltimore, Maryland

JONATHAN A. FLICK, M.D.

Associate Professor of Pediatrics, Temple University School of Medicine; Chief, Section of Gastroenterology and Nutrition, St. Christopher's Hospital for Children, Philadelphia, Pennsylvania

ARLENE A. FORASTIERE, M.D.

Associate Professor of Oncology, The Johns Hopkins University School of Medicine, Baltimore, Maryland

R. ARMOUR FORSE, M.D., Ph.D.

Associate Professor of Surgery, Harvard Medical School; Chief, Division of General Surgery, Deaconess Hospital, Boston, Massachusetts

LAWRENCE S. FRIEDMAN, M.D.

Associate Professor of Medicine, Harvard Medical School; Associate Physician, Gastrointestinal Unit, Massachusetts General Hospital, Boston, Massachusetts

SCOTT L. FRIEDMAN, M.D.

Associate Professor of Medicine, University of California, San Francisco, School of Medicine; Director, Gastrointestinal Clinic, and Attending Physician, San Francisco General Hospital, San Francisco, California

RICHARD K. FULLER, M.D.

Director, Division of Clinical Prevention and Research, National Institute on Alcohol Abuse and Alcoholism, National Institutes of Health, Rockville, Maryland

GARTH GEORGE, M.D.

Gastroenterology Fellow, University of Miami School of Medicine and Mt. Sinai Medical Center, Miami, Florida

PATRICK D. GERSTENBERGER, M.D.

Clinical Associate Professor of Medicine, University of New Mexico School of Medicine, Albuquerque, New Mexico; Physician, Digestive Disease Associates of the Four Corners, Durango, Colorado

RALPH A. GIANNELLA, M.D.

Mark Brown Professor of Medicine, and Director,
Division of Digestive Diseases, University of Cincinnati
College of Medicine; Staff Physician, VA Medical Center,
Cincinnati, Ohio

FRANCIS M. GIARDIELLO, M.D.

Associate Professor of Medicine, The Johns Hopkins
University School of Medicine, Baltimore, Maryland

YEVGENIY GINCHERMAN, B.A.

Research Fellow, Harrison Department of Surgical
Research, University of Pennsylvania School of
Medicine, Philadelphia, Pennsylvania

NORMAN M. GITLIN, M.D., F.R.C.P. (Lond),
F.R.C.P.E. (Edin)

Professor of Medicine and Chief of Hepatology, Emory
University School of Medicine, Atlanta, Georgia

MAE F. GO, M.D.

Assistant Professor of Medicine, Baylor College of
Medicine; Staff Physician, Digestive Diseases Section,
VA Medical Center, Houston, Texas

JOHN S. GOFF, M.D.

Clinical Professor of Medicine, University of Colorado,
Denver, Colorado

JOHN L. GOLLAN, M.D., Ph.D.

Associate Professor, Harvard Medical School; Senior
Physician, Brigham and Women's Hospital, Boston,
Massachusetts

ENOCH GORDIS, M.D.

Director, National Institute on Alcohol Abuse
and Alcoholism, National Institutes of Health,
Rockville, Maryland

DAVID Y. GRAHAM, M.D.

Professor of Medicine and Molecular Virology, and
Chief, Gastroenterology Section, Baylor College of
Medicine; Chief, Digestive Disease, VA Medical
Center, Houston, Texas

RICHARD J. GRAND, M.D.

Professor of Pediatrics, Tufts University School of
Medicine; Chief, Pediatric Gastroenterology and
Nutrition, New England Medical Center, Boston,
Massachusetts

ADRIAN J. GREENSTEIN, M.D.

Professor of Surgery, Mount Sinai Medical Center;
Attending Surgeon, The Mount Sinai Hospital,
New York, New York

WILLIAM G.M. HARDISON, M.D.

Professor of Medicine, University of California,
San Diego, School of Medicine; Staff Physician, VA
Medical Center, San Diego, California

WILLIAM V. HARFORD, M.D.

Assistant Professor of Medicine, University of Texas
Southwestern Medical Center at Dallas, Dallas, Texas

MARY L. HARRIS, M.D.

Assistant Professor of Medicine, Division of
Gastroenterology, The Johns Hopkins University School
of Medicine; Director, Endoscopy Fellowship Training,
The Johns Hopkins Hospital, Baltimore, Maryland

STEPHEN K. HEIER, M.D., F.A.C.P., F.A.C.G.

Chief, Section of Endoscopy, and Associate Professor of
Clinical Medicine, New York Medical College; Medical
Director, Endoscopy Unit, Westchester County Medical
Center, Valhalla, New York

RICHARD F. HEITMILLER, M.D.

Assistant Professor of Surgery, The Johns Hopkins
University School of Medicine, Baltimore, Maryland

VICTOR HERBERT, M.D., J.D.

Professor of Medicine, Mount Sinai School of
Medicine; Attending Physician, Mount Sinai and Bronx
VA Medical Centers, New York, New York

NEIL D. HERBSMAN, M.D.

Fellow, Department of Medicine, Memorial Sloan-
Kettering Cancer Center, New York, New York

H. FRANKLIN HERLONG, M.D.

Associate Professor of Medicine and Associate Dean
for Student Affairs, The Johns Hopkins University
School of Medicine, Baltimore, Maryland

ROBERT E. HERMANN, M.D.

Clinical Professor of Surgery, Case Western Reserve
University School of Medicine; Senior Surgeon and
Past Chairman, Department of General Surgery, The
Cleveland Clinic Foundation, Cleveland, Ohio

PAUL J. HESKETH, M.D.

Associate Professor of Medicine, Boston University
School of Medicine; Clinical Director, Section of
Medical Oncology, Boston University Medical Center,
Boston, Massachusetts

MELVIN B. HEYMAN, M.D., M.P.H.

Associate Professor and Chief, Pediatric
Gastroenterology and Nutrition, University of
California, San Francisco, San Francisco, California

A. CRAIG HILLEMEIER, M.D.

Associate Professor of Pediatrics, University of Michigan Medical Center, Ann Arbor, Michigan

LYN HOWARD, M.B., F.R.C.P., F.A.C.P.

Professor of Medicine, Associate Professor of Pediatrics, and Head, Division of Clinical Nutrition, Albany Medical College, Albany, New York

ANTHONY L. IMBEMBO, M.D.

Professor and Chairman, Department of Surgery, University of Maryland School of Medicine; Surgeon-in-Chief, Department of Surgery, University of Maryland Hospital, Baltimore, Maryland

MILES IRVING, M.D., F.R.C.S.

Professor of Surgery, University of Manchester School of Medicine, Manchester; Honorary Consultant Surgeon and Chairman, Department of Surgery, Hope Hospital, Salford, and Manchester Royal Infirmary, Manchester, England

DENNIS M. JENSEN, M.D.

Professor of Medicine, Division of Gastroenterology, University of California, Los Angeles, School of Medicine, Los Angeles, California

PAUL H. JORDAN, Jr., M.D.

Professor of Surgery, Baylor College of Medicine; Senior Surgeon, Methodist Hospital, Houston, Texas

ANTHONY N. KALLOO, M.D.

Director, Therapeutic Endoscopy, Division of Gastroenterology, The Johns Hopkins Hospital, Baltimore, Maryland

MARSHALL M. KAPLAN, M.D.

Professor of Medicine, Tufts University School of Medicine; Chief, Gastroenterology Division, New England Medical Center Hospitals, Boston, Massachusetts

TRACY STOPLER KASDAN, M.S., R.D.

Nutrition Program Coordinator, Mount Sinai and Bronx VA Medical Centers, New York, New York

DAVID A. KATZKA, M.D.

Attending Physician in Gastroenterology, Graduate Hospital, Philadelphia, Pennsylvania

ROGER G. KEITH, M.D., F.R.C.S.C., F.R.C.S., F.A.C.S.

Professor and Chairman, Department of Surgery, University of Saskatchewan College of Medicine; Chief of Surgery, Royal University Hospital, Saskatoon, Saskatchewan, Canada

QAZI E. KHUSRO, M.B., Ch.B.

Assistant Professor, Loyola University of Chicago Stritch School of Medicine; Attending Physician, Foster G. McGaw Hospital of Loyola University, Maywood, Illinois

MICHAEL B. KIMMEY, M.D.

Associate Professor of Medicine and Adjunct Associate Professor of Radiology, University of Washington School of Medicine; Director, Gastrointestinal Endoscopy, University of Washington Medical Center, Seattle, Washington

RALPH P. KINGSFORD, M.D.

Clinical Fellow, Pediatric Gastroenterology and Nutrition, University of California, San Francisco, San Francisco, California

ANDREW S. KLEIN, M.D.

Associate Professor of Surgery, The Johns Hopkins University School of Medicine; Director, Liver Transplant Program, The Johns Hopkins Hospital, Baltimore, Maryland

TAMSIN A. KNOX, M.D., M.P.H.

Assistant Professor of Medicine, Tufts University School of Medicine; Assistant Physician, New England Medical Center Hospital, Boston, Massachusetts

TIMOTHY R. KOCH, M.D.

Associate Professor of Medicine and Assistant Professor of Physiology, Medical College of Wisconsin; Attending Staff Physician, Zablocki VA Medical Center, Froedtert Memorial Lutheran Hospital, and Milwaukee County Medical Complex, Milwaukee, Wisconsin

A. J. KOVAR, M.S., R.D.

Pediatric Clinical Dietician Specialist, The Johns Hopkins Hospital, Baltimore, Maryland

RICHARD A. KOZAREK, M.D.

Clinical Professor of Medicine, University of Washington School of Medicine; Chief of Gastroenterology, Virginia Mason Clinic, Seattle, Washington

ROBERT C. KURTZ, M.D.

Professor of Medicine, Cornell University Medical College; Attending Physician, and Director, Gastrointestinal Endoscopy Unit, Memorial Sloan-Kettering Cancer Center, New York, New York

MARK J. KUTCHER, D.D.S., M.S.

Associate Professor and Chairman, Department of Diagnostic Sciences, University of North Carolina School of Dentistry, Chapel Hill, North Carolina

JUAN LECHAGO, M.D., Ph.D.

Professor of Pathology, Baylor College of Medicine; Director, Surgical Pathology, The Methodist Hospital, Houston, Texas

GLEN A. LEHMAN, M.D.

Professor of Medicine, Indiana University School of Medicine, Indianapolis, Indiana

JOHN E. LENNARD-JONES, M.D., F.R.C.P., F.R.C.S.

Emeritus Professor of Gastroenterology, University of London; Honorary Consulting Gastroenterologist, The Royal London Hospital and St. Mark's Hospital, London, England

SCOTT D. LEVENSON, M.D.

Clinical Instructor in Medicine, University of California, San Francisco, School of Medicine; Attending Physician, San Francisco General Hospital, San Francisco, California

BERNARD LEVIN, M.D.

Professor of Medicine, and Chairman, Department of Gastrointestinal Oncology and Digestive Diseases, University of Texas M.D. Anderson Cancer Center, Houston, Texas

KEITH D. LILLEMOE, M.D.

Associate Professor of Surgery, The Johns Hopkins University School of Medicine; Active Staff, Department of Surgery, The Johns Hopkins Hospital, Baltimore, Maryland

JOHN A. LoGIUDICE, M.D.

Director of Gastroenterology, West Suburban Hospital Medical Center, Oak Park, Illinois

SUSAN L. LUCAK, M.D.

Assistant Professor of Clinical Medicine, Columbia-Presbyterian Medical Center; Assistant Attending, Presbyterian Hospital, New York, New York

PETER HUGH MacDONALD, M.D., F.R.C.S.C.

Assistant Professor of Surgery, Queen's University Faculty of Medicine; General Surgeon, Kingston General Hosital and Hotel Dieu Hospital, Kingston, Ontario, Canada

ANDREW MacPHERSON, M.A., Ph.D., M.R.C.P.

MRC Clinician Scientist and Senior Lecturer in Medicine, King's College School of Medicine; Honorary Consultant Gastroenterologist, King's College Hospital, London, England

MARGARET MALONE, Ph.D., MRPharm.S.

Associate Professor of Pharmacy Practice, Albany College of Pharmacy, Albany, New York

NORMAN E. MARCON, M.D., F.R.C.P.C.

Assistant Professor of Medicine, University of Toronto Faculty of Medicine; Chief, Division of Gastroenterology, The Wellesley Hospital, Toronto, Ontario, Canada

RONALD E. MASON, M.D.

Clinical Research Fellow and Voluntary Instructor in Medicine, Division of Digestive Diseases, University of Cincinnati College of Medicine, Cincinnati, Ohio

PAUL N. MATON, M.D., F.R.C.P., F.A.C.P.

Oklahoma Foundation for Digestive Research, Oklahoma City, Oklahoma

RICHARD W. McCALLUM, M.D., F.A.C.P., F.R.A.C.P., F.A.C.G.

Paul Janssen Professor of Medicine, University of Virginia; Chief, Division of Gastroenterology, Hepatology, and Nutrition, University of Virginia Health Sciences Center, Charlottesville, and Program Director, Gastroenterology Training Program, Salem VA Medical Center, Salem, and Roanoke Memorial Hospital, Roanoke, Virginia

AIDEEN McGUINNESS, B.Sc.

Clinical Nutritionist/Dietitian, Meath Hospital, Dublin, Ireland

ROBIN S. McLEOD, M.D., F.R.C.S.C., F.A.C.S.

Associate Professor of Surgery, University of Toronto Faculty of Medicine; Staff Surgeon, Mount Sinai Hospital, Toronto, Ontario, Canada

CHARLES E. McQUEEN, M.D.

Assistant Professor of Medicine, Uniformed Services University of the Health Sciences, Bethesda, Maryland; Staff Gastroenterologist, Walter Reed Army Medical Center, Washington, D.C.

PHILIP B. MINER, Jr., M.D.

Professor of Medicine, and Director, Division of Gastroenterology, University of Kansas, Kansas City, Kansas

EMIL P. MISKOVSKY, M.D.

Assistant Professor of Medicine, Division of Gastroenterology, The Johns Hopkins University School of Medicine, Baltimore, Maryland

MACK C. MITCHELL, M.D.

Associate Professor of Medicine, The Johns Hopkins University School of Medicine; Chairman of Medicine, Greater Baltimore Medical Center, Baltimore, Maryland

ROBERT K. MONTGOMERY, Ph.D.

Assistant Professor, Division of Pediatric Gastroenterology and Nutrition, New England Medical Center and Tufts University School of Medicine, Boston, Massachusetts

SANTIAGO J. MUNOZ, M.D.

Associate Professor of Medicine, and Medical Director, Liver Transplantation Program, Jefferson Medical College of Thomas Jefferson University, Philadelphia, Pennsylvania

JOSEPH M. NESTA, M.D.

Assistant Clinical Instructor, Department of Medicine, University of Connecticut School of Medicine, Hartford, Connecticut

JOHN E. NIEDERHUBER, M.D.

Professor and Chairman of Surgery, and Professor of Microbiology and Immunology, Stanford University School of Medicine; Chief, Surgery Service, Stanford University Hospital, Stanford, California

COLM O'MORAIN, Ph.D.

Professor of Gastroenterology, Trinity College; Head, Department of Medicine, Meath-Adelaide Hospitals, Dublin, Ireland

FLOYD A. OSTERMAN, Jr., M.D.

Associate Professor, Director of Cardiovascular Diagnostic Radiology, and Section Chief, Interventional Radiology, The Johns Hopkins Hospital, Baltimore, Maryland

PANKAJ J. PASRICHA, M.D.

Assistant Professor of Medicine, The Johns Hopkins University School of Medicine; Staff, Division of Gastroenterology, The Johns Hopkins Hospital, Baltimore, Maryland

JOHN H. PEMBERTON, M.D.

Associate Professor of Surgery, Mayo Medical School; Consultant in Colon and Rectal Surgery, Mayo Clinic, Rochester, Minnesota

MARK A. PEPPERCORN, M.D.

Associate Professor of Medicine, Harvard Medical School; Director, Center for Inflammatory Bowel Disease, Beth Israel Hospital, Boston, Massachusetts

ROBERT E. PETRAS, M.D.

Chairman, Department of Anatomic Pathology, Cleveland Clinic Foundation, Cleveland, Ohio

DOMINIQUE Q. PHAM, M.D.

Fellow in Gastroenterology and Hepatology, VA Medical Center, Washington, D.C.

HENRY A. PITT, M.D.

Professor and Vice-Chairman, Department of Surgery, The Johns Hopkins Medical Institutions, Baltimore, Maryland

DANIEL H. PRESENT, M.D.

Clinical Professor of Medicine, Mount Sinai School of Medicine of the City University of New York, New York, New York

PHILIP PUTNAM, M.D.

Assistant Professor of Pediatrics, Department of Pediatric Gastroenterology, Children's Hospital, Pittsburgh, Pennsylvania

JOHN H.C. RANSON, B.M., B.Ch., M.A.

S. A. Localio Professor of Surgery, New York University School of Medicine; Director, Division of General Surgery, New York University Medical Center, Associate Director of Surgery, Tisch Hospital, and Attending Physician, Bellevue Hospital Center and New York University Medical Center, New York, New York

JEFFREY B. RASKIN, M.D.

Professor of Medicine, Division of Gastroenterology, University of Miami School of Medicine, Miami, Florida

A.J. RATE, F.R.C.S.

Tutor in Surgery, University of Manchester School of Medicine, Manchester; Honorary Registrar in Surgery, Salford Health Authority, Salford, England

DAVID W. RATTNER, M.D., F.A.C.S.

Associate Professor of Surgery, Harvard Medical School, Boston, Massachusetts

WILLIAM J. RAVICH, M.D.

Associate Professor of Medicine, Division of Gastroenterology, The Johns Hopkins University School of Medicine; Director, Gastrointestinal Endoscopy and The Gastrointestinal Diagnostic Laboratory, and Clinical Director, The Johns Hopkins Swallowing Center, The Johns Hopkins Medical Institutions, Baltimore, Maryland

WILLIAM G. RECTOR, Jr., M.D.

Associate Clinical Professor of Medicine, University of Colorado Health Sciences Center, Denver, Colorado

JAMES C. REYNOLDS, M.D.

Associate Professor of Medicine and of Cell Biology and Physiology, University of Pittsburgh School of Medicine; Chief, Division of Gastroenterology and Hepatology, Co-Director, Digestive Disorders Center, and Director, Gastrointestinal Laboratory, University of Pittsburgh Medical Center, Pittsburgh, Pennsylvania

JOEL E. RICHTER, M.D.

Professor of Medicine and Director of Clinical Research, Gastroenterology Division, University of Alabama School of Medicine, Birmingham, Alabama

LAYTON F. RIKKERS, M.D.

M.M. Musselman Professor and Chairman, Department of Surgery, University of Nebraska Medical Center, Omaha, Nebraska

MALCOLM G. ROBINSON, M.D.

Clinical Professor of Medicine, University of Oklahoma College of Medicine; President and Medical Director, Oklahoma Foundation for Digestive Research, Oklahoma City, Oklahoma

JOHN L. ROMBEAU, M.D.

Associate Professor of Surgery, Hospital of the University of Pennsylvania, Philadelphia, Pennsylvania

J. N. ROSENSWEIG, M.D.

Clinical Fellow, Division of Pediatric Gastroenterology and Nutrition, The Johns Hopkins University School of Medicine, Baltimore, Maryland

GAYLE M. ROSENTHAL, M.D.

Staff Physician, West Suburban Gastroenterology, Oak Park, Illinois

JOEL J. ROSLYN, M.D.

Alma Dea Morani Professor and Chairman, Department of Surgery, Medical College of Pennsylvania, Philadelphia, Pennsylvania

BRUCE S. ROTHSCHILD, M.D.

Assistant Professor of Psychiatry, University of Connecticut School of Medicine, Farmington; Director, Consultation-Liaison Psychiatry Services, St. Francis Hospital and Medical Center, Hartford, Connecticut

ANIL K. RUSTGI, M.D.

Assistant Professor of Medicine, Harvard Medical School; Assistant Physician, Massachusetts General Hospital, Boston, Massachusetts

ROBERT A. SANOWSKI, M.D.

Clinical Professor of Medicine, University of Arizona College of Medicine, Tucson; Chief of Gastroenterology, Carl T. Hayden VA Medical Center, Phoenix, Arizona

MICHAEL G. SARR, M.D.

Associate Professor of Surgery, Mayo Medical School; Chairman, Division of Gastroenterologic and General Surgery, Mayo Clinic and Mayo Foundation; Consultant, Gastroenterologic Research Unit, Mayo Clinic, Rochester, Minnesota

SCOTT J. SAVADER, M.D.

Assistant Professor of Radiology and Surgery, The Johns Hopkins Hospital, Baltimore, Maryland

THOMAS J. SAVIDES, M.D.

Assistant Clinical Professor of Medicine, University of California, San Diego, School of Medicine, San Diego, California

I. HERBERT SCHEINBERG, M.D.

Professor of Medicine Emeritus, Albert Einstein College of Medicine of Yeshiva University, Bronx; Attending and Senior Research Associate, St. Luke's-Roosevelt Hospital Center, New York, New York

PAUL C. SCHROY III, M.D.

Assistant Professor of Medicine, Boston University School of Medicine; Assistant Visiting Physician, Boston University Medical Center, The University Hospital, and Boston City Hospital, Boston; Attending Physician, Boston VA Medical Center, Jamaica Plain, Massachusetts

ARND SCHULTE-BOCKHOLT, M.D.

Research Fellow in Gastroenterology, University of Frankfurt and University Hospital, Frankfurt, Germany

MARVIN M. SCHUSTER, M.D., F.A.C.P., F.A.P.A.

Professor of Medicine and Psychiatry, The Johns Hopkins University School of Medicine; Director, Division of Digestive Diseases, Francis Scott Key Medical Center, Baltimore, Maryland

SEYMOUR I. SCHWARTZ, M.D.

Professor and Chair, Department of Surgery, University of Rochester School of Medicine and Dentistry; Surgeon in Chief, Strong Memorial Hospital, Rochester, New York

LEONARD B. SEEFF, M.D.

Professor of Medicine, Georgetown University School of Medicine; Chief of Gastroenterology and Hepatology, VA Medical Center, Washington, D.C.

ELDON A. SHAFFER, M.D., F.R.C.P.C., F.A.C.P.

Professor and Head, Department of Medicine, The University of Calgary Faculty of Medicine; Director, Department of Medicine, Foothills Hospital, Calgary, Alberta, Canada

JAMES V. SITZMANN, M.D.

Associate Professor of Surgery, Director, Division of Surgical Oncology and Nutrition Support Service, and Medical Director, Tumor Registry, The Johns Hopkins Hospital; Consultant Surgeon, VA Hospital, Baltimore, Maryland

LEE E. SMITH, M.D.

Professor of Surgery, and Director, Division of Colon and Rectal Surgery, George Washington University School of Medicine and Health Sciences, Washington, D.C.

ANDREW H. SOLL, M.D.

Professor of Medicine, and Director, Affiliated Training Program in Gastroenterology, University of California, Los Angeles, School of Medicine; Chief, Gastroenterology, Wadsworth VA Medical Center, Los Angeles, California

HANS W. SOLLINGER, M.D., Ph.D.

Professor of Surgery and Pathology, University of Wisconsin School of Medicine, Madison, Wisconsin

JOHN G. STAGIAS, M.D.

Senior Gastroenterology Fellow, Yale University School of Medicine, New Haven, and Griffin Hospital, Derby, Connecticut

RANDOLPH M. STEINHAGEN, M.D.

Assistant Professor of Surgery, Mount Sinai School of Medicine of the City University of New York; Assistant Attending, The Mount Sinai Hospital, New York, New York

IRMIN STERNLIEB, M.D.

Professor of Medicine Emeritus, Albert Einstein College of Medicine of Yeshiva University, Bronx; Attending and Senior Research Associate, St. Luke's-Roosevelt Hospital Center, New York, New York

JAMES M. STONE, M.D.

Assistant Professor, Stanford University School of Medicine, Stanford, California

PAUL H. SUGARBAKER, M.D.

Director, Surgical Oncology, The Cancer Institute, Washington Hospital Center, Washington, D.C.

HATTON SUMNER, M.D.

Clinical Assistant Professor of Pathology, University of Oklahoma College of Medicine; Director, Surgical Pathology, HCA Presbyterian Hospital, Oklahoma City, Oklahoma

UMA SUNDARAM, M.D.

Assistant Professor of Medicine, Yale University School of Medicine; Attending Physician, Yale-New Haven Hospital and West Haven VA Hospital, New Haven, Connecticut

LLOYD R. SUTHERLAND, M.D.C.M., M.Sc., F.R.C.P.C., F.A.C.P.

Professor of Medicine and Head, Divison of Gastroenterology, University of Calgary Faculty of Medicine; Chief of Gastroenterology, Foothills Hospital, Calgary, Alberta, Canada

MARK A. TALAMINI, M.D.

Assistant Professor of Surgery and Director of Minimally Invasive Surgery, The Johns Hopkins Hospital, Baltimore, Maryland

GORDON L. TELFORD, M.D.

Associate Professor of Surgery, Medical College of Wisconsin, Milwaukee, Wisconsin

CHARLES R. THOMAS, Jr., M.D.

Assistant Professor, Division of Oncology, Department of Medicine, and Research Fellow, Division of Experimental Biology, Department of Radiation Oncology, University of Washington School of Medicine, Seattle, Washington

W. GRANT THOMPSON, M.D.

Professor of Medicine, University of Ottawa Faculty of Medicine; Chief, Division of Gastroenterology, Ottawa Civic Hospital, Ottawa, Ontario, Canada

PAUL J. THULUVATH, M.B., B.S., M.D., M.R.C.P. (UK)

Assistant Professor of Medicine, The Johns Hopkins University School of Medicine; Active Staff, Medicine, The Johns Hopkins Hospital, Baltimore, Maryland

GREGORY M. TIAO, M.D.

House Officer, Department of Surgery, University of Cincinnati Medical Center, Cincinnati, Ohio

THOMAS G. TIETJEN, M.D.

Senior Clinical Fellow, Division of Gastroenterology, The Johns Hopkins University School of Medicine, Baltimore, Maryland

JOE J. TJANDRA, M.D.

Consultant Colorectal Surgeon, Melbourne University and Royal Melbourne Hospital, Parkville, Victoria, Australia

MORRIS TRAUBE, M.D.

Associate Professor of Medicine, Yale University School of Medicine; Director, Gastrointestinal Procedure Center, Yale-New Haven Hospital, New Haven, Connecticut

WILLIAM J. TREMAINE, M.D.

Assistant Professor of Medicine, Mayo Graduate School of Medicine; Head, Inflammatory Bowel Disease Clinic, Mayo Clinic, Rochester, Minnesota

SUSAN G. URBA, M.D.

Assistant Professor, Department of Internal Medicine, Division of Hematology/Oncology, University of Michigan Medical Center, Ann Arbor, Michigan

DAVID H. VAN THIEL, M.D.

Medical Director of Transplantation, Baptist Medical Center of Oklahoma, Oklahoma City, Oklahoma

ANTHONY C. VENBRUX, M.D.

Associate Professor, and Associate Director, Cardiovascular Diagnostic Laboratory, The Johns Hopkins Hospital, Baltimore, Maryland

RAMA P. VENU, M.D.

Professor of Clinical Medicine, University of Illinois College of Medicine, Chicago; Consultant in Gastroenterology, West Suburban Hospital Medical Center, Oak Park, Illinois

ARNOLD WALD, M.D.

Professor of Medicine, and Associate Chief, Gastroenterology Section, University of Pittsburgh Medical Center, Pittsburgh, Pennsylvania

DAVID T. WALDEN, M.D.

Assistant Professor of Medicine, and Director of Endoscopy, The University of Texas Medical Branch at Galveston, Galveston, Texas

SHARON WESTERBERG, B.A.

Research Assistant, Jefferson Medical College of Thomas Jefferson University, Philadelphia, Pennsylvania

WILLIAM E. WHITEHEAD, Ph.D.

Research Professor of Medicine and Adjunct Professor of Psychology, University of North Carolina at Chapel Hill, Chapel Hill, North Carolina

PETER F. WHITINGTON, M.D.

Professor of Pediatrics and Medicine, University of Chicago, Pritzker School of Medicine; Director, Section of Pediatric Gastroenterology, Hepatology and Nutrition, and Pediatric Liver Transplant Program, Wyler Children's Hospital, Chicago, Illinois

SIDNEY J. WINAWER, M.D.

Chief, Gastroenterology and Nutrition Service, Memorial Sloan-Kettering Cancer Center, New York, New York

THOMAS N. WISE, M.D.

Professor and Vice Chair, Department of Psychiatry, Georgetown University School of Medicine, Washington, D.C.; Chair, Department of Psychiatry, Fairfax Hospital, Falls Church, Virginia

M. MICHAEL WOLFE, M.D.

Assistant Professor of Medicine, Harvard Medical School; Associate Physician, Brigham and Women's Hospital, Boston, Massachusetts

MARTIN S. WOLFE, M.D.

Clinical Professor of Medicine, George Washington University School of Medicine, and Clinical Associate Professor of Medicine, Georgetown University School of Medicine; Director, Traveler's Medical Service of Washington, D.C.

COL. ROY K.H. WONG, M.D., M.C.

Associate Professor of Medicine, Uniformed Services University of the Health Sciences; Chief of Gastroenterology, Walter Reed Army Medical Center, Washington, D.C.

TIMOTHY A. WOODWARD, M.D.

Mayo Scholar, Mayo Clinic, Rochester, Minnesota; Visiting Clinical Professor, University of Texas M.D. Anderson Cancer Center, Houston, Texas

HARLAN I. WRIGHT, M.D.

Staff, Transplantation Medicine, Baptist Medical Center, Oklahoma City, Oklahoma

CHARLES J. YEO, M.D.

Associate Professor of Surgery, The Johns Hopkins University School of Medicine; Attending Surgeon, The Johns Hopkins Hospital, Baltimore, Maryland

This, the fourth edition of *Current Therapy in Gastroenterology and Liver Disease*, was undertaken because of the continuing changes in the medical, surgical, and nutritional management options for many digestive disease disorders. The third edition, published in 1990 (written in 1989), was very well received. Thirty-five new topics have been added to this edition.

Although there are excellent textbooks on the diagnosis and pathophysiology of gastrointestinal and liver disease, many of these expansive and encyclopedic texts do not provide specific and detailed guidelines for treatment. While reviews of the literature and results of double-blind controlled trials are reported in depth, the reader may not be given an explicit treatment preference or choice of reasonable options for a very specific patient management problem.

The realization that the information on therapy is changing and may be difficult to extract from some comprehensive texts prompted the preparation of the first three editions of this and other books in the *Current Therapy* series.

These books have had broad appeal: in addition to our target audience—physicians experienced in diagnosing and treating digestive and liver disorders, as well as trainees in gastroenterology—internists, primary care physicians, and medical and surgical house officers buy these books because of their value as a terse and authoritative "consultation." Some liken it to having an expert on call at all times. Since each edition is written by new authors (or, as in this fourth edition, world's experts asked to update their contribution to a previous edition), we try to make each edition a "new book." Many readers tell me (as did the *New England Journal* reviewer of an earlier edition) that this book has a prominent spot on their desks, along with the *PDR*, when they are seeing patients. I believe that assembling this book is one of the more useful things I do for patients with digestive disorders.

My sincere appreciation is extended to the contributing authors, who have generously shared their expertise and experience with us. My friend and colleague, Dr. Marshall Bedine, read most of the chapters and provided excellent insight from the vantage of a busy and experienced practitioner. Thanks also to my wife for her tolerance during the editing process; to my secretary, Gayla Roche; and to my editor at Mosby, Lynne Gery. Also, a sentimental thanks to my previous publisher, Brian Decker, and my previous editor, Mary Mansor. To the "authors" who flunked our deadlines, we'll miss your contributions in this edition and will have to rely on the relevant chapters in the third edition. Shame, shame.

Theodore M. Bayless, M.D.

CONTENTS

SMALL INTESTINE

COLON AND RECTUM

THE LIVER

GENERAL TOPICS

PRACTICING GASTROENTEROLOGY IN AN HMO

LESLIE E. CASHEL, M.D.

The basics of gastroenterology practice should be the same no matter in what medical setting the physician and the patient find themselves. Patients either have or perceive they have a gastrointestinal problem. Gastroenterologists endeavor to diagnose and explain the condition to patients and then to cure or, more likely, aid them in coping with a chronic condition in a therapeutic and empathetic fashion. Different medical settings, such as academic hospital practice, fee-for-service (FFS) practice, health maintenance organization (HMO) practice, and clinics, present different environments in which the basic gastroenterology practice occurs. This difference in environment, principally between FFS practice and a staff model health maintenance organization (HMO-S) practice, is the subject of this chapter.

STAFF/GROUP HEALTH MAINTENANCE ORGANIZATIONS

A staff model HMO is a health insurance corporation that owns medical office buildings and hires physicians to work in those buildings and provide health care only to those patients who join that particular health plan. Staff model HMOs vary enormously from one to the other and from one part of the country to another in their organizational structure, both managerially and clinically. For example, the staff model HMOs in the western United States are more likely to have family practitioners as their primary care providers with internists and pediatricians as consultants, while those in the eastern United States are more likely to have internists and pediatricians as their primary care providers.

Small staff model HMOs may hire only primary care providers and contract all specialty care, including gastroenterology, with specialists in otherwise FFS practice. Such gastroenterologists may be asked to undertake clinical sessions in the health plan's medical building for a set fee per session, usually 4 hours, and the health plan pays discounted FFS charges for procedures. However, the originality of possible contract arrangements knows no bounds and they are innumerable.

In general, as an HMO grows in membership, the plan finds that it is more cost effective to hire its own specialists, although this is admittedly controversial and depends on how well the FFS specialist and the plan are able to negotiate mutually agreeable financial arrangements. One rule of thumb is one gastroenterologist per 45,000 members. This is not hard and fast and depends on the demographics of the plan's membership. Plans vary widely in the number of Medicare members they service, and the ratio of gastroenterologist to members is often weighted for age. In our plan, Harvard Community Health Plan of New England (HCHP-NE), every Medicare member counts as four regular adult members to compensate for the extra medical attention the over-65 population needs. This was determined by a time accrual study conducted in our centers and may vary for other HMOs.

Most of my remarks about gastroenterology practice in an HMO-S are based on my experience working at HCHP-NE (formerly Rhode Island Group Health Association). It is not my intent to present an exhaustive culmination of practice experience in all staff model HMOs across the country. There are also many large group practices whose practice milieu may not be dramatically different from those described in an HMO-S. Indeed, it is my feeling that over time the FFS practice environment is becoming more like HMO practice and vice versa, rather than moving further apart. In no way am I trying to say or prove that one medical environment is better than another.

FINANCIAL INCENTIVES

In the 1970s, some of the differences between HMO-S practice and FFS practice were in the division of care and money and the incentives, positive or negative, to hospitalize. Patients paid FFS physicians a fee at the door for that office visit or service. The FFS physician had to worry about comments indicating the patient's perceived direct value of a given visit, such as "I just paid you 80 dollars to tell me to take Maalox?" Patients in an HMO-S paid their premium once a month no matter how many office visits they incurred. Thus, HMO physicians could have patients return to the office every day to check the blood count, for example, without worrying about patient complaints regarding cost, although they might have to answer the question, "Why don't you just put me in the hospital?" FFS physicians would likely put mildly ill patients in the hospital rather than see them in the office every day, because there were monetary incentives and it was more convenient for both patient and physician to do so. The difference in whether a fee occurred at the time of the office visit was felt by some to be more likely to channel chronic complainers to an HMO-S. Without a fee, patients would come in more often for minor complaints, and HMO physicians would see more difficult psychosomatic patients. I have not seen definitive proof either way. At this point, it does not matter, because almost all HMOs are charging co-pays for each visit, often at the behest of the employer, and there are increasingly strict rules governing which type of patient problems warrant hospital admission. So, whether one is in FFS or HMO-S practice, one is dealing with rules for hospitalization and FFS in the office.

Another difference lies in how physicians are reimbursed. HMO-S physicians usually receive a paycheck regularly no matter how many procedures they perform, how many patients are in the hospital, and how many patients cancel or do not show up in the office. HMO-S physicians negotiate their salaries and benefits once a year with one administration. There now exist several surveys of salaried physician compensation, including gastroenterologists, so there are nationwide data with which to compare. FFS physicians salaries depended on their productivity. The more procedures carried out and patients seen, the higher was the remuneration. Remuneration is changing for both physician groups. Some HMOs are beginning to have productivity standards and are instituting monetary incentives of some kind. FFS physicians are entering into capitation agreements with regular payments, often with multiple different insurers.

If an FFS gastroenterologist leaves for a week to take a CME course or go to the AGA meeting, or even take a well-earned vacation, he or she is losing money. The overhead continues and no money is coming in during the period the physician is not seeing patients. HMO-S gastroenterologists do not lose money. They are guaranteed so many weeks per year for vacation, usually 4, and for educational leave, usually 2. In addition, most plans have an educational allowance for each physician, usually around $3,000.

OFFICE SUPPORT STAFF

In FFS, nurses, receptionists, and technicians are hired and managed by the physician(s) or by an office manager who reports to the physician(s). In an HMO-S the support staff is hired and managed by a management structure separate from the physicians. Different HMOs vary in how much interaction there is between the physicians and the management of the support staff. This may include input into evaluations, job interviewing, or participation in disciplinary action. Many HMO-S physicians are relieved not to have responsibility for support staff and decline participation in their management. Other HMO-S physicians feel that not having direct responsibility for support staff changes the attitude of the latter, making them less accommodating. Physicians who work in hospital endoscopy areas where support staff report to a hospital hierarchy often have the same concerns. Support staff in an HMO-S situation may be more likely to lodge a complaint against a physician than if they worked for the physician directly.

OFFICE PROCEDURE

Endoscopy can be performed in an office setting. Dr. Overholt gives an excellent course on how to establish an endoscopy suite. I suspect it is much easier to establish such a suite in an HMO setting than in a private office because of the difference in regulatory requirements. HMOs do not require a certificate of need. I have been performing outpatient endoscopy for over 10 years. Our endoscopy suite is situated next to the "code room" and in the same area where the cardiologists are doing stress tests. Emergency equipment and personnel are readily available. Upper and lower endoscopies, polypectomies, and esophageal dilatations are performed. Fluoroscopy is available in our radiology department, and I simply book the patient in radiology when fluoroscopy is needed. Clearly, a very sick or high-risk patient would be scheduled to be seen in a hospital rather than as an outpatient. The HMO-S gastroenterologist does not personally incur the overhead monetary layout nor the risk of covering initial operational costs; this is borne by the HMO. In addition, physicians in HMOs compete only with themselves for endoscopy time. They usually get to choose the equipment and, since there are fewer people using it, there are fewer breakdowns.

I have also been performing liver biopsies in the center for about a decade. The patient stays in the recovery room the entire day after the biopsy is done early in the morning. Thus, I can check the patient any time during the day while I am seeing other patients. The patient is discharged at the end of the day and returns the following morning to the center for a further check. The savings to the plan are considerable and the outcome is no different than in an outpatient hospital setting. Patients are allowed to bring television sets, headsets, a friend, or anything within reason to keep them from being bored during their stay. I like to be able to see the patient during the day. On rare occasions I have found that a patient whose biopsy was done in a hospital setting has been allowed to get up and walk around or has not had a repeat blood count, despite written orders. When the patient is in my center, I can be assured that I am aware of a problem and that he or she is indeed in bed. Patients who have major risk factors are treated in a hospital setting. Only two of my patients have had to be transported to the hospital after liver biopsy in the center. One patient had very severe pain that stopped as soon as he reached the Emergency Department, and no complications were found. The other patient's blood count dropped, but this was later found to be a laboratory error, and she was fine.*

We have all been faced with a patient who claims to be vomiting and has not kept anything down for days, and yet whose examination does not reveal dehydration and whose basic chemistries are normal. In FFS practice, the physician often has no choice but to hospitalize patients and have the nurses observe if they really are vomiting or having diarrhea. I often have these patients come into the center and spend the day in our recovery room; this way I can check them frequently all day. I can employ a nurse whose sole responsibility is to observe and take care of individual patients without needing to attend to half a floor of patients, as often happens in the hospital. It is cheaper for the plan to pay a nurse overtime to be with the patient one on one in the center than to admit the patient, and it gives me much more clinical information faster. Because other physicians are in the center seeing patients, I can often arrange for a surgeon, a psychiatrist, or whomever else I need to see the patient at some time during the day, and I can personally discuss the case with them. I may even endoscope the patient, if despite the initial normal laboratory tests, the condition progresses and the patient is clearly ill. The patient is promptly sent to the hospital. More often, patients become bored in the recovery room, where it is really quiet, and if they are not symptomatic they want to go home. I had one young man who decided by 2 PM that he really did want a divorce and felt much better.

REFERRAL PATTERNS

Referral patterns are as individual as physicians themselves. FFS gastroenterologists often devote considerable time and energy to establishing a referral practice, and worry about losing referrals as younger gastroenterologists enter the community. More FFS physicians are now participating in health plans with a restricted list of providers, and this has affected some otherwise well established referral patterns that took years to build. In an HMO-S setting, one is guaranteed a practice. The plan would not have hired the physician if the patients were not already there. In the past, FFS gastroenterologists could refer a patient anywhere they wanted while an HMO-S gastroenterologist would only be able to refer to facilities or physicians on a "desig-

nated" provider list. If the HMO-S gastroenterologist wanted to refer a patient for a special test or procedure not on the designated list, the referral would have to be approved by a chief or a medical director. The gastroenterologist may be asked to provide literature or other back-up material showing that this was the standard practice and not an experimental procedure or of unproved benefit. The gastroenterologist can also argue why an exception should be made if there are special mitigating circumstances. Of course, many FFS gastroenterologists now participate in health plans that also have designated provider lists and require preauthorization. The difference sometimes is that the HMO-S gastroenterologist most often has a working relationship with the person doing the authorizing, who is most likely a physician, while the FFS gastroenterologist is often dealing with a nurse over the phone with whom he or she does not have a working relationship.

MILIEU

I have always been amazed at how often I have seen FFS gastroenterologist practices break up and reform. In that sense, FFS physicians hire and fire each other. In large subspecialty groups the hiring and firing process may become more formal. In an HMO-S the hiring and firing process, and certainly the evaluation process, can be very formal. In my HMO-S, physicians are evaluated 3 and 6 months after being hired and annually thereafter. Evaluation forms go to all the primary care providers who refer to the gastroenterologist as a specialist, to the support staff that works with the physician, and to the appropriate management offices to determine what, if any, consumer complaints or legal activity occurred in relation to the physician. Charts are reviewed. Reports from morbidity and mortality reviews and from the risk management department are collected. Physicians who perform procedures have their complication rate reported. The evaluation is conducted between the physician and his or her chief.

We have a very detailed due-process system for physician discipline, be it a question of medical competence or management competence. The due-process system was designed by physicians in the plan. Management competence includes compliance with the policies of the plan and ability to interact appropriately with peers, support staff, or patients. Discipline procedures are carried out by physician chiefs and medical directors, but may involve a physician peer review committee for issues of medical competency. Probably more physicians have asked to leave the plan because of their inability to get along in a group setting than for medical competency issues. FFS gastroenterologists are beginning to deal with discipline issues often designed by government agencies and often by specialties other than gastroenterology that cover gastroenterology practice. This has led to some interesting controversies.

As FFS practices grow larger, they can afford more support staff. A large group of gastroenterologists may

---

*Editor's Note: A recent article on ambulatory liver biopsy reassuringly revealed that the few complaints that would require hospitalization are suspected within the first few hours after biopsy.

employ a nutritionist in their office. In an HMO-S, even though there may be only one or two gastroenterologists, the plan may be able to support a nutritionist who supports not only gastroenterology but also internists, obstetricians, and pediatricians. Many HMO-S practices have consumer relations representatives, who do not have a medical background and are employed as patient advocates. If a patient is displeased about something, it is quite permissible to move them on to the consumer relations representative and out of your office. Often the issue is a misunderstanding, an insurance coverage issue, or an actual error. Sometimes the patient is just belligerent. The consumer relations representatives are trained to allow the patient to ventilate, to determine whether there is a valid solvable issue, and to help the patient resolve the issue. Sometimes the gastroenterologist needs to become involved again; sometimes patients need to change gastroenterologists because there has been a serious breakdown in the patient-physician relationship. Because patients can be heard almost immediately and have someone who is attentive to their concerns, it is my impression that our malpractice claims are lower than would otherwise be expected.

My HMO-S has in-house counsel in our largest center. He is available to any of our physicians for questions or advice, and will read any letter written to a patient to make sure it is legally appropriate. My feeling is that letters written to physicians by a patient's lawyer should be answered by a lawyer, and our lawyer does so. He is a great comfort to our HMO-S physicians. FFS physicians retain lawyers, but pay FFS for services and do not have them "down the hall."

My HMO-S employs continuing care nurses and social workers who analyze the needs of patients in moving from the hospital to the home, or those who are in the home without having gone to the hospital. Often in FFS practice, the hospital social supports follow patients to the hospital door, and patients are then on their own. Our nurses follow through in the home. I never worry about one of my patients going home and panicking about a dressing, an ostomy, or a tube, because our nurses have taken care of these matters or will send the appropriate people (e.g., Visiting Nurse Association, homemaker, ostomy nurse) if necessary.

CLINICAL RESEARCH

There are many examples of clinical research done in an HMO setting. HMOs have a common chart. The internist, the gastroenterologist, the surgeon, and the oncologist have all dictated into the same chart, and all laboratory and other tests ordered by any one of these physicians are in this one chart. HMOs often have multiple computer systems that make long-term follow-up and data retrieval relatively simple. For example, our HMO has an encounter system. Thus, every time a patient sees a physician, that visit, the diagnosis, and often the treatment (e.g., an injection of interferon) are entered in the chart. It then becomes relatively easy to obtain a printout of the records of all patients seen in this particular HMO with, for example, hepatitis C, and to stratify them into those who received interferon and those who did not. This is not commonly available in most FFS offices or indeed in most hospitals, although it clearly exists in some large clinics and group practices. This computer programming is very expensive, and one needs economies of scale to make it feasible.

CLOSING THOUGHTS

In this chapter I have tried to illustrate some of the differences between practicing gastroenterology in an FFS setting and in an HMO-S setting. I hope I have given the impression that there is often overlap, especially in large subspecialty practices, and that the political and social forces today are driving gastroenterologists closer together in their practice concerns no matter in which setting they find themselves. The greatest bond, of course, is that we are all trying to prevent colon cancer, minimize the ravages of inflammatory bowel disease, prolong the lives of patients with end-stage liver disease, and reassure those with irritable bowel syndrome. We are all trying to deliver good health care to our patients no matter what the incentives or the pay structure, and regardless of who is President of the United States.

SUGGESTED READING

Francis AM, et al. Care of patients with colorectal cancer. A comparison of a Health Maintenance Organization and Fee-For-Service practices. Med Care 1984; 22:418–429.

Klatshy AL, et al. Alcohol consumption and blood pressure. N Engl J Med 1977; 296:1194–1200.

Kurata JH, et al. Hospitalization and mortality rates for peptic ulcers: a comparison of a large Health Maintenance Organization and United States data. Gastroenterology 1982; 83:1008–1016.

Maule WF. Nurse performed flexible sigmoidoscopy under medical supervision. HMO Practice 1989; 3:150–151.

Mueller RJ. Colorectal carcinoma: a staff model HMO's experience with screening and hospital use. HMO Practice 1989; 4:130–136.

Overholt BF, Chobanian MD, eds. Office endoscopy. Baltimore: Williams & Wilkins, 1990.

Schoenbaum SC. The quality improvement cycle (QIC) in clinical practice: colorectal cancer detection. HMO Practice 1989; 3:169–172.

Selby JV, et al. A case control study of screening sigmoidoscopy and mortality from colorectal cancer. N Engl J Med 1992; 326:653–702.

RISK MANAGEMENT FOR THE GASTROENTEROLOGIST

PATRICK D. GERSTENBERGER, M.D.

Malpractice actions, litigation, and risk management are unavoidable elements of modern health care delivery. Even though gastroenterology is not a high-risk specialty, tort law pervades our professional and personal lives. To respond effectively, we must understand the basics of tort law, reduce the frequency and cost of preventable patient injuries, and improve our defenses against patient injuries that are unavoidable consequences of illness. Medical liability is a clinical and business problem, and we should draw remedies from both disciplines.

Risk management must identify liability risks specific to our specialty and implement systematic strategies to manage these risks. Properly applied, this process is highly compatible with quality patient care. This chapter summarizes basic tort law and consent issues, reviews malpractice claim data pertinent to gastroenterology and gastrointestinal endoscopy, and provides recommendations for practical risk management.

TORT LAW: THE ELEMENTS OF A MALPRACTICE CASE

A patient injured by the actions of a physician who fails to meet the standard of care may sue for compensation under the law of medical malpractice. Medical malpractice law is a particular application of tort law, which regulates civil injuries arising from the breach of a noncontractual legal duty. A cause of action under a negligence rule of liability must prove four elements to exist: duty, breach of duty, causation, and damages. The plaintiff must show that the preponderance of evidence (rather than the criminal standard of "beyond all reasonable doubt") supports the allegations. If successful, the injured party is entitled to compensation for damages within the limits of statute. In principle, physicians are liable only for those adverse outcomes due to negligence. Adverse outcomes resulting from the normal risk of illness and medical care are, in theory, the encumbrance of the patient.

Understanding these elements is a critical first step in planning risk management strategy (Table 1). This discussion emphasizes duty and breach of duty, the elements most relevant to risk management systems.

Duty

The duty to exercise reasonable care in providing medical treatment ordinarily derives from the physician-patient relationship. Be aware, however, that a duty may be established without the patient actually seeing the physician (accepting a referral, scheduling an appointment, or prescription of a bowel cleansing preparation for an anticipated procedure may establish duty). The physician's duty has been broadly interpreted by the courts and may extend to injured third parties never seen as patients. Examples of such expanded duty include a potential liability to nonpatient sexual partners of patients with infectious illnesses such as viral hepatitis, and to nonpatients injured by medicated patients driving while impaired, such as after conscious sedation.

As a party to the duty, the physician is in a position to delineate the extent of duty. This is especially true for the gastroenterologist acting as a consultant. When a consultation or procedure is completed, you have the opportunity to define and document your role in subsequent management. The record should reflect who will do what. Enumerating a set of recommendations (no matter how appropriate) could conceivably increase your liability exposure if responsibility for carrying out such recommendations is not clearly defined. From a risk management perspective, you should limit your duty to the narrowest extent possible.

Once established, duty may endure until it is specifically terminated. Either the physician or the patient may conclude the doctor-patient relationship, thus terminating a duty. When the physician acts to terminate a duty, certain steps should be taken to avoid liability for abandonment. Advice should be obtained regarding specific state laws. General recommendations are reviewed in Table 2.

Breach of Duty

A physician's duty is to practice within a reasonable standard of care. Specialists are judged against a national standard, reflecting standardization of training and certification, and widely accessible medical literature and continuing medical education. From a legal perspective, the standard of care and whether or not a physician has violated it is determined by the court, usually after hearing expert testimony. Professional custom is the benchmark for this determination. Thus, the standard of care in gastroenterology is the practice that is customary among reasonably trained gastroenterologists who are in good professional standing and are practicing with reasonable diligence. The standard of care generally does not represent optimal practice as viewed from an individual or social cost-benefit perspective. When more than one standard of care is applicable, practicing within the "majority" standard is the safest course from a liability standpoint. If a physician chooses an accepted but less popular approach (conforming to a "minority" standard of care), special documentation giving the reasons for such an approach should be included in the medical record.

Practice parameters (standards, guidelines, practice options, advisories) developed by specialty societies, federal agencies, and other organizations codify commonly held beliefs and customs and serve as evidence of

Table 1 Elements of a Malpractice Case

	Preventive Actions
Duty A duty of care must exist.	*Recognize your potential duty to nonpatients* Implement office policies to track and advise those who fail appointments and referrals. Implement office policies to provide for basic preprocedure medical assessments of patients you have not yet seen. Document advice to potentially infectious patients concerning their risk for transmitting disease to others, and comply with relevant reporting requirements. Document "not to drive" instructions given after conscious sedation. *Limit your duty* When acting as a consultant, define and limit the scope of your care consensually with the patient and referring physician. When seeing a patient without referral, define and limit the scope of your care. Do not unwittingly assume the comprehensive responsibilities of a primary care physician. *Terminate your duty properly* When it is necessary for you to terminate the doctor-patient relationship, do so formally, avoiding liability for abandonment (see Table 2). When patients elect not to follow up as recommended, ensure that they have been advised about the nature of their condition and the risks involved in not continuing care. Document informed refusal and termination of the doctor-patient relationship. Avoid ambiguous noncommunicative lapses in the doctor-patient relationship resulting from failed appointments. When the patient's intent to terminate your duty is unclear, require clarification for the record. *Limit your potential vicarious liability*
Breach of duty A standard of reasonable care was violated, either by action or by failure to act.	*Reflect current standards of care in your practice* Participate in continuing medical education programs regularly, especially those of a national scope. Monitor practice parameters (see Appendix). Document your reasons for deviating from an established practice parameter.
Causation The breach of duty was the proximate cause of the damages.	
Damage The plaintiff suffered a compensable injury.	*Maintain appropriate professional liability insurance* Understand and comply with the terms of your coverage.

the standard of care. Practice parameters that simply state common practice are not likely to affect the outcome of a malpractice case, but parameters encouraging a significant change in customary practice may lead to a shift in the way reasonable specialists practice, in fact establishing a new standard of care. Although important, practice parameters are not conclusive evidence of the standard of care. The weight of a parameter in the court's view will reflect the sponsoring organization's expertise and prestige, the nature and purpose of the parameter, conflicting statements by other authorities, and the direct applicability of the parameter to the case under consideration.

In the current era of cost control, keep in mind that parameters focusing principally on cost constraint may offer little support to a physician being judged according to a standard of care defined by traditional patient care considerations. A parameter primarily reflecting fiscal considerations is likely to be accorded less evidentiary weight than a parameter specifically intended to embody prevailing professional standards. Physicians complying with such "cost-containment" parameters (until such time that a corresponding shift in the customary reasonable standard of care follows) bear the risks of liability from any resulting injuries. Courts have been reluctant to hold that cost constraints may be taken into account in determining the extent of the physician duty.

Gastroenterologists should be familiar with the published parameters pertinent to their specialty, and when appropriate, clearly document the reasons for deviating from an established parameter (see Appendix).

Causation and Damages

The plaintiff must prove that the claimed damages resulted from the breach of duty. Frequently, this is the

Table 2 Guidelines for Physician-Initiated Termination of the Doctor-Patient Relationship

Provide written notification, by return receipt mail
Provide a reason for termination
Agree to continue providing treatment for a reasonable period (15–30 days), while the patient is arranging for care with another physician
State the date on which termination will be effective
Provide information to aid the patient in identifying other physicians of similar specialty
Offer to provide care in an emergency for a defined period after termination
Include these items in the letter of termination

Adapted from American Medical Assocation Specialty Society Liability Project. Risk Management: principles & commentaries for the medical office. Chicago: American Medical Association; 1990; with permission.

most difficult element to prove in a medical malpractice case. Proving that the standard of care was violated and that damages were incurred is insufficient: the damages must derive from the negligence. Damages may include economic losses (medical bills; loss of income; added expenses for the past, present, and future) and pain and suffering. Such losses are often limited by statute as a result of tort reform. These damages, and defense expenses, are generally covered by medical malpractice insurance to the policy limits. Punitive damages may be awarded in cases of gross negligence, when intentional or reckless conduct is shown. Punitive damages are meant to punish the defendant and serve as an example to others. These are not covered by insurance.

INFORMED CONSENT

The legal process of informed consent embodies the ethical principle of self-determination. Informed consent is the result of effective communication between the patient and the physician and should reflect a genuine process of disclosure and discussion. In essence, competent patients are legally entitled to deliberate and decide voluntarily about undertaking recommended procedures or treatments, after the disclosure of material risks. Failure to obtain informed consent constitutes a form of medical malpractice and is subject to the law's negligence standards. Although required, this process is one of our most powerful risk management tools. It provides an opportunity to build a strong doctor-patient relationship, and shift risk to the patient. A patient informed about the risk of perforation who decides to undergo endoscopy bears that risk, and so indemnifies the endoscopist (who is nevertheless obligated to perform the procedure within a reasonable standard of care).

Informed consent is required for procedures and treatments known to involve significant risks. In most instances the patient consents, but in circumstances of legal incompetence or inability to consent (and when no advance directive is in force), authority may pass to someone else who is legally authorized to provide consent. Specific rules in these instances are evolving and vary from state to state. Practitioners unfamiliar with their own jurisdiction's requirements should seek assistance from legal counsel.

Disclosure

How much should be disclosed? There is no national standard for disclosure. In some states the legislature has defined requirements, while in others the courts have provided guidance. Generally, gastroenterologists are held to one of the following standards, which dictate that we provide the amount of information that

1. A reasonable prudent gastroenterologist in a similar situation would disclose, or
2. A reasonable prudent person in the patient's position would want to know, or
3. The actual patient wants to know.

A conservative approach should be adopted if you are unsure about your own jurisdiction's requirements. The general types of information that must be disclosed include

1. The nature and purpose of the proposed procedure or treatment.
2. The probable risks and benefits of the proposed procedure.
3. Alternatives.
4. The probable risks and benefits of the alternatives.
5. Remote risks involving severe injury, disability, or death.
6. The risk of refusing the proposed procedure.

Documentation

Documentation of the informed consent process should reflect the process described above and not merely the signing of a form. Many institutions rely on standardized consent forms, but they have the potential to supersede the communication process essential to a truly informed consent. Gastroenterologists perform a limited number of procedures that carry significant risk and should consider using *procedure-specific consent documents* written in simple language detailing the nature, risks, and benefits of the proposed procedure and alternatives. This type of document provides more complete evidence of the process than standard forms, but informed consent will not occur if the patient fails to read or understand the information. It is helpful to use procedure-specific forms as teaching aids during the disclosure process, ensuring that all intended issues have been covered. Written or dictated notes in the medical record describing and documenting the informed consent process serve as further evidence of disclosure, if entered before the planned procedure. Witnessing of the entire informed consent process (rather than witnessing of a signing alone) should be considered in high-risk situations. When a patient refuses to undergo a recommended treatment or procedure after appropriate disclosure, document that the refusal was in fact informed.

Exceptions

Informed consent is not required in these instances:

1. *Emergencies,* when the patient has a serious condition requiring immediate care and cannot participate in the consent process, and there is no time to obtain consent from an authorized representative.
2. *Therapeutic privilege:* If the physician believes that disclosure is likely to cause significant emotional or physical harm to the patient.
3. *Compulsory* (legally required) *treatment.*
4. *Waiver,* if a patient waives the right to disclosure.

These exceptions occur infrequently in clinical practice and require particularly careful documentation.

VICARIOUS LIABILITY

Liability is vicarious when it is imposed on one party as a result of the wrongful conduct of another. In other words, the liability derives not from one's own conduct but from the relationship one has with the individual who acts negligently and causes an injury. Generally, vicarious liability is an issue in relationships where one party is in a position to control (or appear to control) the acts of another. Vicarious liability is an increasingly utilized technique, because it allows recovery from a "deep pocket" who does not need to be proven negligent. Consider your added liability when acting as employer, partner, instructor, proctor, endoscopy unit director (administrator), or medical staff officer.

CLAIM AND SUIT DATA: HOW CAN THEY GUIDE US?

Specialty-specific risk management techniques should be based on an understanding of patient injury and claim experience. Studies of claims and suits suffer from the exclusion of patient injuries that fail to result in a demand for compensation. Claim data thus incompletely describe the true scope of patient injuries related to gastroenterology or endoscopy. Nevertheless, they are the best available source for specific risk management information.

Relative Malpractice Claim Risk of Endoscopic Procedures

Comparing procedure-specific claim frequencies with the relative frequency with which these procedures are performed suggests that the relative risks of a malpractice claim arising from the performance of sigmoidoscopy, esophagogastroduodenoscopy, endoscopic retrograde cholangiopancreatography, and colonoscopy are similar (Table 3).

These comparable relative claim risks contrast with reported rates of serious procedural complications for the same procedures that differ 100-fold. This disparity may be partly due to inconsistent use of the informed consent process. Endoscopists are more likely to carefully disclose the risks involved in the most hazardous procedures, spending less time and effort reviewing the potential complications of less hazardous procedures.

Endoscopists should treat even low-risk procedures (e.g., sigmoidoscopy) as important liability events. The informed consent process helps establish a strong positive doctor-patient relationship and should be utilized before every procedural encounter. A well-informed patient who participates in decisions about undertaking an endoscopic procedure is probably less likely to pursue a malpractice action in the event of a poor outcome.

Another factor contributing to the disparity between malpractice and complication rates is likely to be the relative skills of practitioners undertaking these procedures. Sigmoidoscopy is frequently performed by providers without the formal training and experience of endoscopists undertaking the more difficult procedures. Less experienced practitioners may be more likely to perform procedures incorrectly and inappropriately, and may experience more frequent complications and diagnostic errors.

Primary Allegations Against Endoscopists

As expected, the most frequent allegation in endoscopy-related malpractice actions is improper performance. Interestingly, diagnosis error follows in frequency and constitutes a substantial portion of claims (Fig. 1). The significant malpractice risk of diagnostic error should be reflected in the informed consent process. Disclosure results in a sharing of this risk between the endoscopist and the patient.*

Failure to diagnose colorectal malignancy is the major single cause of diagnostic error claims. Sixty-one percent of erroneous diagnosis claims result from failure to diagnose malignancy, and colorectal malignancy represents 69 percent of these. In the largest insurance industry study to date, 32 percent of successful claims for failure to diagnose colon cancer pertained to plaintiffs under the age of 50 (52 percent of indemnity payments), with 19.2 percent under 40 years of age (34 percent of indemnity payments). Endoscopists evaluating the lower gastrointestinal tract must consider the adequacy of their evaluation in view of this condition's long asymptomatic phase and its frequency in the general population. Other frequently "missed" conditions leading to claims include abdominal vascular disorders, inflammatory bowel dis-

---

Editor's Note: The relative legal importance of diagnostic error might cause some of us to alter our discussion of informed consent. Despite our best intentions, medicine is not always an exact science.

ease, peptic ulcer disease, esophageal stricture, benign colonic neoplasm, and nonmalignant gynecologic conditions.

Although the potential complications of endoscopy are known to be numerous, the only significant iatrogenic injuries from a claim standpoint are perforation and related direct injuries of the gastrointestinal tract. Standards of practice and statute require disclosure of all important risks through the informed consent process, but the risk of perforation must be emphasized.

Secondary Allegations Against Endoscopists

Problems with informed consent represent the most common associated allegation in endoscopy-related malpractice claims (alleged in 45 percent of claims specifying a secondary allegation), emphasizing the need for more attention to the consent process in endoscopic practice. Other important associated allegations (those representing more than 5 percent of all specified secondary allegations) include problems with adequacy

Table 3 Relative Malpractice Claim Risks

Procedure	Estimated 1987 Medicare Volume	Endoscopy-Associated Claim Files	Relative Risk
Colonoscopy	658,571	208	1.7
ERCP	37,305	11	1.6
EGD	835,887	190	1.2
Sigmoidoscopy	809,298	153	1.0

ERCP = endoscopic retrograde cholangiopancreatography; EGD = esophagogastroduodenoscopy.
From Gerstenberger PD, Plumeri PA. Malpractice claims in gastrointestinal endoscopy: analysis of an insurance industry database. Gastrointest Endosc 1993; 39:132-138; with permission.

of facilities or equipment, records, and billing and collection. Problems with secondary issues alone usually do not precipitate a claim, but attention to these items in daily practice may reduce the probability of a claim otherwise being brought.

Primary Allegations Against Gastroenterologists

When claim data are viewed on a specialty-specific, rather than a procedure-specific, basis, additional concerns emerge. Diagnostic error and performance error each make up over one-fourth of allegations. As in endoscopy-specific claims, failure to diagnose malignancy remains a frequent allegation. There are significant differences, however, in the types of malignancies missed, with less colorectal (19 percent) and more gastric (17 percent) cancers. Of particular concern are a large proportion (39 percent) of *missed nongastrointestinal tract neoplasms* leading to claims against gastroenterologists. Forty-four percent of these claims pertain to gynecologic and female breast cancers, and 31 percent to bronchopulmonary malignancies.

Careful delineation of duty can reduce the malpractice risk of failing to diagnose a malignant condition arising outside one's area of practice. Gastroenterologists wishing to avoid responsibility for the evaluation and monitoring of nongastrointestinal organ systems should limit their duty consensually with the patient and referring physician, document such an understanding, and request appropriate consultation when indicated.

Claims against gastroenterologists alleging *medication error* point out the malpractice risk of treating inflammatory bowel disease. Informed consent should be carefully documented when initiating therapy with *corticosteroids, immunosuppressive agents,* or other drugs that have significant potential for causing serious complications during a lengthy course of treatment.

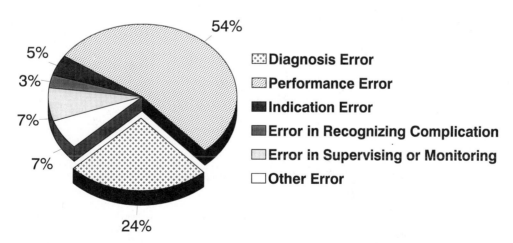

Figure 1 Types of medical misadventures alleged in 496 endoscopy-associated malpractice claims. (Adapted from Gerstenberger PD, Plumeri PA. Malpractice claims in gastrointestinal endoscopy: analysis of an insurance industry database. Gastrointest Endosc 1993; 39:132–138; with permission.)

RECOMMENDATIONS

The possibility of being sued for medical malpractice is an unavoidable risk of doing business in the practice of medicine. Physicians should manage this risk by using good general risk management practices:

1. Develop strong and honest relationships with your patients.
2. Integrate a knowledge of tort law into your daily clinical activities.
3. Define and limit your role.
4. Emphasize informed consent.

In addition, gastroenterologists should add these specialty-specific actions to their risk management armamentarium:

1. Do not underestimate the potential liability of low-risk procedures. Use the protection afforded by the informed consent process before every procedural encounter.
2. Inform endoscopy patients about the risk of diagnostic error. Add this issue to the informed consent process. Consider both clinical and risk management perspectives when evaluating the lower gastrointestinal tract.
3. Emphasize the risk of perforation in the informed consent process.
4. Carefully delineate your duty with regard to nongastrointestinal disease.
5. Increase your attention to the informed consent process when using corticosteroids and immunosuppressive agents.

APPENDIX: *SELECTED PRACTICE PARAMETERS*

The following list was extracted from the American Medical Association's *Directory of Practice Parameters* (October 1990) and the subsequent quarterly issues of the *Practice Parameters Update*. The AMA's Office of Quality Assurance in cooperation with the Practice Parameters Partnership and the Practice Parameters Forum tracks the development and completion of practice parameters by physician organizations.

American Cancer Society   (404) 320-3333
  Summary of Current Guidelines for the Cancer-Related Checkup: Recommendations

American College of Physicians   (215) 351-2400
  Clinical Competence in Colonoscopy
  Clinical Competence in Diagnostic Endoscopic Retrograde Cholangiopancreatography
  Clinical Competence in Diagnostic Esophagogastroduodenoscopy
  Clinical Competence in the Use of Flexible Sigmoidoscopy for Screening Purposes
  Eating Disorders: Anorexia Nervosa and Bulimia: Position Paper
  Endoscopic Sclerotherapy for Esophageal Varices
  Endoscopy in the Evaluation of Dyspepsia
  Guide for Use of American College of Physicians Statements of Clinical Competence
  Hepatitis B Vaccine
  How to Study the Gallbladder
  Management of Gallstones

American Medical Association   (312) 464-5000

  Endoscopic Electrocoagulation for Gastrointestinal Hemorrhage
  Endoscopic Laser Photocoagulation for Gastrointestinal Hemorrhage
  Endoscopic Thermal Coagulation for Gastrointestinal Hemorrhage
  Endoscopic Topical Therapy for Gastrointestinal Hemorrhage
  Garren Gastric Bubble for Morbid Obesity
  Magnetic Imaging of the Abdomen and Pelvis
  Pancreas Transplants
  Rigid and Flexible Sigmoidoscopies

American Society for Gastrointestinal Endoscopy   (508) 526-8330
  Appropriate Use of Gastrointestinal Endoscopy
  Diagnostic and Therapeutic Procedures
  Endoscopic Therapy of Biliary Tract and Pancreatic Diseases
  Esophageal Dilation
  Flexible Sigmoidoscopy: Guidelines for Clinical Application
  Guidelines for Establishment of Gastrointestinal Endoscopy Areas
  Guideline for the Management of Ingested Foreign Bodies*
  Infection Control During Gastrointestinal Endoscopy: Guidelines for Clinical Application
  Informed Consent for Gastrointestinal Endoscopy
  Methods of Granting Hospital Privileges to Perform Gastrointestinal Endoscopy
  Monitoring of Patients Undergoing Gastrointestinal Endoscopic Procedures
  Preparation of Patients for Gastrointestinal Endoscopy: Guidelines for Clinical Application
  Quality Assurance of Gastrointestinal Endoscopy
  Risk Management
  Role of Colonoscopy in the Management of Patients with Colonic Polyps: Guidelines for Clinical Application
  Role of Colonoscopy in the Management of Patients with Inflammatory Bowel Disease: Guidelines for Clinical Application
  Role of Endoscopic Sclerotherapy in the Management of Variceal Bleeding: Guidelines for Clinical Application
  Role of Endoscopy in Diseases of the Biliary Tract and Pancreas: Guidelines for Clinical Application
  Role of Endoscopy in the Management of Esophagitis
  Role of Endoscopy in the Management of the Patient with Peptic Ulcer Disease: Guidelines for Clinical Application
  Role of Endoscopy in the Management of Upper Gastrointestinal Hemorrhage
  Role of Endoscopy in the Patient with Lower Gastrointestinal Bleeding: Guidelines for Clinical Application
  Role of Endoscopy in the Surveillance of Premalignant Conditions of the Upper Gastrointestinal Tract: Guidelines for Clinical Application
  Role of Laparoscopy in the Diagnosis and Management of Gastrointestinal Disease: Guidelines for Clinical Application
  Role of Percutaneous Endoscopic Gastrostomy: Guidelines for Clinical Application
  Standards of Practice of Gastrointestinal Endoscopy
  Statement of Endoscopic Training
  Statement of the Role of Short Courses in Endoscopic Training
  The Appropriate Use of Prophylactic Antibiotics During Gastrointestinal Endoscopic Procedures*
  The Role of Screening Tests Before Gastrointestinal Endoscopic Procedures

Centers for Disease Control   (404) 639-3311
  Universal Precautions for Prevention of Transmission of Human Immunodeficiency Virus, Hepatitis B Virus, and Other Blood-borne Pathogens in Health-Care
  Hepatitis B Virus: A Comprehensive Strategy for Eliminating Transmission in the United States Through Universal Childhood Vaccination

U.S. Department of Health and Human Services, NIH Consensus Development Conference   (301) 469-1143
  Adjuvant Therapy for Patients with Colon and Rectal Cancer
  Therapeutic Endoscopy and Bleeding Ulcers
  Gallstones and Laparoscopic Cholecystectomy

---

*Under development.

U.S. Preventive Services Task Force   (202) 245-0180
  "Screening for Colorectal Cancer" in Guide to Clinical Preventive Services
  "Screening for Hepatitis B" in Guide to Clinical Preventive Services
  "Screening for Pancreatic Cancer" in Guide to Clinical Preventive Services

American Society of Colon & Rectal Surgeons   (708) 359-9184
  Treatment of Anal Fissure
  Antibiotic Prophylaxis in Colon and Rectal Endoscopy
  Detection of Colorectal Neoplasms
  Carcinoma of the Rectum*

American College of Gastroenterology   (601) 984-4540
  Management of Polyps of the Colon*
  Evaluation of Occult Gastrointestinal Bleeding*
  Medical Management of Gastroesophageal Reflux Disease*
  Prophylaxis and Therapy of NSAID-Induced Gastrointestinal Mucosal Disease*
  Evaluation of Cholestatic Jaundice*
  Management of Peptic Ulcer Disease*
  Evaluation of GI Bleeding in Patients with Portal Hypertension*

American Gastroenterological Association   (301) 654-2055
  Detection and Surveillance of Colon Cancer in High Risk Patients*
  Esophageal Manometry*
  Esophageal pH Recording*
  Evaluation of Dyspeptic Syndrome*
  Tube Feeding for Enteral Nutrition*

Society of American Gastrointestinal Endoscopic Surgeons   (310) 479-3249
  The Role of Laparoscopic Cholecystectomy

Guidelines for Office Endoscopic Services
Granting Privileges for Gastrointestinal Endoscopy by Surgeons
Guidelines for Diagnostic Laparoscopy
Granting of Privileges for Laparoscopic (Peritoneoscopic) General Surgery
Summary Statement on Surgical Endoscopic Training and Practice
Guidelines for General Surgery Residency Education in Gastrointestinal Endoscopy*

SUGGESTED READING

Gerstenberger PD. Risk management: concerns in gastroenterology. In Carey WD, Fise TF, eds. Essentials of management of the gastroenterology practice. New York: Igaku-Shoin, 1993.

Gerstenberger PD, Plumeri PA. Malpractice claims in gastrointestinal endoscopy: analysis of an insurance industry database. Gastrointest Endosc 1993; 39:132–138.

National Health Lawyers Association and American Medical Association. Physician's survival guide, legal pitfalls and solutions. Washington, DC and Chicago, 1991.

Plumeri PA. Informed consent and the gastrointestinal endoscopist. Gastrointest Endosc 1985; 31:218–221.

Plumeri PA, Gerstenberger PD, Hughes RW, et al. Risk management: an information resource manual. Manchester, MA: American Society for Gastrointestinal Endoscopy, 1990.

Selby MC, Carroll E, Carter JB, et al. Hospital and physician liability: a legal and risk management overview. Washington, DC: National Health Lawyers Association, 1992.

ENDOSCOPIC SEDATION

M. BRIAN FENNERTY, MD

Conscious sedation is the forte of anesthesiologists but has become an essential skill for gastroenterologists and other practitioners of endoscopy. However, few of us have had formal training in anesthesiology or the principles of administering sedation. We have learned how to sedate patients from mentors in an apprentice system of training, and those mentors in turn learned from others or by hands-on experience. This chapter is intended to shed some light on the science of conscious sedation by reviewing the pharmacology and administration of sedating agents, and the principles and techniques of monitoring patients under sedation.

BACKGROUND

Conscious sedation can be defined as a pharmacologically induced state of depressed consciousness in which the patient's protective reflexes and cooperation are preserved. *Anesthesia* implies a deeper level of depressed consciousness in which protective refluxes are not maintained and the patient's cooperation cannot be expected. These differences between conscious sedation and anesthesia are clinically and medicolegally important because they require different degrees of monitoring and result in differences in procedural safety. However, most endoscopists do not recognize the difference between the levels of sedation, and thus contribute to unnecessary procedural risks to the patient.

The goals of conscious sedation are to alleviate anxiety, provide analgesia if necessary, and (most important) produce antegrade amnesia. Endoscopy can be successfully performed without accompanying sedation, but patient acceptance of the procedure in that setting (in the United States) will be poor. Even the most skilled endoscopists (which we all believe ourselves to be) cannot prevent the discomfort inherent in endoscopic procedures. Also, the quality of examinations without sedation may be suboptimal, and the patient's willingness to undergo subsequent examination will be diminished if the procedure is perceived as being uncomfortable. In the United States patients expect to receive sedation for endoscopic procedures other than sigmoidoscopy, and few physicians feel comfortable performing endoscopy without sedation. Thus, most endoscopic procedures require accompanying sedation.

Endoscopy is remarkably safe. However, the most

common complications accompanying endoscopic procedures are cardiopulmonary events, most of which are related to the sedative medications used to facilitate the procedure. One may conclude from this that it would probably be safer to perform procedures without sedation, but this conclusion is probably erroneous. Although anesthetic-induced hypoxia may contribute to cardiac dysrhythmia and ischemia, these cardiac events may also occur in response to an increased "double product" (heart rate times blood pressure) induced by discomfort or anxiety in the nonsedated patient. However, sedation with narcotics or benzodiazepines results in decreased oxygen saturation, decreased respiration, and altered hemodynamics. These physiologic events are more frequent and severe with deeper levels of sedation, such as in anesthesia. Thus, sedation not only contributes to the ease of performance of endoscopy, but also adds to the risk of the procedure. This leads to the safety caveat that one should administer the lowest effective dose of sedative medication necessary to perform the procedure, and monitoring needs to be commensurate with the level of sedation.

PHARMACOLOGY

Benzodiazepines

All benzodiazepines have similar pharmacologic effects. Their therapeutic use therefore depends on the preparation, side effects, and length of effect versus intrinsic structural differences between the drugs. Benzodiazepines act within the central nervous system (CNS) at specific benzodiazepine receptor sites. Occupation of these receptors results in augmentation of gamma-aminobutyric acid (GABA), which is an inhibitory neurotransmitter resulting in depression of cortical function. Thus, benzodiazepines result in a dose-dependent continuum of effect from mild sedation through drowsiness and sleep to deep anesthesia.

Diazepam gained widespread popularity as the benzodiazepine of choice for conscious sedation because of its availability as an intravenous (IV) agent. Diazepam, like other benzodiazepines, has both behavioral and neurophysiologic effects, including anxiolysis, hypnosis, muscle relaxation, and amnesia. Physiologic effects include a decrease in ventilation (related to decreased respiratory excursions, tidal volume, and increased residual volume) and a mild decrease in blood pressure and left ventricular stroke work. Diazepam reaches steady-state serum levels rapidly, and drug elimination follows in a biphasic pattern, with initial (alpha) rapid phase (drug distribution) followed by a slow (beta) delayed phase (drug elimination), resulting in a half-life of 2 to 4 days. Diazepam is metabolized via demethylation and oxidation to active intermediates, including oxazepam, which accounts for its prolonged pharmacologic effect. Side effects of diazepam administration include occasional paradoxical agitation after administration, pain at the injection site, and phlebitis, which may occur up to 10 days after administration. Pain at the injection site and phlebitis are related to diazepam's inherent non–water solubility requiring a viscid acid vehicle that is the effector of the vessel sensitivity. Pain and phlebitis can mostly be prevented by using the emulsion preparation, but the latter may not be dose equivalent to standard diazepam. The prolonged half-life of diazepam, its inadequate amnesiac effect, and the pain and phlebitis make diazepam a less than ideal (perhaps even inappropriate) choice for endoscopic sedation.

Midazolam is a benzodiazepine containing an imidazole ring that forms water-soluble salts that remain stable in solution. This water solubility accounts for the lack of pain on injection or phlebitis. Midazolam is remarkably stable, with a shelf-life of over 2 years, and is compatible with almost all IV solutions. Its pharmacologic effects are rapid (3 to 4 minutes) and similar to those of the other benzodiazepines, i.e., anxiolysis, hypnosis, and antegrade amnesia. However, midazolam's amnesiac properties (in 70 to 80 percent of patients) are superior to those seen with diazepam (in 20 to 50 percent of patients). Administration of midazolam results in an elimination half-life of 1 to 12 hours compared with the 2 to 4 day half-life seen with diazepam. Midazolam is metabolized to 1-hydroxymethylmidazolam, which is rapidly conjugated in the liver and then excreted renally. Renal insufficiency does not require dose modification. Midazolam's lipophilicity and high clearance rates result in a short duration of action. It was initially reported to be 1½ to 2 times as potent as diazepam on a milligram for milligram basis, but it is more likely 2½ to 4 times as potent as diazepam. Like diazepam, midazolam has great affinity for the benzodiazepine receptor in the brain, and physiologically causes a decrease in respiratory rate and apnea at high doses and a small decrease in mean arterial pressure and stroke volume. Adverse effects of midazolam include nausea and vomiting, hiccups, and cough. The rapid onset of action, short half-life, lack of phlebitis and better antegrade amnesia properties make midazolam the preferred benzodiazepine for conscious sedation. For these reasons, the continued use of diazepam is inappropriate for conscious sedation accompanying endoscopy.

Flumazenil is a benzodiazepine receptor ligand that competitively inhibits the benzodiazepine receptor and therefore has antagonist activity. It has high affinity and great specificity for the receptor and has minimal intrinsic effect, thus acting as a reversal agent for benzodiazepines. Flumazenil's effect is specific for benzodiazepines and has no effect on opiates, ethanol, or IV or general anesthetic drugs. Flumazenil has rapid elimination and a very short half-life of 40 to 80 minutes. It is important to recognize that flumazenil may precipitate acute benzodiazepine withdrawal when given to patients on chronic benzodiazepine therapy. Thus, it is vitally important that chronic benzodiazepine use be recognized in patients before flumazenil is used.

Narcotics

Narcotics affect the CNS via their binding to the μ-opioid receptor, which results in an analgesic effect as well as euphoria. Opiates also cause respiratory depression in a dose-dependent manner that may be reversed by narcotic antagonists. Respiratory depression can occur with doses smaller than the dose needed to achieve altered consciousness. Narcotics depress both the hypoxic and hypercarbic respiratory drive.

In the past, opiate analgesia alone was used by some endoscopists for conscious sedation. Opiates were superior to topical pharyngeal agents and were better accepted by patients. However, because of the superiority of benzodiazepines in producing sedation, opiates are now rarely used alone. When combined with benzodiazepines, opiates result in a potentiation of sedative effect and may be very useful in selected clinical settings.

Meperidine is a synthetic analgesic structurally very dissimilar to morphine, but it has many of the same pharmacologic properties. Meperidine forms a stable water-soluble salt in solution. Like all narcotics, its administration results in mild sedation and euphoria. After IV administration of meperidine, onset of action may be delayed as long as 5 to 10 minutes. Its pharmacologic effect is increased with increasing patient age as well as comorbid medical conditions. Side effects include nausea and vomiting and respiratory depression.

Newer narcotics such as fentanyl, alfentanil, and sufentanil have a greater affinity for the μ-opioid receptor and more rapid onset of action, as well as a shorter duration of action. However, clinical studies have not shown these agents to be superior to meperidine for conscious sedation.*

Narcotic antagonists compete with opioids for the receptor site without causing an opioid effect. *Naloxone* is almost devoid of agonist effects and therefore can be used to reverse opioid-induced CNS and respiratory depression. Its administration results in a prompt reversal of the opioid effect, usually within 1 to 2 minutes. Naloxone is rapidly eliminated via conjugation of the liver. This elimination is more rapid (1 to 4 hours) than that of narcotics and therefore may result in a pharmacologic effect briefer than the effect of the opioid, which can allow later repeat sedation and respiratory depression. Naloxone can precipitate narcotic withdrawal in patients on chronic narcotic analgesia. Withdrawal can be treated by readministration of narcotic.

Neuroleptics

Neuroleptic compounds combined with narcotics produce a state of consciousness termed *neuroleptic analgesia*. *Droperidol* in combination with narcotics and benzodiazepines has been used in this fashion for endoscopic sedation. Neuroleptic analgesia results in a quiescent cataleptic state characterized by indifference to stimulation and immobility. Onset of anesthesia is slow (more than 3 to 5 minutes) and can result in significant hypotension and bradycardia. Respiratory depression may be profound. Recovery from anesthesia is usually rapid, but "slowing" may be seen for up to 24 hours. Because of the significant side effects and physiologic derangements observed with neuroleptic anesthesia, this form of conscious sedation has very little role and offers little, if any, advantage in endoscopic sedation.

TECHNIQUE

Before sedation for endoscopy is initiated, a pre-endoscopic assessment and procedural explanation should be given to the patient. Most patients are referred directly to the endoscopy unit without having been previously interviewed or examined by the endoscopist, and therefore the medical history, medication regimen, and drug allergies are not known to the latter. It is not appropriate to rely on the referral physician's judgment that a patient is fit for the anesthesia and procedure, because he or she may not understand the risk of sedation accompanying these procedures. A brief and directed examination should be performed on every patient. A history or presence of cardiopulmonary and CNS disease should be sought. A useful medical risk classification system is the scheme used by the American Society of Anesthesiology (Table 1). Information on allergies and sensitivities to narcotics, benzodiazepines, and other anesthetics should be elicited. Concurrent medications need to be known in order to avoid drug interactions or withdrawal if reversal of sedation is necessary. Additionally, because of the profound antegrade amnesia seen with midazolam sedation, postprocedure instructions prohibiting driving or operation of dangerous machinery on the day of the procedure, as well as postprocedure dietary instructions, should be given at this time. The preprocedure assessment should then be followed by a careful explanation of the indications, procedure, side effects, and complications of the examination as part of the informed consent process. This assessment and procedural explanation, when conducted in an informative and reassuring manner, results in a more relaxed patient who will be more cooperative and require less sedative medication. The procedure room should be run in a professional manner, with a quiet, harmonious environment allowing the patient to feel confident and relaxed. Extraneous activity and interruptions increase patient anxiety and make for a more difficult procedure.

An indwelling IV canula is required for all endoscopic procedures requiring conscious sedation. It is inappropriate not to have IV access in any procedure in which cardiopulmonary complications occur and resuscitation may be required. The clinical end point of sedation is amnesia and cooperative anxiolysis, which

---

*Editor's Note:** Many centers do use fentanyl, feeling that it is better tolerated than meperidine.

Table 1 American Society of Anesthesiologists (ASA) Classification System for Physical States

I.	Healthy patient
II.	Mild systemic disease (slight functional limitation)
III.	Severe systemic disease (moderate functional limitation)
IV.	Severe systemic disease (threat to life)
V.	Moribund (unlikely to survive 24 hours)

requires uncoupling the higher cortical processing from reflex brain stem functions (i.e., necessitates a depressed CNS). Further degrees of CNS depression (i.e., sleep) do not allow patients to cooperate with verbal instructions and may make them more difficult or combative, as well as increasing the potential for complications. It is important to recognize that increased agitation usually represents oversedation and/or hypoxia and should not lead to increasing the level of sedation. Increased sedation does not increase compliance. A minimal level of sedation is necessary to ensure compliance and permit a relaxed and complete examination, but deeper levels inhibit the ability of the patient to respond to commands and thus should be considered anesthesia (see below).

Meperidine and midazolam are the drugs of choice for conscious sedation. They should be prepprepared and drawn up into labeled syringes whose potencies on a milligram per milliliter basis should never be varied, to prevent inadvertent dosage errors. When meperidine is used in combination with midazolam for conscious sedation, there is up to an eight-fold synergy in their effect. If these agents are used together, opiates should be given first. As the onset of action of opiates can be delayed, 5 to 10 minutes should elapse after opioid infusion before infusion of benzodiazepines. In addition, the usual dose of both meperidine and midazolam should be decreased by one-third to one-half. In aged or infirm patients, further reduction in initial doses of both drugs (one-half to three-fourths) is necessary. Onset of action and patient cooperation are improved with bolus administration, but respiratory depression may be more frequent. However, slow titration also may result in "overshooting" and subsequent prolonged recovery or respiratory depression. A good rule of thumb is to go "low and slow" with small boluses, allowing adequate time between each for the drug effect to be observed. Meperidine, 25 to 50 mg, and midazolam, 1 to 3 mg, are appropriate as initial doses for conscious sedation. In combination with meperidine, or in elderly patients, the dose of midazolam should be appropriately reduced.

There has been no role for routine reversal of conscious sedation. Patients exhibiting significant physiologic compromise, e.g., hypotension, hypoxia, or agitation, should have sedation promptly reversed, with naloxone if meperidine has been given and flumazenil if midazolam has been used. The dose of naloxone is 0.4 mg repeated every 2 to 3 minutes. However, because the dosages of narcotics used in conscious sedation are usually small, the maximal dose of naloxone necessary to reverse narcotic anesthesia is usually 0.4 to 0.8 mg. Flumazenil should be given in doses of 0.2 mg over 20 to

30 seconds, followed by 0.1 to 0.2 mg repeated every 1 to 2 minutes up to a total dose of 1 mg.

There may be an indication for routine use of flumazenil in conscious sedation, because the efficiency of the endoscopy unit can be improved by a rapid turnover of patients. Although flumazenil is relatively expensive, the ability to reverse sedation rapidly obviates the need for a prolonged recovery process and results in earlier discharge of a patient. Thus, routine use of flumazenil increases the efficiency of available personnel and space and may be cost effective. Repeat sedation does not seem to occur with the lower doses of benzodiazepine used in endoscopic sedation. This approach is probably without significant risk and may become more widely practiced.

Monitoring of cardiopulmonary status is discussed in a subsequent paragraph.

PROCEDURES

Upper Endoscopy

The value of topical pharyngeal anesthetic agents such as sprays, solutions, and lozenges in improving patient acceptance of upper endoscopy is unproved. These agents may decrease the amount of coughing and gagging that occurs with upper endoscopic procedures, but their impact is small. This lack of effect may be related to endoscopist's lack of training in proper pharyngeal anesthesia. These agents also prevent the oral intake of fluids and solids for 2 to 3 hours after the procedure because of prolonged pharyngeal anesthesia. I find their use limited and rarely needed for routine diagnostic endoscopy.

Although many endoscopists use a combination of narcotic and benzodiazepine for sedation accompanying upper endoscopy, this practice is probably unnecessary in routine diagnostic cases in which smaller diameter endoscopes are used; this combination of drugs also increases the risk of the procedures. However, for therapeutic procedures, procedures utilizing scopes of larger diameter, or endoscopy coupled with esophageal dilation, a combination of meperidine and midazolam may result in better patient acceptance and improved examination (see above the dose modification for combination therapy). This combination also results in increased respiratory depression, and if deeper levels of sedation occur, higher levels of monitoring are also necessitated. Once again, the lowest effective dose of drug should be given and individualized to each patient.*

Endoscopic Retrograde Cholangiopancreatography

Most patients require a combination of meperidine and midazolam because of the length of these proce-

*__Editor's Note:__ At our institution, most endoscopists seem to employ fentanyl and midazolam for upper endoscopies.

dures, the associated discomfort, and the need for maximal patient cooperation during endoscopic retrograde cholangiopancreatography (ERCP). Thus, many patients require near-anesthesia as opposed to conscious sedation. Not infrequently, 50 to 150 mg meperidine and 5 to 10 mg midazolam are required. These larger doses of sedatives and the increased CNS depression require higher levels of monitoring (see below). Routine reversal of the deeper sedation used with ERCP has not been studied but is widely practiced to reduce recovery time, aspiration risk, and respiratory depression. This reversal from the deeper sedation may result in later repeat sedation because of the larger and repeated benzodiazepine dosages used in ERCP. Prolonged monitoring is still necessary, and early discharge is not appropriate.

Colonoscopy

Again, most patients require a combination of meperidine and midazolam because of the pain associated with colonoscopy. However, the degree of CNS depression is much less than that needed for ERCP, and cooperative anxiolysis should not be exceeded. The endoscopist needs to know when significant pain is occurring in order not to perforate the colon, and increased levels of sedation prevent adequate patient response to pain and also increase the risk of respiratory complications.

MONITORING

All physicians administering endoscopic sedation should be fully trained in cardiopulmonary resuscitation. I believe that certification and training in both basic life support and advanced cardiac life support should be the minimal credentials required for endoscopic sedation. Although rarely needed, adequate resuscitation skills of the physician may be life saving.*

Complications in gastrointestinal endoscopy are rare and death occurs in fewer than one in 10,000 procedures. However, most complications and deaths are related to cardiopulmonary events that are in turn related to the sedation given. As complications and deaths are infrequent, it is unlikely that data on the effectiveness of monitoring in preventing complications will ever be available or adequately studied. Nonetheless, it is accepted that monitoring during conscious sedation is essential, and all patients receiving endo-

scopic sedation require physiologic monitoring to detect cardiopulmonary compromise at the earliest possible time. The degree of monitoring required is dictated by the level of patient sedation.

What degree of monitoring is required? Before the procedure, all patients should have blood pressure, respiratory rate, and pulse determined. During the procedure, these vital signs should be monitored at least every 5 minutes, and the respiratory effort observed visually by someone other than the endoscopist. Patients at increased risk of complications (i.e., those over 60 years of age, those with comorbid medical conditions, and those undergoing procedures requiring increased levels of sedation) should have O_2 saturation determined by automated pulse oximetry. Empiric low-flow supplemental oxygen can be justified in patients over 75 years old, those with significant cardiopulmonary disease, and those undergoing deep sedation and anesthesia. Patients requiring anesthesia (when protective reflexes have been lost and there is a high risk of respiratory depression) probably should have end-tidal CO_2 monitored, because oximetry does not detect significant hypoventilation and hypercarbia. Monitoring guidelines should be established by the department under whose auspices the procedures are being performed.*

SUGGESTED READING

Bartelsman JFWM, Sars PRA, Tytgat GNJ. Flumazenil used for reversal of midazolam-induced sedation in endoscopy outpatients. Gastrointest Endosc 1990; 36:S9–S12.
Bell GD. Review article: premedication and intravenous sedation for upper gastrointestinal endoscopy. Aliment Pharmacol Ther 1990; 4:103–122.
Chokhavatia S, Nguyen L, Williams R, et al. Sedation and analgesia for gastrointestinal endoscopy. Am J Gastroenterol 1993; 88:393.
Fleischer D. Monitoring for conscious sedation: perspective of the gastrointestinal endoscopist (editorial). Gastrointest Endosc 1990; 36:S19–S22.
Keeffe EB, O'Connor KW. 1989 A/S/G/E survey of endoscopic sedation and monitoring practices. Gastrointest Endosc 1990; 36:S13–S18.
McCloy R. Asleep on the job: sedation and monitoring during endoscopy. Scand J Gastroenterol 1992; 27(Suppl 192):97–101.
Porro GB, Lazzaroni M. Premedication for upper gastrointestinal endoscopy: Still a matter for debate? Endoscopy 1991; 23:32–36.
Ross WA. Premedication for upper gastrointestinal endoscopy. Gastrointest Endosc 1987; 35:120–126.
Silvis SE, Nebel O, Rogers G, et al. Endoscopic complications. Results of the 1974 American Society for Gastrointestinal Endoscopy Survey. JAMA 1976; 235:928–930.

*Editor's Note: Certification and recertification in cardiopulmonary resuscitation should probably be part of endoscopy privileges, as stated by the author.

*Editor's Note: The distinction between endoscopy nurses and nurse anesthetists appears to be blurring, at least to this observer. The ASGE guidelines for monitoring are excellent and should be consulted.

ESOPHAGUS AND MOUTH

ORAL DISORDERS OF INTEREST TO GASTROENTEROLOGISTS

MARK J. KUTCHER, D.D.S., M.S.

The gastroenterologist needs to be familiar with a number of oral disorders, if only to be able to differentiate them from the less common oral manifestations of true intestinal or liver disease. Further, the medicinal treatment of gastrointestinal (GI) disease may precipitate unwanted oral consequences. This chapter reviews some common oral conditions and their treatment, focusing on those signs and symptoms necessary to reach a tentative diagnosis, and discusses practical in-office treatment for each. Significant GI diseases with frank oral manifestations are also reviewed and their management discussed.

COMMON ORAL CONDITIONS

Recurrent Aphthous Stomatitis

Aphthous ulcerations are the second most common oral ulcerative disorder after the ulcerations of traumatic origin. Their cause is unknown, but current thought suggests they result from an autoimmune response to the oral epithelium or represent a hypersensitivity reaction to a microorganism such as *Streptococcus*. Their occurrence on oral mucosa has been associated with precipitating factors, including emotional or physical stress, minor trauma to the oral tissues, allergies, acidic foods, hormonal imbalances, and nutritional deficiencies (e.g., vitamin B_{12} and folic acid). There is no known viral etiology for aphthous ulcers, and because of the vast difference in treatment modalities, they must be differentiated from herpetic ulcerations that also occur in the oral cavity.

Clinically, aphthous ulcers begin with little or no prodromal features. Some patients may report the onset of aphthous ulcers concomitant with slight edema of the mucosal area, malaise, low-grade fever, or even submandibular lymphadenopathy. The aphthous ulcer begins as a superficial erosion, usually covered with a grayish-white pseudomembrane. There is no vesicular or bullous stage. Most classically, one to three ulcers exist at one time (see the section on herpes for the differential diagnosis). Aphthous ulcers are round and have a well-circumscribed margin surrounded by a erythematous halo. They vary from 2 to 3 mm to 1 cm in diameter (Fig. 1). The most common sites are the buccal and labial mucosa (cheek or lips) and vestibules, tongue, soft palate, and pharynx. All these areas are those in which the mucosa is not directly bound down to periosteum, in direct contrast to herpes (see next section). Most aphthous ulcers last for 1 to 2 weeks and heal without scarring.

There are no specific curative treatments for recurrent aphthous ulcers. Certainly, if one can identify a recurring source of oral trauma (such as a sharp cusp of a tooth or prosthesis) or a possible acidic food relationship, the etiology can be eliminated. Tetracyclines have been used with some success. Practically, tetracycline elixir can be prescribed as a rinse; patients are instructed to swish vigorously (providing contact with the ulcer) for 2 minutes and then expectorate. The rinse is most appropriate when more than one ulcer is present or the ulcers are positioned posteriorly in the mouth. For one anteriorly located ulcer, the patient can apply a cotton swab soaked in the elixir directly on the ulcer for 2 minutes. Both the rinse and swab should be used four times a day for about a week, and it is best to have the patient eat first, then rinse the mouth with water, before using the antibiotic to ensure maximum coverage of the lesion with the medication. Also, no food or drink for 30 minutes after rinsing will help absorption of the tetracycline. More routinely prescribed by physicians treating aphthous ulcers are the topical steroids. Triamcinolone acetonide (Kenalog) in Orabase, betamethasone valerate (Valisone) ointment, and fluocinonide (Lidex) gel are the most available and easiest to use, and appear to have almost equal success in obtaining an expedient regression of the ulcers. All these topical steroids may be placed on the ulcers after meals and at bedtime. Again, the patient should rinse and clean the mouth before applying the medication.

Patients manifesting numerous oral ulcers that last longer than 2 weeks, are extremely recurrent, heal with scarring, and are refractory to the above treatments may

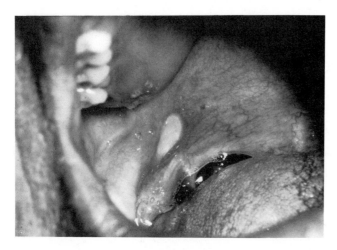

Figure 1 Classically appearing large aphthous ulcer on the lateral aspect of the soft palate; a round ulcer with a halo and grayish-white pseudomembrane covering.

have the more serious counterpart to the common, minor ulcers: called major aphthous (Sutton's disease, or periadenitis mucosa necrotica recurrens). These patients should probably be referred to an ENT, skin, or oral medicine specialist qualified by extensive clinical experience to deal with these serious ulcerations.*

Herpes Simplex Virus Infections

Herpes simplex virus (HSV) causes an initial primary infection and then becomes latent in neural ganglia. Reactivation of the virus is responsible for recurrent disease. Primary infection with HSV typically takes place between 6 months of age and adolescence and is most often subclinical. When clinical signs and symptoms of primary HSV infection are present, the condition is called primary herpetic gingivostomatitis and the child typically manifests fever, malaise, lymphadenopathy, and pain on swallowing. The mouth becomes painful, and almost all the oral tissues (gingival, tongue, palate, buccal mucosa and pharynx) become intensely inflamed. Yellowish, fluid-filled vesicles soon develop panorally and rupture almost immediately, leaving small, shallow, painful ulcerations covered by a grayish membrane and surrounded by an erythematous halo. Individual ulcers may coalesce into larger, ragged-edged ulcerations. Healing occurs over 2 weeks.

Treatment of children (the typical patients with primary herpes gingivostomatitis) is directed primarily toward pain relief and maintenance of general health. Supportive therapy can include bed rest, nutritional supplementation (with milkshakes or liquid "nutra" drinks), and forcing fluids. Remember, the colder (cold acts as an "anesthetic") and blander the food and drink is, the easier it is for the patient to tolerate. Therefore,

---

*Editor's Note: As discussed later, inflammatory bowel disease, especially Crohn's disease, and celiac disease are the GI ailments often considered with recurrent aphthous stomatitis, especially of the major variety.

have the parent chill all liquids and foods, use noncarbonated drinks, and give the child a straw for drinking when possible. Pain relief can be achieved with topical anesthetics such as 2 percent *viscous lidocaine* or a mixture of 50 percent *Benadryl elixir* and 50 percent Maalox. Older children can be instructed to rinse with these anesthetics several times a day; younger children can have their sore areas "painted" with these medications by the parent with a Q-tip. Antipyretics such as acetaminophen are satisfactory for controlling febrile episodes. Antibiotics such as penicillin can be prescribed to treat secondary infection if it develops, but should not be used to treat the primary viral infection. Steroid use is also contraindicated because of the potential to spread the virus on mucosal membranes. Therefore, it is important that the clinician differentiate between herpes simplex lesions and aphthous ulcers (which are treated appropriately by steroids). Acyclovir has not been found routinely effective in treating primary herpes gingivostomatitis, but should be considered for use in an immunocompromised patient. Patients and the parents should be advised to limit autoinoculation to the eyes, face, and genitals by careful hygiene.

Oral HSV infection recurs when the latent virus that resides in the trigeminal ganglion is reactivated. The reactivated virus finds its way to the lips and manifests as herpes labialis (fever blisters) or to the intraoral mucosa, where the lesions are known as recurrent intraoral herpes. Factors that may precipitate recurrences are stress, sunlight, trauma, fever, GI upset, hormonal changes, fatigue, and allergy, all of which are associated with the release of systemic or local prostaglandins. The lip lesions are usually associated with a prodromal stage in which the patient may experience tingling, burning, edema, erythema, or numbness on the lip in the area where the vesicles will develop within 12 to 24 hours. The vesicles are fluid filled, clustered, and on an erythematous base. They develop and rupture in successive crops over several days, then crust and heal without scarring in 10 to 14 days. The fluid weeping from the vesicles contains the intact virus, which can be somewhat easily spread to other areas of the body or to other persons upon direct contact. The intraoral recurrent lesions are less recognized because the episodes are usually asymptomatic. The lesions start as vesicles, but because intraoral vesicles rupture almost immediately, the clinician sees only the ulcers, which classically are small (1 to 3 mm) multiple, shallow, and surrounded by an erythematous halo (Fig. 2). Of great diagnostic importance is the location of these ulcers, which are almost always found on tissues bound firmly to bone, i.e., the gingival tissues around the teeth and the hard palate (see aphthous ulcers above for contrast). These intraoral lesions last for about 1 week and also heal without residual pathology.

Treatment for the intraoral lesions is usually unnecessary because of their asymptomatic nature. If a patient desires more than a brief discussion of the cause of the lesions, a simple nonprescription protective covering can be recommended, such as Orabase. For herpes labialis, the clinician can try several treatment modalities, none

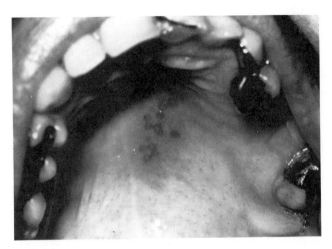

Figure 2 Recurrent intraoral herpes on the hard palate; multiple small ulcerations with halos.

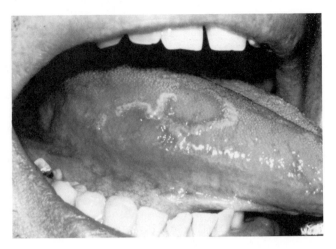

Figure 3 Migratory glossitis (geographic tongue) showing round, bald areas surrounded by slightly raised, whitish borders.

of which are proved efficacious scientifically, but which have had beneficial results in the hands of many practitioners. Generally, the earlier treatment is initiated (during prodrome), the better is the chance of reducing the duration and severity of the outbreak. *Acyclovir* (Zovirax) can be carefully applied five to seven times daily for 1 week. Ice applied for brief periods provides pain relief for some patients. A few steps may be taken to prevent the lip lesions. Herpecin-L or other lip moisturizers or sunguards can be applied to the lips before they are exposed to the elements. Further, prostaglandin inhibitors can be given in an attempt to prevent recurrent episodes. Ibuprofen (Advil, Motrin) can be prescribed in therapeutic doses starting several days before the patient is likely to be exposed to a precipitating factor (e.g., sunlight at the beach, taking an examination) and continued for the period of increased risk.

Benign Migratory Glossitis

Benign migratory glossitis (BMG) is a transitory, inflammatory-appearing condition of the tongue of unknown cause. It is important because of patient inquiries and confusion among clinicians as to its relationship with systemic diseases (there is none!). It is a condition primarily affecting adults, and women more than men. It has been associated with anxiety and emotional distress and with deeply fissured tongues. BMG appears as multiple areas of erythema due to the desquamation of the filiform papillae in irregular circinate patterns, the "bald" areas outlined by a thin, often raised, white-yellow band (Fig. 3). The dorsum and lateral borders of the tongue are most commonly affected. The lesions in one area heal spontaneously while new lesions occur elsewhere on the tongue, giving the impression of wandering or a migratory lesion. The condition may persist for weeks or months, totally regress, and then recur at any time. BMG is almost always asymptomatic, but when burning symptoms are

reported, the clinician may caution the patient to avoid spicy foods, alcohol, and smoking. For the rare, more painful cases, a mixture of 50 percent Benadryl elixir and 50 percent Maalox can be prescribed to coat the painful areas, several times daily. Biopsy is not indicated for the classic appearance of the condition. Malignant transformation has not been reported.

Candidiasis

Candidiasis (moniliasis, thrush) is the most common fungal infection of the mouth. Although most patients harbor *Candida albicans* as host flora, a pathologic overgrowth is favored by numerous factors, including use of broad-spectrum antibiotics, use of steroids, dry mouth, chronically inflamed tissue from denture irritation, poor oral hygiene, and systemic diseases such as diabetes. Today, candidiasis is a common manifestation of immunodeficiency (AIDS). The two clinical presentations encountered most frequently are acute pseudomembranous *Candida* (thrush) and atrophic *Candida* ("denture sore mouth"). Acute pseudomembranous candidal infections are characterized by white, superficial, curdlike patches that are easily scraped off the tissue with a tongue depressor, often leaving a raw, erythematous base (Fig. 4). Atrophic *Candida* infection has little of the white, hyphal masses but appears primarily as a mucosal erythema, especially in a denture-bearing area. Candidiasis is frequently found on the buccal mucosa, tongue, palate, and oropharynx. Diagnosis can usually be made in the office and treatment initiated based on the history and clinical appearance. If a definitive diagnosis is necessary, a cytologic smear can be evaluated for the organisms, or culture on a selective medium performed.

The objectives of treatment are to remove or treat the underlying causes of the fungal overgrowth and to employ antifungal agents. Either oral or systemic antifungals can be used. My decision is based on patient

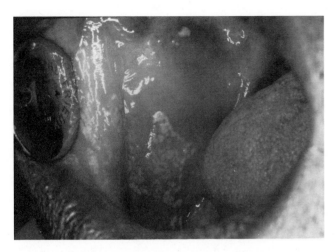

Figure 4 Pseudomembranous candidiasis of the buccal mucosa with small, white, curdlike areas of fungus that can be scraped off with a tongue depressor.

compliance, the extent of the disease, and the patient's ability to afford the newer, more expensive medications. A generic liquid such as nystatin suspension can be prescribed with instructions to swish with one teaspoon thoroughly for 2 minutes, three to four times daily for about 2 weeks. For patients who find this inconvenient, I prescribe clotrimazole (Mycelex) troches, which usually come in packets of 70. Patients let one tablet dissolve slowly on the tongue five times daily for 2 weeks. Those who wear dentures must treat these as well, because the dentures act as a nidus for candidal growth, and recurrence can be expected unless they are also treated with an antimicrobial. Nystatin ointment can be used and applied to the "tissue" surface of the denture after meals (after first rinsing the denture). Further, the patient must remove the denture at night and, after a thorough scrubbing with water, soak it overnight in a commercially available denture cleanser (or 1 teaspoon of nystatin liquid added to the water in the denture cup).

Systemic antifungals cure oral candidal infections as well as the topicals and have the added advantage of once-a-day dosing. Ketoconazole (Nizoral) tablets, one taken with breakfast for 10 to 14 days, are effective, and because of the short period of dosage, no liver dysfunctions have been reported. A newer medication, fluconazole (Diflucan), can also be prescribed. Typically, eight tablets are dispensed and the patient initially takes two with a meal, and then one tablet in the morning with breakfast for the remainder of the week. The systemics also have the advantage of being therapeutic for candidal infections that may be harbored elsewhere.

A fungal infection related to oral candidiasis, and often seen along with the oral condition in patients both immunocompetent and compromised (HIV positive), is angular cheilitis (AC). AC consists of fissuring and cracking at the corners of the mouth. The lesions may have an erythematous base, and patients usually complain of soreness when they speak or eat. Predisposing factors include habits such as lip smacking and drooling,

oral overclosure, vitamin deficiencies, and immunodeficiency. The condition is usually a mixed infection of streptococcal, staphylococcal, and candidal organisms. An ointment that contains multiple agents, such as Mycolog II, can be prescribed; this is available in 15 g tubes and is applied gently four or five times a day until healing occurs. If the patient with AC may possibly benefit from vitamin supplementation, I also prescribe multivitamins, once daily. These can do no harm, and in my opinion often appear to expedite healing of the commissural lesions. Remember that AC will not resolve if the patient has untreated oral candidiasis.

Lichen Planus

Lichen planus (LP) is the most common dermatologic disease with oral manifestations. Although of unknown cause, it is often seen in patients who are high strung or anxious and therefore may also suffer from GI disturbances. Two forms are prevalent. The reticular form occurs frequently on the buccal mucosa, tongue, and floor of the mouth and is for the most part asymptomatic. It may be recognized by the presence of fine, lacy, white lines (striae of Wickham) that are slightly raised, on a nonulcerated but sometimes erythematous mucosa. The painful form is the erosive type, which manifests as erosions and ulcerations of the tissues; however, the striae are often present at the periphery of the lesion and are significant as an identifying sign (Fig. 5). Studies have failed to show that LP is a premalignant condition, but when the clinician is unsure of the diagnosis, a biopsy is recommended. Pain can be severe and patients seem to benefit most from topical steroid therapy. I start by dispensing a tube of Kenalog in Orabase or Valisone ointment and have the patient apply the steroid to affected areas after meals and before bed, for several weeks. Slightly more potent and used for more extensive lesions, *Lidex gel* can be given with the same instructions. Be sure to tell patients to rinse the mouth before applying any medication to oral mucosa to ensure maximal contact of the medication with the lesion.

Food and Drug Allergy

Food constituents and spices can act as allergens, and certainly most medications, in any given individual, can cause oral allergic manifestations. The oral untoward responses are varied in appearance but most frequently present as ulcerations, a lichenoid reaction, or erythema multiforme. The oral reactions may become widespread, unrelenting, and severely painful. It is stressed that even the most benign medication or a simple dosage change can cause an oral response. Therapy is directed toward identification of the offending agent as well as pain relief and treatment of the lesions. The *Physicians' Desk Reference* is a useful source for determining whether a medication produces oral side effects. A careful history to evaluate allergies, diet, and the chronologic events associated with occurrence of the

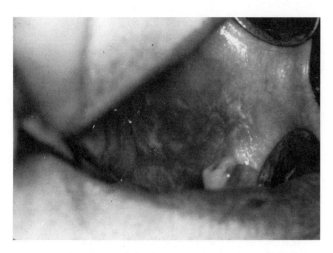

Figure 5 Erosive lichen planus of the buccal mucosa. The ulcerated and eroded area has a peripheral border manifesting the striae of Wickham.

lesions may be necessary to identify the offending agent. A topical steroid such as *Lidex gel* is useful in achieving resolution of the oral lesions, and pain can be relieved with lidocaine viscous 2 percent as a rinse (the patient is cautioned not to swallow). A mixture of 50 percent Benadryl elixir and 50 percent Maalox also gives temporary pain relief and is especially useful if used as a "swish and swallow" at mealtimes to ensure proper nourishment.

Xerostomia and Burning Mouth

Dry mouth results from decreased salivary flow. The decrease may be total or slight, but symptoms do not follow along with actual decrease, but instead are driven by the patient's perception of dryness. Factors predisposing to xerostomia include aging, dehydration, stress, salivary gland and duct disease, diabetes, Sjögren's syndrome, radiation therapy, and, very commonly, medications. Keep in mind that many of the anticholinergic therapies employed to treat GI disorders can cause xerostomia. The oral mucosa becomes pale and dry or red and atrophic in appearance. The tongue may lose its papillae and appear fissured and erythematous. Patients with dry mouth complain of soreness, burning, taste changes, and difficulty in eating and swallowing. Dry mouth quickly leads to candidiasis as well as tooth decay and a breakdown in oral health.

If dry mouth has a cause that cannot be eliminated (e.g., necessary medication, radiation therapy), replacement therapy using saliva substitutes is recommended. Commercial products such as Xero-Lube can improve taste perception, moisten oral tissues, reduce soreness and burning, and (because it contains fluoride) help remineralize tooth surfaces. Having the patient stimulate whatever saliva can be produced by sucking on sugarless, citrus (lemon) candies, or chewing gum is helpful. Sipping water or sucking on ice chips is also

beneficial. Xerostomic patients suffer rapid breakdown of the teeth, so referral to a dentist for fluoride treatments is appropriate. Candidiasis needs to be treated with antifungal agents (see earlier). If one sees a patient who complains of a sore, burning mouth or tongue, and if the clinical examination is within normal limits and history negative for organic causes, the burning may be of psychological origin. A 2 week trial of chlordiazepoxide (Librium) or diazepam (Valium) is helpful in many of these cases. Depending on the individual patient, 5 mg three times daily is enough to alleviate the symptoms in patients who are experiencing oral discomfort due to stress or anxiety.

Halitosis

Bad breath is all too common and makes life unpleasant both for the offender and for persons who must interact with them. Patients with chronic bad breath tend to find their way to the gastroenterologist because of the belief that halitosis is frequently due to stomach problems or digestive disorders.

The quality and intensity of breath normally changes with age, time of day, foods ingested, amount of saliva, and oral hygiene practices. Pathologic conditions affecting the nose, pharynx, or tracheobronchial tree that lead to the growth of gram-negative or anaerobic microorganisms will produce an objectionable odor. Breath odors may also result from pulmonary excretion of odorous substances dissolved in the bloodstream. Aromatic metabolites from ingested foods, the products of digestion, and excretion products of cell metabolism find their way into the pulmonary air. A good example is the detection of garlic in expired air after ingestion of this very aromatic food. The odor is independent of oral or upper aerodigestive conditions. However, impaired digestion of certain foods may be a cause of halitosis. For example, patients fed a diet high in milk fat for peptic ulcer disease sometimes develop bad breath. Nonetheless, the stomach plays virtually no part in the production of halitosis unless eructation or vomiting has occurred, and constipation also does not cause halitosis. Aromatic substances are absorbed from the small intestine, not the stomach or lower intestinal tract.

Extraoral factors, however, cause less than 10 percent of cases of halitosis, which originates from the oral cavity in over 90 percent of cases. The primary cause of halitosis is the growth of gram-negative anaerobic bacteria that produce the malodorous volatile compounds methyl mercaptan and hydrogen sulfide through their putrefactive action on sulfur-containing amino acids, peptones, and proteins. The growth of the causative microorganisms can be traced to poor oral hygiene, periodontal disease, tooth decay, abscesses, dry mouth, food impaction, unclean dentures, hairy tongue, oral infection, malignancy, and diet. Even very small areas of infection or microbial growth in the mouth can cause severe halitosis.

To diagnose the problem of halitosis, the clinician

must tactfully evaluate the smell. A small card waved in front of the patient's mouth can be used to direct the exhaled air toward the examiner. A careful history and examination of the head and neck and oral cavity to rule out the conditions discussed above is mandatory. Review the diet for contributory food products. The gastroenterologist should certainly consider abdominal cramps or diarrhea that suggest malabsorption. If extraoral causes are ruled out, it is reasonable to assume that the problem has an oral etiology. Referral to a dentist resolves the problem in most cases. Remember that many dentists are not aware that very minute areas of oral infection or conditions that promulgate food impaction can cause bad breath. Therefore, the referring gastroenterologist should firmly insist that everything possible be done to ensure that the patient is infection free and placed on a meticulous home care regimen. This includes having the patient brush the tongue daily to remove desquamated epithelial cells and food debris.

There are several helpful steps the clinician can try to alleviate malodor in the short term. First, promote production of saliva and tongue action by encouraging patients to chew fibrous vegetables and fresh fruits. Sugarless gum is also helpful. Hydration should be emphasized, but not rinsing with tap water, which will wash away the protective salivary coating. One can also prescribe chlorhexedine (Peridex), which is one of the few mouthrinses found to reduce malodor. Peridex is available in labeled bottles, and typically the patient is instructed to rinse twice a day with the measured capful amount for 30 seconds. **Caution:** this chemical easily stains the teeth brown (this can be removed by a dentist) and is not to be used in the long term. Another step is to use a masking agent such as oil of peppermint, which follows the same metabolic route as garlic. This can be prescribed as follows: oil of peppermint (⅛ oz) added to glycerin (USP) to fill small eyedropper bottle (dispensed with "dropper" cap), patient to place two drops on tongue, then coat mouth several times a day as needed.

Referral to a dentist and the use of palliative agents are predicated on the clinician actually detecting malodor from the patient's mouth. If no odor is detected, there are at least two other possible explanations for the complaint. First, the patient may be "tasting" an unpleasant sensation, one that is not volatile and therefore not on the exhaled breath. This could be due to vitamin deficiencies, xerostomia, the side effect of a medication, a dental material, or a galvanic reaction. It is necessary to distinguish with the patient between breath and taste changes. Second, the patient in whom you smell no offensive odor may have a psychological problem. In this case, obtaining a history of a chronologic connection between the patient's experiencing the "odor" and times of stress, anxiety, or depression may lead to the correct diagnosis. Also, questions about social, family, financial, and sexual problems may uncover the psychological cause of perceived halitosis. A patient with a suspected psychological problem should be referred to an appropriate health care provider.

SEXUALLY TRANSMITTED DISEASES

An in-depth discussion of the oral manifestations of sexually transmitted disease is outside the scope of this chapter. The frequency of such manifestations is increasing, and the clinician should consider performing an oral examination when appropriate by history or systemic signs, and be vigilant about infection control procedures in the office. The oral lesions of herpes were discussed earlier, and AIDS is the focus of the next section. The primary and secondary lesions of syphilis typically present as singular, clean ulcerations with minimal associated pain. Gonorrhea can manifest as ulcerated gingiva but most commonly as gonococcal pharyngitis. Warts can be sexually transmitted to the oral cavity and appear as typical, small, verrucous lesions or tissue-colored papillary growths. The malignant potential of oral papillomavirus lesions is probably similar to that of genital lesions, and a patient with suspected oral warts, especially one who smokes or drinks, should have these lesions biopsied.

Oral Manifestations of AIDS

The gastroenterologist may be the first medical specialist to interact with a patient with undiagnosed human immunodeficiency virus (HIV) infection when that person is evaluated for such problems as diarrhea and anal warts. A suspicion of HIV infection can sometimes be confirmed by quickly examining the oral cavity for some of the early manifestations of infection with this virus, thus leading to earlier referral and management.

One of the earliest oral manifestations of HIV infection is candidiasis. This fungal infection takes one of three forms: pseudomembranous, erythematous, or angular cheilitis. The pseudomembranous form and AC were described earlier in this chapter; the erythematous form is seen most commonly on the palate of HIV-infected patients. The treatment of oral candidal infections in patients with HIV disease is similar to that described in the candidiasis section, with the proviso that the systemic antifungals discussed should not be used in conjunction with certain other medications such as cyclosporin A, rifampicin, phenytoin, digoxin, coumarin, and oral hypoglycemics.

Oral hairy leukoplakia (OHL) is a unique condition often seen in HIV-infected patients. It consists of a white lesion found predominantly on the lateral borders of the tongue and rarely on the buccal or labial mucosa. It is keratotic and therefore does not rub off like pseudomembranous *Candida*, another leukoplakic-appearing lesion that must be differentiated from OHL. Clinically, this white lesion has a smooth to corrugated appearance; it may be small and faint to the eye or thick, extensive, and bilateral (Fig. 6). When the condition becomes extensive and symptomatic, it can be treated with high doses of systemic acyclovir (2,000 + mg daily) or retinoids (tretinoin [Retin-A]),

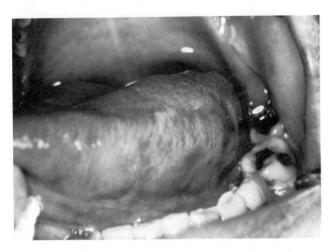

Figure 6 Hairy leukoplakia of the lateral border of the tongue in an HIV-positive patient. Note the white, somewhat corrugated surface of this hyperkeratotic lesion. (Courtesy of Dr. Lauren Patton, University of North Carolina.)

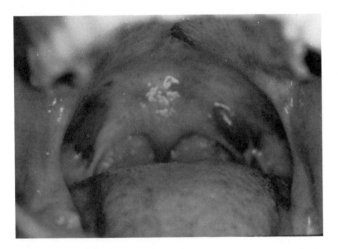

Figure 7 Kaposi's sarcoma in an HIV-positive patient on the hard and soft palate. The multiple vascular lesions were macular at first and are now beginning to ulcerate. (Courtesy of Dr. Lauren Patton, University of North Carolina.)

which usually cause remission of the lesion. However, OHL most likely will recur and need to be retreated.

Kaposi's sarcoma (KS) is the most common oral malignancy in HIV-infected patients. It may occur intraorally alone or simultaneously with skin and lymph node lesions. The first lesions of KS are often seen in the mouth, and most cases have been in men. The oral site most commonly affected is the hard palate, but any region of the mouth may be involved. KS is a vascular lesion that appears reddish-blue, purple-brown in color and may be either flat or raised, smooth-surfaced or botryoid (Fig. 7). The lesion may be solitary or multiple and widespread. The smaller lesions are asymptomatic, but when they are large and exophytic, patients experience discomfort, bleeding, and secondary infection.

Treatment, most appropriately administered by oncologists, includes intralesional or systemic chemotherapy, radiation therapy, surgical debulking, or the use of sclerosing agents.

There are separate chapters on infectious esophagitis and on gastrointestinal manifestations of HIV infection.

ALCOHOLIC LIVER DISEASE

Oral signs and symptoms of alcoholic liver disease range from the classic fetor hepaticus to spontaneous oral bleeding resulting from the depression of liver-dependent coagulation factors. Petechiae may sometimes be observed on the soft tissues in the mouth, especially the ventral surface of the tongue, floor of the mouth, or hard or soft palate. Blood may be observed oozing or crusted around the necks of teeth. Patients may report frank hemorrhaging when they brush their teeth, or may relate awakening with blood in the mouth or on the pillow. Candidiasis may be present in alcoholics owing to poor oral hygiene, poor nutrition, or dehydration. Treatment with ketaconazole may be contraindicated in these patients because of the potential for hepatotoxicity. Alcoholics may also present with bilaterally enlarged parotid glands caused by fatty infiltration. They should be evaluated for oral cancer, since the prevalence of oral malignancy increases greatly in people who drink heavily. Any suspicious lesions (leukoplakia, erythroplakia, or unexplained ulcerations) need to be biopsied. Nutritional deficiencies in these patients can also result in glossitis and loss of tongue papillae, along with AC. Patients complaining of a sore, burning tongue and in whom the clinician sees denuded and erythematous glossal areas usually benefit from multivitamins, while the soreness may be handled with the use of Xylocaine viscous 2 percent as a rinse. Again, exercise caution with this topical anesthetic in these uncompliant, neglectful patients. The dentists of patients who have alcoholic liver disease or who are alcoholic need to be reminded of their patients' bleeding tendencies, especially when invasive dental procedures are being contemplated, and of the impaired healing that can be expected. Lastly, but significantly, dentists must be cautioned about prescribing certain medications for these patients whose drug metabolism may be markedly diminished and unpredictable.

UPPER GASTROINTESTINAL TRACT DISEASES

Plummer-Vinson Syndrome

The oral manifestations of Plummer-Vinson syndrome are primarily the result of iron deficiency anemia. The clinician is therefore likely to find pathologic changes of the tongue, which will appear atrophic, bald, and erythematous. AC may be present, as may a thinning of the vermilion border of the lips and leukoplakic areas of the tongue. The risk of developing oral carcinoma is higher in these patients, and a thorough oral, pharyngeal, and esophageal examination is necessary to rule out malignancy.

Once the iron deficiency anemia has been eliminated, the oral complications usually abate. The glossal pain can be relieved by use of Xylocaine viscous 2 percent as a rinse, typically 1 teaspoon to coat sore areas several times daily. Another helpful agent is a mixture of 50 percent Benadryl elixir and 50 percent Maalox used as a rinse three to four times daily. Artificial saliva substitutes (see the section on xerostomia) can be used to moisten oral tissues and make swallowing easier. Mycolog II (see the section on candidiasis) can be prescribed for AC. Biopsy of leukoplakia to rule out cancer is also indicated.

Peptic Ulcer Disease

The oral cavity can provide the gastroenterologist with important information as patients are evaluated for peptic ulcer disease (PUD). Dietary factors predisposing to or exacerbating PUD can be assessed by looking for staining from coffee or tobacco. Loss of the enamel from the "backside" of the teeth (perimylolysis) may indicate a history of chronic gastric reflux into the mouth. Also, alcohol can be detected on a patient's breath, a precipitating factor to be eliminated. Medical-dental communication may be meaningful, since treatment of PUD includes antacids, anticholinergics, and H_2-receptor antagonists, all medications with possible dental treatment complications. Antacids chelate tetracyclines, which are commonly prescribed for oral infection; anticholinergics may result in xerostomia; and cimetidine may cause thrombocytopenia. Caution is needed by the dentist if narcotic pain medication or anxiolytic drugs are prescribed for a patient receiving cimetidine, because of its effect on hepatic microsomal enzymes.

LOWER GASTROINTESTINAL TRACT DISEASES

Crohn's Disease

The oral cavity is affected in 6 to 20 percent of patients with Crohn's disease. The oral lesions can precede the intestinal radiographic lesions and may manifest as aphthous-like ulcerations, lip edema, and cheilitis or a cobblestone architecture of the gingiva, which is also inflamed and edematous. Mucosal granulomas are usually present only in patients with other extra-abdominal signs of disease. Oral manifestations tend to resolve as the bowel disease is treated.

The pain associated with oral ulcerations can be relieved with a Benadryl and Maalox (50 percent each by volume) rinse or Xylocaine viscous 2 percent. Healing of the oral ulcers can be expedited by prescribing topical steroids such as Lidex gel or Kenalog in Orabase or

Valisone ointment, all to be applied three to four times daily for 1 to 2 weeks.

Ulcerative Colitis

In a significant minority of patients with ulcerative colitis (UC), there are oral lesions consisting most commonly of large, aphthous-like ulcerations. These tend to present initially with the onset of the GI symptoms and persist until the intestinal disease is under control. Patients with UC may also manifest pyostomatitis vegetans of the cheek and lip mucosa with deep fissure-like ulcerations that have a papillary architecture. Further, the anticholinergic medications given to reduce cramps can lead to xerostomia, while use of systemic steroids and sulfasalazine (Azulfidine) may result in candidiasis.

Palliation of the pain may be achieved with Xylocaine viscous 2 percent, Benadryl elixir, or the more powerful analgesic dyclonine. If a topical steroid is used to expedite regression of the oral ulcerations, either Lidex gel or Kenalog in Orabase can be employed. A hint: the patient using Orabase products should be instructed to gently "pat" on the thick emollient and not rub it into the tissues, which causes the material to become gritty and lose its ability to adhere to the oral mucosa.

GASTROINTESTINAL POLYPOSIS SYNDROMES

Gardner's Syndrome

The oral manifestations of Gardner's syndrome consist of osteomas and odontomas of the jaw bones and, rarely, supernumerary (extra) teeth. The jaw lesions do not have malignant potential but may require dental attention. Patients suspected of suffering from Gardner's syndrome, as well as relatives at risk, should undergo jaw radiography, because the bony lesions may be visualized before the intestinal polyps develop.

Peutz-Jeghers Syndrome

Classically, the oral and paraoral signs of Peutz-Jeghers are the multiple small areas of pigmentation of the face, oral cavity, and (most commonly) lips. The pigmented spots on the lips and oral mucosa are present from birth but appear to become more prominent with age, whereas those on the face fade with time. The pigmentations have no malignant potential.

Cowden's Syndrome

Besides the GI, breast, and thyroid abnormalities, this autosomal dominant disease can present with facial trichilemmomas and oral lesions. The oral pathology consists of pebbly, papilloma-like lesions and multiple small fibromas on any of the soft tissues, especially the gingiva.

SUGGESTED READING

Langlais RP, Miller CS. Color atlas of common oral diseases. Philadelphia: Lea & Febiger, 1992.

Little JW, Falace DA. Dental management of the medically compromised patient. 4th ed. St. Louis: Mosby, 1993.

Regezi JA, Sciubba J. Oral pathology: clinical-pathologic correlations. 2nd ed. Philadelphia: WB Saunders, 1993.

Rose LF, Kaye D. Internal medicine for dentistry. 2nd ed. St. Louis: Mosby-Year Book, 1992.

Shafer WG, Hine MK, Levy BM. A textbook of oral pathology. 8th ed. Philadelphia: WB Saunders, 1983.

Sonis ST, Fazio RC, Fang C. Principles and practice of oral medicine. Philadelphia: WB Saunders, 1984.

Wood NK, Goaz PW. Differential diagnosis of oral lesions. 4th ed. St. Louis: Mosby-Year Book, 1991.

GASTROESOPHAGEAL REFLUX: MEDICAL THERAPY

JOEL E. RICHTER, M.D.

Gastroesophageal reflux, with its major symptom, heartburn, is the most common disorder of the esophagus, the major indication for antacid consumption in the United States, and probably the most prevalent clinical condition originating from the gastrointestinal tract. In fact, most healthy persons intermittently reflux gastric contents into the esophagus. Such episodes occur in the postprandial period, are short-lived, rarely cause symptoms, and almost never take place at night. This has been designated *physiologic reflux* in contradistinction to *pathologic reflux,* which is commonly associated with esophageal symptoms (heartburn, regurgitation, dysphagia, or water brash) and/or esophageal mucosal damage. The extent of mucosal damage is variable, ranging from histologic esophagitis to erosions, ulcerations, strictures, or Barrett's esophagus. Although symptoms are common, some patients have no complaints, especially those with Barrett's esophagus and extraesophageal manifestations of reflux disease. The latter presentations include oropharyngeal complaints such as hoarseness, sore throat, and cough as well as respiratory problems including asthma, aspiration pneumonia, bronchiechasis, and chronic bronchitis. The term *gastroesophageal reflux disease* (GERD) has been coined to encompass the constellation of problems and presentations associated with pathologic acid reflux.

In the past two decades, a consensus has developed that GERD is a multifactorial process whose pathogenesis may vary in a given patient. The major predictor of esophageal symptoms and damage is prolonged contact of refluxed gastric acid with the esophageal epithelium. In healthy individuals, the esophagus is protected from prolonged acid contact by a three-tiered defensive system: the antireflux barrier provided by the lower esophageal sphincter (LES) and crural diaphragm, acid clearance mechanisms (peristalsis, saliva, and gravity), and the intrinsic resistance of the esophageal mucosa to damage. Conceptually, GERD occurs when the noxious gastric contents, especially acid and pepsin, overwhelm the esophageal defense mechanisms. This usually takes a long time, and consequently GERD is characteristically a slowly progressive mucosal disorder in which acute life-threatening events are rare. Medical therapy alleviates symptoms and heals esophagitis, but the disease usually recurs when drug therapy is stopped. GERD is therefore a chronic disease, especially in patients with esophagitis.

MEDICAL TREATMENT

Medical management of GERD can be divided into two types: lifestyle modifications and drug therapy. Both of these work to improve GERD either by reducing acid secretion or by enhancing the protective mechanisms of the esophagus.

Lifestyle Modifications

Lifestyle modifications remain the cornerstone of effective antireflux treatment for all GERD patients. The cost is low and the short- and long-term benefits are great. Time spent by the physician explaining the nature of GERD and the reasons for the various therapeutic maneuvers helps enhance treatment compliance. The following maneuvers will produce a response in most patients with mild to moderate symptoms (Table 1).

Elevation of the head of the bed is simple, time-honored, and effective therapy for GERD. Findings from several studies confirm that the use of bed blocks improves acid clearance time and reduces esophageal exposure to acid. Moreover, a recent study found an additive effect in reducing symptoms and healing esophagitis when elevation of the head of the bed was combined with an H_2 blocker (ranitidine, 150 mg twice daily). The preferred way to elevate the head of the bed is on 6 to 8 inch blocks or bricks. An alternative

Table 1 Lifestyle Modifications

Elevate head of bed (>6 inch)
Dietary modifications
  Avoid:
    Foods that decrease LES pressure: fats, chocolate, alcohol,
      carminatives
    Irritants: citrus, tomato, coffee
    Smaller, more frequent meals
    Avoid meals 2 hours before retiring
    Reduce weight (if overweight)
Decrease or stop smoking
Avoid excessive alcohol
Avoid:
  Medications that decrease LES pressure (see text)
  Direct esophageal mucosa irritants

LES = lower esophageal sphincter.

procedure employs a firm, 10-inch wedge, particularly if the patient has a water bed. Using several pillows to elevate the head is not recommended, since the patient usually rolls off them while asleep.*

Particular foods may precipitate reflux symptoms and should be avoided. Liquids with low pH or increased osmolarity (e.g., citrus juices, tomato-based products, and coffee) can evoke heartburn in patients with an acid-sensitive esophagus. Carminatives and certain food ingredients (garlic, onions, peppermint, and some after-dinner liqueurs) lower LES pressure and facilitate belching, often accompanied by reflux. Foods high in fat content and chocolates decrease LES pressure and delay gastric emptying. Patients should refrain from overeating, because increased gastric volume increases the frequency of spontaneous transient LES relaxations and associated reflux. For similar reasons, patients should not eat for several hours before retiring so as to avoid supine reflux. Patients often identify a period of weight gain that coincides with the appearance or exacerbation of reflux symptoms. Although the mechanism remains unclear, weight loss of only 10 to 15 pounds may have a dramatic effect on symptoms. Smoking and excessive alcohol use promote gastroesophageal reflux. Smoking reduces LES pressure, delays esophageal acid clearance, and increases distal esophageal acid exposure. Excessive alcohol reduces LES pressure and prolongs nocturnal acid exposure; the latter may be due to a diminished arousal response after reflux episodes.

Review of concomitant medications is crucial. Many drugs, including theophylline preparations, calcium channel blockers, nitrates, anticholinergics, antidepressants, and progesterone, reduce LES pressure. Calcium channel blockers, nitrates, and anticholinergics may also reduce esophageal contraction pressures, and the latter agents reduce salivary flow. One must also consider drugs that possibly cause esophageal mucosal irritation independent of GERD, such as doxycycline, tetracycline, quinidine, slow-release potassium chloride, iron salts,

and nonsteroidal anti-inflammatory drugs (NSAIDs). One recent surgical series found that 20 percent of patients initially referred for antireflux surgery had drug-induced lesions.*

Drug Therapy

Drug therapy is usually reserved for patients with symptomatic disease not responding to lifestyle modification, or for individuals with esophagitis. Drugs may act by decreasing or neutralizing acid secretion, promoting motility, or improving esophageal mucosal resistance. A list of drugs and their suggested dosages is provided in Table 2.

Antacids

Used on an as-needed basis, antacids are the mainstay for rapid, safe, effective relief of heartburn symptoms. Antacids primarily work by neutralizing acid, albeit for relatively short periods. Therefore, patients need to take these agents frequently, usually 20 to 30 minutes after meals and at bedtime, depending on the severity of the symptoms. Liquid forms are preferable to tablets, although the latter are the most popular preparation of this medication. Antacids are effective in relieving mild to moderate heartburn symptoms. They are particularly useful in patients with situational episodes of heartburn brought on by lifestyle indiscretions or pregnancy. Antacids, even in high doses, are not predictably effective in healing reflux esophagitis.

Excessive use of antacids may be associated with side effects. Magnesium-containing antacids produce diarrhea, and aluminum-containing agents cause constipation. The potential for magnesium or aluminum toxicity further limits their use in patients with significant renal disease, and low sodium antacids (e.g., magaldrate [Riopan]) are preferable for individuals on salt-restricted diets. In pregnant patients, adverse effects of antacids include interference with iron absorption, and metabolic alkalosis and fluid overload, in both fetus and mother, with ingestion of sodium bicarbonate.

Gaviscon

Containing alginic acid and antacids, Gaviscon is a popular drug for treating heartburn. The active component of this medication, alginic acid, interacts with saliva to form a highly viscous solution that floats on the surface of the gastric pool, acting as a mechanical barrier. The barrier reduces the number of reflux episodes and diminishes esophageal acid exposure. Recent studies using radionuclide scintigraphy and 24 hour pH monitoring confirm that Gaviscon effectively prevents episodes of upright acid reflux but is not effective at night. Evidence concerning the clinical

*__Editor's Note:__ Asking about recent weight gain, use of a water bed, or consumption of carbonated beverages may uncover the cause of a relapse or exacerbation.

*__Editor's Note:__ NSAIDs, especially ibuprofen, are commonly the cause of an exacerbation of esophagitis. Finding that a patient takes medications in bed may also implicate drug-induced esophagitis.

Table 2   Drug Therapy for GERD

Drugs	Dose
Antacids	

Mylanta II, Maalox TC
    Tums, Rolaids
	15 ml, 1–2 tablets 30 min after
	    meals and q.h.s.

Gaviscon	2–4 tablets q.i.d., p.c. and q.h.s.
Prokinetic drugs	
Bethanechol (Urecholine)	25 mg q.i.d., 30 min a.c. and q.h.s.
Metoclopramide (Reglan)	10 mg q.i.d., 30 min a.c. and q.h.s.
Cisapride (Propulsid)	10 mg q.i.d., 30 min a.c. and q.h.s.
Sucralfate (Carafate)	1 g q.i.d., 1 hr p.c. and q.h.s.
H_2-receptor antagonists	
Cimetidine (Tagamet)	800 mg b.i.d., AM and 30 min after dinner
Ranitidine (Zantac)	150 mg b.i.d., AM and 30 min after dinner
Famotidine (Pepcid)	20 mg b.i.d., AM and 30 min after dinner
Nizatidine (Axid)	150 mg b.i.d. AM and 30 min after dinner
Omeprazole (Prilosec)	20–40 mg qAM

efficacy of Gaviscon is similar to that for antacids. Although Gaviscon is safe, it contains aluminum, magnesium, and sodium; therefore, the same precautions listed for antacids apply.

Prokinetic Drugs

Drug of this class available in the United States for treating GERD include bethanechol, metoclopramide, and (most recently) cisapride. Bethanechol is a cholinergic agonist that works by increasing LES pressure, improving esophageal peristalsis, and increasing salivary flow, which in turn improves esophageal acid clearance. In contrast, metoclopramide, a dopamine antagonist, works primarily by improving gastric emptying. Cisapride is a prokinetic agent that increases gastric emptying and LES pressure by enhancing the release of acetylcholine from the myenteric plexus.

Multiple studies show that both bethanechol and metoclopramide effectively relieve heartburn symptoms, but their efficacy in treating esophagitis is equivocal. Some physicians prefer to use these prokinetic drugs in treating patients with mild to moderate persistent reflux symptoms. However, I consider their side effect profile, especially that of metoclopramide, to be very bothersome. I therefore currently use bethanechol and metoclopramide only if there is a history of symptoms related to delayed gastric emptying (i.e., after a large meal) or possibly as adjunctive therapy with H_2-receptor antagonists when patients are not responding to acid inhibition alone. European studies have found cisapride, 10 mg four times a day, to be more effective than placebo

and equal to H_2-receptor antagonists in controlling reflux symptoms and esophagitis. Studies in the United States suggest that its efficacy lies primarily in the treatment of reflux symptoms, especially those occurring at night.

Common side effects associated with bethanechol include flushing, blurred vision, headaches, abdominal cramps, and urinary frequency. It is contraindicated in a number of common disorders such as asthma, peptic ulcer disease, ischemic heart disease, and obstructive disease of the intestine or urinary tract. Cisapride is associated with minimal side effects, the most common being abdominal cramps, borborygmus, and diarrhea. The most worrisome feature of metoclopramide is its profile of possible side effects. Fatigue, lethargy, and mood and extrapyramidal problems occur with the full recommended dose (10 mg before meals and at bedtime) in 10 to 30 percent of patients. These effects are reversible on cessation of drug therapy, although tardive dyskinesia may persist. The dopamine antagonist property of metoclopramide may lead to hyperprolactinemia and glactorrhea. It is possible to decrease the frequency of side effects by lowering the dose, giving a larger dose only before troubling meals (such as the largest meal of the day) or at bedtime, or using a sustained-release tablet. Of the prokinetic drugs, only metoclopramide is safe to use during pregnancy.

Sucralfate

This drug is the basic aluminum salt of sucrose octasulfate. Sucralfate acts topically, binding to acid, pepsin, and bile. European studies have found sucralfate to be superior to placebo and equivalent to H_2 antagonists and antacid-alginate in the treatment of GERD. U.S. trials have shown only marginal benefits from sucralfate, although, interestingly, patients with the more severe erosive disease appear to benefit most from its use. This inconsistency may reflect the greater retention of sucralfate within the esophagitis of patients with erosive or ulcerative disease. Sucralfate can be used as adjunctive therapy with H_2 antagonists because, at standard doses, H_2 antagonists do not raise gastric pH high enough to prevent the acidic refluxate from activating sucralfate.

Sucralfate is a safe drug because it has limited systemic absorption, and it may therefore be used during pregnancy. The most common side effect is constipation, a reflection of its aluminum content. Since some of the aluminum may be absorbed, sucralfate should be used cautiously and at reduced dosage in patients with renal disease.*

H_2-Receptor Antagonists

This family of drugs achieved the first real breakthrough in the treatment of GERD and have largely

---

*Editor's Note: Anecdotally, some patients report better results after suspending sucralfate in a small amount of liquid.

supplanted antacids for long-term relief of symptoms and healing of esophagitis. Despite advertising to the contrary, all the H_2 antagonists are equally effective when used in proper doses. H_2 antagonist therapy for GERD differs from that for peptic ulcer disease in two ways. A greater amount of acid suppression is required to control GERD than to control peptic ulcer disease, and acid suppression is needed around the clock or at least during the periods of increased reflux.

To control acid reflux, H_2 antagonists are usually given once or preferably twice a day. Recent data on patterns of acid exposure show that the bulk of acid reflux occurs during the early evening hours after dinner and decreases markedly during the sleeping hours. It may be preferable, therefore, to advise the patient to take a dose of an H_2 antagonist *30 minutes after the evening meal* rather than at bedtime. Clinical trials in patients with GERD show that heartburn (during both day and night) can be significantly decreased by H_2 antagonists in comparison with placebo, although symptoms are rarely abolished. Recent reviews found that overall esophagitis healing rates with H_2 antagonists rarely exceed 60 percent after up to 12 weeks of treatment, even when higher than standard doses are used. Healing rates differ in individual trials, depending primarily on the degree of esophagitis before therapy. Grades I and II esophagitis heal in 75 to 95 percent of patients, whereas grades III and IV esophagitis heal in only 40 to 50 percent of patients. In view of these data, I prefer to use H_2 antagonists in treating patients with moderate to severe reflux symptoms and those with grades I and II esophagitis. On the other hand, the more severe grades of ulcerative esophagitis are best treated with omeprazole.

H_2 antagonists have been used safely for nearly 20 years. Side effects, although infrequent, differ among agents. Cimetidine may cause gynecomastia, impotence, hypospermia, mental confusion, and drug interactions. Ranitidine, generally free of the antiandrogenic and central nervous system effects and drug interactions associated with cimetidine, may produce a higher incidence of hepatic injury than cimetidine. Famotidine and nizatidine are the newest members of the H_2 antagonist category; both appear to have side effect profiles similar to that of ranitidine. Although these agents are not recommended in pregnancy, there is a large human experience with safe use of both cimetidine and ranitidine during gestation. Less common side effects are described in the *Physicians' Desk Reference*.

Omeprazole

A substituted benzimidazole, omeprazole is a potent and long-acting inhibitor of both basal and stimulated gastric acid secretion. It acts by selective, noncompetitive inhibition of the H^+/K^+-ATPase pump located in the secretory membrane of the parietal cell. A single 20 mg morning dose maintains gastric pH at 5 or more for almost 24 hours and decreases gastric volume by over 60 percent. Omeprazole has no effect on LES pressure.

Controlled studies show that omeprazole, 20 mg in the morning, completely abolishes reflux symptoms in most patients with severe GERD, usually within 1 to 2 weeks. Complete healing of esophagitis occurs after 8 weeks in more than 80 percent of patients. In those who do not heal after this time, prolonging therapy with the same dose or increasing the dose usually result in nearly 100 percent healing. Comparison studies consistently show that omeprazole is superior to ranitidine (150 mg) or cimetidine (800 mg) twice a day in relieving symptoms and healing esophagitis. Peptic strictures associated with esophagitis heal faster and require fewer dilatations when treated with omeprazole than with H_2 antagonists.

Side effects of omeprazole are minimal with short-term use, but the safety of its long-term use is not established. The profound hypoacidity produced by omeprazole stimulates gastrin release, promoting the proliferation of enterochromaffin-like (ECL) cells in the gastric fundus. Prolonged therapy with high-dose omeprazole causes a disturbingly high frequency of carcinoid tumors in rats with gastrin concentrations exceeding 1,000 pg per milliliter but not in similarly treated mice or dogs. In humans, extreme hypergastrinemia (over 1,000 pg per milliliter) secondary to the achlorhydria of pernicious anemia is associated with ECL proliferation, but fewer than 5 percent of patients develop gastric carcinoid tumors. However, gastrin concentrations rarely exceed 500 pg per milliliter during routine omeprazole therapy. By removing the acid barrier to ingested organisms, omeprazole may also increase the potential for gastrointestinal infections or gastric carcinoma due to bacterial overgrowth converting food components into carcinogens. For these reasons, Food and Drug Administration regulations specify that omeprazole should not be used for more than 8 to 12 weeks. Obviously, omeprazole is not safe for use during pregnancy.

GENERAL APPROACH

In many patients, the history of heartburn and regurgitation is sufficiently typical to permit a 6 to 8 week trial of therapy without the need for diagnostic tests. Patients failing initial empiric therapy should undergo endoscopy. This procedure is indicated to rule out other diseases (e.g., peptic ulcer disease), assess for the presence and severity of esophagitis, identify potentially complicating Barrett's esophagus or peptic strictures, and guide further treatment. Patients with dysphagia and normal endoscopy may require barium esophagography with a solid-bolus challenge (tablet, marshmallow, food) to help define mildly obstructive rings or strictures.

Endoscopy permits patients with symptomatic reflux disease to be subdivided into three groups (Table 3). Those with symptoms but no gross evidence of esophagitis can be considered at low risk of developing complications such as strictures, ulcers, bleeding, or Barrett's esophagus. The primary goal of therapy in these patients is the control of symptoms, and endo-

Table 3 General Approach to Short- and Long-Term Management of GERD

	Symptoms Without Esophagitis	Mild Esophagitis (Grades I–II)	Severe Esophagitis (Grades III–IV) or Intractable Symptoms

Acute	1. Lifestyle changes
	2. PRN medications
	    Antacids
	    Gaviscon
	    Prokinetic drugs
	    Sucralfate
	    H_2 antagonists
	        ↓
		1. Lifestyle changes
		2. Daily medications
		    H_2 antagonists b.i.d.
		      Regular dose
		      High dose
		    H_2 antagonist + prokinetic
		        ↓
			1. Lifestyle changes
			2. Strong acid suppression
			    Omeprazole, 20–60 mg
			
			        ↓

Chronic	1. Medications usually not needed
	
	2. Follow-up endoscopy not necessary
		1. H_2 antagonists b.i.d., sometimes only in evening
		2. Cisapride, 20 mg b.i.d.
		3. Endoscopy to ensure healing
			1. Full-dose omeprazole
			
			2. Lower-dose omeprazole, 10–20 mg
			3. High-dose H_2 antagonist ± prokinetic
			4. Antireflux surgery
			5. Endoscopy to ensure healing
			6. If long-term medical therapy:
			    Gastrin levels (?)
			    Surveillance endoscopy (?)

scopic follow-up is generally unnecessary. On the other hand, patients with esophagitis, with or without symptoms, are at high risk of developing complications accounting for the major morbidity and, in some cases, mortality from GERD. As already discussed, these patients represent two groups, with those having the more severe grades of esophagitis (III and IV) requiring more aggressive acid suppression to heal the mucosal lesions. Regardless of the degree of esophagitis, the ultimate goal is to heal or minimize the mucosal damage while attempting to prevent further complications. Since symptom relief does not always parallel the improvement in esophagitis, endoscopic follow-up is required to ensure healing.

Initial therapy for all groups is based on lifestyle modifications as outlined in Table 1 and selective use of the drugs listed in Table 2.

Symptoms Without Esophagitis

Patients with mild to moderate symptoms without esophagitis often experience marked symptom improvement with lifestyle changes only. Others may intermittently require antacids, prokinetic drugs, sucralfate, or H_2 antagonists. Only patients with more resistant symptoms require long-term therapy, usually with H_2 antagonists but occasionally with omeprazole.

Mild to Moderate Esophagitis

Patients with mild to moderate esophagitis (grades I and II) are best treated with H_2 antagonists, at least twice daily, until the esophagitis is healed. Some may require higher doses of H_2 antagonists to heal the esophagitis. This may be accomplished by doubling the dose of H_2 antagonists (e.g., ranitidine, 300 mg twice daily; famotidine, 40 mg twice daily), although recent studies suggest that more frequent dosing (e.g., raniti-

dine, 150 mg four times a day) may be a better approach. Other alternatives are to add a prokinetic drug or possibly sucralfate to the H_2 antagonist. Subsequently, an attempt can be made to decrease the drug to an after-evening-meal dose, but only if symptoms and esophagitis are kept under control. Chronic therapy is often required to keep these patients' esophagitis in remission. In these situations, twice daily H_2 antagonists are usually needed; most patients relapse if only an evening dose is given. Recent studies from Europe suggest that cisapride, 20 mg twice daily, may be an alternative effective therapy. Continued endoscopies are not required unless there are important changes in symptoms (dysphagia, weight loss) or evidence of bleeding.

Severe Erosive-Ulcerative Esophagitis

Patients with severe erosive-ulcerative esophagitis (grades III and IV) or intractable symptoms require strong acid suppression to control the disease in both the short and long term. Although higher doses of H_2 antagonists improve the healing rates of severe esophagitis, I believe the expense and inconvenience may not be worth the minimal gain. For this reason, omeprazole has replaced H_2 antagonists for treating the more severe forms of GERD. Omeprazole, 20 mg every morning, heals over 80 percent of patients with erosive esophagitis, but 40 to 60 mg doses may be needed for more recalcitrant patients. With this approach, almost all cases of acute esophagitis can be healed, but maintaining these patients in remission is a major problem because nearly 80 percent relapse within 1 year of discontinuing therapy. Not surprisingly, the major predictors of relapse are low LES pressure and the initial severity of esophagitis. After the esophagitis has healed, an attempt should be made to switch the patient to a maintenance regimen consisting of a high-dose H_2 antagonist, possibly in addition to cisapride. Unfortunately, many patients experience a recurrence of symptoms and esophagitis requiring reinstitution of omeprazole. Some of these may be controlled at a lower maintenance dose such as 10 to 20 mg every morning. The follow-up of these patients is not well defined. I prefer to obtain a serum gastrin level at the end of the first year. If the value is greater than 500 pg per milliliter, intermittent surveillance endoscopy should be considered to look for carcinoid tumors. Because of the potential long-term risk of omeprazole, this treatment should currently be reserved for patients with severe esophagitis who are not surgical candidates.*

Atypical Presentations

Patients with atypical reflux presentations or difficult management problems may require further esophageal testing. The acid perfusion test can be helpful in these cases. If acid but not saline infusion brings on the symptoms, acid reflux is the likely cause. A negative test, however, does not preclude GERD, and these patients should have prolonged pH monitoring. Ambulatory, 24-hour esophageal pH monitoring allows for accurate quantification of acid reflux throughout the circadian cycle as well as correlating symptoms with acid reflux episodes. After the pH electrode has been placed 5 cm above the manometrically determined LES, this study can be performed in the patient's home or work environment, thereby increasing the opportunity of replicating the symptoms. I most commonly perform 24 hour pH monitoring in patients presenting with noncardiac chest pain, suspected pulmonary or ENT complications of GERD, and intractable reflux symptoms associated with a negative work-up who are not responding to H₂ antagonists or omeprazole. In the last group, about two-thirds of the patients do not have acid reflux on pH testing, suggesting that their symptoms are functional in origin. The other third have an excessive amount of acid reflux often requiring higher doses of acid-suppressing medications.

Antireflux Surgery

Although most patients with GERD can be managed medically, approximately 5 to 10 percent require antireflux surgery. In the past, the primary indication for surgery was failure of medical therapy, but this is now extremely rare with the availability of omeprazole. Surgery should still be considered in younger patients with severe GERD who otherwise would require lifetime medical therapy. Other indications for antireflux surgery include recurrent difficult-to-dilate strictures, nonhealing ulcers, severe bleeding from esophagitis, and reflux-related complications of the respiratory tract or ear,

nose, and throat not responding to medical therapy. The presence of Barrett's esophagus alone is not an indication for antireflux surgery. This is discussed in another chapter.

Antireflux surgical procedures are currently performed through the abdomen or chest. All use crural-tightening after reducing the hiatus hernia and returning the esophagogastric junction to the abdomen, as well as varying degrees of fundoplication. Two factors are paramount to successful antireflux surgery. First, is the preservation of esophageal function confirmed by esophageal testing before surgery. This evaluation should include endoscopy, esophageal manometry, and ambulatory esophageal pH monitoring. Older patients with recent onset of ulcerative esophagitis and strictures should be evaluated especially carefully because some may have drug-induced disease in which the esophageal pH studies will be normal. Esophageal manometry is performed primarily to assess the functional motor capacity of the body of the esophagus; measuring the LES pressure is of secondary importance. Nonspecific disturbances of motility, such as low-amplitude peristaltic contractions and intermittent simultaneous contractions, are not contraindications to antireflux surgery because these disorders are probably secondary to the reflux disease itself. On the other hand, it is important to identify aperistalsis, whether this be a manifestation of achalasia, scleroderma, or severe end-stage reflux disease.

The second factor is the skill and experience of the surgeon, which generally is reflected by the frequency with which this operation is performed. In the hands of experienced surgeons who perform careful esophageal preoperative testing, the results of antireflux operations are generally good but not perfect: up to 80 to 90 percent of patients have good long-term outcomes.

Acknowledgment. The author thanks Mrs. Linda Pugh for her secretarial assistance in the preparation of this manuscript.

SUGGESTED READING

Hogan WJ. Gastroesophageal reflux disease: an update on management. J Clin Gastroenterol 1990; 12(Suppl 2):21–28.
Kitchin LI, Castell DO. Rationale and efficacy of conservative therapy for gastroesophageal reflux disease. Arch Intern Med 1991; 151: 448–454.
Koelz HR. Treatment of reflux esophagitis with H₂ blockers, antacids, and prokinetic drugs. An analysis of randomized clinical trials. Scand J Gastroenterol 1989; 24(Suppl 156):25–36.
Maton PN. Omeprazole. N Engl J Med 1991; 324:965–975.
Mattox HE, Richter JE. Prolonged ambulatory esophageal pH monitoring in the evaluation of gastroesophageal reflux disease. Am J Med 1990; 89:345–356.
Ramirez B, Richter JE. Promotility drugs in the treatment of gastroesophageal reflux disease. Aliment Pharmacol Ther 1992 (in press).
Spechler SJ. Department of Veterans Affairs Gastroesophageal Reflux Disease Study Group. Comparison of medical and surgical therapy for complicated gastroesophageal reflux disease in veterans. N Engl J Med 1992; 326:786–792.

*Editor's Note: Some physicians utilize a gastric analysis while trying to switch to H₂ antagonists to be sure adequate suppression is allowed. This is usually in patients with Barrett's esophagus.

EXTRAESOPHAGEAL MANIFESTATIONS OF REFLUX DISEASE

WILLIAM J. RAVICH, M.D.

Gastroesophageal reflux disease typically presents with symptoms related to esophageal irritation, such as retrosternal burning, chest pain, and dysphagia. In recent years there has been increased recognition of reflux disease as a cause of extra-esophageal symptoms, such as *sore throat, hoarseness, cough,* or *dyspnea.* Reflux disease is now often diagnosed by otolaryngologists and pulmonologists. It is increasingly common for patients with chronic pharyngitis and laryngitis, recurrent pulmonary infections, and asthma to be referred for reflux testing and treatment. Previous under-awareness of reflux as a possible cause of these problems may have been replaced by a zealous tendency to leap at the diagnosis of reflux. The elicitation of occasional episodes of heartburn may be considered enough evidence for the unwary physician to "confirm" the diagnosis of reflux disease.

In developing an approach to patients with possible extraesophageal manifestations of reflux disease, a number of problems must be appreciated:

1. Extra-esophageal manifestations may occur in the absence of typical reflux symptoms. A paucity of esophageal symptoms does not rule out reflux disease. This is unexpectedly common for patients referred to a gastroenterologist by otolaryngologists and pulmonologists, presumably because more obvious symptoms of reflux would have resulted in an earlier direct referral from the primary physician or self-referral by the patient.
2. The sensitivity and specificity of objective reflux testing, including continuous pH monitoring (CpHM), for patients presenting with extraesophageal manifestations is unknown. Reflux disease is sufficiently common that its confirmation by pH studies in patients presenting with extraesophageal symptoms or findings does not prove that reflux is responsible. Conversely, studies suggest that the pharynx, larynx, trachea, and bronchi are more sensitive to contact with gastric contents than is the esophagus. It is therefore possible that infrequent, short-duration reflux episodes, insufficient to reach the criteria for pathologic reflux by CpHM, might produce reflux-related problems.
3. The effect of antireflux therapy in refluxers presenting with extraesophageal manifestations has not been adequately studied. It is my impression that standard medical therapy is less effective and takes longer to achieve a positive effect

in patients with extraesophageal manifestations than in those with more typical reflux symptoms.

DIAGNOSIS

My initial approach to diagnosis is to evaluate patients by means of a barium cineradiography or videoradiography. This allows the clinician to rule out pharyngeal dysfunction causing aspiration as an alternative explanation for many of the same symptoms. Although barium studies are not a quantitative means of documenting reflux, substantial reflux observed during the study may be accepted as objective confirmation of reflux. However I require confirmation if the radiologist's comments suggest that the amount of reflux observed is only modest.

In the absence of substantial reflux on barium studies, I perform a continuous pH monitor study, preferably using a dual-channel pH probe system with the distal lead located 5 cm above the manometrically determined lower esophageal sphincter and with the proximal lead in the cervical esophagus or pharynx. A positive study in either lead confirms reflux. In general I emphasize the duration of acid exposure in the interpretation of pH probe studies over more complicated methods for determining the significance of reflux. In patients with intermittent symptoms, I also pay attention to the temporal relationship of symptom episodes with reflux events.

Most studies suggest that for a probe located in the distal esophagus, the normal amount of time the esophagus spends at a pH less than 4 is under 4.5 percent for the total, 6 percent for the upright, and 3 percent in the supine study periods. Information about normal and pathological reflux at the level of the cervical esophagus and pharynx is limited, but suggests that normal controls spend less than 2.6 percent of time with a pH less than 4 in the cervical esophagus and that any reflux into the pharynx may be abnormal. More studies are needed to confirm these findings. Although the addition of a proximal probe may increase the number of positive tests, the increment is relatively small and the absence of proximal reflux does not rule out reflux-induced extraesophageal disorders.

A negative pH study does not completely exclude reflux as a cause of extraesophageal manifestations, and either a barium study demonstrating reflux or a temporal association of symptoms with meals or lying down is sufficient to justify a vigorous trial of reflux therapy. However, failure to document reflux should prompt the clinician to review the patient's previous evaluation to assure that alternative causes of symptoms have been pursued with sufficient thoroughness.

In my experience, erosive esophagitis is the exception rather than the rule in patients in whom extraesophageal manifestations predominate. Therefore, I do *not* perform endoscopy in most of these patients unless the severity of typical reflux symptoms or the results of objective testing suggest a high probability of esophageal mucosal injury.

MANAGEMENT

As mentioned, reflux disease is sufficiently common that its presence in patients with extraesophageal manifestations does not prove that reflux is responsible. In this group of patients, the line between diagnosis and therapy is blurred, and a trial of antireflux therapy often serves as a final test of causality. The situation is further complicated by the relative resistance of extraesophageal manifestations to antireflux therapy. In patients with extraesophageal manifestations, I tend to initiate more intensive antireflux therapy from the outset than I do in those with typical presentations of reflux. One should reassess the clinical response at monthly intervals. Failure of symptoms to respond requires modification in drug therapy, at least until improvement is obtained or "maximal" therapy has been utilized (Fig. 1). Unless this aggressive approach is taken, a great deal of time, money, and patience can be exhausted without a resolution of the issue of causality.

In patients with extraesophageal manifestations, the elements of antireflux therapy are the same as for reflux disease in general: antireflux dietary and lifestyle changes, acid-suppressive drugs, prokinetic agents, and

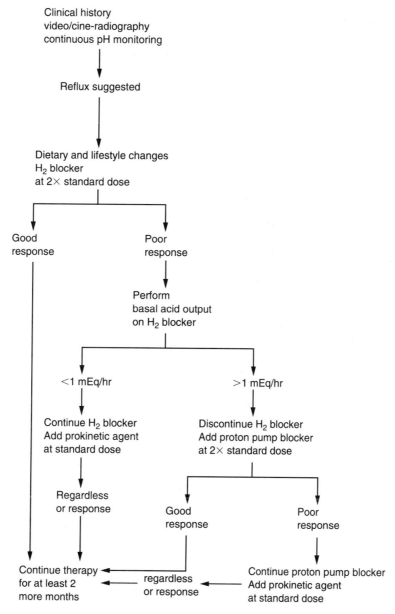

Figure 1 Algorithm for management of extraesophageal symptoms.

surgery. However, the presence of extraesophageal manifestations alters their application. While H_2 blocker therapy accompanied by modest changes in daily habits is usually sufficient to dramatically control typical reflux symptoms, this may not be true in the case of extraesophageal manifestations where even small amounts of refluxed gastric contents, including dilute acid and bile, can cause injury that can take time to repair. Control of acid alone is therefore less often effective in patients with extraesophageal manifestations.

Even more than for typical refluxers, I attempt to emphasize the importance of the usual antireflux dietary and lifestyle modifications, especially during the period in which we are trying to establish whether reflux is responsible for symptoms. I particularly emphasize the importance of small meals, avoidance of lying down after eating, and elevation of the head of the bed, measures that minimize the volume of reflux. (Additional details are presented in the preceding chapter.)

As with the usual approach to drug therapy for reflux disease, I initially concentrate on *acid suppression.* I prefer to start with H_2 blockers at twice the standard dose, using longer-acting formulations and increased dose frequency to provide a more uniform control of gastric acidity (Table 1). If after 1 month of this regimen, the patient indicates a substantial improvement in symptoms, this regimen is continued for a minimum of 2 additional months, with the response assessed at monthly intervals.

If there is little symptomatic improvement after 1 month, a fasting morning basal gastric analysis on acid-suppression therapy is obtained. The patient takes the usual dose of H_2 blockers on the day prior to the test. On the day of the test, the patient fasts and the morning dose is withheld. After intubation, the gastric residual is removed and a 1-hour basal collection is obtained to determine the basal acid output (BAO). The BAO is used to determine the subsequent adjustment in medical therapy, either intensification of acid suppression or addition of a prokinetic agent.

The interpretation of gastric analysis results is based on the work of Colleen and co-workers. In their study of patients with typical refluxers (in whom both symptoms and esophagitis were present), responders had a BAO on standard drug therapy of less than 1 mEq per hour, while refractory patients had a BAO of greater than 1 mEq per hour. Furthermore, those who were initially refractory became responders when acid suppressive therapy was intensified to achieve a BAO of less than 1 mEq per hour.

Based on this information, and cognizant of the dangers of extrapolating these results to patients with atypical presentations, a BAO of less than 1 mEq per hour suggests adequate acid suppression and should prompt one to continue the current acid suppression regimen and add a prokinetic agent, such as *metoclopramide* or *cisapride* at their usual recommended dosage (Table 1). A BAO of greater than 1 mEq per hour is considered evidence of inadequate acid suppression. The H_2 blocker is discontinued and the proton-pump

Table 1 Drug Therapy for Extraesophageal Manifestations of Reflux Disease

Drug	Dose/Frequency
H_2 blockers*	
Cimetidine (Tagamet)	600 mg po qid
Ranitidine (Zantac)	150 mg po qid
Nizatidine (Axid)	300 mg po bid
Famotidine (Pepcid)	40 mg po bid
Proton-pump blocker*	
Omeprazole (Prilosec)	20 mg po bid
Prokinetic agents†	
Metoclopramide (Reglan)	10 mg po qid
Bethanechol (Urecholine)	25 mg po qid
Cisapride (Propulsid)	10 mg po qid

*The doses of H_2 blockers and of omeprazole listed here are twice the standard recommended doses. Once symptomatic control has been obtained, efforts are made to decrease the intensity of drug therapy. Because of cimetidine's relatively short duration of action and side effects at higher doses, other H_2 blockers are preferred.
†Despite its relatively high incidence of side effects, metoclopramide has been my preferred prokinetic agent for extraesophageal manifestations of reflux disease. Bethanechol may provoke bronchospasm and is therefore specifically contraindicated for patients with asthma. The use of erythromycin, an antibiotic with prokinetic properties, has not been reported in reflux disease. Cisapride has just been released for use in the United States. Because of its reported efficacy in reflux disease and low incidence of side effects, it is likely to become the preferrred prokinetic agent for the treatment of reflux disease.

blocker omeprazole is begun at twice the standard dose. If in this latter group there is no substantial improvement after another month, one can then add a prokinetic agent (metoclopramide or cisapride).

OUTCOME OF MEDICAL THERAPY

Information on the efficacy of medical management for the extraesophageal manifestations of reflux disease is limited. In my experience, patients fall into three categories, with a good, fair, and poor probability of response to medical therapy, depending on their clinical presentation and results of objective testing.

Patients with clinically significant typical reflux symptoms and documentation of reflux by either barium or pH probe studies have a good chance of improvement in their extraesophageal symptoms, although the response is less certain than for patients presenting with typical reflux disease. Not infrequently, the typical symptoms respond but the extraesophageal symptoms do not, leaving the question of the relationship between those symptoms and reflux unresolved. In those without significant typical reflux symptoms but with confirmation of reflux by objective testing, the prospect of improvement is fair. Presumably most failures represent patients in whom reflux is incidental to their presenting complaints, although the possibility that reflux-related extraesophageal manifestations are simply refractory to therapy is difficult to exclude. In patients without significant typical reflux symptoms or objective confirmation of reflux, the probability of response is poor. Yet even in this category, a few patients respond dramatically to medical therapy against reflux disease, suggesting that a negative objective testing does not rule out reflux-related manifestations.

The final drug regimen is continued, along with strict antireflux dietary and lifestyle changes, for at least 2 months before I decide on the effectiveness of antireflux therapy. Once a satisfactory response is obtained, the intensity of drug therapy is gradually decreased to establish the regimen required to maintain control of reflux. Symptom breakthrough is common, however, and long-term high-dose H_2 blocker therapy, omeprazole therapy, or combination therapy with acid-suppressors and prokinetic agents are often required for continuing medical management.

ANTIREFLUX SURGERY

Although one should not be reluctant to continue intensive therapy, surgical intervention should be considered if successful. Whereas I rarely advocate antireflux surgery in typical "refluxers" unless symptoms and gross esophagitis cannot be controlled on reasonable doses of drug therapy, I am prepared to do so in patients with severe extraesophageal manifestations even without esophagitis. The rationale includes the frequent need for intensive therapy to maintain control of symptoms in this group of patients as well as the more complete control of reflux that can be obtained with effective antireflux surgery. In a sense, in patients with extraesophageal presentations, the goal of medical therapy is often to establish the causal relation between reflux and their symptoms to permit a more confident recommendation about the appropriateness of surgical intervention.

Failure to respond to the intensive approach to treatment outlined here would appear to constitute strong, but not absolute, evidence *against* reflux as the cause of extraesophageal problems. A decision to recommend surgery is difficult to make under these circumstances unless the suspicion on clinical grounds or objective testing is especially strong.

Antireflux surgery has a high probability of success in those whose symptoms respond well to intensive medical therapy. In some patients, the response to intensive medical therapy is substantial but incomplete. For these patients there is an option of extending treatment for up to 4 months or more to observe whether continuing improvement is observed. Alternatively, one can stop drug therapy to determine whether symptoms exacerbate again.

In these patients, surgical intervention has a lower probability of producing a complete remission of extraesophageal symptoms than in those whose response is more complete and is more likely to produce an incomplete response. This may be due to a multifactorial origin of pulmonary symptoms. For example, a patient with asthma may be more likely to reflux due to altered transdiaphragmatic gradients which could in turn exacerbate the severity of bronchospasm. However, that patient would continue to have asthma after anti-reflux surgery. In this group surgical intervention may still be appropriate, but the patient should not be given unreasonable assurances that it will cause complete symptom resolution.

SUGGESTED READING

Collen MJ, Lewis JH, Benjamin SB. Gastric acid hypersecretion in refractory gastroesophageal reflux disease. Gastroenterology 1990; 98:654–661.

Jacob P, Kahrilas PJ, Herzon G. Proximal esophageal pH-metry in patients with 'reflux laryngitis'. Gastroenterology 1991; 100:305–310.

Koufman JA. The otolaryngologic manifestations of gastroesophageal disease (GERD): a clinical investigation of 225 patients using ambulatory 24-hour pH monitoring and an experimental investigation of the role of acid and pepsin in the development of laryngeal injury. Laryngoscope 1991; 101(Suppl 53):1–78.

McNally PR, Maydonovitch CL, Prosek RA, et al. Evaluation of gastroesophageal reflux as a cause of idiopathic hoarseness. Dig Dis Sci 1989; 34:1900–1904.

Sontag SJ, O'Connell S, Khandelwal S, et al. Effect of positions, eating, and bronchodilators on gastroesophageal reflux in asthmatics. Dig Dis Sci 1990; 849–856.

Wiener GJ, Koufman JA, Wu WC, et al. Chronic hoarseness secondary to gastroesophageal reflux disease: documentation with 24-h ambulatory pH monitoring. Am J Gastroenterol 1989; 84:1503–1508.

SURGERY FOR GASTROESOPHAGEAL REFLUX DISEASE

PETER F. CROOKES, M.D.
TOM R. DeMEESTER, M.D.

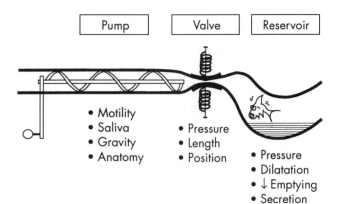

Figure 1 Mechanical model of the antireflux mechanism. The esophagus can be visualized as a propulsive pump, the stomach as a reservoir, and the lower esophageal sphincter as a valve. Esophageal clearance of refluxed gastric juice is determined by the esophageal motor activity, salivation, gravity, and the presence of a hiatal hernia. The competency of the lower esophageal sphincter depends on its pressure, overall length, and length exposed to abdominal pressure. Gastric function abnormalities causing gastroesophageal reflux include increased intragastric pressure, gastric dilatation, decreased emptying rate, and increased gastric acid secretion.

Gastroesophageal reflux is a normal phenomenon, typically occurring in short episodes after eating. Gastroesophageal reflux disease (GERD) is the condition where the degree of exposure of the esophageal mucosa to gastric contents is greater than normal. This excessive exposure has several consequences. The patient's symptoms include heartburn and regurgitation, and later there may be dysphagia. Other effects of GERD include respiratory symptoms such as coughing and wheezing and an asthma-like picture, or hoarseness and laryngitis. Pathologically, GERD is often complicated by esophagitis, which may progress to stricture formation. Barrett's esophagus (columnar lining of the lower esophagus) may develop, and this in turn may be complicated by a Barrett's ulcer which heals with a stricture. Barrett's epithelium is a premalignant condition, with a tendency to lead to dysplasia and adenocarcinoma.

The normal mechanisms to protect the esophagus against GERD can be visualized in the mechanical model summarized in Figure 1. The *pump* includes the peristaltic function of the esophageal body, the effect of gravity in the upright position, and the neutralizing effect of saliva. All these mechanisms tend to clear the esophagus of refluxed acid and limit the exposure time. The *valve* function is the lower esophageal sphincter (LES), the efficacy of which is related to the resting pressure, the total length over which the pressure is exerted, and the length of the portion exposed to intra-abdominal pressure. All the measurements of pressure along the entire length of the LES can be integrated into a 3-dimensional model, the volume (the vector volume) of which is a measure of the resistance exerted by the LES against the reflux of gastric juice. The *reservoir* function of the stomach predisposes to GERD when there is delayed gastric emptying, hypersecretion of acid, or gastric dilatation. In normal people, acid is often refluxed back into the esophagus during short periods of transient LES relaxation. Such episodes are recognized by a drop in the luminal pH from the normal range of 5 to 7 pH to below 4. These episodes tend to occur in the upright position after meals and typically are associated with belching. They are rapidly cleared by a swallow-induced peristaltic wave, which returns most of the acid to the stomach, and carries saliva to neutralize any residual acid. The commonest reason for pathologic esophageal acid exposure is mechanical deficiency of the LES. This is measured manometrically as a defect in pressure (<6

mm Hg measured in midinspiration at the respiratory inversion point), overall length, (<2 cm) or abdominal length (<1 cm) or a subnormal vector volume.

The gastric causes of GERD include hypersecretion and delayed gastric emptying. The identification of these states require gastric acid analysis with pentagastrin stimulation, and radionuclide assessment of emptying of a solid meal. Primary abnormalities of the esophageal body (motility disorder, hiatal hernia, lack of saliva) may cause increased esophageal acid exposure. It is important to identify these gastric and esophageal causes before considering surgical treatment, as they may influence the type of operation performed, or even the decision to operate at all.

INVESTIGATION OF PATIENTS WITH SUSPECTED GERD

Four investigations are key to understanding GERD: endoscopy, barium videoroentgenography, esophageal manometry, and 24 hour pH monitoring. Endoscopy will exclude other serious pathology in the upper gastrointestinal tract causing symptoms, and will identify complications of GERD and hiatal herniation. Barium videoesophagography gives some idea of the adequacy of peristalsis and can distinguish reducible hiatal hernias (disappear after a swallow in the upright position) from nonreducible hernias. When the patient presents with dysphagia, it is wise to obtain this investigation as a "road map" before any instruments are inserted into the esophagus. Ambulatory pH monitoring is vital for defining the disease and manometry is the best

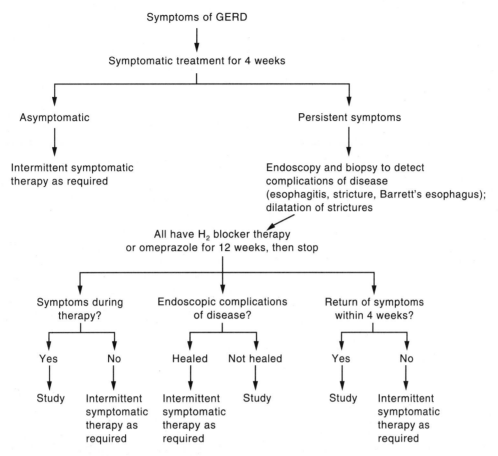

Figure 2 Algorithm showing medical management and indications for functional studies (i.e., 24-hour pH monitoring and manometry) in patients with symptoms of gastroesophageal reflux disease (GERD).

way of assessing the functional status of esophageal body and the LES. More detailed information on the efficacy of esophageal peristalsis and clarification of motor disorders comes from prolonged ambulatory manometry, which can be performed at the same time as 24 hour esophageal pH monitoring. The algorithm outlining when patients should be studied physiologically is shown in Figure 2.

THE PLACE OF MEDICAL TREATMENT

By the time a patient with symptoms of GERD is referred to a surgeon, various medical regimens will have been tried without complete success. The logic behind most medical treatment is reducing the acidity of the refluxed gastric juice. Accordingly, it works best in the long term where the underlying cause is chemical, i.e., where there is acid hypersecretion. Omeprazole, 20 to 40 mg, daily is by far the most effective agent both for symptomatic relief and for healing of esophagitis, but up to 20 percent of treated patients will have persistent esophagitis. The safety of long-term omeprazole is not yet determined, and current guidelines still recommend

restricting continuous treatment to a 12 month period. Therefore, deciding to treat a patient with omeprazole must acknowledge that surgery is likely to be necessary in the future. Other views of the management of esophageal reflux are presented in two other chapters on gastroesophageal reflux and a chapter on Barrett's esophagus.

Prokinetic agents aimed at increasing LES tone and esophageal body peristalsis give little additional relief and are often limited by serious side effects.* Many lifestyle modifications commonly advised for GERD represent good common sense, such as weight reduction and avoiding heavy meals late at night. However, when patients must abstain from coffee, tea, alcohol, tobacco, peppermint, and rich or spicy food, sleep propped up in bed, and wear only loose clothes, they often regard the restrictions as burdensome and do not comply. The goal of surgical therapy is to relieve symptoms and prevent complications without requiring long-term medications or imposing unrealistic lifestyle restrictions.

---

*__Editor's Note__: Cisapride may prove to be helpful and with less side effects.

WHO BENEFITS FROM SURGICAL TREATMENT?

The first requirement prior to consideration of surgical treatment is objective documentation of the disease. This means documenting excessive acid exposure on 24-hour pH monitoring. Very occasionally, the acid exposure may be normal in a patient with typical symptoms and esophagitis on endoscopy: in this situation, review the circumstances of the pH test. An undilated stricture may prevent the refluxed acid from reaching the probe, or the damaging agent may be alkaline duodenal contents in a hypochlorhydric patient. Some patients have prolonged hypochlorhydria after stopping omeprazole, and a history of recent ingestion of this should be sought. However, not all patients with esophagitis or stricture have GERD. Infective esophagitis, caustic injuries, and pill-induced injury are important nonreflux causes for which antireflux therapy is inappropriate.

Uncomplicated Reflux

Many internists and surgeons are reluctant to advise surgery in the absence of demonstrable esophagitis. However, one should not be deterred from considering antireflux surgery in a symptomatic patient when the disease process has been objectively documented by 24 hour pH monitoring. Critical to the decision is the status of the LES. If a defective LES is present, the patient is likely to be condemned to a lifetime of medical therapy, and relapse and progression is common. These patients do well after Nissen fundoplication. If the LES is normal, evidence of gastric hypersecretion or delayed gastric emptying should first be sought. We are cautious about performing fundoplication in patients with a normal LES. Such patients are often "upright" refluxers who are chronic air swallowers. This is the cause of the higher incidence of bloating and fullness after surgery. In the absence of primary gastric pathology, the stimulus to swallow is removed by surgical control of reflux and the problem gradually resolves.

Complicated Reflux

Factors which encourage the development of complications are the presence of a defective LES, defective esophageal clearance, the presence of a hiatal hernia, and the coexistence of duodenal contents in the refluxate. The presence of these factors may modify the operative approach.

Esophagitis is visualized endoscopically and usually classified by some modification of Savary and Miller's grading system. Grade 1 (nonerosive changes, mucosal erythema) is usually disregarded as it is too subjective. Erosive esophagitis may be Grade 2 (isolated erosions) and Grade 3 (confluent erosions). Grade 4 esophagitis (stricture) is discussed below. Patients with esophagitis commonly have a defective LES, and many have some evidence of diminished peristalsis in the distal esophagus as a result of acid exposure. The fact that this rarely reverts to normal following successful acid suppression therapy suggests that prolonged acid-induced damage to esophageal muscle is permanent, and should encourage the surgeon to intervene before this has occurred.*

Stricture is the result of more severe transmural damage, and by definition represents a failure of medical therapy. The recent Veterans Affairs cooperative study on GERD noted that 8 percent of patients free of stricture on entry developed a stricture during the study despite medical therapy. We have noted the development and progression of strictures even in patients taking omeprazole.

A stricture is present if the narrowing is sufficient to prevent the passage of a 12 mm endoscope, or a 12 mm barium tablet. The prevalence of a defective LES and defective esophageal body peristalsis is even higher than in esophagitis, and a hiatal hernia is commonly present. Esophageal shortening, best detected manometrically, is common. Although some very frail patients may be satisfactorily controlled on Omeprazole and dilatations, the majority are best served by combining dilatation with an antireflux procedure. After dilating the stricture to 60 Fr, biopsies and brushings are taken to exclude malignancy. Manometry is then performed to identify defects in the LES and distal esophageal body peristaltic contractions. Twenty-four hour pH monitoring usually shows very high esophageal acid exposure. If the patient's acid exposure is normal as mentioned previously, a drug-induced stricture may be responsible, and the history should be reviewed. Pure alkaline reflux, such as may happen after total gastrectomy, may cause a stricture. However, excessive alkaline reflux is rare on its own, and is generally associated with excessive acid reflux. Surgical correction will generally require an incomplete fundoplication (Belsey), since transmural injury usually has reduced contraction amplitude to below the 5th percentile and increased the prevalence of dropped and interrupted waves. Patients whose dysphagia is initially relieved by dilatation to 60 Fr can be expected to have a good result. If the symptomatic response to adequate dilatation is poor, or if the stricture cannot be satisfactorily dilated at all, or if several unsuccessful antireflux operations have been done in the past, esophageal replacement will be needed.

Barrett's esophagus is the condition where metaplasia in the lower esophagus results in a lining with columnar epithelium. There is a separate chapter on this subject. The intestinal ("specialized") epithelium is the form likely to lead to malignant transformation. It is now widely recognized that neither medical nor surgical treatment leads to appreciable regression of the Barrett's epithelium. Some reports of carcinoma developing years after antireflux surgery have appeared, but in very few did the authors confirm by pH monitoring that the operation had controlled reflux. Surgery offers the best protection against malignant transformation but does

---

*Editor's Note: It is important to rule out drug-induced esophageal ulceration before deciding to refer the patient for surgery.

not completely abolish it. We believe that for relief of symptoms and reduction of further complications in Barrett's esophagus, surgery should be performed. The presence of low grade dysplasia in the epithelium is a strong indication to proceed to antireflux surgery. High grade dysplasia is equivalent to carcinoma-in-situ, and if diagnosed by a knowledgeable pathologist and confirmed by another opinion, is an indication for esophagectomy as 50 percent of the patients will show invasive carcinoma. Since some of these patients have involved lymph nodes, there is even an argument for performing en bloc esophagectomy. Perhaps improvement in endoscopic ultrasound will help make this decision in the future, but at present the extent of surgery for high grade dysplasia is controversial.

WHAT OPERATION SHOULD BE DONE?

Nissen Fundoplication

Patients with uncomplicated reflux do best with a transabdominal Nissen fundoplication. The Nissen operation is the most effective in controlling reflux and has the best record of long term durability. It may be performed transthoracically if the patient is very obese or if a simultaneous procedure on the lung or esophageal body needs to be performed. The important points of technique are (1) obtaining good exposure of the hiatus by use of a sternal retractor with the patient in the reverse Trendelenburg position, (2) exposing the crura and approximating them with nonabsorbable sutures, and (3) mobilizing the fundus by division of the short gastric arteries. If this is done correctly, bringing the fundus behind the esophagus allows it to sit without tension, so that simply pushing the esophagus posteriorly causes it to become "enveloped" in the fundus. A 60-Fr bougie is then passed into the esophagus, and a short (1.5 cm) wrap is then made and secured with a horizontal 2/0 Prolene suture reinforced by Teflon pledgets. The principles are the same when the operation is done laparoscopically. It is easiest to approach the right crus and esophagus through the transparent part of lesser omentum superior to the hepatic branch of the anterior vagus nerve. Keeping the dissection above this level protects against creating a wrap around the upper stomach. Although long-term studies of the physiologic and clinical outcome of laparoscopic fundoplication are not yet available, the laparoscopic operation so closely resembles the standard open procedure that similar long-term results are likely, provided the operation is done by an experienced surgeon. The earliest laparoscopic antireflux procedures used a ligamentum teres sling round the angle of His, but such procedures are unlikely to be popularized now that the laparoscopic Nissen has become readily available.

Outcome

Almost all patients experience increased abdominal bloating and flatulence after Nissen fundoplication, but in most it is a minor phenomenon. The cessation of heartburn is immediate and gratifying. Some patients experience temporary dysphagia which clears in a few weeks. If patients are selected in accordance with the criteria indicated previously and the operation performed as described, our experience indicates that more than 90 percent can be expected to have long term (10 year) control of reflux.

Complications

Complications of the Nissen operation occur because of technical errors or inappropriate patient selection. Too tight a wrap causes dysphagia from the outset. If the wrap is imperfectly fixed it may disrupt, causing recurrent reflux. The wrap may come to lie around the upper stomach if unrecognized esophageal shortening led to excessive tension. This situation, often called the "slipped Nissen," is more often created at the outset when the surgeon inadvertently wraps the fundus round the upper stomach. In either case, the patient experiences predominantly dysphagia and, to a lesser degree, heartburn. Vagal injury may cause gastric retention, which is particularly serious if the patient cannot vomit. Herniation of the repair may occur if the crura are not closed, and is prone to the same complications as a spontaneous paraesophageal hernia, namely incarceration, bleeding, and strangulation. Finally, there are rare reports of infective complications which arise because of local sepsis around the wrap or in the subphrenic space, leading to gastropleural or gastrobronchial fistulae.

The common causes of inappropriate patient selection are:

1. Creating a wrap in the presence of defective peristalsis. This will lead to dysphagia if the esophagus cannot propel a bolus through the newly constructed valve. The peristaltic defect may be secondary to prolonged reflux. Some mild improvement is often noted after reducing a hiatal hernia and abolishing reflux, but it is rarely adequate. If the peak amplitude of contraction in the distal esophagus is less than 20 mm Hg, a complete wrap should not be done. (See the following section). The most disastrous situation occurs when a Nissen fundoplication is performed in a patient with unsuspected achalasia. This can be entirely prevented by performing careful motility studies on all patients preoperatively.

2. Performing the operation in the absence of documented disease. At best, this adds flatulence and distension to the unrelieved symptoms: at worst, severe dysphagia or esophageal injury because of unrecognized nonreflux disease may cause disaster leading ultimately to the need for esophagectomy.

3. The patient has a normal LES, and the primary problem is in the stomach. This may produce

marked bloating and distension. Nevertheless, if the wrap is created in the manner described, the resistance to reflux is not so great that belching is impossible, and the true "gas bloat" syndrome described by Woodward is rarely seen nowadays. This is probably due to the acceptance of the shorter fundoplication.

4. Performing a Nissen fundoplication when the chief symptom is cough is not always followed by total relief. Some of these patients have a defect in proximal esophageal motility causing retrograde transport towards the pharynx. Despite reflux control, they may continue to aspirate swallowed food and saliva. The best results are obtained when a clear correlation between esophageal acidification and the respiratory symptom is observed on 24-hour pH monitoring and the patient has a normal esophageal motility study.

Belsey Operation

The transthoracic Belsey operation is an incomplete (270°) fundoplication where the wrap is fixed to the esophagus and to the diaphragm. It is best suited to patients with defective peristalsis (peak amplitude in the distal esophagus < 20 mm Hg) and esophageal shortening, since it imposes less outflow resistance, and the thoracic approach allows for more extensive mobilization of the esophageal body. Its ability to protect against reflux is somewhat less than that of the Nissen procedure and the incidence of late recurrent reflux higher.

The principles of the operation involve mobilizing the entire cardia, and placing two rows of three sutures to fix the wrap to the lower esophagus in the first row, and to the esophagus and under surface of the diaphragm in the second row. The long-term outcome is similar to the Nissen procedure, but the lower incidence of side effects related to the wrap must be offset against a small but definite incidence of post-thoracotomy pain and a higher incidence of long-term recurrence of reflux.

Esophageal Lengthening Procedures

As reflux disease advances, esophageal shortening and fixed hiatal herniation make it difficult to reduce the cardia below the diaphragm. Forcibly placing the wrap under tension leads to wrap disruption. If despite careful mobilization of the thoracic esophagus, the cardia will not lie in the abdomen without tension, an esophageal lengthening operation should be done. This is done by placing a 45 Fr bougie in the esophagus and along the lesser curvature of the stomach. The GIA stapler is placed and fired alongside the gastric portion of the bougie to produce a 5 cm length of "neoesophagus". This maneuver, known as the Collis gastroplasty, was originally proposed as an antireflux measure in its own right, but is only used now when combined with a Nissen or Belsey wrap. Usually when it is required, the esoph-

ageal motility is also impaired, so the Belsey partial fundoplication is added.

Other Antireflux Procedures

Because of reports of complications after the Nissen operation, some workers have revisited partial fundoplications in an attempt to reduce the side effects related to the total wrap. The Toupet posterior 270° operation and the hemifundoplication of Watson have both been recommended as the operation of choice. The problem with partial fundoplications has always been lack of durability, and only the Belsey operation has stood the test of time in this regard. At this time there is insufficient evidence that any of them has a significant advantage over the Nissen and Belsey operations.

The median arcuate ligament cardiopexy of LD Hill may be useful in a patient with a previous partial gastrectomy. The gastroesophageal junction is "imbricated" and fixed to the median arcuate ligament. Intraoperative manometry is necessary to ensure a satisfactory rise in LES pressure. There is a risk of damage to the celiac axis during the insertion of the sutures into the median arcuate ligament.

The Angelchik prosthesis, a Silastic-filled "donut" which is tied around the gastroesophageal junction, is generally an effective antireflux measure, but has a high incidence of complications severe enough to require removal of the prosthesis. These include migration of the device into the chest or peritoneal cavity, or erosion into the gastrointestinal tract. It has no advantage except ease of insertion, and cannot be recommended as an ideal antireflux procedure.

ANTIREFLUX SURGERY IN SPECIAL SITUATIONS

Motility Disorders

Patients with achalasia are at risk of reflux after myotomy. The further onto the stomach the myotomy extends, the greater the risk of reflux. Trying to avoid this by limiting the distal extent of myotomy creates the risk of incomplete myotomy and persistent dysphagia. Our preference is to add a Dor anterior hemifundoplication, i.e., by bringing up a tongue of gastric fundus to be sutured to the cut edges of the myotomy. This involves minimal disruption of the diaphragmatic attachments, and has the dual advantage of protecting the mucosa and preventing rehealing of the myotomy. Recently, the advent of thoracoscopic myotomy has allowed the creation of a myotomy, the distal limit of which is controlled by the magnified thoracoscopic image and simultaneous intraoperative endoscopy. No antireflux procedure is added. Although the early results are very encouraging, it would be premature to recommend wholesale adoption of this technique. The use of balloon dilatation and of botulinum toxin injection into the LES is discussed in a separate chapter.

When other motility disorders and reflux coexist, it

is vital to decide if the motility disorder is primary (such as diffuse esophageal spasm) or secondary to prolonged reflux. The former is likely to require a long myotomy and Dor procedure, whereas a reflux-induced motor disorder requires only a fundoplication—whether complete (Nissen) or partial (Belsey) depends on the peristaltic amplitude. Crucial to the difference between primary and secondary motility disorders is the status of the LES. It is unusual to have a defective LES in a primary motor disorder, whereas it is almost always present when secondary to reflux. Reflux secondary to scleroderma presents a special case, since destruction of muscle tissue in the esophageal body and LES leads to both an aperistaltic esophagus and a severely defective LES. The situation is often compounded by severe failure of gastric emptying, and often the best way to protect the esophagus and allow food to reach the jejunum is to perform total gastrectomy and reconstruction via a Hunt-Lawrence jejunal pouch.*

Combined Procedures

Gastric hypersecretion is sometimes associated with GERD, but unless an active, or recently active, duodenal ulcer is documented, we do not recommend adding highly selective vagotomy to the fundoplication. The morbidity of the combined operation is higher than fundoplication alone, and includes an increased risk of disruption of the repair, and to a lesser extent, necrosis of the lesser curve. When it is necessary to perform both procedures, we only divide the short gastric vessels in the upper leaf of the gastrosplenic ligament to avoid fundic ischemia.

Gallstones are commonly found during the work-up. Cholecystectomy may promote duodenogastric reflux and is best avoided unless it is obvious that the gallstones are symptomatic.†

Reoperation for Failed Antireflux Surgery

Failures due to inappropriate patient selection should be preventable by a careful work-up which includes not just structural information from endoscopy and a barium esophagogram, but also physiologic information from manometry and pH studies. The best decisions will be made by surgeons who endoscope their own patients, and who can interpret their own motility and pH studies. After a technical failure, if a reason for the failure can be identified, and the patient has had only one antireflux operation in the past, a good result from redo surgery may be expected. Generally, it is best to approach these patients through the chest. In the case of a slipped Nissen, esophageal shortening which caused the problem in the first place generally requires a Collis-Belsey operation. Patients with several previous antireflux operations are generally better served by esophageal replacement.

Esophagectomy for Reflux Disease

Sometimes because of severe advanced disease or multiple previous unsuccessful antireflux operations, the esophagus must be removed. Reconstruction can be made with colon, jejunum, or stomach, but colon provides the most durable result. It is hard to preserve the vagi in reoperative cases, and leaving denervated floppy stomach leads to epigastric discomfort and nausea after eating, and a high risk of regurgitation. Consequently, the proximal stomach should be removed and the colon graft anastomosed to the antrum.

SUGGESTED READING

DeMeester TR, Attwood SEA, Smyrk TC, et al. Surgical therapy in Barrett's esophagus. Ann Surg 1990; 212:528–542.

DeMeester TR, Bonavina L, Albertucci M. Nissen fundoplication for gastroesophageal reflux disease—evaluation of primary repair in 100 consecutive patients. Ann Surg 1986; 204:9–20.

Spechler SJ and the Veterans Affairs Gastroesophageal Reflux Disease Study Group #277: Comparison of medical and surgical therapy for complicated gastroesophageal reflux disease in veterans. N Eng J Med 1992; 326:786–792.

Stein HJ, Barlow AP, DeMeester TR, et al. Complications of gastroesophageal reflux disease: Role of the lower esophageal sphincter, esophageal acid and acid/alkaline exposure, and duodenogastric reflux. Ann Surg 1992; 216:25–43.

Stein HJ, DeMeester TR. Indications, technique, and clinical use of ambulatory 24-hour esophageal motility monitoring in a surgical practice. Ann Surg 1993; 217:128–137.

Stein HJ, DeMeester TR, Naspetti R, et al. Three-dimensional imaging of the lower esophageal sphincter in gastroesophageal reflux disease. Ann Surg 1991; 214:374–384.

Zaninotto G, DeMeester TR, Bremner CG, et al. Esophageal function in patients with reflux induced strictures and its relevance to surgical treatment. Ann Thorac Surg 1989; 47:362–370.

---

*Editor's Note: It is hoped that omeprazole and octreotide may lessen the need for this latter type of surgery.

†Editor's Note: I hope many general surgeons hear this message.

BARRETT'S ESOPHAGUS, DYSPLASIA, AND CARCINOMA

ROBERT E. PETRAS, M.D.

Barrett's esophagus, the eponym given to an esophagus lined with columnar epithelial cells, is acquired through chronic gastroesophageal reflux. For purposes of this discussion, Barrett's esophagus is defined as the presence of a columnar epithelium lining of the tubular esophagus above the lower esophageal sphincter.

Barrett's esophagus would be little more than a medical curiosity if not for its complications: ulcer, stricture, bleeding, and carcinoma. It is the association with carcinoma that has brought Barrett's esophagus so much attention. Although the exact risk is unknown, the high prevalence and dismal outcome of carcinoma complicating Barrett's esophagus have caused most gastroenterologists to investigate patients with reflux symptoms for the presence of Barrett's epithelium. Once Barrett's esophagus has been diagnosed, it is prudent to place such patients into a cancer surveillance program.

CANCER RISKS AND SURVEILLANCE

The prevalence rate for carcinoma complicating Barrett's esophagus is usually reported to be 10 to 15 percent. These figures probably overestimate the true prevalence rate for several reasons. Barrett's esophagus itself is often asymptomatic, so that the total number of patients with Barrett's epithelium (the denominator in the determination of prevalence) is unknown. Patients with "symptomatic" Barrett's esophagus are likely to have symptoms related to carcinoma. Patients reported in hospital or autopsy series more often represent those with severe disease. Other complicating risk factors, such as cigarette smoking and alcohol consumption, are both strongly associated with esophageal carcinoma and are rarely taken into account in cancer prevalence studies related to Barrett's esophagus.

Cancer prevalence rates reflect patients in a population already determined to have carcinoma. The true problem in assessing the need for cancer surveillance involves patients with Barrett's esophagus who do not yet have carcinoma. What is their risk of developing carcinoma (incidence), and does that risk justify the cost of a cancer surveillance program? Several retrospective studies have addressed these questions and have estimated the incidence rates to be 30 to 40 times higher than the rate of esophageal carcinoma in the general population. Recent prospective studies have confirmed high cancer incidence rates in patients with Barrett's esophagus and have estimated incidence rates 125 to 350 times the rate of esophageal carcinoma in the general population.

Although most clinicians agree that Barrett's esophagus places patients at risk for esophageal adenocarcinoma, no consensus has emerged as to whether the increased risk justifies the cost of a cancer surveillance program. Although the matter is controversial, I think that in the absence of a definitive study to the contrary, it is prudent to place patients with Barrett's esophagus into a cancer surveillance program. The surveillance goal is prevention or early detection of carcinoma. The marker currently used as the end point for cancer surveillance programs is the presence of high-grade epithelial dysplasia in a biopsy specimen.

Dysplasia, the presumed precancerous epithelial lesion, has been regularly recognized in esophageal specimens adjacent to and distant from Barrett's-associated adenocarcinomas. Circumstantial evidence suggests that dysplasia not only may be a marker for carcinoma but may itself be the early carcinomatous change that can progress to invasive carcinoma. All grades of dysplasia have the potential to give rise to invasive carcinoma, and epithelial changes need not go through a recognizable carcinoma in situ phase before being associated with invasion. Although the circumstantial evidence for the dysplasia-carcinoma sequence is compelling, the progression of dysplasia to carcinoma is still largely unproved and the time course unknown. The potential benefits (largely unknown) of removing a dysplastic esophagus must be weighed against the high mortality associated with esophagectomy alone (estimated to be 5 to 15 percent) and a dismal outcome in patients who present with invasive adenocarcinoma of the esophagus (34 percent survival at 2 years and 14.5 percent at 5 years).

DYSPLASIA IN BARRETT'S ESOPHAGUS

Histologic Diagnosis, Significance, and Proposed Patient Management

Dysplasia is recognized histologically, and criteria for identifying these changes in ulcerative colitis can be used in studying Barrett's epithelium. The term "dysplasia" in Barrett's epithelium should be used to described a change that is unequivocally neoplastic. As with inflammatory bowel disease, dysplasia in Barrett's epithelium can be closely mimicked by reparative epithelial changes associated with active inflammation and ulceration. The histologic features of repair and dysplasia in columnar epithelium are compared in Table 1.

Both dysplasia and repair are associated with nuclear enlargement and hyperchromasia, increased mitotic figures, and decreased intracellular mucin. However, some histologic features are more characteristic of repair than of dysplasia. The nuclei of repair are often round or oval with smooth external contours, are evenly spaced, do not overlap, contain granular chromatin with single or multiple chromocenters/nucleoli, and are remarkably similar to one another in both size and

Table 1 Histologic Features Differentiating Dysplasia From Repair in Barrett's Esophagus

Feature	Dysplasia	Repair
Nuclear enlargement	+ to + + +	+
Nuclear hyperchromasia	+ to + + +	+
Nuclear pleomorphism	+ to + + +	0 to +
Irregular nuclear contours	+ to + + +	0 to +
Chromocenters/nucleoli	0 to +	+ + to + + +
Irregular nuclear crowding	+ + to + + +	0 to +
Nuclear stratification	0 to + + +	0 to +
Loss of nuclear polarity	0 to + + +	0
Increased mitoses	+ to + + +	+ +
Inflammatory milieu	0 to + +	+ +
Decreased intracellular mucin	+ to + + +	+ +
High nuclear–to–cytoplasmic size ratio	+ + to + + +	0 to +
Cytoplasmic eosinophilia	0	0 to +
Distortion of mucosal architecture	0 to + + +	+ to + +
Villous configuration	0 to + + +	+ to + +

0 = not present; + = present and mild; + + = present and moderate; + + + = present and severe.

appearance. In contrast to dysplasia, the nuclear–to–cytoplasmic size ratio in reparative cells is often decreased, especially in cells adjacent to ulcerated areas. Nearby active inflammation helps to confirm a diagnosis of repair. Features that favor dysplasia over repair are (1) variable nuclear hyperchromasia associated with pleomorphism, (2) irregular nuclear contour, (3) marked nuclear stratification with crowding and overlap, (4) loss of nuclear polarity, and (5) nuclear and architectural abnormalities that are visible at low magnification.

Some Barrett's-associated dysplasias can look similar to colonic or small intestinal adenomas, but in my experience the majority do not. To avoid confusion that may arise from the relatively benign connotation of the word "adenoma," I agree with those authors who state that the term "adenoma" should be avoided in reference to these lesions in the esophagus because they represent Barrett's-associated dysplasia, usually of high grade, and indicate a high likelihood that infiltrating adenocarcinoma already exists.

Dysplasia has been reported in all major types of Barrett's epithelia. It is certainly more frequent in areas of specialized columnar epithelium (incomplete intestinal metaplasia), and it is unlikely that cancer occurs in the absence of specialized columnar epithelium. It is, however, often difficult or impossible to ascertain epithelial types in mucosa totally replaced by dysplasia or carcinoma.

Currently, a modification of the Inflammatory Bowel Disease–Dysplasia Morphology Study Group Classification is used in assessing Barrett's epithelium. Under this three-tiered system, biopsy findings are classified as negative for dysplasia, positive for dysplasia, or indefinite for dysplasia. Biopsy specimens interpreted as positive for dysplasia are further subdivided into either low-grade or high-grade dysplasia, based on the degree of cytologic change present. In low-grade epithelial dysplasia, the abnormal nuclei are limited to the basal

half of the cells. In high-grade dysplasia, more severe cytologic and architectural alterations are present. Hyperchromasia and pleomorphism are more marked. Nuclear crowding and stratification are often present. Nuclei may be found in the luminal half of the cells. No distinction is made between high-grade dysplasia and carcinoma in situ in this system. If equivocal changes are present, they are usually due to epithelial repair associated with active inflammation. In this setting, the specimen is best classified as indefinite for dysplasia. I consider that true dysplasia can be reliably detected by an experienced surgical pathologist, but because of marked interobserver variation in differentiating low-grade dysplasia from changes indefinite for dysplasia, I have reluctantly followed the recommendations of Reid and colleagues and adopted a similar management for either diagnosis. My current management plan based on this histologic classification is outlined in Table 2.

During surveillance endoscopy, four biopsy specimens at 2 cm increments are obtained throughout the entire extent of the Barrett's epithelium. Because the operative mortality and morbidity rates of esophagectomy are high, it is prudent to confirm a diagnosis of high-grade dysplasia before considering esophagectomy. Immediate repeat endoscopy with multiple biopsies should be performed. A second finding of high-grade dysplasia is considered adequate confirmation. This repeat biopsy approach has the added advantage that intramucosal or invasive carcinoma may be detected with careful endoscopic re-examination and extensive rebiopsy, thus making the decision for esophagectomy easier. If, after an original diagnosis of high-grade dysplasia, the follow-up endoscopy with biopsy is negative, the original specimen should be reviewed again and the diagnosis ideally confirmed by another experienced pathologist. If high-grade dysplasia is again confirmed in the original specimen, esophagectomy is recommended.

Dysplasia can be focal. Because dysplasia is considered neoplastic, it is unlikely that it ever resolves spontaneously. Therefore, gastroenterologists and surgeons must never be lulled into a false sense of security by negative follow-up examinations once true dysplasia has been identified, because such results probably stem from a sampling error.

Dysplasia is relatively rare in patients with Barrett's esophagus, but data suggest that when biopsy specimens are positive for high-grade dysplasia, the likelihood of infiltrating carcinoma is high. Falk et al. recently reported 16 patients who underwent esophagectomy for high-grade dysplasia. Early carcinomas were found in six (38 percent of the resection specimens). Other investigators have also found a high prevalence of infiltrating adenocarcinomas in esophagectomy specimens containing high-grade dysplasia.

Although it is tempting to conclude that patients whose carcinomas were detected early by surveillance endoscopy have benefited from early resection, the enthusiasm for these apparent successes must be tempered by the realization that in at least one series the operative mortality was 25 percent. One must also

Table 2 Dysplasia in Barrett's Epithelium: Management Plan Based
on Histologic Interpretation

Histologic Interpretation	Management
Negative for dysplasia	Yearly endoscopic surveillance
Indefinite for dysplasia or positive for low-grade dysplasia	Medical therapy for reflux, repeat biopsy in 3–6 mo If repeat biopsy is negative, repeat endoscopy at 3–6 mo intervals until two consecutive negative interpretations are encountered, then return to yearly surveillance If definite or low-grade dysplasia persists, continue 3–6 mo surveillance until dysplasia progresses
Positive for high-grade dysplasia	Confirm,* then consider esophagectomy

*See text.

critically consider the number of patients who underwent surgery for high-grade dysplasia and in whom only high-grade dysplasia was identified in the resected specimens. There is no conclusive evidence that invasive carcinoma would ever develop in such patients, and if it did the time course from dysplasia to carcinoma is unknown. Finally, it is necessary to prove that 5 year and long-term survival rates are significantly better in patients in whom cancers were found or not allowed to develop (resection for dysplasia) as a result of surveillance endoscopy programs than in patients in whom adenocarcinomas were discovered outside such programs.

Management recommendations for indefinite or low-grade dysplasia must be considered preliminary, as no long-term follow-up studies have yet been reported. I recommend repeat endoscopy every 2 to 6 months. If two consecutive follow-up studies are negative, I return to yearly endoscopic surveillance. If low-grade dysplasia or indefinite changes persist, I continue 3 to 6 month surveillance until the dysplasia progresses.

Role of Deoxyribonucleic Acid (DNA) Analysis

Several groups have reported their experience with DNA analysis by flow cytometry in patients with Barrett's esophagus. Carcinoma and dysplasia in biopsy specimens are highly correlated with either DNA aneuploidy or high proliferative rates. Furthermore, a progression of DNA abnormalities occurs with increasing histologic atypia in these patients. Some investigators, however, have shown some discordance between DNA abnormalities and dysplasia. It is possible that flow cytometry will be a useful adjunct to the standard

histologic assessment in cancer surveillance of patients with Barrett's esophagus, but more study is necessary. Because some examples of Barrett's-associated adenocarcinoma and dysplasia lack DNA abnormalities as determined by flow cytometry, this technique should not be used alone in a surveillance program. The role of DNA analysis may lie in identifying a group of Barrett's patients requiring less frequent surveillance, since few, if any, patients with a negative histologic appearance and a normal DNA content progressed to adenocarcinoma.

SUGGESTED READING

Achkar E, Carey W. The cost of surveillance for adenocarcinoma complicating Barrett's esophagus. Am J Gastroenterol 1988; 83: 291–294.
Falk GW, Rice TW, Achkar E, Petras RE. High-grade dysplasia in Barrett's esophagus is associated with early cancer (abstract). Gastroenterology 1992; 102:A355.
Hameeteman W, Tytgat GNJ, Houthoff HJ, van den Tweel JG. Barrett's esophagus: development of dysplasia and adenocarcinoma. Gastroenterology 1989; 96:1249–1256.
Hamilton SR, Smith RRL. The relationship between columnar epithelial dysplasia and invasive adenocarcinoma arising in Barrett's esophagus. Am J Clin Pathol 1987; 87:301–312.
Petras RE, Sivak MV Jr, Rice TW. Barrett's esophagus: a review of the pathologist's role in diagnosis and management. Pathol Annu 1991; 28:1–32.
Rabinovitch PS, Reid BJ, Haggitt RC, et al. Progression to cancer in Barrett's esophagus as associated with genomic instability. Lab Invest 1988; 60:65–71.
Reid BJ, Blount PL, Rubin CE, et al. Flow cytometric and histological progression to malignancy in Barrett's esophagus: prospective endoscopic surveillance of a cohort. Gastroenterology 1992; 102: 1212–1219.
Spechler SJ, Goyal RK. Barrett's esophagus. N Engl J Med 1986; 315:362–371.

BARRETT'S ESOPHAGUS: MANAGEMENT DECISIONS

JOHN G. STAGIAS, M.D.
MORRIS TRAUBE, M.D.

Barrett's esophagus is an acquired complication of gastroesophageal reflux disease (GERD) in which columnar mucosa replaces the normal stratified squamous mucosa of the esophagus through the process of metaplasia. It is found in up to 10 percent of patients with symptoms of GERD who undergo endoscopy, and autopsy series have estimated that for every case of Barrett's esophagus that is clinically diagnosed, 20 remained unrecognized. Although there have been several reports of "familial" clustering and of its development as a sequela of chemotherapy, most cases of Barrett's esophagus result from GERD.

Barrett's mucosa alone does not produce symptoms; most patients present with symptoms or complications of GERD, including heartburn, dysphagia from stricture, bleeding, or adenocarcinoma. However, in 10 to 20 percent of patients who present with dysphagia, there is no history of heartburn.

The recognition of Barrett's esophagus is clinically important because of its malignant potential. The diagnosis is usually made at endoscopy by finding characteristic velvety, salmon-pink mucosa that extends at least 2 to 3 cm proximal to the lower esophageal sphincter (LES). When fundic or junctional gastric mucosa is seen histologically, it is often difficult to ascertain whether this represents metaplasia or a gastric lip, but in the setting of chronic symptoms, it is appropriate to consider this to be Barrett's mucosa. With specialized columnar mucosa, even smaller segments are diagnostic of Barrett's esophagus.

The proper management of patients with Barrett's esophagus should be individualized according to the severity of symptoms and the endoscopic findings. It involves the control of symptoms of underlying GERD and regular endoscopic surveillance for detection of early, curable neoplasms. However, there are currently no conclusive data to suggest that optimal medical or surgical control of GERD will reduce the risk of progression to dysplasia and adenocarcinoma or lead to regression of the Barrett's epithelium.*

MEDICAL THERAPY

Asymptomatic

In asymptomatic individuals, it is wise to recommend lifestyle changes to reduce reflux. These include eleva-tion of the head of the bed, cessation of smoking or drinking of alcohol, and avoidance of foods that predispose to reflux. It is difficult to categorically recommend antireflux medications. If they are given to asymptomatic patients, it seems appropriate to give only standard doses of H_2-receptor antagonists (e.g., cimetidine, 400 mg twice daily; ranitidine, 150 mg twice daily; famotidine, 20 mg twice daily; or nizatidine, 150 mg twice daily), but not higher doses or omeprazole, the powerful proton pump inhibitor.

Mild to Moderate Esophagitis

In mild to moderate esophagitis (endoscopic-histologic), therapy should be focused mainly on relief of symptoms, even though this may not be a reliable indicator of healing. While lifestyle changes and H_2-receptor antagonists are an important starting point, up to 85 percent do not have symptomatic relief and require higher doses of H_2-receptor antagonists or omeprazole, 20 mg or more per day. Although one study showed a good correlation between basal acid output and the dose of ranitidine required to heal esophagitis (and alleviate pyrosis), we generally use symptoms rather than gastric analysis to guide therapy.† When symptoms, or endoscopic findings, indicate lack of response, it is more practical to increase the dose or begin therapy with omeprazole than to first perform gastric analysis. Prokinetic agents (metoclopramide and the newer cisapride, 10 to 20 mg four times per day) have also been added to facilitate esophageal clearance, raise sphincter pressure, or improve gastric emptying, but may find particular use as an adjunct to H_2 antagonists or omeprazole; the combination is more effective than the antisecretory drugs alone. Although many patients experience neuropsychiatric side effects with metoclopramide, cisapride is generally well tolerated.

Severe Esophagitis and Barrett's Ulcers

In severe esophagitis or Barrett's ulcers, therapy should begin with omeprazole, 20 mg per day. However, in some patients with Barrett's ulcer, even 40 to 60 mg per day of omeprazole does not produce complete healing after 4 to 6 months of treatment.‡ Therefore, endoscopy should be repeated at 2 to 3 month intervals until complete healing is documented. A discrete ulcer or otherwise severe esophagitis that persists despite 4 to 6 months of intensive therapy is unlikely to heal with medical therapy alone, and antireflux surgery should be considered, as described below.

---

*Editor's Note: Some "esophagologists" feel there may be some benefit from decreasing or eliminating any ongoing acute inflammation. However, as stated, their data are probably not yet conclusive.

---

†Editor's Note: Some other authors focus on the degree of histologic inflammation because, as stated in this chapter, 10 to 20 percent of patients with Barrett's esophagus may not have a history of heartburn.

‡Editor's Note: A seeming lack of toxicity and neoplastic degeneration with prolonged (years) treatment with omeprazole was stressed by Dent at the American Gastroenterological Association meeting in May 1993.

Strictures

Barrett's strictures, which most commonly occur at the squamocolumnar junction, should be extensively biopsied to exclude malignancy. Once this has been excluded, the stricture can be dilated in the same fashion as other esophageal strictures, and omeprazole given to help prevent restricturing. Occasionally, strictures do not respond to multiple dilations, necessitating surgery.

Regression with Medical Therapy

Complete regression of Barrett's epithelium with medical therapy has rarely been demonstrated. In several trials using standard dose H_2-receptor antagonists, there has been no significant (>3 cm) regression. While case reports have documented regression with high-dose omeprazole therapy (40 to 60 mg per day), no data are available from large controlled trials; we therefore do not advocate routine use of omeprazole in all patients with Barrett's esophagus. Although a recent report has documented squamous cell repopulation after the columnar epithelium was ablated with a laser, there is insufficient evidence to recommend such treatment routinely.

SURGICAL THERAPY

Indications for Surgery

The indications for surgery in Barrett's esophagus are similar to those for GERD without Barrett's mucosa and include persistent symptoms despite maximal medical therapy, strictures unresponsive to dilation, nonhealing ulcers or esophagitis after 4 to 6 months of intensive therapy, uncontrollable bleeding, perforation, and pulmonary aspiration from reflux. Multiple factors must be considered in any decision regarding surgery; these may include the patient's operative risk because of comorbid diseases and the results of esophageal manometry. The surgical options are standard antireflux procedures (e.g., Nissen fundoplication, Belsey cardioplasty, and Hill posterior gastropexy) and involve reduction of the hiatus hernial sac in association with a gastric wrap.

Regression with Surgical Therapy

Although some earlier surgical series reported partial regression of Barrett's esophagus after antireflux procedures, those studies had methodologic flaws, and subsequent surgical series have failed to document significant (>3 cm) regression in most patients, or the prevention of complications, including dysplasia and adenocarcinoma, after surgery. Therefore, surgery should not be performed solely because of a finding of Barrett's esophagus, nor as prophylaxis against the development of carcinoma. Furthermore, patients who have undergone an antireflux procedure should be enrolled in a surveillance program at the same intervals as for other patients with Barrett's esophagus (see below).

DYSPLASIA, ADENOCARCINOMA, AND SURVEILLANCE

The most serious complication of Barrett's esophagus is the development of adenocarcinoma. Multiple studies have shown an incidence of adenocarcinoma at least 30 times that of the general population. Unfortunately, adenocarcinoma is often discovered at presentation, and most of these cases are unresectable for cure. Much interest has therefore focused on identifying at an early stage those patients who may ultimately progress to adenocarcinoma.

It is generally accepted that the development of adenocarcinoma follows the sequence of dysplasia, carcinoma in situ, and finally carcinoma. (The concepts of aneuploidy and p53 protein expression are discussed below.) It has therefore been considered logical to screen patients by endoscopy at set intervals so as to identify those with dysplasia before the development of adenocarcinoma. This approach is further supported by the results of large screening programs in areas of China where squamous cell carcinoma of the esophagus is endemic; these programs have been successful in detecting and curing early squamous cell carcinoma. Nevertheless, several difficulties remain with the assumption that screening is worthwhile and will reduce the frequency of lethal carcinoma: (1) it is unclear whether all patients with dysplasia will ultimately progress to carcinoma, so that dysplasia may not be the ideal marker for progression; (2) the time frame required for dysplasia to progress to adenocarcinoma is currently unknown; (3) areas of dysplasia are often endoscopically indistinguishable from nondysplastic tissue, so that small foci of dysplasia may be missed, and a consequent considerable sampling error arises; and (4) any mass screening program is costly to implement. For example, an evaluation of this cost in 1988 estimated that yearly surveillance would cost $62,000 and 78 lost workdays per diagnosed cancer.

Despite these concerns, screening has become the acceptable approach, and several suggestions have been proposed to overcome some of these problems.

No Dysplasia

Once a patient is found to have Barrett's mucosa, multiple biopsies at different levels are recommended in order to detect dysplasia or adenocarcinoma and to assess the degree of inflammation, if any. At the time of the initial and subsequent endoscopic examinations, the locations of the distal tubular esophagus and of the squamocolumnar junction should be accurately documented to facilitate any further diagnostic studies or repeat biopsy. In the absence of dysplasia or adenocarcinoma, patients should undergo surveillance endoscopy with biopsy at 1 to 2 year intervals, unless comorbid conditions deteriorate and surgery would not be considered, making surveillance pointless. The exact timings of surveillance, whether 1 or 2 years, should be determined after considering various factors, including the length of

Barrett's mucosa, the type of columnar tissue (increased malignancy mainly in those with specialized columnar tissue), and the anxiety level of the patient. The availability of flow cytometry results (see below) as well as future genetic marker alteration results may also influence the decision regarding timing of endoscopic surveillance.

Low-Grade Dysplasia

Dysplasia may be subdivided into low- and high-grade dysplasia. Since it is often difficult for the pathologist (interobserver concordance of about 70 percent) to accurately distinguish low-grade dysplasia from regenerating epithelium with inflammation, these patients should be treated intensively for 8 to 12 weeks with lifestyle changes, omeprazole, and, if symptoms continue, prokinetic agents. The pathologic biopsy interpretation should also be confirmed by an expert pathologist. Follow-up endoscopy should be performed at intervals of 3 to 6 months. Any persistent finding of low-grade dysplasia should be closely followed endoscopically at subsequent 3 to 6 month intervals until there is either progression to high-grade dysplasia (see below) or two consecutive examinations negative for dysplasia. The finding of no dysplasia on two consecutive, very thorough examinations may allow for a less intensive surveillance program, as described above.

High-Grade Dysplasia

High-grade dysplasia is a more reproducible pathologic finding, with an interobserver concordance rate of up to 87 percent. However, any finding of high-grade dysplasia should be confirmed by an expert pathologist, and endoscopy and biopsy repeated if sufficient doubt remains. If high-grade dysplasia is confirmed, surgical resection is generally advised, since esophagectomy specimens often show invasive cancer in association with high-grade dysplasia. All columnar epithelium should be removed, in view of reports of adenocarcinoma developing in the remaining columnar mucosa after incomplete surgical resection. Despite this general recommendation, the final decision regarding surgery must also take into account comorbid conditions and the age of the patient.

Flow Cytometry

Since dysplasia is not an ideal marker for the progression to adenocarcinoma, much recent interest has centered on analysis of the cellular DNA content by means of flow cytometry. The principle behind this technique is that aneuploidy (an abnormal amount of DNA per cell) and also an increased number of dividing cells (cells that are tetraploid or in the cell cycle G2/M) are found in many carcinomas. In several reports the finding of aneuploidy or an increased G2/tetraploidy on flow cytometry correlated with the subsequent development of carcinoma. However, some

carcinomas may be diploid (normal DNA content), and some patients with aneuploidy did not develop dysplasia within the study period. A second approach using flow cytometry involved the identification of p53 protein expression, which is normally found on chromosome 17p and negatively regulates cell division. A mutation of this protein may lead to unregulated cell growth and carcinoma and is the most commonly seen genetic alteration in human carcinomas. One recent study has shown that p53 protein overexpression may occur in Barrett's esophagus even in the absence of dysplasia or carcinoma, but prospective studies of patients with p53 protein overexpression have not been reported. Thus, it is unclear what role such studies will ultimately play in surveillance for the development of adenocarcinoma. At the current time, and until additional information is available, flow cytometry and genetic expression studies should not replace dysplasia in the surveillance for carcinoma.

Brush Cytology

Cytologic brushings that permit a more extensive mucosal survey of the esophagus may be complementary to multiple biopsies in detecting dysplasia and adenocarcinoma. In one retrospective series of 65 concurrent biopsies and cytology specimens, the combination of brush cytology and biopsy was superior for the detection of dysplasia and adenocarcinoma to each technique alone. However, as with dysplasia, accurate interpretation of the cytology specimen is paramount, experience with cytopathologic studies in dysplasia is limited, and prospective data are lacking.

Summary Recommendations for Surveillance

Given the current available data, we recommend surveillance for patients with Barrett's esophagus at 1 to 2 year intervals, with several caveats:

1. Patients with new symptoms (e.g., dysphagia, odynophagia, or weight loss) are obviously evaluated sooner.
2. Patients with comorbid conditions who would not be suitable candidates for operative therapy if a carcinoma or dysplasia were found are excluded (at least until more efficacious nonoperative therapy is available).
3. Although a recent study has revealed the development of Barrett's esophagus in women who received chemotherapy for breast cancer, the limited data are insufficient to warrant screening such patients.
4. The finding of low-grade dysplasia should be confirmed by an expert pathologist, and the patient treated intensively for 8 to 12 weeks. Follow-up endoscopy should be performed at 3 to 6 month intervals until there is progression to high-grade dysplasia (see below) or two consecutive examinations negative for dysplasia, at which

time the patient should be screened at 1 to 2 year intervals.

5. The finding of high-grade dysplasia should be confirmed by an expert pathologist. If it is confirmed, complete surgical resection of all the columna-lined esophagus is generally advised.

6. As new data emerge and newer techniques become available, these recommendations will be modified so that surveillance will concentrate on patients at greatest risk for adenocarcinoma. Such surveillance recommendations may depend on techniques other than examination of tissue for dysplasia.*

---

*Editor's Note: There are hints of the coexistence of carcinoma in Barrett's esophagus and carcinoma of the colon. Whether this association will be substantiated epidemiologically or via genetic linkage remains to be determined. As stated in this chapter, future developments should help to narrow the pool of at-risk individuals who need surveillance. Perhaps widespread use of effective acid suppression and an improved lifestyle will lessen the incidence of Barrett's esophagus, unfortunately only to be offset by wider use of nonsteroidal anti-inflammatory drugs and other environmental irritants.

SUGGESTED READING

Cameron AJ. Barrett's esophagus and adenocarcinoma: from the family to the gene. Gastroenterology 1992; 102:1421–1424.

Levine DS, Reid BJ. Endoscopic diagnosis of esophageal neoplasms. Gastrointest Endosc Clin North Am 1992; 2:395–413.

Spechler SJ, Goyal RK. Barrett's esophagus. N Engl J Med 1986; 315:362–371.

Streitz JM, Williamson WA, Ellis H Jr. Current concepts concerning the nature and treatment of Barrett's esophagus and its complications. Ann Thorac Surg 1992; 54:586–591.

GASTROESOPHAGEAL REFLUX IN INFANTS AND CHILDREN

A. CRAIG HILLEMEIER, M.D.

Gastroesophageal reflux refers to the reflux of gastric contents into the esophagus. During the first year of life, it is common for infants to have problems with "spitting up" or vomiting. The severity of these symptoms varies from an occasional wet burp to persistent emesis. Occasionally, these symptoms are so severe that a causal relationship between the vomiting and other conditions, such as failure to thrive or pulmonary disease, is explored. The precise cause of gastroesophageal reflux in most infants remains unknown, but current evidence suggests that abnormal relaxation of the lower esophageal sphincter (LES) plays a significant role. However, it is important to remember that persistent vomiting in an infant may be a manifestation of other systemic illness such as an anatomic abnormality in the gastrointestinal (GI) tract or a metabolic, infectious, or neurologic disorder.

CLINICAL PRESENTATION

The term gastroesophageal reflux during infancy is often used to describe the frequent vomiting or regurgitation seen during the first year of life. In most of these infants, symptoms appear during the first several months and resolve by 12 to 18 months of life. While most of these infants are healthy and thriving, the wide prevalence of this condition means that some infants probably have concurrent problems such as failure to thrive, recurrent pneumonia, or episodes of apnea. It is sometimes difficult to determine a cause-and-effect relationship between gastroesophageal reflux and these disorders.

In infants and older children with neurologic impairment, there is a markedly increased incidence of gastroesophageal reflux and serious complications from its presence. Children with neurologic disorders may also show evidence of large hiatal hernias on upper GI series and often require more aggressive and/or definitive surgery than other children with gastroesophageal reflux. There is also a group of older children who present with symptoms of gastroesophageal reflux similar to those in adults. These children often have symptoms upon strenuous exercise such as weight lifting, and frequently respond to therapy similar to that for adults.

DIAGNOSTIC EVALUATION

The typical infant who has recurrent spitting up, is growing well, and does not have associated problems such as failure to gain weight or recurrent pneumonia does not require or benefit from extensive diagnostic evaluations. A careful history and physical examination usually confirm that the child has physiologic amounts of gastroesophageal reflux during infancy. Often the infant has a history of spitting up for several hours after a feeding. Although projectile vomiting should cause the physician to consider an anatomic problem such as pyloric stenosis or malrotation, many of these infants also end up with a diagnosis of idiopathic gastroesophageal reflux. Children who have severe reflux symptoms that may be associated with symptoms such as failure to thrive or recurrent pneumonia should undergo a contrast study of the upper GI tract to rule out anatomic obstruction. Other diagnostic tests to consider include a pH probe, which is a very accurate means of quantitating the amount of reflux present. However, this test usually provides little information that one cannot obtain from history and physical examination in the vomiting infant.

Endoscopy and esophageal biopsy remain controversial and I consider that they have no role in the infant who is thriving. However, in addition to the traditional histologic signs of esophageal inflammation, the presence of intraepithelial eosinophils on esophageal biopsy in an infant who is thought to have gastroesophageal reflux is considered histologic evidence of esophagitis. Another test increasingly used in children with severe gastroesophageal reflux is nuclear scintigraphy to evaluate gastric emptying. Occasional infants with severe gastroesophageal reflux may have markedly delayed gastric emptying, and this may be useful information prior to surgical intervention. Scintigraphy has also been used to quantitate the degree of reflux but does not seem to be as sensitive as the pH probe.

The child with severe neurologic impairment may often benefit from having the amount of reflux quantitated before surgical intervention by a pH probe. These children also benefit from an upper GI study to rule out any other anatomic abnormalities. The presence of a pH probe before placement of the feeding gastrostomy in neurologically impaired patients may help indicate which of them will require a fundoplication along with the gastrostomy.

The older child with symptoms of gastroesophageal reflux is often treated with acid reduction therapy to reduce the acid sequel reflux without any diagnostic studies being performed.

THERAPY

I tend to be very conservative in treating an infant who is growing well but has symptoms of gastroesophageal reflux. The traditional therapy of placing a child in an infant seat to reduce the amount of gastroesophageal reflux has been evaluated with pH probe studies and has been shown to be ineffective. Positional therapy has shown that placing the patient head down in an elevated prone position results in fewer and briefer episodes of gastroesophageal reflux, but current controversy about the relationship of this position to sudden infant death syndrome has led me not to recommend this in most situations.

Many infants with significant amounts of gastroesophageal reflux seem to be effectively treated by small and more frequent feedings. This presumably reduces the amount of formula in the stomach that is available for reflux. The ultimate in small, frequent feedings is a continuous nasogastric drip, which has proved to be a successful means of getting adequate weight gain in children who have severe reflux and are suffering from failure to thrive, but for some reason are unable to undergo more definitive therapy such as surgical fundoplication. I often suggest that a 4-month-old infant who is taking 8 ounces of formula every 4 or 5 hours may benefit from perhaps 4 to 6 ounces of feeding every 3 to 4 hours.

Thickened feedings are commonly suggested for children with gastroesophageal reflux, although evidence that it reduces the amount of reflux is scant. Even though thickened feedings do not reduce the total amount of reflux time as measured by a pH probe, it has been shown that infants given thickened feedings have reduced the amount of time spent crying, and this may well be because of the satiety from increased caloric intake. The increased caloric density also remains an effective means of promoting weight gain in a child who is failing to thrive.

Pharmacotherapy

In spite of the fact that gastroesophageal reflux appears to be a physiologic process in most infants that is associated with little morbidity, the widespread nature of gastroesophageal reflux during infancy has led to many attempts to find a drug to suppress its symptoms. In large part, these efforts have been dramatically unsuccessful, probably because the medications have little effect on inappropriate relaxation of the LES.

It has been speculated that since some infants with reflux show histologic evidence of esophagitis, it is reasonable to treat them with acid-neutralizing techniques. While antacids may neutralize acid, and H_2 antagonists have been shown to reduce the amount of acid present in gastric secretions of children, I rarely use these agents in infants because their beneficial effects have not been shown. It is often tempting to use acid-neutralizing therapy in an infant who has excessive irritability and symptoms of gastroesophageal reflux, on the theory that the irritability is caused by inflammatory changes in the esophagus. This supposition is rarely, if ever, true and such therapy is almost never successful. The use of traditional antacids in children must also be re-evaluated in the face of new information regarding the possibility of aluminum toxicity with such agents.

Other pharmacologic agents have similarly proved ineffective in the child with gastroesophageal reflux symptoms who is otherwise thriving. Bethanechol, a muscarinic agonist, has been shown to markedly increase LES pressure in infants who have gastroesophageal reflux. However, since most of these infants do not have decreased LES pressure, the rationale is somewhat shaky. At high doses, bethanechol may somewhat reduce the amount of reflux time seen on pH probes, but these high doses are associated with side effects. Thus, this drug is rarely used to treat reflux during infancy.

Metoclopramide, a dopamine antagonist, is commonly used for gastroesophageal reflux. The rationale behind its use is that it may slightly increase gastroesophageal sphincter tone and increase gastric emptying rates, and therefore reduce the amount of reflux. However, few studies using pH probes to quantitate the amount of reflux have been able to substantiate a significant benefit from metoclopramide, and there is a high degree of side effects. In some studies, up to one-third of children who take metoclopramide have increased drowsiness or restlessness, and not an insignificant number have a dystonic reaction that manifests as neck pain rigidity, dizziness, and an oculogyric crisis. Although in most cases this can be treated by withdrawal of the drug and use of diphenhydramine acutely, it appears somewhat arbitrary to use a drug that has little proven effect and a high degree of side effects in infants.

Domperidone, another dopamine antagonist that reportedly has fewer central nervous system side effects, has also been suggested for gastroesophageal reflux during infancy, but it has not been found to be successful.

Another gastric prokinetic agent, cisapride, has been developed but is not widely available for use in the United States. Cisapride is a noncholinergic, nonantidopaminergic agent that probably works through postganglionic release of acetylcholine. Initial studies suggest that it may have a useful role, but experience is very limited.

Surgery

Surgical procedures to tighten the area at the LES and prevent the reflux of gastric contents have become increasingly more common in children. Fundoplication is a common surgical procedure in most pediatric surgery centers. In general, for the infant or child with gastroesophageal reflux that is thought to be the cause of an unacceptable symptom, there is little doubt that appropriate surgical intervention is an effective way to terminate the reflux. Variations on fundoplication involve wrapping the proximal fundus around the distal 3.5 cm of the esophagus.

I find that the child with severe neurologic impairment often does not respond to conservative medical therapy and may benefit from fundoplication. I usually evaluate gastric emptying before performing a fundoplication, as patients who have delayed gastric emptying will benefit from a pyloroplasty at the same time as the fundoplication.

Unfortunately, fundoplications, particularly in the group of children who have severe neurologic impairment and are likely to benefit from them, are not without significant complications. The incidence of small intestinal obstructions, secondary to adhesion, ranges from 5 to 10 percent in most large pediatric series. Children with severe neurologic impairment who are most likely to undergo fundoplications often have a delayed diagnosis with intestinal obstruction because of their inability to manifest the symptoms.

The placement and use of a gastrostomy feeding tube has been shown to either initiate gastroesophageal reflux or worsen the existing reflux. It has been suggested that almost one-fourth of neurologically impaired patients who show no symptoms of reflux before gastrostomy placement become symptomatic after the procedure.

SUGGESTED READING

Cucciara S, Staiano A, Romaniello G, et al. Antacids and cimetidine treatment for gastro-oesophageal reflux and peptic oesophagitis. Arch Dis Child 1984; 59:842–847.

Euler AR, Ament ME. Detection of gastroesophageal reflux in the pediatric age patient by esophageal intraluminal pH probe measurement (Tuttle test). Pediatrics 1977; 60:65–68.

Fonkalsrud EW, Foglia RD, Ament ME, et al. Operative treatment for the gastroesophageal reflux symptom in children. J Pediatr Surg 1989; 24:525–529.

Hillemeier AC, Lange R, McCallum R, et al. Delayed gastric emptying in infants with gastroesophageal reflux. J Pediatr 1981; 98:190–193.

Orenstein DR, Whitington PF. Positioning for prevention of infant gastroesophageal reflux. J Pediatr 1983; 103:534–537.

Orenstein SR, Magill LH, Brooks P. Thickening of infant feedings for therapy of GER. J Pediatr 1987; 110:181–186.

Orenstein SR. Effects on behavior state of prone versus seated positioning for infants with gastroesophageal reflux. Pediatrics 1990; 1985:764–767.

INFECTIOUS ESOPHAGITIS

SCOTT D. LEVENSON, M.D.
SCOTT L. FRIEDMAN, M.D.

Infectious esophagitis has become increasingly prevalent in the past 10 years. This increase can be attributed to a number of factors: the human immunodeficiency virus (HIV) epidemic, increased use of organ transplantation and associated immunosuppression, more toxic cancer chemotherapy regimens, and more liberal use of broad-spectrum antibiotics. Prompt recognition of esophageal infections is essential because of their severe impact on oral intake and quality of life in most patients.

Esophageal infections arise largely because of alteration of the mucosal barrier and/or weakened systemic defenses. The mucosal barrier may be disrupted by gastroesophageal reflux, preexisting ulcerations or erosions, decreased peristalsis, radiation therapy, or obstruction. Systemic factors include HIV infection, immunosupressant drugs, antibiotics, alcohol abuse, diabetes mellitus, and systemic neoplasia.

Normal hosts may develop infectious esophagitis, but the infections are rare and usually less severe. Most patients diagnosed with esophageal infections have HIV infection; the following discussion therefore addresses the immunocompromised patient, except where noted.

CLINICAL PRESENTATION

Patients with infectious esophagitis may present with odynophagia, dysphagia, nausea, anorexia, or heartburn. The exact frequencies of these symptoms have not been established because many patients with esophagitis are asymptomatic. Moreover, different pathogens may lead to similar symptoms, so the clinical presentation does not suggest a specific cause.

DIAGNOSTIC APPROACH

Upper endoscopy with biopsy is the best means to identify a specific pathogen. Nonetheless, because most symptomatic patients have *Candida* esophagitis alone or in association with other pathogens, empiric treatment for *Candida* esophagitis is appropriate before endoscopy (see below). For patients with persistent symptoms after 7 to 10 days of antifungal therapy, endoscopy is indicated. A large channel (>3.6 mm) endoscope with jumbo (3.3 mm) biopsy forceps is recommended to maximize the diagnostic yield. Snare cautery in the esophagus to achieve larger specimens is not advisable because of the risk of perforation. Biopsies, brushings, and culture are helpful in differentiating among the various causes of esophagitis as well as in trying to distinguish between colonization and invasion by the various pathogens. Overall, the diagnostic yield of endoscopy is 90 percent in acquired immunodeficiency syndrome (AIDS) patients. An infectious etiology is found in most of these patients (Table 1).

TYPES OF INFECTIONS AND SPECIFIC TREATMENTS (TABLE 2)

Fungal

Candida

Fungi are the most common type of esophageal pathogens. *Candida albicans* accounts for most cases; *Candida tropicalis, Candida parapsilosis,* and *Candida krusei* are less prevalent. AIDS is the most common underlying etiology. In addition, transient *Candida* esophagitis may accompany acute HIV infection. Oral candidiasis often indicates concurrent esophagitis, although it is not always present in patients with esophageal infection. *Candida* infection appears endoscopically as friable and hyperemic mucosa with overlying white exudative plaques. Diagnostic biopsies show

Table 1 Etiologies of Infectious Esophagitis in Patients with AIDS

Cause	%
Candida alone	46
Candida and CMV	31
Candida, CMV, and HSV	2.5
CMV alone	10
HSV alone	8
CMV and HSV	2.5

CMV = cytomegalovirus; HSV = herpes simplex virus.
From Bohacini M, Young T, Laine L. The causes of esophageal symptoms in human immunodeficiency virus infection: a prospective study of 110 patients. Arch Intern Med 1991; 151:1567–1572; with permission.

pseudohyphae, with or without budding yeast within the epithelium. Transnasal or transoral brush cytology may provide a less invasive alternative to endoscopy, with a reported sensitivity of 84 percent and specificity of 75 percent. Brush cytology is performed by placing a lubricated sheathed sterile brush through a 16 Fr nasogastric tube. The tube is advanced to 35 cm from the incisors, the sheath extended 2 cm outside the tube, and then the brush pushed out to reach approximately 40 cm from the incisors. The entire assembly is then slowly withdrawn over 20 seconds while moving the brush back and forth. Positive brushings for *Candida* display pseudomycelia. *Candida* serology may be useful in immunocompetent hosts but is of little value in immunocompromised hosts.

The treatment regimen currently recommended for *Candida* esophagitis depends on the severity of the esophagitis. The three categories of drugs currently available include nonabsorbable antifungal agents (clotrimazole and nystatin), oral absorbable antifungal agents (ketoconazole and fluconazole), and intravenous antifungal agents (amphotericin B). Topical nonabsorbable agents include clotrimazole (Mycelex), 10 mg five times a day, and nystatin, 500,000 to 1.5 million units (5 to 15 ml) four times a day. Clotrimazole and ketoconazole are imidazole antifungal agents that inhibit the cytochrome P-450–dependent enzymatic synthesis of ergosterol, a principal sterol membrane component of *Candida*.

Ketoconazole (Nizoral), 200 mg per day, is an inexpensive agent with side effects of nausea, diarrhea, and rash in less than 10 percent. **Warning:** Concurrent use of ketoconazole and terfenidine (Seldane) must be avoided because of a reported risk of serious ventricular arrhythmias. Failure of ketoconazole to clear candidiasis has been attributed to a high prevalence of gastric achlorhydria in AIDS patients, which results in impaired absorption of the drug. H_2 antagonists may have a similar effect and should not be prescribed concurrently with ketoconazole. Ketoconazole metabolism can be accelerated by concurrent administration of either isoniazid or rifampin.

Fluconazole (Diflucan) has greater in vivo activity against *Candida albicans* than ketoconazole. In contrast

Table 2 Recommended Treatment Regimens of Esophageal Pathogens

Pathogen	Drug	Initial Dose	Length	Cure (%) (by EGD)	Cost*
Candida	Fluconazole	100 mg PO q.d.	3–8 wk	90	$7/day
	Ketonconazole	200 mg PO q.d.	3–8 wk	50–70	$2.50/day
	Amphotericin	0.25 mg/kg IV q.d.	1–3 wk	95	$46/day
CMV	Ganciclovir	5 mg/kg IV q12 hr	2–3 wk	80	$70/day
	Foscarnet	60 mg/kg IV q8hr	2–3 wk	80	$220/day
HSV	Acyclovir	5 mg/kg IV q8hr	1 wk	–	$140/day
	Vidarabine	15 mg/kg IV q.d.	1 wk	–	$170/day
	Foscarnet	60 mg/kg IV q8hr	2–3 wk	–	$220/day

EGD = esophagogastroduodenoscopy.
*Based on 1993 University of California, San Francisco, pharmacy charge to the patient.

to ketoconazole, fluconazole's absorption is not pH dependent. Fluconazole is an orally active triazole agent that binds to fungal P-450 enzymes. It is prescribed as a 200 mg initial dose followed by 100 mg orally once daily for 3 to 4 weeks. If a patient remains symptomatic, the dose may be doubled after 1 to 2 weeks. Employing this dose-escalation approach, a multicenter study by Laine and colleagues demonstrated endoscopic cure rates in AIDS patients at 4 to 8 weeks of 52 percent of ketoconazole-treated and 91 percent of fluconazole-treated patients. Resolution of esophageal symptoms was obtained in 65 percent of the ketoconazole-treated and 85 percent of the fluconazole-treated groups. The difference in cure rates between these two drugs may be due to the greater absorption, reduced protein binding, and longer half-life of fluconazole. Sixteen percent of patients experience adverse effects from fluconazole (nausea, headache, skin rash, vomiting, abdominal pain, and diarrhea) requiring discontinuation in only 2.8 percent. Fluconazole's effect on the cytochrome P-450 enzymes may alter the metabolism of other drugs whose metabolism is also P-450–dependent, including phenytoin, warfarin, oral hypoglycemic agents, and cyclosporine.

Low-dose amphotericin B (Fungizone), 0.10 to 0.30 mg per kilogram per day IV, because of intolerable adverse effects (pyrexia, nephrotoxicity, and electrolyte disturbances), should be reserved for patients who fail other drugs or who are unable to take oral medications. Amphotericin requires induction therapy in the hospital; it is a polyene compound that binds to ergosterol. In theory, ketoconazole and fluconazole should antagonize the effects of polyene agents because of decreased ergosterol synthesis, but this interference has not been encountered in clinical use. Although 5-fluorocytosine was previously used, the drug has been abandoned for the treatment of Candida infection because of its hepatotoxicity and a 15 percent resistance rate of Candida isolates.

Eradication of invasive candidiasis does not necessarily prolong survival; thus, resolution of symptoms is a reasonable therapeutic end point. If a patient fails to improve after initial therapy, repeat endoscopy is indicated; if Candida esophagitis remains, prolonged treatment (for at least 8 weeks) with fluconazole is recommended. If symptoms persist despite additional fluconazole therapy, endoscopy should be repeated. If Candida is still present, amphotericin B therapy is appropriate for at least 4 weeks.

Recurrence rates for Candida have not been reported, but symptomatic recurrence is not unusual. Although maintenance therapy seems appropriate for patients with recurrent Candida infection, there are no controlled data examining this option. Topical nonabsorbable agents, ketoconazole, or fluconazole administered at one-half the induction doses may be used for such therapy.

Torulopsis Glabrata

Torulopsis glabrata has been identified as an esophageal pathogen in a few HIV-infected and immunocompromised patients from other causes besides HIV (e.g., after chemotherapy). The endoscopic and histologic appearances of torulopsis are indistinguishable from Candida esophagitis but can be discerned by culture. Because of high resistance rates to ketoconazole, fluconazole, 100 mg orally once daily for 3 to 8 weeks, is recommended.

Histoplasmosis and Coccidioidomycosis

Esophageal histoplasmosis has been described in association with pulmonary and hepatic disease. Diagnosis is established by fungal smear and culture of infected tissue or blood. The infection must be managed with amphotericin B, 0.25 to 0.50 mg per kilogram per day IV for 8 to 12 weeks, since ketoconazole and fluconazole are much less effective. Coccidioidomycosis of the gut is rare and, like histoplasmosis, occurs with systemic infection. Treatment with amphotericin B is indicated after diagnosis by fungal smear and culture.

Viral

Cytomegalovirus

Cytomegalovirus (CMV) is the most prevalent viral pathogen in patients with esophagitis. Patients with

CMV esophagitis usually complain of odynophagia or substernal chest pain, occasionally in association with dysphagia and fevers. CMV esophagitis occurs typically in AIDS patients with CD_4 counts less than 150. CMV infections appear endoscopically as extensive large ulcerations of variable depth that can be solitary or multiple. Association with candidal infection is common. Mucosal biopsies characteristically reveal basophilic intranuclear inclusions and periodic acid–Schiff–positive cytoplasmic inclusions in endothelial cells at the ulcer margin. CMV culture of biopsy specimens is often positive but is less specific than evidence of cytopathic inclusions in tissue sections.

The ideal treatment for viral esophagitis is not as clearly established as that for fungal esophagitis; moreover treatment is generally less effective. For CMV, dihydroxypropoxymethyl guanine (DHPG, ganciclovir, Cytovene) is the preferred agent. This drug is an acyclic nucleoside analog of 2'-deoxyguanosine that requires phosphorylation by viral thymidine kinase to be active. It functions by selectively inhibiting viral DNA polymerase. Despite its apparent efficacy, no consistent survival benefit has been shown. Lack of survival advantage may reflect the high mortality rate in all patients with late-stage AIDS when the risk of CMV infection is greatest. Ganciclovir is administered intravenously in doses of 15 mg per kilogram in divided doses (every 8 to 12 hours based on creatinine clearance) for 3 weeks. Recurrences are common. Patients with documented recurrences should be treated with a second 3 week course of ganciclovir, followed by maintenance therapy, 2.5 to 5.0 mg per kilogram per day or 5 mg per kilogram 3 days a week. **Warning:** Ganciclovir should be administered cautiously in patients treated with zidovudine because marked bone marrow suppression may occur.

In patients with documented CMV infection who fail to respond adequately to ganciclovir, foscarnet (Foscavir) may be effective. This agent is a pyrophosphate analog that does not require phosphorylation to be effective, but also functions by selective inhibition of viral DNA polymerase. Foscarnet is less marrow suppressive than ganciclovir. However, because foscarnet is nephrotoxic, the usual dosage of 60 mg per kilogram IV every 8 hours should be reduced when there is renal impairment. **Warning:** Simultaneous use of foscarnet and pentamidine is contraindicated because of enhanced renal toxicity and profound hypocalcemia.

Herpes Simplex Virus

Herpes simplex virus (HSV) is an occasional cause of esophagitis in AIDS patients and has also been reported as a rare cause of esophagitis in immunocompetent individuals. In healthy patients, esophagitis is usually due to herpes simplex type I; however, AIDS patients may have esophagitis due to either type I or type II herpes. The disease is similar to herpetic infections of other mucosal membranes in that the pathogenic features follow a predictable sequence: discrete vesicles form and shallow ulcers develop, which finally coalesce into regions of diffuse inflammation indistinguishable from those resulting from other causes of esophagitis. It is during this late stage of diffuse esophagitis that most patients with herpes are usually evaluated. Endoscopically, HSV appears as vesicular lesions or small ulcerations with a slightly raised yellow border. Pathology of biopsy specimens obtained from the margin of the ulceration (the sites of active viral replication) may show the characteristic histologic appearance of multinucleated giant cells and eosinophilic intranuclear inclusions found in epithelial cells.

Acyclovir (Zovirax), 15 to 20 mg per kilogram per day IV in divided doses) is the drug of choice for HSV. Acyclovir is a guanine nucleoside analog that requires thymidine kinase for phosphorylation and then selectively inhibits viral DNA polymerase. The choice between oral or intravenous acyclovir is determined by the patient's symptoms. Individuals who have severe dysphagia, high fevers, or upper gastrointestinal bleeding should receive intravenous therapy. Most published reports are of small series of HIV-negative immunosuppressed patients in whom acyclovir therapy for HSV esophagitis appeared extremely effective. Most herpes infections respond to acyclovir, although acyclovir resistance is increasingly encountered; foscarnet may be a suitable alternative in this situation. Repeat endoscopy for additional biopsies for culture and sensitivities is indicated for treatment failures. Foscarnet-treated HSV patients may be placed on maintenance acyclovir therapy, since only small numbers of the initial infecting herpes virus are acyclovir resistant. Intravenous adenine arabinoside (ara-A) is an alternative although more toxic regimen.

Idiopathic

Some AIDS patients may develop large symptomatic esophageal ulcerations in the absence of a causative pathogen. The syndrome may be manifested either coincident with acute HIV seroconversion or after the diagnosis of AIDS has been established. Severe odynophagia is the usual presenting symptom. Typically, these ulcers are in the proximal or middle esophagus. Macroscopically, the lesions cannot be distinguished from CMV-induced ulcerations. Electron microscopy may reveal retrovirus-like particles at the ulcer site but no CMV or herpes inclusions. One study identified HIV in these lesions by in situ hybridization, although it remains to be determined whether the lesion is a direct consequence of HIV. Nonspecific esophageal ulcerations respond to a short course of corticosteroids given either orally, 40 mg per day with a 3 week taper, or intralesionally, performed on serial endoscopies. The basis of the response of these lesions to corticosteroids is unknown; infectious causes should be assiduously excluded before steroids are given in this setting. In patients who develop recurrence during the steroid taper, slower withdrawal or intralesional injections may be necessary. Intralesional injections are administered as methylprednisolone, 40 mg diluted in 10 ml normal saline and injected through a sclerotherapy needle in 1 ml increments tangentially along the ulcer edge. This procedure can be repeated every 2 weeks, as needed.

Bacterial

Bacterial infections of the esophagus are primarily limited to *Mycobacterium* species and usually occur in the setting of a systemic infection. *Mycobacterium avium intracellulare* (now commonly referred to as mycobacterium avium complex) has been cultured in patients with esophageal disease but has not been clearly shown to be pathogenic. However, cases of very deep ulcerations and esophagoesophageal fistulas with cultures positive for *Mycobacterium* species have been reported. Effective medical treatment for such invasive mycobacterial infection is still being developed. Currently recommended therapies include four to five medications: a common regimen is 4 weeks of amikacin, 7.5 mg per kilogram IV; 12 weeks of ethambutol, 1,000 mg orally every day; ciprofloxacin, 750 mg orally twice daily; and rifampin, 600 mg orally every day. Infection with *Mycobacterium tuberculosis* may rarely involve the esophagus with ulcerations in association with pulmonary or miliary disease. Diagnosis is established with acid-fast bacillus (AFB) stain and AFB culture. The disease is responsive to multidrug therapy.

Parasitic

Isolated cases of esophagitis due to cryptosporidiosis have been described. Despite trials with spiramycin, hyperimmune bovine colostrum, and diclazuril, there remains no proven effective treatment of this infection. Improvement in immune function with an increase in CD_4 count holds the most promise for eradication of cryptosporidial infection. Current therapy is supportive, with nonspecific antidiarrheal agents and nutritional support.

SYMPTOMATIC THERAPY

In patients with infectious esophagitis, significant dysphagia or odynophagia may lead to poor oral intake and malnutrition, making symptomatic relief an important factor in reversing this trend. Such relief may be obtained by using oral topical anesthetics such as viscous lidocaine (5 ml orally every 2 hours as needed) or Cetacaine spray (two sprays to the oropharynx every hour as needed). Topical anti-inflammatory therapy such as chlorhexidine (Peridex), 15 ml oral rinse for 30 seconds twice daily will treat pharyngeal lesions. Sucralfate (Carafate) slurry, 1 g diluted in 10 ml water, before meals and at bedtime will coat the ulcerations and may provide relief. Antacids (Maalox or Mylanta alternating with ALternaGEL, 15 to 30 ml orally every 2 hours as needed), high dose H-2 blockers (ranitidine, 300 mg orally twice daily), or omeprazole, 20 to 40 mg orally once daily may also help relieve symptoms and perhaps accelerate healing, but no studies have established their efficacy in this setting.

NUTRITIONAL SUPPORT

Malnutrition is common in patients with infectious esophagitis, as a result of both the underlying disease and decreased oral intake because of odynophagia or dysphagia. The extent to which malnutrition exacerbates the consequences of esophageal infections is unknown.

Consultation with a dietitian familiar with esophageal disease and AIDS can be helpful in patient education and in defining a diet that provides maximal nutrition with minimal swallowing effort. Frequent small feedings and puréed or soft foods are better tolerated in patients with esophagitis. Patients should be cautioned against exclusive use of megavitamin and herbal regimens, which are often calorically inadequate and may be toxic. Commercially available nutritional supplements (e.g., Resource, Ensure) may be incorporated into a dietary plan. When oral intake becomes inadequate to meet the patient's nutritional needs, supplemental nasoenteral or percutaneous gastrostomy tube feeding should be provided with formulas such as Isosource HN or Compleat modified. Some evidence supports use of the progestational agent *megestrol acetate* to improve the appetite and oral intake in AIDS patients. Large trials of the agent are currently under way.

SUGGESTED READING

Bonacini M, Young T, Laine L. The causes of esophageal symptoms in human immunodeficiency virus infection. A prospective study of 110 patients. Arch Intern Med 1991; 151:1567–1572.

Connolly GM, Hawkins D, Harcourt WJ, et al. Oesophageal symptoms, their causes, treatment, and prognosis in patients with the acquired immunodeficiency syndrome. Gut 1989; 30:1033–1039.

Laine L, Bonacini M, Sattler F, et al. Cytomegalovirus and *Candida* esophagitis in patients with AIDS. J Acquir Immune Defic Syndr 1992; 5:605–609.

Laine L, Dretler RH, Conteas CN, et al. Fluconazole compared with ketoconazole for the treatment of *Candida* esophagitis in AIDS. A randomized trial. Ann Intern Med 1992; 117:655–660.

Lopez DM, Mora SP, Pintado GV, et al. Clinical, endoscopic, immunologic, and therapeutic aspects of oropharyngeal and esophageal candidiasis in HIV-infected patients: a survey of 114 cases. Am J Gastroenterol 1992; 87:1771–1776.

Simon D, Weiss L, Brandt L. Treatment options for AIDS-related esophageal and diarrheal disorders. Am J Gastroenterol 1992; 87:274–281.

Wilcox CM, Diehl DL, Cello JP, et al. Cytomegalovirus esophagitis in patients with AIDS. A clinical, endoscopic, and pathologic correlation. Ann Intern Med 1990; 113:589–593.

Wilcox CM, Schwartz DA. A pilot study of oral corticosteroid therapy for idiopathic esophageal ulcerations associated with human immunodeficiency virus infection. Am J Med 1992; 93:131–134.

ESOPHAGEAL STRICTURE

ROBERT A. SANOWSKI, M.D.

Esophageal dilation is an effective means of treating benign and malignant strictures and a variety of other esophageal stenosis. Table 1 lists those lesions that commonly cause dysphagia and that symptomatically improve after dilation. The goal of this therapeutic procedure is to enlarge the obstructed tubular esophagus, relieve distressing symptoms, and afford the patient normal or improved swallowing capacity. How to do this effectively, safely, and with the least stress and cost to the patient is the goal of this presentation.

DILATORS VERSUS STRICTURES

All strictures were not created equal. Since the symptom of dysphagia has multiple possible causes, the etiology must be firmly established before dilation is begun. For example, a benign-appearing reflux-associated stricture may be complicated by Barrett's esophagus and adenocarcinoma for which surgery is indicated, whereas serial dilation for gastroesophageal reflux disease (GERD)-induced stenosis is appropriate.

Table 1 Frequent Causes of Esophageal Strictures

Reflux esophagitis (gastroesophageal reflux disease)
Caustic ingestion (lye, pills)
Radiation
Sclerotherapy
Infections (*Candida*)
Webs and rings
Carcinoma
Extrinsic compression (tumor, infections)
Surgery

A plan of dilation should be determined after review of endoscopy, esophageal biopsies, and x-ray findings. In addition to the etiology, the location, contour, and length of the stricture will determine which dilating system best "fits" the stenosis. For example, the dilator chosen to relieve the obstruction of a tortuous postirradiation stricture of the cervical esophagus complicated by a laryngectomy is different from that used to remedy a straight GERD-induced obstruction. The choice of dilators and the advantages and shortcomings of each are given in Table 2.

After a dilator system tailored to the stricture is chosen, therapy is begun to ensure maximal relief of dysphagia with minimal complications. The "rule of threes" for dilator passage should be prudently followed. This means that only three dilators that meet moderate resistance are passed. If a dilator meets no resistance, it does not count in the dilator total. Since most strictures will have had a gradual onset and may be quite fibrotic, treatment should also be gradual to avoid rupture of a stenotic esophageal segment. Several dilating sessions are usually needed for symptomatic improvement, depending on the nature of the stenosis.

USE OF FLUOROSCOPY

The literature is replete with controversy concerning the use of fluoroscopy during dilation, but it is clearly indicated and helpful in positioning guidewires in the antrum before treating a tortuous stricture. An uncomplicated "straight-on" stricture is easily treated with a Maloney rubber bougie. However, if proximal esophageal diverticular pouches are present, the bougie may curl back on itself, exerting increased force on the walls of the esophagus and thus increasing the danger of perforation. When guidewires are used they should be positioned in the antrum under fluoroscopy or through the endoscope without radiographic guidance. If this is not done, the wire may curl in a hiatal hernia, penetrate a long tumor, or perforate the gastric wall. I recommend

Table 2 Menu of Esophageal Dilators

Mercury-Filled	Guidewire – Thermoplastic	Balloon
Maloney Bougie	*Savary-Gilliard-American*	*TTS, Wire Guided*
Advantages	For tight, irregular strictures	For tight, irregular strictures
Easy to pass		Radial directed force
"Blind" passage		Passed through endoscope
No sedation		Patient usually sedated
Good for straight peptic strictures		
Easy to feel resistance		
Disadvantages		
Requires repeat passages	Repetitive passage	
Small size too flexible	Difficult to feel resistance	Balloons are fragile
	Needs long guidewire	May slip in and out of strictures
	Sharp tip dangerous	

TTS = through the scope.

the use of fluoroscopy in complicated strictures, for wire-guided dilation, and whenever there is any question about the safety of dilation. Perforations can be avoided by judicious use of fluoroscopy.

TECHNIQUES OF ESOPHAGEAL DILATION

Mercury-weighted bougies, wire-guided thermoplastic dilators, and balloons passed through the scope (TTS) or guided by fluoroscopy are the three current choices for dilating esophageal strictures. The Hurst and Eder-Puestow dilators should be abandoned because of their perforation potential. The technique of using the three other dilation systems will be discussed.

The procedure is described to the patient, including the risks and benefits, and informed consent is obtained by the physician.

Bougie Dilation

Initial evaluation ensures that the patient has a benign esophageal stricture suitable for dilation by bougie. The patient fasts the morning of the procedure and is treated on an outpatient basis.

Maloney dilators are still commonly used. The tapered tip dilators are available in even sizes in 2 Fr increments up to 60 Fr (20 mm). However, the 20 to 30 Fr sizes tend to curl back in very tight strictures. I prefer the Maloney dilators to the Hurst because the long, tapered tip of the Maloney easily negotiates a stricture, whereas the blunt tip of the Hurst cannot and predisposes to perforation. At my hospital, the procedure is performed while the patient is seated. This position allows the mercury weight of the dilator to apply dilating force to the stricture passively using the force of gravity. The supine, left lateral decubitus, or standing position may also be used. The posterior oropharynx is anesthetized with topical anesthetic. In tighter, painful strictures an analgesic may be used, but sedation is rarely given. Each dilator is carefully disinfected before use. The distal end is lubricated and the dilator is passed into the posterior pharynx. I use my forefinger and second finger as a guide to direct its passage through the oropharynx. The patient is asked to swallow, relaxing the cricopharyngeus and allowing dilator passage into the tubular esophagus. The dilator engages, is passed through the stricture, and is then smoothly and slowly removed without any pause. The first dilation session need not achieve maximal dilation. The first dilator encountering resistance is the first true dilation. Two larger dilators are then passed to achieve the "rule of three."

Symptomatic relief eventually follows dilation whether the therapeutic approach is conservative or aggressive.

Bougie dilation for benign strictures is safe and effective without fluoroscopic observation and has been performed in this manner for many years. However, several reports have indicated that the flexible tip may curl proximal to the stricture or in a hiatal hernia or diverticulum. If the physician is unsure about the technique or the nature of the stricture, or if the stricture is complicated and the dilation difficult, fluoroscopy should be used.

After an initial successful dilation, some patients will be free of symptoms, but most require repeated dilation. Therapy may be daily, weekly, or less frequent, depending on symptom relief. I have found that dilation to a 40 or 46 Fr is required for relief. For tight, fibrotic cervical esophageal strictures, a 40 Fr dilator may be the largest that can safely be passed, while a 50 to 60 Fr dilation is necessary to relieve symptoms of a Schatski ring.

Complications

Dilation of benign strictures with a Maloney dilator is a safe procedure. The reported incidence of perforation is only 0.04 to 0.2 percent. Since bacteremia following esophageal dilation is surprisingly high (55 to 100 percent), I recommend antibiotic therapy before bougie dilation in patients with prosthetic heart valves, rheumatic valvular heart disease, or a history of endocarditis.

TTS Balloon Dilation

Balloon dilation of esophageal strictures affords the therapist another method that further tailors the dilation method to the stricture. Balloons may be passed over fluoroscopically placed guidewires and are very effective in dilating cases of achalasia. This method was used in treating other strictures of the esophagus, but generally has been replaced by TTS balloon dilators. I have found the method of TTS dilation advantageous in tortuous strictures of the cervical esophagus and other benign strictures discovered during endoscopic evaluation. TTS balloon dilators may be passed through the 2.8 mm device channel of the endoscope. Patient preparation is the same as for Maloney dilators, but this experience is easier for the patients since they have usually received sedation prior to the esophagogastroduodenoscopy (EGD).

The longest TTS (Rigiflex) balloon is 8 cm long and has a soft, tapered tip extending 2 to 3 cm beyond its distal end. The balloon size varies from 5 to 18 mm in diameter. I recommend 15 mm as the end point for dilation to ensure safety from perforation.

The procedure is done as part of routine upper endoscopy. If the stricture can be negotiated with the endoscope, the balloon is passed through the silicon-lubricated device channel and out of the endoscope. The endoscope and balloon are pulled back as a unit and the balloon is situated within the stricture. I move the balloon to and fro until satisfied that it is seated well. The balloon is then inflated with water to a pressure of 40 to 60 pounds per square inch (psi). Pressure in the balloon is maintained for 60 seconds and then deflated. The endoscopy assistant uses the balloon inflation "gun" to expand and deflate the balloon with water. I generally repeat the procedure twice to ensure passage of the 1.5

mm inflated balloon and endoscope through the stenosis. A reasonable starting size of the balloon is 10 mm; I do not use one greater than 15 mm in diameter because of the danger of perforation. If repeat dilation is necessary, I switch to the mercury bougie if possible, because I feel this is easier, faster, and more cost effective than a repeat endoscopy and balloon dilation. If, however, this cannot be done, I repeat the TTS dilation. Various types of benign esophageal stenosis have been treated with balloon dilation, including peptic, postsurgical anastomotic, and caustic (pill-induced) strictures.

Complications

Rupture of the balloon may occur during the procedure, but this is generally not a problem. Reports of perforation of the esophagus and bleeding with this technique have been few. I do not recommend routine use in uncomplicated strictures because it adds the cost of an EGD to the dilation fee. Since conscious sedation is then required, the price of monitoring further increases the cost and complicates a simple procedure that can easily be performed with the Maloney bougie.

Guidewire Dilation

Tight, tortuous, complicated esophageal strictures are best treated by the Savary-Gilliard or American dilator systems. These are sets of tapered, thermoplastic dilators graduated from 15 to 60 Fr and passed over a flexible-tip guidewire. The American dilators are radiopaque, whereas the Savary dilators contain horizontal radiopaque bands in the plastic substance. The flexible tip allows safe placement in the gastric antrum. If the wire cannot be readily passed through a tight or irregular stricture, it may be passed through the device channel of the endoscope and properly positioned under fluoroscopic guidance. The well-lubricated dilators are passed over the wire and observed by radiography. An assistant ensures with fluoroscopy that the spring tip remains in the antrum. After three dilators against moderate resistance, the entire apparatus is withdrawn. It must be stressed that the Savary dilators are never passed without wire guidance, and that fluoroscopy or direct endoscopically guided wire placement of the spring tip in the antrum is mandatory. Serious complications (perforation) have occurred when this warning has been ignored. I find the Savary dilators somewhat stiff, and extra caution should be exercised during esophageal dilation to avoid pharyngeal perforation. In uncomplicated short distal strictures caused by GERD, a maximal lumen size of 52 Fr is a realistic goal. However, in long, fibrotic, tortuous stenosis, one may have to be satisfied with maximal passage of a smaller bougie (46 Fr). In tight cervical strictures this may not be achievable without exposing the patient to increased risk of perforation. In such a case, a 40 Fr may be the maximal safe diameter attained.

Complications

Data on the frequency of perforation with the newer over-the-wire dilators are limited to a few studies showing a perforation rate of 0.0 to 0.6 percent. These figures are comparable with those generated from mercury-filled bougie dilations.

SPECIAL PROBLEMS

Esophageal webs are filamentous structures occurring in the cervical esophagus that may cause dysphagia. The treatment of webs is fairly simple. At times the mere passage of the endoscope will rupture the web and relieve the symptoms. In more persistent webs, dilation with the wire-guided system under fluoroscopy may be necessary. However, the Maloney dilator or any of the systems described can be used with excellent results.

Symptomatic lower esophageal rings (LERs) are best treated with large (52 to 60 Fr) Maloney dilators. The therapeutic objective here is to disrupt the ring, not merely stretch it. Smaller-diameter bougies do not relieve dysphagia as well as the passage of a single large dilator.

LERs are a common cause of intermittent dysphagia and food impaction. These are usually associated with a hiatal hernia. I document their presence by having the patient swallow a 1.2 cm barium-filled capsule. This generally impacts in the ring. Patients having an LER with a diameter of 3 to 12 mm have repeated dysphagia; rings measuring 12 to 20 mm cause dysphagia in about 50 percent of patients; if the ring is 20 to 40 mm, dysphagia is rare. In general, treatment of a mucosal ring is not difficult. A bougienage with a 50 Fr Maloney dilator or a 52 wire-guided Savary dilator is required. Gradual stretching of the ring with smaller dilators usually does not relieve the dysphagia. Perforation after this procedure for LER is rare.

Barrett's esophagus may be associated with ulcers and strictures in the middle third of the esophagus. If multiple biopsies do not demonstrate dysplasia or carcinoma, the stricture is then dilated. Pill-induced strictures may also be seen in the middle third of the esophagus. These tend to be tighter and more fibrotic; if they are associated with proximal pseudodiverticula, wire-guided dilation is appropriate. Caustic-induced stenoses tend to be very long and involve one-third to one-half of the tubular esophagus. These too are dilated with the Savary dilators but frequently are resistant to therapy.

FOLLOW-UP THERAPY

Esophageal strictures, especially those secondary to reflux, tend to recur and require repeat dilation. Once the patient develops symptoms, repeat bougienage is indicated. In the case of a reflux stricture containing Barrett's esophagus, periodic biopsy must be done to rule out the development of cancer or dysplasia.

The techniques and dilators for esophageal stricture therapy have evolved in the past few years to the point where there are now three reliable systems that can be used safely in a variety of challenging strictures with satisfactory relief of dysphagia and a reasonable safety profile. H$_2$-receptor antagonists and hydrogen pump inhibitors — potent acid suppressors — now widely used for treatment of reflux strictures may alter the natural history of the most common type of strictures, and decrease the need for esophageal dilation. Avoidance of procedure-induced perforation is an important concept to develop. Following the guidelines of using the appropriate dilator and the "rule of three" plus judicious use of fluoroscopy should make safe esophageal dilation a reality.*

Editor's Note: The management of esophageal perforation usually involves decision making by the endoscopist, the patient's physician, and a surgeon. Patients with achalasia, the subject of a separate chapter, are treated medically and expectantly after a perforation.

FOREIGN BODY EXTRACTION

MARY L. HARRIS, M.D.

Foreign body ingestion in the digestive tract is a commonly encountered problem in both children and adults. Most objects (80 percent) pass spontaneously per rectum, but 20 percent require endoscopic removal and 1 percent necessitate surgical intervention.

In children, the most commonly ingested foreign bodies are coins, toys, crayons, and ballpoint pen caps. Whenever a foreign body is known to have been ingested, the clinician must consider the possibility of a second foreign body. The pediatric age group accounts for 80 percent of all foreign body ingestions.

In adults, denture wearers are most likely to ingest foreign bodies. Dentures eliminate much of the tactile sensitivity of the palate surfaces, which is necessary to identify small objects that may be included in a bolus of food. Other adults susceptible to foreign body ingestion include patients with esophageal stenoses or strictures; those with a history of previous lye ingestion, psychiatric impairment, cerebrovascular accidents, or alcoholism; incarcerated individuals; and the mentally retarded. Adults commonly tend to have problems with meat and bones, specifically fish bones. Inadvertent ingestion of toothpicks is also seen in adult denture wearers with impaired oral sensation. Recurrent episodes of foreign body ingestion occur especially in prisoners, psychiatric patients, and patients with peptic strictures, with a

SUGGESTED READING

Anand BS. Eder-Puestow and Savary dilators. Hepatogastroenterology 1992; 39:494–496.

Chen Pang-Chi. Endoscopic balloon dilation of esophageal strictures following surgical anastomoses, endoscopic variceal sclerotherapy and corrosive ingestion. Gastrointest Endosc 1992; 38:586–589.

Harrison ME, Sanowski RA. Mercury bougie dilation of benign esophageal strictures. Hepatogastroenterology 1992; 39:497–501.

Kozarek RA. Hydrostatic balloon dilation of gastrointestinal stenosis: a national survey. Gastrointest Endosc 1986; 32:15–19.

Saeed ZA. Balloon dilatation of benign esophageal stenosis. Hepatogastroenterology 1992; 39:490–493.

Sanowski RA. Treatment of difficult esophageal strictures, rings and webs. Endosc Rev 1990; 7:8–23.

Webb WA. Esophageal dilation: personal experience with current instruments and techniques. Am J Gastroenterol 1988; 83:471–475.

recurrence rate of approximately 10 percent. Finally, the literature reports that 80 percent of ingested foreign bodies enter the gastrointestinal (GI) tract, and approximately 20 percent enter the tracheobronchial tree.

The physician must be able to distinguish patients who require observation from those one who need immediate endoscopic intervention. The indications for foreign body removal are based on the type of foreign body, the risk of impaction or perforation, and the possibility of ingestion of a toxic substance.

INDICATIONS FOR OBSERVATION

Foreign bodies that are 2.5 cm or less in diameter, round, or blunt usually do not require endoscopic removal. Although it has been recommended that a foreign body be removed if it has not left the stomach within 72 hours, more conservative management involving a 2 week period of observation may be appropriate. An ingested coin in children rarely causes a problem if it is a dime or a penny; larger coins may become impacted at the cricopharyngeal muscle. Children may be asymptomatic despite the coin lodging in the esophagus or trachea. If a coin becomes lodged in the esophagus, it should be extracted immediately because of the risk of perforation or fistula formation. It is vital that an airway be maintained at all times during extraction of foreign bodies at the level of the cricopharyngeal muscle, and one should consider endotracheal intubation. If an endotracheal tube is not used, the patient should be placed in the Trendelenburg position to keep the coin out of the trachea. Of particular note, the copper penny was replaced by the zinc penny in 1982 because of the increasing cost of copper. Zinc tends to be more corrosive when lodged in the esophagus and is another indication for immediate removal. Prompt removal of a coin impacted in the esophagus is advocated, but once it passes into the stomach, the object will usually pass through the GI tract without difficulty. Nevertheless, the patient should be referred for surgical intervention after prolonged delays of 2 or more weeks with the object in the stomach, 6 days in the duodenum, or 10 days in the small intestine.

Coins and buttons are difficult to remove with the standard endoscopic biopsy forceps because they easily slip off the surface. It is recommended that these objects be grasped with an alligator type of forcep or that a snare be used to capture a coin or button. When the coin or button approaches the proximal esophagus, it should be rotated so that it is oriented in a frontal plane representing the largest diameter of the cervical esophagus and hypopharynx.

ESOPHAGEAL BOLUS IMPACTIONS

Impaction of a foreign body in the esophagus is an indication for immediate removal because of the potential for aspiration and other complications. Large pieces of meat may lodge at the level of the cricopharyngeal muscle with subsequent compression of the adjacent trachea, the café coronary or "steakhouse syndrome." This is an emergency situation because of the resultant respiratory compromise. The Heimlich maneuver is useful for impactions in the proximal third of the esophagus. Obstruction in the distal esophagus usually does not require emergent care but warrants prompt attention.

When there is an obvious history of meat bolus ingestion and impaction, endoscopic retrieval is the procedure of choice. Radiography and other barium diagnostic studies are unnecessary. Delaying the removal of a food bolus makes it more difficult to remove the object in one piece. The most efficient method of removing a bolus is using a snare or a basket. If the bolus cannot be moved in a single fragment, one should consider the use of an overtube to protect the airway during multiple passages of the endoscope. Alternatively, the remaining food bolus can be pushed distally into the stomach under direct visualization. Other alternatives in the past for dealing with an impacted food bolus included blind bougienage or enzymatic digestion with papain. Blind pushing of a meat bolus carries the risk of perforation in view of a relatively high incidence of esophageal stricture or stenosis. Enzymatic digestion may injure the esophageal mucosa, placing the patient at risk for perforation. These two alternatives are not recommended. Finally, glucagon decreases lower esophageal sphincter pressure and has been used to relieve meat impaction in the distal two-thirds of the esophagus. However, glucagon has no effect on the motility of the esophagus at pharmacologic doses.

POINTED AND ELONGATED FOREIGN BODIES

Toothpicks, pins, nails, bones, and unfolded paper clips or stiff pieces of wire are associated with a high incidence of perforation. Mucosal laceration and/or free perforation may occur from pointed, sharp foreign bodies. Elongated foreign bodies do not negotiate fixed curves in the duodenum and may become impacted in either the gastric or duodenal wall. Penetration of the bowel wall by the end of a pointed or elongated foreign body is not a contraindication to endoscopic removal unless free perforation is obvious.

There are several techniques for successful extraction of open safety pins from the upper digestive tract with the flexible endoscope. The key issue is to remove the sharp point trailing distally to avoid mucosal laceration or perforation. If the sharp end of the open safety pin is pointing proximally in the esophagus, the safety pin can be grasped with closed biopsy forceps and carried into the stomach, then turned so that the sharp point trails distally during endoscopic extraction. An overtube provides an additional aspect of protection with large safety pins and is advocated on a routine basis. Some endoscopists have attempted to close a safety pin before extraction. This is a difficult maneuver with a snare and often unsuccessful, but it can be practiced on a similar safety pin before endoscopic intubation and attempted closure and extraction.

Regardless of the position of an elongated foreign body, the endoscopic snare is the instrument of choice for extraction. If the elongated object is impacted against the gastric wall or resting horizontally in front of the pyloric channel, there must initially be adequate insufflation of the stomach so that it can be snared. It may be necessary to use a two-channel endoscope to grasp an object with forceps, pull it away from the wall, and then allow for a snare to be passed through the second channel to retrieve the foreign body. When an elongated foreign body is grasped and extracted, the snare should grasp the object in a cephalad point so that the long axis of the object can be aligned with the axis of the esophagus. This also allows for direct visual guidance during removal. If the elongated object is grasped near the center, blind extraction may increase the risk of imbedding in the wall of the upper digestive tract. To maintain the esophagus and hypopharynx in alignment with the endoscope and the foreign body, it is recommended that the patient's head be tilted backward while extending the neck forward in order to create a straight passage. If the elongated object is firmly imbedded in the gastrointestinal wall, surgical intervention may be necessary owing to the risk of perforation.

RAZOR BLADES

Razor blades are usually ingested by adults with psychiatric disturbances or by adults incarcerated and seeking transfer from the penal system to the hospital setting (especially at holiday times). The single-edged blade or the injector type are more commonly swallowed than the double-edged blade. At presentation, the razor blades are usually found in the stomach or small intestine after they have rapidly passed through the esophagus. Surprisingly, they rarely cause mucosal laceration. An overtube should be preloaded over the endoscope before intubation. Once the razor blade has been grasped with standard forceps, the overtube is advanced over the entire foreign body. This allows for protection of the gastric and esophageal mucosa during extraction of the endoscope. If multiple razor blades or sharp objects have been ingested, the overtube may be left in place, which protects the hypopharynx and cricopharyngeal region during successive reinsertion of the endoscope. Patients with razor blades that have passed beyond the pylorus into the duodenum should be observed, as spontaneous passage usually occurs. There is a surprisingly low incidence of perforation once razor blades have reached the duodenum. Because of the angle of the duodenal sweep, the overtube is not useful in the duodenum.

COCAINE AND OTHER TOXIC FOREIGN BODIES

Accidental or intentional drug ingestions are not uncommon causes of visits to the Emergency Department. Cocaine is the drug most commonly ingested in an effort to conceal possession of this illegal material. The management of cocaine "body packers" who deliberately smuggle illicit drugs in the GI tract should be differentiated from that of the cocaine "body stuffer." The body packers are specifically hired to smuggle drugs that are carefully packed and wrapped in containers designed to survive GI tract transit. The smuggling business dictates that it is most efficient for large quantities of drug to be carried by each body packer. Cocaine is typically wrapped in Latex, sometimes condoms, with or without a covering of aluminum foil. A body packer may ingest multiple packages containing cocaine. A condom usually holds 3 to 5 g of cocaine. The ingestion of 1 to 3 g of cocaine in powdered form can be fatal, and thus rupture of even one package carries the risk of death. Radiography will demonstrate the packets 70 to 90 percent of the time in patients in the Emergency Department with a history of ingesting cocaine. A toxicology screen should also be obtained. The usual methods of decontaminating the GI tract (ipecac syrup, carthartics, or enemas) should be avoided because of the risk of packet rupture. Ideally, the safest means of removing the packet is by surgery. Under no circumstances should the endoscopist try to extract the latex packets from above with the gastroscope or from below with a colonoscope. Patients at risk of toxicity from cocaine have often passed broken containers, are symptomatic, or have GI tract obstruction. Surgical intervention is indicated only for intestinal obstruction or significant clinical deterioration. Management of the asymptomatic body packer who has ingested cocaine is difficult; these patients are usually uncooperative. The packets are usually resistant to disruption, and should be carefully monitored and managed medically with follow-up bowel movements and radiography.

The typical body stuffer may ingest cocaine that either is not wrapped or is contained in aluminum foil or an open and relatively porous container such as a sandwich bag. Glass or plastic crack vials are sometimes swallowed as well. In the body stuffer presentation, large quantities of cocaine are most often not involved. Nevertheless, owing to the poor wrapping, a lethal exposure may occur. Radiographic detection of these containers may be more difficult in body stuffers than in body packers, in whom the carefully wrapped packages are more likely to provide air liquid or air solid interfaces. Both body stuffers and body packers are typically uncooperative and equally unlikely to give an accurate history of ingestion.

Other toxic foreign bodies, such as button batteries, are commonly ingested by children and should be removed promptly to avoid corrosive injury to the GI tract and systemic toxicity. The three most commonly involved battery systems are the manganese dioxide, silver oxide, and mercuric oxide. Each of these systems contain a disc alkaline electrolyte that is usually a 25 to 45 percent solution of potassium hydroxide or sodium hydroxide. Corrosive injury may occur rapidly with transmural liquefaction necrosis and subsequent perforation. If the battery lodges in the esophagus, emergent endoscopic extraction is indicated because of the rapid action of alkaline substances and the risk of perforation or esophagotracheal or esophagoaortic fistula. As discussed, it is important to provide protection of the airway by general endotracheal anesthesia. The battery is too smooth to be grasped with the foreign body forceps, and thus the most successful approach is a through-the-scope balloon under direct visualization. The deflated balloon may be passed distal to the battery and subsequently inflated. The inflated balloon, battery, and endoscope are then removed simultaneously. Another alternative is to push the battery into the stomach and then extract it with a polypectomy snare or basket. However, once the battery reaches the stomach, it usually passes without difficulty. This foreign body may be followed daily with radiography and removed endoscopically only if it remains longer than 36 to 48 hours, or if the patient becomes symptomatic. If the battery reaches the duodenum, it cannot be retrieved endoscopically. It also will usually pass without difficulty. Surgical intervention may be considered if the patient becomes symptomatic.*

RECTAL AND COLONIC FOREIGN BODIES

Rectal and colonic foreign bodies may be inserted through the anal canal or via the peroral route. Most

---

*Editor's Note: I am sure there are a number of jokes and puns about swallowed batteries (i.e., "cheap charge," "light at end of tunnel"), but we will leave those for another volume (a gut joke book?).

frequently the foreign bodies lodge at the level of the ileocecal valve when ingested from above. However, various items such as dentures, needles, safety pins, and water-filled balloons or condoms have all been successfully removed from the colon with a flexible scope. The endoscopic snare is the most useful instrument, and it is important that the appropriate length is available since the colonoscopes are longer than the upper endoscopes. Foreign bodies inserted through the anal canal may be difficult to extract without the use of local anesthesia to relax the anal sphincter. If foreign bodies are not passed after 24 to 48 hours of observation and cannot be grasped with a snare, general anesthesia should be administered to relax the abdominal wall and anal sphincter. If it is impossible to manipulate the foreign body manually into the rectum, surgery should be performed.

ENDOSCOPIC TECHNIQUES

Successful removal of foreign bodies in the GI tract is directly dependent on a cooperative patient who understands the procedure and receives adequate medication. Intravenous fentanyl and midazolam are the medications of choice to be administered before the procedure. Glucagon, as mentioned, may be useful during the procedure to relax smooth muscle. General anesthesia is an option for children or uncooperative

patients. Appropriate postprocedure radiographs should be obtained, and an observation period is required to watch for symptoms of perforation, fever, tachycardia, dyspnea, chest or abdominal pain, or even subcutaneous crepitance. Other potential complications of flexible endoscopic foreign body extraction include hemorrhage, impaction of the foreign body, and pulmonary aspiration. In European and American studies, morbidity rates are well below 1 percent with both rigid and flexible endoscopes. Individual training and experience are also important in maintaining a low level of morbidity.

SUGGESTED READING

Cockerill FR III, Wilson WR, Scoy RE. Travelling toothpicks. Mayo Clin Proc 1983; 58:613–616.
Herranz-Gonzalez J, Martinez-Vidal J, Garcia-Sarandeses A, Vazquez-Barro C. Esophageal foreign bodies in adults. Otolaryngol Head Neck Surg 1991; 105:649–654.
Pollack CV Jr, Biggers DW, Carlton FB Jr, et al. Two crack cocaine body stuffers. Ann Emerg Med 1992; 21:1370–1380.
Rogers BH, Kot C, Meiri S, et al. An overtube for the flexible fiberoptic esophagogastroduodenoscope. Gastrointest Endosc 1982; 28: 256–257.
Spitz L. Management of ingested foreign bodies in childhood. Br Med J 1971; 4:469–472.
Webb W. Management of foreign bodies of the upper gastrointestinal tract. Gastroenterology 1988; 94:204–216.

ESOPHAGEAL MOTOR DISORDERS AND CHEST PAIN

DAVID A. KATZKA, M.D.
DONALD O. CASTELL, M.D.

Because of the fear of myocardial infarction and sudden death, chest pain is usually taken as a very serious symptom in an adult. Once patients with a new presentation of chest pain have been thoroughly evaluated to rule out a life-threatening cause, however, they become categorized as having "chest pain of undetermined origin." Although this term is nonspecific, it has become synonymous with, or certainly defined to a large degree by, possible esophageal causes of chest pain. This has resulted from observations that once coronary artery disease has been eliminated, the esophagus is the next most likely cause of the pain. In this chapter, we review the diagnosis and treatment of one diagnosis group that is included in esophagus-derived chest pain, specifically, primary esophageal motility disorders. Gastroesophageal reflux disease, the other main cause of esophageal

chest pain of undetermined origin, is discussed in three other chapters.

DEFINITIONS

"Esophageal motility disorders" is a loose term usually interpreted to include the following manometric patterns: (1) diffuse esophageal spasm, (2) nutcracker esophagus, (3) hypertensive lower esophageal sphincter (LES), (4) nonspecific motor disorder, and (5) achalasia. Although the differentiation between these disorders may sometimes be made clinically, they are best defined manometrically (Table 1). *Diffuse esophageal spasm* (DES) is most suggested by an increased frequency of simultaneous contractions during wet swallows (>10 percent) or the presence of frequent triple-peaked contractions. Less specific but consistent manometric changes include markedly prolonged contractions, high-amplitude nonperistaltic contractions, and incomplete LES relaxation. Because in many patients with motility disorders there may not be chest pain or manometric findings during stationary manometry, a provocative agent may be used, edrophonium (Tensilon), 1 mg administered intravenously during manometry to precipitate spasm. If typical chest pain occurs during the

Table 1 Manometric Criteria for Esophageal Motor Disorders

Diffuse esophageal spasm
Diagnostic:
  Increased, prolonged, simultaneous contractions. May be of long
    duration, repetitive, spontaneous or high-amplitude contractions
Suggestive:
  Multiple peaked contractions
  Multiple repetitive or simultaneous contractions
  Retrograde contractions
  Elevated LES pressure and/or incomplete relaxation

Nutcracker esophagus
Diagnostic:
  High-amplitude (>180 mm Hg), sometimes prolonged but
    peristaltic contractions

Hypertensive LES
Diagnostic:
  LES pressure >45 mm Hg; normal peristalsis

Nonspecific motor disorder
Suggestive:
  Increased number of nonperistaltic contractions
  Prolonged, low-amplitude, or spontaneous contractions
  Hypertensive and/or incompletely relaxing LES but with intact
    peristalsis

LES = lower esophageal sphincter.

pharmacologically increased contractions, the test is diagnostic of an esophageal cause of the pain. Unfortunately, the literature quotes only a maximal 40 percent positive response rate to Tensilon. An occasional patient has spontaneous chest pain during the manometry with manometric change also confirming the diagnosis, but this is unusual.

Nutcracker esophagus is defined more specifically by high-amplitude, sometimes prolonged, but peristaltic contractions. A *hypertensive LES* is defined by elevated resting LES pressure with normal esophageal body. Their roles as causes of chest pain have been debated but they are a factor in some cases.

A *nonspecific motor disorder* is defined by some of the same criteria as DES, but without enough manometric change to be highly suggestive or diagnostic of DES. For example, a finding of isolated prolonged or nontransmitted contractions, retrograde contractions, and incomplete LES relaxation but intact peristalsis is consistent with this diagnosis. Like nutcracker esophagus, it is sometimes difficult to reliably attribute chest pain to these findings, but no doubt it does play a role in some patients with chest pain of undetermined origin.

Achalasia is strictly defined by elevated LES pressure with incomplete relaxation and complete esophageal aperistalsis. It is rarely a diagnostic consideration in patients with unexplained chest pain.

CLIINICAL MANIFESTATIONS

As defined by this chapter, all patients with these disorders may present with chest pain. The quality of the chest pain may be indistinguishable from classic angina, described as a crushing, substernal chest pain. It may occur during rest as well as during exercise. Although usually substernal, esophageal motility disorders may also radiate to the jaw, to the back, and even down the left arm. Esophageal pain may be relieved by sublingual nitroglycerin. To complicate matters further, recent studies suggest that microvascular angina and esophageal motility disorders may be related, so that both may occur simultaneously. The bottom line is that one cannot rely on any particular characteristic of the chest pain in differentiating esophageal from cardiac pain. Some descriptions that may be helpful include chest pain occurring at rest and lasting for hours, or pain brought on by eating. In our experience, one characteristic that is helpful in differentiating an esophageal from a cardiac cause of chest pain is the lack of some of the other symptoms often associated with myocardial ischemia. For example, frank diaphoresis, syncope, urge to defecate, and shortness of breath are uncommonly associated with an esophageal motility disorder. One exception to this rule, however, is the panic attack, which is important to recognize for two reasons: (1) it may manifest with chest pain, shortness of breath, and syncope (from hyperventilation); and (2) some authors suggest that patients with esophageal motility disorders have a remarkably high incidence of psychiatric disorders (up to 80 percent in some series). Important clues to panic attacks may be age under 40 years, a history of psychiatric illness, and a family history of panic disorders.

One way of finding further support for an esophageal cause of the chest pain is to elicit other esophageal symptoms, particularly dysphagia or regurgitation. All causes of chest pain secondary to dysmotility may include dysphagia or regurgitation among the symptoms. This may be attributable to the presence of nonperistaltic contractions and/or incomplete LES relaxation. Although some of these disorders are more likely to present with chest pain (e.g., DES) and others with dysphagia (e.g., achalasia), there is a large overlap. Toward this end, some authors have even described patients who over a period of years changed both symptomatically and manometrically from a pattern of DES to one of achalasia. When dysphagia is described by these patients, it is more typically for both solids and liquids as opposed to primarily solid food dysphagia as reported by patients with mechanical obstruction (e.g., esophageal carcinoma or stricture). Nonetheless, in our experience, patients with motility disorders may still have more difficulty with solids than with liquids. Others describe a sensitivity to cold or hot ingestants, but this has not been shown manometrically to slow esophageal transit.*

---

*Editor's Note: Drinking ice water for several minutes can decrease progressive peristalsis, even simulating aperistalsis.

DIAGNOSIS

At present, diagnosis of these esophageal motor disorders is best established by esophageal manometry with the criteria already described. Barium esophagography may be helpful. A good-quality cine esophagram with a barium-coated marshmallow shows good correlation with manometric findings, but an experienced radiologist must perform the examination. Endoscopy assists in ruling out other esophageal diseases, but is not helpful in diagnosing motility disorders other than possibly achalasia. One method currently being investigated is prolonged ambulatory esophageal pressure monitoring. In some patients with normal stationary manometric examination results, prolonged monitoring may document increased esophageal pressure events concordant with pain, but at this time its yield is considered low and it is by no means a substitute for stationary manometry. One important principle to keep in mind with all these tests however, is that there is still no "gold standard" for esophageal motility disorders, as many of the abnormalities found may not be symptomatically or pathophysiologically related to the chest pain. Prolonged esophageal pH monitoring is also necessary in these patients. Although the primary reason for this is the high frequency of gastroesophageal reflux as a cause of chest pain of undetermined origin, a secondary reason is the overlap between reflux and motor disorders, particularly as found on combined prolonged esophageal pH and pressure monitoring. Some authors have also shown that a positive Tensilon test is more common in patients with reflux and may reflect an overall esophageal hypersensitivity phenomenon.

An algorithm for the diagnosis of esophageal motility disorders is shown in Figure 1.

TREATMENT

Treatment of esophageal motility disorders other than achalasia focuses on two strategies: *reduction of esophageal smooth muscle tone* through either pharma-

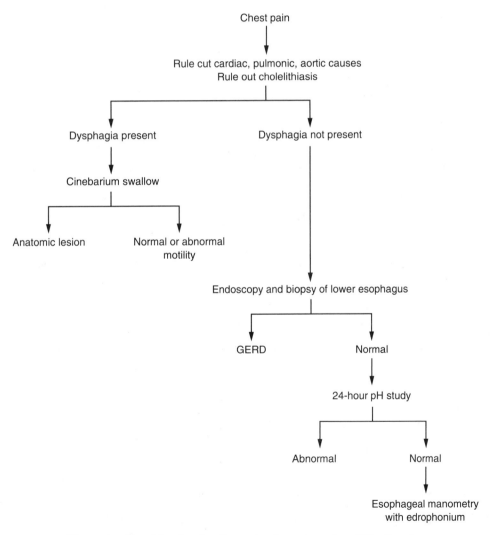

Figure 1 Algorithm for the diagnosis of esophageal motility disorders.

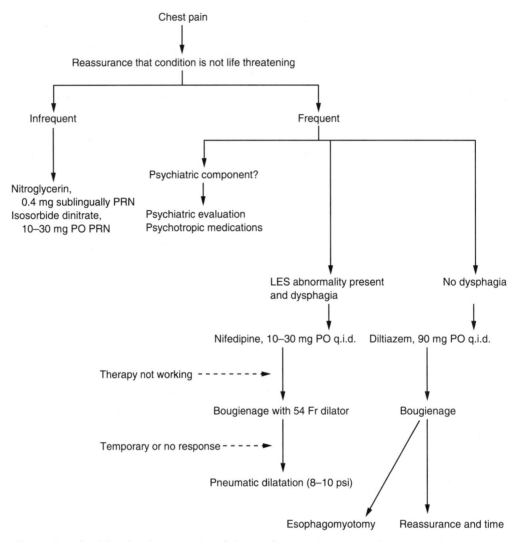

Figure 2 Algorithm for the treatment of chest pain secondary to esophageal motility disorder.

cologic or mechanical means and *treatment of contributing psychiatric components*. It is important to keep in mind that patients with chest pain secondary to esophageal motility disorders can be very difficult to treat and are often refractory to medical therapy.*

An algorithm for the treatment of chest pain secondary to esophageal motility disorders is shown in Figure 2.

Reduction of Esophageal Tone by Drugs

Nitrates

Nitrates relax esophageal smooth muscle probably through a cyclic guanosine monophosphate (GMP) mechanism. In patients with DES, nitrates have been shown to lower both esophageal contraction amplitude

and LES pressure. They may be administered in the form of isosorbide dinitrate (Isordil), 10 to 30 mg four times daily orally or sublingually), or nitroglycerin, 0.4 mg sublingually as needed. The major limitations of nitrates are their side effects, particularly headache and light-headedness, and overall lack of clinical efficacy. We tend to use them on an as-needed basis in patients who have occasional single episodes of esophageal spasm of short duration.

Anticholinergics

Anticholinergics relax esophageal smooth muscle by inhibiting direct stimulatory cholinergic effects on the smooth muscle membrane as well as through cholinergic neural pathways. In vivo, they decrease esophageal contraction amplitude and LES pressure. In patients with chest pain from esophageal motor disorders, hyoscyamine sulfate (Levsin, 0.125 to 0.25 mg orally four times a day or Levsin SL, 0.375 mg orally daily), dicyclomine (Bentyl, 10 to 40 mg orally four times a day),

*Editor's Note: "Very difficult to treat" and "refractory to medical therapy" are the name of the game for most of us in tertiary care centers, regardless of subspecialty.

or propantheline bromide (Probanthine, 15 to 30 mg orally four times a day) may be tried. Limitations of anticholinergics are the high frequency of side effects (dry mouth, dizziness, blurred vision, nausea, lightheadedness, drowsiness, weakness, and nervousness) and their limited efficacy. A good randomized clinical trial establishing their effectiveness in chest pain of esophageal origin has *not* been published. They are *not* a first-line drug in our opinion.

Calcium Channel Antagonists

Calcium channel antagonists are the first-line treatment for patients with frequent chest pain requiring other than occasional as-needed therapy. They inhibit smooth muscle contraction by blocking entry of calcium ions through voltage-dependent calcium channels in the smooth muscle membrane. In the esophagus in vivo, they have been shown to decrease both esophageal contraction amplitude and LES pressure. In humans, the effects of this class of compounds is variable, but diltiazem (Cardizem) has been shown to inhibit contraction amplitude and symptoms in patients with nutcracker esophagus. Nifedipine (Procardia) has also been shown to decrease contraction amplitude and LES pressure in normal volunteers. Verapamil (Calan) has been shown to decrease LES pressure and contraction amplitude in animals but not in humans. Therapeutically, we start using diltiazem at a dose of 90 mg four times a day, since this is the only drug that has been proved experimentally to help patients with esophageal motor-derived chest pain. A moderately high starting dose is recommended, since lower doses have proved ineffective. Diltiazem may also have the benefit of *not* lowering LES pressure as much as the other calcium channel antagonists, thereby theoretically avoiding gastroesophageal reflux. Nifedipine, (10 to 30 mg orally three times a day) on the other hand, is preferred for achalasia because it has been shown to lower LES pressure, and clinical trials have demonstrated efficacy in this patient group. It may also be helpful in patients with DES or other motility abnormalities with hypertensive and/or incompletely relaxing LES pressure accompanied by dysphagia. It can also be used if diltiazem is ineffective. Verapamil is the third-line drug in this group, since it has not so far been demonstrated to be clinically effective for chest pain from esophageal motor disorders. A starting dose of 40 mg orally four times a day is recommended. Limitations of calcium channel antagonists in the treatment of esophageal motor disorders are also side effects (constipation, dizziness, hypotension, and exacerbation of congestive heart failure) and a substantial failure rate in controlling symptoms.

Reduction of Esophageal Tone by Mechanical Methods

Bougienage

Esophageal dilation with a bougie dilator has been reported anecdotally to be useful in some patients with a motility disorder poorly responsive to medical therapy. It may help patients who have dysphagia in addition to the chest pain. Studies have been limited, with only one uncontrolled study showing benefit. Although a large (54 Fr) bougie dilator is generally used, one study showed no difference in clinical response rate between 24 and 54 Fr dilators, suggesting that it may be largely a placebo effect. In any case, it is worth trying in patients refractory to medical therapy, but with the caveats that the therapy is not well tested and the relief experienced is often temporary.

Pneumatic Dilatation. A physician considering this approach in a patient with a nonachalasic esophageal motility disorder must remember that the reported rate of esophageal perforation with pneumatic dilatation is 3 to 5 percent in most series and that specific relief of chest pain occurs in less than 50 percent. Given these warnings, pneumatic dilatation may be useful in the subset of patients who have dysphagia accompanying chest pain and an elevated LES pressure. The balloon should be inflated to a pressure no greater than 10 psi for a 45 to 60 second duration. In our opinion, only patients who have had a temporary but symptomatic response to previous bougienage should be included. The technique is most useful in patients with a nonspecific or spastic motility disorder that may progress to achalasia.

Esophagomyotomy. An esophageal myotomy is performed by making a longitudinal incision through the serosa up to (but not through) the mucosa, starting at the LES and extending up to the level of approximately the midesophagus. The result of the myotomy is a reduction in esophageal contractile amplitude and LES pressure, with esophageal clearance sacrificed. As a result, myotomy is sometimes combined with a fundoplication to prevent reflux. The surgery is performed through a left thoracotomy. Needless to say, this procedure is used rarely and only for patients with debilatating refractory chest pain thought secondary to the motility disorder. Published results with myotomy for chest pain are fair, with improvement of symptoms in up to 70 percent but complete relief of symptoms in only 50 percent. One small series of 14 patients showed improvement in symptoms in 90 percent, but five of 14 still had persistent severe symptoms. The decision to perform an esophageal myotomy in a patient should be weighed against the fact that one study of long-term (> 10 years) outcome of patients with chest pain from esophageal motility disorders demonstrated that spontaneous resolutions of chest pain may occur in time. One potentially exciting new option with esophagomyotomy, however, may be the ability to perform this procedure laparoscopically. No studies have been published on this subject to date.

Treatment of Psychiatric Components

As discussed above, psychiatric disorders are often found in patients with esophageal motility disorders (anxiety and affective disorders being most common). Furthermore, patients frequently report stress as a precipitant of the chest pain. Consequently, attention to the psychological needs of the patient is of great importance. Some patients may need psychiatric evaluation, but most may be treated by the primary care physician.

Reassurance

A close relationship between physician and patient is mandatory for chest pain of esophageal origin. Some studies have suggested that this relationship is more important than any pharmacologic manipulation. Reassurance alone that the problem is not cardiac or life threatening has been shown to result in a decrease in pain frequency and hospital visits.

Psychotropic Medications

Trazadone (Desyrel) is a nontricyclic, non–monoamine oxidase inhibitor antidepressant. Clinical trials have shown that in doses of 100 to 150 mg per day, patients with DES report global improvement in symptoms without manometric changes. Alprazolam (Xanax) is a benzodiazepine analog. At a mean oral dose of 3.66 mg, it has been shown to decrease panic scores and chest pain in a small group of patients; manometry was not performed. Limitations of psychotropic medications are the side effects as well as dependency. In our opinion, psychotropic medications should not be dispensed without a formal psychiatric evaluation. This is true also for evaluation of other potentially beneficial treatment options such as psychotherapy, biofeedback, behavioral modication modification, and use of relaxation exercises.

SUGGESTED READING

Breumelhof R, Nadorp JHS, Akkermans LMA, Smout AJPM. Analysis of 24-hour esophageal pressure and pH data in unselected patients with noncardiac chest pain. Gastroenterology 1990; 99: 1257–1264.

Castell DO, ed. Chest pain of undetermined origin. Proceedings of a Symposium. Am J Med 92 (Suppl 5A).

London RL, Ouyang A, Snape WJ, et al. Provocation of esophageal pain by ergonovine or edrophonium. Gastroenterology 1981; 81: 10–14.

Katz PO. Disorders of increased esophageal contractility. In Castell DO, ed. The esophagus. Boston: Little, Brown, 1992.

Vantrappen G, Janssens HOJ, Hellemans J, Coremans G. Achalasia, diffuse esophageal spasm, and related motility disorders. Gastroenterology 1979; 76:450–457.

ACHALASIA

COL. ROY K. H. WONG, M.D., M.C.

ETIOLOGY AND PATHOGENESIS

Achalasia is a neuromuscular disorder of the esophagus characterized by symptoms of dysphagia to solids and liquids. An incidence of 1:100,000 has been reported and most patients present between the ages of 30 and 50 years. The cause of achalasia is unknown, but there is evidence of viral, autoimmune, degenerative neurologic diseases and familial origins in a few patients. In over 99 percent of cases, the etiology is idiopathic; less than 1 percent of case reports describe familial achalasia and degenerative neurologic disorders. Familial achalasia has been reported in parent-child relationships, in siblings, and in monozygotic and fraternal twins of both sexes. Multiple congenital disorders associated with achalasia have been noted in certain family pedigrees, especially where consanguineous marriages are involved. Parkinson's disease and neurofibromatosis have also been reported in achalasia, with evidence of primary anatomic lesions in the brain to account for the pathology.

CLINICAL PRESENTATION

Initially, patients present with symptoms of dysphagia with solids and liquids, weight loss, and nonspecific symptoms of chest pain or heartburn. The symptoms of heartburn and chest pain are not necessarily related to meals, prompting the astute clinician to question a neuromuscular disorder of the esophagus. Historically, dysphagia with solids only, or a combination of solids and liquids, may be the primary presenting symptom, although heartburn, chest pain, and regurgitation are noted in 30 to 60 percent of patients. Other common presenting symptoms include morning regurgitation of white froth from pooled saliva in the esophagus, frequent esophageal belches of swallowed air, and sudden awakening because of choking or coughing episodes associated with esophageal contents being regurgitated into the pharynx. Some patients see undigested food on the pillow. Most patients progress to a characteristic clinical and radiographic picture of achalasia and present to the gastroenterologist within 6 months to 1 year of the onset of symptoms.

DIAGNOSIS

The diagnosis of achalasia is usually made radiographically by noting a dilated, aperistaltic esophagus with a narrow, smoothly tapered "bird-beak" distal esophagus. Early in the disease process, the esophagus may be only slightly dilated with minimal delay in esophageal emptying and some tertiary contractions. Barium should be administered in the supine position to test for peristalsis or gastroesophageal reflux to differentiate among achalasia, esophageal spasm, and scleroderma. Administration of amyl nitrate helps differentiate achalasia from adenocarcinoma, as no improvement in esophageal emptying is usually noted with adenocarcinoma. Upper gastrointestinal endoscopy is usually normal except for a dilated, atonic, fluid-filled esophagus with hyperkeratosis in severe cases. Specific endoscopic features of carcinoma or hiatal hernia should be noted, because esophageal perforation during pneumatic dilation is more likely to occur in patients with hiatal hernias. A retroflexed view of the cardia is essential.

In most instances, esophageal manometry reveals (1) elevated lower esophageal sphincter (LES) pressure; (2) incomplete, short-duration LES relaxation upon deglutition; and (3) absent esophageal peristalsis. In less than 30 percent of cases, findings of normal LES pressure with short but complete LES relaxation are noted, although aperistalsis remains a constant manometric finding. Older patients with a short history and weight loss or with significant tobacco and alcohol consumption, and patients with family histories of early gastrointestinal cancer, should be screened carefully for carcinoma. Submucosal infiltrating lesions are probably best diagnosed by endoscopic ultrasonography rather than computed tomographic (CT) scanning.

MEDICAL THERAPY

Pneumatic Dilation

Principles

Any form of therapy that significantly decreases LES pressure will improve esophageal emptying in patients with achalasia. In my experience, exceptions include patients with very large megaesophagus and, possibly, those with severe distal esophageal spasm.

Many unanswered questions remain regarding the most efficacious technique of pneumatic dilation. The major concern is esophageal perforation, but there are no predilation data or patient characteristics to predict which patients are more likely to suffer perforation during pneumatic dilation, except those with obvious hiatal hernia. However, recent studies from our institution at Walter Reed Army Medical Center (WRAMC) and Brooke Army Medical Center provide solid information concerning how to perform a pneumatic dilation safely and effectively. These data indicate that the *size* of the dilator is the most important factor affecting esophageal perforation and not the *rate* of inflation or pressure employed during dilation. Because dilator size is the most important safety factor, the initial dilation should be performed with the

smallest available balloon diameter. Use only one dilator size per session and do not bypass intermediate sizes for a larger size. If the patient remains symptomatic, repeat dilations can be performed after 1 month using the next available size offered by the manufacturer.

Pneumatic dilators manufactured before the advent of polyvinyl balloons are not well standardized and may have balloons of varying sizes even when purchased from the same manufacturer. Diameters may range from 3.0 to 5.0 cm (90 to 150 F), making it imperative that the physician know the dilator size before dilation. When only a single large dilator is available to perform all dilation, inflation pressure (psi) becomes an important variable, because a fully expanded balloon may result in perforation. Unfortunately, it is impossible to know exactly how much pressure should be employed to inflate a specific balloon, as sphincter characteristics vary between patients. With large dilators (3.5 to 5.0 cm), extreme caution should be taken not to fully inflate the bag during the first dilation session. In these circumstances, the technique of pneumatic dilation becomes an art mixed with good or bad fortune because the physician must monitor the inflation pressure, the fluoroscopic waist deformity, and the patient's discomfort.

Comparison of Rigiflex and Hurst-Tucker Dilators

My experience in pneumatic dilation is with the Hurst-Tucker dilator (outside diameter 2.7, 3.3, 3.7, 4.1 cm), which is no longer available, and with sizes that were specially manufactured for my use, and also recently with the Rigiflex achalasia dilator (outside diameter 3.0, 3.5, 4.0 cm), which is currently available and used by most gastroenterologists today. Both dilators have similar overall efficacy, although the Hurst-Tucker dilator is a softer, more compliant bag than the Rigiflex polyvinyl balloon, which is very stiff and hard when inflated to similar pressures. The Hurst-Tucker is similar to older dilators such as the Brown-McHardy and Mosher bags and is intubated directly into the mouth, while the Rigiflex balloon requires initial endoscopy for guidewire placement into the stomach. A radiopaque outer sheath surrounds the Hurst-Tucker dilator, which allows easy identification of the LES waist defect on the bag. The inability to easily identify the LES waist defect on the Rigiflex balloon is the most difficult aspect of using this dilator.

Dilation Technique

The patient is kept NPO for 12-16 hrs before dilation, but if previous endoscopic or manometric experience indicates a large esophageal residual, clear liquids are recommended for 1 to 2 days before dilation. The entire procedure is performed under fluoroscopic guidance with the table at 10 degrees and the patient on his or her back. Oral suction is kept available at the head of the fluoroscopy table.

Balloon Characteristics of Rigiflex Achalasia Dilator

The balloon on the Rigiflex dilator is 13.5 cm long with radiopaque markers on the inner shaft where the balloon is situated. These markers help the operator guide the balloon into position, because the polyvinyl balloon itself is not fluoroscopically visible. Careful inspection indicates that the inner markers are not always positioned exactly in the center of the balloon. Hence, the physician should measure and locate the balloon center, noting the closest radiopaque marker.

Generally, 120 ml of air is required to fully inflate the balloon, but the total amount varies with the size and pressure employed. A similar volume should be aspirated before safely withdrawing the balloon from the esophagus.

Rigiflex Dilation Technique

The patient is sedated with meperidine, 50 to 75 mg, plus either diazepam (Valium), 5 to 10 mg, or midazolam, 2 to 4 mg, intravenously, and the endoscope is intubated. With minimal air insufflation, all esophageal contents are aspirated. As the distal tip of the endoscope reaches the squamocolumnar junction, the fluoroscopic position of the distal tip should be noted with the patient flat on his or her back. This position represents the proximal boundary of the LES and is an important landmark in centering the balloon during dilation. In most instances, this location is a few centimeters proximal to the convergence of the hemidiaphragms. This fluoroscopic image can be distorted by gastric distention that may raise the left hemidiaphragm, while gas in the esophagus, stomach, and small bowel can obscure the convergence of the hemidiaphragm and make it difficult to determine the position of the balloon. After the stomach is entered, air and gastric contents should be completely aspirated and the guidewire passed into the distal stomach. Following removal of the endoscope, the Rigiflex dilator is intubated over the guidewire under fluoroscopic guidance so that the center of the balloon is 1 to 2 cm proximal to the convergence of the hemidiaphragms. This position should correspond to the fluoroscopic location of the distal tip of the endoscope. Once positioned, the balloon is gradually insufflated with air, carefully noting the fluoroscopic image of the balloon and the LES waist deformity (Fig. 1). If the LES waist deformity is not in the center of the balloon, it should be deflated and repositioned appropriately. Because air is not dense, it is difficult to fluoroscopically visualize the air-filled balloon as it expands, and approximately 75 percent of the balloon needs to be inflated before the balloon and the waist deformity is noted. In most cases, the balloon must be deflated and repositioned two to five times before the LES is correctly centered on the balloon. Although this procedure requires time, it is critical, because the LES high-pressure zone spans at least 4 cm and interdigitates further into the distal esophagus and proximal stomach. If not all of the LES muscle fibers are dilated,

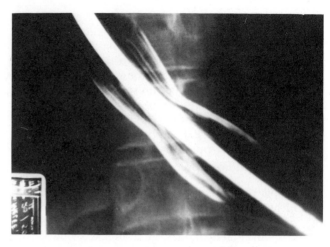

Figure 1 Fluoroscopic image of an inflated Hurst-Tucker dilator with lower esophageal sphincter (LES) waist deformity centered on the radiopaque bag. A similar image is noted with the radiolucent air-filled Rigiflex balloon.

the dilation may be inadequate, and further dilations with larger balloon sizes may result in esophageal perforation. Once centered, the balloon should be fully inflated and the LES waist deformity obliterated. Different inflation pressures are required because of variations in LES pressures, but approximately 8 to 10 psi is required to fully inflate the Rigiflex balloon.

Hurst-Tucker Dilator Technique

Two to three minutes after administration of 75 mg meperidine, a 50 Fr Maloney dilator is passed under fluoroscopic guidance to (1) familiarize the patient with the actual dilation procedure, (2) determine the amount of esophageal residual contents and the need for esophageal lavage, and (3) ensure an unobstructed passage through the distal esophagus. If all of these concerns are met, the Hurst-Tucker dilator is passed and positioned so that the center of the bag is at the convergence of the hemidiaphragms and the bag is gently inflated. The radiopaque lining of the bag allows for easy identification of the waist deformity at lower insufflation volumes of air, since no esophageal or gastric air shadows are present as a result of endoscopy. Once centered, the bag is fully inflated with 10 to 15 psi (X = 12 psi) to obliterate the LES waist deformity.

Similarities of Dilation Technique with Both Dilators

At this point, the dilation techniques are similar for both types of dilators (Table 1). The balloon is fully inflated and deflated after 60 seconds but kept in the same position. To note the reinflation pressure required to obliterate the waist deformity, the balloon is quickly reinflated and deflated. A decrement of 3 to 4 psi is usually noted between the first and second dilations. The dilator is removed and checked for blood.

Table 1 Dilation Technique

Utilize sequential dilation technique beginning with smallest dilator
Use one-size dilator per dilation session
Position LES waist deformity in center of balloon
Fully inflate dilator to obliterate LES waist deformity
Maintain balloon pressure for 60 sec, then deflate
Reinflate balloon noting pressure, then deflate

LES = lower esophageal sphincter.

Table 2 Postdilation Radiographic Technique

Table elevated 45 degrees
30 ml Gastrografin administered orally with anterior and lateral films
If no perforation noted with Gastrografin, 90 ml barium administered orally with anterior and lateral films

Postdilation Radiographic Studies

Thirty ml of Gastrografin is then administered with the x-ray table rotated 45 degrees. Fluoroscopy is performed in the anterior and lateral positions for evidence of perforations, with x-ray films obtained in both views. If no free perforation is noted, 90 ml of barium is administered using the same technique noted above. Barium is heavier and exerts more pressure against the mucosa, revealing small mucosal or muscular perforations not visualized with Gastrografin. Perforations reported in the literature that are not detected by postdilation radiographic studies may result from insufficient administration of contrast material. Using this technique at WRAMC (Table 2), we have not missed a clinically important esophageal perforation in over 100 pneumatic dilations. Before we instituted the technique of graduated pneumatic dilations, perforations noted by using this radiographic technique included a free perforation, gastric and esophageal diverticula formation, and mucosal tears.

Esophageal Perforations

In over 90 percent of patients, dilation-induced chest pain resolves within 5 to 10 minutes of the procedure. Mild residual pain may persist and occasionally require nitroglycerin or nifedipine to relieve it. If no perforation is noted on postdilation radiographic studies, any residual chest pain will resolve within 12 hours. Patients with free esophageal perforation missed on postdilation radiography will continue to have severe chest pain, which will intensify within the first few hours after dilation (Table 3). Pain, diaphoresis, tachycardia, fever, and shock are hallmarks of free esophageal perforation and warrant an emergent Gastrografin swallow, with immediate surgical intervention within 12 hours of the dilation. Small mucosal tears require no follow-up studies and patients are usually asymptomatic. Patients who develop diverticula resulting from deep muscular wall tears, but intact mucosa, should probably be kept NPO, on intravenous (IV) antibiotics, and monitored for 1 day. If the patient remains asymptomatic with normal vital signs, oral antibiotics can be continued for 7 to 10 days. Patients with esophageal mucosal tears that penetrate just beyond the esophageal wall, but are contained, should be kept NPO and on IV antibiotics for several days before radiographic reassessment and institution of oral antibiotic therapy. Isolated case reports of larger perforations in extremely poor surgical candidates treated with potent antibiotics indicate that conservative management is possible. However, the morbidity and mortality rates of early surgical intervention are very low, and surgery should remain the treatment of choice for free esophageal perforations.

Postdilation Prognosis

In my experience, the intensity of pain experienced during dilation, the amount of blood on the dilator, and the degree of esophageal emptying of oral contrast immediately after dilation do not predict a successful outcome. The only consistent predictors for successful dilation include the age of the patient and whether there is a hiatal hernia. Older patients (over 50 years of age) do significantly better than younger patients, who tend to require a greater number of dilations. Between 2 and 5 percent of patients with achalasia have obvious hiatal hernias, and these individuals do exceedingly well with one dilation. However, in my opinion these patients are at greater risk for esophageal perforation and should be sent to surgery if a small balloon is not available. Of two patients with a hiatal hernia who were dilated with a 2.7 cm Hurst-Tucker bag at WRAMC, one developed a small mucosal tear, but both did exceedingly well, with postdilation radionuclide emptying studies resembling normal controls, which is very unusual. Before we instituted the graduated dilation technique, a patient was dilated with a Hurst-Tucker dilator of unknown size (3.5 to 4.0), resulting in perforation with multiple diverticula on the gastric side of the LES.

Efficacy of Pneumatic Dilation

As noted in Table 4, 82 to 93 percent of patients do well after a pneumatic dilation utilizing sequential graduated pneumatic dilations. No perforations were noted in 59 achalasia patients with this technique. At smaller balloon diameters (2.7 to 3.3 cm), both dilators had similar efficacy (Hurst-Tucker 62 percent vs Rigiflex 67 percent). However, at larger diameters, the Rigiflex (3.5, 4.0 cm) seems to be slightly more effective than the Hurst-Tucker (3.7, 4.1 cm), 31 percent and 17 percent, respectively. The overall success rate between dilators did not significantly differ, although more patients in the Hurst-Tucker group required surgery to relieve symptoms (five vs one). This difference is probably related to the less compliant, stiffer polyvinyl Rigiflex balloon as opposed to the rubber Hurst-Tucker bag, which can be fully expanded but may not completely obliterate the LES waist deformity.

Table 3 Treatment of Perforations

Type of Perforation	Treatment
Free esophageal	Emergent surgery
Contained perforation: minimal contrast localized outside esophageal muscular wall	NPO, IV antibiotics for 3 days, BAS in 3 days; if negative, continue oral antibiotics; if positive, IV antibiotics for 7 days
Diverticular formation	NPO, IV antibiotics for 1–2 days; if afebrile and asymptomatic, PO antibiotics for 7 days
Small mucosal tear	None, in most cases; if persistent fever or back pain, consider oral antibiotics

Table 4 Efficacy of Sequential Dilation: Hurst-Tucker versus Rigiflex

Size (cm)	Hurst-Tucker (%) (n = 30)	Rigiflex (%) (n = 29)
2.7	40	–
3.0	–	62
3.3	27	–
3.5	–	17
3.7	10	–
4.0	–	13
4.1	7	–
Total Efficacy	82	93

Other Forms of Medical Therapy

Pharmacologic agents that decrease LESp can improve esophageal emptying and dysphagia. Nifedipine is probably the most potent and widely used agent, although long-acting nitrates have proved equally effective. These agents are best used for short-term relief of symptoms until dilation or surgery can be performed. Intriguing studies utilizing transcutaneous nerve stimulation show improvement in dysphagia with concomitant increases in plasma vasointestinal polypeptide levels.

In a recent case report, a novel approach involving injection of botulinum toxin into the LES of a patient with achalasia produced significant short-term clinical improvement.*

SURGICAL THERAPY

Several large surgical series indicate that, in an experienced surgeon's hands, modified Heller myotomy is an excellent form of primary or alternative therapy, with improvement in dysphagia ranging from 70 to 100 percent. Intuitively, one would think that the surgeon, having the benefit of direct vision and control of the length and depth of myotomy, would have a better chance of relieving dysphagia. Unfortunately, this form of therapy is still an art with a delicate balance between an adequate and an overzealous myotomy resulting in a higher incidence of gastroesophageal reflux (5 to 20 percent) and postoperative stricture formation. To overcome this problem, some surgeons advocate the addition of an antireflux procedure to the standard Heller myotomy. Although several studies report good results, dysphagia is a complication of a tight antireflux wrap, which is accentuated with an aperistaltic esophagus.

Considering the low rates of esophageal perforation (0 to 5 percent) after pneumatic dilation and the excellent results of graduated pneumatic dilation, surgical intervention should be reserved for patients who fail this form of therapy. Since 80 to 90 percent of patients have an excellent result from pneumatic dilation, approximately one in ten will ultimately be surgical candidates.

CANCER SURVEILLANCE

While there is a small but increased risk of squamous cell carcinoma throughout the esophagus in patients with achalasia, routine upper endoscopy with random mucosal biopsies is not advocated. Studies indicate that despite successful medical or surgical therapy, squamous cell carcinoma can still arise in asymptomatic patients. As in most premalignant disorders, the likelihood of malignant degeneration probably increases with the duration of disease.

SUGGESTED READING

Eckardt VF, Aignherr C, Bernhard G. Predictors of outcome in patients with achalasia treated by pneumatic dilation. Gastroenterology 1992; 103:1732–1738.
Ellis FH, Crozier RE, Watkins E. Operations for esophageal achalasia. Results of esophagomyotomy without an antireflux operation. J Thorac Cardiovasc Surg 1984; 88:344.
Kadakia SC, Wong RK. Graded pneumatic dilation using Rigiflex achalasia dilators in patients with primary esophageal achalasia. Am J Gastroenterol 1993; 88:34–38.
Van Goidsenhoven GE, et al. Treatment of achalasia of the cardia with pneumatic dilations. Gastroenterology 1963; 45:326.
Wong RKH, Maydonovitch CL. Achalasia. In Castell DO, ed. The esophagus. Boston: Little, Brown, 233–260.

*__Editor's Note:__ Pashrika, Kalloo, Ravish, and Hendrix described 10 patients at Johns Hopkins treated with botulinum toxin who showed improvement in LES function. The longest follow-up was 1 year. (*Gastroenterology* abstracts, May 1993). It will be interesting to see if botulinum toxin injection becomes a safe procedure with a long enough duration to make it another therapeutic alternative.

NEUROGENIC DYSPHAGIA

DAVID W. BUCHHOLZ, M.D.

RECOGNITION

The most common error in the management of neurogenic dysphagia is failure to recognize the existence or magnitude of the problem until complications, such as aspiration pneumonia or asphyxia, intervene. Recognition of neurogenic dysphagia begins with an understanding of the circumstances in which it may arise.

Causes

Any neurologic disorder capable of impairing oropharyngeal motor and/or sensory function is capable of causing neurogenic dysphagia (Table 1). The oral and pharyngeal stages of swallowing are much more vulnerable to neurologic disease than is the esophageal phase, because the former two are dependent on voluntary cerebral and involuntary brainstem control, respectively, whereas the esophageal phase is primarily governed by an intrinsic neural network. Many neurologic diseases can involve the brain and brainstem (and the cranial nerves and muscles with which they interact) and thereby cause oropharyngeal dysphagia, but the myenteric plexus and smooth muscle of the esophagus are infrequently impaired by neurologic disease.

Among central nervous system (CNS) disorders, the one most commonly associated with neurogenic dysphagia is stroke. Brainstem stroke and bilateral cortical or subcortical strokes are especially likely to do so, but even unilateral cortical stroke can result in neurogenic dysphagia. The diagnosis of stroke is usually apparent by virtue of the abrupt onset of multiple neurologic deficits, but neurogenic dysphagia related to stroke can arise gradually or as an isolated problem. Slowly progressive neurogenic dysphagia due to stroke probably represents gradual confluence of tiny subcortical (periventricular) infarcts resulting from small vessel disease, usually associated with hypertension and aging. Isolated neurogenic dysphagia is occasionally caused by a very discrete brainstem stroke, and the diagnosis may be easily missed because of the absence of other neurologic findings or a magnetic resonance imaging abnormality involving the brainstem, on account of the small size of the lesion.

Other CNS disorders frequently associated with neurogenic dysphagia include traumatic brain injury, Alzheimer's disease (primarily oral phase impairment), Parkinson's disease, other movement disorders, motor neuron disease (amyotrophic lateral sclerosis [ALS]), multiple sclerosis, and neoplasms. Peripheral neurologic disorders such as cranial neuropathies, myasthenia gravis, and a variety of myopathies may produce oropharyngeal muscle weakness and consequent dysphagia.

Table 1 Causes of Neurogenic Dysphagia

Central nervous system
Stroke
  Especially brainstem and bilateral cortical or subcortical strokes
Traumatic brain injury
Alzheimer's disease
  Primarily oral phase impairment
Parkinson's disease
Other movement disorders
  Huntington's disease
  Dyskinesias and dystonias
Motor neuron disease
  Amyotrophic lateral sclerosis (ALS)
  Poliomyelitis
Multiple sclerosis

Peripheral nervous system
Cranial neuropathies
  Base of skull and retropharyngeal neoplasms
  Chronic meningitis
  Guillain-Barré syndrome
Myasthenia gravis
Myopathies
  Polymyositis, dermatomyositis, and sarcoid
  Myotonic and oculopharyngeal dystrophy

Symptoms and Complications

The manifestations of neurogenic dysphagia (Table 2) relate to inadequate performance of the oral and pharyngeal phases of swallowing, which are intended to rapidly propel an entire bolus from the oral cavity to the esophagus without penetration into either the nasopharynx or the larynx. If the muscles of the lips, tongue, palate, pharynx, or larynx are weak or incoordinated, resultant symptoms may be drooling, difficulty initiating swallowing, nasal regurgitation, retained secretions or food in the mouth or pharynx, coughing or choking episodes, laryngospasm, or bronchospasm. The voice may be "wet," hoarse, or weak. More serious complications may ensue, such as aspiration pneumonia, asphyxia, dehydration, and malnutrition, and the physician's task is to avoid these consequences of neurogenic dysphagia by responding effectively to the early warning symptoms.

This task of recognizing neurogenic dysphagia sooner rather than later is made more difficult because neurogenic dysphagia may be relatively "silent" until it causes a complication. One reason for this is the ability of individuals to compensate for neurogenic dysphagia, often unknowingly, by learned behaviors such as chewing more thoroughly, eating more slowly, avoiding difficult-to-swallow items, double swallowing, and flexing the head during swallowing. Accordingly, a history of such compensatory feeding behavior should be sought from at-risk patients with predisposing neurologic disorders. The other reason for "silent dysphagia" is impairment of the laryngeal cough reflex resulting in reduction of the normal cough or choke response to laryngeal penetration. Impairment of the reflex may be due to either laryngeal sensory loss secondary to certain underlying

Table 2 Manifestations of Neurogenic Dysphagia

Symptoms	Complications
Drooling	Aspiration pneumonia
Difficulty initiating swallowing	Asphyxia
Nasal regurgitation	Dehydration
Retained secretions or food in mouth or pharynx	Malnutrition
Cough or choke episodes	
Laryngospasm	
Bronchospasm	
Compensatory feeding behaviors	

neurologic diseases or desensitization of the reflex in the face of chronic laryngeal penetration.

EVALUATION

Candidates for evaluation of suspected neurogenic dysphagia include those with a neurologic disorder (see Table 1) or a history of symptoms or complications of neurogenic dysphagia (see Table 2). Patients with a history of symptoms or complications consistent with neurogenic dysphagia, but without a known underlying neurologic disorder, should undergo formal evaluation by a neurologic consultant.

Physical Examination

Physical examination, in addition to neurologic examination, should attend to evidence of dehydration, malnutrition, and respiratory status. Among neurologic findings, there has conventionally been over-reliance on the gag reflex as an indicator of swallowing function. It is true that neural control of the gag reflex is in proximity to neural control of swallowing, and studies have correlated a decreased gag reflex (as well as dysphonia and decreased level of consciousness) with increased risk of aspiration. Nonetheless, swallowing may be grossly abnormal in the face of a normal or increased gag reflex, and swallowing may be normal despite an abnormal gag reflex.

The patient at risk for neurogenic dysphagia should be observed during feeding, beginning with thick liquids and purées, which tend to be tolerated better than thin liquids and solids. If symptoms of neurogenic dysphagia (see Table 1) are provoked, it is prudent to withhold oral feeding until the patient can be further assessed with videofluoroscopy. Even if cough or choke episodes are absent, the possibility of "silent dysphagia" should be kept in mind, and neurogenic dysphagia should be suspected if any hint of complication arises, such as otherwise unexplained fevers that may indicate airway contamination.

Videofluoroscopy of Swallowing

Further assessment of the patient with neurogenic dysphagia entails consultation with a swallowing thera-

pist (usually a speech-language pathologist or an occupational therapist) and referral for videofluoroscopy of swallowing. A routine barium swallow is inadequate to detect impairment of the rapidly occurring oral and pharyngeal stages of swallowing. Instead, it is necessary to be able to record and then review at slow speed the images obtained as barium traverses the upper aerodigestive tract. However, esophageal imaging should not be neglected, because neurogenic dysphagia may coexist with contributory, treatable abnormalities of esophageal structure and function. Ideally, the study should be performed by a radiologist experienced in videofluoroscopy of swallowing and attended by the swallowing therapist. The initial study may not only be diagnostic of neurogenic dysphagia but also provide an opportunity to modify bolus consistency and head and neck positioning, as directed by the therapist, in an effort to determine potentially useful treatment approaches.

Videofluoroscopic findings characteristic of neurogenic dysphagia include difficulty initiating swallowing, nasal regurgitation, delayed or diminished pharyngeal contraction (leading to retention of barium in the valleculae and pyriform sinuses), laryngeal penetration during swallowing, and aspiration of retained barium after swallowing. The presence or absence of a cough response to laryngeal penetration or aspiration is an important observation. Although there are no data to quantitatively correlate videofluoroscopic findings with complications of neurogenic dysphagia, the consensus is that patients with more than mild laryngeal penetration or aspiration and those with a defective cough reflex are especially at risk, and therefore may be best managed by avoidance of oral feeding.

A common videofluoroscopic finding in patients with neurogenic dysphagia is prominence of the cricopharyngeus muscle at the pharyngoesophageal junction. This is often misinterpreted as cricopharyngeal spasm, and unnecessary procedures such as dilation or cricopharyngeal myotomy may result. The combination of simultaneous pharyngeal manometry with videofluoroscopy has demonstrated that the failure of the pharynesophageal segment to open in most cases of neurogenic dysphagia is due to weakness of the suprahyoid muscles (which pull the segment open) and the muscles of the tongue and pharynx (which push the bolus through the segment), rather than to failure of relaxation or increased tone of the cricopharyngeus muscle. In such cases, myotomy is misguided.

Additional Evaluation

Other studies of value in the management of neurogenic dysphagia include body weights, calorie counts, measurements of fluid intake and output, and blood studies to assess hydration and nutritional status, ideally under the supervision of a nutritionist. Gastroenterologic or otolaryngologic consultation is indicated if clinical or videofluoroscopic findings suggest a concurrent problem such as a structural lesion, gastroesophageal reflux, or esophageal dysmotility that may be independently contributing to the dysphagia and may be directly treatable. The usefulness of a team approach to neurogenic dysphagia should be obvious, preferably involving dedicated individuals from neurology, gastroenterology, otolaryngology, radiology, swallowing therapy, rehabilitation medicine, and nutrition.

MANAGEMENT

Oral Versus Tube Feeding

The first decision to be made in managing neurogenic dysphagia is whether a patient can safely be fed orally. No scientific data exist to guide this judgment, but a number of clinical and videofluoroscopic findings can be taken into account to make a reasonable estimate of a patient's risk of respiratory complications from oral feeding (Table 3). If a patient with neurogenic dysphagia is fed orally, the clinician must be vigilant for warning signs such as cough, bronchospasm, or fever, which may indicate a need to withdraw oral feeding.

There are two reasons for a patient to be fed by tube: (1) if oral feeding is thought to pose an unacceptable risk of respiratory complications (Table 3) or (2) if oral intake capability is insufficient to maintain adequate hydration or nutrition as determined by body weights, calorie counts, fluid intake and output, and blood studies reflective of hydration and nutritional status. If the patient has a reasonable chance of overcoming the need for tube feeding within 1 to 2 months, a temporary nasogastric or nasoduodenal tube should be utilized, if the patient can tolerate it. If the patient is unlikely to recover substantially, a gastrostomy or jejunostomy should be performed, preferably by the percutaneous endoscopic method. There is a separate chapter on this technique.

Swallowing Therapy

When a decision is made to feed a patient with neurogenic dysphagia orally, or when a patient being tube fed has a reasonable prospect of recovering the ability to accept oral feeding, it is advisable to consult a swallowing therapist to help manage feeding and to attempt rehabilitation. The therapist can advise optimal dietary consistencies, based on clinical and videofluoroscopic observations, to promote safety, ease, and efficiency of oral feeding. Certain head and neck postures may facilitate swallowing, such as flexing the neck (to help protect the larynx) or rotating the head toward the side of pharyngeal weakness (to divert the bolus to the other side). Patients can be taught to double swallow in order to clear pharyngeal residue or to inhale before swallowing, and then cough after swallowing to clear laryngeal contamination. Other techniques may be helpful, such as the Mendelsohn maneuver to prolong laryngeal rise and thereby avoid laryngeal penetration. In addition to these compensatory strategies, some therapists utilize exercises of the orofacial, lingual, and laryngeal musculature in an effort to enhance recovery of voluntary functions. Stimulation techniques, such as

Table 3 Findings For or Against Safe Oral Feeding

For	Against
History and physical findings	
Stable or resolving neurologic disease	Unstable or worsening neurologic disease
Normal consciousness	Lethargy or altered consciousness
No difficulty with secretions	Difficulty with secretions
Intact pulmonary reserve	Impaired pulmonary reserve
No cough or choke episodes	Cough/choke episodes
No laryngospasm or bronchospasm	Laryngospasm or bronchospasm
No aspiration pneumonia	Aspiration pneumonia
Videofluoroscopic findings	
No aspiration	Aspiration, especially if substantial
Presence of cough reflex	Absence of cough reflex

an iced mirror applied to the oropharynx to help trigger a delayed or diminished swallowing reflex, are also available.

Although swallowing therapy for neurogenic dysphagia has become routine within recent years, there are no controlled data demonstrating its efficacy. Nonetheless, the same is true for most other forms of neurologic rehabilitation, and common sense and experience suggest that not only physical therapy, occupational therapy, and speech therapy but also swallowing therapy are worthwhile when used thoughtfully. The attending physician should not abdicate responsibility for management of neurogenic dysphagia to the swallowing therapist, and the indications for and goals of therapy should be periodically reassessed by the two caregivers together. In patients with profound neurogenic dysphagia, especially those with progressive disease, the role of swallowing therapy is limited. Other patients may not be candidates for therapy because of cognitive impairment, although it may be beneficial to educate their family members or other caregivers regarding management of feeding.

Medications

Medications have four roles to play in the treatment of neurogenic dysphagia. First, some underlying neurologic disorders including stroke, Parkinson's disease, multiple sclerosis, myasthenia gravis, and polymyositis, are preventable or treatable with medication. Second, difficulty managing oropharyngeal secretions may be aided by reducing the volume of secretions with an anticholinergic agent, although some patients have more rather than less difficulty because of the increased viscosity of their secretions. There are many anticholinergic options, but consideration should be given to a tricyclic antidepressant such as amitriptyline, since it may relieve not only difficulty managing secretions but also depression, which commonly accompanies neurogenic dysphagia. Indeed, depression is usually overlooked and undertreated in this setting, and should be aggressively pursued.

The third role of medication in the treatment of neurogenic dysphagia pertains to coincident gastroesophageal reflux and esophageal dysmotility, which may independently contribute to swallowing disability. Depending on the findings of videofluoroscopy, endoscopy, pH monitoring, and manometry, the patient with neurogenic dysphagia and superimposed esophageal dysfunction may benefit from trials of H_2 blockers, omeprazole, smooth muscle relaxants, or prokinetic agents. Structural lesions that appear obstructive should be dilated or otherwise corrected.

Finally, the fourth aspect of medications with regard to neurogenic dysphagia is the potential for some agents to exacerbate swallowing dysfunction. Sedatives such as benzodiazepines and anticonvulsants can impair cognition, arousal, protective reflex activity, and oropharyngeal muscle performance. Neuroleptic agents and metoclopramide may result in dyskinesias and dystonias that interfere with positioning and muscle function of the upper aerodigestive tract. A multitude of drugs are associated with myopathy, which may result in pharyngeal weakness; these include corticosteroids, colchicine, lipid-lowering agents, and zidovudine. Neuromuscular junction transmission in the oropharynx can be compromised not only by systemic medications such as aminoglycosides but also by local injection of botulinum toxin for the treatment of torticollis and other movement disorders. Topical anesthetics applied to the pharynx for endoscopy may temporarily predispose the patient with neurogenic dysphagia to silent aspiration. Any nonessential medication that falls into one of these categories should be eliminated in the setting of neurogenic dysphagia.

Surgery

Cricopharyngeal myotomy is intended to promote pharyngeal clearance in the face of suspected cricopharyngeal spasm. As mentioned previously, the finding of cricopharyngeal prominence by videofluoroscopy is much more likely to be related to suprahyoid, lingual, and pharyngeal muscle weakness than to increased cricopharyngeal tone; accordingly, myotomy is usually ill-advised. The procedure should be reserved for patients in whom (1) videofluoroscopy demonstrates obstruction of pharyngeal drainage at the pharyngoesophageal segment (not merely retention of barium in the valleculae and pyriform sinuses), and (2) manometry

(ideally performed simultaneously with videofluoroscopy) reveals cricopharyngeal hypertonicity and failure of relaxation. Substantial gastroesophageal reflux is a relative contraindication to myotomy, because postoperative deficiency of the upper esophageal sphincter may predispose to gastropharyngeal reflux and aspiration.

In cases of neurogenic dysphagia, *tracheostomy* may be indicated for issues of upper airway control and ventilatory assistance, but should not be performed for management of neurogenic dysphagia itself. The presence of a tracheostomy tube impairs laryngeal reflexes and laryngeal elevation, thereby interfering with laryngeal protection. A cuffed tracheostomy tube is not absolute protection against airway contamination from seepage around the tube, and a cuffed tube is even more restrictive of laryngeal motion.

Laryngeal closure or diversion is appropriate when patients being fed solely by tube suffer recurrent respiratory complications despite thorough medical efforts to prevent aspiration of oropharyngeal secretions or refluxed tube feedings. Vocal function, if still intact, is generally sacrificed, so the procedure is a last resort in such cases.

Vocal cord medialization, whether by injection (such as with Teflon) or by laryngoplasty, is more useful to enhance speech than to inhibit laryngeal penetration in patients with vocal cord paralysis, largely because airway contamination typically results from defects in addition to impaired vocal cord apposition, including decreased laryngeal elevation, defective downtilting of the epiglottis, and diminished cough reflex. Other surgical procedures for neurogenic dysphagia such as *prosthodontics* and *laryngeal suspension* are largely investigational and cannot yet be routinely recommended.*

SUGGESTED READING

Groher ME, ed. Dysphagia: diagnosis and management. 2nd ed. Boston: Butterworth-Heinemann, 1992.
Jones B, Donner MW. Normal and abnormal swallowing: imaging in diagnosis and therapy. New York: Springer-Verlag, 1991.
Linden P. Videofluoroscopy in the rehabilitation of swallowing dysfunction. Dysphagia 1989; 3:189–191.
Logemann J. Evaluation and treatment of swallowing disorders. San Diego: College-Hill Press, 1983.
Logemann JA. Treatment of aspiration related to dysphagia: an overview. Dysphagia 1986; 1:34–38.

***Editor's Note:** A superb trip through neurogenic dysphagia, led by an experienced and thoughtful neurologist. Any one who did not learn something was sleeping.

SCLEROTHERAPY AND BANDING OF GASTROESOPHAGEAL VARICES

JOHN S. GOFF, M.D.

Varices may form in almost any part of the gastrointestinal tract. They are usually the result of portal hypertension but may sometimes be present for other reasons. The varices that occur at or near the gastroesophageal junction are the most common and frequently lead to severe bleeding that can be life threatening. They usually bleed because they rupture rather than being eroded into by ulceration of the surface epithelium. Bleeding in patients with severe liver disease is complicated by associated coagulopathy and thrombocytopenia. These factors must be kept in mind when managing the bleeding. Bleeding often precipitates or worsens encephalopathy, which further complicates the management of these patients.

THERAPEUTIC ALTERNATIVES

There are many ways to control bleeding varices. Initial management can include intravenous vasopressin or somatostatin and blood products as needed. Tamponade of the varices can be accomplished with a Sengstaken-Blakemore tube or a similar variation of this device. However, to achieve more permanent control of bleeding, one must permanently decrease portal pressure or eliminate the varices from the lower esophagus or stomach so that they will not be able to rupture again. Portal pressure can be reduced with shunt surgery, but the morbidity and mortality rates of shunt surgery, especially in the emergent setting, are extremely high. Alternative shunting procedures are being developed and hold much promise for nonsurgical lowering of portal pressure (see the chapter *Transjugular Intrahepatic Portosystemic Shunting*). Another surgical option that may be considered in certain patients is esophageal transection (Sugiura procedure). Transection is technically easier than shunt surgery and less stressful on the patient, but may not be as effective over the long term in preventing further bleeding as is shunting.

Endoscopic management of bleeding varices through sclerotherapy (EST), tissue glue injections, and more recently endoscopic banding or ligation (EVL) has regained popularity with the increased use and safety of the flexible fiberoptic endoscope.

After the acute bleeding has been controlled with one or more of the above treatments, it is necessary to determine the best approach for long-term management. Propranolol has been shown to decrease the risk of rebleeding if given for prolonged periods at doses sufficient to decrease the patient's pulse by 25 percent.

EST and EVL when performed repeatedly (five or six sessions) will eradicate esophageal varices and thus prevent future bleeding once the varices are fully eradicated. After controlling the patient's acute bleeding, one can opt for elective shunt surgery, which has almost 50 percent less risk of morbidity and mortality. Radiologic embolization procedures or shunting (transjugular intrahepatic portosystemic shunts [TIPS]) are alternative approaches. The embolization methods for access to the superior mesenteric vein, either via the liver or via a minilaparotomy, are effective but have a high recurrent bleeding rate, probably because of recanalization of the varices. TIPS are very effective at lowering portal pressure, but there are no long-term data on their efficacy. There is a separate chapter on this topic.

PREFERRED APPROACH

Medicomechanical

If varices are known or strongly suspected as the bleeding source, and if the patient is not elderly or known to have significant cardiac or vascular disease, vasopressin should be started, 0.1 units per minute, increased by 0.1 to 0.2 unit per minute every 20 minutes until bleeding stops, unacceptable vascular side effects develop, or a dose of 0.8 unit per minute is reached. Somatostatin (octreotide) can be substituted, 25 to 50 µg per minute. Somatostatin has been less well studied than vasopressin, but it seems to reduce portal pressure with fewer cardiovascular side effects and so may be the drug of choice in patients with relative contraindications to the use of vasopressin. If the patient cannot be stabilized, balloon tamponade should be considered to temporarily control the bleeding. However, use of a Sengstaken-Blakemore tube in a patient without first confirming that the source of bleeding is due to varices is likely to lead to failure in well over 50 percent of cases, since up to 50 percent of bleeding patients with known portal hypertension are bleeding from a nonvariceal source. Thus, emergent endoscopy should be performed to try to determine the source of bleeding and control the hemorrhage. If the patient is encephalopathic or otherwise mentally compromised at the time of endoscopy, it is imperative that he or she be first intubated with an endotracheal tube to prevent aspiration.

Endoscopic Sclerotherapy

EST is best done with a short (4 to 6 mm), 25 gauge needle. The sclerosants that are most effective with the fewest side effects are 1 percent sodium tetradecyl sulfate and 5 percent ethanolamine oleate. One or the other is injected into the patient's varices in 1 to 2 ml aliquots just above the gastroesophageal junction. Each varix is injected at least once, but it may be injected twice or more if it is the source of bleeding or is very large. Ideally, injection is made just below the point of bleeding if one is fortunate enough to locate the exact site. Care should be taken to try to place the sclerosant within the varix, as injection into the perivariceal tissue is responsible for many of the complications of EST. A maximal dose of 20 ml is recommended to minimize complications, and injections should not be made above 30 cm from the teeth, to avoid spinal cord injury. Large fundic varices can be sclerosed using nearly the same technique, but larger volumes (up to 5 ml per injection) may be needed to have the same effect as the smaller amounts of sclerosant in the esophagus. Fundic varices are much harder to control endoscopically than esophageal varices.

EST is repeated in about 7 days initially and then every 2 weeks until all the varices are eradicated from at least the distal 5 cm of the esophagus. The same technique is used, except one must try to avoid injecting sclerosant near an ulcer caused by previous EST. On average it takes five sessions to rid a patient's esophagus of varices that can be appreciated by visual inspection. If a patient develops significant esophageal ulcerations (and many of them do), treatment with sucralfate slurries, 1 g dissolved in 30 ml water four times a day, is instituted. Acid-suppressing agents are indicated if there is more diffuse inflammation of the distal esophagus, which suggests a problem with gastroesophageal reflux of acid. If there is rebleeding before a scheduled repeat EST session, emergent EST is carried out in the usual fashion. Once the varices are eradicated, a follow-up examination is scheduled in 1 month and then every 3 months for about a year. Any recurrent varices are injected at the time of follow-up endoscopy. If the patient continues to bleed despite two or more EST sessions, one of the other treatment options, such as portosystemic shunting, must be taken up.

Endoscopic Variceal Ligation

EVL can be used as the primary treatment or can be combined with EST to treat esophageal or fundic varices. If EVL is planned, it is best to backload the overtube onto the endoscope before the endoscopy so that the patient will require only one intubation. The overtube is necessary to facilitate endoscope insertion and removal when reloading the banding device. Alternatively, one can reintubate the patient with the overtube loaded over a 46 Fr Maloney dilator after the diagnostic endoscopy has been performed. The recommended overtube is about 25 cm long and has a built-in mouthpiece. Once the overtube is in place, the endoscope is removed and loaded with the banding device. A small extending cylinder is loaded onto the tip of the endoscope, and the trip wire is passed down the biopsy channel. The internal cylinder with its preloaded band is hooked to the trip wire and placed inside the extending cylinder at the tip of the endoscope. The instrument is inserted via the overtube to the distal esophagus. A varix is identified at the gastroesophageal junction, and the tip of the endoscope is brought into close apposition. Suction is applied to draw the tissue into the dead space created by the banding device on the tip of the

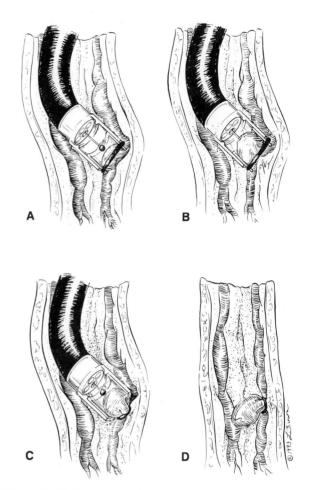

Figure 1 Endoscopic variceal ligation technique. *A,* The endoscope with banding device is advanced to the distal esophagus and brought into close contact with the mucosa containing a varix. *B,* Suction is applied to aspirate the tissue into the chamber at the end of the endoscope. *C,* The trip wire is pulled while maintaining suction in order to strip the band off the inner cylinder and allow it to close around the aspirated tissue. *D,* The end product, a varix, is entrapped in the band, producing a polypoid projection into the esophageal lumen.

endoscope (Fig. 1). The tissue is aspirated into the dead space, creating a red-out appearance. Before the suction is released the trip wire is pulled, which draws the inner cylinder into the outer cylinder and thus strips the band off onto the aspirated tissue. Suction is stopped and a puff of air is used to fully release the tissue from the cylinders at the end of the endoscope. The endoscope is then removed and a fresh internal cylinder with its band is loaded onto the endoscope. The banding process is repeated until all the varices are ligated. If the exact bleeding site can be identified, it should be treated first. The band is placed directly over the bleeding point or just below it, but *never above* the bleeding point, *before* treating at or below the source of bleeding. If the chamber at the end of the endoscope is not fully filled with tissue and thus there is no red-out appearance, there may be inadequate tissue to be secured by the band. A red-out is not mandatory, as there can be enough

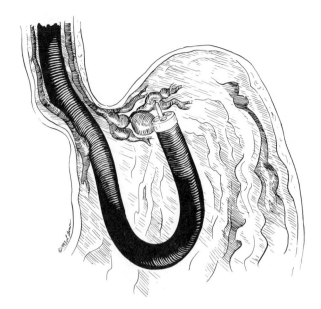

Figure 2 Combination treatment of gastric (fundic) varices. A band has been applied just below the gastroesophageal junction with the endoscope in the retroflex position. Once all the varices are banded, sclerosant is injected, as shown, into the varix a little more distally in the stomach.

tissue aspirated without a full red-out, but caution must be exercised when less tissue is aspirated into the banding cylinders. Misfiring, releasing the band over too small a piece of tissue, can strip off some of the mucosa and create some bleeding, but does not usually induce variceal rupture. Tissue aspiration becomes harder after several bands have been applied at one session or after several sessions when the submucosa has become more fibrotic.

EVL can be performed during active bleeding or electively. As in EST, a band is applied to each varix just above the gastroesophageal junction, and more than one band can be placed on large varices. All varices are banded at least once, but usually two or more bands are applied to large varices at the initial session if EVL is the only treatment being used. The bands are applied in a circumferential manner, starting at the gastroesophageal junction and moving upward from there, because it can become difficult to pass the endoscope past previously applied bands. Like EST, EVL is repeated in 7 days and then every 2 weeks until the varices are eradicated. Long-term follow-up is very similar to that with EST. It takes four or five sessions to eradicate the esophagus of varices with EVL.

Combination Therapy

A combination of EST and EVL can be used to treat esophageal or gastric varices. If one is treating esophageal varices with combination therapy, a band is applied to each visible varix as near to the gastroesophageal junction as possible, and sclerosant is then injected into each varix just above the banded site. The preferred

sclerosants are 1 percent sodium tetradecyl sulfate or 5 percent ethanolamine oleate; only 1 ml of sclerosant is injected per varix. The retreatment protocol is the same as outlined above. Combination therapy is particularly helpful for patients with fundic varices. In the gastric fundus the bands are applied to grossly visible varices just below the gastroesophageal junction, usually with the endoscope in the retroflex position. This is easiest when there is minimal or no blood in the stomach, since visualization of the fundus is severely impaired when there is limited light reflection and a large pool of liquid is present. After a band is applied to each varix around the gastroesophageal junction in the fundus, EST is performed by injecting 1 to 2 ml of sclerosant into the varices just distal to the banding site (Fig. 2). When banding and sclerosing the fundus of the stomach, it is imperative that gastric acid output be totally suppressed after the treatment. Thus, patients should be placed on 20 to 40 mg omeprazole daily, or twice the standard dose of H_2 antagonist. The acid suppression must be maintained until the varices are eradicated.

PROS AND CONS OF TREATMENT

The advantages of endoscopic management of bleeding varices are that it is relatively simple, relatively safe, and effective. EST and EVL have both been shown to control active variceal bleeding better than any other medical means of treatment, and when performed repeatedly they have been shown to effectively reduce the rebleeding rate. They both compare very favorably to shunt surgery, even though the rebleeding rate is higher than with a shunt because of the excess morbidity and mortality rates of the surgery compared with those related to EST or EVL. EVL has far fewer complications than EST. Patients frequently experience fevers, chest pain, pleural effusions, mediastinitis, perforations, bleeding, and stricture formation after EST. Except for some transient dysphagia after the banding session, these complications are virtually eliminated by using EVL. Both EVL and EST take about five sessions to eradicate the varices, but the combination procedure appears to need fewer sessions (average of three) and the combination protocol keeps the complications of sclerotherapy to a minimum by using very small volumes of sclerosant. The combination therapy also enables one to deal more easily with small, but still troublesome, esophageal varices that can be difficult to aspirate into the banding device owing to thickening and scarring of the esophageal mucosa by injecting them with only small amounts of sclerosant.

Initial use of EVL is advantageous in patients who are actively bleeding because of the ability to almost blindly treat the esophagus without fear of causing major complications, as one might with blind (especially blind high-volume) sclerotherapy. Bands can be applied to the gastroesophageal junction without positively identifying where a varix is located. The bands slow flow in all varices if applied circumferentially, and one can then concentrate on applying the second set of bands directly on the now more visible varices, owing to slowing of the bleeding, slightly more proximal in the esophagus. There is no worry about placing a band around esophageal tissue that does not contain a varix, since it will necrose and slough off in the same manner and is not prone to any other specific complications. The distinct disadvantages of EVL when a patient is bleeding are the tunnel vision created by the banding device on the end of the endoscope, and the filling of the chamber at the end of the endoscope with blood, which is rather more difficult to clear than when there is no device on the tip. This can be avoided by trying not to aspirate the blood in the esophagus on the way in to place a band. Once a band is placed, one should attempt to remove some of the blood or clots when removing the endoscope. The endoscope can then be rinsed in water outside the patient before reloading and repassing the endoscope through the overtube. Another advantage of the overtube is that it directs any blood vomited or regurgitated up from the stomach onto the bed rather than into the patient's oropharynx, which may help prevent aspiration.

SUGGESTED READING

Cello JP, Grendell JH, Crass RA, et al. Endoscopic sclerotherapy versus portacaval shunt in patients with severe cirrhosis and acute variceal hemorrhage. Long-term follow-up. N Engl J Med 1987; 316:11–15.

Goff JS, Reveille RM, Stiegmann GV. Three years' experience with endoscopic variceal ligation for treatment of bleeding varices. Endoscopy 1992; 24:401–404.

Health and Public Policy Committee, American College of Physicians. Endoscopic sclerotherapy for esophageal varices. Ann Intern Med 1984; 100:608–610.

Infante-Rivand C, Esnaola S, Villeneuve JP. Role of endoscopic sclerotherapy in the long-term management of variceal bleeding: a meta-analysis. Gastroenterology 1989; 96:1087–1092.

Lieberman DA. Sclerotherapy for bleeding esophageal varices after randomized trials. West J Med 1986; 145:481–484.

Stiegmann GV, Goff JS, Michaletz-Onody PA, et al. Endoscopic sclerotherapy as compared with endoscopic ligation for bleeding esophageal varices. N Engl J Med 1992; 326:1527–1532.

STAGING OF UPPER GASTROINTESTINAL TRACT LESIONS: THERAPEUTIC IMPLICATIONS

MICHAEL B. KIMMEY, M.D.
CHARLES R. THOMAS, Jr., M.D.

Selection of the best treatment for patients with esophageal or gastric cancer is facilitated by an assessment of the local, regional, and distant spread of the malignancy. The TNM staging system (Table 1) has been applied to gastrointestinal (GI) cancer for this purpose.* This staging system is useful because it can be applied to the results of preoperative imaging as well as to surgical and pathologic findings. The prognosis of patients with esophageal and gastric carcinoma has also been linked to the results of preoperative, surgical, and pathologic staging.

The close relationship of tumor stage to prognosis suggests that treatment decisions for individual patients and enrollment in multicenter treatment trials should take advantage of the most accurate assignment of the TNM stage of the tumor whenever possible. We will review the accuracy of currently available imaging methods for staging esophageal and gastric cancer and outline how this information directs the treatment of patients with these diseases.

STAGING METHODS

Upper GI Radiography and Endoscopy

Most patients with esophageal or gastric cancer undergo one or both of these tests for evaluation of symptoms and for the purposes of a tissue diagnosis by endoscopic biopsy. Both tests provide information about the extent of the tumor within the lumen, the presence and degree of obstruction, and the presence of ulceration or bleeding. Unfortunately, the luminal extent of tumor does not correlate with important prognostic factors such as the depth of invasion, regional lymph node involvement, or the presence of distant metastases. Approximately 80 percent of patients with an impassable stricture or infiltrating type of esophageal cancer have a T3 or T4 neoplasm, but lymph node involvement is not predictable by routine endoscopy. The main benefit of contrast radiography and upper endoscopy is to confirm the need for palliative treatment of symptoms of obstruction and bleeding and to provide a tissue diagnosis of the neoplasm.

Computed Tomography

Computed tomography (CT) is the most accurate imaging tool for detecting liver, lung, and adrenal metastases in patients with esophageal and gastric

---

*Editor's Note: The TNM staging system is used in several chapters. Table 1 is similar to that in another chapter, but gastroenterologists are just becoming familiar with the system, and thus the repetition.

Table 1 TNM Staging System

Site	Stage	Criterion
Primary Tumor (T)	TX	Not assessed
	T1	Invades lamina propria or sub-mucosa
	T2	Invades muscularis propria
	T3	Invades adventitia or serosa
	T4	Invades adjacent structures
Lymph nodes (N)	NX	Not assessed
	N0	No lymph node involvement
	N1	Regional lymph nodes involved*
Metastases	MX	Not assessed
	M0	None present
	M1	Present

*Regional lymph nodes vary with the location of the primary tumor.

cancer. The detection of celiac axis lymph node enlargement in patients with obstructing esophageal tumors impassable by an ultrasound endoscope also requires CT imaging. CT is less reliable than endoscopic ultrasonography for detecting depth of tumor invasion and regional lymph node metastases. Newer CT scanners that obtain rapid images by using a spiral technique are able to detect the bolus of contrast material as it traverses the visceral vasculature and may prove to be useful in detecting major vessel involvement by tumor.

Endoscopic Ultrasonography

Endoscopic ultrasonography (EUS) is a technique that uses the improved resolution of tissue detail allowed by high-frequency ultrasound. Lesser degrees of tissue penetration inherent in these high-frequency transducers are acceptable because the transducer is taken close to the tissue of interest by putting it on or within an endoscope. The GI wall is imaged as a five-layered structure that closely correlates with the histologic layers. This makes EUS an ideal method for detecting the depth of tumor invasion into the layers and therefore in assigning T stage.

Studies using EUS that compare the preoperative staging of esophageal cancer and gastric cancer to the pathologic stage of the resected cancer have shown an accuracy of 70 to 90 percent in determining depth of tumor invasion. Most important, in determining whether a patient is in a favorable category for primary surgery, the accuracy of predicting that the cancer has not spread outside the esophageal or stomach wall is about 90 percent, with few false-positive results. EUS overstaging of GI malignancies is usually caused by inflammatory reaction around a tumor, especially if an ulcer is present. The involvement of contiguous organs (T4 stage) such as the trachea, aorta, pericardium, pleura, diaphragm, and liver can also be accurately detected by preoperative EUS.

Lymph nodes as small as 2 mm in diameter adjacent to the GI wall can also be imaged with EUS. The distinction between benign and malignant lymph nodes can be problematic, but it is clear that the shape and echo pattern of the node is more important than its size. Rounded, hypoechoic nodes with an echogenicity similar to that of the primary neoplasm are more likely to be malignant than hyperechoic nodes and those with indistinct boundaries. False-negative EUS findings of lymph node involvement are usually due to the presence of microscopic malignant foci within nodes, or involved nodes that cannot be imaged by EUS because the endoscope cannot be passed through a tight stricture. False-positive results are caused by enlarged inflamed nodes, especially when there is concomitant anthracosis. The overall accuracy in detecting regional lymph node involvement varies from 50 to 90 percent in reported series.

EUS imaging is not sufficient for detecting distant metastases other than celiac node involvement. The liver and adrenals are incompletely imaged because of limited penetration of the EUS beam. The lungs are also not imaged with EUS because of the poor conduction of US through air.

EUS staging of esophageal and gastric carcinoma has been compared with CT staging in several studies. EUS was found to be superior to CT in determining the depth of invasion in most series. The superiority of EUS to CT is no surprise, given the lesser resolution of CT compared with EUS and the dependence of CT on detecting disruption of fat planes by malignant invasion. Some patients, especially after weight loss, have little periesophageal and perigastric fat. The advantage of EUS over CT in detecting the depth of invasion is most pronounced with gastroesophageal junction tumors, where problems of partial volume artifacts occur with CT because of the posterolateral angulation of the distal esophagus.

EUS and CT are complementary in detecting regional lymph node involvement. EUS is more reliable in detecting malignant nodes immediately surrounding the esophagus and stomach and for detecting nodes less than 1 cm in diameter in the celiac and left gastric areas. CT is useful for detecting more distant nodes and those separated from the GI tract by air-filled structures such as the pretracheal nodes.

EUS is more accurate than CT in determining tracheal and aortic involvement in patients with esophageal cancer. CT criteria for detecting aortic involvement require that the fat plane between the aorta and esophagus be obliterated over a 90-degree arc; EUS can detect much more focal aortic involvement by the cancer. CT is more useful than EUS for detecting liver, lung, and adrenal metastases and for detecting celiac node enlargement when the ultrasound endoscope cannot be passed through tight malignant strictures.

Other Staging Methods

Magnetic resonance imaging does not provide significant advantages over CT for staging esophageal and gastric cancer. Imaging to date has been limited by the lack of an adequate luminal contrast agent and by long-image acquisition times that result in motion artifacts. Both of these limitations are expected to improve in the future.

Bronchoscopy and laparoscopy may be useful in staging selected patients with esophageal and gastric cancer. When tracheal involvement with esophageal carcinoma is suspected from CT or EUS findings, bronchoscopy may provide confirmation. Involvement of the serosal surface of the stomach with neoplasm can be difficult to assess with EUS unless ascites is present. Laparoscopy can detect serosal invasion with a high degree of accuracy and should be used if nonsurgical treatment options are being considered.

APPROACH TO THE PATIENT WITH ESOPHAGEAL CANCER

Esophageal carcinoma remains a disease with a dismal prognosis for most patients. Overall 5 year survival rates are only about 5 percent. Nevertheless, advances in potentially curative combination chemotherapy and radiation therapy regimens, with or without surgical resection, have offered hope and a chance of cure for many patients. Simultaneous advances in nonsurgical palliation measures have also been made. The need to select the best form of treatment for individual patients has thus become increasingly important. Accurate preoperative staging currently offers the most rational approach to the choice of treatment for individual patients.

Our approach to the staging and management of patients with esophageal carcinoma is outlined in Figure 1. Patients with biopsy-proved esophageal carcinoma are first evaluated clinically for symptoms that require immediate palliation, and for the presence of concurrent debilitating diseases that would preclude further treatment. Those who are candidates for further treatment undergo a chest and abdominal CT scan to look for metastases. If none are present and if other mediastinal organ involvement is not detected, EUS staging is performed. Patients with disease confined to the esoph-

ageal wall (T1 and T2) and no lymphadenopathy (N0) undergo primary surgical resection to avoid the toxicity of neoadjuvant treatments. Those with T3 and or N1 lesions are offered entry into clinical trials of neoadjuvant chemotherapy and radiation followed by repeat CT staging and surgery if metastases are not detected. EUS has not proved reliable in the detection of residual cancer after neoadjuvant therapy. Patients with T4 lesions are offered various forms of palliation, depending on the predominant symptom present.

Special Situations

A major limitation in the application of EUS imaging to patients with esophageal carcinoma has been the inability to pass the endoscope through malignant esophageal strictures in up to 50 percent of cases. Some information about T stage can usually be obtained by imaging from above a stricture, but the ability to detect descending aortic, pericardial, and celiac node involvement is limited when the stricture cannot be passed. Previous esophageal dilation has not been very useful in permitting subsequent passage of the blunt-tipped echoendoscope, which cannot be maneuvered through irregularly placed lumens because of its oblique viewing optics. Forceful passage of the endoscope is discouraged because esophageal perforation has been reported to occur in this setting.

EUS has been proposed for the detection of cancer in patients with Barrett's esophagus. The results of EUS staging of adenocarcinoma arising in Barrett's esophagus parallel the staging results of other esophageal carcinomas. Similarly, EUS can detect esophageal wall thickening by a Barrett's cancer invading the submucosa, but an endoscopic nodule, mass, or ulcer is usually present, making this situation analogous to the role of EUS in staging other esophageal cancers. There is no compelling evidence demonstrating that EUS can detect high-grade dysplasia or intramucosal carcinoma in patients with Barrett's esophagus when no endoscopically visible abnormality other than Barrett's epithelium is present.

APPROACH TO THE PATIENT WITH GASTRIC CANCER

There are fewer treatment options for gastric cancer than are available for esophageal cancer. Neoadjuvant radiation and chemotherapy for gastric cancer have not been as extensively studied and are not as promising as in esophageal cancer. Furthermore, nonsurgical palliative measures for bleeding and obstruction are not as effective, so that surgery is needed in many patients. Thus, there is a lesser need for accurate preoperative staging in patients with gastric cancer. Nevertheless, efforts to improve the therapies for gastric cancer should be directed by accurate pretreatment staging in order to ensure uniform comparisons of various forms of treatment.

Most of the recent efforts to improve the outcome of

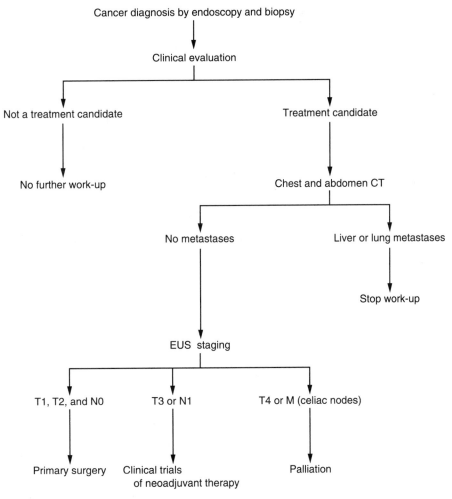

Figure 1 Algorithm for the staging of esophageal cancer.

patients with gastric cancer involve either neoadjuvant therapy or surgery with radical lymph node dissection. Patients with suspicious regional lymph nodes on CT or EUS staging are candidates for neoadjuvant combined modality phases I and II trials, in an attempt not only to decrease the bulk of the primary lesion and thereby increase the chance for surgical resection, but also potentially to sterilize sites of microscopic nodal disease. Responders to neoadjuvant treatment are more likely to realize increased local control and possibly survival benefit after surgical resection, compared with surgical resection alone. Moreover, through the administration of neoadjuvant therapy in a protocol setting to patients with T3 and/or N1 stage, biologically aggressive tumors are likely to declare themselves by developing measurable metastatic disease at the time of restaging. This would save such patients the potential inconvenience and risks of an incurable laparotomy. In short, patients with subclinical metastatic disease can be selected and not taken to surgery.

Our practice plan for patients with gastric cancer is outlined in Figure 2. All patients who show no evidence of metastatic disease after a history and physical examination, chest radiography, and liver function blood tests and with a normal serum creatinine level undergo a dynamic-bolus abdominal CT scan. Patients without clear metastases are then imaged with EUS. Patients with disease outside the gastric wall (T3 or T4) or those with suspicious regional nodes (N1) are offered enrollment in phase I or II combined modality clinical trials. After completion of neoadjuvant combination chemotherapy, those without evidence of extraregional tumor spread on repeat CT scanning are surgically explored. A subtotal or radical gastrectomy and lymph node dissection is performed, followed by a 15 to 20 electron cGy fraction of intraoperative radiation therapy. Adjuvant concomitant external-beam radiation therapy and 5-fluorouracil–based chemotherapy is begun 3 to 6 weeks postoperatively. Patients with metastatic disease on initial staging or after chemotherapy are treated with palliative measures directed at the predominant symptom.

PROS AND CONS OF THIS APPROACH TO STAGING

The staging algorithms outlined in Figures 1 and 2 assume that established treatments and experimental

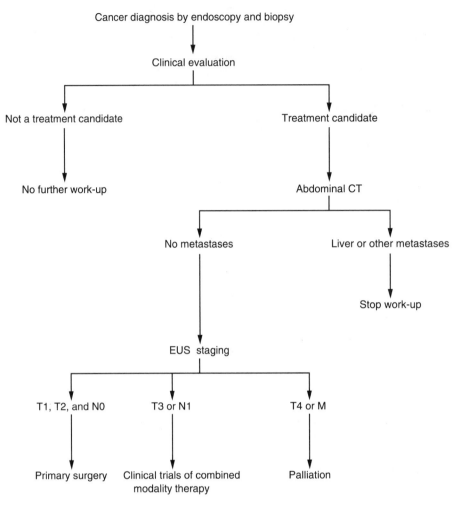

Figure 2 Algorithm for the staging of gastric cancer.

protocols are available based on staging results. If staging will not change how the patient is to be managed, staging tests will not benefit the patient and will only contribute to increased costs.

The impact of preoperative tumor stage on the results of neoadjuvant or primary radiation and chemotherapy is currently being studied, and randomized trials of the impact of tumor staging on overall patient survival and outcome are needed. Nevertheless, given the impact of tumor stage on patient survival, it is logical that current treatment trials and the selection of treatment for an individual patient should be directed as much as possible by the most accurate preoperative staging available.

SUGGESTED READING

Beahrs OH, Henson DE, Hutter RV, et al, eds. Manual for staging of cancer. 3rd ed. Philadelphia: American Joint Committee on Cancer, JB Lippincott, 1988.

Botet JF, Lightdale CJ, Zauber AG, et al. Preoperative staging of esophageal cancer: comparison of endoscopic US and dynamic CT. Radiology 1991; 181:419–425.

Botet JF, Lightdale CJ, Zauber AG, et al. Preoperative staging of gastric cancer: comparison of endoscopic US and dynamic CT. Radiology 1991; 181:426–432.

Halvorsen RA, Thompson WM. Primary neoplasms of the hollow organs of the gastrointestinal tract. Staging and follow-up. Cancer 1991; 67 (Suppl. 4):1181–1188.

Siewert JR, Holscher AH, Dittler HJ. Preoperative staging and risk analysis in esophageal carcinoma. Hepatogastroenterology 1990; 37:382–387.

Takashima S, Takeuchi N, Shiozaki H, et al. Carcinoma of the esophagus: CT vs. MR imaging in determining resectability. AJR 1991; 156:297–302.

Zuccaro G, Sivak MV, Rice TW. Endoscopic ultrasound and the staging of esophageal and gastric cancer. Gastrointest Endosc Clin North Am 1992; 2:626–636.

CANCER OF THE ESOPHAGUS

RICHARD F. HEITMILLER, M.D.

Carcinoma of the esophagus is a devastating disease because of its poor survival statistics even with therapy, and because of its adverse affect on swallowing and therefore the patient's quality of life. The goals of any therapy designed to manage patients with esophageal cancer are to relieve the dysphagia and treat the underlying cancer itself. An ideal therapy would accomplish both goals effectively and safely. Currently there are three main treatment strategies: (1) local control; (2) single modality therapy (e.g., surgery, radiation, or chemotherapy); and (3) combination therapies. Because of its effectiveness in both relieving dysphagia and treating esophageal cancer, surgery (either alone or as a combined therapy) should be considered for all patients with local or local-regional disease. This chapter therefore focuses on preoperative surgical evaluation, surgical techniques, and results. Combination therapy techniques are covered in a separate chapter.

Although esophageal cancer continues to be an aggressive malignancy that usually presents in an advanced stage, significant advances have been made in its treatment. These include (1) increased treatment options, (2) decreased surgical morbidity and mortality, (3) the development of more effective chemotherapies, and (4) improvements in prevention through identifying patients at risk as well as premalignant pathologic lesions.

SYMPTOMS

Dysphagia is the most common presenting symptom. It is usually of 3 to 4 months' duration and is associated with weight loss that is often out of proportion to the degree of dysphagia. Patients with esophageal cancer near the gastroesophageal junction often complain of a new epigastric burning sensation. Persistent back pain unrelated to swallowing suggests adjacent mediastinal or vertebral invasion. Respiratory symptoms (most frequently cough) are a sign of airway invasion in patients with middle or proximal third lesions. Symptoms associated with metastatic disease vary according to the metastatic site.

PRETREATMENT EVALUATION

The pretreatment work-up requires establishing a diagnosis, staging the cancer, and optimizing the patient's nutritional and pulmonary status.

The diagnosis is strongly suggested on the basis of a barium esophagogram demonstrating an "apple core" obstructing lesion within the esophagus. Although these are not necessary for diagnosis, it is my practice to use cine radiographic techniques for evaluating patients preoperatively because they provide much greater information on a patient's pharyngeal and esophageal function than standard single film contrast techniques. I have found this information helpful in the postoperative management of these patients. Regardless of the radiographic findings, the diagnosis must be confirmed by endoscopy with samples obtained for both cytologic and pathologic evaluation. In addition to establishing tissue for biopsy, the following endoscopic information is helpful in planning treatment: (1) the specific location of the tumor and its length (recorded in centimeters from the incisors); (2) whether or not there is Barrett's esophagus, and if so its extent; and (3) determination as to whether there is gastric invasion.

Once the diagnosis has been established, the tumor is staged. There are a number of staging systems for esophageal cancer, including the American Joint Committee on Cancer Staging (AJCCS TNM), the Japanese and the International Union Against Cancer (UICC), and the WNM (based on wall penetration, nodal status, and metastasis) systems. The disadvantage of all these systems has been the lack of clinical applicability because of the difficulty in establishing the depth of esophageal wall tumor invasion and the status of regional lymph nodes. I prefer the Japanese and UICC system as it is based on proved prognostic factors and correlates well with survival rates.

As mentioned, however, it is very difficult to accurately stage esophageal cancer patients before surgery. This has significant implications when patients are treated nonoperatively. Oral and intravenous contrast-enhanced chest and abdominal computed tomography (CT) is the best overall screening test. The size of the primary tumor and the presence of mediastinal invasion are determined. Chest magnetic resonance imaging is helpful if there is any question of aortic, pericardial, or vertebral invasion. Any esophageal tumor that lies adjacent to the trachea or mainstem bronchus requires flexible bronchoscopy regardless of the patient's symptoms or the radiographic findings. CT poorly assesses the depth of esophageal wall invasion, on which the "T" status is based.

Transesophageal ultrasonography, however, accurately determines the depth of tumor invasion and the size of regional lymph nodes (and therefore the probability of nodal metastasis). The drawbacks are that transesophageal ultrasonography requires equipment that is not available at all institutions and an experienced operator to achieve accurate results. In addition, the transesophageal echo probe must be able to pass through the narrowed esophageal lumen in order to image the tumor.*

Nodal status is best screened by CT. Supraclavicular, mediastinal, and paragastric lymphadenopathy suggests

---

*Editor's Note: There is a separate chapter on staging upper gastrointestinal tract tumors, including information on endoscopic ultrasound.

nodal metastasis. Transesophageal ultrasonography provides additional information about regional paraesophageal lymph nodes. Appropriate biopsies can be obtained if necessary. CT of the brain and technetium-labeled bone scans complete the metastatic work-up. More recently, both video-assisted thoracoscopy and laparoscopy are being studied as a means of providing an accurate pretreatment pathologic staging.

Before any treatment, especially surgery, is considered, it is important to optimize the patient's nutritional and pulmonary status. If surgery is planned, it is essential to consult the operating surgeon before placing any endoscopic feeding tubes, as this may significantly affect plans for esophageal reconstruction.

TREATMENT OPTIONS

My opinion is that surgery should be considered for all patients with local or local-regional esophageal cancer. The precedent for resecting obstructing gastrointestinal (GI) tumors, even in the setting of locally advanced disease, has been well established in the management of patients with obstructing small or large bowel tumors. The same principles apply to the treatment of patients with obstructing esophageal carcinoma. Local tumor control, with relief of dysphagia, is best accomplished surgically. This is especially true now that the surgical risks and length of hospitalization have decreased to acceptable figures. If disease recurs after surgery, it rarely involves the reconstructed esophagus, and therefore mechanical dysphagia does not recur. In contrast, local control failure with recurrent dysphagia is a common drawback of nonoperative forms of treatment (e.g., endoscopic Nd:YAG laser therapy and radiation therapy). For patients with early staged tumors, surgery alone yields excellent survival statistics. For patients who present with locally advanced tumors (stage III), which are considerably more common, there is much room for improvement in survival regardless of the therapy selected. Despite the development of new treatment modalities, I believe that surgery will continue to play a central role in the management of these difficult patients. Local control measures as the sole mode of therapy, such as Nd:YAG laser therapy, intraluminal funnel tubes, and radiation therapy, should be reserved for patients who are not candidates for surgery or combined modality therapy.

I determine the therapeutic approach on the basis of the patient's clinical stage and operability.

Localized Disease, Operable

I recommend surgery for all patients with localized disease, even if there is evidence of regional lymph node metastasis, provided that the medical condition permits. There are two surgical options: (1) surgery alone or (2) surgery as part of a combined therapy. Recent published results from simultaneous neoadjuvant chemotherapy and radiation therapy have shown encouraging improve-

ments in the time to recurrence and survival compared with historical controls. Combination therapy is covered in greater detail in a separate chapter. The surgical techniques are the same whether performed alone or as part of a combined approach.

Partial Esophagogastrectomy

Unlike the situation in the rest of the GI tract, it is not possible to resect segments of the esophagus and reconstruct it by joining the proximal and distal ends back together again. This is because the esophagus has no mobile mesentery. Therefore, resecting an esophageal pathologic condition necessitates excising the lesion and all the distal esophagus. Usually a portion of the proximal stomach is removed in continuity in order to include the lesser curvature and the left gastric lymph nodes that drain the lower esophagus. The surgical resection is therefore properly termed a partial esophagogastrectomy. Depending on the tumor location and the incisional approach used, different lengths of esophagus are resected. In all cases, however, the operation performed is a partial esophagogastrectomy (Fig. 1). The resected esophagus is replaced with segments of the abdominal GI tract, which are mobilized along with their blood supply, and then transposed into the chest (or the neck) and anastomosed to the remaining proximal esophagus. There is no prosthetic

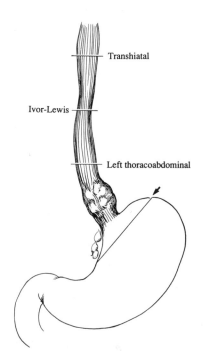

Figure 1 A distal third esophageal cancer is shown. Regardless of the incisional approach used, the operative procedure performed to resect the tumor is a partial esophagogastrectomy. A portion of the proximal stomach is resected (as indicated by the arrow) and, depending on the incisional approach used, different lengths of proximal esophagus are resected as indicated.

esophagus. A number of incisional approaches are used to perform a partial esophagogastrectomy, including transhiatal, Ivor-Lewis, left thoracoabdominal, and three-incision techniques (Fig. 2). In the past, proponents have argued in support of their preferred technique, giving the impression that these were uniquely different procedures. All the techniques are partial esophagogastrectomies, and in the proper hands they yield similar results in terms of both surgical morbidity and mortality and survival. The only variables in performing a partial esophagogastrectomy are which incisions to use, how much esophagus is resected, and what is used to replace the esophagus.

Transhiatal partial esophagogastrectomy (THE) is an increasingly popular surgical approach that does not require a thoracotomy. It places the esophagogastric anastomosis in the neck, where the consequences of an anastomotic leak are minimized. The intrathoracic esophagus is mobilized "bluntly" from above through the cervical incision, and from below through the esophageal hiatus. The esophagus is usually reconstructed with stomach, which is mobilized and passed up through the chest into the neck (a gastric pull-up), where it is anastomosed to the remaining esophagus. The exposure given by a THE approach necessitates removing all but the proximal 3 to 4 cm of esophagus.

The Ivor-Lewis partial esophagogastrectomy has traditionally been the standard surgical approach, although in my practice it has been largely replaced by THE. The Ivor-Lewis approach was designed to optimize surgical exposure of the intrathoracic esophagus, which passes through the upper two-thirds of the chest along the right posterior mediastinum. Therefore, a midline abdominal incision is used to mobilize the stomach and lower esophagus, the abdominal incision is closed, and the patient is repositioned for a right thoracotomy. The involved intrathoracic esophagus is mobilized, the stomach is pulled into the right chest, a partial esophagogastrectomy is performed, and the esophagus is reconstructed by esophagogastric anastomosis high within the chest, usually at or above the level where the azygos vein enters the superior vena cava.

The left thoracoabdominal partial esophagogastrectomy utilizes a single incision that extends from the left chest onto the abdomen and provides excellent exposure of the upper abdomen and lower third of the esophagus. This technique is ideal for patients with esophageal tumors near the gastroesophageal junction, especially when the extent of gastric involvement is unclear, because it yields superb exposure and maximizes reconstructive options for the lower third of the esophagus.

Three-incision techniques seek to combine the

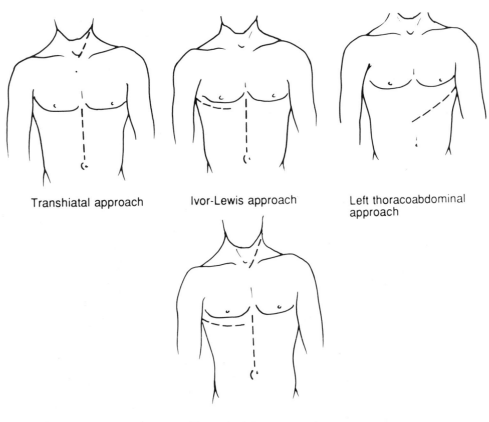

Transhiatal approach   Ivor-Lewis approach   Left thoracoabdominal approach

Three- Incision approach

Figure 2 The different incisions used to perform a partial esophagogastrectomy. (From Reichle RL, Fishman EK, Nixon MS, et al. Evaluation of the postsurgical esophagus after partial esophagogastrectomy for esophageal cancer. Invest Radiol 1993; 28:247–257; with permission.)

safety of intrathoracic esophageal mobilization under direct vision with the excellent functional results obtained from a THE and gastric pull-up. In patients with a middle third lesion lying adjacent to the airway or the aortic arch, the intrathoracic esophagus is first mobilized via a right thoracotomy. Once it is determined that the lesion is resectable, the chest incision is closed and the patient returned to the supine position, where a transhiatal gastric pull-up and cervical esophagogastric anastomosis are completed.

Localized Disease, Inoperable

Most patients with localized disease are surgical candidates. In some, however, local invasion of mediastinal structures such as the airway, aorta, or vertebral bodies prevents surgical resection. In others, poor pulmonary function, significant medical illness, advanced age, extreme malnutrition, or systemic steroids increase surgical morbidity and mortality rates to prohibitive levels and therefore render the patient inoperable. These patients are best given palliative therapy by endoscopic Nd:YAG laser treatments to open the esophageal lumen and by external beam radiation. Systemic chemotherapy can also be considered, but this is contraindicated in many of these patients for the same reasons that make them inoperable. Endoscopically placed salivary bypass tubes (funnel tubes) are optimally reserved for patients who cannot tolerate or who fail the above-mentioned therapy. There is a chapter on various mechanical palliative measures.

Patients with tumors that invade contiguous mediastinal structures represent a particularly difficult treatment subgroup. In these patients, either inadequate or overzealous nonoperative treatment results in fistulization into adjacent structures, with life-threatening consequences. Some authors have advocated planned incomplete surgical resection for these patients, especially those with airway invasion, to achieve local control and prevent tracheoesophageal fistulization (TEF). In general, for these patients, I have advocated radiation therapy at reduced daily doses (often with chemotherapy), with frequent sequential studies to assess treatment response.

Malignant Tracheoesophageal Fistula

Patients who present with a malignant TEF are among the most difficult to treat. Treatment options are further limited by pneumonitis and malnutrition, the inevitable consequences of TEF. In addition to nutritional support and treatment of the respiratory infection, management options include (in order of increasing invasiveness) (1) placement of intraluminal salivary bypass tubes, alone or with gastrostomy tube placement; (2) esophageal exclusion with cervical esophagostomy, draining gastrostomy, and feeding jejunostomy; and (3) esophageal resection, surgical repair of the TEF, esophageal reconstruction, gastrostomy, and feeding jejunostomy. The specific method chosen is based on the patient's age, nutritional status, degree of respiratory compromise, and tumor stage.

Metastatic Disease

Survival in patients with metastatic esophageal cancer is short (months not years, usually), and the emphasis of treatment is on palliation. Surgery is not advocated for these patients. Palliation of dysphagia is best achieved endoscopically with Nd:YAG laser; external beam radiation therapy can also be added. Endoscopically placed salivary bypass tubes are used in patients who will not tolerate or who fail laser or radiation therapy. There is little role for systemic chemotherapy in the palliation of these patients.

OUTCOME

Surgery has still not achieved widespread acceptance as treatment of patients with esophageal carcinoma. This reluctance no doubt reflects the results of earlier surgical series that demonstrated low resectability rates, significant complications, and an operative mortality as high as 33.3 percent. Given such high morbidity and mortality, any potential benefits of surgery would justifiably be overlooked. Nonetheless, these data ignore more recent surgical developments and are not remotely representative of current surgical results. Current surgical mortality rates of approximately 5 percent or less are considered standard regardless of the surgical technique used. Mortality rates as low as 2 to 3 percent have been reported in large series, which is remarkable given the patient's underlying disease, age, associated medical illness, and nutritional deficiencies. In practice, there is a wide variation in surgical results depending on a surgeon's training and the volume of esophageal surgery performed. The recommendations made in this chapter are reasonable only if the surgery is performed by surgeons experienced in this work.

In my experience at Johns Hopkins with 106 esophagectomies for carcinoma, operative mortality has been 5.4 percent. Morbidity has included pneumonia in six patients (5.5 percent; two of these were culture negative and appeared to have adult respiratory distress syndrome), supraventricular tachyarrhythmias in 16 (14.5 percent), cerebrovascular accident in one (0.9 percent), abdominal wound seromas requiring local drainage in 16 (14.5 percent), postoperative hoarseness in ten (9 percent overall, four mild, one recurrent laryngeal nerve sacrificed intentionally), and one patient with a delayed anastomotic leak (0.9 percent). The standard length of hospitalization at our institution varies according to cell type. Patients with adenocarcinoma have a mean hospital stay of approximately 11 days, in those with squamous tumors it is about 15 days. On discharge, patients are eating a six-meal regular diet. With time, patients invariably return to a three-meal-per-day regimen and can maintain their weight with this. Nutritional supplements, either oral or enteral tube feedings, are infrequently required. Postvagotomy symptoms develop in 15 to 20 percent of patients and are successfully managed medically.

SUGGESTED READING

Ellis FH Jr, Gibb SP, Watkins E Jr. Esophagogastrectomy: a safe, widely applicable, and expeditious form of publication for patients with carcinoma of the esophagus and gastric cardia. Ann Surg 1983; 198:531–540.

Heitmiller RF. Results of standard left thoracoabdominal esophagogastrectomy. Semin Thorac Cardiovasc Surg 1992; 4:314–319.
Mathisen DJ, Grillo HC, Hilgenberg AD, et al. Transthoracic esophagogastrectomy: a safe approach to carcinoma of the esophagus. Ann Thoracic Surg 1988; 45:137–143.
Orringer MB, Forastiere AA, Perez-Temayo C, et al. Chemotherapy and radiation therapy before transhiatal esophagectomy for esophageal carcinoma. Ann Thorac Surg 1990; 49:348–355.
Reichle RL, Fishman EK, Nixon MS, et al. Evaluation of the post-surgical esophagus after partial esophagogastrectomy for esophageal cancer. Invest Radiol 1993; 28:247–257.

CANCER OF THE ESOPHAGUS: COMBINED MODALITY THERAPY

ARLENE A. FORASTIERE, M.D.
SUSAN G. URBA, M.D.

Esophageal cancer comprises 1.5 percent of invasive cancers diagnosed annually in the United States. There has been little change in survival over the past three decades, and less than 10 percent of individuals are alive 5 years after diagnosis. The prognosis for newly diagnosed patients is poor even when the disease appears to be clinically localized, because occult spread to regional lymph nodes and distant sites occurs early in the course of the disease. The most common presenting symptoms, dysphagia and odynophagia, do not occur until the esophageal lumen is narrowed to one-third to one-half of its normal size, and tumor may penetrate the muscular layers to involve contiguous structures before the lumen becomes obstructed. Because the esophagus has an intercommunicating submucosal lymphatic network, metastatic spread to lymph nodes or distant sites may occur before symptoms lead to the diagnosis.

Esophageal carcinoma occurs most commonly in older men who have a long history of alcohol intake and cigarette smoking. Recent epidemiologic data indicate that 71 percent of esophageal cancers are squamous cell, 17 percent are adenocarcinoma, and 12 percent belong to a miscellaneous group that includes malignant melanoma, sarcomas, and small cell neuroendocrine tumors. Although squamous cell carcinoma is most common, the incidence of adenocarcinoma of the distal esophagus and gastric cardia is rapidly increasing by approximately 10 percent per year. Since 1987 there has been a greater than 100-fold increase in adenocarcinoma in men, so that now this is the most common histologic subtype of esophageal cancer in white males under age 50. This same epidemiologic pattern is also being observed in Great Britain and the Scandinavian countries. The only identified risk factor is dysplastic Barrett's epithelium associated with chronic gastroesophageal reflux.

THERAPEUTIC ALTERNATIVES

Treatment options and prognosis are determined by the extent of disease at diagnosis. Localized disease is confined to the esophagus, and regional involvement occurs with tumor invasion of surrounding lymph nodes. The standard treatment for local-regional disease consists of surgical removal of the tumor with lymph node dissection. Unfortunately, the 3 year survival rate is only 18 percent for patients with localized disease and 11 percent if regional lymph nodes are involved. Some institutions report similar results with primary radiation therapy. These figures remain unchanged if radiation therapy is added either before or after surgery. Because of this poor outcome, several investigational approaches are under evaluation: (1) preoperative and/or postoperative chemotherapy, (2) preoperative combined chemotherapy and radiation therapy, and (3) combined chemotherapy and radiation without surgery.

If the patient has local-regional disease but is not a surgical candidate because of medical risks, or because the disease invades or is adherent to critical structures in the mediastinum (i.e., aorta, bronchus, pericardium), radiation therapy is the standard treatment. Recently, investigators evaluated the use of combined chemotherapy and radiation therapy in patients with locally advanced disease, and results showed an improvement in survival.

Metastatic disease is incurable, with a median survival of 6 months and a 3 year survival rate of 4 percent. The most common sites of metastases are distant lymph nodes, lung, liver, and bone. Treatment recommendations depend on the patient's overall medical condition and performance status, and require informed discussion between the patient, family, and physician. The options include supportive care with emphasis on pain control and nutrition, radiation therapy for particularly painful or problematic tumor sites, or systemic chemotherapy. Because treatment with standard chemotherapeutic agents has not altered survival rates, experimental protocols should be considered

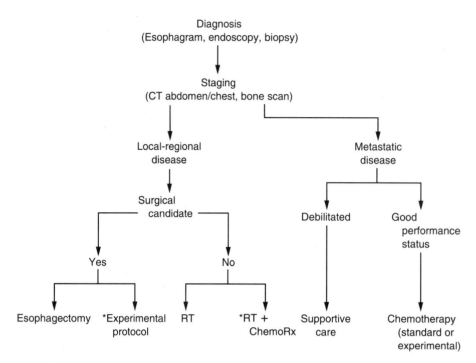

*Preferred Treatment

Figure 1 Decision-making schema for esophageal cancer management. RT = radiation therapy; ChemoRx = chemotherapy.

if available. An algorithm for the management of esophageal cancer is shown in Figure 1.

PREFERRED APPROACH

Local-Regional Disease

After the diagnosis of esophageal cancer is established by endoscopy and biopsy, an evaluation of extent of disease that includes barium esophagography, computed tomographic (CT) scan of the chest and abdomen, and bone scan should be performed. These studies allow the physician to distinguish patients with local-regional disease that is potentially curable with surgery or experimental multimodality treatment from those who have metastatic disease or extensive, unresectable local-regional disease that is incurable. There are two major limitations to the use of current staging procedures: (1) the depth of tumor invasion into the esophageal muscle cannot be determined by routine radiographic studies and endoscopic biopsy, and (2) CT cannot distinguish whether enlarged regional nodes (diameter greater than 1 cm) contain tumor or represent nonmalignant change only.

Pathologic staging, as defined in the American Joint Committee on Cancer Manual for Staging of Cancer, correlates with prognosis and is based on depth of invasion and nodal involvement. Techniques such as endoscopic ultrasonography and laparoscopy that may provide more accurate information on the depth of invasion and nodal status are under investigation.

However, until these methods become widely available, patients with regional node involvement, as determined by CT, are approached as having disease that is potentially resectable for cure. Therefore, if disease is localized, or if lymph node involvement is limited to regional lymph nodes, surgery is the standard treatment. Most patients experience weight loss as a result of dysphagia before diagnosis, and may have a long history of cigarette smoking and associated chronic pulmonary disease. Therefore, preparation for surgery includes dietary counseling and high-calorie liquid nutritional supplements, enteral or parenteral feeding if necessary, and pulmonary toilet with incentive spirometry and bronchodilators.

Surgery

Our preferred surgical approach is transhiatal esophagectomy with thoracotomy. This procedure has two advantages. First, it avoids the major thoracic and abdominal incisions used in the more traditional thoracotomy and laparotomy, which can be physiologically stressful in the elderly population in which this disease most often occurs. Second, transhiatal esophagectomy uses a cervical esophageal anastomosis that minimizes the risk of mediastinitis and sepsis. This can occur when patients who have an intrathoracic esophagogastric anastomosis experience a postoperative disruption of the suture line as a complication.

The transhiatal esophagectomy employs an upper midline abdominal incision to enter the peritoneal cavity, and a 5 cm oblique cervical incision parallel to the anterior border of the sternocleidomastoid muscle. Blunt finger dissection of the esophagus from the mediastinum is carried out, and when the entire intrathoracic esophagus is freely mobile, it is delivered into the cervical or abdominal wound. The esophagus is ligated and removed, and the stomach is introduced into the posterior mediastinum to replace the esophagus in the chest. The abdominal wound is closed, a cervical esophagogastric anastomosis is performed, and then the cervical wound is repaired. Although it is not possible to do a formal en bloc dissection of contiguous lymph nodes, all accessible nodes are removed by blunt dissection along with the esophagus. Survival data for patients who undergo thoracotomy with formal lymph node dissection (Ivor-Lewis approach) are nearly identical to those obtained for patients treated with transhiatal esophagectomy.

Potential intraoperative complications include entry into the pleural cavity requiring chest tube placement, or (rarely) tracheal laceration. Postoperatively, recurrent laryngeal nerve paralysis can occur, which is usually temporary. As surgical technique and retractor placement have been meticulously studied and refined, this complication has become infrequent. Esophagogastric anastomotic leaks can occur but usually heal without serious sequelae.

Preoperative Multimodality Treatment

Because of the generally poor survival rates of patients treated with standard surgery, various combinations of radiation therapy, chemotherapy, and surgery have been investigated in patients with operable local-regional disease. No randomized trial has shown a survival benefit for preoperative radiation therapy compared with surgery alone, although local control of disease and resectability may be improved.

Another investigational approach involves preoperative cisplatin-based chemotherapy. The results of several trials in patients with squamous cell carcinoma of the esophagus in which one to three cycles of chemotherapy were administered before esophagectomy suggested improved survival rates. However, two randomized trials comparing preoperative chemotherapy with surgery alone failed to show a survival advantage for chemotherapy-treated patients. A large multi-institutional randomized trial is in progress, comparing treatment with esophagectomy alone versus three cycles of preoperative cisplatin and 5-fluorouracil (5-FU), esophagectomy, and two additional cycles of postoperative chemotherapy. This trial includes patients with adenocarcinoma of the distal esophagus and cardia as well as those with a squamous cell histologic appearance. Most commonly, chemotherapy regimens for esophageal carcinoma include various combinations of cisplatin, bleomycin, vinblastine, and 5-FU. The toxicity of cisplatin, the most frequently used chemotherapeutic agent in this disease, includes nausea and vomiting, renal dysfunction, ototoxicity, and peripheral neuropathy. Bleomycin can cause mucositis and pul-

monary toxicity, and 5-FU is often associated with stomatitis and diarrhea. All these drugs can cause myelosuppression.

An alternative approach is to combine chemotherapy and radiation therapy before esophagectomy. The most studied regimen consists of administration of two to three courses of cisplatin, 100 mg per square meter on day 1, and 5-FU, 1,000 mg per square meter per day for 4 to 5 days every 3 to 4 weeks, concomitant with radiation therapy (3,000 cGy) followed by surgery. Median survivals reported from several studies ranged from 14 to 18 months. At the University of Michigan, we evaluated an intensive 21 day regimen of preoperative chemoradiotherapy. Radiation was given to a total dose of 4,500 cGy over 3 weeks, and the chemotherapy consisted of cisplatin as a continuous infusion on days 1 to 5 and 17 to 21, vinblastine on days 1 to 4 and 17 to 20, and 5-FU as a continuous infusion during the entire 21 days of radiation therapy. The results of this trial suggested improved survival (median, 29 months), with 44 and 35 percent of patients alive at 3 and 5 years, respectively. These observations must be confirmed, and a prospective randomized trial is in progress to compare this preoperative regimen with the use of esophagectomy alone. The results will not be available for several years. Our preferred approach for patients with local-regional, resectable esophageal cancer is combined chemotherapy and radiation therapy followed by surgery in an experimental protocol. If an organized research protocol is not available or not desired by the patient, we recommend immediate esophagectomy.

Radiation Therapy Alone

If a patient with local-regional disease is not a surgical candidate for medical reasons, primary radiation therapy can be used effectively. The outcome is highly dependent on established prognostic factors that include tumor length, location in the esophagus, degree of obstruction, and total radiotherapy dose. Thus, tumors less than 5 cm in length, located in the upper one-third, causing either mild or no obstruction, and treated with high doses (e.g., 6,600 cGy) have the best prognosis. Five year cure rates of 15 to 20 percent for highly selected patients have been reported. Definitive radiation can be administered in doses ranging from 5,000 cGy, given over 5 weeks, up to 6,600 cGy, given over 7 weeks. Complications of therapy include esophagitis, radiation pneumonitis, pericarditis, and esophageal stricture. The most frequent postirradiation complication is esophageal stricture, which occurs in approximately 40 percent of patients. Repeated esophageal dilatation is often required. The spinal cord should be shielded with doses higher than 4,500 cGy, its maximal radiation tolerance, to protect it from injury. Responses to treatment can be assessed by barium esophagogram and endoscopy.

For patients with unresectable local-regional disease caused by tumor invasion into mediastinal structures that precludes surgical removal, radiation therapy is used primarily to palliate symptoms of dysphagia. Approximately two-thirds of patients achieve some palliation that can last on average 3 to 10 months. However, with radiation alone, only 50 percent of irradiated patients maintain swallowing function to the time of death. Laser endoscopic surgery should also be considered as an alternative to help restore swallowing function in these incurable patients.

Radiation Therapy and Concomitant Chemotherapy

Clinical trials have been conducted to evaluate the combination of chemotherapy and concomitant radiation therapy without surgery. A large prospective multicenter randomized study compared radiation therapy alone, 6,400 cGy, with combination therapy. The combined treatment consisted of radiation to a dose of 5,000 cGy and four courses of concurrent cisplatin and 5-FU chemotherapy during weeks 1, 5, 8, and 11. An interim analysis showed a significant difference in survival at 2 years — 38 versus 10 percent — and a median survival of 12.5 months versus 8.9 months in favor of the combined modality treatment. This large trial establishes chemotherapy plus radiation therapy as the preferred treatment over radiation therapy alone for patients with unresectable local-regional disease.

Metastatic Disease

Decision making for the treatment of metastatic esophageal carcinoma should take into account that the disease is incurable, the median survival for this group of patients is a dismal 6 months, chemotherapy has not been shown to prolong survival, and patients will want to make choices regarding their quality of life. Palliation of symptoms and restoration of swallowing function to allow patients to handle secretions should be the primary goals of treatment, if patients choose not to enroll in investigational chemotherapy trials.

Supportive Care

One reasonable treatment option is supportive care only, particularly for patients who are debilitated. This care may include radiation therapy for the primary tumor or laser endoscopy to allow patients to feed themselves and handle secretions for as long as possible. Radiation can be delivered effectively in doses ranging from 4,000 cGy, given in 200 cGy fractions over a period of 4 weeks, to 6000 cGy given over 6 weeks. Thus, the complication of aspiration pneumonia common in patients with an obstructed esophageal lumen can be avoided.

The placement of a prosthetic tube into the lumen of an esophagus that is obstructed by tumor or in which a tracheoesophageal fistula is present is another approach to restoring swallowing function. Although this may be successful for 4 to 6 months, it is infrequently used as a palliative procedure because of mortality rates of 10 to 40 percent associated with tube placement.

Complications consist of esophageal perforation, mediastinitis, and aspiration of gastric contents when tubes are placed for distal lesions. In about 25 percent of patients the tubes become dislodged, and they frequently become obstructed by food as well. Candidates for this procedure have advanced cancer for which there is no other therapeutic alternative.

Our preferred method of restoring swallowing function is laser endoscopic surgery. Depending on the degree of obstruction, laser treatment can provide an adequate lumen for patients to aliment themselves and prevent aspiration of secretions. Because patients with metastatic disease usually experience some degree of anorexia as well, laser treatment coupled with gastrostomy tube placement can be an effective way of restoring swallowing function and providing adequate caloric intake.

Other effective supportive care measures involve the aggressive use of narcotic analgesics and enteral nutritional supplements. Radiation therapy alone, delivered to symptomatic sites of disease such as bone metastases, can often reduce symptoms and lead to a short-term improvement in quality of life.

Experimental Protocols

If the patient has a reasonable performance status and desires treatment, the best option is an experimental protocol. Patients offered such therapies should be ambulatory and capable of all self-care, but may or may not be able to carry out work activities. They should be up and about more than 50 percent of waking hours. This definition of functional capability or performance status serves as a reliable indicator to help physicians guide patients and families toward supportive care only or potentially life-prolonging investigational chemotherapy. Current chemotherapy regimens have not been shown to improve survival, and therefore more active drug combinations need to be identified. Some investigative approaches include new chemotherapeutic agents, biologic response modifiers, and radiation or chemotherapy sensitizers.

Standard Chemotherapy

If no protocols are available for the patient who desires treatment and has a reasonable performance status, the recommended treatment is systemic chemotherapy. The most commonly used chemotherapy regimen is cisplatin, 100 mg per square meter IV on day 1, and 5-FU, 1,000 mg per square meter per day given in a continuous IV infusion on days 1 to 5, every 28 days. Patients should have a creatinine clearance of at least 60 ml per minute, because cisplatin is a nephrotoxin. The chemotherapy is strongly emetogenic, and pretreatment with antiemetic agents is therefore mandatory. Currently, the most effective antiemetic is ondansetron, a serotonin antagonist. Other potential toxicities of this chemotherapy regimen include peripheral neuropathy, ototoxicity, diarrhea, stomatitis, and myelosuppression.

Tumor response should be assessed after every two cycles of treatment.

SUGGESTED READING

Blot WJ, Devesa SS, Kneller RW, Fraumeni JF. Rising incidence of adenocarcinoma of the esophagus and gastric cardia. JAMA 1991; 265:1287–1289.

Forastiere AA. Treatment of loco-regional esophageal cancer. Semin Oncol 1992; 19(Suppl 11):57–63.

Forastiere AA, Orringer MB, Perez-Tamayo C, et al. Pre-operative chemoradiation followed by transhiatal esophagectomy for carcinoma of the esophagus: final report. J Clin Oncol 1993 11:118–1123.

Herskovic A, Martz K, Al-Sarraf M, et al. Advantage of chemoradiotherapy compared to radiation alone in randomized phase III trial for patients with esophageal cancer: an intergroup study. N Engl J Med 1992; 326:1593–1598.

Orringer MB. Transhiatal esophagectomy without thoracotomy for carcinoma of the thoracic esophagus. Ann Surg 1984; 200:282–288.

Roth J, Putnam JB Jr, Lichter A, Forastiere AA. Esophageal cancer. In DeVita V, Hellman S, Rosenberg S, eds. Cancer, principles and practice of oncology. 4th ed. Philadelphia: JB Lippincott, 1993:776.

LASER USE AND PHOTODYNAMIC THERAPY FOR GASTROINTESTINAL CANCER

STEPHEN K. HEIER, M.D., F.A.C.P., F.A.C.G.

The options available for the treatment of gastrointestinal cancer (Fig. 1, top section) have increased markedly over the past decade, particularly when combinations for multimodal therapy are considered. Each option has its proponents, most options address certain circumstances better than other alternatives, and all have their limitations. Numerous factors influence the selection of therapy (those of greatest weight presented in Fig. 1, bottom section) and dictate that we avoid regimentation in our approach, select with patient input from the array of options, and be ready to alter the management plan with often-changing clinical circumstances and research data. Two noninvasive therapies that are proving most versatile are neodymium:yttrium-aluminum-garnet (Nd:YAG) laser therapy and photodynamic therapy (PDT). After a discussion of their use, some other endoscopic therapies will be briefly critiqued.

At the end of this chapter, our approach to esophageal cancer is reviewed, emphasizing multimodal therapy. This disease entity was selected because it highlights the use of endoscopic laser therapies through an integrated program and best demonstrates the complexity of therapy selection.

Nd:YAG LASER THERAPY

Nd:YAG laser therapy uses an invisible infrared beam that destroys tumor tissue by penetrating the tumor surface and converting to thermal energy, result-

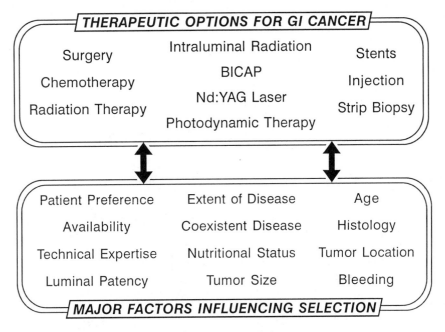

Figure 1 Selection of therapy.

ing in cell vaporization and coagulation of feeding tumor vessels. Preferred parameters for tumor treatment include maximal power output (i.e., 90 watts or greater) and a continuous pulse length setting. The duration of the pulse is then controlled by a foot pedal, with the total energy delivered determined by visible tissue changes. The end point is generally a charred surface. Energy delivered beyond the point of charring results in excess smoke generation and high surface temperatures with little additional efficacy. By continuously moving the endoscope tip during pulse delivery, one can treat large tumor areas efficiently.

The laser fiber is extended so that the fiber tip is seen protruding from the endoscope, to prevent endoscope damage. Both torque and endoscope tip deflection can result in the fiber retracting into the endoscope, necessitating constant attention to fiber position. The laser beam exiting the fiber tip has an 8- to 10-degree angle of divergence. Therefore, the farther the fiber tip is from the targeted tissue, the larger is the beam spot size on the tissue and the less is the energy delivered per unit tumor surface area. The fiber tip is usually positioned about 1 cm (range of 0.5 to 2 cm) from the tumor surface. If the tip is too close to the tissue, excess tissue penetration and fiber damage may result; if the tip is too far from the tissue, the tissue response is inadequate. The angle at which the laser beam enters the tissue also affects the amount of light reflection and the depth of light penetration. Torquing the scope and deflecting its tip to aim the beam across the visual field, attempting to approximate a perpendicular angle to the targeted tissue, maximizes tumor destruction. However, tumor regions requiring less transaxial necrosis, such as a superior margin of esophageal tumor close to the normal esophageal wall, are treated with the laser beam aligned along the luminal axis.

Three possible adverse effects of Nd:YAG laser therapy are patient pain, tissue edema, and smoke generation. Pain most commonly occurs with treatment of esophageal tumors, especially near their superior margins, and rectal tumors. The high intrathoracic and pelvic temperatures can be diminished by allowing time for heat dissipation. This is accomplished by slowing the pace of therapy through shorter duration pulses and longer time gaps between pulses. Pain is less common during the treatment of gastroduodenal and proximal colonic tumors and is considered a warning signal that transmural injury may be occurring.

Edema of normal tissue adjacent to tumor results from heat transmission and can obscure the definition of the tumor margins. The field of laser therapy may then be inadvertently and progressively extended beyond the actual tumor margins, further worsening the edema and promoting stricture formation. By clearly demarcating the tumor margins early in the therapy with a series of carefully delivered laser pulses, tumor zones are precisely outlined and normal tissue injury can be minimized. Significant edema may take one to several days to resolve and limits dietary advancement even after

luminal patency has been achieved within the borders of the tumor.

Smoke is generated in copious volumes both when the tumor tissue becomes carbonized and when the laser beam hits blood. Smoke generation can be reduced by avoiding overtreatment of tumor regions and by prompt treatment of any points that start to bleed during therapy. Nevertheless, gaseous overdistention can result from smoke generation and from the coaxial air flow around the laser fiber; this can be prevented by frequent suctioning beyond the tumor. Suctioning is performed by passing the scope into the stomach when treating esophageal tumors, or by advancing the scope to the transverse colon when treating rectosigmoid tumors. Intraluminal smoke can also deposit a residue, both on the light bundle and on the microchip lenses, which can be easily cleaned off after temporary scope withdrawal. Eructated smoke is unpleasant to personnel, and rooms with the highest frequency of air exchanges are chosen for the therapy, with micropore masks made available for personnel.

The therapy is usually performed in a retrograde fashion relative to the direction of scope advancement, so that edema and char do not interfere with access to and visualization of tumor regions. At times, however, prograde therapy gives clearer access beyond ledges or allows easier passage of the scope through tight tumor segments that are visibly short in length.

Laser sessions are usually spaced at least 2 days apart to allow maximal necrosis from previous coagulation of feeding vessels. When the goal is to establish luminal patency, 2 day intervals are usually chosen. However, when the goal is bleeding control or curative ablation, and sufficient tumor bulk has been ablated, longer intervals may be chosen to better assess the response to therapy. In the colon, dead tumor tissue often self-debrides by the time of a subsequent endoscopy, but in the esophagus mechanical debridement with the tip of the endoscope is often necessary.

Esophageal Cancer

Delivery of Therapy

An endoscope can usually be passed through even tightly obstructing lesions to perform retrograde laser therapy. However, on occasion limited dilatation may be necessary, with a bougie over an endoscopically placed and fluoroscopically confirmed guidewire. Excessive dilatation may add an element of risk beyond the laser therapy itself. Dilatation used as monotherapy is usually of only transient aid, with additional dilatations resulting in progressive tumor compression, incrementally shorter relief, and an added measure of difficulty in applying laser therapy.

Since palliative Nd:YAG laser therapy destroys only the obstructing intraluminal component of the tumor, gradual regrowth results in reobstruction. Our randomized trial of Nd:YAG laser therapy versus PDT documented by Kaplan-Meier analysis that about 50 percent of patients maintain an adequate duration of response for 6 to 7 weeks after Nd:YAG laser therapy. However, outside the trial situation, pragmatic timing is to repeat therapy after about 4 weeks, before the patient develops significant symptoms and requires more extensive therapy. Subsequent follow-up can be individually tailored after noting regrowth patterns at the time of the first follow-up therapy.

Patient Instructions

Peristalsis is ineffective through an esophageal tumor lumen, and use of gravity in conjunction with dietary guidelines is necessary after re-establishment of luminal patency. Instructions include avoidance of hard food, chewing well, following bites with liquid to flush the lumen, and eating in an upright position. If lower esophageal sphincter function is compromised, antireflux precautions are warranted. If symptoms return before the scheduled follow-up visit, patients should report promptly to avoid functional deterioration and other complications.

Effects of Therapy

Laser therapy relieves dysphagia in most patients, decreases the rate of nutritional deterioration, improves functionality, prevents aspiration, and may reduce the rate of spontaneous fistula formation resulting from blocked pulsion forces penetrating through a weakened esophageal wall. Several studies have documented improved quality of life, and two studies have suggested prolongation of survival. Complications are few (2 to 4 percent) but may include fistula, hemorrhage, fever, luminal plugging with tumor debris, and stricture formation.

Limitations of Therapy

Re-establishment of luminal patency cannot be expected to correct tumor-induced anorexia, so it is not surprising that technical improvement does not always translate into functional improvement. Factors correlated with less optimal functional results include poor performance status at onset, long tumors (larger than 5 to 10 cm), and cervical tumors (due to decreased

Table 1 Frequent Indications for Nd:YAG Laser Therapy

Obstructing tumors
  Esophagus
  Gastroduodenal
  Colon

Bleeding tumors
  Single vessel
  Diffuse bleeding

Curative ablation
  Early cancer
  Adenomas not amenable to polypectomy

proximal peristalsis and possible nerve involvement, as well as technical difficulty). Laser therapy is contraindicated in the presence of fistulas, except as needed to facilitate prosthesis placement. With continued progression of disease, the response to repeated laser therapy may also diminish. Options in patients with poor initial or subsequent responses include prosthesis insertion or percutaneous endoscopic gastrostomy (PEG). At times, hospice care may be more appropriate than additional procedures. Prostheses and PEG placement are discussed in separate chapters.

In spite of the limitations of Nd:YAG laser therapy, its utility for palliating esophageal cancer prompted its application in other gastrointestinal afflictions (Table 1), some of which are discussed below.

Gastroduodenal Cancer

Treatment of patients with proximal gastric cancer affecting the gastric cardia involves an approach similar to that outlined for those with esophageal cancer.

Patients with distal gastric cancer are most often candidates for either curative or palliative surgical intervention. For patients with gastroduodenal cancer who are not surgical candidates, or for patients with recurrent gastric cancer, effective palliation can be achieved with laser therapy. However, technical difficulties in the treatment of gastric tumors include tumor bulk, disruption of antral emptying, and definition of pyloric anatomy. Difficulties with duodenal tumors include the curve of the sweep, small luminal caliber, and the tendency for concurrent biliary obstruction.

We reported the palliative laser therapy for noncardiac gastroduodenal tumors, some with concurrent biliary obstruction. Symptoms, including dysphagia, vomiting, abdominal pain and jaundice, were relieved in all patients. Despite greater technical difficulty in treating the duodenal tumors, survival in this group was 394 ± 212 days (range 158 to 677 excluding one benign villous adenoma) compared with 117 ± 89 days (9-221) for patients with gastric cancer. The only complication was anticipated cholangitis in one patient with pre-existing biliary obstruction, successfully treated by stent placement after debridement allowed identification of the exit of biliary effluent.

Laser therapy for the cure of benign villous adenomas of the ampulla of Vater has also been reported by Ponchon and colleagues in a small group of patients in 1989, with no evidence of recurrence on endoscopic follow-up from 14 to 53 months.

Colon Cancer

Most patients with colon cancer are candidates for curative or palliative resection or diverting colostomy. However, the frequency of this disorder, its spectrum of presentations, and human factors combine to give rise to several indications for laser therapy. The earliest indication, formulated by Kiefhaber, was for the relief of obstruction preoperatively, thus obviating a two- or three-stage operation and allowing for primary resection and anastomosis. For patients with incurable cancer due to metastases or local invasion, laser therapy offers an alternative to colostomy or resection. This option is particularly important for patients who are not good surgical candidates and who refuse, or may have difficulty coping with, colostomy. In addition, laser therapy may relieve symptoms of bleeding and of tenesmus due to tumor bulk, symptoms that would not be addressed by colostomy. Finally, in selected patients, laser treatment has been used as curative therapy for colon cancer. Patients in this category have mostly been poor surgical candidates for whom abdominoperineal resection was the alternative.

Laser therapy has been used for these indications both above and below the peritoneal reflection, although most therapy has been delivered for rectosigmoid cancers. Palliation has been effective in 80 to 90 percent of patients, with complications in 3 to 10 percent (consisting of perforation, bleeding, and sepsis) and death in 0 to 2.5 percent. Therapy may not be technically possible or effective with tumor encroachment on the anal canal, sphincter dysfunction, or pain due to sacral plexus involvement.

Bleeding Tumors

Laser therapy, as noted above, has been used to control bleeding from tumors. We analyzed the laser therapy of bleeding tumors in 32 patients with acute blood loss evidenced either by transfusion requirements (22 patients requiring over 6 units per patient) or a fall in hematocrit greater than 6 (two patients), or with chronic disabling hematochezia (eight patients). Tumors were located throughout the intestinal tract, and histologic diagnoses included adenocarcinoma, squamous cell carcinoma, lymphoma, renal cell carcinoma, melanoma, and two villous adenomas. Laser therapy was used because of metastatic disease in 20, recurrence after surgery in six, and severe coexistent disease in ten patients. Six patients had spurting arterial bleeding. Therapy was localized in the case of spurting arteries, or aimed at significant tumor debulking in the case of diffusely bleeding lesions. Failure to initially control bleeding occurred in only one patient. Bleeding recurred in another seven patients a mean of 90 days after initial control. Survival overall averaged 279 days and there were no complications from the laser therapy. Laser therapy was effective for tumors with either single-vessel or diffuse bleeding, including those with diffuse bleeding from extensive surfaces (e.g., tumors of greater than 8 cm in length). However, patients with large transfusion requirements (more than 4 units) and younger patients (under 65 years old) had a higher incidence of subsequent rebleeding.

Adenomas Not Amenable to Polypectomy

Impediments to successful polypectomy of sessile adenomas include certain surface characteristics (large size, flat, and soft, so that the snare "shaves" but does not grasp the tissue) and inadequate accessibility behind folds and flexures. Laser therapy may be considered for such polyps, particularly in the setting of multiple recurrences or recurrence after surgical resection. The decision to institute laser therapy should weigh factors such as risk of invasive carcinoma, adequacy of tissue sampling, age, and coexistent illness. If instituted, laser therapy is performed in conjunction with partial polypectomy of amenable portions. This technique is repeated until re-epithelialization with negative biopsies is documented, and is followed by close surveillance (with random biopsies) at incrementally longer intervals. In one of 39 patients we treated with this approach, partial polypectomy during therapy revealed an invasive cancer. In another 94-year-old nonoperative candidate, metastatic disease was discovered during therapy. These findings emphasize the importance of adequate tissue sampling (and resampling), careful patient selection, and informed consent that explains that the tissue ablated by laser therapy is not available for histologic examination. Our complications included bleeding requiring transfusion (5 percent) and a nonobstructing cecal stricture. Perforations and symptomatic stenoses have also been reported by others, and the complication rate may be proportionate to the size and circumferential extent of the tumor.

PHOTODYNAMIC THERAPY

PDT is still investigational. Destruction of tumor results from a photochemical reaction, initiated when nonthermal laser light activates drug that has concentrated within the tumor. The drug currently used is dihematoporphyrin ethers (DHE, Photofrin), which is injected intravenously 2 days before endoscopy and light application. This allows time for drug clearance from the normal tissues surrounding the tumor, thus limiting normal tissue toxicity.

An argon dye laser is used to generate the 630 nm red light necessary for drug activation. Laser fibers with a focusing microlens tip can be used to deliver a forward beam spot of light to a tumor, but fibers with a cylinder diffusing tip are more commonly used. These fiber tips deliver light circumferentially over the length of the tip and are available in tip lengths ranging from 1.0 to 2.5 cm in 0.5 cm increments. Thus, tumor segments can be treated circumferentially during a light application. A series of fiber tips of appropriate lengths are selected to cover the entire length of a tumor, treating tumor segments in a retrograde sequence.

When activated by light, the drug generates reactive singlet oxygen, which destroys tumor cells. Much of the tumor damage is vascular. Few changes are visually apparent during the light application except, at times, a barely perceptible cyanotic hue. Two days later the dead tumor tissue is debrided, and any areas with a less than optimal response can be treated with a second light application.

Table 2 Photodynamic Therapy for Early Cancer

Investigator	Site	No. of Patients	Duration Follow-Up	Complete Response (%)
Lambert (France)	Esophagus	65	21 mo	71
Oguru (Japan)	Esophagus	11	>1 yr	82
Tian (China)	Esophagus	13	24.7 mo	100
Oguru (Japan)	Stomach	30	>1 yr	93
Hayata (Japan)	Stomach	16	20.3 mo	56
Monnier (Switzerland)	Esophagus	15	20.1 mo	80

The only systemic toxicity of the drug is skin photosensitivity, which lasts about 1 month and requires patients to take precautions against sun exposure.

Esophageal Cancer

Tumors throughout the body have been treated with PDT, but in the gastrointestinal tract most attention has focused on esophageal cancer.

Light Dosimetry

At New York Medical College, we performed a light dosimetry analysis, evaluating the effects of varying quantities of light on the depth of tumor necrosis from PDT. This analysis factored in the distinction between the light dose delivered from the fiber tip (measured in joules per centimeter length of cylinder diffusing fiber tip) and the tissue dose of light (measured in joules per square centimeter of tumor tissue exposed). When the light dose is held constant, tighter tumor areas receive a more concentrated tissue dose of light and therefore undergo a greater depth of necrosis. Conversely, those areas within a tumor length that are wider (e.g., an ulcerated depressed area) and perhaps thinner walled will undergo less necrosis. The end result of therapy is a more patent and even lumen.

We found that a standardized light dose could therefore be used. The light dose selected, 300 joules per centimeter length of cylinder diffusing fiber tip, resulted in an effective range of tissue doses. Furthermore, this light dose was significantly lower than those generally used previously, minimizing the risk of fistula formation because thin-walled areas would likely be exposed to very low tissue doses.

Comparison with Nd:YAG Laser Therapy

In our randomized comparison of PDT with Nd:YAG laser therapy, the most important finding was that the duration of clinical response was longer after PDT, averaging 84 days compared with 57 days. This longer response was associated with a greater increase (at 1 month after therapy) in Karnofsky performance status and esophageal grade. Other advantages of PDT included more comfortable treatments (no burning sensation) that did not generate volumes of smoke. The nonthermal laser powers used did not damage endoscopes. The tumor selectivity of the therapy and the standardized light delivery contributed to its ease of application.

Skin photoreactions were few and relatively mild after PDT. New photosensitizers associated with shorter-duration skin sensitization are being developed.

Early Cancer and Other Gastrointestinal Cancers

The most significant clinical impact of PDT may be in the noninvasive treatment of early cancer. Its theoretic advantages are localized destruction of tumor, little systemic toxicity, and differential drug concentration between neoplastic and normal tissue. Thus, microscopic nests of cancer cells, too small to localize visually, may be efficiently eradicated by exposing the identified region of early cancer to activating light. Early cancer in the esophagus and stomach have responded very favorably (56 to 100 percent complete response rates) (Table 2) according to reports from France, Switzerland, China, and Japan and some limited experience in the United States. Follow-up intervals so far are short and some protocols have employed multimodal therapy. Nevertheless, PDT should be considered an option for the treatment of early cancer in patients who are not surgical candidates.

There have also been anecdotal reports of PDT being used to treat periampullary tumors, colon cancer, and villous adenomas. Data are too limited at this time to define indications or response rates.

BICAP TUMOR PROBE

The BICAP tumor probe delivers electrocoagulation through pairs of bipolar electrodes arranged longitudinally on the surface of an olive-shaped tip. The olives are available in a variety of diameters, and are connected distally to a spring tip and proximally to a 60 cm long shaft. This entire apparatus is then passed over a flexible guidewire. After tumor dilatation, either retrograde or prograde BICAP applications are delivered under fluoroscopic control, using distance markers along the shaft for incremental guidance. The most proximal tumor application is monitored endoscopically to ensure accurate probe placement. The applications result in a 1 to 4 mm depth of coagulation necrosis circumferentially. Debridement is performed about 48 hours later with possible repeat treatment.

Advantages of the BICAP tumor probe include rapid circumferential therapy that is particularly efficient for long tumor segments, and no associated smoke or gaseous distention. The equipment is both of lower cost and more portable than that required for laser therapy. For cervical esophageal cancers, the therapy may be technically easier to perform than laser therapy.

Disadvantages include a potentially significant complication rate, reported to be 25 percent (including 10 percent delayed hemorrhage, 10 percent fistula, and one unexplained death) in a 1987 pilot trial by Johnston and colleagues. Post-therapy strictures may occur in 5 to 13 percent because of the 360-degree burn. The probe is not recommended for asymmetric or noncircumferential tumors because of the increased danger of normal tissue injury, although a probe with a 180-degree treatment surface is available. The therapy requires fluoroscopic monitoring with attendant scheduling difficulties. The probe assembly is rigid and may not be able to negotiate tortuous angulated strictures safely. Finally, because the probes cannot be passed through endoscopes, they can be used only for esophageal and rectal tumors where they can be most easily oriented.

Despite these disadvantages, one retrospective analysis found the probe effective for circumferential esophageal tumors, especially those of considerable length or of the cervical esophagus, and noted a lower complication rate compared with low-powered delivery of laser therapy.

INJECTION THERAPY

Successful palliative esophageal tumor necrolysis with relief of dysphagia has been reported both with 3 percent polidocanol and with dehydrated ethanol injections, two agents also used for injection sclerosis of varices. Both agents are delivered by commonly available sclerotherapy injectors, with small aliquots (0.5 to 2 ml) injected at spaced intervals throughout the tumor, and with injection sessions spaced 1 week apart. Few patients have been treated to date, treatment parameters have not been standardized, and some patients analyzed received multimodal therapy. Response and complication rates remain to be defined. Apparent advantages include availability, simplicity, lack of smoke generation and gaseous distention, and low cost.

Potentially curative injection therapy has been reported by Hagiwara and colleagues. Peplomycin absorbed onto activated carbon particles was injected into superficial esophageal cancers of six patients, five of whom remained without evidence of recurrent cancer for 27 to 72 months, and one of whom has been cancer free for 8 months after a second course for a recurrence (at 27 months). The intent is to avoid systemic toxicity and maximize drug concentration both in the primary tumor and in the regional lymph nodes. Drug distribution to regional nodes was documented in rats and in a group of patients who underwent esophagectomy 1 day after injection therapy.

STENTS

Conventional rigid plastic stents have not gained general favor because of a high mortality rate associated with their passage (4 to 9 percent), a high perforation rate (5 to 18 percent), a high overall complication rate (14 to 44 percent), and the frequent inability of patients to tolerate intake beyond liquids or semisolids. In addition to perforation, acute complications include bleeding from insertion trauma, dyspnea from tracheal compression, stent malposition with occlusion by tumor, and stent migration. Acute complication rates may be lower in centers experienced in stent intubation and may be reduced by gradual dilatation over several sessions prior to insertion. Delayed complications include tissue erosion with bleeding or perforation, tumor overgrowth, stent migration, and food impaction. Stents are probably contraindicated for cervical esophageal cancer and asymmetric exophytic intraluminal tumors.

However, stents are the preferred therapy for an esophageal fistula. Furthermore, stents require a single endoscopy for placement, patients do not usually require subsequent endoscopies, and dysphagia is rapidly improved. Stents may therefore be practical when laser therapy is not possible because of extrinsic tumor compression, when the response to laser therapy is less than adequate owing to long tumors, or when further laser therapy is inappropriate because of progressive clinical deterioration.*

Cuffed stents consist of a foam rubber wrap around the proximal shaft of a conventional stent, the cuff being contained within a thin outer sheath of silicone rubber. The cuff is deflated before and during stent insertion by syringe suction through a plastic cannula that inserts into the cuff. The cuff self-inflates upon placement when the cannula is removed with a tug. These stents are useful when there is no tumor ledge to hold a conventional stent in place, as with a postradiotherapy fistula. A unique problem is that the cuff may expand through a fistula into a lung passageway, causing acute bronchial obstruction and dyspnea. We have had several of the cuffs deflate within several months, perhaps from debris trapped in the plastic cannula insertion site resulting in a one-way valve mechanism (so that the cuff may deflate with coughing but inflation is prevented). We therefore reserve these stents for special circumstances.

Self-expanding metal stents, still investigational, are available in three types: Z stents (Gianturco), Wallstents, and Nintinol mesh. Because of problems with tumor ingrowth after deployment, the first two types are currently being made with a silicone membrane. These metal stents may result in easier and less traumatic intubation because they can be compressed and deployed by small-diameter delivery tubes. Also, dysphagia may be more effectively relieved because of the stents' larger inner diameters after expansion (15 to 20 mm). Metal stents are more expensive than their plastic

---

***Editor's Note:** The chapter following this one also includes an informative discussion of stents.

counterparts. Complications have included perforation, migration, tumor overgrowth, food impaction, and torn silicone membrane with tumor ingrowth. These stents, which are currently undergoing evaluation and design modifications, are also discussed in the next chapter.

ESOPHAGEAL CANCER: SELECTION OF THERAPY*

The overall 5 year survival rate of patients diagnosed with esophageal cancer is only 6 percent. It is unfortunate that many patients presenting with dysphagia due to this disease are not good surgical candidates, often because of a combination of unresectability, coexistent disease, and poor nutritional status. In those patients selected for surgery, multiple series have documented substantial operative mortality (3 to 33 percent), considerable morbidity, and low 5 year survival (3 to 25 percent) even when lesions are deemed resectable for cure intraoperatively. Only earlier detection and perhaps improved staging will improve these dismal statistics.

If a computed tomographic (CT) scan shows no distant metastases, we continue the staging evaluation with endoscopic ultrasonography and consider bronchoscopy for proximal lesions. Although endoscopic ultrasound results have been reported to both under-stage and over-stage, it is more accurate for local assessment (i.e., depth of invasion and nodal involvement) than CT. In patients with a nontraversable lumen, the endoscopic ultrasound examination is limited to an evaluation above the obstruction. This is because sufficient predilatation of the lumen may carry inordinate risk, whereas evaluations performed after laser therapy has established luminal patency are unreliable owing to therapy-related inflammatory alterations. However, it has been demonstrated that almost 90 percent of patients with nontraversable lesions have T3 or T4 tumors.

For the patient with early esophageal cancer, surgery is the prime modality, with PDT an option for patients who refuse or are poor candidates for surgery. However, since PDT is a local therapy, it must be used in a multimodal fashion (e.g., in conjunction with radiation and chemotherapy) if regional adenopathy is documented or even likely. Thus, stage T2 patients and probably T1 patients should receive intensive adjunctive therapy even in the absence of overt adenopathy, whereas patients with carcinoma in situ may be considered for PDT alone.

Radiation therapy alone has been suggested as an alternative to surgery for many patients, since the 6 percent 5 year survival rate is similar to that reported after surgery, but without operative mortality. Furthermore, for a small group of patients with resectable tumors, Earlam and Johnson (1990) reported a 5 year

survival rate of 14 percent after radiation therapy alone. Herskovic and colleagues compared radiotherapy (5000 cGy) combined with chemotherapy (fluorouracil and cisplatin) to radiotherapy (6400 cGy) alone in 129 patients mostly with squamous cell cancer (88 percent). These patients had local regional disease as defined by CT using the old TNM classification system (none with distant metastases and only 15 percent with regional adenopathy, 88 percent T1 or T2). The study documented a modest survival advantage for combined therapy (median survival 12.5 versus 8.9 months), but at the expense of substantial toxicity. Increased survival at 2 years was emphasized, although this was based on excluding the ten patients (of the 61 receiving combined therapy) who died during the 100 day course of chemotherapy, while including another 16 patients who did not complete the chemotherapy but presumably survived at least 100 days. Only ten patients reached 2 year follow-up. The authors commented on the small fraction of patients with esophageal cancer eligible for enrollment in their study, and cautioned against extrapolating their results to the larger population of patients with this disease. Perhaps by initiating combination therapy with local ablation using PDT, the outcome of patients with local regional disease could be further improved. Using PDT in a multimodal approach, Lambert reported a 65 percent 2 year survival for patients with superficial squamous cell carcinoma.

By combining an intensive preoperative regimen of chemotherapy (cisplatin, vinblastine and 5-fluorouracil) with concurrent radiotherapy (4500 cGy), followed by transhiatal esophagectomy, Orringer and colleagues achieved a median survival of 29 months in a group of 43 patients with local regional disease (almost 50 percent had adenocarcinoma). But a more recent study by the same group (Urba and colleagues) failed to detect any increase in survival by combining a single-drug preoperative regimen (5-fluorouracil) with radiotherapy (4900 cGy) in patients with local regional adenocarcinoma, and noted marked toxicity. Preoperative radiation therapy alone has been demonstrated not to be beneficial for esophageal cancer in several randomized trials, but preoperative chemotherapy and chemoradiotherapy regimens require further evaluation.

For many patients, attempts at curative surgical resection are not warranted. This group includes patients with either invasion of adjacent structures (T4) or metastatic disease (M1 or stage IV), or with regional adenopathy (N1) associated with lesions above the carina or extensive adenopathy with lesions below the carina. These patients benefit from endoscopic therapies aimed at the rapid relief of dysphagia. We initiate therapy with PDT because of its efficacy, its ease of application, patient tolerance, and its duration of response. However, if skin photosensitivity would adversely affect an outdoor occupation or recreational lifestyle, we initiate Nd:YAG laser therapy. Furthermore, although we did not combine PDT and Nd:YAG laser therapy in our protocols, portions of those tumors with a less than optimal response to PDT may

*Editor's Note: This section provides the group's overview of available modalities, which are discussed in separate chapters in this edition.

benefit from limited Nd:YAG laser therapy. Conventional stents are reserved for patients with fistulas, deteriorating clinical status, or a poor response to either PDT or Nd:YAG laser therapy. Metal mesh stents, when improved to reduce complication rates, may ultimately achieve safe, rapid, and prolonged relief of dysphagia.

A pilot trial by Sargeant and colleagues of patients with adenocarcinoma and squamous cell carcinoma used Nd:YAG laser therapy followed by 30 Gy or 40 Gy external beam radiation. The lower dose of radiation, compared either with higher-dose radiation or with historical controls treated by laser therapy alone, was associated with prolongation of palliation and survival, warranting prospective evaluation. In a randomized study by Sander and colleagues, Nd:YAG laser therapy followed by afterloading with iridium-192 (compared with laser therapy alone) was helpful, but only in patients with squamous cell carcinoma and a high performance status. However, the authors did not recommend afterloading, as the benefit was limited to prolongation of the first dysphagia-free interval, and at the expense of shorter subsequent dysphagia-free intervals, additional endoscopies (for the afterloading therapies), prolongation of hospitalization, esophagitis, mediastinitis, and dysmotility.

The role of radiation therapy or chemotherapy for adenocarcinoma in particular, and of chemotherapy for advanced disease in general, remains unclear. Chemotherapy is generally avoided in patients with advanced cancer, because response rates are lower and these patients are less able to tolerate the associated toxicity. Nevertheless, Coia and colleagues relieved dysphagia in 23 of 30 patients with stage III or IV disease by combining radiotherapy with a single-bolus intravenous injection of mitomycin and intermittent 96 hour infusions of 5-fluorouracil (until evidence of disease progression). However, patients frequently experienced nausea, vomiting, and esophagitis. When radiotherapy or chemotherapy is planned, laser therapy is often useful initially for establishing luminal patency and subsequently for treating recurrent esophageal obstruction.

In summary, PDT and Nd:YAG laser therapy can play important roles in the schema for managing esophageal cancer, although often as part of a multimodal program. Specifically, PDT can be a noninvasive option for early cancer, and either PDT or Nd:YAG laser therapy can be a primary modality for advanced cancer. However, the best approach to esophageal cancer is individualized, with awareness of the multiple tools, improved staging, continued innovation, and an emphasis on investigational protocols.*

---

*Editor's Note: Because of the timeliness of this chapter, the novelty of some modalities, and the excellent overview of esophageal cancer management, we have included a large number of references. Some might add: The longer the reference list, the smaller the chance of one best answer.

SUGGESTED READING

Barr H, Krasner N, Raouf A, Walker RJ. Prospective randomized trial of laser therapy only and laser therapy followed by endoscopic intubation for the palliation of malignant dysphagia. Gut 1990; 31:252–258.

Brunetaud JM, Maunoury V, Cochelard D, et al. Endoscopic laser treatment for rectosigmoid adenoma: factors affecting the results. Gastroenterology 1989; 97:272–277.

Coia LR, Engstrom PF, Paul AR, et al. Long-term results of infusional 5-FU, mitomycin-C, and radiation as primary management of esophageal carcinoma. Int J Radiat Oncol Biol Phys 1991; 20:29–36.

Earlam RJ, Johnson L. 101 oesophageal cancers: a surgeon uses radiotherapy. Ann R Coll Surg Engl 1990; 72:32–40.

Fleischer D, Sivak MV. Endoscopic Nd:YAG laser therapy as palliation for esophagogastric cancer. Parameters affecting initial outcome. Gastroenterology 1985; 89:827–831.

Hagiwara A, Takahashi T, Kojima O, et al. Endoscopic local injection of a new drug delivery format of peplomycin for superficial esophageal cancer: a pilot study. Gastroenterology 1993; 104: 1037–1043.

Heier SK, Leibowitz KA, Rothman K. Palliative endoscopic laser therapy of noncardiac gastroduodenal tumors. Gastrointest Endosc 1990; 36:192.

Heier SK, Chang P, Rothman K, et al. Laser therapy for the control of tumor bleeding: results and factors influencing outcome. Gastrointest Endosc 1991; 37:283.

Heier SK, Bigornia E, Antonelle R, et al. Laser therapy of adenomas not amenable to polypectomy. Gastrointest Endosc 1993; 39:297.

Heier SK, Rothman K, Heier LM, Rosenthal WS. Randomized trial and light dosimetry of palliative photodynamic therapy. Gastrointest Endosc 1992; 38:279.

Herskovic A, Martz K, Al-Sarraf M, et al. Combined chemotherapy and radiotherapy compared with radiotherapy alone in patients with cancer of the esophagus. N Engl J Med 1992; 326:1593–1598.

Jensen DM, Machicado G, Randall G, et al. Comparison of low-power YAG laser and BICAP tumor probe for palliation of esophageal cancer strictures. Gastroenterology 1988; 94:1263–1270.

Johnston JH, Fleischer D, Petrini J, Nord HJ. Palliative bipolar electrocoagulation therapy of obstructing esophageal cancer. Gastrointest Endosc 1987; 33(5):349–353.

Kozarek RA, Ball TJ, Patterson DJ. Metallic self-expanding stent application in the upper gastrointestinal tract: caveats and concerns. Gastrointest Endosc 1992; 38:1–6.

Lambert R. Endoscopic therapy of esophago-gastric tumors. Endoscopy 1992; 24:24–33.

Loizou LA, Grigg D, Atkinson M, et al. A prospective comparison of laser therapy and intubation in endoscopic palliation for malignant dysphagia. Gastroenterology 1991; 100:1303–1310.

Orringer MB, Forastiere AA, Perez-Tamayo C, et al. Chemotherapy and radiation therapy before transhiatal esophagectomy for esophageal carcinoma. Ann Thorac Surg 1990; 49:348–355.

Payne-James JJ, Spiller RC, Misiewicz JJ, Silk DBA. Use of ethanol-induced tumor necrosis to palliate dysphagia in patients with esophagogastric cancer. Gastrointest Endosc 1990; 36:43–46.

Ponchon T, Berger F, Chavaillon A, et al. Contribution of endoscopy to diagnosis and treatment of tumors of the ampulla of Vater. Cancer 1989; 64:161–167.

Sander R, Hagenmueller F, Sander C, et al. Laser versus laser plus afterloading with iridium-192 in the palliative treatment of malignant stenosis of the esophagus: a prospective, randomized, and controlled study. Gastrointest Endosc 1991; 37:433–440.

Sargeant IR, Loizou LA, Tobias JS, et al. Radiation enhancement of laser palliation for malignant dysphagia: a pilot study. Gut 1992; 33:1597–1601.

Schaer J, Katon RM, Ivancev K, et al. Treatment of malignant esophageal obstruction with silicone-coated metallic self-expanding stents. Gastrointest Endosc 1992; 38:7–11.

Urba SG, Orringer MB, Perez-Tamayo C, et al. Concurrent preoperative chemotherapy and radiation therapy in localized esophageal adenocarcinoma. Cancer 1992; 69:285–291.

PALLIATION OF ESOPHAGEAL CANCER: DILATATION, STENTS, AND OTHER MODALITIES

MOUNES DAKKAK, M.D., Ph.D., M.R.C.P.
JOHN R. BENNETT, M.D., F.R.C.P.

Carcinoma of the esophagus becomes symptomatic late in its natural history. Consequently, many patients on initial presentation are unsuitable for curative treatment or unfit for radical surgery. Recent developments of more sophisticated imaging (endoscopic ultrasonography, magnetic resonance imaging) only help in accurate selection of the few patients who may benefit from curative treatment, but the fact remains that most patients are in need of palliation.

Untreated carcinoma of the esophagus inevitably leads from progressive dysphagia to dehydration and malnutrition. Therefore, the principal aim of palliative therapy is to provide adequate nutrition, usually by creating and maintaining a patent esophageal lumen.

Over the years, several methods have emerged. Some, such as intracavitary irradiation and laser therapy, are discussed in other chapters.

SIMPLE DILATATION

The advantage of simple dilatation is its simplicity, since it can be performed during the initial diagnostic procedure. A variety of instruments can be used, including bougies (Eder-Puestow, Tridil, Celestin, Savary-Gilliard, or Key-Med Advanced dilators) and hydrostatic balloons. The maximal diameter of each of these dilators is 17 to 20 mm. Patients are usually kept under observation for a few hours after the procedure.

The risk of perforation, although higher than in dilatation of benign strictures, is relatively small. The disadvantage of this method is its short longevity: repeat dilatation is usually required within 2 to 3 weeks, which creates great inconvenience for the patient, is a great burden on the endoscopist, and multiplies the risk of perforation. In certain cases, when the tumor may be growing slowly, it may still be a viable option. We often use a few bougie dilatations with the Key-Med Advanced or Savary-Gilliard dilators, but if the need for repeat dilatation arises within 2 to 3 weeks we do not persist.

ENDOPROSTHESES (STENTS)

One of the first attempts to create an endoprosthesis for esophageal tumors may be that of the Frenchman Leroy d'Etiolles in 1845, who used decalcified ivory to make short tubes, but his effort was doomed to failure. The first success did not come until 1885 when Sir Charter Symonds successfully inserted a 6 inch tube surgically under direct vision, but it was not until 1914 that tubes were inserted surgically with the aid of an introducer. Over the following years, a variety of stents were designed for surgical or endoscopic insertion (Table 1).

Purely palliative intubation via surgical gastrostomy caused a disproportionate number of deaths (up to 15 percent). During the late 1960s and the 1970s, when endoscopy became more widespread and flexible fiberoptic instruments became available, the emphasis changed from surgical toward endoscopic placement of stents, thereby reducing morbidity and mortality rates.

Selection of Stents

After years of experimentation with different materials, stents are now made of inert material resistant to denaturation and to both gastrointestinal secretions and irradiation, even if they remain in place for more than 2 years. The currently popular materials are silicone rubber (Atkinson tube), Tygon (used for self-made tubes in Amsterdam), and reinforced silicone (Wilson-Cook). Latex, which is now available in a new reinforced design (Celestin-Medoc), is still tarnished with earlier problems of denaturation and release of the coil. In reality, stents now outlive patients.

The diameter of commercially available stents is 11 to 12 mm. The length of the stent to be inserted will depend on endoscopic measurement of the length of the tumor. The stent should be 4 cm longer than the tumor, allowing 2 cm above and 2 cm below. All currently available stents have shoulders or corrugations to prevent proximal migration, and all have individually designed introducers and a pushing extension (Fig. 1).

We use the Atkinson tube with the Nottingham introducer, but other stents and introducers follow broadly the same basic principles. The Nottingham introducer is one of the few that can also be used for withdrawing or extracting the prosthetic tubes, while other systems require an alternative arrangement such as a balloon or snare.

Stents for Tracheoesophageal Fistulas

There are stents surrounded by a cuff of polyurethane sponge material that can be used to close a tracheoesophageal fistula associated with an esophageal tumor. No other treatment is suitable for this hazardous situation.

Procedure

The procedure is usually performed with the patient under sedation with a benzodiazepine, occasionally supplemented with an opiate. On rare occasions, general anesthesia is used. Although the procedure is endoscopic, the use of radiologic screening is essential.

After bougie dilatation of the tumor to 18 mm (54 Fr), the prosthetic tube, mounted on the introducer, is

Table 1 Palliative Stents

Stent	Year	Material
Symmonds	1885	Boxwood and ivory
Guisez	1914	?
Souttar	1924	Gold plated/German silver
Brown	1949	Silver
Kropff	1954	Polyethylene/Resinyl
Mackler	1954	Polyvinyl
Coyas	1955	Polyvinyl
Holinger	1955	Polyvinyl
Mousseau-Barbin	1956	Neoplex
Carter	1957	Polyethylene
Sachs	1959	Nylon
Celestin	1959	Polyethylene/spiral reinforced latex rubber
Weisel	1959	Polyethylene
Gourevitch	1959	Latex rubber
Coni	1964	Polyethylene
Haring	1964	Latex rubber with stainless steel
Stirnemann	1965	Porflex
Procter-Livingston	1968	Armored latex rubber
Palmer	1970	Tygon
Collis	1971	Stainles steel
Didcott	1973	Expanding stainless steel covered with rubber
Tytgat	1976	Tygon
Atkinson	1978	Silastic rubber
Jaeger	1979	Tygon
Frimberger	1983	Expanding metal mesh
Wilson-Cook	?	Silicone reinforced with metal spiral
Buess	1988	Silicone with embedded metal spiral
Domschke	1990	Self-expanding steel mesh
Kozarek	1992	Steel mesh with or without silicone cover
Schaer	1992	Steel mesh covered with silicone
Ultraflex	1992	Steel mesh with dissolvable gelatine

inserted under radiologic guidance. The desired position is obtained using a combination of endoscopic measurement and radiologic screening, before the stent is released. It is good practice then to use a narrow endoscope to inspect the esophagus, passing through the stent to the stomach to ensure a satisfactory position.

Complications

Perforation. This is the greatest hazard and the most immediate. The figures are variable, but 9 percent, which is quoted in one large survey, is representative. The more skillful and careful operators are not immune, but they may have a lower rate of complications (our perforation rate over the last 5 years is 4 percent). Prophylactic intravenous antibiotics at the time of the procedure, early recognition of the leak, and active conservative management ensure the survival of most patients who sustain perforation.

Aspiration. This may occur during the procedure or afterward as a result of heavy sedation or nursing of patients in the supine position. Adequate care during and after the procedure would reduce this risk.

Migration. With modern stents this happens, only occasionally in either a proximal or distal direction, because of the special features designed to reduce this

possibility. Displaced stents are repositioned or removed and then reinserted.

Bolus Obstruction. This can be avoided if the patient is provided with satisfactory diet advice, particularly as regards drinking plentifully with meals.

Reflux. This occurs when the stent is in the lower esophagus as a result of bridging of the gastroesophageal junction. Advice on posture and symptomatic treatment are usually adequate. Survival is rarely long enough for significant esophagitis to develop.

Overgrowth of Tumor. This necessitates replacement with a longer stent. Endoscopic therapy (by laser or alcohol injection) needs to be applied to the overgrowing tumor before extraction of the stent. A longer stent will then be required as a replacement.

Erosion of the Esophageal Wall. Erosion leading to a fistula or bleeding is another rare complication.

Limitations of Stents

Angulated Tumors. These lead to bending of the stent, which may partially block its lumen or promote its migration.

Problems of Anatomy. Once in place, the stent may have its distal end opening against the gastric wall. This tends to be a problem with patients who have had

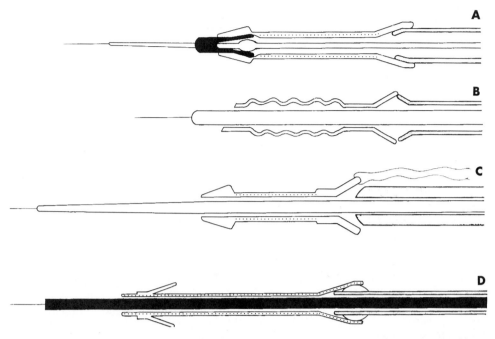

Figure 1 Esophageal stents and their delivery system. *A,* Nottingham introducer and Atkinson tube. *B,* Amsterdam metal introducer and Tygon tube. *C,* Dumon-Gilliard introducer and Wilson-Cook tube. *D,* Medoc introducer and Celestin tube. (From Atkinson M. Endoscopic intubation of oesophageal malignant obstruction. In Bennett JR, Hunt RH, eds. Therapeutic endoscopy and radiology of the gut. London: Chapman and Hall, 1990; with permission.)

a partial or total gastrectomy, but it also occurs when a stent is angulated through the cardia against the greater curvature of an intact stomach.

Tumors of the Upper Esophagus. When the upper margin of a tumor is within 5 cm of the cricopharyngeal sphincter, it is unlikely that a stent will be tolerated, despite some modification of its funnel.

Restricted Diet. Patients are forced to accept some limitation of diet to avoid bolus obstruction.

Advantages

Advantages of stenting include the following: (1) it is better than thermal techniques for nonexophytic tumors and external compression, (2) no further procedure is required in most cases, (3) hospitalization is limited to a few days after the procedure, and (4) economically, it is much cheaper than other methods of palliation.

NEW STENTS

More than one attempt has been made over the last 20 years to introduce expanding metal mesh stents (Didcott in 1973 and Frimberger in 1983), but these never achieved popularity. Over the last few years, the interest has re-emerged, and a few reports have been published concerning metallic self-expanding stents in esophageal neoplastic strictures, after their introduction

for biliary strictures. These are made of surgical-grade stainless steel alloy filaments woven in a tubular mesh; some are covered with silicone. The metallic stent is delivered to its intended position folded and compressed in a plastic sheath, before it is released. It expands when the constraint is removed, or (in some versions) when a gelatine layer is dissolved by moisture.

These stents are now available commercially but are several times more expensive than the traditional stents. They may prove superior in being better tolerated in the upper esophagus and in permitting patients to avoid diet restriction. It is also claimed that they are less likely to migrate or cause perforation, but all these claims remain to be substantiated in randomized trials. One drawback is that a metal stent cannot be removed after insertion, but another one could be inserted to overlap the first stent if there were tumor overgrowth.

ELECTROCOAGULATION (BICAP)

The BICAP tumor probe system consists of a series of staffs with different-sized metal olives through which thermal energy is delivered by in-built electrodes. The probe is passed over a guidewire, and electrocoagulation is applied (circumferentially or noncircumferentially) at several levels of the tumor. There are very limited data to allow comparison between BICAP and laser therapy, but BICAP is easy to use, substantially cheaper, and more portable than laser. Their efficacy is probably

Table 2 Palliative Modalities

	Dilatation	Stent	Met. Stent	Laser	BICAP	Alcohol
Approximate number of procedures	+ + + +	+	+	+ + +	+ + +	+ + +
Cumulative hospital stay	+ + +	+ +	? +	+ + +	+ + +	+ + +
Diet restriction	+	+ +	+	+	+	+
Complications	+	+ + +	?	+	+ +	+ +
Cost	±	+	+ +	+ + +	+	±
Need for special endoscopic training	+	+ +	+ +	+ + +	+ +	+ +

± indicates that the cost above basic endoscopy is very minimal.

equivalent, but there may be more complications such as fistula formation, particularly when the tumor is asymmetric. Hemorrhage has also been reported, but we have not encountered this. Like laser, BICAP has the disadvantage of requiring repeated applications.

We use the BICAP probe, often in conjunction with ethanol injections, for predominantly exophytic tumors.

INJECTION THERAPY

Injection of dehydrated ethanol can induce considerable tumor necrosis. This can be done endoscopically using a needle passed through the operative channel of the endoscope. The method is cheap and effective and may not be less safe than laser or BICAP, but it also tends to require repeated applications. There is a lack of comparative trials to evaluate this method against other techniques, although one comparative study showed endoscopic tumor injection with polidocanol to be as effective as laser therapy. Injection therapy may prove to be a complementary rather than primary therapy.

Results from pilot studies of cytotoxic agents such as 5-fluorouracil injected endoscopically into tumors are not encouraging.

OTHER METHODS

Laser therapy and irradiation are discussed in earlier chapters. Percutaneous endoscopic gastrostomy may occasionally be used as a method to provide nutrition in selected patients.

COMMENTS

The ideal palliative technique for esophageal carcinoma would provide normal swallowing for the patient's remaining days by a method that is quick, safe, and painless, needing only a short inpatient stay and having a low complication rate. There is now a wide choice of

techniques (Table 2). None of these is ideal, but there is an opportunity to select the most appropriate for individual patients. Palliative techniques can be complementary, and although studies are needed to compare different techniques, they should not necessarily be seen to be competitive. Different luminal palliative techniques can also be offered in conjunction with irradiation, either intracavitary (brachytherapy) or external beam. Unfortunately, comparative trials remain scanty and inadequate in numbers and design and are sometimes clouded by enthusiasm for a specific method.

SUGGESTED READING

Angelini G, Fratta Pasini A, Ederle A, et al. Nd:YAG laser versus polidocanol injection for palliation of esophageal malignancy: a prospective, randomized study. Gastrointest Endosc 1991; 37: 607–610.

Bown SG. Palliation of malignant dysphagia: surgery, radiotherapy, laser, intubation alone or in combination. Gut 1991; 32:841–844.

Cox J, Bennett JR. Light at the end of the tunnel? Palliation for oesophageal carcinoma. Gut 1987; 28:781–785.

Cox JGC, Dakkak M, Buckton GK, Bennett JR. Dilators for esophageal stricture: description of a new bougie and a comparison of current instruments. Gastrointest Endosc 1989; 35:551–554.

Dakkak M, Bennett JR. Balloon technology in endoscopy. Baillieres Clin Gastroenterol 1991; 5:195–208.

Jensen DM, Machicado G, Randall G, et al. Comparison of low-power YAG laser and BICAP tumor probe for palliation of esophageal cancer strictures. Gastroenterology 1988; 94:1263–1270.

Johnston JH, Fleischer D, Petrini J, et al. Palliative bipolar electrocoagulation therapy of obstructing esophageal cancer. Gastrointest Endosc 1988; 33:349–353.

Kozarek RA, Ball TJ, Patterson DJ. Metallic self-expanding stent application in the upper gastrointestinal tract: caveats and concerns. Gastrointest Endosc 1992; 38:1–6.

Loizou LA, Grigg D, Atkinson M, et al. A prospective comparison of laser therapy and intubation in endoscopic palliation for malignant dysphagia. Gastroenterology 1991; 100:1303–1310.

Payne-James JJ, Spiller RC, Misiewicz JJ, et al. Use of ethanol-induced tumor necrosis to palliate dysphagia in patients with esophagogastric cancer. Gastrointest Endosc 1990; 36:43–46.

Schaer J, Katon RM, Ivancev K, et al. Treatment of malignant esophageal obstruction with silicone-coated metallic self-expanding stents. Gastrointest Endosc 1992; 38:7–11.

STOMACH AND DUODENUM

LAPAROSCOPIC SURGICAL PROCEDURES: PRESENT AND FUTURE

MARK A. TALAMINI, M.D.

General surgery and alimentary tract surgery has traditionally been a conservative specialty. For many years, surgeons practicing in this area have stood on the sidelines and watched while other specialties took full advantage of technologic advances. The advent of laparoscopic cholecystectomy changed this situation. This single procedure took the world of general surgery by storm. Within a span of two years, nearly the entire general surgery work force had been retrained in this procedure. Within that time interval, it has become the standard of care. The creative process of extending this technology to other areas of the abdomen and the gastrointestinal (GI) tract began as soon as surgeons became comfortable with the laparoscopic view of the abdomen.

The laparoscopic revolution has provided tremendous benefits for patients. The amount of pain is diminished, hospitalization is reduced, scars are less disfiguring, and the physiologic insult to the body as a whole is significantly diminished. However, some key elements of open surgery are missing in laparoscopic surgery, creating at least a marginal detriment. The surgeon cannot use the normal tactile sensation in his fingers to evaluate tissue directly. Similarly, the entire abdomen cannot be viewed at once, diminishing the ability to compare one piece of bowel to another. Perhaps most important, the normal three-dimensional relationships of tissues, as seen in the open abdomen, are absent, forcing the surgeon to evaluate in a two-dimensional plane, using other cues to gain three-dimensional information. All of these detriments are slowly being overcome by the application of technology. The defense industry and the space industry have made use of the significant advances in electronics to enhance human sensory abilities in situations such as air-to-air combat and tank warfare. We are now seeing the beginning of an era where these applications are being used to enhance minimally invasive surgery. Progress may be somewhat inhibited by budget restrictions, which are becoming more limiting each day. It does appear, however, that the use of such technology will make current laparoscopic procedures safer and allow us to broaden our abilities and approach new problems with minimally invasive surgery.

The issues of training and credentialing have indeed been troublesome. Fortunately, these issues will fade as we train new generations of laparoscopic surgeons in surgical training programs. The primary challenge is training the existing fleet of general surgeons with these new technologies. The advanced procedures discussed in this chapter are considerably more difficult than laparoscopic cholecystectomy. Advanced procedures, such as laparoscopic colectomy, should not be undertaken by surgeons who have not had a significant period of adjustment with a simpler procedure such as laparoscopic cholecystectomy or laparoscopic appendectomy. It appears that the best method for training currently practicing general surgeons involves the use of a proctoring period. In this setting, a surgeon skilled in laparoscopic surgery assists a learning surgeon until the trainee surgeon demonstrates safe handling of the instruments and equipment, as well as appropriate surgical judgement when using laparoscopic equipment.

It is the purpose of this brief chapter to review the current state of laparoscopic GI surgery and to make some predictions regarding the future of this tremendously exciting new avenue open to surgeons (Table 1).

LAPAROSCOPIC CHOLECYSTECTOMY

Laparoscopic cholecystectomy led the laparoscopic surgery revolution for a number of reasons. First, it is a relatively easy procedure to perform, making it feasible for large numbers of general surgeons to learn rapidly. Second, it is the most common intraabdominal operation performed in the United States, and therefore there was no shortage of clinical material. Third, the advantages for patients undergoing this procedure are obvious. Hospital stay is reduced from 5 days to 1 day, and the period of disability is reduced from 6 weeks to around 1 week.

Table 1 New Laparoscopic Procedures

Biliary Tree
Cholecystectomy
Laparoscopic management of common bile duct stones
Common bile duct exploration

Acid reduction
Anterior seromyotomy, posterior truncal vagotomy
Anterior highly selective vagotomy, posterior truncal vagotomy
Traditional highly selective vagotomy

Antireflux surgery
Nissen fundoplication
Toupet procedure

Bowel surgery
Small bowel resection
Feeding-access procedures
Crohn's resection
Resection of difficult polyps
Resection of adenocarcinoma

Hernia
Transperitoneal herniorrhaphy
Pro-peritoneal herniorrhaphy

As the saying goes, "There is no free lunch." This is true with respect to laparoscopic cholecystectomy. The price of laparoscopic cholecystectomy has been an increase in the incidence of common bile duct injury relative to injury from open cholecystectomy. Although precise numbers are difficult to obtain, it appears that the duct injury rate in open cholecystectomy is somewhere between one in 500 and one in 1,000. In the early series of laparoscopic cholecystectomy, the duct injury rate appears to be between one in 250 and one in 500. There is no question that for patients undergoing cholecystectomy in this country, laparoscopic cholecystectomy has been a tremendous advance, retaining countless potential lost work hours in the economy and eliminating many thousands of hours of patient discomfort and pain. The other side of the coin, however, is the incidence of a few patients who suffer bile duct injuries requiring extensive reconstructive surgery. The more recent series have had a lower duct injury incidence, suggesting that some of the early high numbers were related to a "learning curve."

Several controversies exist regarding laparoscopic cholecystectomy. Perhaps the most intensively debated issue is the issue of routine interoperative cholangiography. Routine cholangiography was debated in the era of open cholecystectomy. In recent years, fewer routine cholangiograms (without specific indications such as duct size or elevated liver function tests) have been performed, primarily because of the efficacy of endoscopic retrograde cholangiopancreatography (ERCP), sphincterotomy, and endoscopic stone extraction. The technology for laparoscopic cholecystectomy has re-opened this debate. It has been claimed that routine cholangiography in laparoscopic cholecystectomy has the additional benefit of revealing the ductal anatomy, potentially reducing the possibility of ductal injury.

It has *not* been our practice to perform routine cholangiography at Johns Hopkins. We have followed a protocol of preoperative screening of patients using liver function chemistries. Those suspected of having common duct stones undergo ERCP and papillotomy with stone extraction, if indicated, preoperatively. Stones found intraoperatively or postoperatively have been managed with postoperative ERCP and papillotomy. Using this protocol, we have always been able to clear a patient of common duct stones and have not had to perform a single surgical bile duct exploration. Given the current state of technology, we believe this protocol to be superior to laparoscopic common bile duct exploration. In terms of duct injury, the technique of laparoscopic cholangiography requires clipping of the structure in question followed by incision and placement of a catheter for the cholangiogram. If the common duct has been mistaken for the cystic duct, an injury will have occurred owing to the performance of the cholangiogram. It is our contention that the existence of confusing or ambiguous anatomy should indicate the necessity of open laparotomy, rather than cholangiography.

A recent review of the experience with laparoscopic cholecystectomy in the state of Connecticut revealed that a cholangiogram was performed in only 15 percent of cases. This suggests that most surgeons are not performing routine cholangiography during laparoscopic cholecystectomy.

A separate chapter on laparoscopic cholecystectomy appears later in this volume.

COMMON BILE DUCT EXPLORATION

Many laparoscopic surgeons have moved aggressively in the field of laparoscopic common bile duct exploration. This category of therapy encompasses a spectrum of procedures. On the simple end of the spectrum is fluoroscopically guided manipulation of the biliary tree through the cystic duct. With this approach, the cystic duct is dilated progressively with a series of wires and dilators until a basket catheter or a choledochoscope can be placed through the cystic duct into the common bile duct. Stones can then be successfully extracted from above. Other surgeons have performed actual choledochotomy using laparoscopic equipment, followed by placement of a T-tube and closure of the common duct with laparoscopic suturing. Both of these approaches require sophisticated equipment and an additional increment of skill with regard to laparoscopic manipulation.

At Johns Hopkins, our approach to laparoscopic duct exploration has been conservative. Our patients have been well served, thus far, by a protocol of preoperative or postoperative ERCP, papillotomy, and stone extraction in the event of common duct calculi. Furthermore, we have utmost respect for surgical manipulation of the common duct and believe that this will probably be one of the later areas of laparoscopic procedure in our experience. Such an approach may make good sense in a patient with long-standing duct obstruction and a large dilated common duct with thick walls. In such a case, operating on the common duct would not be dissimilar to laparoscopic bowel surgery. On the other hand, a 3- to 5-mm thin-walled common duct must be treated with the utmost surgical respect, and, in our judgement, that requires an open surgical procedure.

UPPER GASTROINTESTINAL TRACT SURGERY

Many of the surgical procedures performed for benign disease of the upper GI tract have fallen into disuse over the last decade, as medical therapeutics have advanced. Surgery for symptoms of ulcer disease, for instance, has become a rare procedure, even in large centers. Similarly, surgery for esophageal reflux has dwindled away as antiacid medications have made symptoms less and less severe. The advent of laparoscopic procedures for these types of diseases may change this equation. There will probably be a set of patients who would prefer undergoing a minimally invasive surgical procedure rather than taking long-term, expensive medications with frequent physician visits and endoscopic procedures. We will probably not know the ultimate place of these new laparoscopic techniques until the procedures have been perfected, until large series have been published and followed, and until the gastroenterologists have become familiar with these procedures and their potential benefits.

A number of procedures have been pursued for symptomatic ulcer disease. In Europe, the seromyotomy approach has been used in open surgery. A laparoscopic approach using this technique consists of a posterior truncal vagotomy and anterior seromyotomy. In this country, Zucker and Bailey have pioneered the use of a posterior truncal vagotomy combined with an anterior highly selective vagotomy. Lately, many surgeons have moved toward performing a standard highly selective vagotomy along both the anterior and posterior trunk of the vegas nerve. This has become possible as instruments and surgical techniques have improved over the ensuing 3 years of laparoscopic surgical experience. One of the difficulties with all of these procedures is that, thus far, patients have been few and far between, not allowing any one surgical group to gain extensive experience. Another difficulty is evaluating the success of these procedures. It is difficult enough to convince a patient to undergo gastric acid analysis before surgery; it is nearly impossible to convince them to repeat the analysis after surgery.

One potential problem is mild gastric atony from the posterior complete truncal vagotomy. In our patients this has not been a long-term problem. It has resolved over time through the use of promotility agents, and in most instances even these agents have been stopped, eventually. The patients that have undergone this procedure have been able to stop taking their proton pump inhibitors or H_2 blockers and have been grateful.

Laparoscopic *antireflux procedures* hold great promise for the future. The availability of an antireflux procedure that creates a minimal amount of pain and only a few days' hospitalization would be of tremendous benefit for many patients who suffer from this vexing problem. A laparoscopic approach to this problem is very similar to cholecystectomy in that the identical operation is being performed. The esophagus is dissected clean for a length of 4 to 5 cm. The short gastric vessels on the fundus of the stomach are ligated and divided, and a bougie dilator is placed in the esophagus so that the wrap is not too tight. The vagus nerves are protected. The fundus is wrapped around the esophagus onto itself and secured with sutures. Finally, the diaphragmatic defect is closed.

A series of 16 laparoscopic Nissen fundoplications was reported at the 1993 American Gastroenterological Association meeting. Patients were discharged at an average of 3.5 days after surgery. Eighty-eight percent reported a "cure" with regard to their symptoms. Additional series have been presented with similar results.

SMALL BOWEL PROCEDURES

The small bowel tasks that can be approached laparoscopically consist primarily of procedures for feeding. Laparoscopically assisted Roux-en-Y feeding jejunostomies have been performed with good success, causing a minimum discomfort and difficulty for the patient. Experience is also growing with resection of small bowel affected by Crohn's disease. In our hands, a number of patients have undergone resection of the terminal ileum with ileo-ascending colostomy. These patients have done well, with rapid discharge from the hospital. One significant advantage of this approach is that it leaves the remainder of the abdomen largely unaffected by adhesions for potential future procedures. With current laparoscopic instrumentation, it is possible to evaluate the entire small bowel with an appropriately gentle bowel instrument.

With all bowel procedures, there are a number of options available for reanastomosing the bowel. Technologies are available to actually suture an anastomosis within the abdominal cavity using laparoscopic instruments. In the case of Crohn's disease, the technical aspects of the reanastomosis must be perfect. For this reason, in our series we have performed laparoscopically assisted procedures where the ends of the bowel have been sewn together on the abdominal wall through a 3-cm incision at the umbilicus. Therefore, the patient has only a 3-cm umbilical incision, two 1-cm port incisions (usually above the symphysis pubis and in the upper midline), and one 5-mm incision that simply needs to be taped closed.

COLON AND RECTUM

The most common surgical procedures performed on the colon and rectum are for tumors. Herein lies a significant controversy with respect to laparoscopic surgery. Most laparoscopic surgeons believe that they can perform just as complete a cancer operation using the laparoscope as can be performed open. There are challenges, however, such as removing the specimen without allowing tumor cells to spread in the peritoneal cavity, or performing a careful palpation examination of the remainder of the colon. These issues are troublesome. A number of prospective randomized studies are currently being carried out to compare 5-year survival rates and recurrence rates with laparoscopic versus open techniques. In the interim, patients desiring these procedures must be fully informed of the potential risks and the newness of the procedures.

On the other hand, there is no doubt that patients who can have surgical procedures performed using minimally invasive techniques suffer less pain, are out of the hospital more quickly, and seem able to return to a regular diet more rapidly. It is not clear why there should be less of a postoperative ileus when an abdominal procedure is being performed through keyholes rather than through an incision, but this does appear to be the case.

There are situations where malignancy is not pertinent. For instance, individuals with large unresectable polyps in dangerous areas of the colon, such as the cecum, are excellent candidates for a laparoscopic approach. Similarly, individuals with colon cancer in the setting of known incurable metastatic disease are excellent candidates. The surgical portion of the therapy will be less disruptive to their quality of life.

There are a variety of methods for reanastomosing the bowel. Totally intracorporeal anastamoses are the most difficult. Low anterior resections have been accomplished using a stapling device placed transanally. The more commonly used laparoscopically assisted approach consists of dissecting the colon from surrounding tissues, freeing it so that it is tethered only by the mesentery. A small 2- to 3-cm incision is then made that includes one of the port entry sites. The colon is extracted through this incision, and the bowel is then resected and sewn back together. The patient has only three puncture sites and a 2- to 3-cm incision. As technology continues to advance, I believe the laparoscopic approach to reanastomosing the bowel will become more and more sophisticated, virtually removing the need to sew the bowel together using a small incision. A problem with all of these approaches is the safe and efficient removal of the specimen. Some surgeons have actually removed low-colon specimens through the rectum prior to anastomosis. The more commonly used approach is to place the specimen in a plastic bag while inside the abdomen, and then remove the plastic bag through a small incision. In this case, compressing the tissue will not result in tumor spread throughout the peritoneal cavity.

A series of 40 prospectively studied laparoscopically assisted colectomies was recently reported in the *Lancet.* Thirty-five of these patients had colorectal cancer, five had benign conditions. Resection margins

and lymph nodes in resected specimens (average, 10) all seemed acceptable. Postoperative stay averaged 8 days (range, 5 to 14). This and other series suggest that this procedure is possible, safe, and probably does not compromise traditional resection objectives for cancer surgery. It was emphasized, however, that obesity can make the procedure difficult, and tumor fixation may make it impossible.

HERNIA REPAIR

Hernia repair is one of the most commonly performed general surgical procedures. For this reason, it was an early and obvious target for a fresh laparoscopic approach. Once again, the effort focused upon providing a less painful procedure that allows an early return to normal activity more quickly. This procedure has had a significant evolution as laparoscopic surgeons have progressed in their experience. Early on, hernia defects were "stuffed" with polypropylene mesh and covered with a patch. Currently, the most commonly performed procedure includes approaching the hernia through the peritoneal cavity. A trap door or window of peritoneum is dissected from the area of the hernia. The hernia sack is either divided or dissected out from the defect. The key structures, Cooper's ligament, the iliopubic tract, and the transversus abdominis arch are identified clearly. A piece of synthetic mesh is placed over the defect and stapled in place. This is similar to covering a pot hole with a sheet of steel in the winter time. Care must be taken to protect the vas deferens and the spermatic vessels that comprise the cord structures. Once the patch is in place, it is covered once again with peritoneum to avoid adhesions between the mesh and bowel from the abdominal cavity.

Early experience with this procedure has been quite favorable, with low recurrence rates and superior patient comfort, even when compared with outpatient tension-free repairs. There are a number of prospective randomized trials currently being performed. A recently reported series by Corbitt discussed 180 patients with a recurrence rate of 1 percent. Another series, presented recently at a meeting by Arregui of Indianapolis, discussed 678 patients from a number of centers with a recurrence rate of 0.5 percent. Both of these series are early with an average 2 years of follow-up. A hernia repair is generally judged to be successful only when we know 10-year recurrence rates, and these are obviously not available at this time. The clear disadvantages of this procedure are that it requires invasion of the peritoneal cavity and general anesthesia. Most standard hernia repairs are now done with local anesthesia and sedation techniques, or a regional technique.

It is extremely important that patients desiring this procedure have the risks, benefits, and the newness of the procedure explained to them in great detail before they agree.

Table 2 Laparoscopic Procedures: The Future

Esophagectomy
Hepatico jejunostomy
Whipple procedure
Distal pancreatectomy
Gastrectomy
Cystectomy and ileal conduit
Ileo-anal pull-through

Table 3 Laparoscopic Procedures: Areas of Controversy

Routine versus selective cholangiography during laparoscopic
  cholecystectomy
Role of ERCP with laparoscopic cholecystectomy
Adequacy of cancer procedures via laparoscopy
Training and credentialling of surgeons
Expense of disposable materials

ERCP = endoscopic retrograde cholangiopancreatography.

THE FUTURE

General surgeons have spent much of the last three years experimenting with this brand-new minimally invasive technology in a quest to answer the question, "What can we do?" Recent poster presentations at national meetings have demonstrated that we can do virtually any procedure using laparoscopic equipment (Table 2). For instance, laparoscopic Whipple procedures and laparoscopic hepatojejunostomy have been reported. Laparoscopic esophagectomy has also been performed. It is now time for us to determine which of these procedures should be performed. This is a much slower and more deliberative process that will require well-designed clinical trials carried out by skilled surgeons. This new area of general surgery has provided tremendous benefits to patients in terms of reduced pain and disability. We hope to see these advantages extended to many other disease processes and many additional patients. It is imperative, however, that patient safety comes first, and that careful prospective randomized trials provide the answers as to which procedures should move forward (Table 3).

SUGGESTED READING

Bittner HO, Brazer SR, Myers WC, et al. Laparoscopic Nissen fundoplication: Operative results and short term follow up. SSAT May 17–19, 1993. Boston, Massachusetts.
Monson JRT, Darzi A, Carey PC, et al. Prospective evaluation of laparoscopic-assisted colectomy (LAC) in an unselected group of patients. Lancet 1992; 340:831.
Orlando R III, Russell JC, Lynch J, et al. Laparoscopic cholecystectomy: A statewide experience. Arch Surg 1993; 128: 494–499.
Zucker KA. Surgical laparoscopy update 1993.

HELICOBACTER PYLORI GASTRODUODENAL DISEASE

MAE F. GO, M.D.
DAVID Y. GRAHAM, M.D.

Helicobacter pylori is a gram-negative spiral bacterium whose natural niche is the human stomach. Although it was isolated only a decade ago, much is known about the bacterium and the effects of *H. pylori* infection on the human host. *H. pylori* infection is now accepted as the most common cause of gastritis. Before the isolation of *H. pylori*, gastritis was known to be associated with peptic ulcer disease (both gastric and duodenal ulcer), gastric carcinoma, and pernicious anemia. It was also known that gastritis was more prevalent in individuals of lower socioeconomic groups, and the frequency differed between ethnic groups. Histologic gastritis was not associated with gender, smoking, use of nonsteroidal anti-inflammatory drugs (NSAIDs), or alcohol. With the exception of pernicious anemia, all of these pre–*H. pylori* gastritis associations have now been transferred to *H. pylori*. The identification of *H. pylori* as a cause of gastritis, and thus possibly of peptic ulcer and gastric cancer, has led to a virtual explosion of investigations of *H. pylori* in gastroduodenal diseases. There are separate chapters on gastritis and on peptic ulcer that also discuss *H. pylori*.

Soon after the original isolation of *H. pylori*, it was shown that treatment of *H. pylori* infection led to marked improvement or even complete resolution of gastritis. These findings suggested that eradication of *H. pylori* infection may influence the natural history and course of *H. pylori*–associated diseases. It has since become clear that most peptic ulcers are a manifestation of an *H. pylori* infection and should be thought of and treated as an infectious disease.

EPIDEMIOLOGY

H. pylori infection appears to be spread by the fecal-oral route. It does not seem to be very infectious. The prevalence of *H. pylori* infection is dependent on factors that affect sanitation and socioeconomic class. In developing countries, most of the population is infected before age 20 years. In developed countries, *H. pylori* infection is infrequent in those of high socioeconomic class, whereas the poor have a rate of acquisition similar to that seen in a developing country. Acquisition of this infection appears to be greatest in children. After childhood the rate of acquisition varies from about 2 percent per year in developing countries to 0.5 percent or less in higher socioeconomic classes in developed countries. *H. pylori* infection clusters within families with children, and it has been suggested that infants may act as the source of infection of the uninfected spouse.

H. pylori infection is present in approximately 95 percent of patients with duodenal ulcer and 60 to 90 percent of those with gastric ulcers, irrespective of age. This infection is the most common, but not the only, cause of these diseases. One can make an analogy with pneumonia. *Streptococcus pneumoniae* is found in most cases of bacterial pneumonia, but as there are other causes of pneumonia, it is not universally present. The likelihood of finding *H. pylori* in patients with ulcer or gastritis depends on the prevalence of other causes of these diseases in the population. For example, gastric ulcers in a population selected from the highest socioeconomic class, where *H. pylori* is infrequent, but in which NSAID use may be common, might be predominantly due to NSAID use. In contrast, in the lower socioeconomic class, *H. pylori* infection is likely to be present even in a patient whose ulcer was caused by NSAID use.

DETECTION

Most methods to detect *H. pylori* are directly or indirectly based on the urease produced by the organism. The noninvasive tests include serologic and urea breath tests. Both first-generation (Pyloristat) and second-generation (HM-CAP) serologic tests for anti-*H. pylori* IgG are commercially available, and a number of rapid, in-office, tests are under development. One product of urease activity, CO_2, can be collected in the breath. If isotopically labeled urea is given, the breath can be directly assayed to confirm the presence of gastric urease activity. Use of the naturally occurring stable isotope ^{13}C, which is not radioactive, allows the test to be done repeatedly and even in pregnant women and infants. Kits containing all the material for the ^{13}C-urea breath test should be readily available in the near future.

Invasive tests are based on obtaining gastric tissue or juice for study. Gastric biopsies can be incubated in a gel or liquid containing urea and the presence of *H. pylori* determined by a color change produced by a pH indicator. Such rapid urease tests are often useful to guide decisions about therapy at the time of endoscopy. Biopsies can also be sent for culture or histology. The histologic appearance is currently the "gold standard" for diagnosing *H. pylori* infection. We recommend that two antral biopsies and one gastric corpus biopsy be taken from every patient with peptic ulcer disease who undergoes endoscopy. The biopsies should be taken from normal-appearing mucosa. The criteria for *H. pylori* infection include the presence of an acute-on-chronic

gastritis, the presence of the organism, or of both. *H. pylori* can be seen on hematoxylin and eosin (H & E) stains but can be better seen with the use of special, especially silver, stains. We currently use the Genta stain, which is a combination of a Steiner stain, H & E, and Alcian blue, pH 2.5. This stain has an advantage because it preserves the gastric mucosal structure while enhancing visualization of the microorganism. The histologic features of *H. pylori* infection are epithelial damage and the presence of polymorphonuclear leukocytes superimposed on chronic inflammation with lymphocytes and plasma cells. The presence of lymphoid follicles should alert the pathologist to the presence of chronic gastritis and *H. pylori* infection. Lymphoid follicles are not present in normal gastric mucosa and persist after *H. pylori* eradication, providing evidence of current or previous infection.

We do not recommend culture for *H. pylori*. This is best reserved for the research laboratory, since *H. pylori* is often difficult to culture in the routine laboratory owing to the fastidiousness and slow growth of the organism. Culture is expensive and the data obtained are currently not clinically useful.

Although endoscopy is also currently expensive, it uniquely allows visualization of the upper gastrointestinal tract for the presence of lesions and simultaneously provides the ability to collect tissue for analysis by rapid urease tests, culture, or histology. Histology provides a permanent record for later comparison.

The endoscopist can also obtain a sample of gastric juice for analysis of pH, urea, and ammonium concentrations. Ammonium is one breakdown product of urea, and a high ammonium-urea ratio has been known to be a surrogate for gastric urease activity for more than 50 years.

THERAPY

Eradication of *H. pylori* infection leads to resolution of gastric inflammation and a change in the natural history of *H. pylori*–related diseases. Because *H. pylori* infection is frequently asymptomatic, two questions frequently asked are whom to treat and which are the best therapies. *H. pylori* is difficult to eradicate. It is largely "outside the body" in an acidic environment that is hostile to the action of most antimicrobial therapies. Initial treatment studies showed that the results of in vitro sensitivity tests did not predict in vivo effectiveness. A decade of work has led to antimicrobial regimens that are well tolerated and will eradicate most *H. pylori* infections. Currently, therapy is primarily targeted toward patients with *H. pylori* infection and peptic ulcer disease.

Peptic Ulcer Disease

Peptic ulcer disease has a multifactorial pathogenesis. Conventional treatment has had two objectives: acceleration of ulcer healing and prevention of ulcer relapse. Initial therapy to accelerate ulcer healing has consisted of inhibition of acid secretion for 4 to 8 weeks with antisecretory drugs such as the H_2 antagonists; the proton-pump inhibitor omeprazole; or the use of topical therapies such as sucralfate. These therapies are effective in accelerating ulcer healing but do not change the natural history of the disease; 60 to 80 percent of ulcers relapse in the first year without maintenance antisecretory therapy. Maintenance therapy can substantially reduce ulcer recurrence, but the relapse rate returns to premaintenance levels when therapy is discontinued. Eradication of *H. pylori* held the promise of cure of the disease, and that promise has now been realized.

Until recently, it was most important to identify which of our effective therapies was best for a particular patient and whether maintenance therapy was needed. The question has now changed to "What is the etiology of the ulcer?". We now recognize three major categories of ulcer disease: *H. pylori* infection, NSAID use, and pathologic hypersecretory states such as the Zollinger-Ellison syndrome. It is now clearly established that eradication of *H. pylori* infection alters the natural history of peptic ulcer disease; it results in more rapid ulcer healing, prevents ulcer relapse, and prevents ulcer complications. This is true for both duodenal and gastric ulcers and includes "resistant" ulcers (defined as ulcers that failed to heal with 12 or 16 weeks of traditional therapy). Ulcer recurrence after anti–*H. pylori* therapy is primarily due to failure of *H. pylori* eradication, recurrent *H. pylori* infection, or the use of NSAIDs.

Early attempts to eradicate *H. pylori* infection typically resulted in treatment failure. Monotherapy, dual therapy, and triple therapy have been used in attempts at eradication. Bismuth subcitrate was one of the first monotherapies. Initially, its usefulness for healing ulcers was ascribed to cytoprotective effects, binding to the ulcer base, to mucus, or bile acids. Colloidal bismuth may also decrease pepsin output and increase local prostaglandins and alkali secretion. Patients treated with bismuth were found to have lower ulcer relapse rates than those given H_2 antagonists. Bismuth is now known to kill *H. pylori,* and a synergistic effect is seen when it is used in combination with other antimicrobial agents.

Triple therapies using bismuth, metronidazole, and tetracycline or amoxicillin have been the most successful anti–*H. pylori* therapies (Tables 1 and 2). We have found that the most effective therapy with the fewest side effects consists of triple therapy: bismuth subsalicylate (Pepto-Bismol), two tablets four times daily; metronidazole, 250 mg three times daily; and tetracycline hydrochloride, 500 mg four times daily for 2 weeks. This regimen is well tolerated and has few side effects. We find that tetracycline is as effective as amoxicillin and has fewer side effects such as rash. In countries where bismuth is not available, recent data suggest that dual therapy with metronidazole, 500 mg three times daily, and amoxicillin, 750 mg three times daily, is successful.

The nitroimidazoles are an important component of

Table 1 Approach to the Patient With an Ulcer

1. Ulcer suspected based on symptoms, signs, or history
2. Presence of ulcer is documented
3. Exclude other causes of ulcer; confirm *H. pylori* infection (gastric biopsy, *H. pylori* serology, urea breath test)
4. Treat with antisecretory drug for 6 wk; triple antimicrobial therapy for first 2 wk
6. Confirm *H. pylori* eradication
7. If infection not eradicated, may re-treat with alternative triple therapy

Table 2 Triple Therapy

Drugs:
   Pepto-Bismol tablets, 2 q.i.d. with meals and at bedtime
   Tetracycline, 500 mg q.i.d. with meals and at bedtime
   Metronidazole, 250 mg t.i.d. with meals
Duration: 14 days

anti–*H. pylori* therapies. However, metronidazole resistance has become an increasing problem; the organisms may be resistant because of previous use of the drug. If metronidazole resistance is frequent in a population or is suspected, or if a patient fails traditional triple therapy, we recommend replacing metronidazole with clarithromycin, 500 mg three times daily. New therapies continue to be investigated, e.g., the combination of proton-pump inhibitors with antimicrobials. The most common antibiotic used with the proton-pump inhibitor omeprazole is amoxicillin. Current studies suggest that amoxicillin, 500 mg four times daily, and at least 40 mg omeprazole daily for 14 days are required. Even with these dosages and treatment periods, eradication rates have generally been lower than we have come to expect from triple therapies. Proton-pump inhibitors have a theoretical advantage over other antisecretory drugs, as they both directly inhibit *H. pylori* growth and reliably increase pH so that the antimicrobials are potentially more effective. Antisecretory therapy is not required for *H. pylori* eradication, and eradication can be included as part of the regimen to accelerate ulcer healing, or after the ulcer is healed. It is usually convenient to accomplish both goals at the same time.

Because the treatment regimen is complicated, the patient must be made aware of the importance of following instructions. Poor compliance is the most common cause of failed eradication. Complications occur in about 15 to 20 percent but generally are mild, and the patient usually must be questioned to elicit this information. The most common side effects are loose stools and nausea.

Nonulcer Dyspepsia

The relationship between *H. pylori* and nonulcer dyspepsia remains controversial. The prevalence of *H. pylori* infection in patients with nonulcer dyspepsia ranges from 39 to 87 percent and is generally identical to that of the general population being studied. A direct association between *H. pylori* infection and dyspeptic symptoms has not been demonstrated. Since the prevalence of this infection in these patients is no greater than in the general population and since symptoms are generally not relieved by anti–*H. pylori* therapy, routine treatment of these patients cannot be recommended. Studies are needed to determine whether there are subsets of these patients who should be given anti–*H. pylori* therapy.*

Gastric Cancer

Atrophic gastritis is a precursor lesion for the most common form of gastric cancer. As *H. pylori* is the most common cause of gastritis, it is only logical that there should also be an association between *H. pylori* and gastric cancer, and there is increasing evidence of such a link. For example, three recent case control studies have found that *H. pylori* infection is associated with a greater risk of gastric cancer. The frequency of *H. pylori* infection is higher in lower socioeconomic classes, a group also known to be at increased risk of developing gastric cancer. The chronic gastric inflammation caused by *H. pylori* infection precedes gastric cancer, and may also contribute to its development by reducing acid secretion and limiting access of the antioxidant ascorbate to gastric juice. The role of *H. pylori* in the development of gastric cancer is the subject of prospective studies in several developing countries. There are so far no guidelines to determine which, if any, U.S. population should undergo *H. pylori* eradication in an attempt to prevent gastric cancer. We believe that eventually we will want to eradicate *H. pylori* infection from the entire U.S. population, but the means and the cost effectiveness of such a program are for future studies.†

Follow-up of *H. pylori* Treatment

H. pylori eradication is defined as absence of evidence of *H. pylori* 4 or more weeks after the end of antimicrobial therapy. The gold standard is endoscopy with biopsy, but this is expensive. Prospective studies have demonstrated that in developed countries, *H. pylori* eradication is infrequently followed by reinfection. Most studies have confirmed eradication by histologic or appearance urea breath test, but guidelines for those in whom eradication must be confirmed and those in whom this may be optional are not available. The decision to confirm eradication is influenced by the severity of the disease, the natural history of the untreated disease, and the availability of methods for follow-up. The widespread availability of the urea breath test will make follow-up easy, rapid, and reliable. Until then, we believe that it is critical to confirm *H. pylori* eradication in every patient who has suffered a major ulcer complication such as bleeding. Confirmation of eradication may be less necessary for the patient with mild duodenal ulcer disease, as one can wait for the return of symptoms or wait the 6 months to 1 year required for the serologic tests to become negative.

Eradication of *H. pylori* infection is the only medical treatment program that has been shown to alter the natural history of peptic ulcer disease. Cure of the disease is cost effective, and we believe that an attempt to eradicate *H. pylori* infection should be made in every patient with this infection and a peptic ulcer. We also recommend attempted eradication of *H. pylori* in ulcer patients who also take NSAIDs, because elimination of *H. pylori* also removes one possible cause of their ulcer disease. The only reasons to deny therapy are that the patient refuses or is allergic to the medications. Failure to eradicate the infection is not a major problem, as one can fall back on traditional antisecretory therapies, attempt eradication with a newer therapy, wait until more effective therapies are introduced, or employ any combination of these options. The major factor preventing use of *H. pylori* eradication therapy for all ulcer patients is the general failure to recategorize peptic ulcer disease as an infectious disease. Many still hold to the belief that one should treat only those with severe ulcer disease, with recurrent disease, or with complicated ulcer disease. Once *H. pylori* ulcer is recategorized as an infectious disease, use of antisecretory therapy alone makes as much sense as the use of methenamine or phenazopyridine hydrochloride, or similar symptomatic or suppressive therapy, for a patient with dysuria and *Escherichia coli* cystitis. The decision to use antimicrobial agents is based on our ability to cure and not on whether there are a number of effective symptomatic or suppressive therapies. We cannot guarantee to the patient with cystitis that we can cure the infection or that it will not recur in the future.

We can tell the peptic ulcer patient that we believe we can cure the current infection and that to do so will change the natural history of their disease. *H. pylori* ulcer is an infectious disease in which alternative noncurative therapies are available. The ulcer is a manifestation of a disease: the wound should be healed and the underlying disease eliminated. In the past our option was less acid, less ulcer. Now we can offer, "No *H. pylori*, no ulcer."

---

*Editor's Note: Patients with histologic evidence of active gastritis are one group in which a decision regarding treatment is needed, as outlined in the next section.

†Editor's Note: The issue not discussed is whether anyone with chronic antral gastritis with intestinalization (metaplasia) who also has *H. pylori* should be kept free of the organism by means of therapy (eradication). Since an early study showed that most of the endoscopists in our unit had antibodies to *H. pylori*, one wonders how many of "us" are infested? How many have chronic gastritis and intestinal metaplasia?

Editor's Note: The gauntlet is thrown! The issue of peptic ulcer and *H. pylori* is discussed in other chapters. The more insidious problem of chronic gastritis and the even hazier issue of premalignancy are also addressed in the chapters *Chronic Gastritis* and *Premalignant Conditions of the Stomach.*

We have included a relatively long list of Suggested Reading because of the controversial nature of this subject.

SUGGESTED READING

Alpert LC, Graham DY, Evans DJ, Jr, et al. Diagnostic possibilities for *Campylobacter pylori* infection. Eur J Gastroenterol Hepatol 1989; 1:17–26.

Borody TJ, George LL, Bandl S, et al. Smoking does not contribute to duodenal ulcer relapse after *Helicobacter pylori* eradication. Am J Gastroenterol 1992; 87:1390–1393.

Börsch GMA, Graham DY. *Helicobacter pylori*. In Benjamin SB, Collen MJ, eds. Handbook of experimental pharmacology. Vol 99. Pharmacology of peptic ulcer disease. Berlin: Springer-Verlag, 1991: 107–148.

Dooley CP, Cohen H. *Helicobacter pylori* infection. Gastroenterol Clin North Am 1993; 22:1–206.

Graham DY. *Campylobacter pylori* and peptic ulcer disease. Gastroenterology 1989; 96(Suppl):615–625.

Graham DY. *Helicobacter pylori:* its epidemiology and its role in duodenal ulcer disease. J Gastroenterol Hepatol 1991; 6:105–113.

Graham DY. Treatment of peptic ulcers caused by *Helicobacter pylori.* N Engl J Med 1993; 328:349–350.

Graham DY, Lew GM, Evans DG, et al. Effect of triple therapy (antibiotics plus bismuth) on duodenal ulcer healing. Ann Intern Med 1991; 115:266–269.

Graham DY, Lew GM, Klein PD, et al. Effect of treatment of *Helicobacter pylori* infection on the long-term recurrence of gastric or duodenal ulcer. Ann Intern Med 1992; 116:705–708.

Graham DY, Lew GM, Malaty HM, et al. Factors influencing the eradication of *Helicobacter pylori* with triple therapy. Gastroenterology 1992; 102:493–496.

Hentschel E, Brandstatter, Dragosics B, et al. Effect of ranitidine and amoxicillin plus metronidazole on the eradication of *Helicobacter pylori* and the recurrence of duodenal ulcer. N Engl J Med 1993; 328:308–312.

Mitchell HM, Li YY, Hu PJ, et al. Epidemiology of *Helicobacter pylori* in southern China: identification of early childhood as the critical period for acquisition. J Infect Dis 1992; 166:149–153.

Parsonnet J, Friedman GD, Vandersteen DP, et al. *Helicobacter pylori* infection and the risk of gastric carcinoma. N Engl J Med 1991; 325:1127–1131.

PEPTIC ULCER DISEASE

ANDREW H. SOLL, M.D.

The normal gastric and duodenal mucosae have a remarkable ability to defend against injury from the acid or peptic activity in gastric juice. In fact, peptic ulcers would be rare if mucosal defense mechanisms were not disrupted by exogenous factors. It is now clear that the two most important factors associated with peptic ulcer are infection with *Helicobacter pyloric* (HP) and use of nonsteroidal anti-inflammatory drugs (NSAIDs). Ulcers occurring in patients under protracted physiologic stress represent a distinct form of peptic ulcer. Uncommon causes of peptic ulcer include extreme acid hypersecretion (e.g., gastrinoma), rare abnormalities of the duodenum (e.g., annular pancreas), and possibly other infections (herpes simplex virus type I). Uncommonly, ulcers may reflect underlying disease processes, such as Crohn's disease or neoplasia. With clarification of the role of HP and NSAIDs, idiopathic ulcers have become the exception.

Despite the fact that most gastroduodenal ulcers are due to NSAIDs or HP, they remain peptic ulcers. With HP and NSAID ulcers, antisecretory agents accelerate healing and refractory ulcers respond to higher doses of potent antisecretory agents. The observation that continued NSAID therapy impairs healing in response to moderate acid inhibition (H_2 receptor antagonists [RA]), but not to marked acid inhibition with 40 mg of omeprazole, suggests that NSAID ulcers are superpeptic ulcers. The terms "peptic/HP ulcer" and "peptic/NSAID" ulcer are preferable.

Although understanding of pathophysiology and therapy is still incomplete, therapy must be adapted to the underlying cause of peptic ulcer. A generic approach to treating peptic ulcer disease (PUD) is no longer appropriate. Therapy will certainly be refined as understanding of pathophysiology and of the impact of therapy on natural history is advanced.

CLINICAL APPROACH

Especially with the present focus on cost effectiveness, the clinical history provides critical information for developing appropriate differential diagnosis and plans for assessment and management. In addition to the common functional disorders discussed below, it is important to exclude drug-induced dyspepsia (e.g., NSAIDs, digoxin, and theophylline) and disorders such as gastric cancer, pancreatic, or biliary tract disease. Especially with the initial presentation of gastric ulcer (GU), gastric carcinoma must be excluded.

Differentiating Gastric Ulcer and Gastric Cancer

Gastric cancer can masquerade as benign GU; however, visual inspection and adequate biopsy detects greater than 98 percent of gastric cancer on the first endoscopy. A thorough initial evaluation obviates the necessity of a second endoscopy to monitor ulcer healing in patients who are responding well to therapy. However, if the ulcer is giant (>2 to 3 cm) or if there were suspicious features on the initial endoscopy or inadequate biopsy, a second endoscopy is warranted. To insure adequate biopsy, the policy at UCLA is to use large biopsy forceps and train technicians to discriminate an adequate tissue sample from debris; four such adequate biopsies have proved to be sufficient to exclude carcinoma (personal communication, W. Weinstein).

Differentiating Peptic Ulcer From Other Common Functional Disorders

Common disorders that frequently overlap with PUD must be identified (Table 1). Acid dyspepsia is an upper abdominal burning discomfort that generally occurs on an empty stomach and is relieved with food, antacids, or antisecretory agents. Although these symptoms are the classical presentation for PUD, two-thirds of such patients do not have ulcers identified. In addition to the typical nonulcer acid dyspepsia, it is useful to distinguish a second form of nonulcer dyspepsia, which I call "dysgastria," referring to symptoms of belch-bloat symptoms of indigestion (Table 1).

Although not documented by formal study, clinical experience indicates that these several function disorders occur together in an overlapping pattern that will confound the uninitiated observer. It is my belief that this overlap reflects common underlying mechanisms, such as hypersensitivity of the afferent sensory nerve pathways. This phenomenon was first recognized in the colon in patients with the irritable bowel syndrome in whom the threshold for distension was markedly reduced compared to control subjects. A similar pattern also holds for two other of the functional bowel disorders (FBD)—the irritable esophagus and irritable stomach.

Overlap of PUD and FBD

Patients with PUD frequently (40 to 60 percent) complain of symptoms atypical for "classic" peptic ulcer, such as nausea, exacerbation by eating, belching, bloating, and fatty food intolerance. These symptoms are indicative of FBD and suggest a possible association between PUD and functional disorders outlined in Table 1. The first patient who taught me about this overlap presented initially with the classic symptoms of duodenal ulcer (DU), which responded well to H_2 RA therapy. However, after a few weeks he returned with a recurrence of epigastric pain, loss of antacid relief, and pain radiation to his back. At endoscopy his ulcer had healed, and subsequent physical examination revealed a paraspinous trigger point that reproduced his pain. Trigger

Table 1 Differential Diagnosis of Peptic Ulcer

Clinical Entity	Symptom Complex	Precipitating Factors	Timing and Relation to Meals	Response to Intervention
Acid dyspepsia	Epigastric burning pain		Usually >2 h postprandially or in the evening or early nighttime hours.	By definition, relief with food, antacids, or antisecretory agents
"Dysgastria"	Indigestion: belching, bloating, early satiety, nausea, and epigastric pain	Often specific food triggers, especially fatty foods. Dysgastria may occur with or without gastroparesis. Must be distinguished from gastric outlet obstruction produced by ulcer or neoplasia.	Usually occurs with or shortly after eating	Decreasing gastric distension with belching or vomiting often decreases symptoms
Esophageal reflux	Epigastric burning pain with substernal radiation	Occurs with increased abdominal pressure (e.g., bending over, with late stage pregnancy) or when the protective effects of gravity are reversed (supine posture, especially soon after eating)	Occurs with a full stomach (i.e., after meals or with delayed gastric emptying)	Relief is generally achieved with antacids or antisecretory agents.
Irritable bowel syndrome	Periumbilical or lower abdominal crampy pain associated with alteration in bowel pattern (diarrhea and/or constipation). Frequently associated with a complaint of abdominal distension and a sensation of incomplete evacuation.	Symptoms usually peak with the urge to move (colonic spasm ± distension). Usually a chronic, undulating syndrome precipitated by stress. Balloon studies reveal a low threshold to distension, i.e., the irritable bowel.	Often worse in the postprandial period, the misnamed "gastrocolic reflex"	Colonic decompression usually reduces symptoms.
"Back-gut" syndrome	Pain and tenderness of paraspinous, intercostal, or abdominal muscles	Symptoms may be exacerbated by twisting or tensing abdominal or rectus muscles and the pain (or a component thereof) may be reproduced by pressure on trigger points.	No direct relation to meals, but overlaps with other functional syndromes	Relief often produced by well-targeted local anesthesia

point injection brought sustained relief. It appeared that the musculoskeletal symptoms developed as a spinal reflex in response to the initial visceral insult. I now try to detect such clues during my initial clinical evaluation.

Patients with intractable peptic ulcer also underline the potential overlap between PUD and FBD. Before the advent of endoscopy and effective medical therapy for PUD, such patients were frequently operated upon, often with a poor outcome. This point was highlighted in a study of patients undergoing proximal gastric vagotomy; when the indication was refractory ulcer, recurrent symptoms occurred in 40 percent, but recurrent ulceration was found in only 4 percent. In contrast, in patients operated for relapsing PUD that remained responsive to medical therapy, recurrences of both symptoms and ulcers occurred in less than 5 percent. Symptoms associated with PUD may reflect mechanisms in addition to acid bathing an ulcer crater and I suspect that many of these atypical cases reflect an overlap of PUD with FBD. Peptic ulcer may serve as one of several triggers for induction of the afferent neuronal hypersensitivity that appears to bridge these overlapping functional disorders. Alternatively, peptic ulcer may result from mechanisms triggered by neuronal dysfunction associated with these other FBD syndromes.

It is essential that the clinician learn to discriminate these overlapping symptom patterns; a detailed history generally reveals clues that allow the overlap to be appreciated. Dissecting out these elements greatly simplifies diagnosis and management. Although endoscopy is the most effective approach for diagnosing PUD, for grading esophagitis, and confirming the presence of gastritis and HP, it cannot replace an expert clinical evaluation. Obviously, before concluding that symptoms are due to functional disorders, it is essential to look for "alarm" markers of serious underlying disease, such as anemia, GI blood loss, anorexia, weight loss, or liver function abnormalities.

Finding a DU in a patient who is not consuming NSAIDs is amongst the most sensitive "diagnostic" tests for HP. However, in patients in whom a DU is identified, HP testing may still be useful; a negative HP test shifts attention to other potential causes for ulcers such as unrecognized aspirin use or gastrinoma, and precludes therapy directed at HP eradication. It is important to recall that several medications (H^+/K^+-ATPase inhibitors, bismuth, sucralfate, antacids, and antibiotics) can suppress HP and lead to negative cultures, biopsies without organisms, and negative breath tests. The finding of chronic active gastritis without HP suggests a false negative for HP, whereas the absence of antral gastritis confirms the absence of HP infection.

A careful history is required to assure that NSAID consumption is detected; NSAID abuse, particularly with aspirin, has been frequently associated with refractory peptic ulcer. Some patients are reluctant to admit NSAID use and this factor deserves consideration especially when peptic ulcers fail to heal. When faced with a slowly healing HP-negative ulcer, measurement of salicylate levels should be considered.

HP AND PEPTIC ULCER THERAPY

Although a tight epidemiologic link was quickly established between HP and peptic ulcer, the relevance of this association was unclear because HP is a very common infection, but only a small proportion of subjects infected with HP develop PUD. In contrast, Koch's postulates have been fulfilled for HP infection as the cause of the very common antral predominant chronic, active gastritis (type B). Proof that HP is a causal factor for peptic ulcer has rested upon the numerous studies indicating that eradication of HP in patients with PUD markedly reduces the otherwise high rate of recurrences. The causal factors that distinguish the small proportion of individuals with HP at risk for PUD remain to be elucidated.

The eradication of HP modestly accelerates initial DU healing rates, compared to standard H_2 blocker therapy. Enhanced healing per se would be a weak justification for eradicating HP at the time of initial treatment. However, it is now very clear that HP eradication decreases subsequent recurrences and the associated costs and risks, and therefore becomes a cure for what otherwise would be a chronic, relapsing disease. In the five available randomized, controlled trials, the yearly ulcer recurrence rate of DU decreased from 84 percent in patients remaining HP positive to only 5 percent in patients with successful HP eradication. Numerous other trials support this conclusion, and, to my knowledge, no data to the contrary have been presented! Fewer data are available to assess the impact of HP eradication on the natural history of GU, but the response appears similar to DU; HP should be treated in patients with GU who are HP positive.

Why not treat HP? Reasons not to treat in the past have included the complexity of the regimens for HP eradication, concern about patient compliance and emergence of resistant organisms, and the uncertainty about long-range benefits. However, in developed countries, once HP eradication is confirmed 4 weeks after the end of therapy, the reinfection rate is very low (<0.5 percent per year). As regimens for eradication are refined and shortened and patient compliance improved, HP eradication with initial therapy will become the indicated approach for all peptic ulcers occurring in the setting of HP infection. I find that the decision is often made by the patient; once informed they have an infection that is a major determinant of the risk of ulcer recurrence, they request antibiotic therapy. Before you elect not to treat HP in the setting of PUD, make sure the patient is informed about and agrees with this decision.

Although uncommon, ulcers may recur after HP eradication and can reflect NSAID use or uncommon disorders, such as gastrinoma.

Specific Regimens

The combination of a proton pump inhibitor (e.g., omeprazole, 20 mg three times a day) with a single antibiotic (amoxicillin 500 to 750 mg three times a day or clarithromycin 500 mg three times a day) for 10 to 14 days is certainly the easiest, but most expensive, regimen. Another good option is the combination of an H_2 RA with metronidazole (250 mg three times a day) and amoxicillin (750 mg three times a day). Studies are needed to confirm the efficacy and establish the proper dose and duration of these therapies. I find triple therapy (bismuth subsalicylate, metronidazole, and tetracycline) to be cumbersome, especially when primary treatment for ulcer healing necessitates additional use of H_2 RA. (See the chapter on *Helicobacter pylori* for a more detailed discussion.) I look forward to evidence that short (3 to 5 day) treatment periods are nearly equally effective.

HP and Recurrent, Refractory, or Complicated Peptic Ulcer

Eradication of HP, if present, is the first step in preventing ulcer recurrence. Although the data are still preliminary, HP eradication reduces the recurrence of ulcer complications and will facilitate healing of refractory ulcers. There is no justification for not eradicating HP in patients with recurrent, refractory, or complicated ulcer disease!

In individuals with a history of ulcer complications, frequent or troublesome recurrences, or refractory ulcer, maintenance therapy with H_2 blockers is indicated until HP eradication is confirmed via a negative urea breath test (which will soon be widely available) or a marked decrease of the titers of HP antibodies after 6 to 12 months. Repeat endoscopy cannot be justified simply to confirm HP eradication. In this high-risk subgroup of ulcer patients, one cannot be faulted for continuing maintenance therapy for another 6 to 12 months, but sustained maintenance therapy is not necessary in most patients.

CONVENTIONAL ULCER THERAPY

Conventional ulcer therapy is indicated for HP-negative ulcers, for healing of HP-positive ulcers, and for maintenance of HP-positive ulcers pending or with failed HP eradication.

Regimens for Initial Therapy

Uncomplicated ulcers can be treated by a variety of safe and effective therapies (Table 2), including antacids, sucralfate, H_2 RA, and proton pump inhibitors (PPI, presently only omeprazole). The rate of healing of DU correlates with the potency, duration of action during the day, and length of therapy with antisecretory agents. For example, healing is more rapid with omeprazole at 40 mg per day and to a lesser extent with the 20 mg per day dose than with conventional doses of H_2 RA. However, with the exception of somewhat more rapid symptom relief, the benefits of this more rapid healing on clinical

outcome are of little clinical importance in uncomplicated ulcer and cost is a more relevant factor.

For healing GU, full doses of H_2 blockers provide effective initial therapy. PPI (omeprazole, 20 mg) are also clearly effective alternatives but are not yet approved for GU therapy in the United States. Although GU respond to antisecretory agents, the variable of most importance is the length of therapy; therefore, with the exception of continued cotherapy with NSAIDs, the most cost effective approach is to treat with the least expensive agent for a longer time. In one study, an advantage of omeprazole over H_2 blockers was evident in subjects continuing NSAID use; in the absence of NSAIDs, ranitidine and the 20 mg dose of omeprazole produced apparently comparable healing. Sucralfate also appears to effectively heal GU, but this is not yet an approved indication.*

The clinical approach to prepyloric ulcers, which occur in the antrum within 2 to 3 cm of the pylorus, falls between that for DU and GU. Prepyloric ulcers frequently coexist with DU and, in contrast to more proximal GU, are generally associated with high normal or elevated levels of acid secretion. However, a risk of neoplasia exists for prepyloric ulcers and adequate biopsy is indicated during the initial endoscopy. Although prepyloric ulcers may differ somewhat in their response to therapy, existing data do not warrant altering management from that outlined for DU.

Therapy on Demand

The advent of over the counter availability of H_2 blockers in the near future highlights the need for a risk to benefit analysis of "on demand" antisecretory therapy. In reality, many patients treat themselves on an "as needed" basis. However, in the HP era, this approach is not appropriate for PUD. If symptoms are recurrent due to PUD and HP is present, the organism should be treated rather than continuing intermittent therapy.

Conventional Maintenance Therapy

Maintenance therapy is currently indicated for patients pending HP eradication, in whom HP eradication has failed, or who have HP-negative ulcer disease. After initial ulcer healing, continued treatment with several medications (Table 2) reduces the high spontaneous recurrence rate found in placebo-treated patients. The goals of maintenance therapy are prevention of symptomatic recurrences and complications. Even in patients compliant with maintenance therapy, asymptomatic recurrences are frequent, but usually remain clinically silent. Therefore, with the possible exception of patients with a prior history of complications, there is no

---

*****Editor's Note:** There is some suggestion that sucralfate may protect a fibroblast growth factor from acid degradation as one mode of ulcer healing.

Table 2 Therapies for Peptic Ulcer

Drug	Mechanism of Action	Dosage Regimen: Ulcer Healing	Dosage Regimen: Maintenance	Side Effects
H_2 receptor antagonists	Inhibit acid secretion by blocking parietal cell H_2 receptors			Cardiac conduction abnormalities, idiosyncratic hepatic injury, immune hypersensitivity reactions, and thrombocytopenia
Cimetidine (Tagamet)		400-600 mg b.i.d. or 800 mg hs	400 mg hs	Gynecomastia, P450-mediated drug interactions with warfarin, diazepam, and phenytoin, theophylline, nifedepine, and flosequinan†
Ranitidine (Zantac)		150 mg b.i.d. or 300 mg hs	150 mg hs	Weak drug interactions, headaches, rare hypersensitivity
Famotidine (Pepcid)		20 mg b.i.d. or 40 mg hs	20 mg hs	
Nizatidine (Axid)		150 mg b.i.d. or 300 mg hs	150 mg hs	
Omeprazole (Prilosec)	Inhibits the parietal cell H^+/K^+-ATPase. Requires pH partition into the stimulated parietal cell; effectiveness markedly compromised in resting or inhibited parietal cells*	20 mg q.AM, 30 min before first meal	10-40 mg, depending on specific circumstances	P450-mediated drug interactions with warfarin, diazepam and phenytoin; rare hepatitis
Sucralfate (Carafate)	Topical action that enhances healing; many theories such as binding growth factors and inhibiting pepsin diffusion	1 g q.i.d. or 2 g b.i.d.	1 g b.i.d.	Aluminum loading in renal failure
Antacids	Acid neutralization and possible topical action of Al-OH complexes	280-1,000 mEq daily		Aluminum loading in renal failure, diarrhea with Mg, constipation with Al

*Effectiveness of omeprazole is markedly inhibited in fasting patients, or in patients on other secretory inhibitors, such as H_2RA or somatostatin.
†Central nervous system side effects in the intensive care unit have been reported more frequently with cimetidine than with the other H_2 blockers; however, this apparent difference has not been tested in controlled trials and may reflect usage patterns and reporting biases with the first drug in a series.

justification to pursue asymptomatic recurrences in patients with a good clinical response to maintenance therapy.

Patient Selection

Since peptic ulcer is a recurrent disease, the challenge for the physician is to base therapy on a prediction of the natural history of ulcer disease in the individual patient. Accurate predictions are difficult in individual patients, but several factors are associated with future recurrences, the most important of which is a prior history of ulcer complications. Recurrent DU hemorrhage has been observed at a rate of 1 percent per month in patients with prior GI bleeding from a DU and this rate was markedly suppressed by maintenance H_2 blocker therapy. Other factors favoring recurrence include frequent prior ulcer recurrences, a history of refractory ulceration, continued cotherapy with NSAIDs, smoking, a deformed duodenum, and age greater than 65 years. Patients with recurrent or refractory ulcers warrant consideration for an acid hypersecretory syndrome, which can be idiopathic or secondary to gastrinoma. It is clear that persisting HP-positive status is a major determinant of recurrent ulceration.

Specific Regimens

Surprisingly, there are no data available to guide decisions regarding the optimal regimen for maintenance therapy in the subgroup who will now be treated (patients with HP-negative ulcers, or HP-positive ulcers failing eradication). The greatest experience is with H_2 RA, so that these agents are my first choice. If the patients fails maintenance doses or has a history of troublesome disease, I favor sustained full dose H_2 RA therapy. Omeprazole is another effective alternative, which is appropriate for the very small group of high-risk patients who have not responded to H_2 RA therapy and are either HP negative or have failed HP eradication.

Duration and Sustained Efficacy*

In the patients who have been studied (mostly HP positive), maintenance therapy continues to be safe and effective for the 3 to 5 years. In fact, ulcer recurrences often decrease in frequency over the course of follow-up. I favor continuing therapy for at least 3 years in high-risk patients before attempting to discontinue. There are conflicting views on the natural history of peptic ulcer—some cases seem to burn out over time, while others continue to be symptomatic for decades. We now need to reassess this situation based upon the behavior of this new subset of patients being treated.

Refractory Ulcers

It is essential to distinguish patients with intractable symptoms associated with refractory ulceration from those with intractable symptoms without active ulceration. A great advantage of current medical management is that refractory ulcers (or their absence) can be identified and virtually all such ulcers can be healed, thereby revealing symptoms due to mechanisms other than refractory ulceration and avoiding unnecessary antiulcer therapy or surgery. Two elements that are critical to the evaluation of refractory ulceration are expert clinical evaluation and endoscopy. Refractory GU require adequate biopsies to identify neoplasia and the several infectious and inflammatory conditions that can mimic peptic ulcer. With refractory DU, particularly in the absence of HP or NSAID use, endoscopic biopsy should be considered to exclude unexpected pathology.

Once it is clear that a refractory peptic ulcer is the problem at hand, factors that can potentially delay healing deserve consideration (these factors are generally similar to those precipitating ulcer recurrences). Obviously patient understanding of and compliance with therapy should be assessed. Aspirin abuse is surprisingly frequent in the setting of refractory and recurrent ulceration, including ulcers recurring after surgery. Clinical evaluation should include salicylate levels, a history from family members, or even a room search since patients frequently decline to admit this habit.

Of the available treatment options, only maximal acid inhibition with a regimen such as omeprazole 40 mg daily or therapy with colloidal bismuth subcitrate (not available in the United States) offers advantages over continued therapy with standard regimens. No difference was found when patients with DU refractory to 6 weeks of H_2 blocker therapy were randomized to subsequent therapy with omeprazole at a daily dose of 20 mg or to therapy with ranitidine (150 mg twice daily).

*Editor's Note: Jensen et al conclude (N Engl J Med 1994; 330:382–386) that long-term ranitidive therapy reduces the risk of recurrent bleeding in patients whose duodenal ulcers healed after severe hemorrhage.

However, 96 percent of the ulcers refractory to 3 months of H_2 RA therapy healed with 8 weeks of omeprazole (40 mg per day), while only 57 percent healing was found with continued ranitidine therapy (300 mg daily). Thus, omeprazole will heal ulcers refractory to standard doses of H_2 blockers but a 40-mg dose appears necessary for a predictable advantage over continued H_2 RA therapy.

Many refractory ulcers are HP positive and although data are preliminary, there is little doubt that eradication of HP will facilitate healing and reduce the strong tendency for ulcer recurrence.

The use of drugs with different modes of action does not enhance healing of uncomplicated or refractory ulcers and the added cost is not justified. In fact, addition of H_2 RA to omeprazole compromises the effectiveness of the PPI (Table 2).

NSAID ULCERS

NSAID use is widespread and endoscopic ulcers are frequent, but clinically significant ulceration occurs infrequently. The pathogenic mechanism(s) distinguishing those few individuals at risk for ulcer complications have not been defined. Differentiating endoscopic from clinical ulcers is critical when interpreting studies. Depending upon the definition, endoscopic ulcers are found at surveillance endoscopy in 10 to 25 percent of patients taking NSAIDs, whereas clinical ulcers present in clinical settings with complications or symptoms at a rate of 1 to 4 percent per patient per year of NSAID use. A selection bias distinguishes the natural history of endoscopic ulcers from clinical ulcers; most endoscopic lesions remain clinically silent. The extrapolation from investigation of endoscopic ulcers to the prevention and treatment of clinical ulcers may be justified but requires caution.

Consumption of NSAIDs appears to be both an independent cause of peptic ulcer and an exacerbating factor for individuals with an underlying ulcer diathesis. The conclusion that NSAIDs are a de novo cause of ulcer is based on the observations that about half of NSAID-associated GU presenting in a clinical setting occur in the absence of HP or its associated antral gastritis.

Prevention and treatment are discussed briefly here and in greater detail in the next chapter.

Treatment

Discontinuation of NSAIDs or a reduction in dose should be the first step when possible. If NSAIDs must be continued, uncomplicated ulcers can be treated with twice daily (b.i.d.) dosing of H_2 RA, whereas complicated, large, or slowly healing ulcers warrant high dose (40 mg) omeprazole therapy. More data are needed to allow confident selection and dosing of therapy. Although misoprostol is reasonably effective healing non-NSAID ulcers, there are no data establishing efficacy healing (in contrast to preventing) clinical NSAID ulcers.

Prevention

Preventive co-therapy with antiulcer agents is not indicated for every patient taking NSAIDs, but is appropriate in patients using both NSAIDs and steroids and in patients with a definite history of prior ulcer disease or with serious comorbid conditions that would compromise tolerance to ulcer complications. Age alone appears to be a risk factor for NSAID-induced ulcer disease but the cost of antiulcer cotherapy for all patients over 65 years of age taking NSAIDs is hard to justify with present data. However, patients over 75 to 80 years old probably warrant antiulcer cotherapy while taking NSAIDs. NSAIDs now carry a warning label regarding ulcer complications and any time NSAIDs are used, with or without these risk factors, the patient should be informed about the potential risk of ulcer complications with these drugs.

Misoprostol

Misoprostol is the only drug currently approved for the prevention of NSAID-induced endoscopic ulcers. Preliminary analysis of a recently completed randomized trial with over 9,000 patients indicates that the rate of ulcer complications was reduced by 40 to 50 percent in patients taking misoprostol (200 μg four times a day) plus NSAIDs versus those taking NSAIDs alone. Side effects of abdominal pain and diarrhea limit the use of misoprostol but these are reduced if the dose is gradually increased from 100 μg daily to 200 μg four times a day. Prevention of NSAID-induced endoscopic ulcers is dose dependent; maximal effect observed with 200 μg four times a day. The dose relation for prevention of ulcer complications has not been determined. In light of the available data, misoprostol must be considered the first choice for ulcer prevention due to NSAID use in a high-risk patient.

Omeprazole and H₂ RA

Full-dose H_2 blockers prevent endoscopic DU but probably not GU, and they are a reasonable choice in patients with a history of DU responsive to these agents or in patients who cannot tolerate misoprostol. Omeprazole has not been formally tested for efficacy preventing NSAID-induced ulceration or its complications, although this agent is the only alternative if ulcers developed during full-dose H_2 blocker and misoprostol cannot be tolerated. There are no guidelines for selecting omeprazole doses in this setting. Although a 40 mg daily dose probably produces a more reliable effect, maintenance should be attempted with the 20 mg dose.

Less Toxic NSAIDs

Switching from NSAIDs to acetaminophen or salsalate provides a good alternative with a lower ulcer risk. NSAID prodrugs such as nabumetone or etodolac, which have a reduced risk of endoscopic ulceration, may also deserve consideration; however, no data from controlled trials address the risk of ulcer complications on these regimens especially in patients who have a prior ulcer history.

SIDE EFFECTS OF THERAPY

The untoward consequences of induced hypochlorhydria remain largely theoretical. However, prolonged acid secretory inhibition should be avoided unless the clinical benefit for managing refractory ulceration or esophagitis justifies the costs and exposure to these theoretical risks. Increased risk of enteric infection with organisms such as cholera and salmonella has been reported in subjects with achlorhydria, but these events have been very infrequently reported with antisecretory therapy.

Another potential untoward effect of prolonged antisecretory therapy is the trophic consequences of the elevation of serum gastrin on the gastric mucosa and possibly on other gastrin-sensitive tissues. In rats, extensive studies have established that high-dose antisecretory therapy with omeprazole or other antisecretory agents induces hyperplasia of the histamine-containing enterochromaffin-like (ECL) cells in the oxyntic mucosa and, at the end of their 2-year life span, formation of gastric carcinoids. This sequence of events has been demonstrated to reflect the hypergastrinemia produced by the secretory inhibition. However, carcinoid formation has not been found in other species, with the exception of mastomys. Hyperplasia of ECL cells also occurs in states of extreme and sustained hypergastrinemia in man (gastrinoma and atrophic gastritis). However, carcinoids only occur with gastrinoma plus MEN-I or with chronic atrophic gastritis. Hypergastrinemia alone does not produce gastric carcinoids in sporadic gastrinoma. For most, hypergastrinemia in response to antisecretory therapy may produce modest ECL cell hyperplasia, but dysplasia and tumor formation have not been found during thousands of patient-years of monitoring and use. The risk of carcinoid formation is very remote.

Omeprazole usually produces only modest hypergastrinemia. However, in a few percent of patients, the fasting serum gastrin concentration can exceed 500 pg per milliliter. I am not reluctant to continue omeprazole longer than 8 weeks if the benefit justifies the expense and theoretical risk. However, I favor measuring fasting serum gastrin levels after 6 months and yearly thereafter in an attempt to detect extreme hypergastrinemia. If hypergastrinemia is found, it is safe to assume that secretory suppression is excessive and need for the drug deserves reassessment or the dose reduced.[0]

Editor's Note: This is current therapy of the peptic ulcer patient, not just the ulcer, as of November 1993. This type of useful chapter is why I continue to bring out new editions of this book.

SUGGESTED READING

Cantu TG, Korek JS. Central nervous system reactions to histamine-2 receptor blockers. Ann Intern Med 1991; 114:1027–1034.

Goodman AJ, Kerrigan DD, Johnson AG. Effect of the pre-operative response to H₂ receptor antagonists on the outcome of highly selective vagotomy for duodenal ulcer. Br J Surg 1987; 74:897–899.

Graham DY, Lew GM, Klein PD, et al. Effect of treatment of *Helicobacter pylori* infection on the long-term recurrence of gastric or duodenal ulcer. Ann Intern Med 1992; 116:705–708.

Griffin MR, Piper JM, Daugherty JR, et al. Nonsteroidal anti-inflammatory drug use and increased risk for peptic ulcer disease in elderly persons. Ann Intern Med 1991; 114:257–263.

Kochman ML, Elta GH. Gastric ulcers—when is enough, enough. Gastroenterology 1993; 105:1582–1584.

Mayer EA, Gebhart GF. Basic clinical aspects of visceral hyperalgesia. Gastroenterology (in press).

Mayer EA, Raybould HE. Role of visceral afferent mechanisms in functional bowel disorders. Gastroenterology 1990; 99:1688–1704.

Piper JM, Ray WA, Daugherty JR, Griffin MR. Corticosteroid use and peptic ulcer disease: Role of nonsteroidal anti-inflammatory drugs. Ann Intern Med 1991; 114:735–740.

Schuster MM. Irritable bowel syndrome. In: Sleisenger MH, Fordtran JS, eds. Gastrointestinal disease. 5th ed. Philadelphia: WB Saunders, 1993:917.

Soll AH. Gastric, duodenal, and stress ulcer. In: Sleisenger MH, Fordtran JS, eds. Gastrointestinal disease. Philadelphia: WB Saunders, 1993, p. 580.

Walan A, Bader J-P, Classen M, et al. Effect of omeprazole and ranitidine on ulcer healing and relapse rates in patients with benign gastric ulcer. N Engl J Med 1989; 320:69–75.

NSAID-INDUCED ULCERATIONS

JEFFREY B. RASKIN, M.D.
JAMES CHONG, M.D.

Nonsteroidal anti-inflammatory drugs (NSAIDs) are the principal agents used for treatment of rheumatologic conditions as well as for common aches and pains. It is estimated that up to 15 million patients in the United States are chronically taking NSAIDs and that 70 million prescriptions are written every year. Studies have suggested that peptic ulceration may develop in up to 25 percent of these patients taking NSAIDs chronically. At least 15 percent of patients chronically taking NSAIDs may have a gastric ulcer at any one time, with a prevalence rate five to ten times that of non–NSAID users. The incidence of duodenal ulceration secondary to chronic NSAID use has risen and may approach 10 percent. With these mucosal ulcerations, NSAIDs are associated with the potentially life-threatening complications of bleeding and perforation.

The ulcerative potential of NSAIDs is believed to be due to both direct toxicity and the indirect compromise of the gastroduodenal mucosal barrier from the inhibition of prostaglandin synthesis. NSAIDs are weak organic acids that become concentrated in the mucosal cell as a result of "ion trapping" and cause increased permeability of the cell membranes, allowing for back-diffusion of hydrogen ions. In addition, by inhibiting gastric and duodenal prostaglandin synthesis, NSAIDs may diminish mucosal blood flow, increase gastric acid production, and decrease mucus and bicarbonate secretion. Thus, NSAIDs have been associated with ulcerations occurring throughout the gastrointestinal (GI) tract. With the ever-increasing use of NSAIDs, especially in over-the-counter forms, physicians must be cognizant of the current information available for the prevention and management of NSAID-induced ulcerations.

PREVENTION

Prophylaxis of NSAID-induced ulcerations should be strongly considered in patients at high risk for the development of such ulcers. Patients at highest risk appear to be the elderly on chronic NSAID therapy with concomitant use of steroids. Other risk factors include pre-existing peptic ulcer disease, a history of previous ulcer complications, connective tissue disease, and use of high-dose NSAIDs. With the increasing percentage of the elderly in the general population and the increased use of NSAIDs in this group, more GI complications related to NSAIDs are reported every year. One-quarter of all episodes of upper GI bleeding among the elderly are associated with NSAIDs, resulting in a mortality rate of 10 percent. The elderly are more susceptible to NSAID-induced injury because of reduced drug metabolism, age-related gastric atrophy, delayed gastric emptying, hormonal imbalances, and decreased intestinal blood flow.

Data are available on patients with rheumatoid arthritis followed by ARAMIS (American Rheumatism Association Medical Information System) outlining the potential risk factors for the development of NSAID-induced GI complications resulting in hospitalization or death. Patients on chronic NSAID therapy have a relative risk (R.R.) of hospitalization 6.45 times that of individuals not taking NSAIDs. The risk factors include age greater than 60 years (R.R. 2.6), upper abdominal pain within the previous 6 months (R.R. 1.5), concomitant administration of NSAIDs and corticosteroids (R.R. 2.9), rheumatoid arthritis (R.R. 2.0), and cigarette smoking (R.R. 1.5). It is likely that any patient with three or more of these risk factors will have a relatively high chance of developing a gastroduodenal ulcer complication. The syndrome of NSAID-associated gastropathy may account for at least 2,600 deaths and 20,000 hospitalizations every year among rheumatoid arthritis patients.

Alternatives

There are some useful recommendations for the prevention of NSAID-induced ulcers without resorting to the addition of another pharmacologic agent. These measures include discontinuing NSAIDs and switching therapy to other classes of analgesics, using the lowest effective dosage of the NSAID, selecting enteric-coated aspirin, taking NSAIDs with meals, changing to a nonacetylated salicylate, and using less potent, short-acting NSAIDs. If these measures are ineffective and full therapeutic doses of the NSAIDs are required, the concomitant use of agents that have been shown to be effective in the prevention of NSAID-induced peptic ulcer disease can be considered.

Acid Suppression

Two recent multicenter, placebo-controlled trials conducted in the United States and United Kingdom have shown that ranitidine can effectively prevent the development of NSAID-induced duodenal ulcers, but has no effect on the prevention of gastric ulceration. The U.S. study, comparing 150 mg ranitidine taken twice a day with placebo in patients requiring chronic NSAID therapy, showed that 82 percent of the ranitidine group had no duodenal mucosal damage compared with 65 percent in the placebo group. More specifically, no duodenal ulcers developed in the ranitidine group as opposed to 8 percent in the placebo group.

The occurrence of NSAID-induced gastric ulcers in both treatment groups showed no significant difference (10 and 12 percent, respectively). The U.K. study also compared 150 mg ranitidine taken orally twice a day with placebo in chronic NSAID users. The data were similar to those in the U.S. study in that, after 8 weeks of therapy, only 1.5 percent of the ranitidine group developed a duodenal ulcer compared with 8 percent in the placebo group. Again, there was no difference in the prevention of NSAID-induced gastric ulcers in either group (6 percent in each).

"Cytoprotective" Agents

Misoprostol (Cytotec), a prostaglandin E_1 analog, has several protective effects on the gastroduodenal mucosa, including inhibition of gastric acid secretion, increased secretion of mucus and bicarbonate, and maintenance of mucosal blood flow. In a large multicenter placebo-controlled trial of low-dose misoprostol (100 μg orally four times daily), high-dose misoprostol (200 μg orally four times daily), or placebo for 3 months in chronic NSAID users with osteoarthritis who continued their NSAID use, the incidence of gastric ulceration was significantly decreased in the low-dose (5.6 percent) and high-dose (1.4 percent) misoprostol groups compared with the placebo group (21.7 percent). The incidence of duodenal ulcerations was 4 percent in the placebo group and 2 and 3 percent in the low-dose and high-dose misoprostol groups, respectively. There was no difference in resolution of the baseline NSAID-associated abdominal pain among the treatment groups.

Another study compared misoprostol with placebo in the prevention of NSAID-induced duodenal ulceration. After 3 months, 200 μg misoprostol orally four times daily with concomitant NSAID use resulted in a significantly lower rate of duodenal ulceration in the misoprostol group (1.1 percent) than in the placebo group (6.5 percent). In addition, the incidence of gastric ulceration was also significantly lower in the misoprostol group (1.5 percent) than in the placebo group (9.0 percent).

Sucralfate has been shown to increase gastric mucus secretion while not affecting acid or bicarbonate secretion. A short-duration, prospective, cross-over study among chronic high-dose aspirin (900 mg orally four times daily) users comparing 1 g sucralfate orally four times daily with placebo in the prevention of NSAID-induced gastric erosions showed that after 14 days of follow-up, there was no significant difference in the gastric erosion score between the two groups. In a controlled trial, misoprostol (200 μg orally four times daily) has been compared with sucralfate (1 g orally four times daily) in the prevention of NSAID-induced gastric ulcers. After 3 months, the misoprostol group developed significantly fewer gastric ulcers (1.6 percent) than the sucralfate group (16 percent).

In another multicenter prospective study comparing the efficacy of misoprostol and ranitidine in the prevention of NSAID-induced gastric and duodenal ulceration, patients who received 200 μg misoprostol orally four times daily had significantly fewer gastric ulcers (0.56 percent) than patients given 150 mg ranitidine orally twice daily (5.6 percent). There was no difference between the groups in the development of duodenal ulcers (1.1 percent within each group). The study duration was 8 weeks and patients continued their NSAID therapeutic doses.

Recently, a placebo-controlled study was completed to examine the efficacy and safety of three different dosage regimens of misoprostol (200 μg orally twice, three times, or four times daily) in preventing NSAID-induced gastric and duodenal ulcers in patients chronically taking NSAIDs for a variety of arthritic conditions. The study showed that all misoprostol doses were significantly better than placebo (11.2 percent) in preventing gastric ulcers (6.3 percent twice daily, 3.2 percent three times daily, 3.1 percent four times daily). All dosage regimens of the misoprostol were equivalent to each other and significantly better than placebo in preventing duodenal ulcers (5.5 percent placebo, 2.2 percent twice daily, 2.5 percent three times daily, 0.9 percent four times daily).

In summary, these studies have shown that misoprostol (200 μg orally four times daily) is significantly more effective than ranitidine (150 mg orally twice daily) or sucralfate (1 g orally four times daily) in preventing

NSAID-induced gastric ulcers, and that misoprostol and ranitidine are equally effective in preventing NSAID-induced duodenal ulcers. The efficacy of other agents, including omeprazole, in preventing NSAID-induced ulcerations has not been reported.

Preferred Approach

Currently, no standardized prophylactic therapy can be recommended for chronic NSAID users, since convincing data regarding long-term clinical benefit are lacking. Even though clinical benefit from prophylaxis has not been demonstrated, many studies have not only a definite correlation of NSAID usage and the development of gastric or duodenal ulcer disease, but also a high correlation in patients presenting with peptic ulcer bleeding and perforation. The ARAMIS data have attempted to define patients at high risk for the development of life-threatening complications (bleeding and perforation) from NSAID-induced ulcer disease.

The decision when to treat rests with the clinician, who must consider many factors. If a decision to treat is made, the above data on the agents available and their individual profiles (efficacy, safety, side effects) offer the clinician the following approaches.

For the prophylaxis of NSAID-induced gastric ulcers, only misoprostol (200 μg orally four times daily) has demonstrated a significant reduction in large multicentered trials. The data do not suggest any therapeutic role for the use of H_2 antagonists or sucralfate in the prevention of NSAID-induced gastric ulcers. Although effective in preventing NSAID-induced gastric ulcers, the recommended dose of misoprostol (200 μg orally four times daily) has been associated with a high incidence of abdominal cramping and diarrhea in some studies. These side effects have prompted some physicians to empirically initiate therapy at lower doses and advance the dosage as tolerated by the patient. Giving the medication with meals has also lessened the frequency of these side effects. Recent evidence is now available that supports the use of lower doses of misoprostol in preventing NSAID-induced gastric or duodenal ulcers. A misoprostol dose of 100 μg orally four times daily or 200 μg orally twice daily has been shown to significantly reduce the incidence of NSAID-induced gastric ulceration as compared with placebo. Misoprostol in a 200 μg oral twice-daily dosage has also been shown to produce significantly less diarrhea as a side effect than four-times-daily dosing. Although these two dosage regimens do not compare with the reduction of NSAID-induced gastric ulcerations by 200 μg misoprostol given orally four times daily, 200 μg misoprostol given orally twice daily now offers an efficacious regimen in the initiation of therapy with fewer side effects. In one study, ranitidine (150 mg orally twice daily) was similar to these low-dose misoprostol regimens in preventing gastric ulcer development but not as effective as high-dose misoprostol (200 μg orally four times daily).

As previously mentioned, studies now describe a higher than originally reported incidence of duodenal

ulceration in chronic NSAID users. Both misoprostol (200 μg orally twice, three times, or four times daily) and ranitidine (150 mg orally twice daily) have proved effective in the prophylaxis of NSAID-induced duodenal ulceration. In comparison studies, both medications are equally effective.

In summary, the appropriate therapeutic approach depends on the clinical situation. If the decision is made to begin a prophylactic regimen in a high-risk patient with no history of NSAID-induced ulceration or of ulcer disease, one can begin with a low-dose regimen of misoprostol, 200 μg twice daily. This dosage will be effective in preventing gastric and duodenal ulceration. If no side effects develop (e.g., diarrhea, abdominal cramps), the dose should be increased if tolerated to a maximum of 200 μg four times a day, which will prevent a larger number of gastric ulcers. In patients with previously documented NSAID-induced ulcers that have healed and in whom prophylaxis is desired with reinstitution of NSAID therapy, the prophylactic regimen could vary depending on the location of the previous ulceration. Although this is not guaranteed, ulcers tend to recur in their previous anatomic locations. In a previous NSAID-induced duodenal ulcer, prophylaxis against a recurrence can be accomplished with ranitidine (150 mg orally twice daily) or misoprostol (200 μg orally twice, three times, or four times daily), while a previous gastric ulceration would suggest a need for misoprostol prophylaxis.

In a patient with a history of documented gastric or duodenal ulcer, misoprostol (200 μg orally four times daily) offers the most effective prophylaxis against both ulcers. The exact prophylactic regimen to recommend for a patient who just has a history of ulcer disease is more difficult. Because the pathogenesis and site of the ulcer may be unknown, it is probably more appropriate to use misoprostol with its proved efficacy in preventing an NSAID-induced gastric or duodenal ulcer.

TREATMENT

The discussion that follows assumes that the ulcer is definitely related to NSAID use, and that other causes or associations such as *Helicobacter pylori* have been excluded. A number of therapeutic agents that neutralize or suppress gastric acid have been studied for the treatment of NSAID-induced ulcers. There are, however, only a few reports describing the cytoprotective agents.

Alternatives

Acid Neutralization

In a 6 week prospective study comparing cimetidine (300 mg orally four times daily) plus antacid (845 mEq neutralizing capacity per day) with antacid alone in patients with NSAID- or steroid-induced gastric ulcerations, significantly more patients in the cimetidine plus antacid group (65.7 percent) experienced healing of their gastric ulcer than in the antacid group (25 percent). Of the patients whose ulcers did not heal after 6 weeks with antacid alone, continued antacid therapy for 6 more weeks healed an additional 67 percent of these ulcers. In one retrospective study of patients with rheumatoid arthritis and an equal number of gastric and duodenal ulcers, antacid therapy alone healed all the ulcers in the small group of patients who discontinued anti-inflammatory treatment. Significant ulcer healing (78 percent) was found, however, in the patients who continued anti-inflammatory medications.

Acid Suppression

A number of trials of H_2 antagonists or omeprazole have been reported in the treatment of NSAID-induced gastric or duodenal ulcer disease. Clinical trials with cimetidine have provided conflicting results in the healing of NSAID-induced ulcerations. In one open-label study involving a few patients who were treated with cimetidine (1 g orally every day), ulcer healing was found in 71 percent after 6 weeks of therapy. Sixty-seven percent of the patients continued their NSAID therapy during the study. Of the patients who did not heal after 6 weeks, 6 more weeks of cimetidine therapy healed an additional 33 percent. Of interest in this study was the fact that all the healed ulcers were duodenal while the refractory ulcers were gastric. Another multicenter open-label trial used cimetidine (800 mg orally at bedtime) in the treatment of NSAID-induced erosions or ulcers with continued NSAID usage. Of 187 patients enrolled, the ulcer healing rate after 4 weeks was 49 percent and after 8 weeks 81 percent. More specifically, after 8 weeks of therapy, 74 percent of gastric ulcers and 85 percent of duodenal ulcers healed. After ulcer healing, a maintenance regimen of cimetidine, 400 mg orally at bedtime for 6 months showed a recurrence rate for erosions or ulcers of 12 percent.

Other studies, however, have shown no improvement of gastric mucosal lesions with cimetidine therapy. A study involving patients chronically taking NSAIDs for rheumatoid disorders and who had gastric mucosal lesions (erosions not ulcers) showed that, after 8 weeks of either cimetidine, 300 mg orally four times daily or placebo with continued NSAID use, progression of endoscopically detected lesions occurred in 56 percent of the cimetidine group and 52 percent of the placebo group. Patients in this study were also taking other medications, which may have altered the ulcer healing rate. In addition, the NSAID dosages were adjusted without restrictions. In another 6 week trial of arthritic patients with endoscopically proved peptic ulcer disease, there was no difference between the healing rates of the cimetidine-treated (400 mg orally three times daily) group and those of the placebo group (69 percent and 60 percent, respectively).

Clinical trials using ranitidine as treatment for NSAID-induced ulcers have shown effective rates of peptic ulcer healing even with concomitant use of NSAIDs. One randomized, single-blind study involved patients with rheumatoid arthritis and peptic ulcer disease (75 percent duodenal ulcer, 25 percent gastric ulcer) who were given either ranitidine, 150 mg orally twice daily, or sucralfate, 1 g orally four times daily. NSAID therapy was continued in 50 percent of the patients. After 9 weeks, the healing rates were 84 percent for the ranitidine group and 83 percent for the sucralfate group. There was no difference in the healing rates for either agent if the NSAIDs were continued or stopped. In another open study, patients with rheumatoid arthritis and peptic ulcer disease were treated with ranitidine, 150 mg orally twice daily, while NSAID therapy was continued. After 12 weeks, gastric ulcers healed in 90 percent of patients and duodenal ulcers in 85 percent.

The healing rates in these two studies are similar to those of peptic ulcers not induced by NSAIDs. A large multicenter prospective trial examined the effect of ranitidine, 150 mg orally twice daily, on the healing rates of gastric and duodenal ulcers in patients randomized to continue or discontinue NSAID therapy. After 8 weeks of therapy, gastric ulcers healed in 63 percent of those continuing the NSAID and 95 percent of those who stopped NSAID treatment. For duodenal ulcers after 8 weeks, the healing rate was 84 percent in those who continued the NSAID and 100 percent in the patients who stopped the NSAID. After 12 weeks of ranitidine therapy, 79 percent of the gastric ulcers and 92 percent of the duodenal ulcers healed in the group who continued NSAIDs. A 100 percent healing rate was noted for both gastric and duodenal ulcers in the patients who stopped NSAID therapy. The differences in gastric and duodenal healing rates between those who continued and those who stopped NSAID therapy were statistically significant. Although this study showed that discontinuation of NSAIDs resulted in the highest ulcer healing rates, patients who continued to take NSAIDs had substantial peptic ulcer healing when ranitidine therapy was extended for 12 weeks. This study seemed to suggest that, despite the previous H_2-receptor antagonist prophylaxis studies that demonstrated failure of these agents in the prevention of NSAID-induced gastric ulcers, longer periods (12 weeks) of acid suppression may result in healing NSAID-induced gastric ulcers even when NSAID therapy is continued.

Limited data are available on the use of omeprazole to treat NSAID-induced ulcers. The largest trial involved patients with gastric ulcers who were randomized to receive omeprazole (20 mg orally daily), omeprazole (40 mg orally daily), or ranitidine (150 mg orally twice daily). Only 11.3 percent of these patients, however, continued their NSAIDs. After 4 weeks of therapy, the gastric ulcers healed in 81 percent of the omeprazole 40 mg per day group, 61 percent of the omeprazole 20 mg per day group, and 32 percent of the ranitidine group. After 8 weeks, the corresponding healing rates were 95, 82, and 53 percent, respectively. There was a statistically significant advantage for both omeprazole regimens during the 4 and 8 week treatment intervals compared with ranitidine therapy. Gastric ulcers healed equally with or without the continued use of NSAIDs. However, patients receiving ranitidine who continued NSAID use had considerably lower healing rates for gastric ulcers than those who received ranitidine and discontinued NSAIDs.

"Cytoprotective" Agents

Few studies have looked at sucralfate therapy for the healing of NSAID-induced ulcers. As mentioned previously, 83 percent of NSAID-induced peptic ulcers (75 percent duodenal, 25 percent gastric) healed after 9 weeks of sucralfate therapy (1 g orally four times daily). A study comparing sucralfate (1 g orally four times daily) with placebo in patients with upper abdominal complaints and NSAID-induced ulcers or erosions showed that even with continued NSAID therapy, there was a small but statistically significant reduction in the gastric lesion score among the sucralfate-treated group compared with the placebo group. However, the data are difficult to interpret because the placebo group had significantly fewer lesions at baseline.

Although numerous studies have shown the efficacy of misoprostol in the healing of peptic ulcers, data on the use of misoprostol in healing NSAID-induced ulcers are sparse. One multicenter study involving rheumatoid arthritis patients taking high-dose aspirin showed that after 8 weeks of treatment, misoprostol (200 µg orally four times daily) was statistically superior to placebo in healing gastric mucosal (70 percent versus 25 percent) or duodenal mucosal injury (67 percent versus 26 percent) in patients who continued their high aspirin intake (650 to 1,300 mg orally four times daily). The actual number of endoscopic ulcers in this study was small, and no conclusions about ulcer healing can be drawn. In a study of patients chronically taking NSAIDs, misoprostol (200 µg orally four times daily) when compared with placebo significantly accelerated the rate of gastric ulcer healing at both 4 weeks (83 percent versus 61 percent) and 8 weeks (96 percent versus 90 percent). However, patients discontinued the NSAIDs during the study period.

Preferred Approach

The initial clinical presentation of NSAID-induced ulceration can range from typical ulcer symptoms or a complication (bleeding or perforation). However, most NSAID-induced ulcers, whether gastric or duodenal, are "silent" or asymptomatic. The data strongly suggest that ulcers associated with NSAID use will heal more rapidly once the NSAID is discontinued, and this should be encouraged. With continued NSAID use, antiulcer therapy will heal these ulcers, but no data are available on the effects of this approach on ulcer complication rates. Studies in patients who continue using NSAIDs have shown that ulcer healing (especially gastric) usually requires a more prolonged course

of therapy (about 12 weeks) to obtain sustained healing rates. Limited studies suggest that omeprazole therapy may not require a prolonged course.

NSAID-Induced Gastric Ulceration

If NSAIDs are discontinued, gastric ulcer healing can be obtained with any of the antiulcer medications (H_2 antagonists, omeprazole, or sucralfate) using standard dosages. Healing rates (8 to 12 weeks of therapy) with these agents (limited data with sucralfate) are identical to those with non–NSAID-associated ulceration once NSAID therapy is discontinued. The choice and duration of therapy depend on the clinical presentation.

Although the prostaglandin analog misoprostol has been effective in some studies, the prostaglandin analogs have not been approved for this indication and are not recommended. If NSAIDs are continued, gastric ulcer healing rates with omeprazole (20 mg orally every day) are significantly better (4 or 8 weeks of therapy) than those of the H_2 antagonists (around 60 percent healing), which provide an alternative approach. Omeprazole healing rates appear identical (limited data) in patients who discontinue or continue NSAID use. H_2 antagonist therapy also appears to be less effective with larger ulcers.

NSAID-Induced Duodenal Ulceration

The most effective healing rates are obtained if NSAIDs are discontinued. It is interesting, however, that, with extended therapy (8 to 12 weeks) and continued NSAID use, the healing rates of duodenal ulcers are identical to those of non–NSAID-associated duodenal ulcer. The H_2 antagonists and sucralfate have been shown to have equal efficacy in the treatment of these duodenal ulcers even with continued NSAID use. Clinical trials of omeprazole therapy in this clinical setting are lacking.

NSAID ENTEROPATHY AND COLONOPATHY

The pathogenesis of NSAID enteropathy is unknown. It has been suggested that NSAIDs cause specific biochemical changes in the enterocytes during drug absorption. These damaging effects cause an increased intestinal permeability and are mediated by neutrophils. Others postulate that the injury is a vascular event. In 60 to 70 percent of patients taking NSAIDs for more than 6 months, an enteropathy develops. Most are asymptomatic, but a few develop a severe complication such as bleeding, perforation, or stricture or a malabsorption syndrome. Iron deficiency and hypoalbuminemia are common problems in these patients. Colitis mimicking classic inflammatory bowel disease has been reported. Recent NSAID therapy has been reported as a cause for relapses of inflammatory bowel disease and complications (perforation, fistula) of diverticular disease. There is a separate chapter on NSAID injury to the small and large intestines.

Preferred Approach

The severe complications of bleeding, perforation, and stricture are treated in the standard fashion. Discontinuation of the NSAIDs will lead to resolution (clinical and histologic) of NSAID-induced colitis. The activation of quiescent inflammatory bowel disease presents a difficult problem in patients with severe arthritis. The acute bowel flare requires therapy and a decision to stop or continue the NSAIDs. No controlled trials are available in addressing the continuation or cessation of NSAIDs in this clinical situation. Patients with hypoalbuminemia and iron deficiency anemia secondary to an "inflammatory" enteropathy may be helped by sulfasalazine (2 to 3 g orally every day) but will require at least 6 weeks of therapy. Metronidazole (800 mg orally every day) for up to 6 weeks has been used in a few patients. In a small placebo-controlled trial of misoprostol (800 μg orally every day), intestinal inflammation was reduced in the misoprostol-treated patients.

SUGGESTED READING

Agrawal NM, Roth S, Graham DY, et al. Misoprostol compared with sucralfate in the prevention of nonsteroidal antiinflammatory drug-induced gastric ulcer: a randomized, controlled trial. Ann Intern Med 1991; 115:195–200.
Bijlsma JW. Treatment of NSAID-induced gastrointestinal lesions with cimetidine: an international multicentre collaborative. Aliment Pharmacol Ther 1988; 2(Suppl 1):85–95.
Bjarnason I, Hopsinson N, Zanelli G, et al. The treatment of non-steroidal anti-inflammatory drug induced enteropathy. Gut 1990; 31:777–780.
Caldwell JR, Roth SH, Wu WC, et al. Sucralfate treatment of nonsteroidal anti-inflammatory drug-induced gastrointestinal symptoms and mucosal damage. Am J Med 1987; 83:74–82.
Ehsanullah RSB, Page MC, Tildesley G, Wood JR. Prevention of gastroduodenal damage induced by non-steroidal anti-inflammatory drugs: controlled trial of ranitidine. BMJ 1988; 297:1017–1021.
Fries JF, Miller SR, Spitz PW, et al. Toward an epidemiology of gastropathy associated with nonsteroidal antiinflammatory drug use. Gastroenterology 1989; 96:647–655.
Graham DY, Agrawal NM, Roth SH. Prevention of NSAID-induced gastric ulcer with misoprostol: multicentre, double-blind, placebo-controlled trial. Lancet 1988; 2:1277–1280.
Graham DY, Stromatt SC, Jaszewski R, et al. Prevention of duodenal ulcer in arthritics who are chronic NSAID users: a multicenter trial of the role of misoprostol. Gastroenterology 1991; 100:A75.
Jaszewski R, Graham DY, Stromatt SC. Treatment of nonsteroidal antiinflammatory drug-induced gastric ulcers with misoprostol. A double blind multicenter study. Dig Dis Sci 1992; 37:1820–1824.
Lancaster-Smith MJ, Jaderberg ME, Jackson DA. Ranitidine in the treatment of non-steroidal anti-inflammatory drug associated gastric and duodenal ulcers. Gut 1991; 32:252–255.
Manniche C, Malchow-Moller A, Andersen J, et al. Randomized study of the influence of nonsteroidal anti-inflammatory drugs on the treatment of peptic ulcer in patients with rheumatic disease. Gut 1987; 28:226–229.
Raskin JB, White R, Jaszewski R, et al. Misoprostol and ranitidine in the prevention of NSAID-induced gastric and duodenal ulcer disease: a multicenter trial. Gastroenterology 1992; 102(Suppl):A151.
Raskin JB, White R, Sue SO. Efficacy and safety of three dosage regimens of misoprostol in the prevention of NSAID-induced gastric and duodenal ulcers: a multicenter trial. Gastroenterology 1993; 104(Suppl):A177, 223.
Robinson MG, Griffin JW, Bowers J, et al. Effect of ranitidine gastroduodenal mucosal damage induced by nonsteroidal anti-inflammatory drugs. Dig Dis Sci 1989; 34:424–428.
Soll AH, Weinstein WM, Kurata J, et al. Nonsteroidal anti-inflammatory drugs and peptic ulcer disease. Ann Intern Med 1991; 114:307–319.
Walan A, Bader JP, Classen M, et al. Effect of omeprazol and ranitidine on ulcer healing and relapse rates with benign gastric ulcer. N Engl J Med 1989; 320:69–75.

SURGERY FOR PEPTIC ULCER DISEASE

PAUL H. JORDAN, Jr., M.D.

Operative treatment of duodenal ulcer has been restricted to the small proportion of ulcer patients who have had complications from ulcers or to those who do not respond to medical therapy. In spite of improved medical treatment, there are still patients who fall into the second category. The principal surgical procedures used include different types of gastric drainage, gastric resection, and gastric denervation or various combinations of these procedures. Initially, the primary objective of ulcer surgery was to prevent recurrent ulcer. Currently, the objective of operation is to cure an ulcer without a recurrent ulcer or any other undesirable sequelae developing as a result of altered gastric physiology. Perhaps no operation will satisfy each of these conditions for every patient. Parietal cell vagotomy without a drainage procedure, the latest contribution to ulcer surgery, has been studied intensively for 23 years. An operative mortality rate of 0.26 percent, a recurrence rate of 4 to 11 percent, and the virtual absence of significant side effects have made it the operation of choice for a growing number of gastric surgeons.

ELECTIVE SURGERY FOR DUODENAL ULCER

Selection of Operation

The indications for elective operation in patients with intractable peptic ulcer disease cannot be defined rigidly. Severity and duration of symptoms, response to medication, patient compliance, frequency of recurrence, and past complications all contribute to this decision.

The intent of each new surgical procedure has been to improve the clinical results of operation. Controlled clinical trials of the commonly used procedures suggest that, with the exception of the persistence or recurrence of ulcers, there is little to recommend one operation over another. In the case of the newest operation, parietal cell vagotomy without drainage, the complications of gastric operations are almost eliminated while an acceptable rate of recurrent ulcer is maintained. This operation has become the procedure of choice in many parts of the world, particularly England and the European continent, yet it has been accepted less well in the United States because it has been feared that the rate of recurrent ulcer will be too high. In fact, I believe that most surgeons who refuse to use the operation do not want to take the time to learn the procedure or to expend the time and patience required to execute it.

Technical factors resulting from inflammation in the area of the duodenal ulcer may dictate the advisability of one type of operation rather than another. However, most surgeons perform a particular operation in preference to another because of personal bias. In fact, a given operation may be best for a specific surgeon to use because he or she is more experienced and skilled with a certain procedure and therefore performs it with greater safety. It would be ideal if it could be determined that one operation was more suitable for a given patient than any other. Although there are claims that such discrimination is possible, the evidence is not convincing.

Operations

Gastrojejunostomy

For the first 30 years of this century, gastrojejunostomy was the operation of choice for duodenal ulcer in the United States. Slowly it was appreciated that there was a high recurrent ulcer rate after gastrojejunostomy, and curiously it sometimes required many years for these ulcers to develop. Eventually, by the middle 1930s, the prominence of this operation began to decline in favor of gastric resection. Nevertheless, gastroenterostomy is still a viable option in special circumstances, e.g., the elderly poor-risk patient with an obstructing duodenal ulcer.

Distal Subtotal Gastrectomy Without Vagotomy

After the era of gastroenterostomy, gastric resection was used extensively to treat duodenal ulcer. After resection, gastrointestinal continuity can be restored by gastroduodenostomy (Billroth I), or gastrojejunostomy (Billroth II). Undesirable postoperative sequelae increase as greater amounts of the stomach are removed to prevent recurrent ulcers. Some of the complications of distal partial (two-thirds to three-quarters) gastrectomy

and gastroenterostomy do not develop if a gastroduodenostomy is performed instead. The high recurrent rate that occurs with the Billroth I method of restoring gastrointestinal continuity precludes its use unless vagotomy is added.

The recurrent ulcer rate reported after distal gastrectomy ranges from 1.2 to 12.7 percent, and the variations are probably related to different amounts of stomach removed by different surgeons. The use of high subtotal gastrectomy without vagotomy is diminishing because of the clinical evidence that it is desirable to preserve as much gastric reservoir as possible, and the persuasive logic that there is little to recommend the operation over vagotomy and antrectomy, which is safer for most surgeons.

Truncal Vagotomy and Drainage

Vagotomy removes the effect of vagal stimulation of the parietal cells and reduces the sensitivity of parietal cells to gastrin. For these reasons, vagotomy has exerted a profound influence on the treatment of duodenal ulcer. The initial operation of Dragstedt and Owens was transthoracic vagotomy alone, but this was abandoned because it was associated with postoperative gastric retention. They modified their procedure to a transabdominal vagotomy and included a gastroenterostomy to facilitate gastric emptying. Transthoracic vagotomy is now performed only in certain circumstances for the treatment of recurrent ulcer.

Because gastroenterostomy was considered a less than ideal drainage procedure, the Heineke-Mikulicz pyloroplasty was widely substituted and became the most popular drainage procedure. Nevertheless, many surgeons think that stasis is not prevented satisfactorily by this type of pyloroplasty even when the single-layer closure technique is used. The significance of poor gastric emptying as a cause of development of a gastric ulcer after Heineke-Mikulicz pyloroplasty has been emphasized. Rather than risk resection or resort to gastroenterostomy, other types of gastroduodenostomy have been recommended to promote satisfactory gastric drainage after vagotomy. Nevertheless, gastroenterostomy is still held in high esteem in the British Isles. Some consider it the drainage procedure of choice because in patients who develop significant dumping, the gastroenterostomy may be dismantled after the stomach has regained the tone lost by vagotomy without fear of gastric retention. The number of recurrent ulcers is greater after vagotomy and drainage (4 to 27 percent) than after high subtotal gastrectomy (4 percent) or vagotomy and antrectomy (1 percent).

Because antrectomy successfully treats most patients with a recurrent ulcer after they have undergone an adequate vagotomy, one can postulate that the higher recurrent ulcer rate after vagotomy and pyloroplasty than after vagotomy and antrectomy is the result of a continued influence by the retained antrum on acid secretion.

Truncal Vagotomy and Antrectomy

Currently, vagotomy and antrectomy is the most popular operation for treatment of duodenal ulcer. Surgeons utilizing this procedure remove 20 percent (antrectomy) to 50 percent (hemigastrectomy) of the stomach. The procedure was introduced independently in the 1950s by Farmer and Edwards because they thought it would produce achlorhydria effectively and at the same time preserve a larger gastric reservoir than that left after high subtotal gastric resection.

Later, the operation was modified by Harkins and colleagues so that reconstruction was by means of gastroduodenostomy rather than gastroenterostomy. They expected fewer patients to experience dumping symptoms and weight loss with this type of reconstruction. Overall good results of 94 percent with a recurrence rate of 0.5 percent and a mortality rate of 1.0 percent were reported for nonbleeding patients. The low mortality was attributed to the selective use of gastroenterostomy for reconstruction, rather than gastroduodenostomy, in patients in whom inflammation involving the duodenum created unusual technical difficulties and made the latter procedure hazardous.

The consensus of many who favor vagotomy and antrectomy is that the clinical results and mortality rate are equal to or better than those obtained with vagotomy and drainage. In my experience, when the two operations were studied prospectively, the principal difference after 5 years was a recurrent ulcer rate of 8.3 percent for vagotomy and pyloroplasty and 1.1 percent for vagotomy and antrectomy. When choosing between these two commonly performed procedures, it seems that the only justification for subjecting healthy persons to the high risk of recurrent ulcer and possible need for reoperation by performing vagotomy and pyloroplasty is the presence of excessive inflammation surrounding the duodenum, which would make resection unduly dangerous.

One of the early frustrating complications associated with vagotomy and antrectomy is delayed gastric emptying. Fortunately, a stomach that has been slow to empty usually regains its ability to do so if given adequate time and if there is no organic obstruction. A less than perfect stoma and a degree of gastric vagal paresis, neither by itself sufficient to interfere with emptying, may delay gastric emptying when combined. By use of contrast studies and endoscopy, the adequacy of a gastric stoma can be determined early and reoperation performed to correct existing mechanical problems rather than waiting long periods for the "stoma to open."

Selective Vagotomy

Since denervation of all intra-abdominal viscera, as occurs with truncal vagotomy, seemed neither necessary nor desirable for treatment of duodenal ulcer, Jackson and Frankson independently introduced selective vagotomy, which denervates only the stomach. Evidence suggests that sacrifice of the extragastric vagi at the time of truncal vagotomy adversely affects small bowel and pancreatic function and causes bile to become lithogenic. Retention of the extragastric vagi has been credited with preventing postvagotomy diarrhea. An enteropancreatic reflex important for pancreatic exocrine and endocrine function also is dependent on the extragastric vagi.* Selective vagotomy has been used in combination with antrectomy or pyloroplasty in the belief that the clinical results achieved were superior, particularly in reducing the frequency of diarrhea, to those obtained with truncal vagotomy.

Parietal Cell Vagotomy Without Drainage

This operation is the newest of the definitive techniques for treatment of peptic ulcer disease. Its synonyms are proximal gastric vagotomy and highly selective vagotomy. Parietal cell vagotomy without drainage was performed first in humans by Amdrup and Jensen and by Johnston and Wilkinson.

The principle of the operation is to section all branches of the anterior and posterior vagus nerves that supply the fundic gland area of the stomach while preserving the hepatic, celiac, and antral branches. The extent of the denervation that one should strive to achieve is generally agreed upon. There is little support for the need to denervate the greater curvature by cutting the right gastroepiploic vessels. Determination of the distal limit of dissection on the lesser curvature remains the most controversial aspect of the operation. Visual assessment of anatomic landmarks is used by most surgeons to make the determination of the antrofundal junction, which is the boundary between innervated and denervated stomach. Preservation of the motor nerve branches to the antrum makes it unnecessary to resect, destroy, or bypass the pylorus in order to ensure satisfactory gastric emptying. It would be desirable to have more accurate and less cumbersome techniques than those currently available to determine the adequacy of vagotomy intraoperatively.

The dumping syndrome is related indirectly to total vagotomy. It is more the result of gastric incontinence that follows destruction or bypass of the pyloroantral pump by pyloroplasty, antrectomy, or gastroenterostomy. Diarrhea after gastric operations is attributed to truncal vagotomy and/or loss of pyloric function. The cause of vagotomy diarrhea is uncertain, while diarrhea resulting from loss of the pylorus is attributed to unregulated gastric emptying. It was expected that preservation of pyloric function and antral innervation associated with parietal cell vagotomy would reduce dumping by permitting nearly normal gastric emptying, and that preservation of the extragastric vagi would reduce the frequency of diarrhea. These predictions are supported by the study of Jordan and Thornby, which showed no significant difference in the frequency of diarrhea

---

*__Editor's Note:__ Perhaps the steatorrhea that occasionally occurs after esophagectomy is due to the severing of vagal feeders to the pancreas.

between parietal cell vagotomy and selective vagotomy and antrectomy, the extragastric vagi being preserved in both operations. Dumping, on the other hand, was virtually eliminated after parietal cell vagotomy because of pyloric preservation.

The mortality and immediate postoperative morbidity rates have been less than with other gastric procedures. The absence of an anastomosis eliminates anastomotic leaks and afferent and efferent loop syndromes. The mortality in several series of patients has been zero. In a survey of 4,557 patients operated on by 40 different surgeons, the mortality was 0.26 percent.

Unlike truncal vagotomy without a drainage procedure, gastric stasis after parietal cell vagotomy has not been a problem. A potential disadvantage of parietal cell vagotomy was the possibility that retention of an innervated antrum would be a potent stimulus for acid secretion. Acid production in response to a test meal, however, is no greater in patients with a vagally innervated antrum than in those with a vagally denervated antrum. It can be reasonably concluded that the retained gastric antrum need not be vagally denervated in the duodenal ulcer patient, provided that it is well drained and in continuity with the acid-secreting portion of the stomach. Nevertheless, antral preservation after parietal cell vagotomy is undesirable in some patients, which is demonstrated by the fact that some recurrent ulcers can be treated successfully by antrectomy. Why antrectomy is required to control ulcerogenesis in some patients and not in the majority is unknown.

Deaths, immediate postoperative complications, and late complications of dumping, diarrhea, and bilious vomiting are fewer after parietal cell vagotomy without drainage than with any other operation used for the treatment of duodenal ulcer. The recurrent ulcer rate associated with this operation is debated. In reports of patients studied 5 to 10 years after parietal cell vagotomy, the recurrent ulcer rate was 4 to 11 percent. In other studies the recurrence rate was reported to be as high as 26 percent.

The discrepancies between the recurrence rates reported by different investigators are the result of variations in the operative technique used and the experience, training, and skill of different surgeons. This is not an easy operation to perform. The recurrence rate is highest for the first patients operated on by any surgeon and is related to a steep learning curve. In one study, the recurrence rate after parietal cell vagotomy was 33 percent for pyloric and prepyloric ulcers and only 15 percent for duodenal ulcers. This has been the experience of numerous authors, but has been denied by others. The evidence is sufficiently convincing for me to abstain from performing parietal cell vagotomy in patients with pyloric or prepyloric ulcer except in unusual circumstances. The inclusion of pyloric and prepyloric ulcers in reports of the results for duodenal ulcers will influence the rate of recurrence after parietal cell vagotomy for duodenal ulcer.

Although the recurrence rate is debatable, the benefits derived from parietal cell vagotomy so outweigh the possibility and consequences of a recurrence that it is my operation of choice for all patients treated electively in whom the pylorus is adequately patent. Whether or not a surgeon elects to perform parietal cell vagotomy depends on his or her preference for a procedure that avoids mortality and serious sequelae, accepting the fact that reoperation for a recurrent ulcer may occasionally be required.

OPERATION FOR BLEEDING DUODENAL ULCERS

Patients operated on to control bleeding represent increased operative risks. It is important that a clinical judgment be made to operate before vital organ functions deteriorate as a result of poor arterial perfusion.

For surgeons who must operate on patients urgently, an accurate diagnosis of the bleeding source is important. Since we cannot predict which patients will fail to stop bleeding or which will rebleed, it is desirable to diagnose the cause of bleeding by endoscopy at a convenient time after the patient has been stabilized.

In the selection of operation for a patient with a bleeding duodenal ulcer, the basic choice is between truncal vagotomy and antrectomy or truncal vagotomy, oversewing of the bleeding ulcer, and pyloroplasty. Although the mortality rate is lower with the latter, which is my preference, opinions differ regarding the effectiveness of vagotomy, oversew, and pyloroplasty to prevent rebleeding, particularly with large, calloused ulcers.

Foster and colleagues, who earlier reported a mortality rate of 28.5 percent after resection, later reported a mortality rate of 9 percent and a rebleeding rate of 8 percent after vagotomy, oversewing the ulcer, and pyloroplasty. This was less than for any other type of procedure, irrespective of the patient's age, and was their procedure of choice for both gastric and duodenal ulcers, unless technical reasons necessitated resection to control bleeding. All reports are not so favorable. I restrict the emergency use of parietal cell vagotomy for bleeding to younger, less critical patients in whom it has been possible to ligate the bleeding ulcer through a duodenotomy and yet preserve the pylorus (Table 1). This method is gaining wider acceptance.

OPERATION FOR PERFORATED DUODENAL ULCERS

Few physicians treat perforated duodenal ulcers by nonoperative means except in very special circumstances in which an operation is contraindicated or in selected patients in whom it is perceived that the ulcer already has sealed spontaneously. Simple closure of an ulcer with an omental patch continues to be widely practiced and considered by many to be the method of choice whenever it can be used. It is also the treatment for perforated "acute" ulcers preferred by some surgeons

Table 1 Summary of Results of Parietal Cell Vagotomy for Duodenal Ulcer

	No. of Cases	Operative Deaths	No. Followed 2–18 Yr	No. of Recurrent Ulcers	Recurrent Ulcers Treated by Surgery	Medicines
Duodenal ulcers	300	2	249	26	8	18
Pyloric and prepyloric ulcers	45	0	39	13	5	8
Obstructing DU	11*	0	11	1	0	1
Bleeding DU	24	1	19	1	0	1
Perforated DU	106	1	89	5	2	3

*Five patients required a drainage procedure.
DU = Duodenal ulcers.

who advocate definitive therapy for perforated chronic ulcers. Definitive treatment refers to operative procedures that not only deal with the emergency aspects of perforation but also attempt to prevent persistent or recurrent ulcer.

When truncal vagotomy was introduced, its adoption for treatment of perforated ulcer was slow because of the fear of causing mediastinitis. This complication did not materialize, and truncal vagotomy combined with pyloroplasty or antrectomy became the accepted treatment of perforated duodenal ulcers for patients who have an ulcer history, have no purulent peritonitis or abscess at the time of operation, and have not been in shock.

One cannot predict with accuracy at the time of operation for perforation those patients who will require a subsequent operation for recurrent ulcer if a definitive procedure is not performed at the time of perforation. Nevertheless, a definitive operation for all patients must provide protection against recurrent ulcer without risking undesirable gastric sequelae or morbidity, particularly for those patients who would not have had further ulcer problems had a definitive operation not been performed.

Absence of debilitating symptoms and a low recurrent ulcer rate (8.0 percent) associated with parietal cell vagotomy for elective treatment of duodenal ulcer suggested that this operation, combined with patch closure of the ulcer, might be an ideal definitive treatment of perforated duodenal ulcer. We performed this procedure in 110 patients with perforated duodenal ulcer, and there was one operative death. Our results make it the operation of choice when it can be performed (see Table 1).

OPERATION FOR OBSTRUCTING DUODENAL, PYLORIC, OR PREPYLORIC ULCERS

Patients who appear to have gastric outlet obstruction may not have cicatricial obstruction, but instead may have functional obstruction due to pylorospasm. The distinction between obstruction and spasm can be determined preoperatively by endoscopic examination and verified at operation by guiding a tapered 40 Fr dilator passed by the anesthesiologist through the

stomach and pylorus and into the duodenum. If this cannot be done easily without force, parietal cell vagotomy should not be used because of the risk of gastric retention associated with the operation performed in this setting. The recurrence rate after parietal cell vagotomy for pyloric and prepyloric ulcers is so high that the operation should not be used for ulcers in these locations, and certainly not when they are responsible for obstruction. Obstruction due to ulcers is best treated by truncal or selective vagotomy and antrectomy.

Gastric ileus, a potential complication of gastric operations, can be potentiated if an operation is performed on the obstructed and grossly dilated stomach. Patients with gastric outlet obstruction should be operated on after several days of preparation. This time is used to correct electrolyte and metabolic imbalances and to give the stomach, decompensated by distention, an opportunity to regain its muscular tone by gastric decompression. The results of operation when gastric outlet obstruction is present are usually excellent.

Balloon dilatation has enjoyed some popularity with gastrointestinal endoscopists in the treatment of pyloric obstruction. There are no long-term follow-up reports evaluating this form of therapy. Further, we have no knowledge of the degree of fibrosis and stenosis present in ulcers said to be treated successfully by this means. The method appears dangerous, time consuming, and of extremely limited value in the management of cicatricial pyloric obstruction.

GASTRINOMA*

Patients with gastrinomas can be divided into those associated with multiple endocrine neoplasia (MEN) I syndrome and sporadic gastrinomas. Gastrinomas in patients with MEN I originate from multiple sites and are malignant in 50 to 75 percent of patients when first recognized. It is generally agreed that, except for special circumstances, all patients with the diagnosis of gastrinoma should be explored; usually, multiple tumors can be identified. The distribution of gross tumors supports the view that MEN I patients preferentially should be

---

*Editor's Note: This subject is also discussed in two separate chapters.

subjected to a distal 70 to 80 percent pancreatic resection together with enucleation of caput tumors and clearance of regional lymph nodes as well as accessible liver metastases. Approximately 10 percent of patients are resectable for potential cure of the neoplasm. Total gastrectomy, formerly the primary form of surgical therapy, has been challenged, but it remains the treatment of choice for patients in whom all tumor cannot be removed.

Sporadic gastrinomas are primarily found to the right of the superior mesenteric artery in the head of the pancreas, duodenum, or surrounding lymph nodes, i.e., within the gastrinoma triangle. These lesions are also frequently multiple but less malignant than gastrinomas associated with MEN I syndrome. This suggests that the process of development and differentiation of the two types of gastrinoma cells is different. Actually, it has been suggested by Passaro that there are two populations of sporadic gastrinoma: one to the right, which is three times more common than those to the left of the superior mesenteric artery. In his experience, the cure rate of those to the right is 43 percent; sporadic tumors to the left of the superior mesenteric artery are almost always intrapancreatic, most will have metastasized when first discovered, and the cure rate is only 6 percent. It was Passaro's opinion that these differences also reflected different etiologies for the two groups of tumor. Some have said that the sporadic gastrinoma in the head of the pancreas has the same malignant potential as the gastrinoma associated with the MEN I syndrome. In my experience, the behavior of sporadic duodenal and sporadic pancreatic gastrinomas in the head are the same and have a lower malignant potential than those associated with MEN I syndrome.

The goal of surgery is removal of all gastrinoma tissue. Since it cannot be ascertained at operation whether this has been achieved, it is my policy to perform a highly selective vagotomy in all patients after resection of tumor and also in patients in whom a tumor is not found. This procedure, which is without morbidity, not only reduces acid secretion but also changes the pharmacodynamics of H_2 blockers so that they are more effective at lower doses. Total gastrectomy for gastrinoma should not be the initial operation of choice unless there is residual, unresectable, extensive tumor.

LAPAROSCOPIC VAGOTOMY

Truncal vagotomy, when indicated as an independent operation for recurrent ulcer, can be performed satisfactorily by the thoracoscopic approach.

Several groups have performed the classic type of parietal cell vagotomy by the laparoscopic approach. The number of patients reported was small and the follow-up inadequate to enable conclusions to be drawn. The technique was described as laborious, technically demanding, and requiring excessive time. The procedure

has been abandoned by some of the ardent advocates of laparoscopic surgery.

An alternative method consists of posterior truncal vagotomy and anterior seromyotomy. The longest follow-up for this procedure by the laparoscopic route has been 2 months in ten patients. This operation has also been performed by an open technique. The procedure is not a parietal cell vagotomy by definition. Whether it can be performed as well by laparoscopic surgery as by the open technique can be determined only by proper testing and evaluation.

Laparoscopic surgery is in its infancy. The equipment available is improving at an exponential rate and will eventually exceed our imagination. In my opinion, the surgical community must monitor and evaluate new laparoscopic procedures with the scientific criteria and care that has become expected of us. Acceptance of a laparoscopic procedure must depend on whether it is better than its counterpart performed by open operation. This judgment must be based on critical evaluation of the results and not on the fact that it is possible to perform an operation by the laparoscopic technique.

RECOMMENDATIONS

Parietal cell vagotomy is an ulcer operation that gives patients a high probability of cure with almost no risk of mortality or morbidity. Patients with duodenal ulcer disease who are noncompliant, are resistant to drug therapy, are prone to recurrence, or have a chronic calloused ulcer should have the option of surgery as well as the option of continued medical treatment associated with recurrent cycles of pain and disability.

Editor's Note: The author and the editor eagerly await the day when scientific data will emerge from the "I can do it!" school of laparoscopic surgery for peptic ulcer disease.

SUGGESTED READING

Donahue PE, Richter HM, Liu Katherine JM, et al. Experimental basis and clinical application of extended highly selective vagotomy for duodenal ulcer. Surg Gynecol Obstet 1993; 176:39–48.

Emas S, Gupcev G, Erikson B. Six year results of a prospective, randomized trial of selective proximal vagotomy with and without pyloroplasty in the treatment of duodenal, pyloric and prepyloric ulcers. Ann Surg 1993; 217:6–14.

Howard TJ, Sawicki MP, Stabile B, et al. Biologic behavior of sporadic gastrinoma located to the right and left of the superior mesenteric artery. Am J Surg 1993; 165:101–106.

Johnston D, Blackett RL. Recurrent peptic ulcers. World J Surg 1987; 11:274–282.

Jordan PH Jr, Thornby J. Should it be parietal cell vagotomy or selective vagotomy-antrectomy for treatment of duodenal ulcer? A progress report. Ann Surg 1987; 205:572–590.

Koruth NM, Dua KS, Brunt PW, Matheson NA. Comparison of highly selective vagotomy and truncal vagotomy and pyloroplasty: results at 8–15 years. Br J Surg 1990; 77:70–72.

Lunde OC, Liavag I, Roland M. Proximal gastric vagotomy and pyloroplasty for duodenal ulcer with pyloric stenosis. World J Surg 1985; 9:165–170.

ZOLLINGER-ELLISON SYNDROME

PAUL N. MATON, M.D., F.R.C.P., F.A.C.P.

In 1955 Zollinger and Ellison described two patients with extreme acid hypersecretion, ulcers in unusual sites, and a tumor in the pancreas. We now know that the clinical spectrum is much broader and that many patients with Zollinger-Ellison syndrome (ZES) have a simple single bulbar duodenal ulcer, and some have no peptic ulceration at all; some have only a modest increase in acid secretion; and only a minority have a tumor in the pancreas. Nevertheless, ZES is rare, with an incidence of about one case per million per year, and can occur at any age, from under 5 to over 70 years. ZES occurs in two forms; sporadic ZES accounts for about 75 percent of cases in most series. These patients have no family history of ZES and no other endocrine diseases, although advanced metastatic gastrinoma can occasionally produce additional hormones, particularly ACTH resulting in Cushing's syndrome. Patients with multiple endocrine neoplasia type I (MEN I) account for about 25 percent of cases of ZES, and ZES occurs in about 50 percent of patients with MEN I. MEN I is an autosomal dominant condition in which virtually all those affected develop parathyroid hyperplasia and hyperparathyroidism; about 80 percent develop islet cell tumors, of which gastrinoma is the most common; and 50 percent develop pituitary tumors.

CLINICAL SETTING

Partly because of the rarity of ZES and partly because the clinical manifestations are broader than the original description of the syndrome, the possibility of ZES is often overlooked, and many patients have had symptoms for years before the diagnosis is made. Although the most common manifestation of ZES is a duodenal ulcer, it is not appropriate to measure gastrin in every such patient. However, the diagnosis of ZES should be considered in any patient with resistant or recurrent ulcers, ulcers in unusual sites, or an ulcer complication; with ulcers and diarrhea or malabsorption, ulcers and kidney stones, or a family history of MEN I; or undergoing peptic ulcer surgery, or with recurrent ulcers after gastric surgery. Furthermore, ZES is a possibility in any patient with watery diarrhea or malabsorption; up to 25 percent of patients with ZES have no ulcer symptoms or endoscopic findings and have only diarrhea. It is unusual for patients with ZES to have only gastric ulcers or only esophagitis, and such patients are more likely to have normal or low acid output.

DIAGNOSTIC TESTS

Serum gastrin is the first test to perform and should always be measured in the fasting state. Ideally, the patient should be taking no antisecretory medications, but circumstances may delay measurement under these conditions (see below). In the most frequently used assay, the upper limit of normal is 100 pg per milliliter. No particular level of gastrin is diagnostic. Patients with ZES have been described with fasting serum gastrin levels as low as 110 pg per milliliter, or greater than 300,000 pg per milliliter. A markedly lipemic serum can give rise to falsely high levels.

If the serum gastrin is elevated, the most important test to perform next is measurement of acid output. This is essential to exclude hypochlorhydric states that can cause hypergastrinemia, and to identify and quantitate the gastric hypersecretory state. The patient must be adequately hydrated and passing urine with a specific gravity of less than 1020, as fluid depletion reduces gastric secretion. Some patients may require intravenous (IV) hydration before the test can be performed. Upper limits of normal for basal acid output are 10 mEq per hour for men and 7 mEq per hour for women. Diagnostic values for ZES are greater than 15 mEq per hour, or greater than 5 mEq per hour if the patient has had gastric surgery. Nevertheless, a raised gastrin level with a normal acid output still suggests ZES, and acid output testing should be repeated or the patient referred to a specialist center if such values are obtained. Maximal acid output has no diagnostic significance but can be measured after administration of pentagastrin.

Many facilities no longer measure acid output, but measurement of gastric pH is simple. If pH is more than 3.5 (less than 0.3 mEq per liter), the hypergastrinemia is due to hypochlorhydria. If the pH is low and gastrin level greater than 1,000 pg per milliliter, ZES is likely. If the tests are equivocal and acid output cannot be measured reliably, the patient should be referred to a center where this can be performed, because knowledge of acid output is crucial to the diagnosis and management of ZES.

Although the secretin test is widely used, it is important to remember that it is not completely reliable, and false-positive and false-negative results can occur. Furthermore, the secretin test is less useful than those for serum gastrin and acid output. If gastrin is elevated but the patient is achlorhydric, the secretin test will not be helpful because the diagnosis is clearly hypergastrinemia due to hypochlorhydria (due to pernicious anemia, gastric atrophy, antisecretory therapy, chronic renal failure, pheochromocytoma, or a previous vagotomy). If gastrin and acid output are elevated, a secretin test will help only if it is important to exclude the retained antrum syndrome, G cell hyperplasia, gastric outlet obstruction, or ZES in a patient with a previous vagotomy or gastric resection. However, these diagnoses can largely be excluded on the basis of the history. The meal stimulation and calcium infusion tests no longer have a place in the routine diagnosis of ZES.

127

INITIAL MANAGEMENT STRATEGY

Because patients with ZES can suffer major ulcer complications with little or no warning, acid output should be controlled as soon as possible, even if this delays definitive diagnostic tests for a few days. On the day the diagnosis is suspected, blood should be drawn for measurement of serum gastrin and the patient given medication. Omeprazole is safe, and the expense of the drug given for the time it takes to establish a definitive diagnosis is small compared with the risks to an untreated patient. Once acid output is under control, the tests to establish the diagnosis of ZES can be planned in a logical and safe manner. The rest of the work-up, the diagnosis of sporadic ZES or ZES with MEN I, and the assessment of tumor extent can usually be delayed even for weeks without detriment to the patient.

Fasting serum gastrin levels should be measured when the patient is not taking H_2 antagonists or omeprazole. However, if the patient is taking medication when first seen, it is safest to obtain a gastrin level at that time, in the knowledge that if the result is equivocal the test can be repeated later off drug. If the patient is stable, oral omeprazole, 60 mg per day, should be given immediately. Many studies have shown that reduction of acid output to less than 10 mEq per hour allows healing of ulcers and prevents complications in most patients with ZES. Acid output should therefore be checked daily and the dose of omeprazole increased until acid output is less than 10 mEq per hour in the last hour before the next dose.

If the patient has a complication from an ulcer or is in the postoperative period when first seen, immediate control of acid output can be achieved by giving ranitidine as an IV bolus of 100 mg together with a continuous infusion of 0.5 mg per kilogram per hour. Acid output should be measured and the dose increased every 4 hours until acid output is less than 10 mEq per hour. A dose of 1 mg per kilogram per hour controls acid output in 70 percent of patients, but occasionally doses as large as 4 to 5 mg per kilogram per hour are required. IV drug dosing should be continued for 24 hours after starting the oral drug. When switching to oral H_2 antagonist, a good estimate of the dose required is obtained by giving 150 percent of the total daily IV dose split into four equal 6 hourly doses. However, the efficacy of this oral dose should still be measured directly.

Once satisfactory control of acid secretion has been achieved and the patient is stable with normal mucosal appearances on endoscopy, other investigations can be performed. To determine basal and stimulated acid outputs and fasting gastrin measurements faithfully with the patient off all antisecretory drugs safely, the patient should stop omeprazole 1 week before the test, switch to a dose of oral H_2 antagonist that reduces acid output to less than 10 mEq per hour until 30 hours before the test, and then be given continuous IV H_2 antagonists, stopping 12 hours before testing.

DIFFERENTIAL DIAGNOSIS OF TYPE OF ZOLLINGER-ELLISON SYNDROME

It is important to determine the type of ZES, especially with regard to tumor management, so that patients with ZES and MEN I avoid unnecessary or ineffective surgery. In every patient with ZES a history or a family history of renal stones, pancreatic tumors, or pituitary tumors should be sought. However, in some patients with MEN I there is no family history, and although most patients with MEN I develop hypercalcemia and kidney stones first, ZES occasionally is the first manifestation. Therefore, in every patient with ZES, plasma calcium, parathormone, prolactin, luteinizing hormone–follicle stimulating hormone, and growth hormone should be measured, and a computed tomographic (CT) or magnetic resonance imaging (MRI) scan of the pituitary should be performed. Despite all these investigations, the diagnosis of MEN I sometimes becomes evident only years later. Now that the MEN I gene is known to be on chromosome 11, genetic analysis should soon make a definitive diagnosis easy and reliable. If the patient proves to have MEN I, tests for other peptides produced by islet cell tumors (VIP, growth hormone–releasing hormone, somatostatin, glucagon, pancreatic polypeptide) should be performed.

CONTROL OF ACID HYPERSECRETION

Long-Term Control

It is essential that control of acid output be measured directly, because symptoms are not a reliable guide to the presence of mucosal disease, and the dose required has to be determined in each patient. In patients with ZES, omeprazole is now the drug of choice for lóng-term control of acid secretion. It is very effective, has a low incidence of side effects and drug interactions, and has proved safe when taken for prolonged periods. Omeprazole given once or twice a day controls acid secretion effectively in all patients. It should be given once a day up to a dose of 120 mg per day. If acid output is still greater than 10 mEq per hour with 120 mg once a day, the dose should be split and given as 60 mg every 12 hours. Such a dose should be sufficient for any patient with ZES. The full effect of omeprazole is not seen for several days, and acid output may continue to fall for a few days with no increase in drug dose. It may be possible to reduce the dose subsequently, but because of the long duration of action, dose reductions cannot be made more often than once a week. The adequacy of control of acid secretion should be checked at least annually, as drug requirements may change.

Although omeprazole has been largely free of side effects, some concerns about long-term use remain. When given to rats for most of their life, omeprazole produces gastric carcinoids as a consequence of achlorhydria and hypergastrinemia. Patients with ZES are already hypergastrinemic, and those with MEN I especially are at increased risk of developing gastric carcinoids. However, studies of patients with ZES given continuous omeprazole for 7 to 10 years have shown no definite increase in the precursor cells of gastric carcinoids or in gastric carcinoid tumors.

If for some reason the patient cannot take omeprazole, H_2 antagonists should be used. Acid hypersecretion can be controlled with H_2 antagonists in nearly all patients if sufficient drug is given, but most patients need these agents every 6 or even every 4 hours. As with omeprazole, the dose required cannot be predicted and has to be determined empirically. Most patients with ZES who have taken both omeprazole and H_2 antagonists say that omeprazole provides better symptom relief. Furthermore, it is very difficult to control acid stringently enough with H_2 antagonists in patients with a gastric resection or esophageal stricture. Dose requirements of H_2 antagonists tend to rise with time, and many patients taking these drugs need annual increases in dosage as determined by gastric analysis. Of the available H_2 antagonists, there has been most experience with ranitidine, some with cimetidine and famotidine, and least with nizatidine. A typical daily dose of ranitidine is 600 mg every 6 hours, but it has been used in doses as high as 9,200 mg per day without problems. Cimetidine in the large doses often required in ZES often causes impotence and gynecomastia in men and should be avoided. Each of the H_2 antagonists is equally effective if equipotent doses are used. If it is necessary to switch from one H_2 antagonist to another, the potency ratio by weight of cimetidine-to-nizatidine-to-ranitidine-to-famotidine is 1:4:4:32.

Some patients who require large doses of H_2 antagonists are able to reduce the dosage by taking anticholinergics that potentiate the H_2 antagonists. However, many patients develop side effects on such a regimen. Octreotide acetate, the somatostatin analog, can reduce acid output satisfactorily, but there is no indication for its use in ZES as there are good alternative drugs with fewer side effects that do not have to be given by injection.

Special Circumstances

Two subgroups of patients with ZES require more profound inhibition of gastric acid secretion than the less than 10 mEq per hour that is sufficient for most patients. Patients who have had a previous partial gastrectomy and especially a Billroth II gastrectomy are sensitive to the effects of acid; they should have acid output reduced to less than 5 mEq per hour, and then further increase drug dose until the gastric and duodenal mucosa are normal at endoscopy. About 5 percent of patients with ZES continue to have recurrent esophageal strictures despite acid output being reduced to less than 10 mEq per hour. If acid output is reduced to less than 1 mEq per hour, there is a marked reduction in the need for

dilatation. In most patients, 60 mg omeprazole twice a day is needed to reduce acid output to this level.

A total gastrectomy should be reserved for the rare patient who is unable to tolerate oral medication, and partial gastrectomy should never be performed in a patient with ZES because it exacerbates peptic ulceration. However, other surgical options for reduction of acid output can be considered in selected patients. A highly selective vagotomy has been shown to reduce acid output and drug requirements, although it does not abolish the need for medication. In patients with ZES and MEN I, hyperparathyroidism exacerbates the manifestations of ZES. A total parathyroidectomy that results in normocalcemia reduces gastrin, acid output and drug requirements. Occasionally, parathyroidectomy results in a normal gastrin level and acid output.

Patients who are undergoing surgery of any type, who are having chemotherapy, or who have gastroenteritis or other condition that might interfere with absorption of oral medication may require an IV antisecretory drug. Patients who cannot take oral drug for more than a day if taking omeprazole, or more than 12 hours if taking H_2 antagonists, should receive a continuous IV H_2 antagonist as described above. In patients undergoing surgery, acid output should be rechecked in the immediate postoperative period, since many require a short-term increase in dose.

CONTROL OF GASTRINOMA

Management of the gastrinoma in patients with ZES has changed in recent years because of increasing knowledge of tumor pathology. Gastrinomas were thought to be islet cell tumors and therefore pancreatic in origin, but recently it has become clear that this is not so. Since the management of gastrinoma differs in patients with sporadic ZES and ZES as part of MEN I, they are discussed separately.

Sporadic Zollinger-Ellison Syndrome

Most gastrinomas are small, have typical endocrine cell histology, and arise within an area bordered by the hilum of the liver, the lateral border of the second part of the duodenum, and the head of the pancreas, the "gastrinoma triangle." Rarely, gastrin-producing tumors occur in the ovary, but these are large, low-grade, malignant adenocarcinomas with gastrin-staining epithelial cells. Recent studies have shown that about 40 percent of primary gastrinomas arise in the submucosa of the duodenum, about 10 to 20 percent in the lymph nodes, and only a minority in the pancreas. Gastrinomas usually spread first to lymph nodes, then to liver, and then to many tissues, especially bone.

Preoperative Tumor Assessment

Imaging of gastrinomas is performed for two reasons: (1) to identify patients with hepatic metastases who are not candidates for surgery and (2) to attempt to identify the primary tumor. Careful prospective studies of various imaging modalities (ultrasonography, MRI, CT, and angiography) have identified the best approach to imaging both primary and metastatic gastrinomas. CT scan with IV contrast is the single best screening test for metastatic disease, but detects hepatic metastases in only about 80 percent of patients. However, subsequent selective hepatic angiography will detect virtually all hepatic metastases missed by CT. For identifying the primary tumor, the best noninvasive tool, CT (which should include the ovaries as well as the pancreatic area), identifies only 40 percent, and angiography identifies only 60 percent of primary tumors in patients subjected to surgery. Furthermore, the addition of venous sampling of portal vein radicals for gastrin, and measurement of gastrin levels after intra-arterial secretin, as performed in specialist centers, have not proved generally useful and are technically difficult and expensive. Therefore, a rational approach to the preoperative assessment of gastrinomas is for every patient to undergo CT scan followed by selective angiography to identify small hepatic metastases missed by CT and possibly to identify the primary tumor.* Patients with no evidence of hepatic disease should then undergo surgery, while those with metastases will require a blind or CT-guided liver biopsy to confirm the diagnosis, together with CT scan of the chest and a bone scan to establish the extent of the disease.

Localized Gastrinoma

Advances in intraoperative techniques by surgeons experienced in operating on patients with ZES have led to major improvements in identifying primary gastrinomas. Since preoperative imaging studies are not very effective, it is important that patients with ZES are operated on by a surgeon experienced with the disease. (Please see the chapter *Endocrine Tumors of the Pancreas*) Every patient with sporadic ZES and no hepatic metastases should undergo an extensive exploratory laparotomy that includes a detailed examination of the pancreas and duodenum, including kocherization of the duodenum to examine posterior aspects of the duodenum and pancreas. The remainder of the abdomen, including gallbladder, liver, omentum, small intestine, kidney, and ovary (all sites where gastrinomas have been found), should be examined carefully. Intraoperative ultrasonography should be performed, as it may identify small tumors within the pancreas that palpation has missed, and endoscopic transillumination of the duodenum to look for submucosal gastrinomas, which are manifested by a failure to transilluminate. Finally, a duodenotomy should be performed to identify tiny gastrinomas on the pancreatic aspect of the duodenum. All visible tumor should be removed, including peripancreatic lymph nodes. Frozen section of these may result

in more extensive node removal. In early series, cures were achieved in only 5 percent of patients. Preoperative imaging and a detailed laparotomy led to tumors being found in about 60 percent of patients and a cure in 30 to 40 percent. With the addition of endoscopic transillumination, tumors are found in 90 percent and cure is achieved in about 50 percent of patients. The addition of a duodenotomy may increase the cure rate further.

If no tumor is found, a blind resection of the body and tail should not be performed, because gastrinomas are distributed in the duodenum and in the pancreatic head region. Some authors have advocated performing a highly selective vagotomy to reduce acid output and drug requirements in those who are not cured. This seems appropriate, but the long-term efficacy of this approach is unknown.

Follow-up After Surgery

Even if all visible tumor is removed after surgery, it is not possible to be certain whether all tumor has been removed and whether the patient is cured. Therefore, the safest approach is to continue with the dosage of IV antisecretory drug that was established preoperatively and then switch to the preoperative oral dose of antisecretory medication and reassess the patient 2 to 3 months later. Tests should be performed for fasting serum gastrin, secretin, and acid output while the drug is being taken and after controlled cessation of the drug (see above). CT and selective angiography should be done to define the postoperative anatomy (which may have been changed by surgery) and set a baseline to assess possible tumor recurrence (if the patient has been cured) or further tumor growth (if the patient is not cured). Even if the patient is cured, acid output may not return to normal. Many of these patients remain mild gastric acid hypersecretors and need small doses of medication.

Of those patients who are cured at the first postoperative assessment, about 50 percent have a biochemical recurrence, and in some recurrent imageable tumor, within 5 years. Thus *all* patients should have *annual* serum gastrins, secretin tests and measurements of acid output. Long-term follow-up studies show that over 90 percent of patients with no hepatic metastases at the time of surgery, and in whom no tumor is found or all visible tumor is removed, even if not cured, have a 10 year survival and live for many years.

Metastatic Gastrinoma

Metastases to local lymph nodes should be removed at laparotomy, but the ideal management of hepatic metastases has yet to be determined. In a small minority of patients who have metastases limited to one part of the liver, resection of all metastases may be possible and may prolong life. Rarely, resection of a single hepatic tumor, has led to complete cure, presumably because the hepatic tumor was the primary. However, most patients with metastatic disease are not surgical candidates, and

---

***Editor's Note:** Endoscopic ultrasound is being assessed in patients with ZES and may prove useful.

these have only a 20 to 30 percent 5 year survival rate. It is important to remember that even patients with extensive metastatic gastrinoma are often asymptomatic if acid output is controlled, and thus any potential benefit of antitumor therapy needs to be balanced against side effects. Published studies have not shown encouraging results. The reports show that none of the modalities used (hepatic arterial embolization, chemotherapy, octreotide, or interferon) prolongs life, and all have significant side effects. At present it is not clear whether any therapy is of benefit for metastatic gastrinoma, other than radiotherapy for bone metastases. Management of these patients should be tailored to the individual.*

Zollinger-Ellison Syndrome as Part of MEN I

In patients with MEN I, local resection of a gastrinoma, or even resection of 90 percent of the pancreas, never leads to a cure. Furthermore, gastrinomas differ from other islet cell tumors in patients with MEN I that are curable by local resection. Recent studies have shown that this is because 50 percent of primary gastrinomas in MEN I arise in the duodenum and only 10 percent in the pancreas. However, unlike patients with sporadic ZES who usually have a single duodenal tumor, most patients with MEN I have multiple duodenal tumors.

Tumor Assessment

All patients with ZES as part of MEN I should undergo a CT scan of the abdomen to assess the pancreas, liver, and surrounding structures. Selective angiography should also be performed to detect any hepatic metastases missed by CT and to examine the pancreas. If the patient has hepatic metastases, a liver biopsy and bone scan should be performed.

Localized Gastrinoma

These patients should not be operated on routinely. Any tumors within the pancreas identified by nonoperative imaging studies are likely to be other types of islet cell tumors, with or without any functional tumor production. Most patients have small (<0.5 cm) submucosal duodenal gastrinomas that can only be identi-

fied at laparotomy with endoscopic transillumination or duodenotomy. Because the only operation likely to lead to cure of ZES (total pancreatic and duodenal resection) carries unacceptable morbidity, the role of surgery in these patients remains uncertain. It may be that they should never undergo surgery, or only have resection of large pancreatic tumors, not to produce a cure but in an attempt to prevent metastases. It may be that detailed localization studies will lead to the development of approaches that avoid a Whipple procedure yet offer a chance for cure. These questions can be answered only in specialized centers with prospective studies.*

Metastatic Disease

Some studies, but not others, suggest that the tumors in patients with MEN I are less aggressive than those that occur in patients with sporadic ZES. Nevertheless, some patients with ZES as part of MEN I die of metastatic islet cell tumors. Whether these are always gastrinomas, or are metastatic nonfunctioning islet cell tumors in patients who also have ZES, has not been studied systematically. In the few studies of chemotherapy or other therapy for metastatic islet cell tumors that included patients with MEN I, the patients were combined with non–MEN I patients. Since ZES with MEN I is rarer than sporadic ZES, there are even fewer data on the treatment of metastatic gastrinoma in patients with MEN I, and management remains problematic.

SUGGESTED READING†

Donow C, Pipeleers-Marichal M, Schroder S, et al. Surgical pathology of gastrinoma: site, size, multicentricity, association with multiple endocrine neoplasia type 1, and malignancy. Cancer 1991; 68: 1329–1334.

Maton PN, Gardner JD, Jensen RT. Recent advances in the management of gastric hypersecretion in patients with Zollinger-Ellison syndrome. Gastroenterol Clin North Am 1989; 18:847–864.

Norton J, Doppman J, Jensen R. Curative resection in Zollinger-Ellison syndrome: results of a 10-year prospective study. Ann Surg 1992; 215:8–18.

Vinayek R, Frucht H, Chiang H-CV, et al. Zollinger-Ellison syndrome: recent advances in the management of the gastrinoma. Gastroenterol Clin North Am 1990; 19:197–218.

Wolfe MM, Jensen RT. Zollinger-Ellison syndrome. N Engl J Med 1987; 317:1200–1209.

---

*Editor's Note: The results of Moertle et al with hepatic artery occlusion and with sequence chemotherapy for patients with hepatic dominant metastases of islet cell carcinoma and carcinoid tumor are reviewed in Ann Intern Med 1994; 120:302–309.

---

*Editor's Note: As mentioned, there is a chapter on surgery of endocrine tumors of the pancreas in another section of the book.

†Editor's Note: There are other pertinent references in the chapter on surgery of endocrine tumors of the pancreas.

UPPER GASTROINTESTINAL BLEEDING

JOHN BAILLIE, M.B., Ch.B., F.R.C.P. (Glasg.)

Acute upper gastrointestinal (GI) hemorrhage is a life-threatening emergency. Early recognition and prompt and appropriate management of this condition will avoid unnecessary deaths. Mortality from GI bleeding can be divided into *avoidable* and *unavoidable* deaths. Avoidable causes of death include delayed or otherwise inadequate resuscitation, aspiration, transfusion reaction, and complications of attempted therapy (e.g., tamponade tube placement). It is particularly tragic when errors of commission or omission result in a needless death from GI bleeding, especially in a young person.*

Most deaths from GI hemorrhage are unavoidable. Patients with liver disease may have GI bleeding as the agonal event. Arterial or variceal hemorrhage may be the lethal event in patients with progressive, multisystem failure. It has long been said that the mortality rate from acute GI bleeding remains static at around 10 percent. Clearly, this figure is lower and falling owing to advances in resuscitation and the benefits of diagnostic and therapeutic GI endoscopy. In many countries, gastroenterologists and surgeons jointly manage GI hemorrhage. In large, specialist referral centers, this may occur in designated GI bleeding units. The advantages of a multidisciplinary approach to GI bleeding are obvious. It is a great pity that "turf" issues in the United States have rendered such obviously appropriate collaboration difficult or impossible in many centers. To ensure the best outcome for every patient, collaborative management is essential. A clear understanding of end points, defining failure of medical management, should result in the patient proceeding without delay to radiologic or surgical intervention. Although this discussion focuses principally on upper GI hemorrhage, the general principles apply to all causes of GI bleeding.

CAUSES

With few exceptions, massive bleeding from the upper GI tract is arterial or variceal in origin (Table 1). Severe erosive disorders such as esophagitis, gastritis, and duodenitis may occasionally cause significant fresh hemorrhage, but the "industrial strength" bleeding that is truly life-threatening suggests that an "arterial pumper" or varix is hemorrhaging. There is an important lesson to be learned from this. One should be skeptical about accepting the diagnosis of, say, "gastritis" in a

*__Editor's Note:__ These avoidable deaths used to be seasonal (July and August) as new house officers learned by trial and error.

Table 1 Causes of Upper Gastrointestinal (GI) Bleeding

Common Causes of Profuse Upper GI Bleeding
 Duodenal ulcer
 Gastric ulcer
 Esophageal varices
 Dieulafoy's lesion*

Common Causes of Acute Upper GI Bleeding, But Rarely Profuse
 Esophagitis
 Gastritis
 Gastric erosions
 Duodenitis
 Mallory-Weiss tear

Uncommon Causes of Profuse Upper GI Bleeding
 Aortoduodenal fistula
 Esophageal ulcer
 Hemobilia
 Vascular malformation
 Malignancy (carcinoma, lymphoma)
 Pseudoaneurysm in pancreatitis†
 Generalized hemorrhagic states (e.g., ITP, DIC)
 Duodenal–small bowel varices
 Ulcerated diverticulum

Common Causes of Chronic GI Bleeding (May Present as Anemia)
 Gastric ulcer
 Duodenal ulcer
 Esophagitis, gastritis, duodenitis
 Vascular malformation‡
 Malignancy (carcinoma, lymphoma)

Uncommon Causes of Chronic GI Bleeding
 Diffuse vascular ectasia ("watermelon stomach")
 Polyps
 Ampullary carcinoma
 Crohn's disease

*Arterial "point" bleeder.
†Splenic artery or pancreaticoduodenal artery.
‡Telangiectasia.
ITP = idiopathic thrombocytopenic purpura; DIC = disseminated intravascular coagulation.

patient with obviously massive hemorrhage. Small arterial bleeding points (e.g., Dieulafoy's lesion) are easily missed by the inexperienced endoscopist. One must always be prepared to reassess the patient who suffers bleeding out of proportion to the apparent endoscopic diagnosis. If necessary, several endoscopies may be necessary to establish the true cause of bleeding. Although duodenal and gastric ulcers are the prime causes of upper GI arterial bleeding, acute esophageal ulcers and Mallory-Weiss tears can also produce this dramatic effect. Indeed, the original description of the Mallory-Weiss lesion was published as an autopsy series. Immunodeficient and immunosuppressed patients, such as those with AIDS, may develop deep, penetrating esophageal ulcers secondary to infection with cytomegalovirus or herpesvirus. A special case is the patient who has undergone previous surgery for aortic aneurysm. Infection of prosthetic aortic grafts can cause aortoenteric fistulas, which mimic acute ulcer hemorrhage. Failure to make the diagnosis of aortoenteric fistula after the initial hemorrhage often results in death (the second or subsequent hemorrhage is usually fatal). Hemorrhage from esophageal, gastric, or duodenal varices is rarely less than spectacular and often life-threatening. The reluctance of varices to stop bleeding (until portal venous pressure has dropped sufficiently low) is due in part to the lack of a muscular arterial wall that can contract and contain bleeding. With the widespread use of endoscopic sclerotherapy, gastric (and more distal) varices have become more common; obliterating esophageal varices by sclerotherapy (or other endoscopic techniques) simply shifts the venous pressure problem "downstream."

As previously stated, "-itis" rarely causes life-threatening hemorrhage. However, esophagitis, gastritis, or duodenitis coupled with a clotting disorder may render a relatively benign condition more serious. Patients on anticoagulant therapy may bleed profusely from relatively unimpressive lesions. Similarly, hemorrhage in the setting of disseminated intravascular coagulation (DIC) or other coagulopathy may be brisk and difficult to contain. Chronic (often occult) upper GI blood loss may result from esophagitis, gastritis, or duodenitis as well as from ulcers, polyps, and telangiectasia. "Watermelon stomach," named after its endoscopic appearance, is a peculiar and sometimes dramatic form of vascular ectasia. A broad spectrum of disorders ranging from burns, trauma, and sepsis to the stress of the perioperative period contribute to acute gastric erosions and ulceration. These may present with acute hemorrhage. It is common in intensive care unit (ICU) practice to suppress acid with continuous infusion of antacids through a nasogastric (NG) tube or intravenous (IV) administration of H_2 blocking agents such as ranitidine or cimetidine. For reasons that are poorly understood, these prophylactic measures are often unsuccessful. Presumably, some defect in mucosal resistance must be involved in stress ulceration.

Benign and malignant tumors of the upper GI tract can cause bleeding that is usually slow, resulting in progressive anemia or iron deficiency. Massive bleeding from an upper GI tumor is most unusual. However, eroding tumors (e.g., carcinoma in the pancreas) or large friable tumors (e.g., ampullary carcinoma) present a major management problem, as they may be resistant to the usual hemostatic measures. Hemorrhage from eroding tumors is often a terminal event. Foreign bodies rarely cause GI bleeding. However, sharp objects (e.g., chicken bones, toothpicks) have been reported to cause life-threatening hemorrhage by perforating the esophagus, creating a fistula into the thoracic aorta. Finally, it should not be forgotten that a story of hematemesis or hematochezia (passing blood per rectum) may be *factitious;* i.e., this may be an invention to gain sympathy or hospital admission in patients with psychiatric illness or those who are seeking shelter and food (which are usually available in hospitals). Prison inmates may claim to have vomited or passed blood and not infrequently swallow foreign bodies (e.g., a razor blade with tape covering the sharpened edge) in an attempt to gain

prison hospital privileges or a brief sojourn in a pleasant hospital environment.

CLINICAL PRESENTATION AND MANAGEMENT

When acute upper GI bleeding presents as hematemesis (vomiting of blood), there is little doubt about the diagnosis. Hematemesis must be distinguished from hemoptysis. This is usually evident from a careful history. Unexplained syncope should always raise suspicion of occult GI bleeding, especially in the elderly. A large volume of blood may be lost into the GI tract without immediate hematemesis or passage of fresh (or altered) blood per rectum. Blood in the GI tract constitutes a protein load that is partially digested and absorbed. Elevated blood urea nitrogen (BUN) is a manifestation of this phenomenon. The protein load may be sufficient to "push" a patient with hepatic insufficiency into encephalopathy. Any stable cirrhotic patient who develops encephalopathy without obvious reason should be suspected of having had occult GI bleeding and appropriately investigated.

A careful history often suggests the underlying diagnosis. For example, repeated retching followed by hematemesis, particularly in the setting of excessive alcohol intake, is a common presentation of a Mallory-Weiss tear. An elderly patient who has been using nonsteroidal anti-inflammatory drugs (NSAIDs) may well have a lesser-curve gastric ulcer. Known liver disease or portal hypertension should raise suspicion of esophageal, gastric, or other varices as the source of a major bleed. Patients with tumors involving or impinging on the GI tract may bleed as a complication of their disease. Chronic renal failure and aortic valve disease predispose to angiodysplasia, which can cause troublesome acute or chronic GI bleeding. An appropriate history and physical examination will reveal the patient with hereditary hemorrhagic telangiectasia (Osler-Weber-Rendu disease). A detailed physical examination may be impractical or undesirable when resuscitative efforts demand immediate attention. A brief but focused initial examination suffices in these circumstances.

The management of massive, acute upper GI hemorrhage is quite different from that of chronic GI blood loss, with or without anemia. Patients with massive upper GI bleeding present sooner or later to an emergency room. Initial evaluation is very important. The number one priority in managing patients with massive GI bleeding is *resuscitation.* There is little point in having the intern (or medical student) take a wonderfully detailed history as the patient becomes dangerously hypovolemic. This is not to say that the history is unimportant, but immediate and vigorous resuscitation is the key to a favorable outcome. When the acutely bleeding patient arrives in the emergency room, at least two large-bore IV cannulas should be placed for venous access. If the patient is markedly hypotensive, it is advisable to place him or her in a head-down position to maintain cerebral perfusion. However, the patient should not be left supine, as this favors reflux of gastric contents and aspiration. If not significantly orthostatic, the patient should preferably be nursed with the head of the bed elevated, to reduce the risk of free reflux of gastric contents into the esophagus and hypopharynx.

While blood is being cross-matched and prepared for transfusion, the circulating volume should be replaced, preferably by colloid (e.g., plasma protein solution, dextran) rather than crystalloid (e.g., saline solution). However, if only standard IV solutions are available, these are certainly better than nothing. The patient who has lost a significant amount of circulating volume is often confused and agitated owing to the effects of reduced cerebral perfusion. Providing supplemental oxygen by nasal cannula or face mask is a simple measure that may improve the patient's mental state. It is a sensible precaution to pass an NG tube for aspiration of stomach contents in patients with acute bleeding. However, care should be taken to ensure that the tip of the tube is well down in the stomach before it is attached to suction. Injury to the distal esophagus when mucosa is sucked into the holes of the NG tube is common and may compound the bleeding problem.

Hemodynamic Status

It is not enough to monitor peripheral blood pressure in patients with acute GI hemorrhage. Baroreceptor reflexes will maintain blood pressure until the circulating volume drops to a dangerously low level. At this point, the reflexes channeling blood away from the periphery to maintain perfusion of vital organs can no longer cope, and circulatory collapse rapidly ensues. This phenomenon can be particularly dramatic in young patients, who are often assumed to be more resistant to the effects of hypovolemia than they actually are. The status of circulating volume can easily be assessed by simple bedside maneuvers such as measuring orthostatic changes in blood pressure (e.g., with the patient lying and sitting, or before and after raising the legs). Where available, a central venous pressure (CVP) line should be placed. CVP is an accurate reflection of circulatory return to the heart; a progressively falling value should alert the physician to volume depletion. ICUs frequently use an indwelling arterial blood pressure monitor, which is a very sensitive method for following the patient's progress.

A risk that is not often considered in resuscitating patients with acute GI hemorrhage is the possibility of overtransfusion. This is particularly problematic in patients with variceal bleeding, who should not be transfused up to their normal hematocrit volume. Restoring the normal circulating volume will elevate portal venous pressure, which may precipitate further bleeding. It is advisable to limit blood transfusion in patients with varices to that required to bring the hematocrit up to around 30 percent. Excessive infusion of colloid or crystalloid solution may push even fit young patients into pulmonary edema. I have seen a fit sailor in his twenties develop gross pulmonary edema after rapid transfusion of 4 L of physiologic saline. This was "treatment" for a syncopal episode, which was wrongly attributed to occult GI bleeding. Not all patients with active bleeding can be stabilized by initial resuscitation. Investigation should not be unduly delayed in the face of persistent hemodynamic instability.

From time to time, a patient with massive bleeding from an upper GI source presents with syncope but no overt bleeding. When bleeding is suspected, an NG tube should be passed and the stomach lavaged to assess the return. If blood is recovered, this is a useful diagnostic test. However, a negative gastric aspirate and lavage means nothing; blood gushing from a duodenal ulcer may not reflux through the pylorus if spasm is present. It is even possible for a pool of blood lying in the dependent area of the stomach to be missed if the NG tube coils in the fundus. If upper GI hemorrhage is sufficiently rapid, the patient may pass fresh bloody stool. This raises the difficulty of distinguishing upper from lower GI hemorrhage. Again, NG aspiration and lavage, if possible, is helpful. Although most fresh rectal bleeding arises within a short distance of the anus, the possibility of an upper GI source should always be considered.

Initial Management

Patients with acute GI bleeding should be kept fasting so that endoscopy can be undertaken when appropriate. Antacids and other liquid preparations (e.g., sucralfate) should not be given, as they obscure the endoscopic view. There is absolutely no place for barium studies in the assessment of acute upper GI bleeding. A baseline electrocardiogram and chest x-ray are useful. Particularly in patients over the age of 50, the hypovolemic insult of hemorrhage may precipitate ischemic events, including myocardial infarction. Amidst the turmoil that accompanies acute GI bleeding, these events may be "silent." The patient who remains persistently hypotensive and tachycardiac despite apparently adequate volume replacement should be assessed for possible myocardial infarction. Baseline chest radiography is helpful should the patient later require evaluation for possible aspiration.

Serial estimations of hemoglobin or hematocrit provide data regarding the efficacy of transfusion. However, in the early stages of significant GI bleeding, the patient can be hypovolemic with a *normal* hematocrit volume. It is a wise precaution in all patients with massive GI bleeding to check basic blood clotting parameters such as prothrombin time, partial thromboplastin time, and platelet count. When appropriate, a screen for DIC is worthwhile. Vitamin K acts too slowly to be of use in the acute situation for correction of a prolonged prothrombin time (e.g., in patients with liver disease). Fresh frozen plasma infusion is preferable, although significantly more expensive. Platelet infusions are rarely indicated unless the peripheral platelet count is exceedingly low (e.g., less than 10,000 per cubic millimeter). Patients who have been therapeutically anticoagulated with sodium warfarin require prompt reversal of this in the face of major hemorrhage.

Empiric use of vasopressin, metoclopramide, or other agents thought to be useful in the management of variceal bleeding is not recommended without confirmation of the diagnosis. Although vasopressin infusion has been used for over 30 years in acute variceal hemorrhage, there is still no well-designed study available to confirm its efficacy. Metoclopramide and somatostatin analog have been used with reported benefit in acute variceal bleeding. Gastric lavage with ice-cold water should be avoided altogether. Thirty years ago there was a vogue for this procedure, as it was felt that cold water would cause a bleeding artery to go into spasm and stop bleeding, but this simply does not work. Gastric lavage with ice-cold water is an excellent way to render a patient hypothermic. In addition, the enzymes of the blood clotting cascade are rendered inactive at 4°C. In short, gastric lavage with ice-cold water is potentially dangerous and has no role in modern management of GI bleeding.

INVESTIGATION OF UPPER GASTROINTESTINAL BLEEDING

Endoscopy is now firmly established as the "gold standard" for the investigation of upper GI bleeding. Contrast studies have little to offer in the acute setting, and barium effectively obscures the endoscopic view. Radioisotope scans and angiography have an important role in carefully selected cases. Endoscopy in the setting of massive upper GI bleeding is one of the most demanding procedures (perhaps *the* most demanding) performed by gastroenterologists. The patient is often restless despite sedation. The endoscopic view may be suboptimal; the presence of blood and clot obscures common landmarks in the upper GI tract and may quickly disorient the inexperienced endoscopist. Accordingly, endoscopy in this setting should be performed by the most experienced endoscopist available.

If the patient has been difficult to resuscitate and remains hemodynamically unstable, it is likely that there is continuing arterial or variceal hemorrhage. Despite attempts at gastric lavage, preferably using a large-bore (e.g., Ewald) tube, the stomach and esophagus may contain a significant amount of blood. A patient with this amount of active hemorrhage is at significant risk from reflux of gastric and esophageal contents and subsequent aspiration. This risk is increased by sedating the patient for endoscopy and suppressing the gag reflex with pharyngeal anesthesia. It is strongly recommended that a cuffed endotracheal tube be placed before endoscopy in this setting. Even an apparently well sedated patient may become agitated during attempts to pass an endotracheal tube. For this reason, it is wise to enlist the help of an anesthesiologist. Endotracheal intubation is particularly useful for endoscopy in patients with acute variceal hemorrhage, when attempts may be made to perform variceal sclerotherapy. It is most important for the anesthesiologist to understand that the endotracheal tube should not be removed before withdrawal of the endoscope. Indeed, it should remain in place with the cuff inflated for at least 5 minutes after the endoscopy has finished. Unfortunately, anesthesiologists without experience of managing patients in these circumstances may follow their usual operating room practice, which is to attempt extubation just as the surgeon is finishing wound closure. If the endotracheal tube cuff is deflated and the tube withdrawn as the endoscope is being removed, the patient may still regurgitate (or vomit) and aspirate, thereby negating any benefit prior to airway protection. If endotracheal intubation is not available, it is worth considering the use of an endoscopic overtube, through which an endoscope can be repeatedly advanced and withdrawn while maintaining access to the esophagus. This affords a degree of protection against aspiration.

Endoscopy should be performed with a large-channel therapeutic gastroscope whenever possible. If food debris or blood clots are present, the suction channel of a standard endoscope quickly becomes blocked. When a large amount of particulate matter is encountered, the endoscope should be withdrawn and a large-bore aspiration tube passed for further gastric lavage. It can take a long time to render the esophagus, stomach, and duodenum sufficiently clean to obtain a satisfactory endoscopic view. Repeated aspiration of blood and washing with sterile water or saline will eventually yield results unless there is continuing massive hemorrhage. It may be necessary to turn the patient to move a pool of blood and visualize a previously obscured part of the stomach. These manipulations are rendered considerably safer when endotracheal intubation has been performed and the patient is adequately sedated or anesthetized. Sometimes it is impossible to identify the source of acute upper GI bleeding at endoscopy because of a persistently obscured view. This is particularly problematic in the patient with a bleeding lesion close to the gastroesophageal junction in the fundus of the stomach, where blood tends to pool.

When the diagnosis cannot be made at endoscopy, the alternatives are to await further stabilization and (hopefully) cessation of bleeding. Alternatively, the patient may proceed to a selective angiographic study by an interventional radiologist. It is always impressive how much better the endoscopic view is once bleeding has stopped and some hours have passed, allowing blood and clot to move "downstream." Great care must be taken to avoid attributing massive hemorrhage to a relatively insignificant finding. For example, one must be skeptical of a diagnosis of esophagitis or gastric erosions when bleeding clearly appears arterial or variceal in origin. If necessary, the patient should undergo further endoscopy, preferably by a more experienced endoscopist, whenever doubt remains.

ENDOSCOPIC THERAPY

Endoscopy affords the opportunity to apply therapy in suitable circumstances. There are chemical, thermal, mechanical, and topical means of hemostasis at our disposal (Table 2). Since the decision to attempt

Table 2 Endoscopic Therapy for Upper GI Hemorrhage

Chemical
  Epinephrine solution (usually 1:10,000)
  Hypertonic (1.8%) saline
  Sclerosants
    Ethanolamine oleate
    Sodium morrhuate
    Absolute alcohol

Thermal
  Monopolar, bipolar, and multipolar electrocautery
  Microwave coagulation
  Laser (carbon monoxide, Nd-YAG)

Mechanical
  "Endoscopic sewing machine"
  Clips
  Banding (varices)

Topical
  Ferromagnetic
  Clotting factors
  Cyanoacrylate (SuperGlue)

endoscopic therapy has to be made at the time of the procedure, the necessary equipment should be available. For this reason, endoscopy carts that are used to transport equipment to ICUs and other sites of emergency procedures should be suitably equipped for therapeutic intervention.

Injection

Injection of chemicals that cause vasoconstriction (e.g., epinephrine) or an intense inflammatory reaction (e.g., sclerosants) is achieved using a thin needle housed within a plastic catheter. This so-called sclerotherapy needle can be used to inject agents other than sclerosants. As with all modes of endoscopic therapy, successful application requires access to the bleeding site. If the bleeding varix or artery can be identified and targeted, injection is usually straightforward. The current trend is to use larger volumes of epinephrine solution and smaller volumes of sclerosant agents. Although epinephrine (usually given as a 1:10,000 solution) has vasoconstrictive properties, increased tissue pressure due to the volume of injection may be equally important in hemostasis. There is considerable variation in injection technique for bleeding ulcers. However, it is common practice to make a number of injections around the bleeding point before making a final injection directly into it. The risk of systemic upset from epinephrine injection is more theoretical than real.

A number of sclerosant agents are available for endoscopic use; the most commonly used in the United States are ethanolamine oleate, sodium morrhuate, and absolute alcohol. These chemicals share the property of producing an intense inflammatory reaction at the site of injection. A common by-product of this phenomenon is local ulceration, which may be responsible for delayed complications, such as bleeding and perforation. Particular risk factors for complications of endoscopic

sclerotherapy include repeated treatments at intervals of only a few days, and a sclerotherapy needle length greater than 5 mm. Certain sclerosant agents, such as absolute alcohol, may be particularly prone to cause ulceration.

Sclerotherapy

The technique for endoscopic sclerotherapy varies considerably and is usually a matter of personal preference. However, most endoscopists now prefer to inject directly into the varix (intravariceal) rather than between the varices (paravariceal), as the latter is associated with significant risk of ulceration. It is often difficult to be certain that the tip of the needle is inside the varix. For this reason, some endoscopists perform sclerotherapy under fluoroscopy using radiopaque contrast media mixed with the sclerosant to help visualize the local venous anatomy. If the injection is truly intravariceal, the sclerosant will opacify and outline the venous system of the varix. Another way to monitor this therapy is to connect a manometric (pressure measuring) system to the sclerotherapy needle. There is a separate chapter on management of bleeding esophageal varices.

Ulcer Injection

There is also no "correct" technique for injection therapy of bleeding ulcers. One commonly used technique is to make injections in a ring around the offending vessel before attacking the center. As stated previously, volume may be as important as chemical content when using injection therapy for hemostasis. Accordingly, a total of 5 to 10 ml of epinephrine solution (or sclerosant) may at times be appropriate. Care should be taken when using a sclerotherapy needle in the stomach, particularly proximal to the antrum, as the wall is thin compared with the esophagus. I have seen one elderly patient develop acute abdominal pain immediately after epinephrine injection into a high, lesser-curve ulcer. As there was no evidence of perforation, the pain was probably due to serosal or peritoneal irritation from a transmural injection.

Thermal Energy

A variety of methods of applying thermal energy to coagulate or vaporize tissue have been developed for use through an endoscope. These include monopolar, bipolar, and multipolar (heater) probes, microwave probes, and, of course, laser. Electrocautery probes (e.g., the heater probe) are metal-tipped catheters through which current can be applied to heat tissue. The depth of penetration of this thermal energy varies with the design of the probe. Clearly, it is wise to avoid uncontrolled, deep tissue coagulation because of the risk of perforation. For this reason, monopolar probes have fallen out of favor, as their depth of penetration is significant and difficult to control. To facilitate washing the target lesion and prevent adherence of coagulum, most modern electrocautery probes incorporate a water jet. A high-powered jet of water can be extremely useful when attempting to dislodge blood and clot from an ulcer. The ability to coagulate an ulcer base for hemostasis depends on suitable access. It is sometimes impossible to achieve direct or even tangential contact with the target using a heater probe.

A potential means of applying thermal energy from a distance is by use of a laser. Although so-called "contact" lasers have been developed, these have not proved particularly useful or effective for GI bleeding. The most commonly used laser for endoscopic work, including hemostasis, is the neodymium-yttrium argon garnet laser (Nd-YAG) system. This has the desired tissue penetration, although the surface tends to vaporize at higher energy levels. A modification of the standard Nd-YAG laser is the "water-guided" laser, which uses a jet of water as a conduit for the light beam. The water cools the surface sufficiently to prevent vaporization and its attendant problems. The laser is theoretically more flexible than the electrocautery probe, because it can be used from a distance, but in practice there is little difference. The bleeding site must be clearly targeted before the laser can be used effectively. One disadvantage of the laser compared with the electrocautery probe is that it cannot be applied tangentially. The laser also has the disadvantages of being very expensive and not easily portable. In particular, it is difficult to transport a laser system to the ICU for emergency treatment. In view of this, most endoscopy emergency carts are equipped with an electrocautery device (e.g., a heater probe) and some form of injection system for epinephrine or sclerosants.

Mechanical Devices

A variety of ingenious mechanical devices have been developed for hemostasis at endoscopy. These include the so-called endoscopic sewing machine, in which an ingenious device attached to the tip of a standard gastroscope provides the means to insert a running suture across the base of an ulcer or other bleeding site. Despite the obvious attractions of such a system, the endoscopic sewing machine remains experimental. A modified endoscopic catheter allows the placement of small metal clips at the bleeding site. The tissue to which these clips are attached eventually sloughs, releasing the clips, which are passed through the gut in the normal way. Again, despite the simplicity and effectiveness of such clips when accurately targeted, this technique has yet to catch on. Rubber-band ligation of hemorrhoids has been around for a long time. Recently, this inexpensive and apparently low-risk therapy has been applied to esophageal and gastric varices. A small banding device is attached to the tip of a standard gastroscope. The offending varix is identified and sucked into the lumen of the banding device. With the varix snugly seated, the device is triggered by the endoscopist. A small rubber band is released over the "neck" of the varix, constricting it; the varix subsequently thromboses and sloughs off. This seems to be a simple and so far relatively uncomplicated technique, particularly when compared with its "rival," variceal sclerotherapy. (The chapter on bleeding esophageal varices provides details on banding varices as well as sclerotherapy.) For bleeding varices that do not respond to sclerotherapy and banding, a variety of surgical devascularization and ligation procedures are available. However, as expected, when these procedures are used in high-risk patients (e.g., those with Child's class C), the morbidity and mortality rates are significant.

Topical Treatment

Topical treatments for acute upper GI bleeding have been introduced and evaluated, but none have stood the test of time. In general, they are cumbersome to apply and have uncertain results. The application of SuperGlue (cyanoacrylate) to an ulcer base or other bleeding diathesis is an attractive concept but a nightmare in practice. Despite every effort to avoid contaminating the endoscope channel, this is all but impossible. At best, getting SuperGlue in the endoscope channel necessitates an expensive repair. Apart from the technical difficulty, the tendency for cyanoacrylate to fall off the treated surface is a problem. There has also been at least one report of SuperGlue embolism associated with intravascular injection of the compound. A variety of blood clotting factors have been applied to bleeding sites in the hope of stimulating clot formation; again, the results are unpredictable. Finally, the ferromagnetic treatment is, if nothing else, interesting! Iron filings are liberally applied to the bleeding site, usually an ulcer. These are then drawn tightly into the base of the ulcer with a powerful external magnet, and the patient appropriately positioned. Needless to say, this particular technique has failed to gain widespread acceptance.

MANAGEMENT OF CONTINUED HEMORRHAGE

Mortality from upper GI bleeding has fallen in the last 20 years, thanks to early and effective resuscitation followed by endoscopic diagnosis and therapy. In particular, surgical morbidity and mortality has decreased because few patients now undergo exploratory surgery for bleeding without a probable site having been identified by endoscopy or vascular radiology. One cannot overemphasize the need for prompt and adequate resuscitation of patients with acute GI hemorrhage. Endoscopy is a useful diagnostic and therapeutic tool, but it is a mistake to rush into an endoscopic procedure before the patient has been stabilized. Sometimes it is impossible to stabilize a patient who has profuse arterial or variceal bleeding. In these circumstances, the risks of uncontrolled volume depletion outweigh those of endoscopy in the hypotensive patient. Endoscopy is not necessarily the appropriate first-line management for acute GI bleeding. For example, if the bleeding source is known (e.g., from a previous endoscopy) or strongly suspected (e.g., hemobilia in a patient with hepatoma), endoscopy may be superfluous and may delay appropriate management, such as angiography with embolism or surgery. As is true in medicine in general, each case needs to be managed on the basis of the best information available.

Interventional Radiology

If an artery is actively bleeding, it may be possible to define the site of the diathesis by angiography. Vascular radiologists are specialists in this technique, which requires placement of an arterial imaging catheter, usually by the femoral route. Extravasation of contrast material injected through the catheter into the lumen of the bowel is good evidence of an active bleeding site. Selective catheterization of the celiac axis and mesenteric arteries often identifies the source of a persistent arterial hemorrhage. Once the site has been defined, an infusion of vasopressin may be effective in stopping the hemorrhage. This treatment is not without risks, as vasopressin acts by causing local vasospasm and therefore ischemia. The risk of intestinal (and cardiac) ischemia must always be considered, especially in arteriopathic patients. Infusion of vasoactive substances is a purely temporizing maneuver. If a more permanent "fix" is desired, a variety of materials can be injected into the artery to embolize the bleeding site. Homologous blood clot can be used if the effect is not intended to be permanent. The thrombolytic system of the body will reverse the effect of clot embolus within hours to days. A foreign material that resists digestion, such as Gelfoam or metal springs, will permanently block the vessel. Again, the risks of ischemia and infarction must be considered. In addition, embolization beyond the intended site is a potential risk.

What should be done when acute GI bleeding is intermittent? This is always a difficult problem. If a bleeding site cannot be identified by endoscopy, the vascular radiologist is often invited to perform a study. However, the yield of such a study will be low if the artery is not actively bleeding. For this reason, the vascular radiologist may defer angiography until a radionuclide (e.g., technetium-labeled red cell) scan has been performed. Radionuclide scans are relatively insensitive but are often positive if bleeding exceeds 1 to 2 ml per minute. A positive radionuclide scan gives the vascular radiologist some confidence that the study will have a chance of detecting the offending vessel. If angiography is performed and a bleeding vessel cannot be defined, one alternative is to leave the catheter in place for 24 to 48 hours. This catheter can subsequently be used to perform angiography should the bleeding site "open up." In this event, it is also useful for therapy (vasopressin infusion or embolization).

Surgery for Bleeding

No surgeon likes to open a patient's abdomen to search for a source for bleeding without some idea of the task involved. Even if the exact bleeding site has not been identified, the endoscopist (or radiologist) may be able to give the surgeon a good idea of the rough vicinity of the lesion. For example, repeated pooling of blood in the gastric fundus is highly suggestive of a lesion within a few centimeters of the gastroesophageal junction. However, blood and clot may often defeat the most aggressive therapeutic endoscopist. Surgery for acute bleeding should not only address the immediate problem but prevent a recurrence. For example, if the likely cause of the bleeding is a peptic ulcer, the surgeon may wish to perform a definitive ulcer operation (e.g., including vagotomy or antrectomy). It is very rare now for a patient to undergo total gastrectomy because a bleeding site cannot be identified. This is a major operation with considerable physiologic sequelae.*

For everyone involved in managing patients with acute GI bleeding, a small bowel bleeding source may be the most challenging. It is fortunate that few patients with acute upper GI hemorrhage have a source in the small bowel, as this is undoubtedly a blind area for imaging of all kinds. It is rare for small bowel bleeding to be acute, although occasionally a tumor (usually benign) may ulcerate. The legendary bleeding Meckel's diverticulum is a rare beast indeed. In my experience, a Meckel's isotope scan usually gives a false-positive result.

Intraoperative endoscopy may be of considerable help in identifying the source of small bowel bleeding. The operating room is a rather hostile environment for the gastroenterologist, so some understanding and cooperation between gastroenterologist and surgeon are essential. Using gas-sterilized equipment, a long endoscope (usually a colonoscope) can be advanced all the way down the small bowel through a high enterostomy incision. This is often made distal to the ligament of Treitz. The endoscope is advanced by the surgeon, who threads it through the loops of bowel by hand, from the outside; it usually is possible to reach all the way to the ileocecal valve. It is a wise precaution to have the surgeon cross-clamp the ileocecal valve or cecum itself to prevent massive inflation of the colon during endoscopy. This makes returning the bowel to the abdomen difficult and will win no friends in the operating room. When the endoscope is withdrawn, gas can be aspirated and the small bowel returned to the abdomen.

Intraoperative enteroscopy provides two benefits. First, abnormalities may be seen directly using the endoscope; a pathologic condition usually is more easily seen when the endoscope is withdrawn. Second, light from the endoscope transluminates the bowel wall, making it relatively simple to identify vascular abnormalities such as a large telangiectasia. Whenever an abnormality is seen by either the endoscopist or surgeon, a suture should be placed in the bowel wall at that site. After the procedure, the enterostomy incision is repaired. If an abnormality has been discovered, this may

---

*Editor's Note: One still encounters some surgeons who insist on major gastric resections because of continued acid production despite the use of H_2-receptor antagonists, e.g., cimetidine. Hopefully, omeprazole usage will permit less radical surgery in the future.

be dealt with in a variety of ways. Vascular lesions may be simply oversewn or, if they are multiple, a segment of bowel may be resected with an end-to-end anastomosis. Similarly, a small bowel tumor or Meckel's diverticulum may be dealt with by segmental resection.

Peroral enteroscopy is an evolving technique that requires a particularly long endoscope. (There is a separate chapter on enteroscopy.) The so-called sonde-type enteroscope is weighted, and once positioned in the proximal small bowel is left, often for many hours, to progress by peristalsis. When fluoroscopy reveals that the enteroscope has reached the distal ileum, it is withdrawn by slow traction and the bowel inspected. Sonde enteroscopy is time-consuming and rather unpleasant for the patient, and so-called "push" enteroscopy has come into favor. It is said that in cases of occult GI bleeding, "push" enteroscopy will yield a diagnosis in 30 percent. At present, enteroscopy is limited to specialist centers only, in view of the expense of the equipment involved and the expertise required. However, as endoscope technology continues to advance, it is likely that whole bowel endoscopy will become a reality in the not too distant future.

Practical Suggestions for Management

Some deaths from GI bleeding are unavoidable. For example, acute GI hemorrhage may be the agonal event in a patient with liver failure or multisystem disease. In these circumstances, the patient may have a "living will" or similar document indicating that they do not wish to have their lives unduly prolonged. These wishes must be respected. Short of this, it is sometimes appropriate to limit the volume of transfusion. Great care has to be taken when this is done to ensure that everyone involved in the patient's care, including the family, is comfortable with the decision.

SUGGESTED READING

Baillie J, Yudelman P. Complications of endoscopic sclerotherapy of esophageal varices. Endoscopy 1992; 24:284–291.

Fullarton GM, Birnie GG, MacDonald A, Murray WR. The effect of introducing endoscopic therapy on surgery and mortality rates for peptic ulcer hemorrhage: a single center analysis of 1125 cases. Endoscopy 1990; 22:110–113.

Fusamoto H, Hagiwara H, Meren H, et al. A clinical study of acute gastrointestinal hemorrhage associated with various shock states. Am J Gastroenterol 1991; 86:429–433.

Laine L, El-Newihi HM, Migikovsky B, et al. Endoscopic ligation compared with sclerotherapy for the treatment of bleeding esophageal varices. Ann Intern Med 1993; 119:1–8.

Lin HJ, Perng CL, Lee FY, et al. Endoscopic injection for the arrest of peptic ulcer hemorrhage: final results of a prospective, randomized comparative trial. Gastrointest Endosc 1993; 39:15–19.

Loizou LA, Bown SG. Endoscopic treatment for bleeding peptic ulcers: randomized comparison of adrenaline injection and adrenaline injection + Nd:YAG laser photocoagulation. Gut 1991; 32:1100–1103.

Oxner RB, Simmonds NJ, Gertner DJ, et al. Controlled trial of endoscopic injection treatment for bleeding from peptic ulcers with visible vessels. Lancet 1992; 339:966–968.

Panes J, Viver J, Forne M. Randomized comparison of endoscopic microwave coagulation and endoscopic sclerosis in the treatment of bleeding peptic ulcers. Gastrointest Endosc 1991; 37:611–616.

Sung JY, Chung SCS, Low JM, et al. Systemic absorption of epinephrine after submucosal injection in patients with bleeding peptic ulcers. Gastrointest Endosc 1993; 39:20–22.

Swain CP. Operative endoscopy in acute upper GI bleeding—indications, techniques, prognosis. Hepatogastroenterology 1991; 38:201–206.

STRESS-RELATED EROSIVE SYNDROME

M. MICHAEL WOLFE, M.D.

Stress-related erosive syndrome (SRES) is a widely recognized cause of upper gastrointestinal (GI) hemorrhage, whose clinical features have been well characterized since the original endoscopic description by Lucas in 1971. Stress-related lesions in the stomach and duodenum can be detected endoscopically within several hours of a stressful injury or illness as multiple punctate subepithelial hemorrhages, erosions, or superficial ulcerations. Mucosal injury occurs in 70 to 100 percent of critically ill patients admitted to an intensive care unit (ICU); the risk of developing these lesions appears to be directly correlated with the severity of the underlying illness. Although most individuals with stress-related mucosal injury remain asymptomatic, 10 to 20 percent of those who do not receive prophylactic therapy experience GI hemorrhage of an occult or overt nature. Owing to improvements in the perioperative management of patients, the incidence of clinically overt GI hemorrhage appears to have declined in recent years. Nevertheless, mortality rates in critically ill patients with gross hemorrhage are still 50 to 80 percent. Most of these deaths are not directly attributable to the hemorrhage itself, but rather reflect the nature and severity of the underlying illness.

The precise pathophysiology of SRES is not firmly established. However, it is clear that gastric acid and pepsin play an integral role in the erosive process. Despite normal or subnormal rates of acid and pepsin secretion, with the exception of central nervous system injury, in which gastric acid hypersecretion is often observed, gastric acid is believed to play a primary role in the pathogenesis of SRES. As with other acid-peptic–related disorders, SRES appears to result from an imbalance between aggressive and defensive factors. The most critical defensive "loss" in the pathogenesis of SRES appears to be mucosal ischemia. Gastric mucosal cells are highly susceptible to diminished blood flow, which promotes intramural acidosis, the production of oxygen-derived free radicals, increased cell permeability, and diminished acid-buffering capacity. In addition, mucosal ischemia leads to diminished mucus and bicarbonate secretion and defects in epithelial cell restitution after injury, all of which contribute to the back-diffusion of hydrogen ions into the gastroduodenal mucosa. Back-diffusion of acid is believed to be central to the disruption of the surface epithelial barrier, with subsequent erosive change resulting in clinically significant GI hemorrhage.

Most patients in an ICU are at risk for SRES, and those most susceptible to gastroduodenal mucosal injury are patients with extensive burns (Curling's ulcers), intracranial hypertension (Cushing's ulcers), major trauma, sepsis, respiratory failure necessitating ventilatory support, renal failure, liver dysfunction, coagulopathy, multiple organ failure, or shock. Because most patients are asymptomatic, stress-related bleeding is generally not recognized until overt bleeding occurs. Owing to the prognostic implications of the progression of SRES, the cornerstone of therapy has been prophylaxis rather than active treatment.*

MEDICAL TREATMENT

Principles of Therapy

The risk of overt GI hemorrhage and subsequent death due to SRES is most closely correlated to the underlying disease. The major thrust of therapy must therefore be directed at treating the underlying cause of physiologic stress. Sepsis must be treated aggressively with appropriate antimicrobial therapy, abscesses drained surgically or percutaneously, metabolic abnormalities corrected, ventilatory support optimized, and adequate nutrition instituted. Nevertheless, in spite of such efforts, prophylactic regimens are generally employed to diminish the probability of GI hemorrhage due to SRES and to affect associated high rates of morbidity and mortality should bleeding develop. Various approaches for preventing GI bleeding due to SRES are in use. However, the method used most extensively has been to decrease the concentration of hydrogen ions in the stomach. When intragastric pH is increased to 3.5 to 4.0, the conversion of pepsinogen to pepsin is decreased;

proteolytic activity in the stomach is subsequently diminished. Moreover, when intragastric pH approaches 7.0, pepsinogen is irreversibly denatured and clotting factors become operable, enabling the clotting cascade to proceed. Finally, platelet aggregation, which occurs only at a pH greater than 5.9, also contributes to successful hemostasis and subsequently to prevention of bleeding due to SRES. For these reasons, it has been postulated that maintenance of intragastric pH at 7.0 or above would constitute optimal prophylaxis. However, most studies have aimed at maintaining intragastric pH above 3.5 to 4.0 and have indeed demonstrated this pH to be effective in preventing gastroduodenal hemorrhage.

Antacids

Initial studies by Hastings and colleagues demonstrated that antacids were effective in decreasing the incidence of stress-induced GI hemorrhage. However, as noted in this and subsequent studies, the dose of antacid required to maintain intragastric pH near 4.0 is significant, and antacids are cumbersome to administer. Other problems include the increased incidence of diarrhea caused by the high magnesium concentration found in many high-potency antacid preparations. In addition, the need for nasogastric intubation with its inherent complications, the requirement for increased nursing time, the occurrence of metabolic alkalosis, the price of antacids themselves when used in high doses, and other costs associated with their administration have all led to diminished use of these agents in prophylaxis of SRES.

Despite their shortcomings, antacids provide effective prophylaxis of SRES. In a meta-analysis, data from eight prospective studies compared antacid with placebo or no therapy. This analysis found that only 3.4 percent of patients receiving antacids had clinically significant bleeding, while 17.5 percent of those receiving placebo or no therapy bled. When occult bleeding was used as the minimal criterion for bleeding, only 3.7 percent of antacid-treated patients showed evidence of bleeding, whereas 27.3 percent of those receiving placebo or no therapy had such evidence. Thus, the bulk of evidence favors the conclusion that antacids are superior to no therapy in the prevention of GI bleeding due to SRES.

Several intricate protocols designed to maintain intragastric pH above 3.5 to 4.0 have been devised involving the use of antacids in SRES prophylaxis. In general, 30 ml of a high-potency antacid (e.g., Maalox Plus, Mylanta II) should be administered either hourly or every 2 hours. Should diarrhea develop, as it often does, the high-potency antacid may be alternated with an antacid containing aluminum hydroxide only (e.g., Amphojel), provided that the necessary dosage corrections are made for differences in acid-neutralizing capacity. Intragastric pH should be monitored to make necessary dosage adjustments and as discussed in detail below, gastric residual should be assessed to avoid the possibility of distention and subsequent tracheopulmonary aspiration.

---

*Editor's Note: Cook et al (N Engl J Med 1994; 330:377–381) question prophylaxis except in patients with coagulopathy or who require mechanical ventilation, because they think few critically ill patients have clinically important GI bleeding.

Histamine-Receptor Antagonists

Numerous placebo-controlled trials have established the efficacy of H_2-receptor antagonists in preventing stress-induced bleeding. Early comparisons of antacids and cimetidine for stress ulcer prophylaxis reported superior results with antacids. Detection of occult blood in nasogastric aspirates was considered the minimal criterion for bleeding in these studies. However, occult bleeding is no longer considered a reliable indicator of treatment failure; recent observations indicate that only a minority of patients with occult bleeding secondary to SRES develop clinically significant hemorrhage. Recent studies defining prophylactic failure as "overt bleeding" have therefore concluded that H_2-receptor antagonists and antacids are equivalent in their ability to prevent stress-related hemorrhage. Shuman and colleagues reviewed 16 studies (2,133 patients) that compared intravenous cimetidine with placebo or oral antacids in the prevention of stress-related bleeding. They found cimetidine and antacids to be equally effective in preventing overt hemorrhage, and both regimens to be far superior to placebo. The incidence of overt bleeding was 11 of 402 (2.7 percent) in the cimetidine-treated, 25 of 458 (3.3 percent) in the antacid-treated, and 108 of 720 (15 percent) in the placebo-treated patients. Other H_2-receptor antagonists, including famotidine and ranitidine, have not been investigated as extensively. In two nonplacebo controlled studies, ranitidine has been shown to be comparable to cimetidine in the prevention of stress-related hemorrhage.

Dosing regimens for H_2-receptor antagonists initially consisted of intermittent IV administration at fixed doses. Using fixed-dose bolus IV H_2-receptor antagonist administration, ranitidine appears to be at least equivalent to cimetidine in maintaining intragastric pH above 4.0. However, newer regimens using continuous infusions with cimetidine and ranitidine have been shown to raise intragastric pH continuously and more reliably than intermittent infusions, eliminating the peaks and troughs observed in gastric pH with intermittent therapy. To date, two trials have established the clinical efficacy of continuous cimetidine infusion not only in increasing intragastric pH, but also in preventing stress-related hemorrhage. In light of the reduced costs, the convenience, and the potentially superior therapeutic efficacy compared with intermittent IV administration, suggested regimens include continuous infusion therapy with cimetidine, 37.5 to 100 mg per hour, or ranitidine, 6.25 to 12.5 mg per hour, with or without initial loading doses of 300 and 150 mg, respectively. Optimal therapy would include regular monitoring of intragastric pH, with dose increments as necessary to maintain intragastric pH above 4.0. Currently, insufficient information is available regarding the safety and efficacy of parenteral famotidine, and nizatidine is not commercially available for IV use.

Cimetidine and ranitidine are physically compatible and chemically stable with standard IV electrolyte solutions, as well as conventional total parenteral nutrition (TPN) solutions for at least 24 hours. Their inclusion in these solutions allows single daily infusion set-ups, thereby reducing nursing time and pharmacy expenses. Additional benefits of administering H_2-receptor antagonists via TPN include the reduction in fluids required for drug delivery from 250 to 500 ml per day to 5 to 10 ml per day, and a reduction in risks associated with peripheral IV catheterization, such as phlebitis and peripheral line sepsis.

Concern has been raised about the increased potential for nosocomial pneumonia in mechanically ventilated patients receiving stress ulcer prophylaxis. The elevation in intragastric pH allows bacterial colonization of the stomach and tracheobronchial tree, and in theory a greater frequency of nosocomial pneumonia due to aspiration of infected gastric contents. An early retrospective study evaluating the risk factors for nosocomial pneumonia in 233 ICU patients receiving continuous mechanical ventilation reported an association with cimetidine treatment, with an odds ratio of 2.1. The authors appropriately acknowledged, however, that the association may merely reflect the use of cimetidine in the most severely ill patients, who are at greatest risk for pneumonia. Subsequent prospective clinical trials have not supported a role for H_2-receptor antagonists in the development of nosocomial pneumonia. A meta-analysis of eight randomized controlled trials involving 535 patients found a trend in favor of a reduced incidence of pneumonia with H_2-receptor antagonists, concluding that prophylaxis for stress ulcers with antisecretory therapy did not increase the incidence of pneumonia compared with placebo. A subsequent report by Driks and colleagues concluded that sucralfate was preferable to prolonged acid suppressive therapy, with 23 percent rates of nosocomial pneumonia in a group of patients receiving "antacids or H_2-receptor antagonists," but only 12 percent in the sucralfate-treated patients. This conclusion, however, was misleading and invalid with regard to H_2-receptor antagonists. Patients on antacids had a 23 percent incidence of pneumonia, whereas only 5.9 percent of those treated with H_2-receptor antagonists developed pneumonia, the lowest risk of all three treatment strategies. Therefore, it seems likely that the risk of nosocomial pneumonia is *not* increased by H_2-receptor antagonist therapy compared with placebo or sucralfate.

Substituted Benzimidazoles

Substituted benzimidazoles ("acid pump blockers") are potent antisecretory agents that are very effective in the treatment of several acid-peptic disorders, including ordinary peptic ulcer, gastroesophageal reflux disease, and Zollinger-Ellison syndrome and other hypersecretory states. However, substituted benzimidazoles such as omeprazole and lansoprazole are less effective in patients who are not eating. The reason is that these agents are prodrugs and must be activated to their active moieties before they can inhibit acid secretion by gastric parietal cells. The drugs can be activated only in an acidic milieu (pH < 4), which occurs only in the secretory canaliculus of *activated* parietal cells. Omeprazole, as well as other substituted benzimidazoles, is absorbed systemically and reaches the secretory canaliculus, which has a pH of 1 to 2 when stimulated with a meal. Within the secretory canaliculus, omeprazole is protonated by H^+ ions to form a sulfenamide, which then forms a disulfide bond with H^+/K^+ ATPase, the "acid pump," thereby irreversibly inactivating it.

In addition to omeprazole's not being available in an IV form in the United States, its ability to prevent stress-induced GI hemorrhage has not been evaluated adequately, and its prophylactic use in SRES therefore cannot be recommended at present. Many clinicians have adopted the practice of opening omeprazole capsules and instilling the granules through a nasogastric tube and into the stomach of patients who are not eating. Omeprazole granules have an enteric coating that has been designed to dissolve in alkaline pH. If the capsules are instilled through the tube in a nonacidic compound, the enteric coating is disrupted and the drug may be protonated by acid present in the stomach. This method has not been assessed in any reliable or organized fashion and it cannot therefore be recommended as effective therapy in the prevention of GI hemorrhage due to SRES.

Sucralfate

Sucralfate is a basic aluminum salt of sucrose octasulfate that has proven efficacy in the treatment of duodenal ulcer disease. It does not inhibit gastric acid secretion, and its ability to neutralize acid is minimal. Its postulated mechanisms of action are primarily mucosal protective, and include formation of a protective barrier and stimulation of the synthesis and release of endogenous prostaglandins. Sucralfate's stimulatory effects on prostaglandins are believed to account for the stimulation of bicarbonate and mucus secretion by gastroduodenal mucosa. Because most ICU patients have reduced gastric mucosal blood flow as well as decreased mucus and bicarbonate secretion, the ability of sucralfate to reverse these effects indicates a theoretical therapeutic role for this agent in the prophylaxis of SRES. However, a potential therapeutic role for sucralfate in critically ill patients is controversial. Tryba reviewed the efficacy of sucralfate in SRES in comparative studies with antacids and H_2-receptor antagonists. Although some studies demonstrate a beneficial effect of sucralfate in the prevention of SRES, others do not. Widely varying formulations and doses of sucralfate were employed in these studies, and until a large, prospective, randomized trial is conducted, it seems prudent to withhold judgment regarding the efficacy of sucralfate in SRES prophylaxis.

As stated, some earlier studies reported a beneficial effect of sucralfate in SRES prophylaxis and suggested a decreased incidence of nosocomial pneumonia in ICU patients treated with sucralfate compared with those treated with antacids or antisecretory agents. More recent data do not support this latter contention and do not provide a rationale for the use of sucralfate in the

prevention of SRES. Nevertheless, because the agent is nonsystemic, its use may be preferred in groups of patients in whom systemic medication may be contraindicated. The recommended dose of sucralfate in these patients is 1 g in a liquid slurry given through a nasogastric or other feeding tube every 4 to 6 hours. To prevent clogging of the tube, the tube must be flushed regularly with either water or normal saline.

Prostaglandins

Prostaglandins are 20-carbon-chain fatty acid derivatives of arachidonic acid that are produced by cells throughout the GI tract and most other tissues. They have a dual mode of action: at low dose, they are exclusively mucosal protective agents, stimulating mucus and bicarbonate secretion by surface epithelial cells, increasing mucosal blood flow, and enhancing cell restitution. In addition to their protective properties, at higher doses, they also inhibit acid secretion by blocking parietal cell production of cyclic AMP. Although much attention has been given to the mucosal protective properties of prostaglandins, they are clinically effective only in doses at which gastric acid secretion is inhibited. It therefore is not possible to separate the acid-inhibiting properties of prostaglandins from their clinical efficacy.

At present, the only prostaglandin in use is misoprostol, a prostaglandin E_1 analog that has proved effective in the prevention of gastroduodenal ulceration caused by NSAIDs. A few anecdotal reports, as well as a double-blind, nonplacebo-controlled study have shown misoprostol to be as effective as a titrated antacid regimen in preventing overt bleeding and the development of large ulcers in postoperative ICU patients. In a smaller, unblinded study, arbacet, a prostaglandin E_2 analog, was associated with a high rate of treatment failure, defined as occult bleeding or lack of pH control compared with antacid. However, overt bleeding was not seen in either treatment group. Because prostaglandins have not been assessed in a large placebo-controlled, randomized trial, their use in the prevention of gastroduodenal ulceration due to SRES cannot be recommended at this time.*

NONMEDICAL TREATMENT

Endoscopic and Surgical Therapy

Although maintenance of intragastric pH above 4 is effective in preventing overt bleeding in most patients, some develop stress-induced bleeding despite optimal therapy. Treatment of established bleeding due to SRES is similar to that of other nonvariceal upper GI sources and includes appropriate fluid and blood product resuscitation, correction of abnormalities of coagulation factors, correction of qualitative and quantitative plate-

---

*__Editor's Note:__ Information on the usefulness (if any) of prostaglandins in diffuse hemorrhagic gastritis is needed.

let defects, and direct attempts at establishing hemostasis. Endoscopy is required to confirm that stress-induced ulceration is the source of bleeding and to define the bleeding sites precisely. Although there is little published experience regarding the use of endoscopic techniques such as electrocoagulation, thermal coagulation, and intramucosal injection of sclerosing agents, the use of these methods in bleeding due to gastroduodenal ulceration has been demonstrated. If endoscopic measures fail, more invasive techniques are often necessary and include angiography, for both localization and potential treatment of SRES-related bleeding. If a bleeding site can be demonstrated by angiography, intra-arterial vasopressin, 0.2 to 0.4 U per minute, or arterial embolization may be effective in controlling the hemorrhage.

Situations in which surgeons are faced with a patient who is bleeding massively from an unknown source are becoming increasingly rare as diagnostic preoperative precision has improved. Owing to the underlying medical problems that have predisposed patients to SRES, these individuals are particularly poor surgical candidates. Surgical mortality rates in such patients have ranged from 50 to 77 percent. Nevertheless, when all nonsurgical approaches have failed, the diagnostic procedure of choice may still be laparotomy, often accompanied by intraoperative endoscopy. The stomach and duodenum should be inspected carefully for evidence of ulceration or for blood in the stomach. If no evidence of bleeding is found during initial inspection, a large incision extending across the pylorus from the antrum to the duodenum is made, followed by a more proximal gastrotomy, to inspect the stomach for possible lesions in the high fundus or gastric cardia. If, after a thorough inspection, the bleeding site remains undiagnosed, many surgeons suggest that the operation be terminated, as further studies may be necessary. The bleeding rates after vagotomy and pyloroplasty are higher than those after vagotomy and antrectomy. More extensive gastric resection, in particular blind total gastrectomy, should be avoided in all but the most desperate situations, in view of excessively high mortality rates.

ENTERAL FEEDING AND OTHER EXPERIMENTAL APPROACHES

Previous studies have suggested that the incidence of GI hemorrhage in mechanically ventilated patients given enteral feeding is diminished, indicating a potentially protective effect of feeding on gastroduodenal mucosa. Although no prospective studies have been performed to evaluate enteral feeding as a form of prophylactic therapy in SRES, one recent prospective analysis examined the effect of enteral feeding in ICU patients. In this study, 0.9 percent sodium chloride or enteral feeding was administered into the duodenum while intragastric pH was monitored. Intragastric pH was higher throughout the infusion of enteral feeding, although the pH was less than 4.0 for a significant period in both groups. A second study performed in chronically ill patients showed that while both intragastric and intrajejunal feedings *lowered* intragastric pH, the addition of liquid cimetidine to the regimens increased gastric pH to greater than 5.0. Because of the additional benefit of nutritional support provided to these patients, further studies using enteral feedings containing H_2-receptor antagonists are warranted to determine their efficacy in SRES prophylaxis.

Several other agents have been examined in animal studies and may be effective in the prevention of stress-induced hemorrhage. The compounds include lithium chloride, glucagon, epidermal growth factor, fibroblast growth factor, oxygen radical scavengers, and inhibitors of xanthine oxidase. The mechanism of action of these agents is diverse, and before their clinical use, prospective analyses must be undertaken to determine their true clinical value.*

SUGGESTED READING

Ballesteros MA, Hogan DL, Koss MA, Isenberg JI. Bolus or intravenous infusion of ranitidine: effects on gastric pH and acid secretion. Ann Intern Med 1990; 112:334–339.

Driks MR, Craven DE, Celli BR, et al. Nosocomial pneumonia in intubated patients given sucralfate as compared with antacids or histamine type 2 blockers. N Engl J Med 1987; 317:1376–1382.

Fiddian-Green RG, McGough E, Pittenger G, Rothman E. Predictive value of intramural pH and other risk factors for massive bleeding from stress ulceration. Gastroenterology 1983; 85:613–620.

Hastings PR, Skillman JJ, Bushnell LS, Silen W. Antacid titration in the prevention of acute gastrointestinal bleeding. N Engl J Med 1978; 298:1041–1045.

Layon AJ, Florete OG, Day AL, et al. The effect of duodenojejunal alimentation on gastric pH and hormones in intensive care unit patients. Chest 1991; 99:695–702.

Ostro MJ, Russell JA, Soldin SJ, et al. Control of gastric pH with cimetidine: boluses versus primed infusion. Gastroenterology 1985; 89:532–537.

Shuman RB, Schuster DP, Zuckerman GR. Prophylactic therapy for stress ulcer bleeding: a reappraisal. Ann Intern Med 1987; 106: 562–567.

Tryba M. Stress bleeding prophylaxis with sucralfate. Pathophysiologic basis and clinical use. Scand J Gastroenterol 1990; 25(Suppl 173): 22–33.

Wolfe MM, ed. Gastrointestinal pharmacotherapy. Philadelphia: WB Saunders, 1993; 25–137.

Zuckerman GR, Cort D, Shuman RB. Stress ulcer syndrome. J Intensive Care Med 1988; 3:21–31.

*****Editor's Note:** Prevention of upper GI bleeding is reviewed by Peterson in N Engl J Med 1994; 330:428–429.

CHRONIC GASTRITIS: CLASSIFICATION

DONALD A. ANTONIOLI, M.D.

PROBLEMS IN EVALUATION AND CLASSIFICATION

A confusing array of classifications for gastritis has developed over the years. One previous major source of difficulty was a lack of consensus as to what constitutes "gastritis." In the clinical setting, the term has often been used as a synonym for nonulcer dyspepsia, whereas it has been defined radiographically as abnormal mucosal folds noted in contrast studies and endoscopically as erythema, with or without friability. However, it is now agreed that the correct definition is the pathologic one: inflammation of the stomach or, more restrictively, of the gastric mucosa.

Another problem in classification and evaluation has been lack of knowledge concerning the etiology and pathogenesis of many cases of gastritis. The gastric mucosa has a limited repertory of morphologic responses to a presumably large number of damaging agents; thus, diverse etiologies (microbiologic, dietary, chemical) give rise to stereotyped end-organ changes that offer few clues as to causation. However, recent progress in defining the causes of gastritis is clarifying the issue of classification (see later).

Frustrating, also, has been the well-documented lack of correlation between endoscopic and histologic findings. For example, mucosa that is red and friable may be unremarkable histologically, whereas mucosa that is apparently normal endoscopically may show rather severe gastritis at microscopic examination. No satisfactory explanation for these discrepancies has been proposed, but the focal nature of some gastric lesions may make it difficult to obtain precisely targeted biopsy specimens.

The significance of chronic gastritis is the subject of much debate. It is a lesion that increases in frequency with increasing age in the general population, but its relationship, if any, to upper gastrointestinal symptoms is unclear. Particular forms of gastritis (such as granulomatous gastritis or chemical gastritis) may suggest a limited range of etiologic agents. Severe gastritis of the proximal stomach may lead to functional consequences: hypo- or achlorhydria and pernicious anemia. However, the greatest importance of chronic gastritis is that it represents a precancerous condition (Fig. 1). The sequence outlined in Figure 1 is not inevitable, however, particularly for *Helicobacter pylori*–related gastritis and for the chemical-related injuries. Also, the sequence may be modified by environmental and genetic factors. Premalignant conditions of the stomach are discussed further in another chapter.

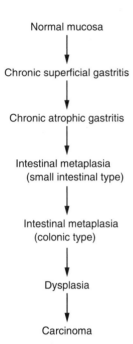

Figure 1 Postulated stages in the development of intestinal-type gastric adenocarcinoma.

A final problem in the evaluation of gastritis lies in defining the significance of minor degrees of chronic inflammation in biopsy specimens. In other words, what is the acceptable extent of chronic inflammation for the histologic picture still to be considered normal? Small amounts of chronic inflammation, particularly if confined to the superficial lamina propria in older patients and not associated with other evidence of injury, are probably a normal variant. However, with the recognition of *H. pylori* as an important factor in the genesis of gastritis, a search for this organism should be made even in the presence of only modest amounts of inflammation.

CLASSIFICATION AND HISTOLOGIC FEATURES

A classification of chronic gastritis, based on current knowledge of etiology and modified from that proposed by Yardley, is given in Table 1. Chemical gastritis is discussed in other chapters; only reflux gastritis is reviewed briefly here. The treatment of chronic gastritis is discussed in the next chapter.

Regardless of the cause, the histologic diagnosis of chronic gastritis encompasses the following features, singly or in varied combinations.

Mononuclear inflammation (lymphocytes and plasma cells) is the single most important requirement for the diagnosis. If the inflammation is confined to the upper portion of the lamina propria and is unaccompanied by other abnormalities, the lesion is termed "chronic superficial gastritis." In more severe chronic gastritis, mononuclear cells occupy the entire thickness of the lamina propria, and lymphoid follicles may form.

Mucosal atrophy consists of a decrease in size and/or

Table 1 Classification of Chronic Gastritis

Helicobacter pylori–related (chronic nonspecific gastritis) (or others)

Metaplastic atrophic gastritis
   Autoimmune (type A)
   Environmental (type B)

Chemical gastritis

Miscellaneous
   Eosinophilic gastritis
   Granulomatous gastritis (including Crohn's disease)
   Lymphocytic gastritis

number of gastric glands; the surface-foveolar compartment is typically not affected. Atrophy is usually accompanied by *metaplasia,* which may take two forms. *Pyloric metaplasia* consists of the conversion of corpus-fundic glandular epithelium into a phenotype reminiscent of pyloric mucosa. Oxyntic and pepsinogen cells are replaced, focally or diffusely, by mucous cells that produce predominantly neutral glycoproteins. *Intestinal metaplasia* may occur in any part of the stomach (but is typically more extensive distally) and develops in two forms, small intestinal and colonic. Small intestinal (complete) metaplasia contains goblet, absorptive, and Paneth cells; the goblet cells contain acidic glycoproteins (chiefly sialomucins). In advanced cases, areas of small intestinal metaplasia may assume a villiform architecture like that of the duodenum. Conversely, colonic (incomplete) metaplasia contains goblet cells but lacks absorptive and Paneth cells. It also contains epithelial cells with partially developed features of both mucous and absorptive cells. Acidic glycoproteins are also produced in incomplete metaplasia, but they are predominantly sulfomucins.

The pathogenesis of metaplasia is unclear. Extensive metaplasia of the corpus is significant because of the potential for developing achlorhydria and pernicious anemia. Intestinal metaplasia, particularly the colonic (incomplete) type, may be significant as a precursor condition in the development of intestinal-type gastric adenocarcinoma (see the chapter on premalignant lesions of the stomach).

Activity in chronic gastritis is defined as the presence of neutrophils in the lamina propria, within gland or surface epithelium, and/or in gland lumens. The term "active" rather than "acute" is used to describe this feature, because neutrophils may be present throughout the course of chronic gastritis and do not connote a brief, self-limited component of the injury. All the features of chronic gastritis described above may be focal or diffuse, either in the stomach or in a particular biopsy specimen.

SPECIFIC FORMS OF CHRONIC GASTRITIS

H. pylori–Associated Gastritis (Synonyms: Chronic Nonspecific Gastritis; Diffuse Antral Gastritis)

H. pylori gastric infection, which is discussed fully in the chapter on that organism, is extremely common,

being noted in 40 to 60 percent of healthy adults over age 50 years in developed countries and, in hospital-based studies, in up to 90 percent of patients with chronic gastritis and almost 100 percent of patients with duodenal ulcer. The prevalence of *H. pylori*–associated gastritis increases with increasing age; in the United States, it is the cause of only 20 percent of gastritis in hospital-based studies of children. Although the relationship of *H. pylori* infection to upper gastrointestinal symptoms is problematic, almost every patient with *H. pylori* has some degree of histologic gastritis.

H. pylori–associated chronic gastritis is typically antral in location and diffuse; however, it often involves the corpus and may even extend to the cardia. Activity is common, with neutrophils characteristically being localized to the lamina propria and epithelium in the glandular neck area. Although the formation of lymphoid follicles is common, atrophy and intestinal metaplasia are absent or inconspicuous, at least in the early stages of gastritis; the natural history of the lesions is still unclear. The organisms can often be recognized as slightly curved or spiral bacteria in routine hematoxylin and eosin–stained slides. The diagnosis can also be made by histochemical stains on tissue sections, culture, and serology, as discussed in the chapter on *H. pylori.*

H. pylori gastritis is being investigated as a possible precursor condition in the development of both intestinal-type gastric adenocarcinoma and low-grade B-cell gastric lymphomas of the mucosa-associated lymphoid system (MALT-omas). Demonstration of a positive correlation between *H. pylori* gastritis and these neoplasms would have obvious implications concerning the treatment of this type of gastritis.

Autoimmune (Type A) Metaplastic Atrophic Gastritis

In its pure form, autoimmune metaplastic atrophic gastritis is a diffuse injury confined to the corpus and fundus. Inherited as an autosomal dominant disorder, this type of gastritis is characterized by the development of autoantibodies (to oxyntic cells and intrinsic factor) and of hypo- or achlorhydria, pernicious anemia, and hypergastrinemia, the last-named sometimes associated with secondary development of endocrine cell hyperplasia or neoplasia in the proximal stomach.

Histologically, autoimmune gastritis shows prominent atrophy and metaplasia (both pyloric and intestinal). In the late stages, the mucosa becomes thin and smooth and chronic inflammation may be modest ("burned-out" atrophic gastritis). Specialized oxyntic and pepsinogen cells may be difficult or impossible to identify. Antral G (gastrin-producing) cells undergo hyperplasia secondary to the loss of feedback inhibition by hydrochloric acid, with development of antral endocrine tumors in occasional patients. In American patients with this type of gastritis, the risk of gastric adenocarcinoma is low, and routine surveillance is not recommended, as discussed in the chapter on premalignant lesions.

Environmental (Type B) Metaplastic Atrophic Gastritis

This type of gastritis shows wide geographic variation in prevalence, being much less common in the United States than in Japan and much of South America. It develops as a result of dietary and environmental factors; diets high in nitrates and salt, and those deficient in green vegetables and fresh fruit, have been implicated. Unlike type A metaplastic atrophic gastritis, environmental gastritis is not associated with the development of autoantibodies or functional abnormalities. Hydrochloric acid production may be decreased in severe cases, but this finding is unusual; pernicious anemia does not occur. Type B gastritis is the setting most frequently associated with chronic gastric (but not duodenal) peptic ulcer disease.

Initially, environmental gastritis develops in multiple separate areas, typically along the junction of the body and antrum adjacent to the lesser curvature. Over time, the antrum tends to become extensively involved, with diffuse inflammation of this portion of the stomach in severe cases. The corpus and fundus may also be involved in advanced disease, but in a multifocal, patchy manner. In biopsy specimens, type B gastritis is commonly focal in distribution. Chronic inflammation and atrophy are variable and activity is usually not identified, but intestinal metaplasia is prominent.

Both types A and B gastritis may be associated with the formation of gastric hyperplastic polyps (common) and adenomas (rare). The risk of malignancy is reviewed in the chapter on premalignant lesions.

Reflux Gastropathy

The features of reflux gastropathy, best defined in patients with gastroenterostomies (e.g., Billroth II procedure), are due to a combination of gastric surface injury from duodenal contents refluxed into the stomach and prolapse of gastric mucosa. The epithelial injury results in surface-foveolar zone vascular congestion and edema, as well as epithelial hyperplasia; inflammation is typically not prominent. Mucosal architecture is distorted by splaying of the muscularis mucosae, with increased numbers of smooth muscle fibers arrayed in the lamina propria, and misplacement of benign gastric glands into the submucosa. In severe cases, one or more polyps of the hyperplastic-inflammatory type may develop at the gastroenterostomy stoma.

Miscellaneous Forms

Eosinophilic Gastritis

Allergic-eosinophilic disease and the mucosal form of eosinophilic gastroenteritis typically involve the antrum (less often the corpus) in a multifocal manner. Chronic inflammation is modest; atrophy and metaplasia do not occur. The major histologic finding is increased numbers of eosinophils in the lamina propria, often associated with eosinophils infiltrating surface and gland epithelium or forming gland abscesses. In allergic disease, antral biopsy specimens are more consistently positive than those from the duodenum, where the lesions may be very focal.

The differential diagnosis of eosinophil infiltrates in the stomach includes allergy, parasitic infections, and resolving peptic injury. Clinicopathologic correlation is necessary to evaluate these various possibilities.

Granulomatous Gastritis (Including Crohn's Disease)

Granulomatous gastritis is an uncommon entity with diverse etiologies (Table 2). Irrespective of the cause, granulomatous gastritis tends to have a stereotyped clinical presentation. Involvement is almost always distal, with thickened mucosal folds, variable erosions and ulcers, and frequent gastric outlet obstruction. The major endoscopic differential diagnosis is infiltrating carcinoma or lymphoma.

Histologically, granulomas are identified in the mucosa or submucosa in a background of chronic gastritis with or without activity, atrophy, or metaplasia. The biopsy findings must be correlated with the clinical data to obtain the correct diagnosis, because the histopathology is not specific. Focal involvement of the biopsy specimen is suggestive of Crohn's disease (even in specimens that lack granulomas), whereas granulomas with central necrosis point to an infectious etiology; however, granulomas with caseation or other types of necrosis are unusual in the stomach, even in infectious cases. Histochemical stains and cultures for organisms should be performed on biopsy tissue; the tissue should also be examined with polarizing lenses to detect any possible foreign material.

After appropriate studies and evaluation of all clinical data, there remains a group of patients with apparently idiopathic, or isolated, granulomatous gastritis. The natural history of these cases is unclear. Some apparently have a self-limited course, but occasionally the gastric involvement may be the first evidence of Crohn's disease.

Lymphocytic Gastritis

A recently described entity, lymphocytic gastritis is characterized by chronic inflammation in the lamina propria and infiltration of the surface-foveolar epithelium by an excess of T lymphocytes. The epithelial cells may have features of injury, such as cytoplasmic vacuolization and loss of normal columnar shape. Endoscopi-

Table 2 Differential Diagnosis of Granulomatous Gastritis

Crohn's disease
Infections
  Tuberculosis
  Fungi
Sarcoidosis
Foreign body
Idiopathic

cally, lymphocytic gastritis has a typical varioliform appearance, but with the increasing recognition of this entity, it is apparent that the gross appearance may be nonspecific. Both the corpus and antrum may be involved.

The significance of this type of gastritis is unclear. Some examples have been identified in patients with untreated celiac disease, and a few in patients with *H. pylori* infection. The resemblance of lymphocytic gastritis to the small intestinal lesion of celiac disease suggests an immune-mediated (possibly autoimmune) injury.

THE SYDNEY SYSTEM FOR THE CLASSIFICATION OF GASTRITIS

At the 1990 World Congress of Gastroenterology in Sydney, Australia, a new classification of gastritis was proposed that encompasses etiologic, endoscopic, and histologic components. One major aim of this proposal is to provide flexibility in accommodating new developments in clinical research on gastritis. The histologic component includes grading of the following variables on a four-point scale (none, mild, moderate, and severe): *H. pylori*, chronic inflammation, active inflammation, atrophy, and intestinal metaplasia. Specific types of gastritis (e.g., granulomatous) are designated as such; nonspecific types are described with an assessment of the variables listed earlier.

The utility of the Sydney System is the subject of much current controversy and its adoption internationally is still unclear. However, it does provide a framework to describe the diverse components of gastritis, to accommodate new entities, and to evaluate the effects of therapy.

COMMENTS

Knowledge of the etiologies and pathogenesis of chronic gastritis continues to increase, and the recognition of *H. pylori* as a major cause of gastritis is a major breakthrough. To obtain the most information on classifying gastritis, multiple biopsies should be taken (even from endoscopically normal mucosa) from both corpus and antrum. In this way, lesions can be defined precisely and the natural history of chronic gastritis determined in serial biopsy specimens.

SUGGESTED READING

Blaser MJ. Hypotheses on the pathogenesis and natural history of *Helicobacter pylori*–induced inflammation. Gastroenterology 1992; 102:720–727.

Correa P. Chronic gastritis: a clinico-pathological classification. Am J Gastroenterol 1988; 83:504–509.

Haot J, Jouret A, Willette M, et al. Lymphocytic gastritis: prospective study of its relationship with varioliform gastritis. Gut 1990; 31:282–285.

Hui PK, Chan WY, Cheung PS, et al. Pathologic changes of gastric mucosa colonized by *Helicobacter pylori*. Hum Pathol 1992; 23: 548–556.

Price AB. The Sydney system: histological division. J Gastroenterol Hepatol 1991; 6:209–222.

Wolper R, Owen D, DelBuono L, et al. Lymphocytic gastritis in patients with celiac sprue or spruelike intestinal disease. Gastroenterology 1990; 98:310–315.

Wyatt JI. Gastritis and its relation to gastric carcinogenesis. Sem Diagn Pathol 1991; 8:137–148.

Yardley JH. Pathology of chronic gastritis and duodenitis. In Goldman H, Appelman HD, Kaufman H, eds. Gastrointestinal pathology (USCAP monographs in pathology, No. 31). Baltimore: Williams & Wilkins, 1990:69–143.

CHRONIC GASTRITIS: MANAGEMENT

ARTHUR J. DeCROSS, M.D.
RICHARD W. McCALLUM, M.D., F.A.C.P., F.R.A.C.P., F.A.C.G.

This discussion of chronic gastritis focuses on the entity of nonerosive, nonspecific gastric mucosal inflammation, which histologically embraces both a superficial epithelial infiltration of inflammatory cells and the deeper inflammation associated with atrophy of the gastric glands, with or without metaplastic epithelium. Excluded from this discussion are the categories of gastritis attributable to specific histologic disease (e.g., granulomatous disease, eosinophilic gastroenteritis, Mé-

netrier's disease), causes of chiefly erosive mucosal injury (e.g., nonsteroidal medications, alcohol, ischemia, radiation, acute stress injury, caustic ingestion), and the rare infectious gastritides (e.g., syphilis, cytomegalovirus, herpes simplex virus, fungi). These more specific forms of gastritis usually require some consideration of the underlying cause in order to address their management.

Let the reader beware: Any current approach to the management of chronic gastritis needs to remain creative and adaptable, for many issues are continuing to evolve. Just consider how the first decade of *Helicobacter pylori* has shaken the foundations of acid-peptic dogma, or consider how advances in the diagnosis and therapy of both gastroesophageal reflux disease (GERD) and gastric motility disorders have refocused more serious attention on the concept of nonulcer dyspepsia. For example, in the first case, we now know that active chronic gastritis can never be healed with acid suppression alone. In the latter case, the differential diagnosis of nonulcer dyspepsia has expanded, and it is no longer tenable to focus narrowly on gastritis as the only reasonable cause of symptoms in nonulcer dyspepsia.

GASTRITIS AND DYSPEPSIA

It must be clear that we are discussing management of the histologic diagnosis of chronic gastritis in the setting of a patient who is complaining of dyspepsia. This presumes two critical points that will be expanded on: (1) the patient has nonulcer dyspepsia, which by definition indicates that he or she has had an upper endoscopy without gross evidence of peptic ulcer disease or GERD; and (2) the physician is attributing dyspeptic symptoms to histologic gastritis, a diagnosis made from gastric biopsy at the time of endoscopy. Our management recommendations are not intended to usurp the traditional empiric approach to the initial presentation of dyspepsia in the primary care setting.

Dyspepsia refers to the symptom complex commonly referred to as "indigestion" or "upset stomach," which generally includes symptoms of epigastric burning, gnawing, or pain; belching; heartburn; nausea; or bloating. These symptoms are generally thought to be referable to the upper gastrointestinal tract, and they are often exacerbated by eating. In the absence of gross endoscopic findings and laboratory evidence of biliary-pancreatic disease, these symptoms are referred to as nonulcer dyspepsia.

There is evidence to support several etiologies of nonulcer dyspepsia. The more common, which are not necessarily mutually exclusive, include GERD (endoscopically negative), gastric motility disorders, irritable bowel syndrome, and chronic gastritis. Chronic gastritis (more specifically, the active chronic gastritis of *H. pylori*) is associated with about 50 percent of cases of nonulcer dyspepsia. This is significantly higher than the prevalence of *H. pylori* among asymptomatic controls. Unfortunately, the successful resolution of gastritis (through eradication of *H. pylori*) does not consistently result in the resolution of dyspeptic symptoms. Nonetheless, as we discuss later, our experience has convinced us that there is a group of nonulcer dyspeptic patients who appear to benefit significantly from the treatment of *H. pylori*–positive gastritis.

It should be noted that chronic gastritis, as a histologic diagnosis, has no correlation with gross endoscopic mucosal appearance. Macroscopic edema, friability, and erythema do not predict the presence or severity of histologic gastritis. Conversely, up to 40 percent of cases of endoscopically normal-appearing gastric mucosa may be involved with gastritis. Consequently, a mucosal biopsy is required for the diagnosis of chronic gastritis. About 80 percent of cases of chronic gastritis are the chronic gastritis of *H. pylori* infection, referred to as "active" chronic gastritis owing to the characteristic presence of neutrophils. The bacteria usually are detected by routine histologic study, but special stains (e.g., Giemsa) for the organism can be

specifically requested. As discussed in another chapter, at the same time that biopsies are being sent for histologic study to assess for gastritis, an extra gastric biopsy may be obtained for a urease test, which is another way to confirm the infection.

MANAGEMENT

When we choose to address chronic gastritis as the most reasonable explanation of a nonulcer dyspeptic patient's symptoms, we find it most useful to separate our management strategies according to whether the patient has *H. pylori*–positive or –negative gastritis (Fig. 1).

Helicobacter Therapy

Although the standard management of *H. pylori* is handled elsewhere in this book, we have been impressed with the efficacy and tolerability of the recent therapies that combine high-dose omeprazole (20 mg twice daily) with either amoxicillin (500 mg four times daily) or clarithromycin (500 mg three times daily) for 2 weeks. These combinations seem to provide more rapid symptom relief, and probably enhanced compliance, compared with our experience with metronidazole-based triple therapy. However, they are more expensive and need to be prescribed cautiously. Amoxicillin is obviously contraindicated in penicillin-allergic patients, and its use may result in *Clostridium difficile* colitis in a few patients. Clarithromycin is a macrolide and thus subject to the drug interactions of that class of antibiotic. Furthermore, *H. pylori* can acquire resistance to the macrolides.

Omeprazole, a proton-pump antagonist, is the most powerful inhibitor of gastric acid secretion available on the American market. Many patients are rendered virtually achlorhydric on this medication. This may be the explanation for its anti-*Helicobacter* properties. Achlorhydria enables the survival of complement-activating IgG immunoglobulins in the gastric lumen, which theoretically could help clear the infection. This class of immunoglobulin is ordinarily destroyed in the acidic gastric juice. Alternatively, the organism's microenvironment, which is ordinarily alkaline as a consequence of its urease activity, may prove to be toxic to the organism in the total absence of neutralizing acid. Omeprazole is virtually free of side effects and is completely safe for short-term use.

If the patient's symptoms are relieved, we do not necessarily pursue documentation that the infection has been eradicated. Should the symptoms persist after therapy, or recur later, the status of the infection must be confirmed as discussed elsewhere in this book. Sometimes, symptoms persist despite successful eradication of the organism. However, as stated earlier, many patients' symptoms are so dramatically improved that we feel a course of anti–*H. pylori* therapy is reasonable for documented *H. pylori* infection when the physician

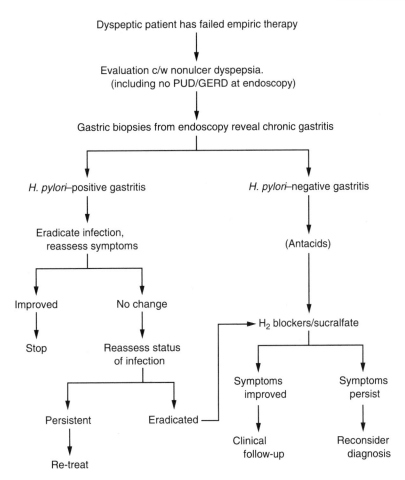

Figure 1 Algorithm for the management of chronic gastritis. GERD = gastroesophageal reflux disease; PUD = peptic ulcer disease.

suspects this as the cause of nonulcer dyspeptic symptoms.

Antacid Therapy

The traditional first line (or phase I) approach to the management of *H. pylori*–negative chronic gastritis in the nonulcer dyspeptic patient is the use of an antacid compound, although the patient will probably have exhausted this option before undergoing endoscopy. There can be no rationale as to the general selection of a particular antacid agent, the dosage, or the timing of the dosage, because the mechanism of dyspepsia in gastritis is mysterious. It is wisest to allow the patient to take antacids as needed within certain parameters (any regimen more aggressive than four tablespoons every 6 hours is probably excessive).

In the healing of peptic ulceration, antacids probably work through mechanisms of cytoprotection, with a minimal component of acid neutralization. Antacids do not resolve histologic gastritis, and the mechanism by which they provide relief in dyspepsia is unknown. However, antacids may cause symptoms of their own: aluminum-based compounds tend to cause constipation, while magnesium-based compounds may result in diar-

rhea. They may also contain a surprising amount of sodium, which may adversely affect salt-restricted patients. Aluminum-based antacids are best avoided in patients with renal insufficiency, who may become hyperaluminumemic. Certain antacid products contain simethicone, which acts as a surfactant to break down gas bubbles and is touted for the relief of excessive gassiness. Although this agent is theoretically attractive, there are no firm data to support its utility. Simethicone is often empirically recommended in a dose of 40 mg three times daily and appears to be free of significant side effects.

Histamine-2 Receptor Antagonist or Sucralfate

A trial of H_2 blockers or sucralfate is the next level (phase II) of therapeutic intensity after antacids. All H_2 blockers work by reducing gastric acid secretion through blocking H_2 receptors on the gastric parietal cells. In the treatment of peptic ulceration, it has become fashionable to take H_2 blockers before bedtime, in keeping with the observation that most acid secretion occurs overnight. This is effective and convenient therapy. However, this regimen fails in the treatment of GERD, for which twice-daily dosing has proved more effective in achieving symptom relief as well as tissue healing. We mention this because there is some evidence that a significant percentage of cases of nonulcer dyspepsia may be associated with acid reflux on esophageal pH monitoring, and so may represent endoscopically negative GERD. It might therefore become confusing if H_2-blocker therapy intended for chronic gastritis were begun with a regimen more appropriate for GERD, because the physician could not then be sure that symptom relief was not a consequence of treating GERD. We therefore suggest initiating treatment with a dose more consistent with peptic ulcer therapy. In fact, if the patient seems to require further acid suppression to achieve symptom relief, this should alert the physician to reconsider the diagnosis of GERD. Although we do not favor one agent over another, cimetidine is probably more troublesome than the others in the patient for whom polypharmacy is a concern. Cimetidine inhibits the P-450 metabolic pathway and can lead to unpredictable fluctuations in the levels of theophylline, warfarin, and anticonvulsants, to name just a few of the more serious interactions. Otherwise, as a class, H_2 blockers have a remarkably good safety profile, the most common adverse reaction being headache in less than 10 percent of patients. Regardless of how H_2 blockers affect dyspepsia, they do not cause resolution of histologic gastritis.

Sucralfate, as mentioned above, is a perfectly acceptable alternative to H_2 blockers. This drug is a sulfated disaccharide complex with aluminum hydroxide that has proved effective in ulcer healing, although its mechanisms of action are not fully understood. The drug is thought to coat ulcer bases and thus provide a cytoprotective function, promoting re-epithelialization. It may function by merely interfering mechanically with continued peptic digestion of the ulcer base, but evidence indicates that this drug may also increase protective prostaglandins, possess some minimal activity against *H. pylori,* and have some poorly understood primary cytoprotective effect related to its aluminum content. It does not resolve histologic gastritis but can provide relief for certain patients with dyspepsia. Although sucralfate is a very safe medication, its size and frequency of dosage (one tablet either twice or four times daily) can be inconvenient.

The physician who has exhausted these options in the approach to *H. pylori*–negative chronic gastritis should stop and seriously consider alternative explanations for the symptoms of nonulcer dyspepsia.

POSTGASTRECTOMY GASTRITIS

We feel that postgastrectomy gastritis merits separate attention, since the concept of alkaline (bile) reflux gastritis still engenders controversy. There is certainly a well-described postgastrectomy syndrome in 5 to 35 percent of patients that takes the form of burning epigastric pain unrelieved with antacids, worsened with meals, and associated with bilious vomiting that does not relieve the pain. This syndrome seems to contrast with the afferent and efferent loop syndromes, in which vomiting does relieve the discomforting symptoms. The dyspeptic symptoms associated with the postgastrectomy state have often been attributed to the gastritis that many believe is a consequence of "alkaline reflux" (the duodenal juice rich in biliary-pancreatic and jejunal secretions that bathes the gastric remnant). There is credible support for this concept. First, chronic exposure of the gastric mucosa to bile can lead to predictable histologic changes of gastritis that include villus-like foveolar hyperplasia, glandular cystification, lamina propria edema, mucosal capillary vasocongestion, and minimal inflammatory cell infiltration. Second, the autologous instillation of either duodenal contents or an alkaline Bernstein test will produce symptoms in patients suspected of having the syndrome, but supposedly not in controls.

Surgical Intervention

A surgical revision intended to divert the alkaline secretions away from the gastric remnant (most commonly represented by the example of converting a Billroth II to a Roux-en-Y gastrojejunostomy) sometimes results in resolution of the gastritis. Unfortunately, the symptom complex is not predictably eliminated by such a procedure, even when the gastritis is shown to have resolved. As expected, such inconsistent results only serve to fuel a controversy over the significance of alkaline reflux gastritis.

Medical Intervention

No single medical therapy has been very successful in the treatment of this entity, and reports have been largely anecdotal. Bile acid resins such as cholestyramine can be tried, although they are not very palatable and often result in bloating and constipation. Other agents that bind bile salts, such as aluminum-based antacids and sucralfate, have not proved effective. Ursodeoxycholic acid has been tried in an attempt to render the composition of the bile less toxic to the mucosa. This drug is generally well tolerated and safe, if only anecdotally effective for this purpose. Misoprostol, a prostaglandin E_1 analog, has also been tried in this syndrome and may be effective for some patients. This agent has significant side effects of cramping and diarrhea and should not be used in women of childbearing potential, as it is an abortifacient. Agents that promote clearance of the refluxate from the gastric remnant—the promotility drugs—have also been reported to have success in relieving symptoms, but it is not clear whether this is achieved through resolution of the gastritis or simply through a reduction in gastric stasis.

Refractory Symptoms

Perhaps 5 to 10 percent of patients with this syndrome are refractory to conservative medical measures as well as being severely debilitated by their symptoms. Malnutrition and weight loss in particular should highlight the failing patient. Nonetheless, in this group, a surgical revision for biliary diversion should be considered very cautiously and with extensive preoperative evaluation. Endoscopic and barium contrast studies are mandatory to exclude mucosal erosive disease or mechanical obstruction as a cause of symptoms. Furthermore, we feel that gastric emptying studies, using radionuclide solid meals, are necessary in the assessment of gastric remnant motility. Surgery for biliary diversion is not going to help patients with gastric remnant dysmotility manifested by stasis and vomiting. In fact, their symptoms after a Roux-en-Y diversion can be worsened.

SUGGESTED READING

DeCross AJ, Marshall BJ. Eradication of *Helicobacter pylori:* which patients, which drugs? Drug Ther 1993; 23(1):25–36.

Hocking MP, Vogel SB. Alkaline reflux gastritis and esophagitis. In Vogel SB, Hocking MP, eds. Woodward's postgastrectomy syndromes. Philadelphia: WB Saunders, 1991:126–127.
Klauser AG, Voderholzer WA, Knesewitch PA, et al. What is behind dyspepsia? Dig Dis Sci 1993; 38:147–154.
Marshall BJ, McCallum RW, Guerrant RL, eds. *Helicobacter pylori* in peptic ulceration and gastritis. Boston: Blackwell Scientific, 1991.
Meyer JH. Chronic morbidity after ulcer surgery. In Sleisenger MH, Fordtran JS, eds. Gastrointestinal disease. Philadelphia: WB Saunders, 1993:731.
Sauerbruch T, Schreiber MA, Schussler P, Permanetter W. Endoscopy in the diagnosis of gastritis. Diagnostic value of endoscopic criteria in relation to histological diagnosis of gastritis. Endoscopy 1984; 16:101.
The Sydney System: a new classification of gastritis. The Working Party Report of the World Congresses of Gastroenterology. J Gastroenterol Hepatol 1991; 6:207–251.
Weinstein WM. Gastritis. In Sleisenger MH, Fordtran JS, eds. Gastrointestinal disease. Philadelphia: WB Saunders, 1993:545.

GASTROPARESIS

MARVIN M. SCHUSTER, M.D., F.A.C.P., F.A.P.A.

ETIOLOGY AND PATHOGENESIS

Gastric emptying disorders may be acute or chronic and the cause may be functional or mechanical. The disorder in emptying may be either excessively rapid or delayed. Rapid emptying results most frequently from gastric surgery (vagotomy, partial gastric resection, pyloroplasty) associated with the dumping syndrome. Delayed gastric emptying can be seen with any of these disorders.

The most common cause of acute alterations in gastric motility and emptying are drugs, gastroenteritis, and metabolic disorders. Metabolic causes include ketoacidosis, hypokalemia, uremia, hepatic failure, hypothyroidism, and hypo- or hypercalcemia. Among the drugs that most commonly produce altered emptying of the stomach are anticholinergics, opiates, psychotropics, ganglionic blocking agents, and dopamine agonists. Infection of volunteers with the Norwalk agent has been demonstrated to produce acute delay in gastric emptying that may extend to a subacute period of 2 to 3 weeks, after which resolution usually occurs. However, there are reports indicating that chronic gastroparesis may also have its onset after an acute infectious (usually "flu"-like) process.

The most common causes of chronic changes in gastric emptying are diabetes mellitus, vagotomy, and partial gastric resection. Gastric dysmotility is seen in 20 to 30 percent of diabetics. Liquids and digestible solid emptying is often normal, whereas indigestible solids empty slowly. Delayed gastric emptying can be an isolated phenomenon or part of a more generalized dysautonomia. Neuromuscular and collagen vascular disorders also may lead to gastric emptying disturbances. Patients with chronic intestinal pseudo-obstruction often have delayed gastric emptying, as do those with anorexia nervosa. Altered gastric emptying may also be seen in pregnancy.

Mechanical obstruction is usually due to peptic disease or cancer, but may also be seen in adult hypertrophic pyloric stenosis.

CLINICAL PRESENTATION

Symptoms of rapid emptying are sweating, weakness, giddiness, tachycardia, and occasionally orthostasis. The earliest symptom of delayed gastric emptying is early satiety, which may be associated with or followed by nausea, bloating, distention, and occasionally dyspeptic symptoms. Later, patients experience vomiting, anorexia, and weight loss.

DIAGNOSTIC TESTS

Upper endoscopy and upper gastrointestinal (GI) x-ray examination with contrast material, while generally inadequate to establish the presence of disordered emptying, may point to underlying etiologic or pathogenetic factors such as ulcer, inflammation, scarring, pyloric hypertrophy, or mechanical obstruction. Tests of gastric emptying rely generally on radionuclide scintigraphy. Gastric manometry with perfused tubes and electrogastrography with surface abdominal electrodes are becoming more useful as experience and technology improve, but are not available to most physicians.

TREATMENT

As previously noted, the optimal treatment involves correction of the underlying disorder. This may not be possible, either because the underlying disorder is unknown or because it is uncorrectable. When this is true, measures are taken to alter the pathophysiology as much as possible and to treat symptomatically.

Treatment is discussed under two broad headings: that of delayed gastric emptying and that of rapid gastric emptying. If the underlying disorder is not amenable to treatment or not immediately responsive, symptomatic therapy is instituted. When the disorder is primary, symptomatic therapy is the only treatment available.

Some disorders are more responsive to treatment than others. For example, gastric stasis associated with hypothyroidism and myxedema responds more rapidly to treatment than stasis associated with diabetic neuropathy. Nevertheless, strict diabetic control may produce some improvement, particularly when this is accompanied by correction of ketoacidosis and electrolytes. Diabetic gastroparesis, for unknown reasons, may appear episodically or even cyclically. Gastric symptoms may be independent of the blood sugar or electrolyte disturbance.

Rapid Emptying

Accelerated gastric emptying is most commonly seen in the dumping syndrome after gastric surgery (either subtotal gastrectomy or truncal vagotomy with pyloroplasty). Subtotal gastrectomy accelerates the emptying of both liquids and solids, whereas vagotomy and pyloroplasty accelerates liquid emptying but has a less predictable effect on emptying of solids. Treatment of rapid gastric emptying involves both dietary therapy and drug therapy.

Dietary Therapy

Dietary therapy involves the restriction of fluids during meals, since fluids tend to empty rapidly. Instead, dry meals, low in simple sugars (which increase osmolarity) and high in complex carbohydrates, are prescribed. In particular, hyperosmolar fluids are interdicted; so is added salt. Soluble fiber, such as psyllium seed compounds and oatmeal, may be beneficial because these can slow down gastric emptying. Pectin is a dietary fiber that has been shown to delay liquid emptying in patients with the dumping syndrome and may provide symptomatic improvement. Small, frequent feedings are recommended.

Drug Therapy

Specific drugs may slow down gastric emptying to a degree but usually are not dramatically effective. When anticholinergic agents are used, they should be given in increasing doses to the point at which side effects appear. They should be administered prophylactically one-half hour before meals to allow time for absorption before intake of food. Opiates may provide some benefit, but their addiction potential generally precludes their use except in severe instances of dumping syndrome.

Octreotide may be effective, particularly in late dumping syndrome, by delaying gastric emptying and inhibiting insulin release in response to a carbohydrate meal. Because serum serotonin has been shown to be elevated in the dumping syndrome, serotonin antagonists such as cyprohepatidine have been prescribed in doses of 4 mg administered 30 to 60 minutes before meals.

Delayed Emptying

Symptomatic Management

Acute or episodic gastroparesis, which can be seen in otherwise uncomplicated diabetes or associated with electrolyte disturbance, ketoacidosis, sepsis, or surgery, should be managed with nasogastric decompression, fluid and electrolyte replacement, and correction of any coexisting sepsis or ketoacidosis. Prolonged aspiration can also be helpful in alleviating chronic distention from accumulation of swallowed air that remains in the stomach owing to the inability to empty it. Decompression of a distended stomach may not provide relief if there is a significant central component to the nausea and vomiting. Gentle intermittent suction is preferred to continuous suction, since the latter often results in occlusion of the aspirating ports. When chronic aspiration is required, a percutaneous endoscopic gastrostomy (PEG) may be performed, or it may be combined with a percutaneous jejunostomy (PEJ) for feeding. This is discussed under diet and nutrition.

Diet and Nutrition

Since the stomach tends to empty liquids more rapidly and easily than solids, the consistency of the diet is often more important than the type of food, with the exception of fats, which may aggravate gastric stasis from any cause because they delay gastric emptying. Fats should therefore be avoided. Hypertonic solutions are not well tolerated, nor are poorly digestible fibers. In fact, the fibrous material can form bezoars that may further obstruct the gastric outlet. Meat impactions of the stomach often can be dissolved with papain (Adolph's meat tenderizer without spice). One teaspoon is mixed in a half-glass of water and sipped slowly for 10 minutes. Phytobezoars do not respond to papain digestion as meat protein does, and therefore fibrous bezoars may have to be removed endoscopically or sometimes even surgically.

The diet should be as liberal as tolerated. The best nutritional substance is food, and the ideal food is the most normal diet that can be tolerated. When only soft foods can be managed, blenderized or baby foods may have to constitute a large part of the diet. When only liquids are tolerated, adequate nutrition can be maintained by liquid formulas such as Sustacal and Ensure. However, when used in full strength, these solutions are hypertonic and therefore delay gastric emptying. Dilution may be necessary.

When gastric stasis is so severe that even liquids fail to empty, a medical trial of enteral feeding directly into the jejunum should be attempted, bypassing the stomach. Often the nasojejunal tube must be passed endoscopically because gastric motility is inadequate to propel it out of the stomach. If jejunal feeding (or direct measurement of intestinal motility) demonstrates good motility and satisfactory tolerance of jejunal tube feedings, a percutaneous jejunal feeding tube can be placed. This can be done in one of two ways. The simplest and generally most effective manner is via a PEG with a double-lumen tube placed so that one remains in the stomach while the other traverses the stomach and passes into the jejunum. The advantage of this approach is that the gastric tube can be used for decompression whenever nausea and vomiting are severe, while the jejunal tube is used for providing nutrition. The jejunal tube, by permitting fluid and electrolyte replacement at home, can diminish the need for hospitalization due to dehydration induced by vomiting. Vitamin supplements are often advisable.

Patients with PEGs and PEJs may wish to try oral liquids, soft foods, or even solids that are well chewed in small quantities to satisfy appetite needs. If these too are not tolerated, patients may derive some benefit from sham feeding (chewing soft foods or drinking liquids and aspirating the swallowed material via the gastrostomy as soon as gastric distention produces nausea and vomiting).

Enteral feeding may not be possible if dysmotility involves the small bowel as well as the stomach. In this case, total parenteral nutrition via a central line may be required. Patients who do not tolerate enteral feeding but have benefited from intermittent gastric aspiration may wish to discontinue the PEJ and keep the PEG for gastric decompression, and to provide the satisfaction that can be obtained from sham feeding.

Drug Therapy

H$_2$-Receptor Antagonists. Inhibition of acid production by H$_2$ blockers or proton-pump inhibitors (omeprazole) may be helpful for dyspeptic symptoms and gastroesophageal reflux of acid that is associated with gastric stasis.

Antiemetics. Symptomatic treatment of nausea and vomiting with phenothiazine drugs and antihistamines may be required intermittently or continuously. Prochlorperazine maleate (Compazine), although one of the more effective antiemetics, carries the risk of producing extrapyramidal symptoms when doses significantly higher than 40 mg per day are required. In rare instances, these side effects are not reversible. The scopolamine patch has the advantage of long-term gradual dosing and is preferred by some patients. Scopolamine, as well as antiemetics (most of which have anticholinergic action), may not only produce uncomfortable dryness, blurred vision, or urinary retention but may also further slow gastric emptying. When nausea and vomiting do not respond to these more common antiemetics, cannabinoids may provide relief.

Promotility Agents. In recent times, a new class of drugs has been developed. The prokinetic (promotility) agents are actually "designer" drugs whose molecular structure is based on that of haloperidol, which was noted to have, in addition to its psychotropic action, a promotility effect. Attempts were then made to design new drugs that would improve motility without producing the central nervous system (CNS) effects of haloperidol. Bethanechol, a cholinomimetic agent, should not be considered a promotility agent, since its effect is massive and uncoordinated. This may be one of the reasons it is also generally ineffective for the treatment of motility disorders, including those involving the stomach.

The first prokinetic agent approved in this country was metoclopramide (Reglan), which unfortunately crosses the blood-brain barrier and can produce hyperkinesia or somnolence in about 30 percent of patients, often to the extent that the drug has to be discontinued. The second-generation prokinetic drug domperidone was designed so that it would not cross the blood-brain barrier, and it therefore does not produce these CNS side effects. For this reason, it can also be tolerated in higher doses. Both metoclopramide and domperidone achieve their promotility effect by inhibiting the dopaminergic nervous system, which inhibits esophageal and gastric motility. Inhibition of the inhibitor results in improved motility and improved antroduodenal coordination, which is important for appropriate gastric emptying. Metoclopramide also releases acetylcholine, which may assist in stimulating GI motility. Unfortunately, however, neither of these drugs is effective distal to the ligament of Treitz, since dopamine nerves begin to disappear at that site.

Domperidone has an antiemetic effect despite the fact that it does not cross the blood-brain barrier and therefore does not enter the vomiting center. The reason is that the chemoreceptor trigger zone (which, like the vomiting center, also controls vomiting) is located in the brainstem outside the blood-brain barrier and is therefore accessible to domperidone. Both domperidone and metoclopramide are best administered one-half hour before meals to allow time for absorption by the duodenum and small bowel, which is necessary for their effectiveness. To facilitate gastric emptying and duodenal absorption, it may be necessary to initiate gastric emptying intravenously (IV) and subsequently follow up with oral administration of these agents. Only metoclopramide is available for parenteral use. A nighttime dose maintains the blood level during the hours of sleep so that the morning dose can then be more effective. Metoclopramide is generally given in doses of 10 mg, although some people tolerate only 5 mg. Domperidone can be administered in 20 mg doses or higher; its main side effect is constipation. Permanent dyskinesia has been reported with metoclopramide in rare instances.

A third-generation drug, cisapride, has become available by prescription. This is a 5-HT3 antagonist and therefore can alter motility throughout most of the GI tract. Experience has shown its effect on colonic motility to be unpredictable and usually disappointing.

Recently, Japanese investigators have demonstrated that erythromycin mimics exogenous motilin in inducing the migrating motor complex in the small intestine in dogs and in humans by competing for motilin receptors in the gut. Belgium workers have demonstrated the stimulation of antral phase III–like contractions in both normal volunteers and patients with diabetic gastroparesis, some of whom had autonomic neuropathy. A dose of 40 mg, which is effective in inducing phase III migrating motor complexes in the small bowel, was also effective in stimulating antral activity in three-fifths of patients, whereas a high dose of 200 to 350 mg was effective in all the diabetic patients. Because this high dosage has less efficacy in the small bowel than a 40 to 70 mg dose, diabetic patients with gastric and small bowel dysmotility would probably respond better to the lower dose of 50 mg (40 to 70 mg). Erythromycin is more effective when given IV but also has efficacy when administered orally 30 to 60 minutes before meals and at bedtime. Because the lowest-dose tablet contains 200 mg, a 50 mg dosage can best be achieved by using the liquid suspension (¼ tsp of the 200 mg per 5 ml strength administered one-half hour before meals and at bedtime). Two preparations of erythromycin that are readily available are ethylsuccinate EES and EryPed.

More recently, octreotide (Sandostatin), a somatostatin analog, has been shown to induce the migrating motor complex in small bowel in patients with scleroderma. However, octreotide has its effect directly on small bowel and does not seem to stimulate gastric acidity; it may actually delay gastric emptying. Octreotide use in scleroderma is discussed in another chapter.

SURGICAL TREATMENT

Experience with operative approaches for both gastric stasis and accelerated gastric emptying has been variable. In my experience, subtotal gastrectomy is of little help in the treatment of delayed gastric emptying, and vagotomy and pyloroplasty often worsens the situation. In drastic situations a total gastrectomy, while carrying its own problems, may improve nutrition and absorption.

The response of the dumping syndrome and other forms of rapid gastric emptying to operative intervention is also unpredictable. Both the Roux-en-Y procedure and interposition of a 10 cm segment of reversed jejunum are used with varying degrees of success.

SUGGESTED READING

Brown CK, Dkanderia U. Use of metoclopramide, domperidone and cisapride in the management of diabetic gastroparesis. Clin Pharm 1990; 9:357–365.
Drenth JPH, Engels LGJB. Diabetic gastroparesis: a critical reappraisal of new treatment strategies. Drugs 1992; 44:537–553.
Geldorf H, Van der Schee EJ, Van Blankenstein M, Grashuis JL. Electrogastrographic study of gastric myoelectric activity in patients with unexplained nausea and vomiting. Gut 1986; 27:799–808.
Janssens J, Peters TL, VanTrappen G, et al. Improvement of gastric emptying in diabetic gastroparesis by erythromycin. N Engl J Med 1990; 322:1028–1032.
Koch KL. Gastric dysrhythmias and the current status of electrogastrography. Pract Gastroenterol 1989; 13:37–44.
Koch KL. Stomach. In: Schuster MM, ed. Atlas of intestinal motility. Baltimore: Williams & Wilkins, 1993:158.

PERCUTANEOUS ENDOSCOPIC GASTROSTOMY

PATRICK G. BRADY, M.D.

Percutaneous endoscopic gastrostomy (PEG) was introduced in 1980 by Ponsky and Gauderer as an alternative to surgical gastrostomy and nasoenteric tubes. Since that time, the technique has become widely accepted, and 50,000 to 74,000 PEG procedures are performed annually in the United States. PEG placement can be accomplished easily and safely and is generally well tolerated. Procedure time is short and general anesthesia is not required. The purpose of PEG is to provide long-term enteral feedings to patients who are unable to maintain sufficient oral intake to meet their nutritional requirements. PEG placement is successful in approximately 95 percent of attempts. This chapter discusses the indications, contraindications, placement techniques, alternatives, and complications of PEG.*

---

*Editor's Note: Dr. Ponsky authored this chapter in the third edition of this book. The current chapter contains more details on placement and on complications management.

INDICATIONS AND CONTRAINDICATIONS

PEG is indicated for long-term nutritional support in patients who are unable to eat but have a functioning gastrointestinal (GI) tract. Specific indications for PEG include neurologic conditions causing impaired swallowing; neoplasms involving the oropharynx, hypopharynx, and esophagus; facial trauma; and as a route to provide supplemental feedings in patients with increased metabolic needs. Placement of a jejunal tube through the gastrostomy tube, percutaneous endoscopic jejunostomy (PEJ), can be used to provide enteral feedings to patients at risk for aspiration of gastric contents, and to patients with gastroparesis or outlet obstruction requiring prolonged gastric decompression. PEJ, however, has not been conclusively shown to reduce the risk of aspiration of gastric contents.

PEG is not indicated in patients who are expected to recover their ability to eat within a few weeks. Likewise, it is not indicated in moribund patients or in those with a rapidly progressive illness whose death is expected in 1 month or less. If enteral feedings are required in these circumstances, a small-caliber nasoenteric feeding tube is the preferred method. Absolute contraindications to PEG are inability to appose the gastric wall to the anterior abdominal wall, as indicated by inability to transilluminate the anterior abdominal wall, and total obstruction of the pharynx or esophagus. Relative contraindications include coagulation disorders, massive ascites, proximal small intestinal fistula, neoplastic or infiltrative disease of the gastric or abdominal wall, and portal hypertension. PEG can be performed in patients with obesity, hepatomegaly, and partial gastrectomy if the endoscopist can adequately transilluminate the anterior abdominal wall. Partial obstruction of the hypopharynx or esophagus is not a contraindication to PEG if the area of stenosis can be dilated sufficiently to allow passage of an endoscope. Previous surgery involving the left upper quadrant is not a contraindication provided that adequate transillumination of the abdominal wall can be achieved. In this situation, the PEG site should be at least 3 cm from surgical scars, since small intestine or colon may be adherent to the abdominal wall at these sites.

Patients with severe malnutrition, particularly those with serum albumin levels of 2 g or less, are at increased risk for complications from PEG placement. These patients should be started on nasoenteric tube feedings, and PEG should be postponed until their nutritional condition has improved. Active ulcers should be treated and healed before PEG, and active infections also should be treated before PEG.

TECHNIQUE

Three basic techniques are used for PEG tube placement; the pull method, the push method, and the introducer method. The pull method is the original one introduced by Ponsky and Gauderer and is the most widely employed technique. These methods all rely on transillumination to identify the site at which the gastric and anterior abdominal walls are apposed. They also allow endoscopic confirmation of proper positioning of the gastrostomy tube. Percutaneous gastrostomy has also been reported with use of a nasogastric tube to insufflate the stomach followed by direct percutaneous catheter placement under fluoroscopic control. This latter method is not recommended, since lack of transillumination makes inadvertent puncture of adjacent viscera more likely.

Pull Method

Once patients' condition has been optimized, they are fasted overnight. A single dose of a parenteral antibiotic is given before the procedure. Cefazolin or a similar cephalosporin is preferred for prophylaxis. Immediately before the procedure, the abdomen is washed with a povidone-iodine (Betadine) solution and then draped with sterile towels. Intravenous sedation is administered, when necessary, immediately before the procedure.

The procedure is performed with the patient in the supine position. Initially a diagnostic endoscopy is performed. When this is accomplished, a site for insertion of the PEG tube is selected. With the room lights dimmed, the endoscope is slowly withdrawn from the antrum into the body of the stomach along the anterior wall. Clear transillumination of the abdominal wall in the left upper quadrant indicates the site where the gastric and abdominal walls are apposed. Finger pressure is then applied to this area and should result in clear indentation of the gastric wall, identifying the site for the endoscopist. Internally the site will lie above the angularis on the anterior gastric wall. The exact location of the site externally is not important, except it should not lie immediately adjacent to the costal margin.

Once the site has been located, the skin is anesthetized with 1 percent lidocaine using a 1½ inch, 25 gauge needle, which can be advanced into the stomach to confirm correct site placement (Fig. 1). A 0.5 to 1 cm incision is then made in the skin with a no. 11 scalpel blade; an incision smaller than 0.5 cm would interfere with catheter withdrawal through the skin. With the stomach fully distended with air, a 16 gauge Medicut catheter is inserted through the skin incision and into the stomach (Fig. 2). A snare is looped around the catheter and tightened. Once the snare is in place, the metal stylet is removed, leaving the plastic cannula in place. A no. 2 silk suture, 60 inches long, is passed through the cannula into the stomach (Fig. 3). The snare is moved from the cannula onto the silk suture, where it is again tightened. The endoscope, snare, and silk suture are then removed as a unit and the cannula is removed. A continuous length of silk suture now enters through the abdominal wall and exits through the mouth. The suture exiting through the mouth is securely tied to the end of a mushroom-tipped catheter that has been fitted with a tapered cannula (Fig. 4). The catheter is pulled retro-

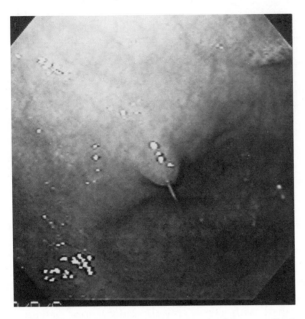

Figure 1 The 1½ inch, 25 gauge anesthetizing needle has been advanced into the gastric lumen.

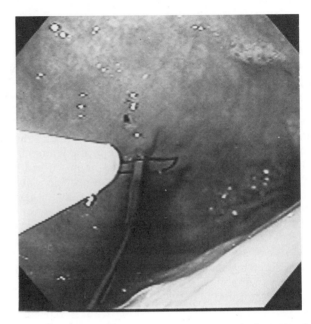

Figure 3 Suture material has been passed through the cannula. The snare is being moved from the cannula onto the suture.

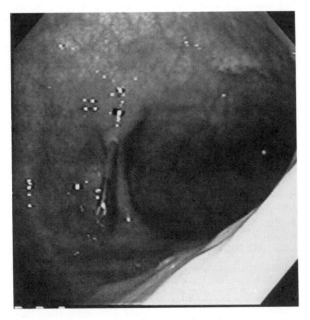

Figure 2 The 16 gauge Medicut catheter has been inserted into the gastric lumen. The metal stylet has not yet been withdrawn.

grade through the esophagus, stomach, and abdominal wall. The tapered cannula leading the catheter should not be grasped, since this will cause it to separate from the catheter. When the catheter itself emerges, it may be grasped and pulled into position. After several inches of the catheter have exited from the abdominal wall, the endoscope is reinserted and the catheter is pulled into position under endoscopic guidance. The catheter is

properly positioned when the inner bumper just contacts the gastric wall (Fig. 5). If the bumper is indented, excessive tension has been applied and may result in necrosis of the underlying tissue. When the catheter has been properly placed, the endoscope is removed. An external bumper and fixation device are applied again, care being taken to avoid excessive tension. A Christmas-tree adaptor is added to the end of the catheter, completing the procedure. The external bumper can be loosened or removed in 1 week. When PEG was originally described, 14 to 16 Fr mushroom catheters were used for PEG tubes. To avoid occlusion and administer medications, larger tubes, up to 20 Fr, have now been used without difficulty.

Push Method

The push method is a modification of the pull method. In the push method, a 0.035 inch, 300 cm long guidewire with a flexible tip is passed through a cannula or needle into the gastric lumen. The guidewire is then grasped with a snare, and the endoscope, snare, and guidewire are removed together, resulting in a continuous length of guidewire entering through the abdominal wall and exiting at the mouth. An elongated gastrostomy tube with a tapered end is then pushed into position over the guidewire while both ends of the guidewire are held firmly. When the tube exits the abdominal wall, it is grasped and pulled into its final position using endoscopic monitoring. When the gastrostomy tube is in position, the excess tubing is cut off to give the desired length. An external bumper is added to maintain apposition of the gastric and abdominal walls. The push and pull techniques have the same success and compli-

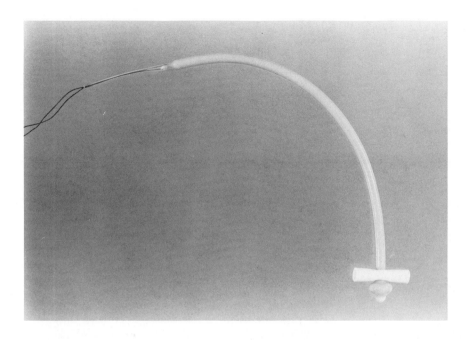

Figure 4 A 16 gauge mushroom-tipped catheter fitted with a tapered cannula, and an internal bumper to allow use as a PEG tube.

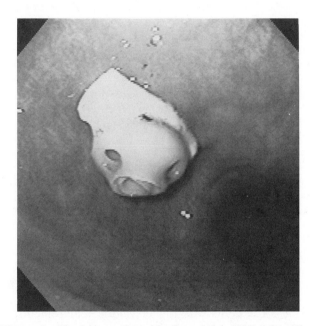

Figure 5 Final internal positioning of the PEG tube. The internal bumper was shortened before insertion because the patient had a stenosis in the upper esophagus. The tip of the catheter has been cut off to allow insertion of a J tube should this become necessary at a later date.

cation rates, and selection of one of these methods is a matter of operator preference.

Introducer Method

In the introducer method, the site is located using transillumination in the standard fashion. The endoscope remains in the stomach throughout the procedure, which is conducted under endoscopic guidance. The site is anesthetized with 1 percent lidocaine and a small incision is made in the skin. After direct puncture of the abdominal wall with a 16 gauge needle, a short guidewire is passed into the gastric lumen. Taking care to maintain the guidewire in a straight position, an introducer with a peel-away sheath is pushed over the guidewire, using a twisting motion. When the endoscopist has confirmed correct positioning, the introducer and guidewire are withdrawn, leaving the sheath in the gastric lumen. A Foley catheter is then passed through the sheath and into the gastric lumen. The Foley balloon is inflated and the sheath peeled away and removed. The catheter is pulled up to the gastric wall, and an external anchoring device is put into place to maintain correct positioning. This method may be associated with a number of technical problems, the most common being failure to keep the guidewire in a straightened position while passing the introducer. This may be associated with failure to enter the gastric lumen, inadvertent withdrawal of the guidewire, and occasionally puncture of an adjacent viscus. A Foley catheter is not ideal for use as a gastrostomy tube since the balloon may rupture, be inadvertently deflated, or be used as a feeding channel by inexperienced nursing personnel. Recently, the technique has been modified to allow passage of a mushroom rather than a Foley catheter. Because of these potential problems, the introducer method should be reserved for patients with severe stenoses of the pharynx or esophagus that permit passage of a small-caliber endoscope, but not a PEG tube.

PERCUTANEOUS ENDOSCOPIC JEJUNOSTOMY

Percutaneous endoscopic jejunostomy (PEJ) was introduced in 1982. It has been used with varying degrees of success for patients with partial gastric outlet obstruction, aspiration, and gastroesophageal reflux. At present, there is no convincing evidence that PEJ reduces the risk of aspiration pneumonia. Since PEJ tubes are more difficult to care for and do not appear to reduce the risk of aspiration pneumonia, their use is rarely required.

A standard PEG can be converted to a PEJ by adding a Y connector to the end of the PEG tube. A Touhy adaptor is added to one arm of the Y connector, and a small-caliber feeding tube that can accept a guidewire (Fredrich Miller or similar tube) is passed through this adaptor and into the stomach. After insertion of a guidewire, the tube can be maneuvered into the duodenum under fluoroscopic or endoscopic control. Tying a piece of silk suture to the end of the feeding tube will allow the endoscopist to grasp the suture with a biopsy forceps and carry the feeding tube into the duodenum along with the endoscope. Before the endoscope is withdrawn, the guidewire is passed through the feeding tube. The guidewire is left in place while the endoscope is withdrawn to prevent retraction of the feeding tube along with the endoscope. The guidewire can be removed after the endoscope has been withdrawn. Feeding is accomplished through the small-caliber feeding tube, using continuous infusion. The other limb of the Y connector can be used for gastric suction if necessary. PEJ requires the use of larger gastrostomy tubes (20 Fr). Commercial kits are now available with all the tubing and adaptors required for PEJ placement. Specific and detailed orders should be left for the nursing staff regarding the care and use of PEJ tubes. Only liquid feedings, liquid medication, and water should be given through the PEJ tube to avoid tube occlusion.

REPLACEMENT OF PEG TUBES

In 4 to 6 weeks, the gastric wall becomes firmly adherent to the anterior abdominal wall. At this time, it is safe to remove the PEG tube. In most cases, this can be done by exerting firm traction on the tube while simultaneously stabilizing the abdominal wall adjacent to the PEG site with the other hand. If an internal cross-bar is present, it will become detached and eventually pass in the stool. A few of the older, commercially available tubes must be removed retrograde with the endoscope. When dealing with an unfamiliar PEG tube, it is wise to read the instructions supplied by the manufacturer before attempting to remove the tube.

PEG tubes can be removed when the patient has resumed an adequate oral intake. Indications for replacement of a PEG tube include deterioration of the tube, obstruction of the tube lumen, or inadvertent removal by the patient or caregiver. If the tube has been removed inadvertently, it should be replaced as soon as possible, since the tract between the stomach and abdominal wall may close in a matter of hours. The tube may be replaced with either a Foley catheter or, preferably, a mushroom catheter. The latter is stretched over a metal stylet to narrow the mushroom sufficiently

to allow it to pass into the stomach. It is important that emergency room and nursing home personnel be aware of the need to replace catheters promptly, and be capable of inserting a Foley catheter to maintain a patent gastrostomy.

The gastrostomy button is an alternative to longer catheters for replacement of a gastrostomy tube. This device has a deformable mushroom on the gastric side and a flat bar on the opposite side that sits flush with the skin. There is an antireflux valve to prevent reflux of gastric contents onto the skin. Since the device is less apparent, it may be useful in confused patients who are prone to pull out their gastrostomy tubes. It is also helpful in patients who have skin irritation because of reflux of gastric contents.

INITIATION OF FEEDINGS

Tube feedings can be safely initiated 2 hours after PEG placement, provided that the patient shows no evidence of an ileus. The ability to resume feedings soon after PEG tube placement is a major advantage of PEG compared with surgical gastrostomy. Feedings may be given either by continuous infusion or by the bolus method through PEG tubes. PEJ feedings can be given only by continuous infusion. Isotonic feeding formulas containing 1 calorie per milliliter are preferred for initiation of feedings. If an isotonic formula is used, the feedings do not require dilution. Feedings by continuous infusion are initiated at a rate of 25 ml per hour; this can be increased to 50 ml per hour after 24 hours and to full volume on the third day. PEJ feedings should not exceed 150 ml per hour.

Bolus feedings are initiated at a volume of 50 ml every 4 hours. After each bolus, the tube is flushed with 50 ml of water. Residual volumes are checked before the next feeding, and if they are less than 100 ml, the volume of the feeding is increased by 50 ml. When a volume of 200 ml of feeding formula is achieved, the frequency of bolus feedings is increased to once every 3 hours, and finally to once every 2 hours. Usually, eight 200 ml bolus feedings are given during the day, and no feedings at night. In patients with higher caloric requirements, a formula with a higher caloric density may be used, or a greater number of feedings may be given.

COMPLICATIONS

Short-term complications of PEG are relatively infrequent. The overall short-term complication rate is approximately 17 percent, with major complications in 3 percent. Long-term follow-up, however, indicates that complications may occur in up to 70 percent of patients, most of them minor (Table 1). Major complications include serious wound infections, intraperitoneal leak of gastric contents, gastrocolic fistula, bowel perforation, GI bleeding, and aspiration pneumonia. Minor complications include peristomal leakage, stomal enlargement,

Table 1 Complications and 30-Day Mortality Rate of Percutaneous Endoscopic Gastrostomy

Author	No. of Patients	Complications (%)	30-Day Mortality (%)
Strodel (1983)	43	12	9
Ponsky (1983)	150	10	–
Larson (1984)	23	10	–
Deutsch (1984)	23	10	10
Russell (1984)	28	9	14
Cohen (1984)	207	15	–
Hogan (1986)	40	17.5	15
Wendel (1990)	42	33	26
Taylor (1992)	97	47	22

tube dislodgment, tube occlusion, minor skin infections, pneumoperitoneum, and subcutaneous emphysema. The most common major complication is wound infection; the most common minor complication is tube dislodgment.

Most wound infections are minor, but major infections such as necrotizing fascitis may also occur. The incidence of wound infection can be decreased by the use of prophylactic antibiotics such as cephazolin. If the initial endoscopic evaluation shows evidence of candidal esophagitis, PEG should be postponed until the fungal infection has been eradicated, to avoid a candidal wound infection. If the skin incision is too small for the gastrostomy tube, excessive tension will be produced at the skin edge, resulting in skin ischemia and poor drainage of fluid from the subcutaneous tissue, changes that favor infection. Making the skin incision slightly larger than the tube prevents these problems and reduces the incidence of infection. If a small peritubal abscess occurs, it can be treated by incising the skin over the abscess, beginning at the catheter rather than at the exit site. This incision can then be irrigated with hydrogen peroxide several times a day until the cavity closes. Necrotizing fasciitis is a severe, rapidly progressive, and potentially fatal infection resulting in necrosis of the subcutaneous tissue and the adjacent fascia. In advanced cases, the muscle itself is involved. Treatment involves broad-spectrum antibiotics and wide surgical debridement.

Purulent drainage around the catheter usually represents a foreign body reaction rather than a true infection. This can be treated by topical cleansing with hydrogen peroxide. The site should be kept dry by exposing it to the air and avoiding occlusive dressings. Rubber catheters incite more of a foreign body reaction than Silastic catheters. In cases that do not respond to local cleansing measures, replacement of a rubber catheter with a Silastic one may solve the problem.

Tube occlusion can usually be rapidly resolved by flushing the tube with water. The problem can be avoided by following each bolus feeding with 50 ml of water. If medications or a blenderized diet are to be given through the gastrostomy tube, larger catheters should be used (18 to 20 Fr).

Tube migration can lead to gastric outlet obstruction or duodenal obstruction. Rarely, a tube can migrate completely through the gastrostomy and cause small bowel obstruction. Distal tube migration can be prevented by leaving an external bumper in place without tension. The tube can also be marked at the level of the gastrostomy, allowing nursing personnel to adjust its position if necessary. Migration is not a problem with the PEG button, which is an advantage of this replacement device. If a tube has migrated through the pylorus, it can usually be repositioned by exerting steady pressure on the end of the tube still protruding through the stoma. If the tube has completely migrated through the stoma, it can be removed with the use of an endoscope if it is still in the stomach or duodenum. If the tube is distal to the ligament of Treitz, endoscopic removal will not be possible and the patient should be observed while waiting for spontaneous passage.

A gastrostomy tube may also migrate into the abdominal wall. This is due to excessive traction on the gastric wall, with subsequent erosion of the internal bumper and end of the tube into the gastric or abdominal wall. Clinically, this will result in inability to infuse feedings and to reposition the tube, and in leakage around the tube. Migration into the abdominal wall can be confirmed by radiography or endoscopy. Treatment of this condition is surgical, with removal of the original tube and replacement with a new tube. If a guidewire can be passed through the gastrostomy tube into the stomach, an incision can be made down to the level of the bumper. The bumper and catheter are then removed, leaving the guidewire in place. A new tube may then be inserted using the introducer technique.

Gastrocolic fistula results from PEG tube placement when the colon is interposed between the stomach and anterior abdominal walls. It can be avoided by proceeding only when clear transillumination is present and by avoiding sites with scars from previous surgery. Gastrocolic fistulas may be asymptomatic for long periods. They can be suspected if feedings rapidly induce diarrhea. Diagnosis is made by instilling water-soluble contrast material through the gastrostomy tube. Most gastrocolic fistulas resolve spontaneously when the gastrostomy tube is removed.

Gastrointestinal hemorrhage from the gastrostomy site is caused by excessive tension on the cross-bar, resulting in ischemic necrosis of the underlying gastric mucosa. This is prevented by avoiding excessive traction on the PEG tube. Likewise, leakage of gastric contents into the peritoneum is related to improper tension on the gastrostomy tube. Inadequate tension does not cause apposition of the gastric and abdominal walls. Excessive tension can result in necrosis of the gastric wall. Water-soluble contrast agents instilled through the gastrostomy tube will demonstrate the leak. Small leaks can be treated by adjusting the tension on the gastrostomy tube and placing the bowel at rest. Larger leaks require surgical correction. Leakage of gastric contents into the peritoneum can also result if the tube is pulled out or dislodged within several days of placement. This usually necessitates surgical correction.

Pneumoperitoneum and subcutaneous emphysema are frequent findings after PEG placement. These are benign conditions that require no therapy if the patient is asymptomatic. Subcutaneous emphysema occurs because the skin incision is too tight to allow intragastric air to escape around the gastrostomy tube. Either finding in the setting of fever and peritoneal signs is more ominous and requires further evaluation. If leakage of gastric contents is suspected, the diagnosis can be confirmed with a contrast study.

OUTCOME

Very few studies have looked at patient outcome after PEG. Taylor and colleagues studied 97 patients from Olmsted County, Minnesota, of whom 23 percent were able to resume oral feedings. The probability of surviving was 78, 35, and 27 percent for 30 days, 1.5 years, and 4 years, respectively. Pneumonia was a major cause of death both before and after 30 days. Survival was better for patients who had a PEG for central nervous system disease, had no evidence of diabetes, and were younger and female. Clarkston and colleagues studied 42 patients who had a PEG; 20 had the PEG tube removed in the first 60 days. Mortality was 43 percent in the first 60 days, and patients with a malignancy had the highest mortality rate. Mortality rates for other studies are given in Table 1.

These studies indicate that many patients regain their ability to take oral feedings within 30 to 60 days after PEG placement, and that 30 day mortality is substantial. Patients who are likely to recover or to die within 30 days can be managed with modalities other than PEG, e.g., small-caliber nasoenteric feeding tubes. In particular, patients with malignancy seem to fare poorly after PEG placement and are not good candidates for this type of supportive therapy unless treatment of the primary problem is feasible. We need to assess patients for PEG placement carefully and select only those who are likely to benefit from the procedure.*

ALTERNATIVES TO PEG

Alternatives to PEG include total parenteral nutrition (TPN); small-caliber, soft, nasoenteric feeding tubes; surgical gastrostomy; and surgical jejunostomy. TPN is best suited to patients whose GI tract is not functional owing to disease or resection. For example, patients with a proximal small bowel fistula, or short bowel syndrome, would benefit from TPN. Patients with a functioning GI tract should be fed enterally.

Initial studies comparing PEG with surgical gastrostomy showed that PEG was less expensive and had a shorter procedure time and fewer complications. A

subsequent study comparing PEG with surgical gastrostomy performed under local anesthesia showed that PEG retained a cost advantage but had a similar complication rate. Gastrostomy can also be done at the time of laparoscopy, but this method has not been critically studied. At present, PEG remains the procedure of choice for placing a gastrostomy tube. Surgical gastrostomy is best reserved for patients who have contraindications to PEG or who have failed PEG placement.

Operative jejunostomy has all the disadvantages of operative gastrostomy. In addition, small-caliber jejunostomy tubes frequently become occluded and are difficult to replace. Compared with PEJ, however, operative jejunostomy does have the advantage of employing a fixed tube that will not migrate back into the stomach. Operative jejunostomy can be performed under local anesthesia. The most frequent use of operative jejunostomy is in patients who require surgical therapy for the primary GI problem and are unable to tolerate gastric feedings.

The choice between a soft, small-caliber, Silastic nasoenteric feeding tube and a PEG tube is a matter of clinical judgment. Disadvantages of the nasoenteric feeding tube include more frequent clogging and displacement, an inability to check gastric residuals, and an inability to give bolus feedings and medications through these tubes. Personnel in long-term care facilities prefer PEG tubes to small-caliber feeding tubes. PEG tubes are also less difficult for a patient and the caregiver to manage at home. A recent randomized trial comparing PEG and small-caliber nasogastric tube feedings found that tube displacement or obstruction occurred in 90 percent of the nasogastric tube group and none of the PEG group; prescribed feeding levels were reached in 55 percent of the nasogastric group and 93 percent of the PEG group. Small-caliber, nasoenteric feeding tubes are best suited for short-term use in patients who are likely to recover the ability to eat, or in patients with a very limited life expectancy. They are also useful in acutely ill patients while awaiting improvement in their condition before placing a PEG.

SUGGESTED READING

Clarkston WK, Smith OJ, Walden JM. Percutaneous endoscopic gastrostomy and early mortality. South Med J 1990; 83:1433–1436.
Di Sario JA, Foutch PG, Sanowski RA. Poor results with percutaneous endoscopic jejunostomy. Gastrointest Endosc 1990; 36:257–260.
Hogan RB, DeMarco DC, Hamilton JK, et al. Percutaneous endoscopic gastrostomy—to push or pull: a prospective randomized trial. Gastrointest Endosc 1986; 32:253–258.
Jain NK, Larson DE, Schroeder KW, et al. Antibiotic prophylaxis for percutaneous endoscopic gastrostomy: a prospective randomized, double-blind clinical trial. Ann Intern Med 1987; 107:824–828.
Park RH, Allison MC, Lang J, et al. Randomized comparison of percutaneous endoscopic gastrostomy and nasogastric tube feedings in patients with persisting neurological dysphagia. BMJ 1992; 304:1406–1409.
Ponsky JL, Gauderer MWL. Percutaneous endoscopic gastrostomy: a nonoperative technique for feeding gastrostomy. Gastrointest Endosc 1981; 27:9–11.

---

*Editor's Note: This seems to be an ideal topic for a demonstrated technology assessment to show that gastroenterologists are capable of utilizing cost-effective methods.

Russell TR, Brotman M, Norris F. Percutaneous endoscopic gastrostomy: a new, simplified and cost effective technique. Am J Surg 1984; 148:132–137.

Stiegmann GV, Goff JS, Silas D, et al. Endoscopic versus operative gastrostomy: final results of a prospective randomized trial. Gastrointest Endosc 1990; 36:1–5.

Taylor CA, Larson DE, Ballard DJ, et al. Predictors of outcome after percutaneous endoscopic gastrostomy: a community-based study. Mayo Clin Proc 1992; 67:1042–1049.

GASTRIC CANCER

MICHAEL G. SARR, M.D.*

Although gastric cancer is known to have decreased in incidence over the last five decades (a fourfold decrease), it still accounts for 20,000 to 25,000 new cases per year in the United States and 3,000 per year in Canada. Currently, it is one of the five most common gastrointestinal (GI) malignancies and the third most common cause of GI cancer-related death, accounting for 3 percent of all cancer deaths. Gastric neoplasms are predominantly adenocarcinomas (95 percent); the remaining 5 percent include leiomyosarcomas, lymphomas, and the more unusual carcinoids, carcinosarcomas, and squamous cell carcinomas. Because these latter lesions behave in a similar fashion to their counterparts elsewhere in the alimentary tract, this chapter focuses specifically on adenocarcinoma. Carcinoma of the cardia behaves more like distal esophageal cancer and is usually managed as such. The chapter *Cancer of the Esophagus* provides relevant information.

EPIDEMIOLOGY

The incidence of gastric cancer varies widely among different countries. In Japan, it is the most common malignancy (100 per 100,000) and accounts for more deaths than any other cancer. It is also particularly common in Chile, Columbia, Hawaii, Iceland, Finland, and adjoining parts of Russia. Because of the unique and disproportionate distribution of gastric cancer across these different cultures and diverse races, an environmental factor has been strongly suspected for several decades. The cause of the increased incidence in these countries is probably multifactorial, but one factor common to each of these countries is the high consumption of smoked fish and meat products that contain increased concentrations of 3,4-benzpyrene, a putative carcinogen. Moreover, in support of an environmental factor, the incidence of gastric cancer decreases in first- and second-generation Japanese who move to the United States. Whether the disease in these countries

represents a different entity from that in the countries where it is less common remains speculative. Some have suggested this concept because, for instance, the biologic behavior of gastric cancer in Japan appears to be somewhat less aggressive; survival data for gastric cancer from Japan are consistently far superior to any experience in American or European centers (see below).

In addition to the decreasing incidence in Western cultures, the anatomic distribution is changing as well. In the past, cancers of the distal stomach predominated, but in the last decade the anatomic location appears to be spread equally between the proximal, middle, and distal stomach. This represents a notable relative increase in cancer of the proximal stomach. The proximal lesions are four times more common in men than in women and appear to carry a worse prognosis.

ETIOPATHOGENESIS

Although the cause of gastric cancer remains elusive, a number of pathologic conditions have been associated with an increased incidence. These include diseases of the gastric mucosa (including atrophic gastritis, pernicious anemia, intestinal metaplasia, and Menetrier's disease), adenomatous gastric polyps, gastric ulcer, the postgastrectomy gastric remnant, lymphocytic gastritis, and the familial polyposis syndromes. A sequence for gastric carcinogenesis has been proposed involving a pathogenesis of primary mucosal injury. The initial, even nonspecific mucosal injury may come from aging or from repeated exposures to aspirin, alcohol, bile, autoimmune factors, or unknown mucosal irritants. Nutritional or undefined other genetic factors impair mucosal repair mechanisms and lead to changes of chronic atrophic gastritis, often with intestinal metaplasia. The associated hypochlorhydria permits the intraluminal bacterial proliferation so common in gastric cancer. Bacterial nitrate reductases convert ingested nitrates to nitrates and nitrosamines, well-appreciated mutagens in experimental models of carcinogenesis. Support for this concept comes from the association of gastric cancer and several forms of atrophic gastritis. Furthermore, one pathologic study found that the associated gastritis increased as the area of invasive malignancy was approached. Recent epidemiologic studies have suggested that infection with *Helicobacter pylori* is associated with an increased risk of certain histologic forms of gastric cancer.

Other disorders purportedly associated with gastric

cancer include adenomatous, but not hyperplastic, gastric polyps, especially so when the polyps are larger than 2 cm. Whether previous gastric surgery predisposes to gastric cancer in the remaining gastric remnant remains controversial; however, the subsequent risk of gastric cancer is not decreased after a previous gastric resection. The time interval to malignant transformation in this setting may be important because, if the risk is increased, it is increased only after 15 to 20 years. Thus, routine endoscopic surveillance screening does not appear to be justified except perhaps in selected patients such as the subgroup of patients with pernicious anemia or severe intestinal metaplasia-dysplasia who have undergone a previous partial gastrectomy, or in patients with adenomatous polyps. There is a separate chapter on premalignant gastric lesions.

Although often discussed, gastric cancer almost certainly does not arise in previously benign gastric ulcers. Malignant gastric ulcers are malignant from the onset. The fact that some of these ulcers "heal" temporarily with optimal medical management has only confounded this issue. "Benign" ulcers that rapidly recur or fail to heal in 6 to 12 weeks of treatment should prompt an aggressive interventional approach with repeated biopsy, cytologic studies, and strong consideration of surgical treatment.

CLINICAL PRESENTATION AND DIAGNOSIS

The clinical presentation of patients with cancer of the stomach can be variable, depending on the histopathologic type of lesion and the stage. Patients with early gastric cancer (disease confined to the mucosa and submucosa) may be asymptomatic and discovered only incidentally or, as in Japan, by mass screening programs. Those with more advanced disease may harbor vague nonspecific complaints of anorexia, fatigue, malaise, and unexplained weight loss. More specific GI symptoms include indigestion, dyspepsia, abdominal pain, or symptoms suggestive of peptic ulcer disease. More advanced lesions can include intraluminal bleeding with melena, hematochezia, or unexplained anemia. Symptoms of gastric outlet obstruction (vomiting or early satiety) are also not uncommon initial complaints, either secondary to mechanical obstruction from a distally located mass or from a nondistensible stomach infiltrated with gastric cancer (linitis plastica).

Diagnosis first requires clinical suspicion. In the past, the diagnosis was most often obtained by a barium meal study, but the sensitivity of this test is only about 75 to 80 percent. Use of an air-contrast technique may further increase the sensitivity. Currently, however, gastroscopy is the "gold standard" with an accuracy of about 85 percent. Use of 10 to 12 biopsies taken circumferentially from the inside edge of the ulcer combined with brush cytology should increase the sensitivity to nearly 100 percent, provided that clinical suspicion is high. Computed tomography (CT) is of little use in terms of diagnostic sensitivity; although CT scans

are obtained as part of the work-up, they have little to offer except possibly showing liver metastases or confirming the presence of ascites in patients with more advanced disease. The exact role of endoscopic ultrasonography has yet to be defined; it may be more useful for staging (depth of invasion, presence of perigastric enlarged lymph nodes). There is a separate chapter on ultrasonography in the diagnosis of upper GI tract cancer.

Gastric ulcers can present a formidable challenge and mandate biopsy and follow-up endoscopy, especially when sited away from the incisura (the most common location of benign gastric ulcers) or when associated with enlarged gastric folds. To maximize diagnostic accuracy, suspicion of malignancy should remain high, and multiple (10 to 12) biopsies should be obtained from the edge of the ulcer and combined with brush cytology. Probably all these patients should undergo repeat endoscopy 6 to 8 weeks later after a trial of medical therapy. Persistent ulcers require further aggressive evaluation and surgical consideration.

MANAGEMENT

No one would argue that gastric cancer is basically a surgical disease. Operative resection offers the only hope for cure. Unfortunately, the disease is rarely diagnosed in its early stages, and in most series only 10 to 20 percent of patients are diagnosed with disease confined to the stomach; locoregional lymph node metastases and extragastric spread are present in over 50 percent of patients at the time of diagnosis, while about 30 percent have distant metastases (peritoneal, liver, or distant lymph nodes). In patients with node-negative disease and carcinoma confined to the mucosa-submucosa, 5 year survival approaches 85 to 90 percent, but invasion of the muscularis and serosa decreases survival to 50 and 40 percent, respectively. Serosal penetration and positive lymph nodes portend a dismal prognosis (5 year survival less than 15 percent). Overall, only 10 to 20 percent of all patients with gastric cancer live 5 years. Obviously, many questions arise as to the appropriate surgical management of the individual patient with gastric cancer.

Preoperative Clinical Staging

An important aspect of initial management of the patient with gastric cancer is clinical staging. Appropriate preoperative evaluation will prevent an unnecessary, nontherapeutic abdominal exploration in up to 20 to 30 percent of all patients presenting with gastric cancer. Certain factors should preclude surgical intervention, because operative "palliation" offers no survival advantage, makes necessary the morbidity of a laparotomy, and provides no effective "palliation." These factors include a palpable rectal shelf (Blumer's shelf) indicative of extensive peritoneal disease, malignant ascites, palpable liver metastases, peripheral lymphadenopathy (supraclavicular nodes), or bony metastases. Possible exceptions include patients who cannot eat and thus maintain fluid and nutritional requirements by mouth, and those with significant intragastric blood loss causing symptomatic, refractory anemia (see Palliation).

Surgical Therapy

Currently, the appropriate operative approach to effect a truly "curative resection" is controversial. How extensive a gastrectomy should be performed? What is the role for formal, extended lymphadenectomy as championed by the extensive Japanese experience? How is operative palliation best provided?

Currently, most American and European surgeons perform a so-called "radical" subtotal gastrectomy (60 to 70 percent of the stomach) for cancers of the distal third of the stomach, a high subtotal resection (90 percent of the stomach) for cancers of the middle third, and a total gastrectomy for proximal tumors, large bulky midgastric lesions, multicentric tumors, or the infiltrative lesions (linitis plastica). These operations are designed to remove the involved part of the stomach with at least a 5 cm proximal gastric margin and a small (at least 1 cm) cuff of proximal duodenum (distal margin), each histologically confirmed by frozen section to be free of disease. The specimen includes the greater and lesser omenta and their associated perigastric nodes. Enteric continuity is restored by gastro- or esophagojejunostomy, depending on the proximal extent of gastric resection. No formal attempt is made to remove the more distant nodes unless they are palpable and easily removed. Extended radical lymphadenectomies have not gained acceptance because of presumed increased morbidity and mortality; a generally poor prognosis when nodal metastases are present; and the increasingly prevalent view (be it right or wrong), as championed with the model of breast cancer, that most malignancies are systemic diseases from the start, and that removal of lymph nodes is nontherapeutic and for staging purposes only.

Controversy has arisen through the many reports from Japan claiming markedly improved survival in patients with gastric cancer undergoing formal, extended lymphadenectomies. Their results have been almost unbelievable, with 5 year survivals of 30 to 50 percent with nodal metastases. These results are far superior to those from any series in Western countries, causing some to question whether gastric cancer in Japan represents a different disease with a less aggressive natural biology.

The ability to understand the Japanese approach requires a basic understanding of the sites of nodal spread favored by gastric cancer and the Japanese terminology of the "radicality" of resection. A detailed discussion of this approach is beyond the scope of this chapter, but briefly, the pertinent lymph nodes at risk for involvement by gastric cancer can be divided into four levels. N1 nodes include the level 1 nodes, i.e., the perigastric nodes along the greater and lesser curvatures of the stomach. N2 nodes are the level 2 nodes that accompany the named arteries to the stomach. N3 nodes (level 3) are one echelon distant (e.g., celiac, base of small bowel mesentery), while N4 nodes include level 4 nodes one further echelon distant (para-aortic). The extent of resection is described as R1, which includes a complete resection of N1 nodes, R2 the removal of all N2 nodes, R3, R4, and so forth. With this approach, Japanese surgeons routinely report 5 year survivals of 30 to 50 percent in patients with involved N1 and N2 nodes, and even extended survivals with more distant nodes resected by R3 procedures. Such an excellent survival rate is unheard of outside the Orient. Although two recent studies suggest a potential benefit of extended lymphadenectomy in selected subgroups of patients with gastric cancer, a dramatic improvement in survival has not been demonstrated convincingly, and most American surgeons have not embraced this approach.

Histopathologic Staging

What accounts for these dramatically different results between Japan and the Western world? In part, some differences can be explained by the different staging systems adopted by each group. In the United States, the clinicopathologic staging system used for gastric cancer is that proposed by the American Joint Committee on Cancer Staging System (Table 1). In contrast, the Japanese staging system is much more rigorous, precise, and scientific and is based on their detailed studies of the spread of gastric cancer in their extended resections. Their system not only emphasizes size and depth of gastric wall invasion and the anatomic level of nodal metastases, but also incorporates features of the primary tumor as described by Borrman and Lauren (Table 2), which also is predictive of survival. These differing staging systems make comparison of results difficult, if not impossible. Moreover, the less "radical" Western resections and the TNM system probably understage patients, since distant nodes are not removed and thus not examined histologically, while the Japanese approach examines all these nodes histologically and thus correctly and accurately stages patients.

What can we conclude from these differing clinical experiences? First, the routine radical subtotal resections are probably adequate for early gastric cancer. Second, extended lymphadenectomies (R2 resections) might benefit selected patients with serosa involvement (T3) and perigastric (N1) nodal metastases. Third, extensive lymphadenectomy has little to offer the patient with more distant locoregional nodal metastases (N3, N4 nodes).

Palliation

Advanced gastric cancer can cause several problems that require symptomatic palliation despite incurability. After all, palliation suggests the relief of symptoms *to improve the quality of life* but without hope or intent of cure. For instance, the most common indications for palliation include bleeding and obstruction. Some ulcer-

Table 1 American Joint Committee on Cancer Staging:
TNM Classification

Stages*			
Stage IA	T1	N0	M0
Stage IB	T1	N1	M0
	T2	N0	M0
Stage II	T1	N2	M0
	T2	N1	M0
	T3	N0	M0
Stage IIIA	T2	N1	M0
	T3	N1	M0
	T4	N0	M0
Stage IIIB	T3	N2	M0
	T4	N1	M0
Stage IV	T4	N2	M0
	Any T	Any N	M1

*Primary tumor (T)
  T1   Invasion of lamina propria or submucosa
  T2   Invasion of muscularis subserosa
  T3   Tumor penetrates serosa
  T4   Extragastric invasion of adjacent structures
Locoregional lymph nodes (N)
  N0   No lymph node metastases
  N1   Metastases in perigastric lymph nodes within 3 cm of primary tumor
  N2   Metastases in perigastric lymph nodes >3 cm from primary tumor, or in lymph nodes along left gastric, common hepatic, or splenic or celiac arteries
Distant metastases (M)
  M0   No distant metastases
  M1   Distant metastases (includes N3 and N4 nodal metastases)

Table 2 Gross and Histologic Classification
of Gastric Cancer

Borrman classification (gross)
  Type I: polypoid mass
  Type II: ulcerated
  Type III: ulcerated with limiting infiltrative characteristics
  Type IV: infiltrating tumor

Lauren classification (histologic)
  Intestinal form: moderately well differentiated
  Diffuse form: infiltrating, less well differentiated

ating gastric cancers can bleed acutely, requiring immediate intervention, or more commonly they cause a chronic blood loss resulting in symptomatic anemia; the latter may occasionally be amenable to endoscopic intervention using laser photocoagulation or even a course of low-dose radiotherapy. Gastric outlet obstruction, either mechanical from an obstructing antral or pyloric tumor or functional from an infiltrating adenocarcinoma restricting gastric distensibility and impeding gastric emptying, prevents the patient from maintaining nutrition or hydration by the oral route. In these patients, operative palliation is indicated. Objective palliation is best obtained by resection of the offending tumor whenever possible, especially for bleeding. Occasionally, resection is impossible owing to local invasion, in which case a proximal gastroenteric bypass can be constructed. Quite often, these palliative bypasses do not work well. A feeding jejunostomy tube allows for provision of fluid, electrolytes, and nutrition, but whether this is good palliation is debatable, especially in the already debilitated patient with extensive disease; this treatment may prolong survival somewhat, but at the cost of a very poor quality of life. Selected individuals with a good performance level and minimal malnourishment who are or will be candidates for chemotherapy might represent exceptions to this concept.

MOLECULAR BIOLOGY OF GASTRIC CANCER

Prediction of the natural biology of gastric cancer will be made possibly only by a better understanding of the molecular mechanisms of gastric carcinogenesis. Although this area remains in its infancy, important advances in our appreciation of the molecular biology of gastric cancer are being made. Specific genes conferring an inherited predisposition to gastric cancer or the genes most susceptible to mutation that directly initiate the malignant transformation have been sought, but not yet identified. Certain associations have, however, been described. In certain gastric cancers and areas of mucosal dysplasia, overexpression of the protein p21, as coded by the ras oncogenes, has been found. This protein may be important in several mechanisms of tissue growth and cell regulation, including signal transduction, differentiation, and cellular proliferation. Mutations in the p53 tumor suppressor gene, similar in concept to changes described in colon cancer, are common in gastric cancer; higher rates of p53 abnormality appear to correlate with stage of disease. Abnormalities in certain growth factors or their cell surface receptors have also been found in gastric cancer. Basic fibroblast growth factor 2, rearranged fibroblastic growth factor receptor gene, and the K-sam oncogene have been amplified in certain undifferentiated diffuse cancers yet not in well-differentiated forms. Although of no current clinical use, these and other as yet poorly understood abnormalities in nuclear and cell surface markers hold the key to an eventual understanding of the molecular basis of malignant transformation. Hopefully, a better understanding of the interaction of oncogenes, tumor suppressor genes, growth factors, and other molecular signaling systems may lead to more directed and effective methods of treatment and possibly prevention.

CHEMOTHERAPY

Although gastric cancer is reputedly one of the most responsive of GI malignancies, the impact of chemotherapy on survival in patients with disseminated gastric cancer remains marginal. Partial responses to single or multiple drug regimens have been reported in 20 to 50 percent of patients, but the responses have been short-lived (less than 6 months) and no study has yet been able to demonstrate convincingly that survival has been extended with a partial response. In contrast, survival can be extended with complete responses, but such a dramatic response occurs in (optimistically) less than 10 percent of patients. Nevertheless, as our understanding of the biology of gastric cancer and the effect of chemotherapy improves, new regimens or treatment designs (adjuvant, neoadjuvant) may prove rational and successful. Single- and multiple-agent regimens are discussed in the next chapter.

Design of future regimens will be built on the experience gained from the therapeutic trials discussed in the next chapter. For patients with primary intraperitoneal disease, some interest has been directed toward regional therapy with intraperitoneal treatment strategies. Either drugs alone or drugs bound to activated carbon particles have had promising results, but further evaluation is necessary.

As with breast cancer and colon cancer, interest has been generated in the potential role of chemotherapy after curative resections for adenocarcinoma of the stomach. Combination of 5-fluorouracil and leucovorin or mitomycin C have been proposed (with or without concomitant radiation therapy—see below), and while the results are promising, the data are not immediately convincing.

Neoadjuvant chemotherapy is a logical extension of the current therapeutic approaches used in breast, colon, and pancreatic adenocarcinomas. The following rationale can be proposed: (1) surgery alone is inadequate in most patients, (2) gastric cancer appears to be susceptible to chemotherapy, (3) preoperative metastatic disease is largely microscopic, (4) the agent can be delivered to the neoplasm preoperatively before the blood supply has been disrupted, and (5) in general, the patient's performance status is best before surgical intervention. Preliminary studies with FAM and EAP

suggest some benefit, but long-term follow-up is necessary. Details are presented in the next chapter.

In summary, the chemotherapeutic approach to advanced gastric cancer continues to evolve with the introduction of new, unique strategies. However, no regimens have produced sufficiently convincing, objective results for any one approach to be considered as routine therapy. Further evaluations of these new approaches should be made in controlled studies with objective end points.

RADIOTHERAPY

Radiation therapy has been used fairly extensively in a postoperative therapeutic setting, but without convincing data demonstrating objective benefit for survival and quality of life. Currently, the only potentially justifiable role of radiation therapy in unresectable or recurrent gastric cancer is as a directed, palliative approach to specific problems related to the tumor. Details of radiation therapy and intraoperative radiation are given in the next chapter.

SUGGESTED READING

Akoh JA, McIntyre IMC. Improving survival in gastric cancer: review of 5-year survival rates in English language publications from 1970. Br J Surg 1992; 79:293–299.

Anderson RF Jr, Chin JL, Au K-S, Simmons J. Radiation therapy for gastric carcinoma. Cancer Treat Res 1991; 55:247–264.

Behrns KE, Dalton RR, van Heerden JA, Sarr MG. Extended lymph node dissection for gastric cancer. Is it of value? Surg Clin North Am 1992; 72:433–443.

MacDonald JS. Gastric cancer: chemotherapy of advanced disease. Hematol Oncol 1992; 10:37–42.

Thompson GB, van Heerden JA, Sarr MG. Adenocarcinoma of the stomach: are we making progress? Lancet 1993; 342:713–718.

Wright PA, Williams GT. Molecular biology and gastric carcinoma. Gut 1993; 34:145–147.

GASTRIC CANCER: NONSURGICAL MANAGEMENT*

JEFFREY S. FEIN, M.D.
ROBERT C. KURTZ, M.D.

At present, surgery is the only treatment with curative potential for gastric cancer. However, most patients in the United States present with advanced, incurable disease. Even among the subgroup of 30 to 40 percent of patients who undergo potentially curative resection, cancer recurrence is common. For all patients with newly diagnosed gastric cancer, 5 year survival is only 5 to 15 percent. As survival is closely matched with stage at presentation (Fig. 1), it is clear that effective forms of treatment in conjunction with surgery are needed.

TREATMENT PLANNING

Once the diagnosis of gastric cancer is made, the initial evaluation of patients includes a physical examination, with particular attention to sites of possible nodal metastases, such as the supraclavicular areas. Liver function tests may give a clue to the spread of disease to the liver. Chest radiography allows for assessment of possible pulmonary metastases. Computed tomography (CT) of the abdomen is an accurate technique for detecting ascites and metastases to the liver and other intra-abdominal organs. Sites of possible metastatic disease should be biopsied. Focal defects in the liver can

---

*Editor's Note: There is some overlap of coverage with the previous chapter, and portions of this chapter have been incorporated there.

be biopsied either by laparoscopy or with CT or ultrasound guidance.

In addition to detecting distant metastases, adequate treatment planning also requires careful staging of local disease. Accumulating data indicate that evaluation by endoscopic ultrasonography (EUS) is more accurate than CT in assessing the depth of primary tumor invasion into the gastric wall (T) and in determining cancer spread to regional lymph nodes (N). However, because of its limited depth of penetration, EUS cannot replace CT for the detection of distant metastases, such as those to the liver.

TREATMENT OPTIONS

Surgery

After staging, patients with localized gastric cancer are candidates for curative surgery, even if there is evidence of regional nodal disease. However, given the grim survival statistics for most patients, effective neoadjuvant and adjuvant therapy for patients with potentially curable disease must be a consideration. Palliative surgical procedures may be important therapeutic options for patients with advanced disease. These aspects are discussed in detail in the preceding chapter.

Chemotherapy

Adjuvant Chemotherapy

To establish appropriate strategies for adjuvant therapy, one must understand the patterns of recurrence in gastric cancer. Most patients develop either local regional recurrence in the gastric bed and surrounding lymph nodes, or relapse within the peritoneal cavity. Distant metastases to areas such as liver, lung, and bone, although common, rarely occur in the absence of concomitant local regional recurrence. Overall tumor stage as determined by the TNM classification (please see Table 1 in the preceding chapter) represents an

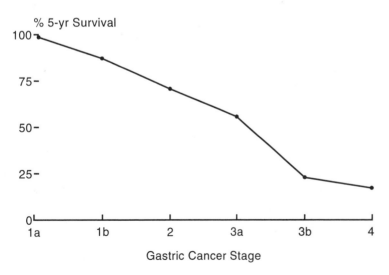

Figure 1 Gastric cancer stage at presentation correlated with 5 year survival. (Data from Jpn J Clin Oncol 1984; 14:385.)

important tool in planning adjuvant therapy. The combination of increasing T and N stages portends a poor prognosis. Advanced-stage patients (T3–4, Nany, and M0) relapse frequently, despite undergoing potentially curative surgery.

A number of chemotherapeutic agents, including mitomycin C, fluorouracil (5-FU), doxorubicin, and cisplatin have been used in adjuvant clinical trials after the surgical removal of all obvious disease. In general, single-agent chemotherapy has yielded low response rates (less than 30 percent), short durations of response (4 to 5 months), and rare complete responses.

The identification of modestly active single agents has led to the development of multidrug regimens, most of which have included 5-FU as a component. Unfortunately, Western trials of adjuvant combination chemotherapy have failed to demonstrate a reproducible survival benefit for patients treated with chemotherapy as compared with untreated controls. In a randomized prospective trial, the Gastrointestinal Tumor Study Group (GITSG) investigated the benefit of adjuvant chemotherapy using 5-FU plus methyllomustine given postoperatively for 18 months compared with no postoperative therapy. A survival advantage was noted in the group that received adjuvant therapy. However, two similar trials failed to confirm the positive results of the GITSG study. A large multi-institutional trial of 5-FU, doxorubicin, and mitomycin C (FAM) also showed no benefit.

Currently, there is no standard proven adjuvant chemotherapy regimen for patients with locally advanced disease that is resected for cure. Patients with early-stage tumors (T1–2, N0, M0), although infrequently seen in the United States (less than 10 percent), have a relatively good chance of long-term survival with surgery alone and should not receive adjuvant therapy. Patients with locally advanced disease should receive adjuvant treatment only in the context of clinical trials.

Neoadjuvant Chemotherapy

Theoretical considerations for neoadjuvant (or primary) chemotherapy in patients with locally advanced but potentially surgically curable gastric cancer are twofold. First, patients with resectable disease might have a greater cure rate after responding to chemotherapy. Second, patients with initially unresectable disease might meet criteria for resectability after downstaging by chemotherapy. At present, the role of neoadjuvant therapy is unproved and remains investigational.

At Memorial Sloan-Kettering Cancer Center, patients with locally advanced gastric cancer (T3–4, Nany, and M0) are offered enrollment in a study to evaluate neoadjuvant FAMTX (5-FU, doxorubicin, methotrexate) chemotherapy, surgery, and postoperative intraperitoneal 5-FU and cisplatin along with systemic 5-FU. The rationale for the use of both systemic and regional therapy is based on the pattern of both intra-abdominal

and distant recurrences seen with gastric cancer. EUS is used for T and N staging, and CT is used to detect distant metastases. Preliminary data in 23 patients suggest that the regimen is reasonably well tolerated and does not increase operative morbidity or mortality. While there have been no operative deaths, two patients have died from chemotherapy-related sepsis. Fifty-six percent of patients underwent curative surgical resection after the neoadjuvant treatment and had negative margins. Resectability rates seem encouraging, but it is much too early to assess the impact of this program on overall survival.

Palliative Chemotherapy

Metastatic gastric cancer remains an incurable disease. The chemotherapeutic standard is single-agent 5-FU, although both duration of response and length of survival are short. Combination chemotherapy regimens have been extensively studied. Regimens that have been shown to have activity include FAM, EAP (etoposide, doxorubicin, cisplatin), and FAMTX. A prospective randomized trial comparing FAM with single-agent 5-FU failed to show a survival advantage for the combination treatment program. In addition, significantly greater toxicity was observed in the patients receiving FAM. More recently, in a randomized trial comparing FAMTX with EAP in patients with unresectable disease, FAMTX was shown to be equally as effective as EAP but significantly less toxic. The major toxicity of EAP was myelosuppression. A randomized, controlled clinical trial comparing FAMTX with single-agent 5-FU has not yet been undertaken.

Radiation Therapy

Adjuvant Radiation Therapy

Gastric cancer is known to be a somewhat radiosensitive tumor. However, radiation therapy alone is not a viable form of treatment because tumor bulk and the low radiation tolerance of the normal adjacent stomach and bowel generally preclude effective tumor control. Owing to the large proportion of patients in whom gastric cancer recurs either locally or intraperitonealy, the potential role of adjuvant radiation therapy has been evaluated. In many of the studies, external beam radiation therapy has been combined with systemic chemotherapy, usually 5-FU. In a randomized trial of 62 patients with locally advanced but resectable disease, Moertel and associates were unable to establish 5-FU and radiation therapy as effective adjuvant therapy. In a nonrandomized study of only 25 patients, Gez demonstrated a median survival of 33 months and a projected 5 year survival of 40 percent in patients who received adjuvant 5-FU and radiation therapy. Another use for radiation therapy is the palliation of gastric cancer complications and symptoms, such as local tumor bleeding and bone pain in advanced metastatic disease.

Intraoperative Radiation Therapy

Intraoperative radiation therapy (IORT) has been studied primarily in Japan. It is less commonly available and is almost exclusively investigational in the United States. The rationale for adjuvant IORT is based on the goal of eradicating residual nests of tumor cells, usually found in regional lymph nodes. The technique permits the retraction of dose-limiting organs from the radiation port. Abe and Shibamoto in Japan prospectively compared tumor bed IORT after both curative and palliative surgical resections with surgery alone in over 200 patients. The most impressive survival difference was in patients with stage IV disease, those with direct extension into an adjacent organ. In 27 patients a 19.5 percent 5 year survival rate was noted. There were no 5 year survivors in the stage IV group treated with surgery alone. IORT may hold future promise.

Endoscopic Therapy

Endoscopic Strip Biopsy for Early Gastric Cancer

In the mid-1980s, Karita and associates in Japan pioneered a new endoscopic technique called "strip biopsy" for the treatment of well-differentiated early gastric cancer confined to the mucosa. The initial report described the technique for lesions up to 2 cm in size, although more recently it has been used to treat early cancers up to 5 cm. The rationale behind strip biopsy is that well-differentiated mucosal tumors are unlikely to have lymph node metastases. Therefore, cure is potentially attainable without the need for surgical intervention and gastrectomy.

The strip biopsy technique requires endoscopic injection of saline under the tumor, producing the appearance of a submucosal mass. With the edge of the mass lifted by a grasping forceps, a snare is placed around the elevated tissue, which includes the cancer. The tumor is then removed by electrocautery. If the mass is too large to be removed in one piece, multiple partial resections using the strip biopsy technique can be performed during the same endoscopic procedure.

In 1992, Karita and Tada reported the results of strip biopsy resection in 12 patients with well-differentiated gastric cancer confined to the mucosa. The technique was successful in producing complete resection in the ten patients with lesions ranging from 2.5 to 5 cm in size, but was unsuccessful in two patients, both with lesions larger than 5 cm. All lesions in this series required multiple partial resections to achieve complete tumor removal. In the successfully treated cases, the depth of invasion was confined to the mucosa based on histologic examination of the resected specimens. EUS may play a role in identifying those few patients in the United States with early gastric cancers amenable to strip biopsy.*

*Editor's Note: The reader is referred to the article by Karita and Tada for more details on this potentially important technique. Efforts to include a complete chapter in this edition were unsuccessful.

Palliative Endoscopic Therapy

Laser. As an alternative to surgical resection or bypass for palliation, endoscopic laser therapy can offer relief of obstruction due to gastric cancer. Encouraging results have been reported, particularly when the obstructing lesion is short, as in the cardia or prepyloric region. The neodymium:yttrium-aluminum-garnet (Nd: YAG) laser is most often used. Fleischer and Sivak treated 15 patients with obstructing lesions of the gastric cardia who had a mean tumor length of 6.3 cm and narrowest lumen diameter of 3.3 mm. After an average of 2.8 treatments over 6 days, the mean diameter of the lumen increased to 12.1 mm. Improved food intake was noted in all patients and there were no major complications from the therapy. Laser photocoagulation may also play a role in treating patients with diffuse bleeding from bulky tumors.

The usefulness of laser therapy and its precise role in the palliative management of gastric cancer await further study in a large number of patients. There is no doubt that certain subsets of patients, particularly those who are poor risks for palliative surgery, will benefit from this treatment.

Percutaneous Endoscopic Gastrostomy. Whatever the treatment plan, maintenance of adequate nutrition is important for success. Since its original description by Ponsky and Gauderer in 1981, percutaneous endoscopic gastrostomy (PEG) has become a routine procedure, performed in an outpatient setting without general anesthesia, in patients unable to take oral feedings and in whom parenteral nutritional support is not feasible. PEG and percutaneous endoscopic jejunostomy (PEJ) placement are rapid and safe and can eliminate the need for long-term nasal feeding tubes. Although the original use of PEG was in neurologically impaired adults and children, the potential of this procedure for cancer patients was quickly realized. In one study of 42 patients with dysphagia and cancers of the head and neck, successful placement of PEG and PEJ occurred in 39. No immediate complications occurred. After a mean follow-up of 4.5 months, only one patient developed pneumonia presumed to be due to aspiration. Complication rates for surgical gastrostomies are reported to be as high as 75 percent.

In patients who have had previous total or subtotal gastric resections, PEJ may be used. Shike and colleagues demonstrated an 83 percent success rate with PEJ. PEJ allowed infusions of significant amounts of fluids and between 900 and 2400 calories per day. There is a separate chapter with details of these endoscopic techniques.

COMMENTS

Gastric cancer management now includes combinations of surgery, chemotherapy, radiotherapy, and endoscopic therapy. Improved patient survival will depend on future close collaboration between investigators in these fields; it remains the major goal of gastric cancer management, but results other than in early-stage disease have been disappointing. Therefore, quality of life issues should be an important component of any treatment plan. Intensive adjuvant or neoadjuvant chemotherapy or radiotherapy programs belong only in well-designed clinical trials.

SUGGESTED READING

Abe M, Shibamoto Y. Radiotherapy in carcinoma of the stomach and pancreas. World J Surg 1987; 11:459–464.

Ajani JA, Ota DM. Current strategies in the management of locoregional and metastatic gastric cancer. Cancer 1991; 67:260–265.

Botet JF, Lightdale CJ. Preoperative staging of gastric cancer. Comparison of endoscopic ultrasound and dynamic CT. Radiology 1991; 181:426–432.

Karita M, Tada M. The successive strip biopsy partial resection technique for large early gastric and colon cancer. Gastrointest Endosc 1992; 38:174–178.

Kelson D. Adjuvant therapy of upper gastrointestinal tract cancers. Sem Oncology 1991; 18:543–559.

Kurtz RC, Sherlock P. The diagnosis of gastric cancer. Semin Oncol 1985; 12:11–18.

Parsonnett J, Friedman GD. *Helicobacter pylori* infection and the risk of gastric cancer. N Engl J Med 1991; 325:1127–1131.

PREMALIGNANT CONDITIONS OF THE STOMACH

JUAN LECHAGO, M.D., Ph.D.

Primary malignancies of the stomach consist largely of adenocarcinomas, carcinoid tumors, lymphomas, and malignant stromal tumors. Some of these lesions appear de novo, without a detectable precursor lesion, whereas others are heralded by conditions amenable to early detection and often curable with timely and appropriate treatment. Such conditions can be categorized, either as lesions associated with an increased risk of cancer development or as precursor lesions directly related to cancer formation. The latter sometimes evolve into early cancer, making it very difficult to ascertain the true biologic nature of the lesion, e.g., dysplastic versus neoplastic. In this chapter, I discuss the precursor lesions for gastric adenocarcinoma, carcinoid tumor, and lymphoma.

Adenocarcinoma is the most common tumor of the stomach and a common malignancy in many parts of the world. However, the overall incidence of gastric adenocarcinoma has declined to variable degrees worldwide, and to a very significant extent during the last 50 years in the United States. Current prevalence rates in this country are below eight cases per 100,000 population; in 1990, the estimated number of new cases was 23,000, and the death rate was 5 percent in females and 8.5 percent in males. Unfortunately, most such tumors are detected clinically at an advanced stage, and the 5 year survival rate of surgically treated lesions, currently estimated at 10 percent, is essentially the same as it was several decades ago. Although several classifications have been proposed for adenocarcinoma of the stomach, one that has retained a good deal of popularity is that of Lauren, which divided such tumors into a diffuse (33 percent) and an intestinal (53 percent) pattern, the remaining 14 percent being unclassifiable. Whereas diffuse adenocar-

cinomas generally do not recognize a precursor lesion and appear de novo, the intestinal type has been associated with a number of precursor conditions, including chronic multifocal atrophic gastritis associated with intestinal metaplasia and gastric dysplasia, gastric polyps, postgastrectomy gastric remnant, and, arguably, Ménétrier's disease. In contrast, chronic gastric ulcer, once it is proved benign, is no longer regarded as a significant premalignant condition. The general decline of gastric cancer, particularly in the United States, has been almost exclusively at the expense of the intestinal type, whereas the diffuse and the cardial varieties have gained in relative incidence. It is believed that this decline in intestinal type of gastric adenocarcinoma is the result of a similar decline in some of these precursor conditions, notably chronic atrophic gastritis.

Another significant development in this area is characterization of the early gastric cancer, first described by Japanese workers. This entity is defined as the presence of adenocarcinoma confined to mucosa and submucosa, regardless of whether or not there is metastatic involvement of the regional lymph nodes. When diagnosed and treated at this early stage, these carcinomas have a 90 to 95 percent 5 year survival rate. Even though the frequency of early gastric cancer is relatively low in the United States, increasing awareness of its existence and of the radiologic and endoscopic parameters leading to its recognition has resulted in their representing 13 to 27 percent of all gastric cancers being diagnosed.

Gastric carcinoid tumors are relatively infrequent lesions accounting for approximately 0.3 percent of all gastric tumors and 3 percent of gastrointestinal carcinoids in some series. These lesions have been further classified as sporadic, with a relatively high malignant potential, and secondary to hypergastrinemic states such as autoimmune (type A) chronic atrophic gastritis associated with pernicious anemia, or with the Zollinger-Ellison syndrome only when it is part of the MEN I syndrome. This second type of gastric carcinoid evolves from enterochromaffin-like (ECL)-cell hyperplasia, dysplasia, and microcarcinoid formation and appears to have an indolent course. The premalignant potential of long-term treatment with proton-pump inhibitors will also be discussed. This last issue is also discussed in the chapter on Zollinger-Ellison syndrome.

Lymphomas constitute approximately 3 percent of all gastric neoplasias, an intriguing statistic considering that the normal gastric mucosa does not contain a lymphoid population comparable with that seen in the small and the large intestine, generally referred to as gut-associated lymphoid tissue (GALT), or mucosa-associated lymphoid tissue (MALT). Most gastric lymphomas present as high-grade, large cell immunoblastic lymphomas, whereas others present as low-grade, small lymphocytic, well-differentiated B-cell lymphomas, categorized as MALTomas by Isaacson and coworkers. Whereas most of the latter tend to be low grade and indolent in nature, some would appear to evolve in later stages into a high-grade type. It has been proposed that such MALTomas arise from the lymphoid follicles that appear in chronic nonatrophic gastritis, often associated with peptic ulcer disease and with *Helicobacter pylori* infection. An interesting entity, sometimes referred to as pseudolymphoma, is currently under scrutiny. Some regard it as merely a benign nodular lymphoid proliferation, often associated with mucosal ulceration, but others believe it to be an early or noninvasive stage of MALToma. Indeed, numerous examples of lymphoma have been reported, seemingly arising from a pseudolymphoma. Whether or not this entity represents an early malignancy, a consensus is progressively emerging in that the term pseudolymphoma lends itself to confusion and should probably be discarded.

METHODS OF CLINICAL EVALUATION

The desirable common denominator of the methods used to evaluate the premalignant conditions of the stomach is that they be able to detect the conditions either before they become invasive or when they are still amenable to successful surgical treatment. Such techniques must possess the ability to identify and characterize subtle changes and to discriminate between lesions with an ambiguous appearance.

Imaging Studies

Radiography of the stomach, including double-contrast studies, is capable of detecting masses, which may be benign or malignant; ulcerations, also benign or malignant; and irregularities of the mucosal surface suggestive of an underlying proliferative process involving the mucosa or submucosa. The value of this approach is largely to call attention to lesions that must then be studied by other means for an ultimate answer. Although radiologic discovery of fungating masses or of large ulcers with deep craters and raised edges strongly points to a possible malignancy, current standards of practice demand that such lesions be further

visualized endoscopically and evaluated by biopsy and/or cytologic studies to establish their precise nature.

Endoscopy, Endoscopic Biopsy, and Cytology

The availability of modern flexible gastroduodenoscopes has provided an enormous boost to the diagnostic capabilities of gastroenterologists. Because these instruments retroflex, they permit a thorough exploration of the stomach. An additional method, little used in Western countries but popular in Japan, involves the application of intravital dyes such as toluidine blue or Congo red to the gastric mucosa. Normal and metaplastic mucosa take up the dye readily, but foci of severe dysplasia and early carcinoma do not and thus stand as gray-white areas next to the colored mucosa. This affords an opportunity to search the mucosa for lesions perhaps too subtle to be detected by routine endoscopic inspection.

It is essential that endoscopist and pathologist function as a team when a biopsy is obtained in order to provide maximal benefit to the patient. The pathologist depends on the endoscopist to (1) obtain the appropriate samples based on his or her observation; (2) handle, label, and deliver the delicate tissue samples adequately and in a timely fashion; and (3) provide the pertinent information regarding the patient and the nature and location of the biopsy samples.

The ideal number of biopsy samples procured during endoscopy varies with the type of lesion. If an ulcer is being investigated, samples must be obtained from the bed, four quadrants of the edges, and the surrounding mucosa. If it is an exophytic lesion, this must be sampled thoroughly from the top, the base or pedicle, and the surrounding mucosa to rule out in situ malignancy. In the case of possible dysplasia or endocrine cell hyperplasia and dysplasia, it is important to take generous samples of antrum, corpus, and fundus, paying special attention to the lesser curvature mucosa and to other features such as areas of granularity, thickening of the mucosal folds, and discoloration. Advanced carcinoma of the stomach is relatively easy to see and sample, but subtler early lesions, including early carcinoma, may require a minimum of eight biopsy samples for 95 to 99 percent rate of positive results.

Endoscopically directed brush cytology is also an important diagnostic tool in the detection of malignant and premalignant lesions of the gastric mucosa. This approach alone provides a positivity rate of 80 to 85 percent of cases of gastric carcinoma. When applied in conjunction with biopsy sampling, it not only yields a positive result in virtually all cases, but also reduces the number of directed biopsies necessary to attain such a result. Another cytologic approach used to explore submucosal biopsies not accessible to brush cytology involves the use of needle aspiration carried with a sclerotherapy cannula passed through the therapeutic port of the endoscope.

EVALUATION AND MANAGEMENT

Chronic Multifocal Atrophic Gastritis, Intestinal Metaplasia, and Dysplasia

Chronic multifocal atrophic gastritis (MAG) is a variant of chronic atrophic gastritis that is relatively infrequent in the United States but very common in areas of the world with a high incidence of gastric cancer such as Japan, China, Colombia, Peru, Chile, Costa Rica, and probably some Scandinavian countries. However, this entity is found in the United States, usually in individuals from disadvantaged socioeconomic strata. It is important that it be diagnosed early, since it carries a definite potential for malignant transformation. The etiology, pathogenesis, and pathology of MAG are discussed in the chapter on gastritis classification under the name of environmental (type B) metaplastic atrophic gastritis. In advanced stages of MAG, foci of type III intestinal metaplasia, also called incomplete or colonic, appear and are characterized by significant amounts of sulfated mucins and of cellular atypia. This type of metaplasia is a statistically significant marker for the development of gastric adenocarcinoma and probably represents a precursor lesion for such malignancy. A further step in the malignant progression of MAG is the appearance of gastric epithelial dysplasia (GED), an incompletely defined change that represents a common denominator with other conditions such as adenomas, gastric remnants, and, rarely, Ménétrier's disease. Mild GED appears to be a relatively banal lesion, and a regression rate of 66 percent has been reported. Severe GED, by contrast, rarely regresses, and progression to carcinoma has been shown to be 75 percent during an 18 month follow-up period.

No medical therapy is available for the intestinal metaplasia and GED associated with MAG. Whereas eradication of *H. pylori* may lead to a marked improvement of the mucosal histologic picture in early cases of MAG and in mild GED, it is improbable that such an approach would substantially change the biologic behavior of severe GED, a lesion probably committed to a malignant evolution. Surveillance of patients with well-established MAG by yearly endoscopy and biopsy is carried out on a cost-effective basis in Japan, where the incidence of this type of gastritis is very high. In the United States, such widespread surveillance is not regarded as time or cost effective because of its low frequency. This underscores the importance of recognizing and properly diagnosing MAG in these relatively uncommon patients; surveillance of this smaller subset of individuals not only becomes cost effective but should result in an improvement in their currently dismal mortality rate when malignant transformation occurs.

Subtotal gastrectomy is indicated for patients with early gastric carcinoma, a multifocal lesion that recognizes a "field effect" biologic behavior. Some also advocate surgical intervention for cases of long-standing severe GED, regarding this condition as part of a continuous spectrum with early gastric carcinoma. How

long one should wait, or how severe GED has to be before surgery is recommended, is unfortunately not settled, depending largely on a subjective threshold that varies with each individual.

Gastric Mucosal Polyps

Gastric mucosal polyps are diagnosed endoscopically in approximately 4 to 5 percent of symptomatic patients. They have a comparable sex distribution and their incidence increases with advancing age, being found in more than 7 percent of patients over 80 years of age. Gastric mucosal polyps can be classified as fundic gland polyps, hyperplastic (regenerative) polyps, or adenomas. Heterotopic pancreas and related hamartomas, carcinoid tumors, and adenocarcinomas may also present as polypoid lesions. The variety of lesions mentioned above indicates that when a gastric polyp is visualized endoscopically it should be removed if small enough, or thoroughly biopsied if too large for complete excision. Microscopic examination will reveal the nature of the lesion and dictate the subsequent therapeutic choice.

Fundic Gland Polyps

Fundic gland polyps, originally described in the stomach of patients with familial polyposis, have later been seen in individuals who have gastritis, who have a gastroenteric anastomosis, or who are treated with proton-pump inhibitors, or in seemingly normal stomachs. These lesions tend to be small (1 to 5 mm in diameter), often multiple, sessile, smooth nodules localized in the proximal gastric mucosa. Generally regarded as malformations, these polyps are composed of normal-appearing oxyntic mucosa exhibiting a normal or shortened foveolar compartment and the presence of small cystic dilatations in the upper portion of individual glands. Although their natural history is unclear, there is no evidence that these lesions possess a malignant potential.

Hyperplastic Polyps

Hyperplastic polyps, by contrast, are more frequently seen in the antrum, in the same way as most adenomas. These lesions are also small (0.5 to 2 cm in diameter), sessile or pedunculated, and often multiple. They are formed by reactive mucinous foveolar-type epithelium, sometimes presenting cystic dilatations, and accompanied by variable degrees of stromal inflammation and even fibrosis. These polyps, by far the most common among such lesions in the stomach, are rarely the origin of a malignancy.

Adenomas

Adenomas are lesions of variable size, ranging from 0.5 cm to 5 cm in diameter when left untreated, composed of proliferating glandular structures that exhibit variable degrees of atypia. The malignant potential of these lesions has been reported to range between 10 and 75 percent, depending largely on the size of the lesions being studied in individual series. With the advent of flexible endoscopy, many adenomas are currently diagnosed when they are 2 cm or less in diameter, and most are therefore benign. Conversely, cancers tend to occur in adenomas measuring 2 cm or more in diameter; such lesions must therefore be either removed on discovery or, failing this, very thoroughly sampled to rule out malignant transformation. Ultimately, unless there is an overriding medical contraindication, all adenomatous lesions of the stomach should be removed, either endoscopically if small enough, or surgically if too large. After resection, a 6.1 percent local recurrence rate has been recorded within 1 year of the original polypectomy. The appearance of new polyps, sometimes hyperplastic and often adenomatous, has been noted in as many as one-third of cases, and malignancy has been encountered in 3.4 percent of patients with gastric adenomas. These figures indicate that endoscopic surveillance in patients after polypectomy for adenoma has a well-defined value.

Postgastrectomy Gastric Remnant

Many studies have shown that adenocarcinomas appear in the gastric remnant after partial gastrectomy. However, it is far less clear whether the incidence of such neoplasias is higher than that in an unoperated comparable population. This may become a moot point in the future, since modern treatment of peptic ulcer disease with H_2 blockers and proton-pump inhibitors has drastically reduced the need for surgical intervention, and particularly for antrectomy. It is important to distinguish between gastrectomy carried out for early gastric cancer, in which recurrence usually takes place within 5 years, and that done for benign peptic ulcer, with a 15 to 25 year lag period. Therefore, for a cancer to be considered as arising de novo in a gastric remnant, it must be diagnosed 5 years or more after gastrectomy to rule out the possibility that the malignancy was already present at a very early stage at the time of surgery. Although statistics as to the true prevalence of adenocarcinoma in gastric remnants are disparate, it is accepted that the highest degree of risk is present in patients in whom surgery takes place at or before the age of 40 and who have been operated on for at least 15 to 20 years. Surveillance of this subset of patients with endoscopy and multiple biopsy may uncover the true incidence of gastric remnant cancer, providing an early diagnosis necessary for a better survival rate after surgical treatment.

Ménétrier's Hypertrophic Gastropathy

Ménétrier's disease is an uncommon condition consisting of generalized hyperplasia of foveolar and surface mucous gastric cells, leading to hypertrophy of the rugal folds mostly in the proximal stomach, and associated with hypochlorhydria and protein-losing enteropathy. Although quite a few isolated reports have appeared claiming that this condition is associated with the development of gastric adenocarcinoma, many of the reports are not well documented enough to firmly establish such association. To further compound matters, many cases of Ménétrier's disease are treated with partial gastrectomy because of the severe clinical manifestations, thus truncating the natural evolution of the lesion and precluding prospective studies. However, there are a few well-documented instances in which adenoma, severe gastric dysplasia, or carcinoma have developed during a prolonged follow-up of Ménétrier's disease.

Surgical removal of the diseased portion of the stomach is carried out to alleviate the severity of the weight loss and the hypoalbuminemia. Although the rationale behind it is not readily apparent, treatment with H_2 blockers such as cimetidine and ranitidine has proved reasonably effective in increasing body weight, normalizing serum albumin levels, and improving the patient's subjective well-being. Recently, omeprazole treatment has been claimed effective in cases in which H_2 blockers had been of little help. With improving medical management of Ménétrier's disease, it may be appropriate to survey such patients by yearly endoscopy and biopsy of suspicious lesions such as nodules, erosions, and ulcerations.

Chronic Atrophic Corporal Gastritis and Pernicious Anemia

This entity, also known as autoimmune or type A gastritis, is seen almost exclusively in association with pernicious anemia. Again, the reader is referred to the chapter on classification of gastritis for a discussion of the etiology, pathogenesis, and pathology of this entity. In patients with pernicious anemia, hyperplasia of the argyrophil ECL-cells may evolve into dysplasia and, in some cases, results in the appearance of carcinoid tumors of the stomach. Although as a rule these tumors exhibit an indolent course, they are capable of invading and metastasizing to both regional lymph nodes and the liver. In younger patients presenting a reasonable surgical risk, these tumors have been removed through partial or segmental gastrectomy. A difficult problem is posed by the fact that these neoplasms occur on a background of ECL-cell hyperplasia, and therefore more recurrences may be noted with time, raising the unpleasant possibility of further segmental gastrectomies. Conversely, a "curative" total or subtotal gastrectomy is associated with significant morbidity and even death and may not be an attractive or sensible alternative in many instances.

Antrectomy, an operation that by removing the main source of gastrin withdraws its potentially carcinogenic influence upon the ECL-cells, has been tried with some measure of success. After antrectomy, it has been seen that the numbers of ECL cells in patients with pernicious anemia are dramatically lowered, with regression of the hyperplasia and even of small lesions categorized as carcinoid tumors. On the strength of these findings, some workers recommend antrectomy in patients with significant ECL-cell hyperplasia and dysplasia, or at the time of segmental gastrectomy for the removal of an invasive carcinoid tumor. However, a thoughtful evaluation of the risk-benefit ratio of such intervention should be carried out for each individual patient, taking into account the morbidity and mortality rates of the procedure against the slow progression and the rarity of fatal outcome that characterize this type of gastric carcinoid.*

Early Scandinavian and American literature revealed an increased incidence of gastric adenocarcinoma in patients with pernicious anemia. However, a more recent Mayo Clinic epidemiologic study failed to find such increased incidence, and current Scandinavian studies note a declining rate of such malignancy. Careful analysis of this apparent discrepancy reveals that some early reports contained many patients in whom pernicious anemia was diagnosed shortly before or concurrently with the cancer, thus raising doubts about their being true cases of pernicious anemia. Moreover, such reports often described a mixture of fundic low-malignancy adenocarcinomas, typical of pernicious anemia, and antral high-malignancy lesions identical to those seen in environmental gastritis, as discussed above. It is probable, therefore, that many Scandinavian pernicious anemia patients may have had MAG secondary to exposure to *H. pylori* and other environmental factors, whereas the patients studied in the Mayo Clinic report did not appear to have such a type of gastritis. It can be concluded that pernicious anemia patients with autoimmune gastritis alone do not appear to have a significantly increased risk of gastric adenocarcinoma. A diminishing number of such patients may also have environmental gastritis, the latter being associated with an increased rate of gastric malignancy. Although no proof is available, some of the evidence to date suggests that pernicious anemia patients with both autoimmune and environmental gastritis may have a somewhat higher risk of developing gastric adenocarcinoma than non–pernicious anemia patients with environmental gastritis alone.

In view of this evidence, should pernicious anemia patients be monitored for malignancy? Upon confirmed initial diagnosis of pernicious anemia, patients should be subjected to gastric endoscopy, and biopsies should be obtained from the corpus, antrum, and lesser curvature, as well as from any endoscopically visible lesions. This initial assessment will provide the baseline data to dictate subsequent evaluation and further treatment. In individuals who have fundal gastritis alone without carcinoid tumors, probably no specific monitoring protocol needs to be instituted. In patients showing intramucosal carcinoid tumors, in contrast, a yearly survey for

evidence of invasive carcinoid should be adopted. If an invasive carcinoid is present, the possibility of appropriate resection should be considered, taking into account the caveats analyzed above. If environmental gastritis is found, on the other hand, a yearly survey to monitor the evolution of the mucosal lesions is deemed prudent by some. In the presence of severe atypia, surgery must be strongly considered.

Zollinger-Ellison Syndrome Associated with MEN I

Patients with the Zollinger-Ellison syndrome, also characterized by massive hypergastrinemia comparable with or higher than that seen in pernicious anemia, generally exhibit significant ECL-cell hyperplasia but, as a rule, do not develop gastric carcinoid tumors. An exception are the patients in whom the gastrinoma is part of the MEN I syndrome, as the ECL-cell hyperplasia has been seen to progress to the formation of carcinoid tumors, strongly suggesting the participation of a genetic factor in their occurrence. In these individuals, the gastrinoma is potentially more malignant and prone to dramatic systemic manifestations. Thus, its surgical removal becomes a priority and should eliminate the trophic influence on the ECL-cells, forestalling the appearance of gastric carcinoids. Should such gastrinoma not be amenable to surgical removal, these patients can often be controlled with long-term acid suppression with proton-pump inhibitors, and they are at risk for the development of a gastric carcinoid. Such uncommon individuals may benefit from endoscopy and biopsy of the stomach at prudent intervals, as recommended for pernicious anemia patients.

Long-Term Treatment with Proton-Pump Inhibitors

Treatment with very potent acid-suppressing agents such as proton-pump inhibitors (omeprazole) causes a profound hypochlorhydria that results in significant hypergastrinemia. Long-term administration of this and other acid-suppressing agents to rats resulted in ECL-cell hyperplasias, dysplasias, and the appearance of invasive carcinoid tumors. Such findings provoked a good deal of trepidation in terms of human administration for fear that such patients may develop carcinoid tumors similar to those seen in pernicious anemia. However, similar long-term administration experiments failed to elicit the appearance of carcinoid tumors in other animal species such as mouse or dog, suggesting that this reaction is idiosyncratic for the rat. Indeed, a number of publications studying humans treated for variable lengths of time with omeprazole has failed to document even the appearance of significant ECL-cell hyperplasia. A recent article from Europe, reporting the experience with patients administered omeprazole for as long as 8 years, demonstrates that the hypergastrinemia that results from such protracted therapy has a moderate range and is self-limiting. In addition, unlike rats, humans seem to exhibit a limited ECL-cell response to the omeprazole-induced hypergastrinemia, falling short

---

*__Editor's Note:__ There was a dramatic fall in serum gastrin levels from 2,000 to 200 μg per deciliter and a decrease in enterochromaffin polyps after antrectomy in our patient, described by Kern and colleagues.

of dysplasia or carcinoid tumor formation. In light of current information, it seems safe to conclude that omeprazole-induced long-term achlorhydria and hypergastrinemia do not represent a significant risk for the appearance of gastric carcinoid tumors.

Currently, patients on long-term omeprazole are systematically surveyed endoscopically with biopsy of their gastric mucosa, partly because it is required by official regulatory agencies, but it does not appear that such a survey will be particularly rewarding. Some evidence has been presented suggesting that patients treated with omeprazole may have a higher incidence of fundic gland polyps than a control population of age- and sex-matched untreated individuals. Although the evidence supporting this association is still being debated, this may well constitute a moot point inasmuch as these polyps have never been seen to evolve into dysplastic or neoplastic lesions.*

Follicular Gastritis and Pseudolymphoma

At times, dense, follicular lymphoid infiltrates appear on a more or less focal basis in the stomach, generally in connection with antral *H. pylori*-associated gastritis (see the chapters on gastritis classification and on *H. pylori* gastroduodenal disease) and/or gastric peptic ulcer. The term pseudolymphoma has been used to describe such infiltrates, denoting their similarity to a lymphomatous infiltration and the difficulty that the endoscopist and the pathologist may experience in arriving at the correct differential diagnosis, especially when dealing with endoscopic biopsies. This is particularly so in cases of well-differentiated small cell lymphomas, also known as MALTomas. Several morphologic parameters have been proposed to help in this distinction: (1) in lymphoid hyperplasia the infiltrate tends to "push" rather than infiltrate the glands forming lymphoepithelial lesions, (2) it is polymorphic rather than monomorphic, and (3) by immunocytochemistry it

is polyclonal rather than monoclonal. Interestingly, some so-called pseudolymphomas have proved monotypic in terms of globulin contents, and examples of true, well-differentiated lymphoma have been reported arising in such lesions. These findings raise the possibility that at least some pseudolymphomas may represent early stages of well-differentiated lymphoma, a theory enthusiastically embraced by Isaacson and collaborators. It is important for the welfare of the patient to make the distinction between focal lymphoid hyperplasia and well-differentiated small cell lymphoma of the stomach. In the latter, radio and chemotherapy tend to be ineffective, whereas surgical resection results in disease-free periods ranging from 1 to 20 years. However, since partial and subtotal gastrectomy are major operations with significant morbidity and mortality rates, it is important to resort to all available technologic approaches, including flow cytometry and B-cell gene rearrangement studies, to firmly establish the diagnosis of malignancy.

COMMENTS

The potentially premalignant conditions discussed herein possess widely variable malignant potential. More significantly, some lack the sensitivity and specificity desirable for use as guidelines for surveillance and treatment. It is important, however, that they all be readily recognized, since their existence presents the treating physician with the need to make a decision that may involve long-range follow-up or the implementation of a treatment with significant cost, inconvenience, or even morbidity. Table 1 summarizes these conditions, their possible outcome, the recommendations for surveillance, and the treatment when available.

---

*Editor's Note: Similar opinions regarding the relative safety of long-term use of omeprazole are expressed in other chapters.

Editor's Note: This excellent chapter complements the chapters on gastritis classification, chronic gastritis, *H. pylori*, Zolinger-Ellison syndrome, and chronic polyposis syndromes. Also, as the author illustrates, it is vital that the clinician act in concert with the informed and interested pathologist. If you have no such relationship, foster one or get outside pathology consultations on problem cases.

Table 1 Recommended Surveillance and Treatment for Premalignant Conditions of the Stomach

Premalignant Condition	Associated Malignancy	Surveillance Recommended	Treatment Available
Chronic multifocal atrophic gastritis (MAG)	Gastric adenocarcinoma (generally in antrum)	Yearly endoscopy and biopsy for dysplasia and early cancer	None for premalignant condition
Adenomatous polyps	Gastric adenocarcinoma	Endoscopy and biopsy to determine nature of polyp	Polypectomy
Postgastrectomy gastric remnant	Gastric adenocarcinoma (postchemical gastritis?)	Late (after 15 yr)?	None for premalignant condition
Ménétrier's hypertrophic gastropathy	Gastric adenocarcinoma?	Yearly endoscopy and biopsy in medically treated cases	Partial gastrectomy, H₂ blockers, omeprazole
Chronic atrophic autoimmune gastritis	Gastric carcinoids / Gastric adenocarcinoma?	Initial endoscopy and biopsy to rule out invasive carcinoid or concurrent MAG	Antrectomy?
Zollinger-Ellison syndrome associated with MEN I	Gastric carcinoids	Endoscopy and biopsy, only if gastrinoma is unresectable	Subtotal gastrectomy?
Lymphoid hyperplasia (pseudolymphoma)	Gastric lymphoma MALToma?	Initial endoscopy and biopsy to rule out lymphoma	None unless lymphoma is present or appears later

SUGGESTED READING*

Antonioli DA. Gastric carcinoma and its precursors. In Goldman H, Appelman HD, Kaufman N, eds. Gastrointestinal pathology. Baltimore: Williams & Wilkins, 1990:144–180.

Bradburn DM, Redwood NFW, Venables CW, Gunn A. Medical therapy of Ménétrier's disease with omeprazole. Digestion 1992; 52:204–208.

Correa P. Human gastric carcinogenesis: a multistep and multifactorial process—First American Cancer Society Award lecture on cancer epidemiology and prevention. Cancer Res 1992; 52:6735–6740.

Furukawa H, Iwanaga T, Hiratsuka M, et al. Gastric remnant cancer as a metachronous multiple lesion. Br J Surg 1993; 80:54–56.

Kern SE, Yardley JH, Lazenby AJ, Bayless TM, et al. Reversal by antrectomy of endocrine cell hyperplasia in the gastric body in pernicious anemia: a morphometric study. Mod Pathol 1990; 3:561–566.

---

*Editor's Note: These references are quite recent and represent the rapid changes in this field; thus, we have included a few more than in most chapters.

Lamberts R, Creutzfeldt W, Struber HG, et al. Long-term omeprazole therapy in peptic ulcer disease: gastrin, endocrine cell growth, and gastritis. Gastroenterology 1993; 104:1356–1370.

Lechago J, Correa P. Prolonged achlorhydria and gastric neoplasia: is there a causal relationship? Gastroenterology 1993; 104:1554–1557.

Rindi G, Luinetti O, Cornaggia M, et al. Three subtypes of gastric argyrophil carcinoid and the gastric neuroendocrine carcinoma: a clinicopathological study. Gastroenterology 1993; 104:994–1006.

Rugge M, Farinati F, Di Mario F, et al. Gastric epithelial dysplasia: a prospective multicenter follow-up study from the Interdisciplinary Group on Gastric Epithelial Dysplasia. Hum Pathol 1991; 22: 1002–1008.

Sjöblom SM, Sipponen P, Järvinen H. Gastroscopic follow up of pernicious anaemia patients. Gut 1993; 34:28–32.

Spencer J, Diss TC, Isaacson PG. Primary B cell gastric lymphoma. A genotypic analysis. Am J Pathol 1989; 135:557–564.

Wotherspoon AC, Ortiz-Hidalgo C, Falzon MR, Isaacson PG. Helicobacter pylori–associated gastritis and primary B-cell gastric lymphoma. Lancet 1991; 338:1175–1176.

FUNCTIONAL AND BEHAVIORAL DISORDERS

FUNCTIONAL DISORDERS OF THE UPPER GASTROINTESTINAL TRACT

WILLIAM V. HARFORD, M.D.

Functional gastrointestinal (GI) disorders can be defined as disturbances of GI function in the absence of pathology demonstrable on customary diagnostic studies such as radiography, endoscopy, or biopsy. The organic basis for some functional disorders may be apparent on more sophisticated studies done principally for research. For example, postprandial antral hypomotility is found during gastric manometric studies in some patients with nonulcer dyspepsia (NUD). However, the pathophysiology of many functional disorders is unclear or unknown.

The physician's approach plays an important role in the success or failure of treatment of functional GI disorders. The absence of objective pathology on standard studies makes it difficult to arrive at a confident diagnosis. Exhaustive and repeated examinations may be made in attempts to find organic pathology. The physician may tell the patient that nothing can be found or may imply that the symptoms are due to psychopathology or hypochondriasis. Most functional symptoms are chronic and respond poorly to medication. Some patients may indeed have contributing psychopathologic conditions or abnormal illness behavior and may be confused, frustrated, and demanding. These factors undermine the patient-physician relationship. A thorough history and physical examination, sensitivity to both physical and psychological symptoms, a rational and limited work-up to screen for organic illness, careful explanation, reassurance, empathy, and patience are the elements of satisfactory treatment of functional GI disorders (please see peptic ulcer chapter for "ulcer-related dysphasia").

NONULCER DYSPEPSIA

Clinical Features

A substantial proportion of the population suffer from symptoms related to the upper abdomen such as epigastric discomfort or burning, fullness, bloating, distention, early satiety, belching, and nausea. These symptoms are often related to food. When no objective cause can be found, these patients are said to have NUD, which has several general patterns. Some patients have prominent associated heartburn and may, in fact, have a component of gastroesophageal reflux. Others have symptoms identical to those of peptic ulcer disease (PUD), but no ulcer can be demonstrated. Other NUD patients have symptoms suggestive primarily of motility abnormalities. There is substantial overlap among these patterns. The GI symptoms of irritable bowel syndrome (IBS) occur commonly in patients with NUD, as they do in the general population.

Pathophysiology

There is no evidence of acid hypersecretion or abnormal acid sensitivity in NUD. In one study, patients with documented acid hypersecretion and NUD were treated with vagotomy. Acid secretion was reduced but symptoms were not. Acid suppression with H_2-receptor antagonists has been of only marginal benefit compared with placebo, with the possible exception of patients with prominent heartburn or ulcer-like symptoms.

Chronic infection with *Helicobacter pylori* (HP) is associated with histologic chronic superficial gastritis and an increased risk of PUD. Some studies have shown an increased prevalence of HP infection in patients with NUD, but others have not. Most individuals infected with HP have no symptoms. There is no evidence that chronic HP infection is associated with any particular symptom cluster. Treatment with bismuth compounds suppresses HP infection and improves symptoms temporarily in HP-positive NUD patients, but bismuth has other beneficial effects on gastric mucosa. There is no strong evidence to date that HP infection causes NUD, or that eradication of HP infection ameliorates the symptoms of NUD. There is a separate chapter on *H. pylori* infection.

As many as 50 percent of NUD patients have symptoms primarily suggestive of a gastric emptying disorder, including epigastric discomfort, bloating, fullness, nausea, and belching after meals. Decreased postprandial antral motility and delayed gastric emptying (particularly of solids) have been reported in this group. It is important to exclude other causes of delayed gastric emptying such as diabetes mellitus and gastric outlet obstruction in such patients. Recently, several studies have shown that some NUD patients have a reduced threshold for discomfort with balloon distention of the stomach, suggesting the possibility of a visceral sensory disorder.

Of the analgesics, only acetaminophen has been associated with chronic NUD. However, it is recommended that patients with NUD who are taking aspirin or other nonsteroidal anti-inflammatory drugs (NSAIDs) discontinue these if possible.

Smoking, alcohol, coffee, and tea have not been shown to be associated with NUD. There is an increased frequency of anxiety, depression, and somatization in patients seeking medical care for NUD, but this is not unique to NUD and is associated with a variety of other conditions such as IBS and noncardiac chest pain.

Diagnostic and Therapeutic Approach

The initial history and physical examination are important to screen for potential organic causes of dyspepsia. Certain symptoms, such as fever, persistent anorexia, or weight loss, for example, would be of concern and suggest a cause other than NUD. The differential diagnosis should include gastroesophageal reflux disease (GERD), PUD, biliary disease, pancreatitis, gastric or pancreatic cancer, malabsorption, giardiasis, diabetes, thyroid disorders, hyperparathyroidism, coronary artery disease, and adverse reactions to medications, among others. Simple screening laboratory studies may be advisable, including a complete blood count, sedimentation rate, chemistry survey, and stool for occult blood.

In patients under the age of 45 who do not take NSAIDs and have no worrisome symptoms, the risk of malignancy is very small. Recently, several authors have suggested that the serum antibody to HP may be used to screen for the risk of duodenal ulcer disease. If the HP antibody is negative, the risk of duodenal ulcer is small. Such patients may not require any further evaluation for NUD, and a therapeutic trial could be initiated. Patients who have NUD and take NSAIDs should be advised to stop the NSAIDs if possible. Sometimes a change from one type of NSAID to another may improve dyspepsia. Patients over the age of 45, those with troublesome symptoms, those who cannot discontinue NSAIDs, and those who are HP antibody–positive should probably all be evaluated further, preferably by upper GI endoscopy, or by upper GI x-ray examination if endoscopy is not available.

When the diagnostic evaluation is negative, a careful explanation of potential causes of NUD, along with reassurance, are important. The physician should be attentive to evidence of psychological distress or an unvoiced concern, such as fear of cancer. If severe psychological distress is suspected, this possibility should be gently explored, as psychiatric referral and treatment may improve the patient's ability to cope with dyspepsia. For most patients, however, explanation and reassurance are sufficient and specific treatment is not required. Few

studies demonstrate that medication relieves symptoms of NUD, beyond the strong placebo effect that has been observed.

In patients with prominent complaints of heartburn or peptic-type pain, a trial of an antacid or standard dose H_2-receptor antagonist for 4 to 6 weeks is harmless. Despite lack of evidence of efficacy in most studies, individual patients may respond. If a clear response is reported, treatment may be continued on an as-needed basis. This approach has the additional benefit of being appropriate for patients who actually have GERD or PUD that was missed on the initial evaluation.

Patients with symptoms suggestive of a gastric emptying disorder may benefit from eating smaller meals more frequently and avoiding fatty foods, which delay emptying. A trial of a prokinetic agent is reasonable. Metoclopramide is a dopamine-receptor antagonist and cholinergic agent with both central antiemetic and peripheral prokinetic effects. In a dose of 5 to 20 mg one-half hour before meals, it has been found to be better than placebo in relieving dyspeptic symptoms. However, up to 20 percent of patients have side effects, including chronic extrapyramidal symptoms, making it unsuitable for chronic use in many patients. Cisapride has recently been approved by the Food and Drug Administration for treatment of reflux esophagitis. It is a prokinetic agent that facilitates acetylcholine release from the myenteric plexus. Unlike metoclopramide, it has no significant central nervous system (CNS) effects. Cisapride has been used for NUD, and a meta-analysis of clinical trials concluded that this agent is significantly better than placebo for this disorder. The usual dose is 5 to 10 mg one-half hour before meals.

Some NUD patients have persistent, troublesome symptoms that are not improved by H_2-receptor antagonists or prokinetic agents. In those difficult patients who are infected with HP, it is hard to resist attempting to eradicate the infection. Although most studies have shown no benefit, individual patients may improve. If a decision to treat is made, a proved regimen should be used, such as two bismuth subsalicylate tablets four times a day, combined with tetracycline, 500 mg four times a day, and metronidazole, 250 mg three times a day, all taken for 2 weeks. Potential adverse reactions as well as the importance of compliance should be reviewed with patients before starting treatment.

NAUSEA AND VOMITING

Vomiting is coordinated by a center in the lateral reticular formation of the medulla. This center receives afferent input from the vagal nerves and GI sympathetic nerves, from the chemoreceptor trigger zone (CTZ) in the fourth ventricle, and from corticobulbar tracts. The CTZ has receptors for dopamine and opiate neurotransmitters.

Some of the causes of nausea and vomiting are outlined in Table 1. It is important to exclude underlying causes that may be corrected. A careful history should

Table 1 Causes of Nausea and Vomiting

Acute
  Gastroenteritis, enterotoxins
  Drugs, including alcohol
  Acute intestinal obstruction
  Visceral pain
  Pancreatitis
  Cholecystitis
  Anaesthesia and surgery
  Metabolic disturbances
    Diabetes
    Adrenal insufficiency
    Uremia
  Hepatitis
  Vestibular disorders
  Motion sickness
  Radiation

Chronic
  Gastric outlet obstruction
    Peptic ulcer
    Gastric cancer
    Pancreatic disease
  Partial small bowel obstruction
  Motility disorders
    Diabetic gastroparesis
    Drug-induced delayed emptying
    Postgastric surgery
    Chronic intestinal pseudo-obstruction
    Idiopathic gastroparesis
  Metabolic disorders
  Pregnancy
  Increased intracranial pressure
  Eating disorders
  Idiopathic cyclic vomiting
  Psychogenic

Table 2 Medications for Nausea and Vomiting

Medications	Indications
Histamine-$_1$ blockers	Motion sickness
Meclizine (Antivert)	Vestibular disease
25–50 mg PO once daily	
Diphenhydramine (Benadryl)	
25–50 mg PO q6–8h	
Anticholinergics	Motion sickness
Scopolamine (Transderm Scop)	
1 patch q3 days	
Phenothiazine derivatives	Various causes
Prochlorperazine (Compazine)	Postoperative
5–10 mg PO q6–8h	
25 mg rectal q12h	
5–10 mg IM q4h (daily maximum 40 mg)	
Promethazine (Phenergan)	
25 mg PO q4–6h	
12.5–25 mg rectal q4–6h	
12.5–25 mg IM q4h	
Prokinetics	Chemotherapy
Metoclopramide (Reglan)	Motility disorders
Motility disorders	
10 mg PO ½ hr before meals	
10 mg IM or IV q6h	
Chemotherapy	
1–2 mg/kg IV q2h × 2 doses, then q3h × 3 doses	
Cisapride (Propulsid)	
5–10 mg PO ½ hr before meals	
5-HT$_3$-receptor antagonists	Chemotherapy
Ondansetron (Zofran)	Radiation therapy
0.15 mg/kg IV ½ hr before, 4 and 8 hr after chemotherapy	Postoperative

include a review of all medications. Physical examination should include neurologic evaluation. Laboratory studies should include tests for metabolic and endocrine disorders. In all women of child-bearing age, a pregnancy test should be made early. If a GI cause is suspected, endoscopy and x-ray studies are helpful. In a few patients, the cause of nausea and vomiting is not apparent even after extensive evaluation. Some of these patients have idiopathic disturbances of gastric motility and emptying that may be documented by radionuclide gastric emptying studies or electrophysiologic testing; others may have psychophysiologic disturbances.

Table 2 lists examples of some of the medications used for nausea and vomiting. Different agents are useful for different situations.

Phenothiazine Derivatives

When it is not possible to correct the underlying condition, the most commonly used medications are the phenothiazine derivatives, which act as dopamine antagonists in the CNS. Promethazine also has antihistaminic properties. Sedation, extrapyramidal reactions, and orthostatic hypotension are the most common adverse effects. Phenothiazines should be given cautiously to the elderly, who are most vulnerable to these effects.

Prokinetics

Metoclopramide is an antagonist of both central and peripheral dopamine receptors and thus has antiemetic effects independent of its prokinetic effects. The prokinetic effects are mediated by an increase in sensitivity of the GI tract to acetylcholine. Metoclopramide is particularly useful for treatment of nausea and vomiting in patients who appear to have a disturbance of gastric motility. In the treatment of gastric stasis, absorption may be delayed, so it may be advisable to prime patients with intravenous (IV) or intramuscular medication. Metoclopramide has also been used, in much higher doses than for motility disturbances, for nausea and vomiting associated with cancer chemotherapy. Metoclopramide may cause sedation and extrapyramidal effects. Contraindications to metoclopramide include evidence of GI obstruction, Parkinson's disease, or the use of other dopamine antagonists such as phenothiazines. Anticholinergics partially antagonize the effect of metoclopramide.

Cisapride does not have antidopaminergic effects and thus does not have either the antiemetic effects or CNS side effects of metoclopramide. It acts primarily by enhancing acetylcholine release in the gut and has strong prokinetic effects, thus ameliorating nausea and vomiting indirectly by improving gastric and small bowel motility.

5-HT$_3$-Receptor Antagonists

Ondansetron is a serotonin type 3 receptor antagonist whose specific site of action is not clear. It acts both on peripheral vagal terminals and in the CNS in the CTZ. It has little effect on GI motility. Ondansetron has been very useful in the treatment of chemotherapy-related nausea and vomiting, especially in cisplatin-based regimens. It has also been used both in postoperative patients and in those undergoing radiation therapy. Adverse reactions are uncommon. Ondansetron is available only in IV form.

Postgastric Surgery Nausea and Vomiting

After vagotomy or partial gastrectomy, patients may develop nausea and vomiting from a variety of mechanical causes, including recurrent ulcer, stenosis of the gastroenterostomy, and afferent loop obstruction. Dumping, bile-alkaline reflux gastritis, and gastric stasis may also cause nausea and vomiting after vagotomy and gastric surgery. Diet changes are the most effective treatment for the dumping syndrome. A number of agents have been tried for bile-alkaline reflux gastritis, including aluminum hydroxide–containing antacids, sucralfate, and cholestyramine, without uniform success. Revision of the gastroenterostomy to form a Roux-en-Y jejunal limb to prevent bile reflux helps some patients but not others, and no method for predicting success has been developed. A number of patients with stasis after vagotomy and gastric surgery improve with metoclopramide. A Roux-en-Y limb does not help these patients, who may require a total gastrectomy if symptoms are severe and unremitting.

RUMINATION

Rumination is the repeated and involuntary regurgitation of recently ingested food, usually one mouthful at a time. Part of the material may be spat out or it may be reswallowed. It usually begins within 15 minutes of eating and may last several hours, but characteristically stops when the food becomes acid to taste. It is effortless and not associated with abdominal discomfort, heartburn, or nausea. It must be distinguished from GERD, vomiting, and bulimia. Rumination is particularly common in institutionalized retarded children. In infants and children, it may be associated with failure to thrive. It may also occur in otherwise normal young people and adults, for whom it does not pose a threat to health but may be a source of concern and embarrassment.

In adults, rumination appears to be a learned habit. Motility studies have shown that episodes of rumination are associated with spike waves seen simultaneously in the esophagus and stomach that are due to sudden increases in intra-abdominal pressure. These increases in pressure are caused by contraction of the abdominal wall muscles and diaphragm. Transient relaxation of the lower esophageal sphincter (LES) may occur during some episodes, facilitating regurgitation.

A careful explanation of the pathophysiology and reassurance are the most important aspects of therapy. Behavior modification has been used. One such method consists of having the patient eat in the presence of the therapist, while being encouraged to refrain from regurgitation. The quantity of food is increased in gradual fashion. Biofeedback and operant conditioning have also been reported. Neither drug therapy nor surgery is indicated.

GLOBUS PHARYNGEUS

Globus pharyngeus is a continuous sensation of a lump or tightness in the throat unrelated to swallowing. It is not dysphagia or odynophagia and may be transiently relieved by swallowing. Up to 45 percent of normal individuals may experience the globus sensation at some time. Typically, a careful examination does not disclose an organic cause for this symptom. The term "globus hystericus" has been used in the past, implying a psychoneurotic cause, but these patients have no higher incidence of psychopathology than normal controls.

Globus pharyngeus probably has multiple causes. A minority of patients have conditions such as sinusitis, pharyngitis, dental infection, a vallecular polyp or cyst, pharyngeal pouch, goiter, cervical bone spur, or (most importantly) squamous cell cancer. There is no evidence of dysfunction of the upper esophageal sphincter (UES). Some uncontrolled studies have found a high incidence of associated esophageal motor disorders, but a cause-and-effect relationship has not been established. Several studies have noted that increased gastroesophageal reflux is found in about 50 percent of globus patients, a significant number of whom do not have heartburn. In one study, 15 percent of globus patients had edema of the arytenoids compatible with reflux laryngitis. Antireflux treatment for globus has been disappointing, but there have been no studies reported in which omeprazole was used.

In young patients with a short history of this condition, reassurance and a brief trial of antacids are indicated. In patients with persistent symptoms, in older patients, and in those with a history of smoking, a careful oropharyngeal examination, laryngoscopy, and fiberoptic esophagoscopy are appropriate. Lateral cervical spine x-ray films may show bone spurs. If available, a 24 hour esophageal pH monitoring study should be conducted if esophageal reflux is suspected. When evidence of abnormal reflux is found, a trial of omeprazole, 20 to 40 mg daily for 12 weeks, may clarify whether the globus symptom is reflux related.

HICCUPS

A hiccup is a sudden contraction of the inspiratory muscles, terminated by abrupt closure of the glottis. Coordination of hiccups occurs in a nonspecific area of the cervical spinal cord between C3 and C5. Areas of the brainstem and midbrain are also involved in the reflex arc. Afferent input occurs through the phrenic and vagal nerves, as well as from sympathetic afferents of segments T6 to T12. Phrenic efferents innervate the glottis, accessory muscles of respiration, and the diaphragm. Vagal efferents may be responsible for the decreased esophageal contractile tone and LES pressure associated with hiccups. Hiccups usually involve one side of the diaphragm, most often the left.

Hiccups may be caused by a wide variety of disorders involving some part of the reflex arc, either central or peripheral. Some of the causes are listed in Table 3. Most transient hiccups have a benign cause and require no treatment. Chronic hiccups often have a discernible cause, and every effort should be made to find this cause and correct it. In addition to the history, physical examination, and screening laboratory, other studies that may be appropriate depending on the clinical circumstances include chest radiography, upper GI endoscopy, abdominal ultrasonography, and computed tomography of the head.

When the cause cannot be found or if it cannot be corrected, a variety of simple physical maneuvers should be tried. Some examples are listed in Table 4. These maneuvers have in common an attempt to disrupt the hiccup reflex arc. If these fail, pharmacologic agents may be required, and Table 4 lists some of those most commonly used. There are scores of anecdotal reports of different drugs, reflecting the inconsistent success of pharmacotherapy. One class of agents that should not be used are the benzodiazepines, which may cause or worsen hiccups. Recently, baclofen, a drug used to treat spasticity, has been reported to relieve hiccups. Several authors have described the successful use of hypnosis or acupuncture. Phrenic nerve block should be considered only for severe and intractable chronic hiccups after all other conservative measures have been exhausted. Fluoroscopy should be used to determine which side of the diaphragm is contracting, and a temporary block should be created before considering phrenic nerve ablation.

AEROPHAGIA AND BELCHING

Normally, 2 or 3 ml of air reaches the stomach with every swallow. Anxiety, and certain activities such as chewing gum or smoking, increase the amount of air swallowed. Carbonated beverages add to the gastric air bubble. Belching occurs when relaxation of the LES and UES allows this air to escape.

Belching may become a dramatic and distressing symptom. It is possible to learn how to take large amounts of air into the esophagus and stomach, up to 250 ml in a fraction of a second. Patients who have learned how to do this can be observed to elevate the chin and extend the neck, which holds open the UES, while making an inspiratory effort with the glottis closed, thus reducing intrathoracic pressure. The swallowed air does not always go into the stomach but may stay in the esophagus, to be subsequently expelled by contraction of the chest wall and diaphragm. In some patients a substantial fraction of air enters the stomach, and from there, the small bowel. Belching may be a learned response or a semivoluntary compulsive tic. Initially, the

Table 3 Causes of Hiccups

Transient Hiccups
  Sudden excitement, emotion
  Gastric distention
  Esophageal obstruction
  Alcohol ingestion
  Sudden change in temperature

Persistent or Chronic Hiccups
  Toxic/metabolic: uremia, diabetes, hyperventilation, hypokalemia, hypocalcemia, hyponatremia, gout, fever
  Drugs: benzodiazepines, steroids, alpha-methyldopa, barbiturates
  Surgery/general anesthesia
  Thoracic/diaphragmatic disorders: pneumonia, lung cancer, asthma, pleuritis, pericarditis, myocardial infarction, aortic aneurysm, esophagitis, esophageal obstruction, esophagitis, diaphragmatic hernia or irritation
  Abdominal disorders: gastric ulcer or cancer, hepatobiliary or pancreatic disease, inflammatory bowel disease, bowel obstruction, intra-abdominal or subphrenic abscess, prostatic infection or cancer
  Central nervous system disorders: traumatic, infectious, vascular, structural
  Ear, nose, and throat disorders: pharyngitis, laryngitis, tumor, irritation of auditory canal
  Psychogenic
  Idiopathic

Table 4 Treatment of Hiccups

Nonpharmacologic methods	*Examples*
Irritation of uvula or nasopharynx	Tongue traction, lifting uvula, swabbing pharynx
Counterirritation of vagal nerve	Carotid sinus massage
Interruption of respiratory rhythm	Breath holding
Counterirritation of diaphragm	Pulling knees up to chest
Relief of gastric distention	Nasogastric aspiration
Pharmacologic agents	*Dosages*
Baclofen	5 mg PO t.i.d., increasing q3 days to 80 mg/day maximum dose if needed
Chlorpromazine	25–50 mg IV q6h 25–50 mg PO q6h
Metoclopramide	10 mg IV q4h 10 mg PO q6h
Phenytoin	200 mg IV 100 mg PO q.i.d.
Quinidine sulfate	200 mg PO q.i.d.

patient may have learned to associate relief of certain symptoms with belching. These symptoms may include dyspepsia from gastroesophageal reflux, peptic ulcer, biliary tract disease, IBS, or even angina pectoris. Nausea or psychological distress may increase the swallowing rate, leading to gas accumulation in the stomach. Belching relieves the distress of gastric distention, and a vicious cycle is initiated. Treatment of the underlying condition may decrease the stimulus to the learned reflex, and belching may stop. However, it may also persist even if the initial condition resolves.

Some patients with aerophagia may retain a significant amount of gastric air without belching, causing the "gas bloat syndrome," or may pass a significant amount of gas into the small intestine, causing additional distention and discomfort. Symptoms in these patients are usually aggravated by meals, especially large meals. The "gas bloat syndrome" may also be a consequence of fundoplication surgery, which may leave the patient unable to belch.

It is irrational, given the pathophysiology of belching, to use antacids, simethicone, charcoal, or pancreatic enzymes, unless these are aimed at some underlying condition. If belching persists once the underlying condition has been treated, careful explanation and reassurance may be helpful. Patients with a strong psychoneurotic component may be difficult to reassure and may not accept the physician's explanation. Some physicians have learned to demonstrate belching at will. This may be an effective technique for educating patients regarding the physiology of belching.

SUGGESTED READING

Allan SG. Antiemetics. Gastroenterol Clin North Am 1992; 21: 597–611.
Kellow JE. Motility-like dyspepsia. Med J Aust 1992; 157:385–388.
Koufman JA. The otolaryngologic manifestations of gastroesophageal reflux disease (GERD): a clinical investigation of 225 patients using ambulatory 24-hour pH monitoring and an experimental investigation of the role of acid and pepsin in the development of laryngeal injury. Laryngoscope 1991; 101:1–64.
Launois S, Bizec JL, Whitelaw WA, et al. Hiccup in adults: an overview. Eur Respir J 1993; 6:563–575.
Physiology of belch (editorial). Lancet 1991; 337:23–24.
Smout AJ, Breumelhof R. Voluntary induction of transient lower esophageal relaxations in an adult patient with the rumination syndrome. Am J Gastroenterol 1990; 85:1621–1625.
Talley NJ. Non-ulcer dyspepsia: myths and realities. Aliment Pharmacol Ther 1991; 5(Suppl 1):145–162.
Timon C, Cagney D, O'Dwyer T, Walsh M. Globus pharyngeus: long-term follow-up and prognostic factors. Ann Otol Rhinol Laryngol 1991; 100:351–354.

OBESITY

LAWRENCE J. CHESKIN, M.D.

THE CLINICAL PROBLEM

Malnutrition is a major health problem worldwide and, as such, is most commonly equated with undernourishment. However, in the developed world, and especially in the United States, malnutrition takes a different form—overnourishment. This type of malnutrition leads to an excess of body fat, also known as obesity, and to its myriad medical complications. Obesity is the most important risk factor in the development of noninsulin-dependent diabetes, and it is a significant risk factor for diseases of virtually every organ system (Table 1), even certain cancers. The risk of most of these complications increases with the degree of obesity, though for some, notably coronary vascular disease and strokes, the risk correlates best with the regional distribution of fat. Abdominal deposition of fat (android or apple-shape pattern), seen commonly in men and less often in women, is associated with a high risk for cardiovascular disease; in contrast, excess fat in the thighs, hips, and buttocks (the gynecoid or pear-shape pattern) is associated with a low risk of such complications.

Moderate to severe obesity also elevates overall mortality, carrying a relative risk of death of almost 1.9 for adult men and women at least 40% over ideal body weight, according to actuarial tables. In addition to the medical risks, and perhaps more motivating for many of those seeking to lose weight, are the unfortunate psychosocial consequences of obesity. Our society fosters widespread prejudice against obese individuals, detectable in the opinions of children as young as 6 years

Table 1 Health Risks of Obesity

NIDDM
Hypertension, CAD
Hyperlipidemia
Strokes
Cancer (endometrial, post menopausal, breast, colorectal)
Sleep apnea
Gallbladder disease
Gastroesophageal reflux disease
Fatty liver
Osteoarthritis
Gout
Infertility
Thromboembolism

NIDDM = non–insulin dependent diabetes mellitus; CAD = coronary artery disease.

Table 2 Grading Obesity by Body Mass Index (BMI)*

Grade	Degree of Obesity	BMI
3	Morbid	>40
2	Moderate to severe	30-40
1	Mild to trivial	25-29.9
0	Not obese	20-24.9

*BMI = weight (kg)/height (m)^2.

Table 3 Metropolitan Height-Weight Table, 1983*

Height	Weight	
	Men	Women
4'10"		100–131
4'11"		101–134
5'0"		103–137
5'1"	123–145	105–140
5'2"	125–148	108–144
5'3"	127–151	111–148
5'4'	129–155	114–152
5'5"	131–159	117–156
5'6"	133–163	120–160
5'7"	135–167	123–164
5'8"	137–171	126–167
5'9"	139–175	129–170
5'10"	141–179	132–173
5'11"	144–183	135–176
6'0"	147–187	
6'1"	150–192	
6'2"	153–197	
6'3"	157–202	

*For individuals 25 to 59 years old.

of age, according to one study. The resulting social and job discrimination contributes to low self-esteem and the high rate of depression among the obese who have sought treatment. Also noteworthy in this vein are the association of childhood sexual abuse with subsequent obesity, the greater social stigma borne by obese women compared with obese men in our society, and the higher prevalence of obesity among those of low socioeconomic status, black men and women, and Native Americans.

What, then, defines this condition, obesity? We all know it when we see it, but a method of standardization is desirable. Obesity is technically defined as an excess of body *fat* (>25 percent of body weight for men and >30 percent for women), rather than an excess of body *weight*. With the exception of very muscular individuals (e.g., certain types of athletes and laborers), relative weight is a reasonable surrogate measure for the less readily obtained measure of adiposity (percent of body weight constituted by fat).

Weight adjusted for height, or *body mass index* (BMI), defined as weight in kilograms divided by the square of the height in meters, is very useful for defining and grading the severity of obesity (Table 2) and attendant risks. Grade 0 is associated with the lowest mortality risk, as derived from life insurance data. These data are most commonly summarized in tables of "ideal" body weight (IBW) for different heights and frame sizes (Table 3), but some caveats are in order. First, at least one third of the adult U.S. population is more than 20 percent over IBW, as are 60 percent of middle-aged black women. The public tends to treat these "ideal" weights as gospel, and much unnecessary deprivation and unhappiness can be attributed to generally unsuccessful attempts to attain and maintain these weights. Second, not only are IBWs unrealistic goals for most obese people, they also apply only to the population from which the data were drawn—upper middle-class whites in their early twenties. This must be considered in light of evidence that the relative weight associated with lowest mortality increases with age (Table 4). Third, although existing evidence is not entirely persuasive, it is possible that "yo-yo" dieting may pose greater health risks than staying at a moderately obese level.

Therefore, it is probably best to steer patients away from IBW tables and to encourage weight loss for medical reasons only in those with grade 2 or 3 obesity, especially if they are young, already suffer from complicating medical conditions, or have a strong family history of diabetes and cardiovascular or cerebrovascular dis-

ease. For those with trivial obesity (grade 1) the benefits of successful weight loss are psychosocial and not medical. These patients should be encouraged to focus on a healthier (low-fat, high-fiber) diet and increased physical fitness (exercise) rather than just the number on the scale.

In the case of abdominal fat deposition, however, even mild excess adiposity may pose a medical problem. A waist-to-hip ratio of more than 1.0 for men and 0.8 for women suggests the diagnosis of abdominal obesity, and can be easily measured with a tape rule around the narrowest point above the umbilicus and the widest point below the hips. Fortunately, this metabolically active abdominal fat is usually first to go with weight loss. The pear shape is both safer and more durable than the apple, as many women who attempt to lose weight have learned. From an evolutionary perspective, lower-body obesity may have conferred a selective advantage by helping to ensure survival through times of food shortage and being easily mobilized only under the hormonal influences of pregnancy and breastfeeding.

Despite the inescapable fact that genetic influences exist (witness various adopted-twin studies), genetics does not appear to account for the majority of variability in BMI seen in the population, nor is it an insurmountable barrier in those who were fortunate (or unfortunate) enough to draw the putative genes leading to metabolic efficiency in the lottery of conception. Both the environment and learned behaviors are supremely important as modifiers of genetic predisposition and are good places to focus treatment.

TREATMENT

Perhaps no other field of medicine today is as subject to the fads, hype, and unreasonable expectations as the

Table 4 Desirable Weight by Age

	20-29 yr	*30-39 yr*	*40-49 yr*	*50-59 yr*	*60-69 yr*
4'10"	84-111	92-119	99-127	107-135	115-142
4'11"	87-115	95-123	103-131	111-139	119-147
5'0"	90-119	98-127	106-135	114-143	123-152
5'1"	93-123	101-131	110-140	118-148	127-157
5'2"	96-127	105-136	113-144	122-153	131-163
5'3"	99-131	108-140	117-149	126-158	135-168
5'4"	102-135	112-145	121-154	130-163	140-173
5'5"	106-140	115-149	125-159	134-168	144-179
5'6"	109-144	119-154	129-164	138-174	148-184
5'7"	112-148	122-159	133-169	143-179	153-190
5'8"	116-153	126-163	137-174	147-184	158-196
5'9"	119-157	130-168	141-179	151-190	162-201
5'10"	122-162	134-173	145-184	156-195	167-207
5'11"	126-167	137-178	149-190	160-201	172-213
6'0"	129-171	141-183	153-195	165-207	177-219
6'1"	133-176	145-188	157-200	169-213	182-225
6'2"	137-181	149-194	162-206	174-219	187-232
6'3"	141-186	153-199	166-212	179-225	192-238
6'4"	144-191	157-205	171-218	184-231	197-244

Adapted from Andres R. Mortality and obesity. In: Hazzard WR, et al, eds. Principles of geriatric medicine and gerontology. 3rd ed. New York: McGraw Hill, 1994:852.

treatment of obesity. Part of the reason lies in the inherent difficulty of reconciling a society whose main fuels are fatty foods and ethanol, with an ideal body form typified by the Barbie doll. Given that our profession is unlikely to have any say in what body form people are striving for, the next best approach is to lobby for reasonable goal weights for our own patients, encourage those who really need to lose weight to do so, and steer them toward safe, comprehensive treatment.

The components of a comprehensive approach to weight loss are listed in Table 5. The omission of any of these items is likely to adversely affect long-term results. The long-term success rate, defined as losing weight and keeping most of it off for 5 years, is quite low, perhaps 5 to 15 percent in the few studies available. Although this rate is clearly poor, it must be viewed in context and compared with our similarly poor success in treating other chronic conditions and addictions, for example, cigarette smoking and drug abuse. In fact, if one views the chronic pleasurable overconsumption of food energy as a kind of addiction, an instructive distinction between food and other reinforcing substances appears. The cigarette smoker need never smoke again; the obese person, however, must learn to coexist with the offending substances in order to live. In this light, the treatment of obesity should be likened not to the cure of an infectious disease but to the *control* of a *chronic condition*. As such, we cannot expect many complete cures and will need to be constantly on the alert for relapses in those who appear to be in remission.

Medical Assessment

The first step in treating the obese patient is the medical assessment. The patient may desire weight loss or may be reluctant. By all means encourage the reluctant patient with medical complications of obesity

Table 5 Components of Comprehensive Weight-Loss Programs

Medical assessment
Behavioral modification
Dietary modification
Exercise modification
Long-term follow-up

to lose weight but recognize that any attempt at weight loss will be almost certain to fail, even in the short run, if the patient is not self-motivated to change.

Begin as always with a thorough history and physical. The *weight history* may be of value in identifying precipitants of weight gain and suggesting fruitful avenues for treatment. For example, a change in job leading to a reduction in physical activity may be detected. Also of interest is whether the onset of obesity was in childhood or later in life. Although only about a fifth of obese adults were obese children, about four-fifths of obese children become obese adults. Obesity in childhood often results in hyperplasia of fat cells, an actual increase in number of cells, while adult-onset obesity results in only an increase in average cell size, not number. Treatment of the hyperplastic form of obesity is said to be more difficult because weight reduction does not greatly reduce the number of fat cells, only their average size.

Other information that can be gleaned from the weight history include postpartum weight gain (the average woman weighs about 10 lb more 2 years postpartum compared with prepregnancy, but the amount is extremely variable), weight gain after smoking cessation (average gain of about 6 lb, again highly variable, and the most common excuse women give for not wanting to quit), and evidence of yo-yo dieting and disorders such as binge eating (consuming inordinately large amounts of food within a specified period twice a week or more in private for over 1 year with loss of control and negative emotional sequelae) and bulimia nervosa (binge eating plus purging by vomiting and/or laxatives or diuretics). When an eating disorder is suspected, prescribing a diet and exercise program will not be helpful and may even be counterproductive. Instead, referral to a center experienced in the treatment of these problems is recommended. There is a separate chapter on eating disorders.

The history should also include questions to help rule out *endocrinologic* causes of obesity such as hypothyroidism, hyperadrenalism, and neuroendocrine tumors, though in adults even the most common of these, hypothyroidism, is rarely a significant factor in causing obesity. Also inquire about *drugs* that may be associated with weight gain (Table 6) and symptoms suggestive of diseases that often complicate obesity, such as diabetes, coronary artery disease, hypertension, arthritis, and sleep apnea. Symptoms and signs of *depression* should also be sought, as depression is a common accompaniment of severe obesity and may require additional treatment. *Childhood sexual abuse* is also common, and must be brought up late in the interview after a rapport has been established. Individual or group counseling may be helpful when sexual or other abuse is detected. The family history is of interest for endocrinologic diseases, obesity, and its complications.

The physical examination may be somewhat limited when the patient is morbidly obese, but it can yield evidence of endocrinological causes and detect complicating conditions. It is necessary to obtain not only an accurate weight and height for calculation of the BMI but also the two simple tape measurements for the waist-hip ratio, an important modifier of risk in obesity, as previously noted.

Laboratory evaluations should serve to screen for the complications of obesity. Blood chemistries should include counts of fasting serum glucose, cholesterol, and triglycerides and liver function tests. In addition, an electrocardiogram should be taken, as well as a complete blood count and urinalysis to establish a baseline prior to beginning treatment. A measurement of thyroid stimulating hormone (TSH) should be obtained if there is any suspicion of thyroid dysfunction, and other endocrine and metabolic tests if indicated.

Behavioral Assessment

It is critical to gain a sense of the behavioral as well as the medical aspects of the patient's situation. This can be accomplished by referral to an appropriately skilled psychologist or through your own guided discussions with the patient.

First, it is important to assess not only specific behaviors but also the impact of these behaviors, and the obesity itself, on the patient's level of functioning and quality of life. It may only emerge with inquiry that the patient has withdrawn from all unnecessary social interactions, or is no longer able to enjoy certain activities or interests because of weight gain, or has

Table 6 Drug Causes of Weight Gain

Steroids
Progestins
Tricyclics
Phenothiazines
Lithium

suffered job discrimination, to name just a few examples.

Also related to quality of life are the patient's expectations about what changes will occur with successful weight control. Although it may be motivating for the patient to believe that life will improve with weight loss, disappointment may follow unless the changes likely to occur have been placed in proper perspective. Medical benefits can certainly be expected with weight loss in the obese suffering from medical complications. For example, diabetics can often discontinue insulin or oral agents, antihypertensive medications may become unnecessary, and sleep apnea usually disappears with as little as a 10 to 15 percent loss of initial weight. On another level, however, although self-assurance often increases, the wallflower does not become the life of the party and the competent worker does not get a promotion upon losing weight. Encourage obese patients toward a balanced view by reminding them that societal prejudices about body weight and character are in no way based on fact, and that they are the same good and worthy people whether they weigh 250 or 125 lb.

In exploring specific behaviors, it is useful to assist the patient in identifying various *eating cues*. These cues are situations or feelings that lead to eating, often in an inappropriate way. It is axiomatic in our society that physical hunger is rarely a significant part of life, even for the poorest among us. In fact, physical hunger is not an eating cue for most obese people, because we rarely let ourselves get to the point of true hunger. Instead, we eat in response to a whole host of other cues, most of which are inappropriate. The most common eating cues cited are: *habit* ("It's 12:30 so I guess I'll have lunch" or "I have a jelly doughnut and coffee in the car on the way to work"), *stress* ("I've got to finish this paper, and eating while I work helps me concentrate"), *boredom* ("There's nothing else to do" [a subcategory is watching television and eating at the same time]), *emotions* ("I eat when I'm depressed or upset"), and *food as a reward* ("After a hard day, I deserve a rich dessert"). Underlying some of these cues is the association of food with love, care, and comfort, which may have its antecedents in early childhood but persists into adult life and pervades our culture.

The patient should be helped to recognize that using food to deal with stress, boredom, and emotions is, at best, ineffective. The stressful situation, for example, does not resolve with eating. In fact, eating may worsen the problem by distracting a person from dealing directly with the situation while adding the stresses of obesity and its sequelae.

Simply telling a patient not to eat when under stress is useless, of course. Instead, use the following three-step approach. First, recommend a period of observation and recording to enable the patient to *recognize the cue.* For instance, one can ask the patient to wear his or her watch upside-down as a reminder to ask "Why am I reaching for the food at this time?" If the patient is not physically hungry, one of the possibly inappropriate cues is most likely in play, and its nature should be guessed at and recorded. Second, suggest the *substitution* of other responses for inappropriate eating. For stress, this might be writing down what the stress is, formulating a plan for doing something about it, doing something (besides eating) to relieve the stress on the spot, or, at the very least, substituting a walk around the block or a call to a friend for the bag of potato chips. The third step is *repetition,* that is, to keep making appropriate responses to the problematic cue and to reap the rewards of the new behavior, which include the positive responses of others to the change in approach, not just to eating, but to life, that the patient makes.

Although some degree of change is necessary and beneficial, not every maladaptive behavior must be completely eliminated nor must every rich food be replaced by celery sticks without dip. While losing a large amount of weight in a reasonable amount of time does require a fairly aggressive diet and exercise program, maintaining a new lower weight does not. If the patient can learn to control even partially a few of the more important inappropriate eating behaviors and to shift to a diet somewhat lower in fat and calories than baseline, that is sufficient to maintain weight in the new, lower range. This is easy to see and difficult to do, but impossible if behaviors are not addressed as part of a comprehensive approach to the treatment of obesity.

Another behavior of interest in obesity is restraint. One can simplistically categorize patients as restrained or unrestrained eaters. Restrained eaters believe that they must exercise a good deal of control over their eating—they are always conscious of what they can and cannot eat. Unrestrained eaters do not control their eating to any great extent. Restrained eating may lead to some paradoxical results—once restraint is relaxed, an exaggerated response may ensue in a frenzy of all or nothing behavior. Such patients may be superb dieters, but are equally superb at overeating once the diet has been "broken." The issue is one of too much of a good thing. Although a certain amount of control and monitoring is necessary for maintaining weight loss, high levels of restraint may be more problematic than low ones in the long run. One solution is to couple the teaching of ways to control inappropriate eating cues with dietary changes that emphasize foods lower in fat and calories, so that lower restraint is required to maintain a given intake. This scheme definitely discourages skipping meals when the patient is physically hungry.

Dietary Assessment

Although as most aspects of diet are more properly characterized as behaviors, the need remains to understand patients' tastes and the macronutrient composi-

tion of their usual array of food choices. This information is a tool for suggesting behavioral changes that will comport with the patient's preferences and lifestyle. Although the physician can and should get some idea of these things in talking with the patient, a formal dietary assessment is best done by a dietitian using either a prospective or retrospective food diary.

The results of such an assessment must be interpreted with caution, as both retrospective underreporting and prospective restrained eating are common. Despite these shortcomings, the information gathered can be very useful. For example, the macronutrient composition of a patient's diet will often be weighted toward fats, protein, and simple carbohydrates. By cutting fat and increasing the intake of complex carbohydrates, such patients can considerably increase the volume of food they consume as they attempt to reach and maintain a lower weight.

A helpful tool in altering the composition of the patient's diet is the technique of gradual change. For example, a patient reluctant to switch from whole milk to skim milk could first try 2% milk (which is actually 38% fat), get used to that in a month or two, and then move on to 1% for another month. At this point, the patient should notice something interesting—the once-favored whole milk will now taste too oily. At some later date, the final step to skim milk can be made with few or no feelings of deprivation, demonstrating that taste preferences are acquired and eminently changeable even in later life.

Recommend scouring the supermarket aisles (at a time when the patient is not hungry) for tasty, fat-free alternatives to favored foods. Encourage the patient to explore the wide variety of fat-free foods now available and to focus on the good taste of the new choice rather than comparing it to the "real thing." The presentation of nutritional information on foodstuffs is changing. The new food labels will list not just grams of fat but also the percentage of the daily dietary fat allotment those grams represent. The patient should be taught (usually by the dietitian) to read both the old and new labels and to stay within a "fat budget."

This is also a good time to be improving the dietary habits of the patient's family, something that is particularly easy to do when the patient is the primary cook and food shopper. Including the family in this process not only improves their diet but also makes it easier for the patient if at least the house can be a temptation-free zone. Even if other members of the family must have junk food, they can be instructed to partake outside the home or to put only individually packaged items in the cupboard. Small-size purchases of rich desserts and the like are desirable in general—the smaller the dietary indiscretion, the less severe the consequences.

Specific recommendation on types of diets are listed under "Types of Diets."

Exercise Assessment

Exercise alone is, unfortunately, not a terribly effective method of losing weight. It is difficult for the untrained person to do enough of it, and most if not all of the expended energy is compensated by increased caloric intake. Exercise is, however, a superb way to *maintain* a lower weight after weight loss, enabling a person to eat somewhat more than a nonexerciser and maintain the same given weight. Regular aerobic exercise will also improve cardiovascular fitness, trim inches, and promote growth of metabolically more active muscle tissue.

An exercise assessment should include a record of the usual degree of physical activity, any limiting factors such as joint disease or previous injuries, types of activity the patient finds enjoyable, and a measurement by an exercise physiologist of the current fitness level. A formal stress test is not required unless active cardiovascular disease is suspected.

The rule of thumb in devising an exercise regimen is the phased-in approach. Most obese patients have a very limited capacity to exercise. Rather than suggesting a type or level of activity that is unlikely to inspire adherence, make sure that the plan fits into the patient's schedule and lifestyle.

The first phase consists of increasing the amount of everyday physical activity, without introduction of a formal exercise regimen. This includes taking the stairs in gradually increasing increments, parking the car farther away from the mall entrance, walking to the mailbox, and the like. This step alone may double the level of physical activity in a very sedentary person.

The next phase is a walking plan. People are most likely to comply with such a plan if the walk is scheduled during a break or lunchtime at work, and/or when the daily energy level is highest, for example, early morning. Having a companion to walk with and a place to walk indoors are also helpful in increasing compliance.

One half hour is the minimum amount of time a patient should make available for each session of exercise. The intensity of the exercise is not critical to the burning of calories—walking at a leisurely pace for one hour is roughly equal to walking briskly for half an hour. Allow the patient to set the pace. Initially, it may be quite slow, but in the absence of pulmonary or cardiovascular disease, most patients soon find the going easier and faster. This reinforcement can be strengthened by goal setting. Have the patient keep a log of the time spent walking and the distance covered after each session. The patient can then see the progress being made and set the goal a bit higher from time to time.

Next, the types of activities performed should be broadened. Walking or jogging can and should remain an ingredient at this stage, but with the addition of other forms of aerobic exercise. Recommend aerobics classes, stationary or outdoor bicycling, swimming, a cross-country skiing machine, or just about anything else that will burn calories and be enjoyable. Team or racquet sports and golf can be suggested to provide social interaction as well as to increase energy expenditure. Again, the most important criterion for a good exercise plan is that it be one that patients are likely to follow and be comfortable with as a habit for the rest of their lives.

Types of Diets

It is best to start by instilling in your obese patients a degree of skepticism about commercially advertised diets that are not part of a comprehensive approach to weight management. Many are based on very limited menus, the rationale being that monotony helps curb consumption. Others involve diuretic agents. In fact, any reduced-calorie diet will initially cause diuresis, which makes the diet seem efficacious. The diuresis will usually result in an approximately 2% to 4% loss of body weight during the first 7 to 10 days, but most of this weight will be regained as soon as the period of severe caloric restriction ends.

After the diuretic phase, the amount of weight loss to be expected on any diet obeys a simple formula. Lipolysis of one pound of adipose tissue yields about 3,500 kilocalories; it is therefore necessary to restrict energy intake and/or increase energy output by about 500 kilocalories per day to lose one pound of fat per week. Because some muscle may also be lost and muscle is poorer in energy than fat, the rate of weight loss may be somewhat higher than predicted. However, two countervailing factors are at work. First, with sustained moderate-to-severe caloric restriction, a modest reduction in metabolic rate occurs. This decrease makes weight loss somewhat more difficult to achieve, but caloric requirement, corrected for the new, lower weight, fortunately appears to return to prediet level within a few months of resuming a balanced diet. Second, because lower weight means reduced caloric need, the same caloric intake will represent less of a deficit as the patient loses weight. A regular program of physical activity can partially compensate for both these factors by helping to blunt the decrease in metabolic rate and by building muscle mass, which is more metabolically active and therefore has a higher caloric requirement than adipose tissue.

How much of a caloric deficit should be recommended, and in what form should the calories be taken? The answer depends on the degree of obesity, the presence or absence of co-morbidities, such as diabetes and hypertension, the results of the behavioral assessment, and, to some extent, the patient's preferences. In any case, it is important to remind the patient that the diet is only part of an overall plan and will fail in the long term unless accompanied by changes in behavior.

For patients with grade 1 obesity, it is best to recommend a caloric deficit of at most 500 to 750 calories per day to achieve 1 to 1.5 pounds of weight-loss per week. The dietitian can design a low-calorie, food-based diet that is either *balanced-deficit* reducing total number of calories while keeping proportions from carbohydrate, fat, and protein roughly the same as before, or *fat-deficit*, with most of the caloric reduction resulting from restriction of fat intake. The latter approach is preferable in light of the typical American diet that is too high in fat (37% of total calories). Also, a greater volume of food can be eaten on a diet that emphasizes complex carbohydrates and reduces fat to 20% of calories consumed. The new labeling regulations will help identify dietary fat.

Patients with grade 2 obesity will also benefit from the safety and nutritional soundness of a fat-deficit diet. It is important, however, to recognize that at this level of caloric restriction it will take more than a year to attain a weight-loss of 50 to 70 pounds. Few patients can sustain this degree of restriction for that long; therefore, for a limited period a *very low calorie diet* (VLCD) (fewer than 800 calories per day) may be needed. The VLCD is justified particularly if the patient already suffers from comorbidities that are likely to be alleviated with significant weight-loss and/or if the patient is near the upper end of grade 2 obesity.

VLCDs can consist of food, commercially available liquid supplements, or a combination of both. With full compliance, the amount of weight lost on a VLCD ranges from 2.5 to 4 pounds per week, depending on body mass and level of physical activity. The initial diuretic phase may be pronounced and accompanied by (usually transient) lightheadedness, headache, or fatigue. Later symptoms may include constipation and intolerance of cold. Electrolyte abnormalities are rare, but serum must be monitored at least monthly and more often during the first month of the VLCD. Renal insufficiency and severe cardiopulmonary disease are relative contraindications to a VLCD.

Gallstones may arise or become symptomatic, probably due to gallbladder stasis, and a decrease in bile acids, which occurs during or immediately after any severely restricted (especially fat-restricted) diet. To prevent stasis, the patient can add to the diet two teaspoons of a fat such as canola oil taken in *one* daily dose, which will allow the gallbladder to contract.

A VLCD should be administered only under a physician's supervision and with full attention to the behavioral changes necessary to sustain the weight loss that this regimen will produce.

In grade 3 (morbid) obesity, corresponding to twice ideal body weight or more, the only practical diet for most patients is a VLCD with careful medical monitoring and long-term follow-up. It should be noted, however, that even a modest weight-loss can yield substantial health benefits for morbidly obese patients. Sleep apnea often disappears with as little as a 10% loss in weight, and hypertension, diabetes and gastroesophageal reflux may also improve significantly. Do not view, nor let your patient view, modest weight loss as a failure or a waste of time. The same is true for lower grades of obesity.

Drugs and Surgery

Adjuvant anorectic medications may be useful for the morbidly obese patient, either from the start, to enhance compliance with the diet or later, when compliance begins to waver or hunger becomes an issue. There is little doubt that such medications are generally safe and substantially increase weight loss during the period in which they are used. Commonly used anorectic drugs include *phentermine, fenfluramine,* and a *combination* of the two. These are controlled substances, but

tolerance probably does not develop and the abuse potential is low. One reasonably effective agent, *phenylpropanolamine,* is even available over the counter. The true amphetamines and thyroid medications should not be prescribed for weight loss.

Whether obesity should be considered a chronic disease and treated on a long-term basis with anorectic drugs is a philosophical issue. In the present climate of medical treatment, these agents are best used only after attempts at dieting have failed in patients who are morbidly obese and/or suffer from comorbid conditions.

The surgical treatment of morbid obesity has improved considerably since the days of the jejunoileal bypass and jaw wiring. There is a separate chapter on obesity surgery. Probably the best procedure currently available is the gastric bypass that combines stapling of the stomach to make a small-capacity proximal gastric pouch with a short-segment bypass of the proximal small bowel created by a Roux-en-Y loop. Results are quite good in the short term. Long-term results, as with all methods of weight loss, depend largely on the patient's ability to make behavioral changes. Therefore, aside from access to a hospital with adequate experience in this procedure, the best chance of long-term success will come with referring the patient to a center that offers and insists upon extensive preoperative evaluation and maintenance therapy of long duration consisting of regular sessions in dietary management and behavior modification. Do not make the mistake of viewing surgery as a treatment that does not require the patient's active involvement—an unmotivated or unguided patient can and will defeat the procedure.

MAINTENANCE

The physician and the patient should both know that the long-term results of attempts at weight loss are often poor. It is therefore important to expose the patient, at the beginning of treatment, to the attitudes and behaviors that are likely to foster long-term maintenance of weight loss (Table 7). These may be summarized as follows.

- Readiness—Correct timing for change is vital. It is folly for your patient to begin a diet when he or she is not yet convinced of the need to do so or is in the midst of a stressful life event such as divorce.
- Setting reasonable goals—Aiming for an attain-

Table 7 Key Ingredients of a Weight Loss Plan

Be ready
Set reasonable goals
Find a reliable support system
Build in maintenance from the outset
Become invested in your goals
Make gradual changes
Keep records (be compulsive)
Make it enjoyable
Be flexible

able rather than an "ideal" body weight is advisable. A reasonable long-term goal might be the lowest weight the patient has successfully maintained for one year or more during the previous ten years.

- Reliable support systems—Obtaining helpful assistance aids in both weight loss and maintenance. This usually involves seeking out a friend or relative who knows how to listen and not just give advice.
- Building in maintenance—Planning and executing behavioral changes from day 1 is essential.
- Becoming invested in one's goals—Learning how to talk to oneself in a positive way in order to enhance commitment to self-set objectives is a useful technique.
- Making gradual changes—Modifying food choices and level of physical activity reduces the sense of deprivation and may make the process of change easier and the changes themselves more likely to be permanent.
- Keeping records—Recording weight, foods eaten, exercise, and precipitants of inappropriate eating is an excellent way to identify problem areas and to spot a relapse before it gets out of hand, thereby improving the chances of long-term success.
- Making it enjoyable—This is self-explanatory. It is much easier to comply with new behaviors if they can be enjoyed. If your patient cannot stand to exercise, do not tell him or her to do it anyway. Instead, suggest taking a child to the park or walking around the mall to people-watch. The achievement of a positive change in lifestyle is, by

itself, very reinforcing and should not be discounted as a source of satisfaction and enjoyment.
- Being flexible—This applies to both the physician and the patient. If an approach that has been given a fair trial is not working, or if the patient's circumstances change (a new job, for example), the weight loss plan may need to change, too.

In closing, it should be obvious that helping patients lose weight and keep it off requires a comprehensive and sustained effort. Although it is true that only the patient can do it, this is one area where the diligent and caring physician can make a real difference.*

SUGGESTED READING

Folsom AR, Kaye SA, Sellers TA, et al. Body fat distribution and risk for death in older women. JAMA 1993; 269:483–487.
Garrow JS. Treatment of obesity. Lancet 1992; 340:409–413.
Kayman S, Bruvold W, Stern JS. Maintenance and relapse after weight loss in women-behavioral aspects. Am J Clin Nutr 1990; 52:800–807.
Must A, Jacques SD, Dallal GE, et al. Long-term morbidity and mortality of overweight adolescents. N Engl J Med 1992; 327: 1350–1355.
Ravussin E, Swinburn BA. Pathophysiology of obesity. Lancet 1992; 340:404–408.

---

*Editor's Note: Specific diets are available from a nutritionist. Earlier editions of this book have had sample diets, but they should not substitute for a nutritionist.

There is an excellent symposium, "Methods of Voluntary Weight Loss and Control," from an NIH Technology Assessment Conference, published in the October 1, 1993, issue of the *Ann Intern Med* 119:641–770.

OBESITY: SURGICAL INTERVENTION

R. ARMOUR FORSE, M.D., Ph.D.

Obesity and medically serious obesity, with their associated co-morbidities, constitute a major medical problem in the United States. It is interesting to note that in other countries both obesity and morbid obesity are increasing. Unfortunately, this appears to be related to the increased consumption of American food as well as to the American lifestyle. In a more generalized assessment, it appears that obesity and morbid obesity are more prevalent in industrialized countries. The morbidity and the mortality rates of obesity are often difficult to numerate, partly because of the poor reporting of

obesity and morbid obesity as a medical diagnosis. With the advent of the weight tables used by the insurance industry, the issue of weight and life expectancy became increasingly and more accurately apparent.

Despite the issues and controversies that arise with the representation of the data, there continues to be evidence that obesity is a major health problem that decreases life expectancy. Obesity is related to cardiovascular disorders, including hypertension, congestive heart failure, arrhythmias, atherosclerotic heart disease, and stroke. It has been established for some time that type II diabetes is very weight dependent. In terms of the gastrointestinal tract, obesity has been associated with cholelithiasis and increased gastroesophageal reflux symptoms. To a lesser degree, obesity has been statistically associated with gastrointestinal malignancies. Abnormal menses are associated with obesity, and there is an association of estrogen-dependent tumors with obesity, including endometrial and breast carcinoma. This is thought to be due to the increased estrogen metabolites with obesity. As another aspect of obesity, the chronic exposure of the weight-bearing joints to the increased weight accelerates degenerative arthritis. Finally, there is a relationship of deep venous thrombosis and chronic venous insufficiency. From the psychosocial perspective, obese people experience loss of self esteem and rejection by others. They are discriminated against both socially and for employment, and often must be loners. There is mounting evidence that the severe forms of obesity, particularly when they occur in childhood, are associated with a history of abuse, including psychological, physical, and sexual abuse. Problems of abuse may persist and require professional help. It is thus not surprising to find that the issue of obesity is now considered a major health problem in America.

The solution to obesity is relatively simple: weight loss. The equation to obtain the weight loss is relatively very simple, in that daily consumption of calories must be less than daily caloric utilization. Despite this, there is still considerable difficulty in achieving weight loss in patients with only mild obesity, and a high failure rate in patients with medically significant obesity. There is also difficulty with weight maintenance for all categories of obese patients.

The long history of poor results from a conservative approach to obesity led to the development of bariatric surgery for obesity. Since the initial operations, there has been considerable improvement in the surgical approach with better long-term results and fewer complications. On the other hand, there has been very little progress with the conservative approach. This was made apparent in two NIH consensus conferences, one dealing with treatment and the other with the surgical approach to obesity. None of the reviews of dietary, pharmacologic, behavior modification, and exercise therapies have been able to demonstrate the magnitude of weight loss or the long-term weight maintenance needed for patients with medically significant or morbid obesity. The conclusions have consistently been that there is still a role for surgery in the treatment of obesity. What is more concerning is the recent evidence indicating that obese patients who try conservative therapy and fail will do so many times, repeating the cycle often under medical advice. There are two problems with this approach. First, there is a period of instability with each weight loss and gain, and this is associated with an increased health risk. Second, these obese patients usually wind up with additional weight gain at the end of the treatment failure, which only aggravates the underlying problem. This has been called the "yo-yo" phenomenon and should be diagnosed and prevented. Thus, conservative therapy has its limitations and significant risks, and patients receiving it must be properly supervised.

ROLE OF SURGERY

Surgery clearly has a limited role and must still be viewed as aggressive therapy, to be used when there is ample evidence of failure of conservative therapy. Patients who are considered for surgery are those who have morbid obesity or what is referred to as medically significant obesity. Such an individual is usually defined by using weight criteria: (1) 100 pounds over his or her ideal weight or (2) a body mass index of 40 or greater. The latter definition is being more frequently used as it corrects the weight for the height and also avoids the use of ideal weight tables. Exceptions to the weight limitations are patients with significant comorbid problems, including sleep apnea, progressive diabetes, and crippling arthritis. The age limitations are usually set at 21 and 55 years of age. There are clearly exceptions to both ends of this range. Young adults with progressive diabetes and severe obesity can be significantly helped with their medical and psychosocial problems by the amount of weight that surgery will induce. At the other extreme are the older patients with crippling arthritis who must achieve control of their weight before joint prostheses can be placed.

PREOPERATIVE EVALUATION

The preoperative work-up of morbidly obese patients must be extensive, in part to determine the degree of the medical problems and to control them for the surgery, and in part to rule out other medical diseases that cause obesity. In the preoperative period, the patient must begin to learn about eating habits and approaches to food and stress. Although this information will have been given before and during conservative therapy, it must now be taught in the context of the limitations that the patient will have with the obesity surgery. The patient must be completely educated about the limitations of the surgery as well as the expected outcome. This will include opportunities to talk with other patients who have had the surgery and interactions with the patient support group. Such groups are very helpful in learning about life after the operations and the expectations and limitations.

There is still controversy over the use of the psychological interview or questionnaire as preoperative assessment. It is used to attempt to identify those individuals who might benefit from preoperative psychological assistance. The psychological information has also provided the health care team with some insight into the patient (e.g., compulsive behavior) and helped the team work with the patient.

The dietitian must ensure that the patient understands the need for good dietary support, and will be a key individual for the patient as he or she learns new eating habits and a new diet. Our dietitian works with patients preoperatively and postoperatively as well as during hospitalization to assist in the early transition and learning of new eating habits.

The surgical procedure itself has evolved over several decades and is now performed with relatively low morbidity and mortality rates. This is due to not only an improved surgical approach but also to these patients being looked after in a center with an established excellence in caring for the morbidly obese. This medical care extends from the nurses and the paramedical personnel to the equipment and the operating room.

PRINCIPLES OF SURGERY

There are two well-established surgical approaches. The primary focus of these operations currently is the stomach. A reduction in the gastric reservoir is one important aspect and a pouch of 50 ml or smaller is necessary. The outlet of the pouch needs to be limited to a diameter of about 1.0 cm. These two aspects of the surgery are the basis for the gastroplasty operation. The one currently used is the Mason vertical-banded gastroplasty, which uses a piece of mesh to reinforce the outlet of the pouch. This operation provided the patient with a sense of early satiety. I have had limited success with this operation; mechanical failures at the staple line or the outlet have been both short- and long-term problems. I have also found that eating is often difficult for the patient undergoing this operation, because the food often has to have a semiliquid or soft consistency.

The other operation is the gastric bypass, which combines the limited gastric pouch with a segment of proximal jejunum being used to drain the pouch, thus adding an element of malabsorption. The patient has a sense of early satiety as well as malabsorption and the "dumping syndrome," which add to the weight loss and are an additional negative feedback to inappropriate eating habits. I have had excellent success with this operation in a large series in Montreal and now in Boston.

Vertical Gastric Bypass

My experience is also based on a prospective randomized clinical study in which the two operations were compared. Another prospective randomized trial was carried out in Adelaide, Australia. In both of these, better results were obtained with the gastric bypass operation, in terms of both mechanical success and the weight loss achieved. As a result of these findings, I now perform the vertical gastric bypass. This specific type of operation involves a dependent outlet from the gastric pouch, with a vertical staple line that is more resistant to the long exposure to enteral stress. The operation is performed through an upper midline incision. A gastrostomy tube is placed in the bypassed stomach for decompression but also to provide enteral support (fluids or nutrition) if there is a delay in processing through the postoperative dietary stages. This has also provided access for medications that are initially difficult to take with the new gastric pouch. If there is evidence of cholelithiasis, a cholecystectomy is performed to reduce the risk of a biliary complication during the weight loss.

PERIOPERATIVE MANAGEMENT

The perioperative management of these patients is very important, good fluid and electrolyte therapy being paramount. All medications, including prophylactic antibiotics, must be provided in a dose that is appropriate for the patient. I have used intravenous protein without glucose as the postoperative fluid after using Ringer's lactate for the first 24 hours. The patient's urine is then monitored for glucose and ketone levels. The presence of ketones without glucose is a sign of recovery and progression to an adaptive fast indicating the lack of a serious infection. The presence of glucose and no ketones indicates a continuation of the surgical stress response and raises a concern about a serious postoperative infection.

Early ambulation and chest physiotherapy are very important. Patient-controlled analgesia has been very helpful, and when possible an epidural analgesic has been used for pain control. The patient is given water on the third postoperative day with advancement through to a liquid diet using Carnation Instant Breakfast for the necessary protein over the next 3 days. The patient is maintained on this liquid diet for about 4 to 6 weeks, and then carefully advanced, through puréed to soft food and then a solid diet. This is all designed to prevent unnecessary vomiting and staple-line trauma and to promote a controlled learning experience of the eating behavior.

POSTOPERATIVE FOLLOW-UP

The postoperative follow-up is monthly until the weight stabilizes, with frequent blood tests to evaluate electrolyte, mineral, and vitamin deficiencies. This operation is associated with a significant incidence of iron, folate, and vitamin B_{12} deficiency, necessitating supplementation. The incidence of other mineral and vitamin or protein deficiencies with this operation is very low. Considerable time is spent by the dietitian and myself educating the patient about eating behavior as well as the dissociation of eating from other behavior. The patient and the family and friends all need to adjust. If there are problems with adjustment, a psychologist or psychiatrist is consulted.

RESULTS

The success of the surgery can be evaluated by the extent of weight loss and the morbidity and mortality rates. In my current experience the vertical gastric bypass provides the best results, with 80 percent of the excess weight lost after the first year. Follow-up of these patients up to 3 years continues to indicate excellent weight control in 80 percent. Similar results are reported by other surgeons using the gastric bypass operation, and in all series the mortality rate is very low (<1 percent).

Another approach to evaluating the success of the

bariatric operation is to determine the outcome of the medical comorbidities. One can now use pooled data from a number of reports to carry out this evaluation. By definition, *cured* means the absence of symptoms with no need for medications, and *improved* means a reduction in the dosage of medications. Hypertension, with a prevalence of 30 to 60 percent in the morbidly obese, is cured in 60 percent and improved in 90 percent of patients postoperatively. This is partly due to the diuresis, the decreased insulin level, and the sympathetic tone. Diabetes, which is present in 20 percent of the patients, is cured in up to 90 percent and improved in 100 percent. Dyslipidemia, with a prevalence of 20 percent, has a 70 percent cure rate and 85 percent improvement. Sleep apnea has also been cured after bariatric surgery in up to 100 percent of patients with this condition. This includes not only increased Po_2 and decreased Pco_2 but a significant reduction in the periods of apnea. Morbid obesity is associated with significant alterations of cardiac function, and there is often obese cardiomyopathy. There is now evidence that cardiac obese cardiomyopathy improves after the surgery, in part because of the magnitude of weight loss but also because of the persistence of the weight loss obtained. The cardiac studies conducted included echocardiography, nuclear multigated angiography scans, and repeat pulmonary artery catheterization. With all tests there has been improvement of cardiac status with a decrease in atrial dilatation, decreased ventricular hypertrophy, and improved hemodynamics to both fluid and exercise challenges.

There are significant changes in patients' self-esteem and psychosocial situation. This results in a positive feedback that helps with the changes needed for adaptation to the eating behavior. Patients are better able to engage in physical exercise, and emphasis is placed on developing programs of activity. Their improved appearance then allows patients to become more extroverted, which has additional positive feedback. These improvements are all directed back to the issues of eating behavior and the need to dissociate food from daily endeavors.

RECOMMENDATIONS

I believe that bariatric surgery continues to play a very important role in the treatment of morbid obesity. The surgery can be performed relatively safely in experienced centers and produces excellent results in most patients. Care of the surgical patient requires close supervision and an active program to deal with eating behavior and diet. Surgical treatment of obesity is associated with significant improvement in the medical comorbidities, and this should be considered during the process of patient selection.

SUGGESTED READING

Deitel M, ed. Surgery for the morbidly obese patient. Philadelphia: Lea & Febiger, 1989.
Gastrointestinal surgery for severe obesity. Ann Intern Med 1991; 115:956–961.
Gastrointestinal surgery for severe obesity: National Institutes of Health Consensus Development Conference Statement. Am J Clin Nutr 1992; 55:615S–619S.
MacLean LD, Rhode BM, Samplis J, Forse RA. Results of the surgical treatment of obesity. Am J Surg 1993; 165:155–162.
Wadden TA, VanItallie TB, eds. Treatment of the seriously obese patient. New York: Guilford Press, 1992.

ALCOHOLISM*

ENOCH GORDIS, M.D.
RICHARD K. FULLER, M.D.

Alcoholism is recognized by its complications, but the treatment of these is not the treatment of alcoholism. Gastroenterologists are familiar with many of the toxic consequences of alcohol abuse. In fact, an estimated 15 to 30 percent of admissions to large urban hospitals are related to the complications of alcohol abuse and alcoholism. The management of these complications is certainly important; however, the treatment of alcoholism means the modification of alcohol-seeking and alcohol-abusing behavior (Table 1). If this behavior is not arrested, the patient goes on to repeated problems from drinking or dies. To treat the hemorrhage or the pancreatitis and not to treat the alcoholism is bad medicine, akin to treating iron deficiency anemia without treating the colon cancer that is causing it.

Physicians, because of their authority and knowledge, are in an advantageous position to begin the management of alcoholism. Nevertheless, many are reluctant to do so. There are several reasons for this reluctance. They may believe that alcoholism is simply a symptom of some underlying psychological problem and that alcoholism itself cannot be addressed directly. They may see alcoholism as a moral, not a medical, issue. They may consider the condition hopeless. These views are almost certainly incorrect. Physicians may also fear that

---

*Editor's Note: This carefully written, detailed, and well-documented chapter is the prototype of the useful manuscript I am seeking for this book. Unless you are skilled and comfortable in dealing with alcoholics, this chapter is "must" reading.

Table 1 Alcoholism versus Complications of Alcoholism

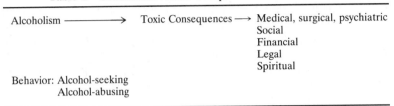

by discussing drinking with a patient, he or she will be offended and find another doctor. This argument has some merit but it obviously cannot justify failing to practice good medicine. Further, if all physicians managed the problem appropriately, they might gain patients, because some who had walked out on other physicians might now be ready for help. Finally, a minority of physicians have problems with alcohol themselves and find it impossible to examine someone else's drinking objectively.

We have written this chapter with the following assumptions. Physicians reading it are busy, and their primary interest is in clinical gastroenterology and its scientific basis. However, they want to practice good medicine and are willing to take a certain amount of time to address the problem of alcoholism. Although many physicians will probably refer the patient to long-term treatment by others, this first step is critical. The reward is the saving of many more lives than can be saved by intimate knowledge of hepatic cytoarchitecture or liberal application of sclerotherapy.*

WHAT IS ALCOHOLISM?

Alcoholism is a chronic relapsing disease characterized by four main clinical features: (1) tolerance, a state of adaptation in which more and more alcohol is needed to produce desired effects; (2) physical dependence, which means that upon interruption of drinking, a characteristic withdrawal syndrome appears that is relieved by alcohol itself (e.g., morning drinking) or by other drugs in the alcohol-sedative group; (3) impaired control, which means that the alcoholic person cannot invariably regulate total alcohol intake at any drinking occasion once drinking has begun; and (4) the dysphoria of abstinence, or "craving," which is the most elusive feature of alcoholism and which leads to relapse. (Formal diagnostic criteria for alcohol use disorders can be found in two major diagnostic systems: The Diagnostic and Statistical Manual of Mental Disorders, Third Edition, Revised (DSM-III-R), published by the American Psychiatric Association; and the International Classification of Diseases, Tenth Revision (ICD-10), published by the World Health Organization.)

*Editor's Note: Touché!

TREATING ALCOHOLISM

Alcoholism treatment consists of (1) recognizing alcoholism, (2) confronting the patient with the problem, (3) safe conduct through withdrawal, and (4) long-term management of the illness.

Recognizing Alcoholism

Recognizing alcoholism is no problem in the acutely ill hospitalized patient who has one of the major alcohol-related medical complications. In the office, things are more difficult. The patient is not acutely ill, will choose to hide or deny the problem, and will prefer that the medical complication be addressed and the drinking overlooked. The denial of the problem is not simply deliberate lying; much of the denial is unconscious because the thought of living without alcohol can be terrifying to one addicted to it. Here the physician must use a combination of clues: clinical, laboratory (well-known abnormalities of bone marrow, liver, and urate metabolism), and social (especially job, marital, and legal problems) to make the diagnosis.

A standard alcoholism-detection questionnaire (e.g., CAGE, Michigan Alchololism Screening Test [MAST], Short MAST) is helpful because it provides a structured and consistent means to detect individuals at risk. This information can then be used as a starting point for helping a patient confront alcohol problems. For example, the CAGE questionnaire (Table 2) is a self-report screening instrument that takes about 1 minute to complete. ("CAGE" is a mnemonic for the four questions that make up the instrument.) It is suitable to a busy medical setting when there is limited time for patient interviews. One "yes" response suggests an alcohol use problem; more than one is a strong indication that a problem exists.

Alcoholics are tolerant of large concentrations of alcohol: they may be ambulatory and coherent with a blood alcohol level that would be lethal to a nondrinker. The small, commercially available breath alcohol meters, no larger than a paperback book, are very convenient and settle doubts and disagreements about recent drinking in a few seconds. When a drinking bout has ended more than 12 hours or so before the consultation, and the blood alcohol level is zero, clues to alcoholism may be provided by tremor, tachycardia, and hypertension in a usually normotensive patient. These are early

Table 2 CAGE Questionnaire

1. Have you ever felt you should **C**ut down on your drinking?
2. Have people **A**nnoyed you by criticizing your drinking?
3. Have you ever felt bad or **G**uilty about your drinking?
4. Have you ever had a drink first thing in the morning to steady your nerves or get rid of a hangover (**E**ye opener)?"

From data in Mayfield DG, McLeod G, Hall P. The CAGE questionnaire: validation of a new alcoholism screening instrument. Am J Psychiatry 1974; 131:1121–1123; and from data in Ewing JA. Detecting alcoholism: the CAGE questionnaire. JAMA 1984; 252:1905–1907.

signs of withdrawal. Gamma glutamyl transpeptidase and mean corpuscular volume abnormalities caused by alcohol use are familiar to gastroenterologists. Newer laboratory tests, such as the carbohydrate-deficient transferrin, which could provide a clinically useful indicator of heavy alcohol consumption and which do not depend on the presence of liver disease, may become available in the near future.

Discussing Alcoholism with Your Patient

Discussing alcoholism with patients must be handled firmly but tactfully. It can be managed as a mutual exploration of the possibility that alcohol is causing many of their troubles. The information gleaned from standardized questionnaires and laboratory tests is helpful, because patients see that their situation is not unique and that they have not been singled out for harassment. If the patient consents to have the physician contact a family member or close friend, the physician can enlist the help of these relatives or friends to join in a meeting with the patient. At this meeting, the others quietly describe to the patient the impact of the drinking on their lives and urge him or her to agree to treatment. The impact of such a meeting is stronger if family or friends state their intent to terminate contact with the patient unless he or she enters treatment.

If the patient agrees to be treated, and if the physician chooses not to manage the alcoholism any further, the patient should be referred immediately to another therapist or agency for help, as well as to Alcoholics Anonymous.

Safe Conduct Through Withdrawal

Many patients are alcohol free at the time they seek treatment for their alcoholism and in no discomfort from withdrawal. For these patients, the approaches described in the section "Long-Term Management" may begin promptly. Patients who still have alcohol in their system, have mild withdrawal symptoms, or are uncomfortable from withdrawal symptoms may need treatment. The aim of treatment is to relieve symptoms and prevent the more serious complications of withdrawal. For clarity, we have divided this discussion into two parts: (1) a description of the withdrawal syndrome and (2) practical details about its treatment.

The Withdrawal Syndrome

Clinical Picture. Upon interruption of drinking, even before the blood alcohol has reached zero concentration, the patient may experience a group of adrenergic symptoms: tremor, sweating, tachycardia, systolic and diastolic hypertension, and irritability (or mild agitation). In addition, the patient may be sleepless. These symptoms vary in intensity and subside within several days or, rarely, 1 or 2 weeks. The diastolic pressure may be as high as 115 mm Hg. We do not recommend treating hypertension below this level, since it usually disappears within a few days as the withdrawal itself subsides. (Some patients, of course, are hypertensive as well as alcoholic and will need treatment while sober. There is no way of knowing this beforehand, however, unless a physician had to treat the patient for hypertension during a previous period of abstinence.) The tremor is a postural tremor at about eight per second; sometimes it is hard to distinguish it from anxiety, but if the fingers continue to shake when the examiner immobilizes the wrist and elbow, it is probably alcohol withdrawal. A tongue tremor, if present, is virtually pathognomonic. The patient may be nauseated and unable to hold food at the beginning of withdrawal. Some patients hallucinate during the first 1 or 2 days. Hallucinations may be visual or auditory, are usually recognized by the patient as abnormal, are not associated with persistent belief (as in delusion), and are not a sign of psychosis.

Hyperglycemia. Hyperglycemia in nondiabetics is often seen in early withdrawal. It is probably more common in malnourished patients, since normal glucose tolerance depends on adequate nourishment. In addition, alcohol is known to blunt the insulin response of the pancreas to a glucose load. With abstinence and eating, this condition rapidly clears and a diagnosis of diabetes should not be made.

Seizures. Patients may experience seizures, usually 2 or 3 days into withdrawal. These are epileptiform, are not characteristically preceded by an aura, are temporally related to the cessation of drinking, and, of course, are accompanied by a brief period of unconsciousness. Results of electroencephalography and brain scans are normal; we order these only once in any patient. Competing causes of seizures (epilepsy, hypoglycemia, an old head injury with organized seizure focus) must be considered but are rarely found.

Delirium Tremens. A minority of patients enter a severe form of withdrawal on about the third day, delirium tremens (DT), characterized by disorientation, agitation, fever, fluid loss, tremulousness, and hallucinations.

Treating Withdrawal Syndrome

Assessment. A rating scale, the Clinical Institute Withdrawal Assessment for Alcohol (revised) (CIWA-Ar), has proved of value in managing alcohol withdrawal in general hospitals. This scale, which takes approximately 2 to 5 minutes to administer, consists of ten items.

The first nine are nausea and vomiting; tremor; paroxysmal sweats; anxiety; agitation; tactile, auditory, and visual disturbances; and headache or fullness in the head. These are graded on a 0 to 7 Likert scale. A tenth item, disorientation and clouding of the sensorium, is scored 0 to 4. The higher the score, the greater is the severity of withdrawal. Scores of 9 or less represent minimal withdrawal, and pharmacotherapy is not necessary. Scores of 10 to 19 represent mild to moderate withdrawal, and 20 or more is severe withdrawal. Since no scaling instrument is infallible, such instruments should be used to complement, not replace, a thorough clinical evaluation of the patient.

Pharmacotherapy. For those who require pharmacotherapy and who can be continually observed (usually on an inpatient basis), we recommend 20 mg diazepam every 1 to 2 hours orally until the symptoms are suppressed, because the benzodiazepines (BZs) have been shown to reduce the occurrence of DT. The longer-acting BZs have an advantage over the shorter-acting variety because the long half-lives of diazepam and chlordiazepoxide and their metabolites enable drug levels to be maintained longer, thereby reducing the necessity of additional doses. The shorter-acting BZs (e.g., oxazepam and lorazepam) are preferable for patients with liver disease because they are glucuronidated rather than oxidized. In addition to their proved efficacy, BZs are quite safe. However, the metabolism of the BZ may be inhibited by cimetidine, isoniazid, disulfiram (Antabuse), and oral contraceptives. BZs should not be administered after the withdrawal syndrome is over because of alcoholics' substantial risk for becoming dependent on these medications.

Propranolol and clonidine control many of the adrenergic manifestations of withdrawal, but we see no advantage in their use, unless the early hypertension is severe. One drug might then control both withdrawal and blood pressure, even though the alpha$_2$ agonists (e.g., clonidine) do not reduce the frequency of seizures. Carbamazepine (CBZ) was initially studied in Europe for treating alcohol withdrawal, and recent American studies have confirmed the earlier results. A recent U.S. study compared CBZ with oxazepam and found them equally safe and effective. An advantage to CBZ is that it does not have the problem of potential abuse. Disadvantages include no parenteral form and occasional serious hematologic (e.g., aplastic anemia) and dermatologic adverse reactions. Other medications have been studied to treat withdrawal. The addition of one such medication, the beta blocker atenolol, to a BZ regimen resulted in smaller doses of BZ being needed to treat withdrawal.

In summary, while other agents are available, BZs have the major advantage that they are established as both safe and effective.

Although safe and comfortable withdrawal can be accomplished by giving tapering doses of alcohol over several days, we do not do this. True, this is the substance the patient is addicted to, and one does not have to rely on other drugs that do not have identical pharmacology; however, the arguments against using alcohol make

sense. First, nurses would be kept busy giving alcohol around the clock. Second, it is hard to maintain an ambiance conducive to serious counseling about sobriety when patients reek of alcohol. Third, there is an ethical question inherent in prescribing a known liver and marrow toxin to patients already sick with these complications. Finally, disulfiram therapy cannot be started while ethanol is used for detoxification.

Sometimes it is safer to let the patient shake rather than risk drug toxicity. Sedation should be avoided, if possible, in patients with chronic obstructive pulmonary disease. With advanced liver disease, we use very little sedative or none, since the metabolism of BZs is retarded in this state. Alcohol and BZs make depression worse, and it is better to avoid sedatives in a severely depressed patient. Note that a mild depression during alcohol withdrawal is expected and appropriate and is almost always self-limited.

Seizures. Whether withdrawal seizures are an indication for phenytoin (Dilantin) therapy in addition to the standard use of a BZ is controversial. We do not recommend phenytoin because we believe that the seizures are controlled for the whole period of withdrawal with adequate BZ therapy. (There is no controversy about the fact that anticonvulsants have no role in long-term management in the abstinent state. The long-term treatment for withdrawal seizures is abstinence.)

Delirium Tremens. If the patient is experiencing DT, it is essential to support the airway and maintain fluid and electrolyte balance. For the patient's safety and that of others, it is important to control the patient's agitation. Administering diazepam intravenously is effective; the dose should be carefully titrated to the level of agitation. The patient should be calm but not somnolent. In one controlled study of DT, the initial doses required for calming varied from 15 to 160 mg, and repeated doses were often required.

Nutrition. The physician should be concerned with nutrition. Middle-class alcoholics are generally not particularly malnourished. Among patients who are, the most common deficiencies are of folate, thiamine, and magnesium. Many physicians routinely administer all three, and this can do no harm. Magnesium deficiency manifested by low serum magnesium levels must be corrected promptly because magnesium depletion lowers the threshold for withdrawal seizures. Claims that magnesium alone is a suitable regimen for withdrawal have not been validated. Thiamine must be administered to malnourished patients before glucose; failure to do so may precipitate Wernicke's syndrome.

Table 3 summarizes management choices based on the condition of the patient when seen in the office. (Patients hospitalized for complications of alcohol may undergo withdrawal at the same time and may need treatment for it.)

Long-Term Management

The goal of long-term management is maximal restoration of physical and social functioning. Complete

Table 3 Office Management of the Alcoholic Patient

Sober (no alcohol present):
  Verify with breath meter

Comfortable, can listen:
  Confrontation; then long-term management (see text), including immediate offer of disulfiram

Uncomfortable, in withdrawal: Administer CIWA-Ar
  Withdrawal mild: Prescribe one day's sedative dosage (e.g., 5–20 mg diazepam) with return to physician next day. Next day, proceed with confrontation and long-term management. The mistake here is to prescribe a whole bottle of diazepam. This accomplishes nothing, and the patient is likely to drink and use the pills together.
  Withdrawal troublesome (or patient has had seizures or DT during a previous withdrawal): admit for detoxification.

Alcohol present:
  Can stop drinking: Return sober next day, continue as under "Sober." It is safer not to offer sedatives to a drinking patient.
  Cannot stop drinking: Admit for detoxification. The gastroenterologist may choose to manage the inpatient withdrawal on a general service or may admit the patient to a specialized unit. Insurance coverage for alcoholism detoxification is now provided in many policies. Do not admit the patient under a false diagnosis such as "gastritis"; this fuels the patient's denial and impedes recovery. The advantage of a specialized detoxification unit is that nonmedical services, such as AA, counseling, and group therapy, are generally available.

CIWA-Ar = Clinical Institute Withdrawal Assessment for Alcohol (revised).

abstinence is the only recommendation that can ethically be made at present. The commonly offered advice, "You should try to cut down on your drinking," is not worth the breath it takes to give it. Nor can the memory of past pains alone be relied on to turn things around. If it could, we would not see relapsing pancreatitis or repeated episodes of hemorrhagic gastritis.

The outlook for recovery from alcoholism may be seen to hinge on the outcome of a struggle between two functional parts of the brain: the part that determines appetite and the part that can understand the consequences of surrendering to that appetite and can decide not to. We have no currently approved therapy to modify the pathologic appetite for alcohol. At present, we can appeal only to the cognitive function of the brain with teaching, persuasion, and coercion. However, research on a number of promising medications (e.g., naltrexone) is under way that will help us to control craving and prevent relapse, thereby filling a major gap in the alcoholism treatment pharmacopeia.

The physician is the most competent person to describe the health consequences of alcoholism, and this should be done in detail. The physician can also counsel, for example, by indicating to the patient those other areas in life that are being damaged by alcohol. For the patient merely to know all this is not enough; he or she must also be persuaded that the struggle for a better life is worthwhile despite the fluctuating discomfort of abstinence. Joining with others in a self-help organization can be a potent force. The largest and perhaps best known of these organizations is the fellowship of Alcoholics Anonymous (AA). AA is neither an encounter group nor a religious denomination. Its sole aim is to help drinkers to stay sober. All patients should be encouraged to attend; although not all will respond to AA's style and message, many benefit from the sense of dignity and personal worth that AA imparts. Every physician should have available the names and telephone numbers of several AA members of diverse backgrounds who, with the patient's consent, can be

called while the patient is in the office. The patient can often be taken to the first meeting that evening.

Disulfiram

Although disulfiram has been used for over 40 years to treat alcoholism, carefully controlled studies of its efficacy have been made only recently. This research indicates that when patients are given disulfiram to take at their discretion, this agent, in addition to standard treatment, does not result in longer periods of abstinence than that achieved by standard treatment alone. This is because compliance with the medication is often poor. However, this same research indicated that more socially stable middle-aged men drink less frequently if prescribed disulfiram. Strategies have been devised to improve compliance with the disulfiram regimen. A recent controlled study has shown that having, for example, spouses or friends observe ingestion of the medication two or three times a week improves its efficacy. Whatever its long-term value, disulfiram buys time initially by putting up a "chemical fence" so that patients know they cannot drink that day, and even for 3 or 4 days after stopping it. Ambivalence about taking disulfiram is common, and the physician can point out that this indicates a less-than-total commitment to sobriety. Such a discussion may help patients overcome their ambivalence and elect to take disulfiram.

Disulfiram can be given as soon as 12 hours after the last drink. Nowadays, the dosage is designed first for safety and then for efficacy. A common routine, which is based more on clinical experience than on pharmacokinetic evidence, is 0.5 g daily for 5 days, then 0.25 g daily. A full-blown alcohol-disulfiram reaction includes immediate flushing of the face and neck (sometimes the rest of the body as well), an initial hypertension, tachycardia, and conjunctival injection. Within minutes the flush resolves, the blood pressure falls, and the patient feels faint, often nauseated, chilled, and generally sick. Convulsions are not part of the usual reaction. Finally, after a variable amount of time, but not more than 2 hours, the patient becomes sleepy and may sleep for several hours. On awakening, the patient is well. Compensated liver disease and diabetes are not contraindications to therapy.

Disulfiram is a safe drug; the most common side effect is sedation, which wears off usually in the first 2 weeks. Other side effects, including a rare but well-documented drug-induced hepatitis, are seen infrequently. Because disulfiram hepatitis is an idiosyncratic reaction that usually occurs early in administration, it is important to obtain liver function tests on a regular basis when first prescribing the drug. A recommended schedule is that liver tests be obtained before treatment, at 2 week intervals for 2 months, and at 3 to 6 month intervals thereafter. Because liver tests may indicate a resumption of drinking as well as incipient hepatitis, a discussion with the patient is necessary. Unless it is evident that the patient has been drinking, the medication should be stopped if deterioration in liver function occurs.

Absolute contraindications to disulfiram are pregnancy, severe depression, organic brain syndrome, severe active liver disease, and cardio- or cerebrovascular disease. The last two are contraindications not because disulfiram is in itself toxic to the heart or the brain, but because the rare patient who drinks while taking disulfiram (most patients stop it several days before drinking) will undergo a hypotensive episode. Disulfiram interferes with the biotransformation of certain medications, including phenytoin, isoniazid, diazepam, chlordiazepoxide, warfarin, imipramine, and desipramine. This has to be kept in mind when prescribing disulfiram. It is emphasized again, however, that for most alcoholic patients, disulfiram is easy and safe to prescribe.

Other Aspects of Patient Care

Patients frequently attribute relapse to stress. In many cases this may be true, but stress is often used as an excuse for drinking. Patients taking disulfiram who relapse have almost all stopped disulfiram several days before the alleged drink-provoking stress occurred. Counseling and social work are valuable because they help the patient undo the damage that drinking has done and adjust to a sober routine. When life has some rewards, the patient is more likely to view the struggle for sobriety as worthwhile.

In general, a psychiatric diagnosis cannot be made while the patient is either drinking or in early withdrawal. Most alcoholics do not need treatment for psychiatric illness; they are drunk, but not mentally ill. Once sober, however, a minority need treatment by a psychiatrist for an affective disorder, a manic-depressive disorder, or panic attacks. In the sober state, they can respond to competent psychiatry as do nonalcoholics.

Insomnia

There is no role for sedation in the long-term management of alcoholism. It does not control the drinking and it sets patients up for a possible second drug habit. Insomnia may persist many months after withdrawal; the sleep electroencephalogram results may not become normal in a year's time. Sleeping pills should not be prescribed. Patients should be told that the condition will improve in time if they do not take pills. The most common cause of insomnia, however, is caffeine, and most cases of insomnia respond to the cessation of all caffeine, including coffee, tea, and cola beverages.

Role of the Physician (Table 4)

We know physicians who genuinely enjoy the long-term management of alcoholism, including nonmedical counseling. Most, however, prefer not to do this and choose to refer their patients to a competently run alcoholism treatment program, where a variety of

---

Table 4   Checklist: What the Concerned Physician Should Know and Have Available in the Practice to Manage Alcoholism

To Know:
1. The pharmacology of alcohol: its distribution, metabolism, tolerance, physical dependence
2. The pharmacology of one sedative, e.g., diazepam and how to use it
3. The pharmacology of disulfiram and how to use it

To Have Available:
1. A supply of disulfiram in the office so that it can be started immediately on acceptance. The remainder of the patient's supply is prescribed in the usual way.
2. A small alcohol breath analyzer. Test for heavy drinking and tolerance.
3. Photocopies of one standard questionnaire (e.g., CAGE, MAST, short MAST, etc.) so the patient can be engaged in a neutral way.
4. The following telephone numbers:
   - Several willing members of AA of both sexes and various ethnic and occupational backgrounds who will respond to a telephone call, if possible while the patient is in the office.
   - The local AA Intergroup Office (see telephone directory) for help in finding AA members as above, and also for other members if those known are unavailable. The AA Intergroup office often knows which detoxification units have available beds.
   - A list (obtained from the telephone directory) of other alcoholism support groups in your area.
   - The local National Council on Alcoholism and Drug Dependence affiliate group for further screening and referral, especially to outpatient services.
   - Three or four of the available public and private inpatient detoxification units.
   - Three or four of the available public and private outpatient multidisciplinary programs.

counseling and social work services are frequently available. Many of these programs also handle the prescription of disulfiram and have AA meetings on their premises. More recently developed techniques, such as cognitive behavioral therapy, which are useful for some patients, are available through these programs. These specialized techniques are usually beyond the available time and expertise of gastroenterologists.

When voluntary approaches fail, coercion may become necessary. Sometimes it has already been applied by others. The spouse may be contemplating divorce. The job may be in danger. There may be court pressure after driving while intoxicated or family violence. In many states, legislation has tightened the requirement for prompt reporting to medical licensing agencies of alcoholic physicians. In these situations, the added use of mandatory disulfiram can be very helpful. Finally, a trusted physician confronted with patients' repeated alcoholic hemorrhage or pancreatitis may tell them that after the acute episode is over, he or she will no longer be responsible for their care if they do not immediately begin disulfiram under supervision and enter treatment for alcoholism. Coercive measures may seem harsh but the stakes are very high: alcoholism is a malignant disease.*

---

*Editor's Note: Bravo! Bravo! (two authors!)

SUGGESTED READING

Ewing JA. Detecting alcoholism: the CAGE questionnaire. JAMA 1984; 252:1905–1907.

Fuller RK, Branchey L, Brightwell DR, et al. Disulfiram treatment of alcoholism: a Veterans Administration cooperative study. JAMA 1986; 256:1449–1489.

Kadden RM, Cooney NL, Geffer H, Litt MD. Matching alcoholics to coping skills or interactional therapies: post treatment results. J Consult Clin Psychol 1989; 57:698–704.

Mayfield DG, McLeod G, Hall P. The CAGE questionnaire: validation of a new alcoholism screening instrument. Am J Psychiatry 1974; 131:1121–1123.

Moore RD, Bone LR, Geller G, et al. Prevalence, detection, and treatment of alcoholism in hospitalized patients. JAMA 1989; 261:403–407.

O'Malley SS, Jaffe AJ, Chang G, et al. Naltrexone and coping skills therapy for alcohol dependence: a controlled study. Arch Gen Psychiatry 1992; 49:881–887.

Sellers EM, Naranjo CA, Harrison M, et al. Diazepam loading: simplified treatment of alcohol withdrawal. Clin Pharmacol Ther 1983; 34:822–826.

Thompson WL, Johnson AD, Maddrey WL, Osler Medical Housestaff, Baltimore, MD. Diazepam and paraldehyde for treatment of severe delirium tremens: a controlled trial. Ann Intern Med 1975; 82:175–180.

Volpicelli JR, Alterman AI, Hayashida M, O'Brien CP. Naltrexone in the treatment of alcohol dependence. Arch Gen Psychiatry 1992; 49:876–880.

Wright C, Vafier JA, Lake CR. Disulfiram-induced fulminating hepatitis: Guidelines for liver-panel monitoring. J. Clinical Psychiatry 1988; 49:430–434.

ANOREXIA NERVOSA AND BULIMIA NERVOSA

BRUCE S. ROTHSCHILD, M.D.
JOSEPH M. NESTA, M.D.

Anorexia nervosa and bulimia nervosa are eating disorders of increasing prevalence, with a female-to-male ratio of 20:1. The rate of occurrence in high school and college age women is 0.5 percent for anorexia and 3 percent for bulimia.

The cause of these disorders is unknown, although a multifactorial perspective taking into account biologic perturbations, societal pressures, and psychological issues is empirically most useful. Briefly, women with these disorders often have a proclivity for weight instability, exist in a social context that overly prizes thinness, and need to cope with destructive personality patterns, family relationships, and/or traumatic life events.

Anorexia nervosa is a disorder of willful and dramatic starvation (Table 1). Patients lose body weight by starvation, compulsive exercise, and, at times, purging, with laxative and diuretic abuse. Their thoughts are marked by an overwhelming fear of fatness, and their perception is altered by a distorted body image. Thus, a 5 ft, 4 inch, 80 pound woman might not recognize the medical danger in which she is putting herself, as insight tends to atrophy along with body fat. Indeed, this difficulty in getting the patient to recognize she has a serious problem is one of the most challenging aspects of the disorder.

Table 1 DSM-III-R:* Diagnostic Criteria for Anorexia Nervosa

A. Refusal to maintain body weight over a minimal normal weight for age and height (e.g., weight loss leading to maintenance of body weight 15 percent below that expected; or failure to make expected weight gain during period of growth, leading to body weight 15 percent below that expected

B. Intense fear of gaining weight or becoming fat, even though underweight

C. Disturbance in the way in which one's body weight, size, or shape is experienced (e.g., the person claims to "feel fat" even when emaciated, believes that one area of the body is "too fat" even when obviously underweight)

D. In females, absence of at least three consecutive menstrual cycles when otherwise expected to occur (primary or secondary amenorrhea if the periods occur only after hormone [e.g., estrogen] administration)

---

*Diagnostic and Statistical Manual of Mental Disorders. 3rd ed. Revised.

Table 2 DSM-III-R: Diagnostic Criteria
for Bulimia Nervosa

A. Recurrent episodes of binge eating (rapid consumption of a large amount of food in a discrete period)
B. A feeling of lack of control over eating behavior during the eating binges
C. The person regularly engages in self-induced vomiting, use of laxatives or diuretics, strict dieting or fasting, or vigorous exercise in order to prevent weight gain
D. A minimal average of two binge-eating episodes a week for at least 3 months
E. Persistent overconcern with body shape and weight

Bulimia nervosa is a disorder of binge eating and purging (Table 2). The diagnosis is made irrespective of body weight and is defined by ingestion of huge amounts of calories in a short period in an uncontrollable fashion. This is usually followed by self-induced vomiting and is often accompanied by laxative or diuretic abuse.

Mortality rates for the two disorders range from 1 to 5 percent. Early detection and treatment by professionals who are informed both psychiatrically and medically improve the prognosis.

The remainder of this chapter focuses on treatment. General aspects of psychiatric treatment are covered, followed by more specific recommendations regarding the gastrointestinal (GI) complications associated with these disorders.

ANOREXIA NERVOSA

The level of severity of illness dictates the treatment setting. The percentage of ideal body weight may be the most important factor in this regard. We believe optimal inpatient treatment occurs with a psychiatric admission to a specialty eating disorder unit. This unit should be in a hospital and have access to experienced medical physicians and ancillary services.

The most basic function of intensive treatment for anorexia nervosa is helping the patient to begin to eat normally again. As anyone who has tried to "kick a habit" will attest, changing basic biologic behaviors is no easy feat. These patients need the imposed structure and support of a well-trained staff knowledgeable in eating disorders. Inpatient treatment is necessary for the most severely ill patients. Day hospital treatment, where available, is a less restrictive approach for patients able to muster some self-control and motivation. Indeed, the day hospital (in which, for example, patients attend a program 7 hours a day, 5 days a week) offers the advantage of providing structure and support for part of the week while allowing the patient to work on "self-feeding" while away from the program.

Weight restoration is the first order of business for the starved patient. Many abnormal eating habits, food preoccupations, rigid thinking patterns, and tendencies to depression can be reversed solely with the approximation of body weight back to the normal range.

What is the proper goal weight range for an individual patient? A combined approach using Metropolitan Life Table data along with the patient's personal weight history, particularly in regard to loss and resumption of menses, is crucial. A goal weight range slightly below normal can be a realistic compromise in that the patient is able to accept it and yet is spared medical complications.

Once a patient is in a safer weight range, treatment can ensue on an outpatient basis. This should occur at least once weekly, and the patient should be weighed regularly by the treating physician. She should be exhorted to refrain from weighing herself, as weight gains can precipitate panic and weight loss can lead to a downward spiral (the new lower weight becomes the maximal weight "allowed").

Psychotherapy usually occurs on a one-to-one basis, although there is evidence suggesting that family therapy is more useful for younger patients. Psychological issues are explored, but never at the expense of attending to weight and medical issues.

The utility of pharmacotherapy for anorexia nervosa is limited. Early trials of neuroleptics targeted at the "delusional" distorted body image proved to be without benefit. The best "antidepressant" for these patients tends to be food and normalization of body weight. Occasional use of a short-acting benzodiazapine, e.g., alprazolam, 0.25 mg 30 minutes before meals, for patients who are extremely anxious around mealtime can be beneficial.

Recently, there has been some suggestion through case reports that the serotonin reuptake blocker fluoxetine can aid anorectic patients with weight gain. This is counterintuitive, given fluoxetine's tendency to promote mild weight loss in several depressed patients for whom it was prescribed. However, it is possible that this agent has the ability to free the patient somewhat from rigid obsessional thinking. A daily dose of 20 mg would be likely, although 10 mg might be safer in a severely emaciated patient. Ultimately, up to 60 mg daily might be needed. Again, support for this approach remains anecdotal, and controlled studies need to be performed.

Finally, what about the patient who is not taking responsibility for getting better? A patient may see her psychiatrist weekly and the internist monthly and still continue to lose weight. The treating physicians can make all the right recommendations, including hospitalization, but it is ultimately the patient's decision whether to follow through with these. It is not in the patient's best interest to continue in therapy indefinitely in the face of noncompliance with the treatment plan of weight gain. If the patient cannot be kept medically safe as an outpatient, hospitalization is warranted. Involuntary psychiatric hospitalization is justified only in very rare circumstances and usually results in little benefit, because treatment alliance between physician and patient is needed to effect behavioral change. Patients who have become significantly medically compromised, but lack the insight or desire to work on their problem, are probably best served by a short-term medical admission to correct medical complications and reverse weight loss. Similarly, in the outpatient setting, if a patient is not able or willing to work on her eating disorder in therapy, the internist may remain involved to provide medical support and surveillance of the patient, e.g., on a monthly basis. Referral back to the psychiatrist for further therapy may be made when the patient is better able to actively work on her problem.

BULIMIA NERVOSA

Although patients with bulimia nervosa tend not to lose weight down to dangerously low levels, their health can be seriously jeopardized by their bulimic behaviors. Significant metabolic abnormalities can result from vomiting, laxative abuse, and diuretic abuse. The most common metabolic abnormality is a hypochloremic metabolic alkalosis. Hypokalemia is also common. Severe disturbances of this kind can lead to seizures, cardiac arrhythmia, and death.

In general, bulimic patients can be treated outside the hospital setting. However, patients who are binge eating and purging numerous times daily, and experiencing frequent medical complications, need inpatient or perhaps day hospital treatment. In ambulatory treatment, laboratories should be checked on a regular basis, depending on the symptoms of the patient. This may range from following electrolytes once monthly to once every 6 months.

Psychotherapy for bulimia often includes the patient's keeping a meal record or a food journal that is reviewed weekly. Along with this focus on food intake, the therapy tries to correct cognitive distortions involving diet, weight, and esteem. Emphasis is placed on improving destructive interpersonal relationship patterns, which usually have a role in initiating and maintaining the disorder.

Comorbid diagnoses are more common with bulimia nervosa than with anorexia nervosa. The experienced clinician will be on the lookout for substance abuse, major depression, or borderline personality disorders in patients with bulimia. These conditions need to be diagnosed, and then properly treated, in order to maximize therapeutic impact.

Unlike anorexia nervosa, there is clearly a strong role for medication in the treatment of these patients. Numerous antidepressant trials have been run, and essentially have all shown effect compared with placebo. Antidepressants of all types are included: tricyclics, monoamine oxidase inhibitors, trazodone, buproprion, and the selective serotonin reuptake inhibitors (SSRIs), such as fluoxetine, sertraline, and paroxetine. These medications are useful independent of a comorbid diagnosis of major depression. Thus, it is important to stress that all the agents marketed as antidepressants are also effective antibulimic drugs.

Which agent to choose? The advent of fluoxetine and the SSRIs that have followed have changed prescription habits immensely. The SSRIs generally do not promote weight gain as most of the other antidepressants potentially do. This is an extremely important selling point in trying to convince a reluctant patient to take medication when she is already overconcerned about body weight. Also, SSRIs tend to be better tolerated in general than the older antidepressants. A special warning should be made for buproprion: it is generally contraindicated in this population, as pretrial studies resulted in a significantly higher incidence of seizures in bulimic patients.

Laboratory tests should be made upon initiating a medication (complete blood count, SMAC, and one set of thyroid function tests should suffice). Fluoxetine is a good first-line drug and is started at 20 mg daily; if, after 1 month, only marginal improvement has occurred, the dosage can be doubled. This is often the maximal dose needed, but some patients require 60 mg daily in a single morning dose. When the medication is effective, patients report a decrease in their desire to binge and general improvement in mood stability.

For patients who do not respond to fluoxetine, it is reasonable to try another SSRI such as sertraline, 50 to 100 mg daily, or a tricyclic antidepressant with a relatively favorable side effect profile such as nortriptyline or desipramine. For example, nortriptyline can be started at 25 mg at bedtime, increased to 50 mg after 4 days, and then increased to 75 mg after another 4 days. This last dose is frequently sufficient to reach the targeted therapeutic blood level (between 50 and 150 mg per milliliter). A blood level should be drawn 5 days after reaching this dose, and future dosing adjustments should be made accordingly. Potential side effects of lightheadedness, dry mouth, and constipation should be discussed with the patient. For patients who are actively bulimic, an electrocardiogram should be obtained either before or at the start of treatment.

Some patients with bulimia represent a significant suicidal risk. All such patients, of course, should be seen concurrently by a psychiatrist. Prescribing for these patients is often best done by the psychiatrist so that the prescription of the medication can be incorporated into the psychotherapeutic process. Two week supplies with one refill are usually a safe way to dispense for this higher-risk population.

GASTROINTESTINAL MANAGEMENT

The gastroenterologist's evaluation of a patient with a suspected eating disorder requires a comprehensive medical assessment, including history, physical examination, laboratory blood studies, and anthropometric measurements. The most useful of these measurements are the patient's height, current weight, and percentage of ideal body weight. The patient's usual weight also has clinical significance. A weight loss greater than 10 percent of usual weight occurring within 1 to 2 months, or a weight less than 70 percent of usual weight, is a concern. Calorie and protein requirements are determined per individual patient. The patient's weight is consistently monitored. A typical initial diet is 1,200 to 1,500 calories per day and 50 to 70 g protein per day. Caloric adjustments are made weekly to ensure a weight gain of 2 to 4 pounds per week. When the goal weight is achieved, a maintenance caloric diet is utilized.

Anorectic patients are fed orally. If they are unable to tolerate regular food, oral liquid nutritional supplements are used. Rare patients who refuse to eat and are medically compromised as a result of this malnutrition, or consistently fail to gain satisfactory weight, may require enteric tube feedings or intravenous (IV) fluids.

GI problems encountered in patients with an eating disorder are reviewed by organ involvement. Bulimic patients, with their characteristic history of ingesting large quantities of food with high carbohydrate content and repetitive volitional vomiting, can develop significant dental disease. Injury to the lingual surfaces of teeth precipitated by the chemical action of the regurgitated gastric contents, and aggravated by the mechanical action of the tongue against the teeth, causes loss of dentin and enamel. This is perimylolysis. Patients with perimylolysis complain of hot and cold temperature sensitivity and have an increased incidence of dental caries. The incidence of dental caries may also be affected by bulimics' high carbohydrate intake. Evaluation by a dentist is recommended when these conditions are present.

Enlargement of parotid glands is commonly noted in patients with eating disorders. It may be painless or painful, and the exact pathophysiology remains unresolved. The observation that benign parotid enlargement occurs in obese patients, and in patients with restrictive diets without anorexia nervosa or bulimia nervosa, has led to the speculation that for bulimic patients, this is secondary to their commonly noted underlying obesity, while for anorectic patients, this is secondary to underlying malnutrition.

Hyperamylasemia is also common in these patients. When the amylase has been analyzed, it is frequently the salivary-type isoamylase. In bulimic patients, this elevated serum amylase has been observed during periods of active purging, with resolution of the hyperamylasemia when this behavior has resolved. It is postulated that repeated vomiting may injure the salivary glands or induce hypersalivation, causing this hyperamylasemic state.

Hyperamylasemia with abdominal pain may also represent acute pancreatitis. Acute pancreatitis, although infrequent, has been documented in patients with anorexia nervosa. When reported, pancreatitis occurs in severely malnourished patients during the refeeding phase of treatment. It responds to conventional therapy for acute pancreatitis.*

Rumination can also occur in patients with eating disorders. Recently ingested food fills the oral cavity 10 to 15 minutes after eating; this can be expectorated, rechewed, or reswallowed, only to reappear in a cyclic fashion. This is an involuntary action that lasts approximately 30 minutes and then ceases. It is not associated with nausea; it can be associated with a neuromotility disorder of the esophagus and stomach. Rumination can be extremely difficult to treat. Biofeedback techniques have been used.

It is not unexpected that symptoms suggestive of esophageal disease are seen in patients with eating disorders. Anorectics, with their delayed gastric emptying, and bulimics, with their frequent purging, may experience heartburn, regurgitation, and chest pain (classic symptoms of gastroesophageal reflux disease). Thus, esophagitis, esophageal erosions, esophageal strictures, and Barrett's esophagus can develop. Gastroesophageal reflux, with its complications, respond in this population to conventional therapy. Bulimics, with their repeated retching and vomiting, are at risk for esophageal rupture (Boerhaave's syndrome), gastric rupture, and Mallory-Weiss tears.

Acute gastric retention can occur with refeeding or binge eating and can result in gastric rupture. The usual clinical presentation for acute gastric retention is rapid onset of nausea, vomiting, and abdominal pain with abdominal distention, with gastric or gastroenteric dilation seen radiographically. This distention responds to making the patient NPO, with nasogastric suction and IV fluids. If peritoneal signs are present, or free air is seen radiographically, IV antibiotics and surgical consultation are indicated.

Gastric motility disorders are very common in anorexia nervosa. Delayed gastric emptying occurs in at least 80 percent of patients with this disease and may involve solid or solid and liquid phase emptying. It is unclear whether this is primary, secondary, or an epiphenomenon of this disorder. The observation that the severity of the malnutrition influences the magnitude of these symptoms, and that refeeding anorectic patients often improves their symptoms, suggests that dysfunctional emptying may be secondary to the anorexia nervosa. The delayed gastric emptying may not be totally reversible after restoration of body weight. Pharmacologic intervention may be required with severe symptoms. Bethanechol, 25 mg orally four times a day, or metoclopramide, 10 mg orally 30 minutes before meals and at bedtime, have been utilized. Both drugs have limitations. Bethanechol can cause abdominal cramping, urinary frequency, and blurred vision in these dosages. Depression and tardive dyskinesia can occur with metoclopramide. Cisapride or domperidone may prove more effective with this population.

Basal and stimulated gastric acid output are decreased in anorexia nervosa, as noted in the limited literature studies, in which both measurements failed to return to control levels with refeeding.

No consistent structural abnormalities of the stomach or small intestine in patients with anorexia nervosa have been seen radiographically.

The most commonly encountered symptoms of colonic dysfunction are constipation and diarrhea. Fre-

---

*Editor's Note: This is reminiscent of the occasional college wrestler who starves to drop a weight class and then binges on steak after weighing in, only to develop pancreatitis.

quently, underlying laxative abuse is the cause. This can occur in an anorectic patient but is more often seen in bulimics. These patients commonly complain of constipation, or alternating diarrhea and constipation, often associated with nausea, vomiting, and weight loss. Concomitant usage of diuretics and vomiting can complicate their management.

Chronic laxative abuse leads to a "cathartic colon": a dilated, hypotonic colon with loss of haustrations, often on only one side. Histologic damage to the ganglion cells in Auerbach's plexus may be seen and can contribute to poor colonic tone and the often present constipation. Chronic ingestion of anthraquinone laxatives can cause a brownish-black discoloration of the colonic mucosa (melanosis coli).

Constipation can be difficult to manage in these patients. It has been our practice to start most eating disorder patients on docusate sodium, 100 mg orally twice a day. Any electrolyte or volume imbalances are corrected. All medications are reviewed. If an agent produces a high incidence of constipation, an alternative is suggested. Consideration is given to exclude other conditions that may present with constipation, such as hypothyroidism. Judicious intake of fluids and exercise is encouraged. Bulk laxatives are initially tried unless the patient has a known cathartic colon or has prominent symptoms of delayed gastric emptying. In these cases, a low-residue diet is employed. If these interventions fail, subsequent therapies include use of osmotic laxatives, enemas, or polyethylene glycol agents. On initial presentation, patients who consume large amounts of laxatives are tapered off these agents. We try to minimize use of stimulant laxatives.

In refractory cases, or cases with alarming presentations such as Hemoccult-positive stools or high clinical suspicion of intestinal obstruction, further evaluation is required. This entails radiographic investigation: abdominal x-rays, barium studies or serial KUBs after ingestion of radiopaque markers, endoscopy, or manometry.

There are isolated case reports of laxative abuse causing protein-losing enteropathy and steatorrhea.

Finally, significant elevations of liver function test results have not been routinely seen in patients with eating disorders. Mild elevations in transaminase may be noted while anorectic patients are refed. This probably reflects mild steatosis or hepatic glycogen deposition, and tends to normalize with time.

It is important to realize that GI complaints are extremely common in patients with eating disorders. Waldholtz and Andersen studied GI symptoms in 16 consecutive anorexia nervosa patients. They noted that, with refeeding and psychiatric treatment, statistically significant symptom improvement occurred in the anorexia, constipation, diarrhea, vomiting, and early and late meal-associated bloating. Abdominal pain, nausea, and heartburn improved, but not to statistically significant levels. This conclusion is confirmed in our clinical experience. Aggressive initial evaluation of all GI symptoms may not be warranted and in fact may be counter-productive to therapy. The fasting required to perform many of these tests, and the additional time needed, can cause these patients to miss meals, which can lead to additional loss of nutritional support. This is not to imply that these symptoms should be neglected. Persistent and unprovoked vomiting, persistent reflux symptoms refractory to conventional therapy, inappropriate weight gain, Hemoccult-positive stools, exacerbation of symptoms associated with well-documented previous GI diseases, and hemodynamically compromised GI bleedings or refractory constipation require further evaluation.

A comprehensive initial evaluation with a conservative approach to medical therapy, combined with medical monitoring for contributory pathologic states, provide the best clinical outcome for patients with eating disorders.

SUGGESTED READING

Comerci GD. Medical complications of anorexia nervosa and bulimia nervosa. Med Clin North Am 1990; 74:1293–1310.

Cuellar RE, Van Thiel DH. Gastrointestinal consequences of the eating disorders: anorexia nervosa and bulimia. Am J Gastroenterol 1986; 7:1113–1121.

Herzog DB, Copeland PM. Eating disorders. N Engl J Med 1985; 313:295–303.

Lucas AR, Callaway CW. Anorexia nervosa and bulimia in Bockus' gastroenterology 1985; 7:4416–4434.

Waldholtz BD, Andersen AE. Gastrointestinal symptoms in anorexia nervosa: a prospective study. Gastroenterology 1990; 98:1415–1419.

Webb WL. A clinical review of developments in the diagnosis and treatment of anorexia nervosa and bulimia. Psychiatr Med 1988; 6:24–38.

Diagnostic and statistical manual of mental disorders. 3rd ed. Revised. Washington, D.C.: American Psychiatric Association, 1987.

CHRONIC ABDOMINAL PAIN IN CHILDREN AND ADOLESCENTS

RALPH P. KINGSFORD, M.D.
MELVIN B. HEYMAN, M.D., M.P.H.

Chronic abdominal pain syndrome in children and adolescents is defined as recurrent or persistent abdominal pain that lasts longer than 3 months. It is one of the most perplexing and difficult problems that confronts practitioners involved in the care of children and adolescents. Chronic abdominal pain is a source of frustration to both patients and families, especially when it interferes with daily activity. Up to 30 percent of school age girls and 12 percent of school age boys are reported to have symptoms consistent with chronic recurrent abdominal pain. Only about 5 to 15 percent of children and adolescents with chronic abdominal pain have a diagnosable organic cause, although this percentage may increase as diagnostic methods evolve and improve. Physicians must convey confidence and trust and approach these children and adolescents with a systematic and thorough investigation of the causes of the symptoms. Consultation with a pediatric gastroenterologist experienced in evaluating and treating affected patients may be helpful in formulating an appropriate management plan.

DEFINITION

Chronic abdominal pain can be classified into two major categories: organic and nonorganic.

Organic Abdominal Pain

Chronic recurrent abdominal pain due to an underlying organic cause is often associated with reproducible and consistent findings on abdominal examination. The pain, usually distant from the umbilicus, frequently awakens the patient from sleep. Other associated complaints may consist of fever, vomiting, diarrhea and/or bloody stools, and weight loss. Laboratory screening may be useful.

The differential diagnosis for organic causes of abdominal pain is extensive. Some of the more commonly encountered conditions are listed in Table 1; readers should refer to appropriate chapters in this book to find more information about the treatment of these specific disorders.

Carbohydrate intolerance, primarily lactose intolerance, is the most common diagnosable cause of abdominal pain in childhood. Cramping pain due to carbohydrate malabsorption is often associated with bloating, flatulence, and diarrhea. Sorbitol, found in some fruit juices and "sugar-free" products, can cause symptoms,

Table 1 Causes of Chronic Abdominal Pain in Children and Adolescents

Gastrointestinal
  Carbohydrate intolerance
  Acid-peptic disease
    Helicobacter pylori
  Irritable bowel syndrome
  Inflammatory bowel disease
  Pancreatitis
  Henoch-Schönlein purpura
  Hemolytic-uremic syndrome
  Appendicitis
  Mesenteric adenitis
  Cholelithiasis

Genitourinary
  Urinary tract infection
  Pyelonephritis
  Pelvic inflammatory disease
  Dysmenorrhea

Miscellaneous
  Musculoskeletal
  Neurologic (migraine-equivalent)
  Metabolic (porphyria)
  Familial Mediterranean fever
  Child abuse (physical or mental)

especially abdominal pain, when ingested in large amounts.

Acid-peptic disease is suggested by epigastric pain, often appearing 60 to 90 minutes postprandially, and is classically described by the cycle of pain relieved by food ingestion followed again by pain. Primary gastritis is rarely (less than 5 percent) associated with *Helicobacter pylori* in younger children, but in adolescents the prevalence approaches that of adults. Upper endoscopy with biopsy can confirm a diagnosis of ulcer disease, inflammatory infiltrates, or *H. pylori* infection. Esophagitis due to gastroesophageal reflux may cause chronic epigastric pain and should be suspected particularly in children and adolescents with chronic pulmonary disease.

Of pediatric patients with inflammatory bowel disease, 50 to 70 percent initially complain of abdominal pain. Abdominal pain is a more frequent symptom in Crohn's disease than in ulcerative colitis. The pain often is postprandial, localized to the right lower quadrant. Fever, weight loss, growth retardation, sexual immaturity, and a variety of extraintestinal manifestations may be present. Ulcerative colitis is almost always associated with bloody diarrhea and symptoms of rectosigmoid disease.

Dysmenorrhea and pelvic inflammatory disease may cause persistent pain in adolescent females. Dysmenorrhea may be suspected when pain is pre- or perimenstrual.

No organic etiology for the abdominal pain is found in up to 95 percent of patients presenting to the physician. Of these, about 50 to 60 percent are eventually evaluated by a pediatric gastroenterologist.

The treatment of organic causes of abdominal pain can be found in the appropriate chapters.

Nonorganic Abdominal Pain

Nonorganic chronic abdominal pain can be sub-classified as (1) dysfunctional abdominal pain and (2) psychogenic pain. Up to 90 percent of children and adolescents with chronic abdominal pain are reported to fall into a dysfunctional category. Most of these patients have altered bowel motility (irritable bowel syndrome [IBS]); a smaller group with epigastric discomfort have nonulcer dyspepsia. Psychological problems account for a few adolescents and, less commonly, children with chronic abdominal pain. Patients in this category have varying levels of complaints that are often difficult to differentiate from organic etiologies, particularly when patients and families have medical knowledge or family members with organic disease.

PATHOPHYSIOLOGY OF NONORGANIC CHRONIC ABDOMINAL PAIN

Little is known about the mechanisms involved in nonorganic chronic abdominal pain. Intestinal mucosa is devoid of nerve endings that serve as pain receptors. However, serosal surfaces contain abundant propriocep-tive receptors that are sensitive to distention of the bowel wall.

Hereditary and familial factors have some causal relationship. The link to altered bowel motility, however, is poorly understood. Studies of older adolescents suggest a hyperactive colonic response to various stimuli, including mechanical distention with a balloon, food stimulation, and emotional arousal. Provocative studies using common neurotransmitters (e.g., catecholamines, serotonin) have not been revealing.

Recent attempts have been made to relate motility disorders to autonomic dysfunction, since many symptoms associated with chronic abdominal pain, such as dizziness and headaches, could be explained on the basis of autonomic dysfunction. Such studies to date have been inconclusive, however.

IBS is characterized by alterations in bowel habits with either constipation or diarrhea; occasionally, both occur in the same patient. Children and younger adolescents have features typical of a childhood-type of IBS, with abdominal pain as the primary manifestation and mild to nonexistent changes in bowel habits. Adolescents and adults present with either prominent constipation or diarrhea.

CLINICAL PRESENTATION

In children with nonorganic chronic recurrent ab-dominal pain, the pain is usually episodic, occurring at least three times during a 3 month span. The pain may be diffuse, localized, or variable in location but is typically described as periumbilical (Apley's rule) and cramping. Activity is usually not disrupted and sleep is not disturbed. Two-thirds of patients complain of other symptoms, including fatigue, nausea, headaches, dizzi-ness, eructation, and flatulence. Weight gain and growth are not affected, unless overzealous dietary restrictions are imposed, often by an overbearing parent. Physical examination is usually unremarkable or inconsistent with the primary complaints, with some nonspecific generalized tenderness on palpation without guarding, rigidity, or rebound. Findings of laboratory investiga-tions, radiologic imaging studies, and endoscopy (if performed) are normal.

Adult-type IBS is occasionally observed in adoles-cents. The pain is often periumbilical and lower abdomi-nal and is relieved by defecation, although many patients complain of a sensation of incomplete evacuation after defecation. The onset of pain is associated with looser stools, increased stool frequency, and abdominal disten-tion. Constipation is more common than diarrhea. Patients with IBS often have obsessive-compulsive personalities and tend to be high achievers.*

Nonulcer dyspepsia is a poorly understood and imprecise term. It can be defined as chronic or recurrent upper abdominal pain or nausea that may or may not be related to meals. Patients may also complain of bloating, early satiety, eructation, and, occasionally, anorexia. The differential diagnosis includes gastroesophageal reflux, gastric motility disorders, and biliary dyskinesia. No discernible laboratory or histologic abnormalities can be found. Chronic pancreatitis is an uncommon condition in the pediatric age group and is sometimes confused with nonulcer dyspepsia.

Psychogenic chronic abdominal pain typically is not associated with an underlying organic cause but often provides some form of secondary gain for the patient. However, patients with significant organic disorders may also realize positive reactions to their complaints, so an appropriate evaluation should be performed as clinically indicated in order not to overlook organic problems that may accompany psychosocial issues. It is easier to diagnose pain of a psychogenic origin when it is accompanied by a psychiatric condition, such as depres-sion or conversion reaction. Helpful diagnostic features include the presence of a personality disorder (e.g., hysteria), a strong family history of psychiatric illness, or an obvious unresolved emotional or stressful situation. Predisposing factors may consist of a recent move or change of school, family dynamics, relations with friends, and serious illness or death of a family member or friend.

DIAGNOSIS

A detailed history and thorough physical examina-tion are essential to obtain useful diagnostic clues that help discriminate between an organic and nonorganic etiology (Table 2). Often, a simultaneous diagnostic and therapeutic approach is the most useful way to approach the problem, expanding the level of investigation on the basis of patient response and degree of abnormality.

****Editor's Note:** As adults, these individuals frequently seem to choose accounting, bookkeeping, computing, or administrative careers. Asking about childhood or young adult abdominal or bowel problems is sometimes helpful when evaluating adults with possible IBS.

Table 2 Clinical Approach to Children and Adolescents with Chronic Recurrent Abdominal Pain Syndrome

Evaluation	Treatment
Initial	
Thorough history and physical examination	Reassurance; be available
CBC, ESR, urinalysis including microscopic evaluation, urine culture	Build trust
Optional	
Stool O&P, C&S, ELISA for *Giardia*	Education
Lead level	Ensure patient expectations are included in treatment plan
Liver enzymes	
Amylase	Avoid medication
Carbohydrate (lactose) hydrogen breath test	Counseling
Abdominal/pelvic sonography	Stress management
Flexible sigmoidoscopy	Psychiatric evaluation
Upper/lower endoscopy including biopsies	
Radiographic studies including abdominal plain films	
Rarely indicated	
Manometry	Temporary separation from family
ERCP	
Laparoscopy/laparotomy	Hospitalization

CBC = complete blood count; ESR = erythrocyte sedimentation rate; O&P = ova and parasites; C&S = culture and sensitivity; ELISA = enzyme-linked immunosorbent assay; ERCP = endoscopic retrograde cholangiopancreatography.

All patients should undergo an initial screening consisting of a complete blood count, erythrocyte sedimentation rate, urinalysis with microscopic examination and possibly a urine culture, and stool for occult blood and white blood cells. Stool for ova and parasites (and enzyme-linked immunosorbent assay [ELISA] for *Giardia*), lead level, blood tests for liver enzymes and amylase, lactose (or other carbohydrate) hydrogen breath tests, sonography, flexible sigmoidoscopy, upper and lower endoscopy, and radiographic studies are obtained if clinically indicated. Invasive studies such as manometry, laparoscopy, and laparotomy are performed only when clearly indicated.

TREATMENT OF NONORGANIC CHRONIC ABDOMINAL PAIN

Excellent communication and trust are important factors in approaching these cases, so that patients and families can direct their attention away from the overt symptoms and focus on the underlying issues. A thorough history and physical examination and screening laboratory studies can help reassure families that while the pain is real, no physical abnormality exists.

The physician should be accessible and have a positive attitude regarding the resolution of symptoms; when an organic etiology is not involved, most symptoms resolve with time. Hence, medications should be used sparingly. Denial and shyness are defense mechanisms and should be approached in a sensitive, but deliberate manner. Terms such as *emotional, psychogenic,* and *stress-related* are interpreted as "imaginary or manipulative" and could alienate the patient and family. The older child's and adolescent's perceptions of his or her symptoms and expectations should be tailored into treatment goals and discussed openly.

Reassurance and education are essential. Patients should be advised to maintain a regular meal pattern. Dietary manipulation is controversial and should be avoided unless specific food intolerances are documented. Dietary fiber additives have been beneficial in only about 40 percent of cases; fiber supplementation can exacerbate flatulence, abdominal distention, and abdominal pain. Unless other diagnoses coexist, medications, including stool softeners, and antispasmodic and antidiarrheal agents, have no role in treating children and adolescents with chronic recurrent abdominal pain. Rarely, intervention with special techniques such as biofeedback, relaxation, and stress management are necessary. These require the input of appropriate professionals. A pediatrician specializing in behavioral issues, a school counselor, or a clinical psychologist can be particularly helpful in evaluating and treating these children. Hospitalization is seldom necessary but may be useful to provide a period of separation of the patient from other family members and to allow objective assessment of the complaints. Patients with significant psychogenic pain may require psychiatric intervention.

For patients with IBS in whom constipation is an associated symptom, mineral oil (plain) or lactulose may prove beneficial. (Please see the chapter *Constipation in Children.*) Suppositories and enemas should be avoided to prevent discomfort and to thwart family struggles that may interfere with subsequent therapy. When gas and distention are predominant symptoms, simethicone and charcoal may be helpful. The diarrhea in these patients may respond to increased dietary or supplemental fiber or antispasmodic agents. Increased physical activity and initiation of a postprandial bowel movement regimen, with a reward system encouraging patient cooperation, may normalize the bowel patterns of patients with IBS and provide symptomatic relief.

SUGGESTED READING

Apley J, Hale B. Children with recurrent abdominal pain: how do they grow up? Br Med J 1973; 3:7–9.

Galler JR, Neustein S, Walker WA. Clinical aspects of recurrent abdominal pain in children. Adv Pediatr 1980; 27:31–53.

Garber J, Zeman J, Walker LS. Recurrent abdominal pain in children: psychiatric diagnoses and parental psychopathology. J Am Acad Child Adolesc Psychiatry 1990; 29:648–656.

Silverberg M. Chronic abdominal pain in adolescents. Pediatr Ann 1991; 20:179–185.

Stickler G, Murphy D. Recurrent abdominal pain. Am J Dis Child 1979; 133: 486–489.

Stone RJ, Barbero GJ. Recurrent abdominal pain in childhood. Pediatrics 1970; 45:732–738.

Walker LS, Greene JW. Children with recurrent abdominal pain and their parents. J Pediatr Psychol 1989; 14:231–243.

IRRITABLE BOWEL SYNDROME

W. GRANT THOMPSON, M.D.

As defined by the Rome criteria (Table 1), the irritable bowel syndrome (IBS) occurs in 10 to 15 percent of adults in Western countries. If other functional bowel syndromes such as functional diarrhea or functional bloating are included, the figure is much higher (Table 2). Fortunately, most individuals with IBS do not seek attention for this chronic, benign disorder, and most of those who do are satisfactorily managed by their primary care physician. The few referred to specialists constitute a large portion of their practice and often present difficult management problems. This chapter provides a management strategy for the gastroenterologist.

PATHOGENESIS

The cause and mechanisms of IBS symptoms are unknown. IBS does not appear to be purely a motility

Table 1 Rome Criteria

At least 3 months of continuous or recurrent symptoms of
1. abdominal pain or discomfort that is
   (a) relieved with defecation
   (b) and/or associated with a change in frequency of stool
   (c) and/or associated with a change in consistency of stool

and

2. two or more of the following at least one-quarter of occasions or days:
   (a) altered stool frequency*
   (b) altered stool form (lumpy/hard or loose/watery stool)
   (c) altered stool passage (straining, urgency), or feeling of incomplete evacuation
   (d) passage of mucus,
   (e) bloating or feeling of abdominal distention

*For research purposes, "altered" may be defined as >3 bowel movements/day or <3 bowel movements/wk.
From Thompson WG, Creed F, Drossman DA, et al. Functional bowel disorders and chronic functional abdominal pain. Gastroent Int 1992; 5:75–91.

Table 2 Functional Disorders of the Intestines

C. *Functional bowel disorders*
  C1 Irritable bowel syndrome
  C2 Functional abdominal bloating
  C3 Functional constipation
  C4 Functional diarrhea
  C5 Unspecified functional bowel disorder

D. *Functional abdominal pain*
  D1 Functional abdominal pain syndrome
  D2 Unspecified functional abdominal pain

From Thompson WG, Creed F, Drossman DA, et al. Functional bowel disorders and chronic functional abdominal pain. Gastroent Int 1992; 5:75–91; with permission.

disorder, since we are unable to measure physiologic events in the gut that are coincident with symptoms. However, the small and large intestines of IBS patients are hypersensitive or hyperreactive to stimuli such as eating, drugs, hormones, intraluminal distention, and emotional and physical stress. The cause of IBS symptoms may some day be found in the enteric nervous system (ENS) and its signals to and from the brain. The ENS or "gut brain" is very complex. It manages gut function through the interaction of gut hormones, neurotransmitters, and nerve plexes, all modified by events in the environment, the brain, and the gut itself. Thus, IBS pain may be as much due to an abnormal perception of normal gut physiologic events as to a normal perception of abnormal gut events. The gut symptoms must therefore be seen in the context of the patient's physical and psychosocial environment.

CLINICAL SETTING

Any management plan must take into account the special circumstances of those who consult gastroenterologists. IBS is a chronic, recurring disorder without cure and without dire consequences. By all physical measures, it is a benign disease. IBS subjects in the community who do not see doctors have a psychological and personality profile similar to that of the unaffected population. Most of those who see a primary care physician are satisfactorily managed there. Why, then, do a small group see specialists? Patients often volunteer that their symptoms are more severe than those suffered by others, and it may be so. However, it is also well-known that IBS patients seen in tertiary care centers have more psychological problems than other patients and normal controls. They are also more likely to have suffered a threatening life event in the months before consultation, such as a death in the family or loss of a job or spouse. Still others resort to illness behavior to achieve some secondary gain with family, employer, or disability insurer.

Some patients may blame psychological difficulties on the physical symptoms. In others, the often unstated psychosocial difficulties constitute a "hidden agenda" (Table 3). The somatic symptoms can be troublesome and severe in their own right, but it is their interaction with the patient's psychosocial environment that complicates management, inhibits acceptance, and prompts referral. A treatment approach that does not include measures to address the hidden agenda is likely to be unsuccessful.

MANAGEMENT STRATEGY

The patient who is referred to a gastroenterologist is one of a minority of sufferers who have sought help from physicians, and a still smaller group who have been unsatisfied by their encounter with primary care. The following approach to such patients includes discussion of the first clinical encounter, the follow-up visit and

Table 3 The Hidden Agenda

Insecurity with diagnosis
    Fear of serious disease
    Cancerphobia

Dissatisfaction with treatment

Threatening life event
    Loss of spouse
    Loss of job
    Death in family
    Physical or sexual abuse

Depression, anxiety, hypochondria, pain, panic.

Secondary gain (illness behavior)
    Dependent relationship
    Manipulation of employer or family
    Disability pension

Table 4 Management Strategy

First clinical encounter
    Confirm diagnosis and convince patient
    Determine previous tests and treatments
    Rational use of tests—ensure clean colon
    Bran
    Determine hidden agenda and advise

Follow-up visit (6–8 wk later)
    Ensure acceptance of diagnosis
    Confirm explanation and compliance with advice
    In unimproved patient:
        Resist temptation to reinvestigate
        Stress management, relaxation (see next chapter)
        Treat depression, anxiety
        Limited use of drugs for specific symptoms (Table 5)

The difficult patient
    Regular, brief visits
    Specific referrals:
        Psychiatrist
        Esteemed colleague
        Behavior and psychology treatments if available
    Ensure continuing care with primary care physician and
        gastroenterologist

establishment of continuing care, and the management of the especially difficult patient (Table 4).

First Clinical Encounter

Positive Diagnosis

The first task is to confirm the diagnosis as firmly and credibly as possible. The symptoms should be reviewed in detail. The Rome criteria in Table 1 serve as a guide to identify IBS features. Some patients do not quite fulfill the IBS criteria and might fit better in one of the other diagnostic groupings suggested in Table 2. History taking should include a search for symptoms that cannot be explained by IBS, such as bleeding, anemia, weight loss, or fever. One should also be suspicious of organic disease if the symptoms occur frequently at night or if they begin late in life.

Many drugs affect the gut. In particular, the physician should inquire about the use of opiates, calcium channel blockers, antibiotics, and laxatives. If diarrhea is a dominant symptom, one should consider the possibility of lactose intolerance or excessive use of caffeine or sorbitol (an artificial sugar used in diet gums). A dietary history is important to exclude fad diets and to establish whether the fiber intake is satisfactory. Beyond these factors, it is unlikely that any dietary factor is the "trigger" of IBS. Physical examination should be thorough and will be negative. These referred patients very often have abdominal scars from the removal of a normal gallbladder, appendix, or uterus.

The patient should be carefully questioned about previous consultations. Often the referred patient has visited many physicians, and tests have been done unnecessarily and repeatedly. It is usually best that they not be repeated.

Ordinarily the gastroenterologist will wish to perform a sigmoidoscopy. This test enables inflammatory bowel disease (IBD) or perianal disorders to be excluded, but most importantly it is of therapeutic benefit. Confidence in the diagnosis of IBS is the foundation of its management, and the patient needs to know that the physician has taken the symptoms seriously enough to look at the bowel.

Special circumstances may indicate further tests, e.g., a family history of IBD, endemic giardiasis, or suspected lactose intolerance (especially in non-Caucasians). In a typical IBS patient without symptoms or signs of organic disease, the tests should not be exhaustive. If not previously given to a patient over 40 years old, a barium enema is prudent. The Rome criteria are not symptoms of colorectal carcinoma, but it is best that the management relationship start with a clean colon.

Reassurance

Once the diagnosis is firm, the physician should set about convincing the patient. The possible reasons for the patient's concerns should be explored: for example, cancer in the family, anxiety, hypochondriasis, or pressure of friends and relatives. Diagnostic tests should be kept to the necessary minimum, since they increase anxiety and insecurity ("If the doctor is uncertain of the diagnosis how can I be otherwise?"). Explaining IBS to a patient is difficult but important. One may start by describing its frequency in the population, its unknown cause, and its benign nature. It may be compared with a headache: just as severe pain can occur in an apparently normal head, severe abdominal pain can occur in an apparently normal gut. The complex gut contractions required to move contents through the long intestinal tract can be explained, along with the functions of the ENS and its obvious connections with the brain. The relation of symptoms to stress and anxiety can be illustrated by having the patient recall the varied gut reactions of classmates before college examinations.

Once convinced of the diagnosis, the patient may be reassured of its benign nature. Reassurance may prove to be the gastroenterologist's most effective therapeutic weapon.

Dietary Fiber

Even if the patient claims to be on a high-fiber diet or is taking a psyllium preparation, it is seldom that enough fiber is ingested to have an impact on gut function. There are no clinical trials that establish the benefit of bran for IBS. Nonetheless, bran is effective in the constipated phase of the syndrome and is a safe and inexpensive way to recruit the 40 to 60 percent placebo response. I usually start the patient on 1 tablespoon of bran three times a day with meals. I explain that the object is to use bran's water-holding capacity to expand the stool, which ensures more adequate stimulation of gut reflexes such as the urge to defecate. The result should be less hard or difficult-to-pass stools and a regularization of bowel action. There may be an increase in flatulence or bloating during the first week of bran ingestion. Commercial psyllium and fiber preparations are satisfactory alternatives, provided that they are taken regularly and in sufficient quantity.

The Hidden Agenda

On this first visit, careful attention should be paid to the hidden agenda. Why has the patient chosen this occasion to visit a specialist? Why is he or she unsatisfied with the care of the primary care physician? Possible answers are dissatisfaction with the diagnosis, fear that some sinister disease is being missed, or the desire for a more effective treatment for the somatic symptoms. Others have mistakenly been put on a low-roughage or unnecessarily restrictive diet, have lost weight, and are sure they have cancer. More subtle, of course, are psychosocial problems. The high likelihood that the patient has suffered abuse or a threatening life event in the months leading up to the consultation indicates that these might be more important than the somatic symptoms themselves. At least, such an event may impair the patient's ability to cope with the symptoms. Many patients suffer depression or anxiety that is amenable to specific management. Although the patient seems convinced that the symptoms cause the psychological distress, it seems more likely that psychological distress complicates or exaggerates the symptoms. The patient's relationships with other family members should be explored. It is also wise to establish whether a disability pension is at issue.

Sometimes the hidden agenda is easily dealt with. A man long suffering from IBS symptoms who has a close relative die of cancer of the colon may need only to be convinced that he has no such disease. Overt depression or extreme anxiety might be managed by pharmacotherapy. Explanation of the interactions of stress with the somatic symptoms may encourage a patient to take appropriate action to relieve the stress. Some patients may benefit from relaxation therapy. This is described in another chapter. Others may require more complex interventions as described later.

THE FOLLOW-UP VISIT

Compliance and Comprehension

It is my practice to see patients 6 to 8 weeks after the initial visit, to establish whether they have understood the explanation and are satisfied with the diagnosis. Those patients who are improved or satisfied can be returned to the care of their family physicians. They should, of course, be warned that IBS is a chronic, remitting condition and that the symptoms will recur from time to time. To deal with recurrences, the measures described above should be reinstituted.

In unimproved patients, the symptoms should be reviewed with other diagnostic possibilities in view. The physician should, however, resist the temptation to do further tests without good reason. One should also ensure that sufficient fiber is being employed and that "gassy" foods are being avoided.

Drug Therapy

In a chronic, benign condition, often beginning in youth and affecting nearly 15 percent of the population, drugs should be avoided when possible. Klein reviewed the controlled clinical trials of drugs used in IBS and found no convincing evidence that any are globally useful. The complex and variable symptoms seem unlikely to be cured by a single agent. In the United States, no drugs are approved for use in this syndrome by the Food and Drug Administration.

Nonetheless, certain drugs may be useful in certain circumstances. If the patient has a single dominant symptom that is causing some disability, it makes sense to use an agent to minimize that symptom (Table 5). For example, some patients have precipitous diarrhea and urgency. While they may not mention it spontaneously, the threat of incontinence can be very troubling, and such patients are reluctant to engage in social activities for fear of embarrassing themselves. Loperamide is an ideal drug for this situation, since it not only inhibits small bowel fluid secretion and gut motility, but also increases tone in the anal sphincter. One or two tablets should be given before a meal, a social engagement, or a stressful event to prevent urgency and diarrhea. Occasionally, a patient with predominant diarrhea responds to cholestyramine. Care should be taken not to use too much of an antidiarrheal drug, because it may exaggerate the constipated phase of IBS. In the United States, a 1 mg over-the-counter loperamide (Imodium) tablet is available and may be adequate.

When abdominal pain regularly follows meals, an anticholinergic drug may be given before the meal to interrupt the gastrocolonic response. This targets the drug for maximal effect at the time of symptoms and minimizes the side effects that a 24 hour anticholinergic

Table 5 Drugs for Certain Circumstances

Indication	Drug	Dose
Dominant diarrhea plus incontinence	Loperamide	1–2 tabs before meals, social engagements or stressful situations
	Cholestyramine	1 scoop hs
Dominant pain		
Postprandial	Anticholinergic Dicyclomine (Bentyl)	10–20 mg 10–15 min before meals
Chronic pain	Tricyclic (amitriptyline)	25 mg hs and increase
Dominant constipation	Bran, psyllium	1 tbsp t.i.d. with meals and increase p.r.n.
	Osmotic laxatives	
	Lactulose	1–2 tsp hs
	Polyethylene glycol solution	8 oz hs
	Mg SO4 (Milk of Magnesia)	1–2 tbsp hs
Gas (flatus)	Simethicone Beano (beta-galactosidase)	

blockade might incur. Some patients with dominant abdominal pain may respond to a tricyclic antidepressant even though depression is not obvious. These drugs affect the afferent nervous system and serotonin activity in the brain.

Symptoms dominated by constipation may be overcome by a bulking agent, either bran or psyllium in doses beyond those hitherto given. Some patients may take up to 10 tablespoons of bran a day before the desired effect is achieved. It is important that the bran be taken every day with ample fluids to prevent, rather than treat, constipation. Should this be ineffective, an osmotic laxative such as lactulose, Milk of Magnesia, or polyethylene glycol–electrolyte solution (Colyte, GoLYTELY) may be given in small doses at bedtime.

For the gas-prone patient, simethicone might be considered a logical placebo. As a surfactant it breaks up gas bubbles, but its efficacy in ridding the gut of gas is questionable. Activated charcoal may be given in capsule form but is awkward, messy, and of doubtful benefit. In patients producing excessive flatus who do not respond to withdrawal of gas-producing vegetables, Beano (beta-galactosidase) has achieved anecdotal success.

Many drugs proposed as IBS treatments have failed to establish their efficacy over time. These include mebeverine, trimebutane, peppermint oil, domperidone, and cisapride. Newer drugs such as the calcium channel blockers, 5-hydroxytryptamine antagonists, and somatostatin should be regarded as experimental. In my opinion, they should not be used for IBS outside clinical trials. They are costly, their efficacy is doubtful, and their use may distract from the more important issues.

Continuing Care

Some patients present more difficult psychosocial problems and need some of the special interventions cited below. In any case, the gastroenterologist and primary care physician should ensure continuing care and make every effort to prevent the doctor-shopping that is so common in IBS patients. Such patients often seek alternative medicine treatments.*

THE DIFFICULT PATIENT

Improve Functioning

Every gastroenterologist's practice has difficult IBS patients who consume much time and challenge his or her skill. Many can be successfully managed by periodic and regular visits to the primary physician and the gastroenterologist to deal with psychosocial difficulties. Such patients demand constant reassurance and are often satisfied when they get it. In such patients, cure is not likely, and improved functioning in society should be the treatment objective. They should be encouraged to engage in social events, become financially independent, and avoid abusive relationships. Those seeking disability insurance payments for IBS symptoms may place the physician in conflict. A disability pension may not encourage the independent living and improved social functioning that such patients need.

Consultative Options

Consultations with other physicians should have a specific objective. If a serious mental illness is suspected, psychiatric consultation will be necessary. If the physi-

---

***Editor's Note:** In one British report, over one-fourth of IBS patients were using alternative health sources, and recent anecdotal figures are higher. Perhaps the hour that some practitioners spend with the patient is helpful.

cian feels that he or she is losing the confidence of the patient, both may benefit from a consultation with a respected colleague. This doctor should confirm the diagnosis and reaffirm the method of treatment, thus making future management easier. There are a number of behavioral and psychological options. Although these have undergone intensive study, controlled clinical trials are obviously difficult. Nonetheless, such treatments as relaxation therapy, biofeedback, hypnotism, stress management, and psychological interventions may be helpful to certain patients if there are suitable experts in the community. Some patients with chronic pain may benefit from the multidisciplinary approach of a pain clinic.

Chronic Care

In all cases the gastroenterologist and the primary care physician should maintain control of the patient's medical care. The psychiatrist, psychologist, and pain clinic personnel are ill equipped to provide such care over the long term. Further discussion of the management of some of these difficult patients is found in the next two chapters.

SUGGESTED READING

Drossman DA, Thompson WG. Irritable bowel syndrome: a graduated, multicomponent treatment approach. Ann Intern Med 1992; 116:1009–1016..

Drossman DA, Sandler RS, McKee DC, Lovitz AJ. Bowel patterns among subjects not seeking health care. Use of a questionnaire to identify a population with bowel dysfunction. Gastroenterology 1982; 83:529–534.

Klein KB. Controlled treatment trials in the irritable bowel syndrome: a critique. Gastroenterology 1988; 95:232–241.

Thompson WG. The irritable bowel. Gut 1984; 25:305–320.

Thompson WG. Irritable bowel syndrome: Pathogenesis and management. Lancet 1993; 341:1568–1572.

Thompson WG. Gut Reactions. New York Plenum 1989.

Thompson WG, Creed F, Drossman DA, et al. Functional bowel disorders and chronic functional abdominal pain. Gastroenterol Int 1992; 5:75–91.

Thompson WG, Dotevall G, Drossman DA, et al. Irritable bowel syndrome: guidelines for the diagnosis. Gastroenterol Int 1989; 2:92–95.

Walker EA, Roy-Byrne PP, Katon WJ. Irritable bowel syndrome and psychiatric illness. Am J Psychiatry 1990; 147:565–572.

Whitehead WE, Winget C, Fedoravicius AS, et al. Learned illness behavior in patients with irritable bowel syndrome and peptic ulcer. Dig Dis Sci 1982; 27:202–208.

STRESS MANAGEMENT IN PATIENTS WITH FUNCTIONAL DISORDERS*

WILLIAM E. WHITEHEAD, Ph.D.

Functional gastrointestinal (GI) disorders are defined as "a variable combination of chronic or recurrent gastrointestinal symptoms not explained by structural or biochemical abnormalities. They include symptoms attributed to the pharynx, esophagus, stomach, biliary tree, small or large intestines, or anorectum" (Drossman and colleagues). GI disorders currently regarded as functional include globus, noncardiac chest pain, diffuse esophageal spasm and nutcracker esophagus, functional dyspepsia, irritable bowel syndrome (IBS), levator ani, proctalgia fugax, and pelvic floor dyssynergia.

For most of these disorders, there is evidence that stress and/or psychological symptoms of anxiety and depression play a role in triggering exacerbations of the disorder. This evidence is most compelling for IBS, in which 84 percent of patients who come to physicians report that stress causes increased abdominal pain or altered bowel habits, and more than 50 percent say that

IBS first appeared during a stressful period in their life. Other functional GI disorders have been less thoroughly investigated than IBS. It is this association of GI symptoms with stress or anxiety that provides the rationale for stress management training as a treatment for these disorders.

Laboratory studies have shown that stress and emotion alter the motility of the esophagus, stomach, small intestine, and colon, and these effects of stress on GI motility are assumed to be the primary mechanism by which stress provokes functional GI symptoms. However, it has also been suggested that stress and negative affect may lower the threshold for awareness of physiologic activity and the threshold for interpreting these sensations as symptoms of disease.

The treatment recommendations given below rely heavily on studies of patients with IBS, because there is an extensive literature on the treatment of this disorder but very little research available on the treatment of other functional GI disorders. It seems reasonable to assume that treatments that are effective for IBS will also be effective for other functional GI disorders, because (1) there is a substantial overlap between the diagnosis of IBS and that of these other disorders and (2) stress and emotional arousal appear to play a similar role as triggers for symptoms in these other disorders.

THERAPEUTIC ALTERNATIVES

Extrapolating from the experience with IBS, approximately 70 percent of patients with functional GI

*****Editor's Note:** Some physicians complain that they don't know what to do with their "problem" patients with functional bowel disease. This chapter provides specific guidelines in clear but scholarly fashion.

disorders do not require stress management training. They can be managed adequately with education, reassurance, and conservative medical therapy (Table 1). Patients who are most likely to benefit from these conservative measures are (1) first time presenters with these complaints, (2) those with mild or infrequent symptoms, and (3) those with little evidence of psychiatric symptoms such as anxiety and depression.

Establishing Trust

The doctor-patient relationship is particularly important to the management of patients with functional GI disorders, because these are chronic, relapsing conditions. Trust in the physician is essential to the patient's acceptance of symptom recurrence as natural to the disorder, and essential to the acceptance of referral for stress management training if this becomes necessary.

Establishment of trust depends on conveying interest and sympathy in the patient's distress. This may be difficult, because physicians are trained in hospital settings to prioritize their time and resources in terms of how potentially fatal a patient's illness or injuries may be. Moreover, patients with functional disorders often approach physicians with a defensive and somewhat hostile attitude because of previous encounters in which their complaints were dismissed as trivial or as purely hypochondriacal. Defensiveness and hostility tend to elicit the same attitude in physicians. The only way one can communicate sympathy and interest is to try to see the illness from the patient's perspective.

The evaluation of a patient with a functional GI disorder should include a screening questionnaire for psychological symptoms, because many patients with these disorders have psychological distress severe enough to warrant referral to a psychiatrist or psychologist. It is preferable to give such a questionnaire as a routine part of registering new patients, because if this is done later, after a negative medical evaluation, it will be perceived as rejection. The SCL-90-R is recommended because it is brief (about 10 minutes) and easily interpreted.

Another important element in establishing and maintaining trust is to schedule patients for follow-up appointments, even if they are currently asymptomatic or have been referred to another provider for stress management training. This demonstrates your continued interest in them, and it is appropriate to the management of a chronic, relapsing disorder.

Education

Patients benefit by learning about the anticipated course of their illness and the types of events that can trigger symptoms. For example, patients with IBS benefit from learning that the disorder is chronic but characterized by periodic exacerbations and remissions. This helps them interpret recurrences of symptoms appropriately as something normally to be expected, rather than

Table 1 Conservative Management of Irritable Bowel Syndrome: Patients with Mild or Infrequent Symptoms

Education
  Natural history of the disorder
  Role of stress and diet

Reassurance
  Address worries about cancer, inflammatory bowel disease

Conservative medical therapy
  Increase fiber
  Decrease foods that trigger symptoms
  Take moderate exercise
  Take antispasmodic medications when needed during
    exacerbations

as evidence that the diagnosis or treatment was incorrect. They may also benefit from learning that stress and certain foods can provoke their symptoms. This helps them learn ways of altering their habits so as to minimize the occurrence of symptoms.

Reassurance

Many patients tolerate the symptoms of a functional GI disorder for a number of years before consulting a doctor. They may consult primarily because they are afraid they have an organic disease such as cancer, peptic ulcer, or inflammatory bowel disease. These fears are often triggered when a relative or friend develops one of these diseases after reporting symptoms superficially similar to those of the patient. These patients may benefit from simple reassurance combined with education about the physiologic basis of their disorder.

Conservative Medical Therapy

Conservative therapy may take different forms, depending on the type of functional GI disorder present. For IBS, conservative management involves (1) increasing the amount of fiber in the diet to approximate 30 g per day; (2) eliminating foods such as dairy, caffeine, and spices identified by the clinical history or specific testing as triggers for symptoms in the patient; and (3) moderate exercise. Anticholinergic medications are often prescribed to be taken as needed for abdominal pain but should not be prescribed on a regular fixed dose. Conservative management for functional dyspepsia may include (1) decreasing or eliminating agents that stimulate acid secretion such as nicotine, alcohol, caffeine, and spices; (2) avoiding binge eating (eating large quantities of food in a short time); and (3) as-needed use of antacid tablets (Table 2).

Tricyclic Antidepressants

Tricyclic antidepressants are useful for chronic pain syndromes (including non-GI pain) and for somatization disorders (a pattern of multiple, unexplained somatic complaints). In patients with IBS, these medications

Table 2 Conservative Management of Functional Dyspepsia: Patients With Mild or Infrequent Symptoms

Education
  Natural history of the disorder
  Role of diet, smoking, alcohol

Reassurance
  Address worries about peptic ulcer, cancer

Conservative medical therapy
  Decrease alcohol, caffeine, spices, other agents that stimulate acid secretion
  Stop smoking
  Avoid binge eating
  Take antacid tablets as needed

have been found to be superior to placebo for reducing abdominal pain and decreasing diarrhea. Controlled trials have not been reported for other functional GI disorders. It is possible that the newer antidepressants that selectively inhibit the uptake of serotonin, fluoxetine (Prozac) or sertraline (Zoloft), will also be effective for functional GI disorders, but there are as yet no published trials with which to evaluate their efficacy. Consequently, the tricyclic antidepressants are currently recommended. Good first choices (because of their relatively low side effect profiles) are nortriptyline (Pamelor), 50 to 75 mg daily, and desipramine (Norpramin), 150 mg at bedtime.

The mechanism of action by which tricyclic antidepressants benefit patients with IBS is disputed. The published trials have been conducted in unselected groups of patients, not all of whom were depressed, and the doses were often too low to be considered effective for the management of depression. This, in combination with the fact that tricyclic antidepressants also have anticholinergic effects, has led some to believe that their benefits are due to peripheral anticholinergic actions in the bowel. However, a central nervous system action through the amelioration of depression has not been ruled out.

Antidepressant medications are not recommended as a first line of treatment in patients for whom other therapies such as stress management training might be effective, because functional disorders are chronic. Antidepressant medications have side effects, may produce physiologic and psychological dependency, and are relatively expensive when taken chronically. One should be reluctant to start a patient on a psychotropic medication such as this if it might have to be taken indefinitely. It is recommended that these medications be reserved for patients who are clinically depressed or who have severe abdominal pain that has failed to respond to stress management training.

Tranquilizers are sometimes suggested for the treatment of functional GI disorders because many of these patients are anxious or have symptoms triggered by stress. However, controlled trials have not shown tranquilizers to be beneficial for functional GI disorders, and

they share with antidepressants a propensity to cause side effects and dependency. They are not recommended.

STRESS MANAGEMENT TRAINING

Several types of stress management training have been tested and found beneficial in patients with IBS. In order of complexity and cost, these are:

1. Progressive muscle relaxation training. This is an arousal-reduction technique in which the patient is taught a set of exercises to perform daily. These exercises involve tensing and relaxing muscle groups while paying attention to the sensations produced. Over 4 to 6 weeks of daily practice, the patient should learn to relax tense muscles voluntarily and quickly. Audiotapes are available to guide these exercises at home.
2. Nonspecific biofeedback training. When used to teach relaxation, biofeedback may involve monitoring skeletal muscle activity with electrodes applied to the skin of the forehead. This activity is amplified and fed back to patients as an auditory or visual signal to help them learn to relax. Alternatively, patients may be taught to relax by learning to warm their hands with the aid of a biofeedback signal related to skin temperature, or to reduce the sympathetic activity related to sweating (galvanic skin responses).
3. Hypnosis and autogenic training. These procedures also aim at arousal reduction but use suggestion or mental imagery to achieve this goal. In hypnosis, a state of hypersuggestibility is induced by any of several techniques, after which suggestions are given to relax tense skeletal muscles and decrease smooth muscle contractions. Autogenic training is similar to hypnosis but relies heavily on mental images to induce relaxation. For example, patients may be asked to imagine their abdomen feeling warm or their bowel flowing like a river.
4. Cognitive behavior therapy. This is a technique for teaching patients to control stress and negative emotions through changes in their habitual thought patterns. For example, patients who become anxious and suffer diarrhea and pain whenever they give a speech may be helped to discover that their anxiety is related to automatic, self-defeating thoughts such as "I am not a very good public speaker; this will probably go badly." They may be taught to detect these automatic thoughts and to substitute more positive thoughts such as "I can give good talks if I prepare and practice."
5. Psychotherapy. Discussions between the therapist and patient are used to (1) identify stressors that trigger symptoms, (2) identify maladaptive ways the patient copes with stress, and (3) teach

more effective coping techniques. Emphasis is usually placed on social interactions or relationships within the family as causes of stress.

Patient Selection

Patients with mild or infrequent functional GI symptoms and those who are first-time consulters are not likely to need stress management training, since approximately 70 percent of them can be expected to respond to conservative management and to education and reassurance. Patients with moderate to severe symptoms should be considered for stress management training (Table 3), and depending on previous experience with IBS, they are most likely to benefit if (1) their symptoms (especially pain) are intermittent rather than continuous, (2) they can relate exacerbations of their GI symptoms to stressful events or to anxiety, and (3) they are anxious or depressed.

A few patients with functional GI disorders appear to obtain some benefit (secondary gain) from their symptoms. Most commonly, this involves increased sympathy and attention from family members and friends, or avoidance of work or unpleasant social interactions. Occasionally, it may involve financial compensation through disability payments or prescriptions for narcotic analgesics or tranquilizers. If the short-term benefits of having symptoms outweigh the discomfort and inconvenience, the patient's motivation for treatment may be compromised. Such patients respond poorly to stress management training. They tend also to be poor candidates for other forms of psychotherapy because they cannot easily accept a psychological perspective for their physical symptoms, but psychotherapy has the best chance of helping these patients.

The assessment of secondary gain requires judgment on the part of the clinician as to (1) whether the disability exhibited by the patient is disproportionate to what is seen in other patients with similar symptoms and (2) whether the response of family and friends to the symptoms is appropriately sympathetic, as opposed to being hostile or overindulgent. The information necessary to make this judgment is best obtained by open-ended questions about how the illness has affected work, social activities, and family life.

Patients whose GI symptoms are more or less constantly present and who cannot relate exacerbations of their symptoms to stressful events are also less likely to benefit from stress management training. This pattern of symptoms is often associated with evidence that the patient obtains secondary gain for the symptoms.

Choice of Technique

In addition to complexity and cost, the stress management techniques outlined above are ranked in terms of how much they require patients to switch to a psychological perspective for an understanding of their GI symptoms. Relaxation training and biofeedback are simple arousal reduction techniques that require very

Table 3 Management of Patients With Moderate to Severe Functional Gastrointestinal Disorders

Establish a trusting doctor-patient relationship

Refer to a psychologist or psychiatrist for stress management
  Choose a treatment based on
    Patient's level of psychological distress
    Patient's ability to take a psychological perspective
  Optimize patient follow-through by
    Being personally familiar with two or three referral sources
    Making the appointment for the patient
    Checking up at the patient's next visit

Schedule periodic follow-up visits

little commitment to a psychological perspective; patients need only believe that stress can trigger occurrences of symptoms in the same way that coffee might trigger them. Hypnosis and autogenic training also require very little commitment to a psychological explanation for symptoms, but they are nontraditional approaches that are often viewed as psychological, and they may be difficult for many patients to accept. Cognitive behavior therapy and psychotherapy require a major shift in the patient's perspective to be effective. The ability to take a psychological perspective should be considered when deciding on which stress management techniques to recommend to the patient.

The patient's degree of psychological distress should also be considered in choosing the best approach to stress management. Patients with relatively low levels of anxiety and depression (but whose symptoms increase in response to stress) benefit more from arousal reduction techniques, hypnosis, and cognitive behavior therapy than do patients with greater psychological distress. On the other hand, patients with high levels of psychological distress are more likely to benefit from psychotherapy than those with low levels, possibly because it is easier for them than for their less anxious counterparts to shift to a psychological perspective. One should also take into account the greater need of the severely psychologically impaired patient, especially the depressed patient, for the more comprehensive approach to psychological treatment to be found in psychotherapy and cognitive behavior therapy.

The patient's age may also influence the choice of treatment. Peter Whorwell, who pioneered the use of hypnosis to treat IBS, reports that patients over age 50 are less likely to benefit. This is probably due to the greater reluctance of older patients to accept treatments they view as untraditional.

Choice of Provider

A few gastroenterologists have acquired training in one or more of these techniques and use them as needed in their clinical practice. However, most primary care physicians and gastroenterologists do not have the time or training to provide stress management training, and elect to refer their patients to a psychologist or psychiatrist.

Patients frequently do not follow up on referrals to psychologists or psychiatrists, so physicians should do anything they can to increase the likelihood that they will do so. For example, consider making the appointment for patients before they leave your office, or personally introducing them to a psychologist working in your clinical setting. Take the time to identify two or three psychologists or psychiatrists who are competent and willing to accept patients with functional GI disorders, so that you can refer your patients to someone you know. Always check, on the patients' next visit, whether they contacted the person to whom you referred them and whether they are benefiting.

SUGGESTED READING

Drossman DA, Thompson WG. The irritable bowel syndrome: review and a graduated multicomponent treatment approach. Ann Intern Med 1992; 116:1009–1016.

Drossman DA, Thompson WG, Talley NJ, et al. Identification of sub-groups of functional gastrointestinal disorders. Gastroenterol Int 1990; 4:159–172.
Greenbaum DS, Mayle JE, Vanegeren LE, et al. Effects of desipramine on irritable bowel syndrome compared with atropine and placebo. Dig Dis Sci 1987; 32:257–266.
Guthrie E, Creed F, Dawson D, Tomenson B. A controlled trial of psychological treatment for the irritable bowel syndrome. Gastroenterology 1991; 100:450–457.
Whitehead WE, Schuster MM. Behavioral concepts and behavioral approaches to treatment. In: Gastrointestinal disorders: behavioral and physiological basis for treatment. Orlando, Academic Press, 1985:13–28.
Whitehead WE, Schuster MS. Irritable bowel syndrome. In: Winawer SJ, ed. Management of gastrointestinal diseases. Vol 2. New York, Gower, 1992:32.1–32.25.

SEXUAL DYSFUNCTION IN PATIENTS WITH GASTROINTESTINAL DISORDERS

THOMAS N. WISE, M.D.

Advances in knowledge of the psychophysiology of the sexual response cycle, and increased attention to quality of life in the medically ill, converge to qualify sexuality in the patient with gastrointestinal (GI) disorders as an area of importance. Sexuality is more than a procreative function; it is a fundamental human experience that offers physical pleasure and emotional sustenance. Failure to address sexuality can exacerbate the poor self-image, discouragement, and depression often found in the chronically ill.

The very nature of GI disease challenges both emotional well-being and sexual functioning. Disorders of alimentation and excretion cause malaise and discomfort that affect an individual's energy level and mood. When excretory function is compromised, the individual may fear incontinence or odor that will affect the physical intimacy inherent in sexuality. Along with the features of the disease itself, the various treatments, i.e., drugs or surgery, can modify sexual function. It is thus necessary for the gastroenterologist to develop a systematic format to understand and ascertain sexual functioning in patients with such diseases.

EVALUATION

The clinician must obtain a sexual history within the context of the patient's disease and life setting. Studies have demonstrated that patients respond well to such an assessment and perceive their physician to be interested in them as unique people who have a life beyond the consulting room. An understanding of the causes of sexual problems is based on a biopsychosocial history wherein patients' level of sexual functioning is understood within the context of their biological, psychological, and social capacities. The most useful method of assessing sexuality is to partition the three dimensions of sexual functioning into *impersonal aspects* due to illness, treatment, and role limitations; *intrapersonal effects* that foster psychological distress; and *interpersonal issues* that affect both patient and sexual partner (Table 1). To

Table 1 Effects of Illness on Sexuality

Intrapsychic
  Shame regarding body image
  Depression

Impersonal
  Erectile dysfunction due to surgery, medication
  Vaginal stenosis due to fistula following surgery
  Malaise, pain due to illness

Interpersonal
  Sexual partner's fear or disgust
  Anger of partner (often seen in spouse of an alcoholic)

achieve this best the clinician must define patients' actual sexual functioning.

SEXUAL RESPONSE CYCLE

Sexuality is a three-phase psychophysiologic response composed of drive, arousal, and release (Table 2).

Drive is an instinctual need for sexual activity that is perceived as sexual arousal in response to cognitive or physical sensation. Sexuality is a motivated behavior in which an internal tension state of erotic tension may foster activity toward the goal of orgasm. Disease states or psychological conditions clearly modify such libidinal feelings. Illness, however, does not completely ablate sexual urges, and denial of such needs can promote frustration or depression.

The next phase of the sexual response cycle is that of arousal, characterized by erection in the male and vaginal lubrication in the female. As arousal increases, there is a concurrent increase in autonomic reactivity characterized by increasing heart rate, increased respiratory rate, a sex flush over the upper chest, and nipple hardening in both males and females. The final phase of the cycle is that of release or orgasm, characterized by emission and ejaculation in the male and orgastic release with vaginal contractions in the female. The release phase is followed by a resolution period that differs in males and females; women are capable of multiple orgasms, whereas men have a refractory period that can last from 30 minutes in the young man to a long hiatus in the older man. A 60-year-old man may not be able to have another

Table 2 The Sexual Response Cycle

Drive
  Subjective urge to relieve sexual tension

Arousal
  Erection in males
  Vaginal lubrication in females

Release
  Orgasm

Table 3 Historical Elements That Help Differentiate Organic From Psychological Impotence

Course of disorder
  Onset of organic impotence is often gradual

Context
  Psychogenic impotence may occur only with a specific partner
  Adequate tumescence during masturbation suggests psychogenic
    etiology

Comorbid medications or diseases foster dysfunction
  Cimetidine, antihypertensive medication, serotonin reuptake
    blockers, colon cancer surgery, alcoholism, diabetes

erection for 12 hours. It is important to understand this three-phase cycle, since it allows the physician to pinpoint the sexual dysfunction. A common diagnostic problem is differentiating organic erectile difficulties from psychogenic impotence (Table 3). Historical elements that help in such a differential diagnosis include whether the disorder occurred gradually in a setting of alcoholism or when a new medicine was introduced, as is often the case in organically caused dysfunctions. Can the male patient develop a functional erection during masturbation or with sexual partners other than his usual mate? These two phenomena suggest psychologically motivated dysfunction. Often the history is not sufficiently clear to definitively label the cause, so that ancillary tests such as endocrine, vascular, or neurologic studies are needed.

BIOPSYCHOSOCIAL FRAMEWORK

After defining the sexual dysfunction, the clinician must place the problem within a tripartite biopsychosocial framework. The clinical problem should be partitioned into the effects of the illness on intrapsychic issues (psychological issues), the interpersonal ramifications of the disease (partner-specific and social factors), and the impersonal aspects of disease and treatment (biologic factors).

In considering intrapsychic issues, the clinician must first attempt to understand the individual's life-stage tasks and personality. Each patient comes to the physician at a specific phase in the life cycle with different life tasks that affect sexual issues. Thus, the adolescent has the task of obtaining an education to allow independence, but must also cope with emerging sexuality and development into an autonomous adult. How will an ostomy affect this? The young mother of two children has the task of caring for her children as well as trying to be a partner in a marriage, whereas the single mother has the increasing burden of raising her children as well as supporting them. How will chronic active hepatitis affect her? The older individual who is retired has the task of maintaining a sense of self-esteem but does not always have the same challenges as younger individuals. Rigid stereotypes of age-related tasks are no longer accurate in contemporary culture. The older male, widowed or single, may find himself in a sexually pressured dating environment and develop erectile dysfunction due to performance anxiety.

What is the patient's basic personality? Is the patient a worrier who tends to be depressed and feel vulnerable? Is he or she conscientious, goal directed, and tidy? Is he or she agreeable and always seeking to please others, or is there a tendency to be aggressive and challenging? Such characteristics can be accentuated in settings of disease and psychological distress. Sexuality is an important variable in this milieu. Thus, the individual who is a worrier will be increasingly self-conscious after an ostomy or prone to depression if the body image changes as a result of steroid treatment. Does the patient have a formal psychiatric disorder such as an anxiety disorder or panic disorder, which often begins during a setting of illness or a mood disorder. Anxiety and depression may modify sexual drive and exacerbate either arousal or release phase disorders. The overanxious male may find himself unable to develop an erection if he has had a few failures in the past, and begins to be a "spectator" of his sexual performance, i.e., focusing on his erectile capacity rather than immersing himself in the sexual act. The depressed female may be sufficiently ashamed of bodily changes after ostomy surgery to avoid coital experiences.

Next, it is essential to understand the interpersonal elements of sexuality. Understanding the reaction of the sexual partner to the patient's disease is important. Thus, review of the frequency and nature of the sexual response as well as satisfaction allow a baseline from which to understand present difficulties. If available, a sexual partner can offer data about premorbid sexual functioning and present sexual issues in the relationship. Discussing sexuality with both patient and spouse offers support that this is an important area of concern.

The impersonal effects on sexual functioning are often unique to each specific disease and are discussed in the following section.

SPECIFIC DISORDERS

Irritable Bowel Syndrome

Irritable bowel syndrome (IBS) occurs commonly in the general population (about 10 to 12 percent), although only a minority of affected individuals seek medical care. From an intrapsychic perspective, people who do seek medical treatment for IBS have an increased tendency to experience anxiety and feel self-conscious. Sexuality in IBS patients is further complicated by a recent finding that women with this syndrome often have histories of sexual abuse. This could cause unique vulnerabilities to sexual difficulties, since sexual abuse causes fearful and negative images of sexuality linked with aggressive and coercive behaviors by older partners. The somatic preoccupation of such patients can create both anger and distancing from the sexual partners. As symptoms often become a consuming focus, they may limit activities such as travel, or going out to restaurants. It is often quite difficult to cope with a partner who is generally not feeling well but has a disorder that has been repeatedly demonstrated not to be life threatening. The focus on dietary changes, however, can create interpersonal stressors, particularly if a partner points out that the IBS patient is frequently drinking coffee or sodas that may make the condition worse. Frequent urgency, tenesmus, and cramping can lower sexual drive. Fear of incontinence is an ever-present reality in many diarrhea-predominant patients with IBS. Patients with constipation-predominant syndromes frequently complain of cramping and a general

sense of malaise, which can further diminish sexual ardor. The medications given for IBS rarely modify sexual functioning.*

Inflammatory Bowel Disease

Inflammatory bowel disease (IBD), both regional enteritis and ulcerative colitis, are serious disorders. The malaise and lowered energy from the active disease diminishes sexual drive. The interpersonal aspects of this disorder can have grave consequences, depending on the individual's stage of life. The child or adolescent with IBD can be isolated from peers owing to frequent absences from school. Adult patients with IBD may be embarrassed to tell their peers or co-workers that they have such a condition. The treatments for IBD affect both emotions and body image, and consequently sexual functioning. Corticosteroids can promote cushingoid body changes that foster shame and sexual avoidance but can also increase sexual drive. If an individual reacts to steroids with renewed energy and increased sexual drive, this can create difficulties due to dramatic changes in libido. Alternatively, an individual may become depressed on steroids, and lowered drive may ensue.

Surgical treatment for IBD seriously affects intrapsychic, interpersonal, and impersonal aspects of sexual functioning. Individuals may feel ashamed of or embarrassed by ostomies. In the adolescent or young adult who is dating, fear of telling partners about the ostomy is often a primary problem. Fear of odor or fecal spillage is an ever-present worry in many patients. Men are far more tolerant of having spouses help with ostomy appliances than are women, who are often ashamed and unwilling to let their spouses help them. In such situations, it is essential to use ostomy therapists and actively link the patient to peer support groups for education and shared support.† Actual sexual function, the ability to have an erection or orgasm, is generally not organically compromised in men with IBD, since the surgery usually spares the posterior nervous plexuses that promote sexual functioning. Surgical complications such as fistulas modify sexual enjoyment and promote vaginal stenosis, causing dyspareunia in women with IBD. Continent ostomies or pull-through ostomies can minimize the psychological hazards of the ostomy and external procedures.

Colon Cancer

Cancer of the colon has unique issues that differ from IBD because of the anxiety and depression that cancer fosters. If the neoplasm is metastatic, fear and depression due to a possibly terminal illness are common. In such settings, sexuality becomes an important

*Editor's Note: The late afternoon–early evening distention and discomfort so common in IBS patients, usually female, can interfere with the desire for and performance of intercourse.

†Editor's Note: It is reassuring to women with an ileoanal pouch to learn of others who have had successful pregnancies.

medium of emotional communication. Carcinoma of the colon often demands a colectomy that causes impotence due to nervous tissue dissection. The physician must point out to the patient and partner that erectile capacity is not the only measure of affection, and educate the patient and his partner about other forms of mutual gratification.

Other Diseases

Peptic ulcer disease (PUD) responds to a variety of H_2 blockers. The main sexual consequence of treatment for PUD is the sexual side effect of H_2 blockers such as cimetidine and ranitidine, which can cause erectile dysfunction in the male. Newer enzyme-inhibiting agents such as omeprazole have fewer sexual side effects.

Liver disease, most commonly hepatitis of either infectious or alcoholic etiology, can seriously affect sexual function. Long-term alcohol use lowers sexual drive, impairs the ability of males to develop an erection, and limits female sexual arousal. When such individuals initiate and maintain sobriety, they must learn to develop a sexual relationship without intoxication. Furthermore, the interpersonal aspects of alcoholism often promote anger in the partner. In essence, the partner must learn to live with a new person in a sober state. The actual impersonal aspects of sexual functioning in the patient with alcoholic liver disease include the elevated estrogen levels in the male due to less androgen that may lower sexual drive and promote body changes such as gynecomastia and testicular atrophy. Alcoholic individuals also have neuropathic changes to ablate erectile capacity. Women with alcoholism often report lower sexual drive and increasing anorgasmia. Individuals with chronic liver disease due to infectious disorders have to cope with the general malaise and concurrent depression that will clearly modify sexual enjoyment and functioning.

TREATMENT

Treatment of the sexual dysfunctions discussed above involves addressing the problem with both the patient and if possible the sexual partner. Thus, the initial steps are listening, permission, and education. Listening involves taking the initial history and discussing the problem. Concurrent with such listening, permission to discuss sexual concerns reinforces the message that sexuality is important. It is also essential to note that sexuality includes nongenital forms of physical pleasure such as hugging, caressing, and verbal communication when full coital functioning is not possible. In such permissive discussions, the fears of each partner can be discovered. Education will depend on the clinical

situation. The fear of contagion in viral hepatitis is important, and use of condoms or alternative forms of gratification such as mutual masturbation may be appropriate. Ostomy patients often fear rejection. It is easy for the physician to suggest garments that cover the ostomy and maximize visual eroticism. Local ostomy groups can provide information regarding such apparel. In patients with long-term steroid use, bodily changes may cause shame. It is important for the partner to still verbalize sexual attractiveness to the mate as well as discuss any fears of hurting him or her, if in fact there have been pathologic fractures in the past due to osteoporosis. Open communication is also important in individuals who are recovering from alcoholism and resultant liver disease. Often, years of anger and blame due to the substance abuse modify sexual interest and drive, and such areas have to be discussed.

When any of these strategies that encourage permission, education, and support appear to be only modestly successful, referral to the appropriate mental health professional is essential. Thus, a variety of strategies may be used, including psychological treatments to modify both depressive and anxiety disorders that limit sexual function, marital therapies to treat long-standing difficulties due to disease states, and organic interventions for the organic sexual dysfunctions. In addition to such verbal strategies, a variety of organic treatments are now available for male sexual dysfunction. Penile injections with prostaglandin as well as vasodilators such as papaverine allow tumescence in the organically impaired individual. Surgical penile prostheses are very successful in men rendered impotent by organic factors such as surgery. Careful evaluation of any medications that may be fostering impotence is also important.

A final element in treatment is referral of such patients to groups of individuals with similar disorders. Support groups such as the United Ostomy Association (UOA) or the Crohn's and Colitis Foundation of America (CCFA) are very helpful in verbalizing common problems and sharing solutions to these difficulties. Areas of sexuality are commonly discussed within such groups, whose address can often be found in a local telephone book or through the local ostomy therapist.

SUGGESTED READING

Kaplan HS, Wagner G. The new injection treatment for impotence, medical and psychological aspects. New York: Brunner-Mazel, 1993.
Wise TN. Gastroenterology. In: Stoudemire A, Fogel B, eds. Principles of medical psychiatry. New York: Grune & Stratton, 1987:571–582.
Wise TN. A model for the assessment of sexual dysfunction etiology. J Clin Psychiatry Monograph Series 1992; 10:11–18.

INFECTIONS, IMMUNE DISORDERS, AND NUTRITION

GASTROINTESTINAL COMPLICATIONS OF HIV INFECTION

RICHARD E. CHAISSON, M.D.

Individuals with human immunodeficiency virus (HIV) infection have a high prevalence of gastrointestinal disorders. Gastrointestinal diseases in HIV infection may range from mild to life-threatening, and may occur at any time during the natural history of HIV disease. Effective therapy for these complications may substantially enhance the quality of life for HIV-infected people and may contribute to prolonged survival. This chapter reviews current therapeutic options for the gastrointestinal complications of HIV infection.*

ORAL DISEASE

Candidiasis

Oral candidiasis (thrush) is a common complication of HIV, occurring more frequently as cellular immunodeficiency progresses. Topical treatment for thrush is highly effective and extremely safe. Clotrimazole troches four to five times daily or nystatin suspension three to four times daily result in resolution of candidial lesions in several days in the majority of cases, although treatment for 1 to 2 weeks is generally recommended. More severe oropharyngeal candidiasis may be treated with oral azole agents, including ketoconazole 200 mg daily or fluconazole 50 to 100 mg daily. Because many patients with HIV infection have gastric achlorhydria, ketoconazole should be taken with an acidic beverage such as orange juice or cola to enhance absorption. Fluconazole is well absorbed in a neutral environment, however, and may be taken with water. In a clinical trial fluconazole was found to result in faster resolution of oral candidiasis by culture than clotrimazole troches, but

the clinical significance of this finding is uncertain. In general, 1 to 2 weeks of treatment for an episode of oral candidiasis is sufficient, though some clinicians prefer to put patients with frequent episodes on chronic suppressive therapy with clotrimazole or fluconazole.

The widespread use of fluconazole for treatment and prophylaxis of candida and other fungal infections has led to the emergence of fluconazole-resistant *Candida*. Treatment of these infections can be challenging. Topical agents such as clotrimazole and nystatin have not been effective in most cases. While cross-resistance is not universal, use of other azoles such as ketoconazole or itraconazole has also generally been ineffective. Some clinicians have reported success with itraconazole solution, but this has not been verified in clinical trials. The most effective therapy is low dose amphotericin B given intermittently for symptomatic relapses. Use of topical gentian violet has also been successful though cosmetically displeasing in some cases. (See the chapter on oral lesions for additional information.)

Herpes Simplex

Oral herpes is also a common problem in HIV infected individuals, and both HSV-1 and HSV-2 are implicated. Painful outbreaks of oral herpes may be treated with oral acyclovir 200 mg five times daily. For patients who have frequent recurrences, acyclovir suppressive therapy 400 mg twice daily is effective. Fortunately, oral cytomegalovirus (CMV) infections are rare.

Oral Hairy Leukoplakia

This disorder is caused by the Epstein-Barr virus and affects the lateral margin of the tongue and the buccal mucosa. The lesion is rarely symptomatic and does not generally require treatment. In severe cases where symptoms prevent eating or impair taste, oral acyclovir may be effective.

Oral Aphthous Ulcers

Painful aphthous ulcers may be present throughout the gastrointestinal tract, but are most common in the oral cavity. The etiology of the lesions is not known. However, drugs such as didanosine and zidovudine, have been associated with oral and esophageal ulcers in

---

*Editor's Note: An important position paper on HIV infection by the American College of Physicians and the Infectious Diseases Society of America appears in Am Intern Med 1994; 120:310–319.

patients with HIV infection. Discontinuation of these antiretroviral agents is appropriate in a patient who has new presumed aphthous ulcers. A number of symptomatic treatments are available for aphthous ulcers, though none have been rigorously tested. Topical treatment includes the use of lidocaine gel or other such preparations, tetracycline oral suspension, topical steroids such as dexamethasone in Orabase, or combinations of topical agents. Popular preparations include solutions of lidocaine, nystatin and Maalox and solutions of tetracycline, Maalox and Benadryl. For severe cases of aphthous stomatitis, systemic steroids may be of enormous benefit. Prednisone 60 mg daily for 1 to 2 weeks followed by a 1 to 2 week taper may provide dramatic relief.

ESOPHAGEAL DISEASE

Candidiasis

Esophageal candidiasis is a common cause of dysphagia, odynophagia, and weight loss in patients with HIV infection. Although this complication tends to occur in more advanced HIV disease, reports of esophageal candidiasis in patients with CD4 counts greater than 500 per cubic millimeter have been published. Diagnosis is often made presumptively when patients have typical symptoms and oral thrush. Endoscopic diagnosis may be necessary if oral thrush is absent. Treatment for esophageal candidiasis should always be systemic, as topical agents are not reliably effective in this disorder. (See the chapter on esophageal infections for more information.)

Oral azole agents are usually adequate to treat esophageal candidiasis. One clinical trial found fluconazole 100 mg daily superior to ketoconazole 200 mg daily resulting in faster resolution of symptoms and endoscopic improvement. However, many clinicians would use a higher dose of ketoconazole, such as 200 mg twice daily. As noted previously, ketoconazole absorption is limited in patients with gastric achlorhydria; consumption of an acidic beverage with ketoconazole is recommended. This may pose a problem for patients with odynophagia, however. Because fluconazole is well-absorbed even in patients with achlorhydria, I prescribe doses of 100 to 200 mg daily for esophageal candidiasis. Fluconazole is virtually 100 percent bioavailable when taken orally so intravenous administration is rarely necessary. In selected patients with severe odynophagia, a single intravenous dose of fluconazole 100 to 200 mg may relieve symptoms sufficiently to permit subsequent oral dosing. For severe and/or refractory cases of esophageal candidiasis, low dose amphotericin B (0.3 mg per kg daily) is usually effective. Many clinicians give chronic suppressive antifungal therapy in patients who have had esophageal candidiasis. My preference is to treat for 3 to 4 weeks with fluconazole and then stop therapy. If the patient relapses, retreatment with fluconazole followed by chronic suppressive therapy of fluconazole 50 mg three times weekly is effective in preventing further recurrences.

Herpes Esophagitis

Herpetic esophagitis is less common in patients with HIV than might be expected, given the frequency with which HSV causes disease in this patient population. Nonetheless, occasional patients will have herpetic ulcers diagnosed endoscopically. Treatment with acyclovir 200 mg five times daily is recommended. Initially, intravenous acyclovir at doses of 5 mg per kg three times daily may be appropriate. High dose acyclovir is not usually required. The duration of therapy is 10 to 14 days and chronic suppressive therapy may be necessary.

CMV Esophagitis

CMV is the cause of severe esophagitis in patients with HIV, associated with marked odynophagia, retrosternal pain, fever, and inanition. Therapy with ganciclovir or foscarnet produces symptomatic relief slowly in the majority of patients. Adequate clinical trials of therapy for CMV esophagitis have not been performed so treatment recommendations are largely empiric. Ganciclovir 5 mg per kg twice daily for 2 to 4 weeks has been effective in a number of patients. Toxicities of ganciclovir include neutropenia and anemia, especially when the agent is coadministered with zidovudine. Alternatively, foscarnet may be given at 90 mg per kg twice daily. Side effects of this agent include multiple electrolyte disorders and nephrotoxicity. Both agents are equally active against CMV, but foscarnet was shown to prolong survival in a trial comparing these two agents for CMV retinitis. The mechanism of this survival advantage is probably the anti-HIV effect of foscarnet. Because patients with esophagitis are not likely to receive lifelong therapy (unlike retinitis patients), the greater cost and toxicity of foscarnet is probably not worthwhile for esophagitis. After several weeks of therapy, patients may continue on high dose oral acyclovir or no therapy. While the evidence is weak that acyclovir prevents relapses of CMV esophagitis, some clinicians find this approach clinically effective. My own practice is to treat esophagitis for at least three weeks and then give no chronic therapy. If patients relapse, retreatment with ganciclovir followed by maintenance therapy (5 mg per kg daily) is given.

STOMACH DISEASES AND ENTEROCOLIDITES

Patients with HIV infection are subject to numerous conventional stomach and small bowel diseases. (See the specific chapters for the management of these diseases.) However, there are a number of opportunistic processes peculiar to HIV.

CMV Gastritis

CMV may cause a severe gastritis associated with focal ulcers and diffuse inflammation. Therapy is similar to that discussed for CMV esophagitis. The duration of initial therapy may need to be 4 to 6 weeks and some clinicians prefer chronic maintenance therapy.

Mycobacterium Avium Complex (MAC)

MAC is a nontuberculous mycobacterium acquired from environmental exposure that causes disseminated disease in patients with advanced AIDS. Many patients have small bowel involvement with acid fast bacilli-laden macrophages in the submucosal areas of the duodenum and jejunum. Recently, therapy of disseminated MAC with the macrolides clarithromycin and azithromycin has been shown to reduce symptoms and clear bacteremia in a large proportion of patients. Emergence of macrolide-resistant isolates with single drug therapy makes the addition of other agents essential. A U.S. Public Health Service Task Force has recommended that patients with disseminated MAC be treated with a macrolide and at least one other agent, such as ethambutol, clofazamine, rifampin, rifabutin, ciprofloxacin, or amikacin. Studies of patients with severe gastrointestinal involvement have not yet been performed. Nonetheless, patients who are not bacteremic but have documented small bowel disease may be treated with similar regimens. Unfortunately, gastrointestinal toxicity from the macrolides is common and may include nausea, vomiting, abdominal pain, and diarrhea. The frequency of such reactions may be minimized by using lower doses of the macrolides, such as clarithromycin 500 mg twice daily. Treatment of MAC is lifelong, as the infection is never eradicated. The risk of MAC infection may be significantly reduced by the use of rifabutin 300 mg daily as prophylaxis. The U.S. Public Health Service Task Force has recommended that patients with HIV infection and a CD4 count less than 100 per cubic millimeter be treated with rifabutin to prevent MAC disease.

Microsporidiosis

Microsporidia are a recently described class of organisms causing small bowel infections in immunocompromised patients, especially those with HIV infection. The diagnosis of these infections is difficult, although stool detection assays have become available recently. Treatment of microsporidiosis with albendazole results in relief of symptoms in some cases, but controlled trials have not been performed. Use of antimotility agents and oral rehydration is helpful.

Cryptosporidiosis

Cryptosporidiosis is a cause of devastating diarrheal disease in patients with HIV infection. In the normal host, cryptosporidiosis may cause a severe but self-limited diarrheal syndrome that resolves over several weeks. In the immunosuppressed patient, however, cryptosporidiosis may produce profound wasting from large-volume watery diarrhea that persists for months. To date, no effective therapy for cryptosporidiosis has been described. Supportive measures, such as hydration, antimotility agents, electrolyte replacement, and bed rest have been shown to reduce the volume of diarrhea in a large proportion of patients. Nonetheless, patients may continue to have 4 to 6 large volume stools per day in spite of these measures and continue to require aggressive care. Anecdotal evidence has shown that octreotide (Sandostatin) may reduce the volume of stool significantly in selected patients. Controlled clinical trials have failed to document the effectiveness of this therapy, however. Several antimicrobial agents have been evaluated as potential therapy for cryptosporidiosis with mixed results. Spiramycin, an oral macrolide antibiotic, was anecdotally reported to have activity in patients with cryptosporidiosis early in the AIDS epidemic. Subsequent clinical trials have documented no activity of this agent against cryptosporidium and have revealed significant toxicity, including toxic colitis. Paramomycin, an oral aminoglycoside, has also been reported in several case series as having activity. Several small clinical trials have also shown a benefit of paramomycin at doses of 500 mg four times daily. Improvement in diarrhea along with reduction in the number of cryptosporidium oocysts in the stool have been reported. My own practice is to manage patients initially with antimotility drugs such as loperamide, hydration and electrolyte replacement. If this is unsuccessful, a trial of paramomycin may be attempted. Clinical trials of newer agents are underway, but a number of new drugs have been studied with disappointing results.

Isospora belli Infection

This protozoan parasite causes a severe enterocolitis in patients with HIV infection, especially in endemic areas. Isosporiasis has been reported commonly in patients with HIV infection from Haiti, the Caribbean, and South America. Treatment of this infection with trimethoprim-sulfamethoxazole is usually extremely effective, though therapy needs to continue for weeks. Patients who do not respond to trimethoprim-sulfamethoxazole or who are unable to tolerate it may be treated with pyrimethamine.

CMV Colitis

CMV colitis is associated with severe small-volume diarrhea, abdominal cramping, abdominal pain, and fever. Documentation of CMV by colonoscopy is required. Although it is clear from clinical practice that patients with CMV colitis respond to antiviral therapy, the optimal management of this infection is not known. One clinical trial comparing ganciclovir to no treatment failed to document compelling differences in outcome. Patients treated with 2 weeks of ganciclovir had better resolution of colonic lesions by endoscopy, but overall outcome was not significantly better. Most clinicians feel that at least 3 weeks of ganciclovir therapy is necessary to achieve a remission of this disease. As with CMV esophagitis, a one time course of therapy is the initial preferred approach. For that reason, ganciclovir is preferred to foscarnet. For patients who relapse after discontinuation of ganciclovir, chronic maintenance therapy may be instituted. Patients who have CMV colitis are at very high risk of developing CMV retinitis. In the study previously mentioned, one quarter of patients randomized to receive no therapy developed retinitis during the followup period. Whether all patients with CMV colitis should be put on preventive therapy with ganciclovir is unclear.

Clostridium difficile Colitis

Pseudomembranous colitis caused by *C. difficile* toxin is a common consequence of antibiotic therapy in patients with HIV infection. The agents most frequently associated with *C. difficile* colitis are ampicillin, cephalosporins, and clindamycin, though the disease has been caused by a wide variety of antimicrobial agents. Patients present with fever, abdominal pain, diarrhea and dehydration. The diagnosis is made by detection of *C. difficile* toxin in stool specimens. Treatment consists of discontinuing antibiotics and instituting anti-clostridial therapy. Vancomycin 125 mg orally every six hours is usually effective, as is metronidazole 250 to 500 mg three times daily. For severe cases, cholestyramine may be administered as a toxin-binding agent. Patients with HIV infection and *C. difficile* colitis tend to respond to therapy more slowly than other patients. Fever may not

resolve for 3 to 5 days and diarrhea may persist for a week. Although a toxic megacolon-like picture may evolve, surgery is best avoided.

SUGGESTED READING

Bonacini M, Young T, Lane L. The causes of Estophageal symptoms in human immunodeficiency virus infection. A prospective study of 110 patients. Arch Intern Med 1991; 151:1567–1572.

Cello JP. Evaluation of AIDS-related diarrhea. Hosp Pract (Off Ed) 1993; 28:95–102.

Dieterich DT, Kotler DP, Busch DF, et al. Ganciclovir treatment of cytomegalovirus colitis in AIDS: a randomized, double-blind, placebo-controlled multicenter study. J Infect Dis 1993; 167: 278–282.

Greenson JK, Belitsos PC, Yardley JH, Bartlett JG. AIDS enteropathy: occult enteric infections and duodenal mucosal alterations in chronic diarrhea. Ann Intern Med 1991; 114:366–372.

Molina JM, Sarfati C, Beauvais B, et al. Intestinal microsporidiosis in human immunodeficiency virus-infected patients with chronic unexplained diarrhea: prevalence and clinical and biologic features. J Infect Dis 1993; 167:217–221.

Smith P-D, Quinn T-C, Strober W, et al. Gastrointestinal infections in AIDS Ann Intern Med 1992; 116:63–77.

SYSTEMIC INFLAMMATORY RESPONSE SYNDROME: PHARMACOLOGIC AND NUTRITIONAL THERAPIES

YEVGENIY GINCHERMAN, B.A.
JOHN L. ROMBEAU, M.D.

Systemic inflammatory response syndrome (SIRS), previously referred to as the multiple organ failure syndrome, is defined as the sequential failure of lungs, liver, and kidneys after multiple trauma, severe burns, hemorrhagic shock, or infections, especially in immunocompromised individuals. Hematologic, neurologic, and cardiovascular dysfunctions are also common sequelae in SIRS. This chapter briefly reviews SIRS, with emphasis on its pathogenesis and on pharmacologic and nutritional therapies.

PATHOGENESIS

The pathogenesis of the syndrome is not well understood, but a number of risk factors are strongly associated with its rapid progression. These include advanced age, sepsis before admission to the ICU, and increased severity of illness as documented by standardized measurements such as the APACHE (Acute Physiology and Chronic Health Evaluation) scores. Many findings of sepsis are commonly observed, including fever, hyperdynamic circulation, fluid retention, hypotension, ileus, and alterations in the number and function of white blood cells. Specific sites of infection can sometimes be found, but in our experience many patients have no documented sites of infection despite imaging studies and bacterial cultures.

It has been proposed that enteric bacteria and the endotoxins released from the bacterial cell walls serve as a trigger for the progression of SIRS. Release of endotoxins culminates in the production of various vasoactive substances and a characteristic picture of SIRS. Recent research has shown that this very attractive hypothesis is only partially correct. It now appears that translocation of bacteria into mesenteric lymph nodes plays a relatively minor role in the progression of SIRS. However, endotoxemia may still be a factor in the syndrome's pathogenesis.

In most healthy individuals, the gut barrier protects the body from the potentially deleterious effects of the enteric flora. The barrier separating the gut from the rest of the body consists of chemical, mechanical, local, and systemic immunologic components. All of these components are significantly distorted in SIRS, resulting in alterations of gastric acidity, breakdown of the mucosal integrity, and bacterial translocation and endotoxemia. The gut-body barrier can be maintained or restored by prescribing both pharmacologic and nutritional therapies.

PHARMACOLOGIC THERAPY

The pharmacologic therapies can be separated into systemic and gut-specific regimens. Systemic treatments include cardiovascular resuscitation to avoid injury due to hypoperfusion, timely surgery to limit the progression of tissue destruction, and early ambulation to mobilize natural defenses. Nonsteroidal anti-inflammatory drugs (NSAIDs) continue to play an important role in preventing systemic inflammatory reactions. Traditional NSAIDs remain a mainstay of therapy, with promising newer approaches, including the use of antibodies and receptor antagonists directed against proinflammatory cytokines, prostaglandins, and leukotrienes.

Gut-specific treatments include a variety of antacids and histamine-2 blockers. This classic approach is designed to preserve the integrity of the gut wall by decreasing the acidity of the stomach. We believe that antacids and H_2 blockers play a role in the modern treatment of SIRS because of their proved ability to decrease the incidence of stress gastritis and ulceration. However, large quantities of antacids may lead to increased proliferation of bacteria in an alkaline environment. Enhanced proliferation of bacteria often results in an increased incidence of upper airway colonization and aspiration pneumonia. Therefore, the amount of antacids used should be carefully monitored in patients with SIRS. Our experience suggests that the use of cytoprotective agents such as sucralfate results in decreased bacterial colonization of the gut and upper airway, with a concomitant decrease in the incidence of bacterial translocation and systemic endotoxemia. The use of broad-spectrum systemic antibiotics is controversial. These agents decrease infections in patients with SIRS and severe burns and reduce the rates of bacterial peritonitis in cirrhotic patients with variceal bleeding. However, the results remain much less persuasive when broad-spectrum antibiotic therapy is prescribed for more generalized ICU populations, particularly when the patient has no readily identifiable sources of infection.

NUTRITIONAL THERAPIES

Preventive and supportive measures such as nutritional therapies are the cornerstones of treatment of SIRS. Few studies are available documenting the effectiveness of nutrition therapy in the critically ill. Criteria commonly used in such studies include 28 day mortality, ventilator days, amount of oxygen support required, duration of antibiotic treatment, rate of wound failure, and rate of systemic infections. Significant improvements in these criteria have been reported with the timely institution of nutritional therapy and are due in part to an enhanced protein synthesis rate with resultant increases in nitrogen retention.

Enteral Versus Parenteral Nutrition

There is considerable controversy over the use of enteral and total parenteral nutrition (TPN) in patients with SIRS. If the gut can be used safely, enteral nutrition is preferable for patients with SIRS. There is a substantial reduction in the infectious complications rate with early institution of enteral feeds containing 1.2 to 1.5 g per kilogram per day of amino acids compared with TPN. There is no difference in mortality rates and length of in-hospital stay in the studies available. There is an increased incidence of abdominal distention and diarrhea in enterally fed ICU patients. Some experiments confirm increased rates of intestinal mucosal wasting and immunologic dysfunction in parenterally fed animals compared with the animals maintained on enteral feeds. If the same is true in humans, it suggests that exclusive use of TPN in SIRS patients would produce an increase in rates of hypermetabolism. It is clear that there is no fixed rule in deciding whether enteral or parenteral nutrition should be used in patients with SIRS. We maintain that enteral nutrition should be initiated first whenever possible. If this cannot meet full nutrient requirements, TPN should be used until complete enteral feeds are tolerated. Many patients need both nutritional therapies concurrently. There is a separate chapter on enteral and parenteral nutrition.

Timing of Enteral Feeding

The timing of initiation of enteral feeds is of paramount importance. Enteral nutrition should be started within the first 4 to 5 hours after injury, because early initiation results in more effective nitrogen retention. Moreover, the stress response is blunted with early enteral feeding. For example, catecholamine excretion and plasma glucagon concentrations are reduced in patients whose enteral feeds are started early. Experience suggests that if enteral feeds are started early in patients admitted to the ICU, the incidence of SIRS development may be decreased.

Delivery Methods of Enteral Feedings

The routes of administration of enteral feeds are important in critically ill patients with SIRS and include nasogastric and nasoenteric tubes as well as feeding jejunostomies. Our experience suggests that the jejunum is the preferred site for nutrient delivery to patients with SIRS. Continuous feeding into the jejunum is reasonably well tolerated, and evidence suggests that the risk of aspirations is decreased. However, other modalities can be used as temporary measures. An important aspect of nutrient delivery, especially in the critically ill patient, is to provide concurrent gastric decompression while feeding into the jejunum. This reduces abdominal distention by decreasing the deleterious effects of swallowed air.

Caloric Requirements

Our experience indicates that there is neither metabolic nor physiologic advantage to giving ICU patients calories in excess of basal metabolic requirements. In fact, excessive caloric input increases glycogen deposition in the liver and contributes to hepatic dysfunction. A proportion of carbohydrate, fat, and amino acids is calculated using the following principles. A carbohydrate infusion rate of approximately 4 mg per kilogram per minute appears best in most patients; this is unlikely to cause hyperglycemia and excessive hepatic retention of glycogen. The nitrogen requirement in patients with advanced SIRS is 350 to 450 mg per kilogram per day; the remainder of the 2,500 to 3,000 kcal per day that severely septic patients require is administered as fat.

Diet Selection

Recent studies indicate that the type of diet may be an important factor in preventing SIRS. Diet selection is based on the ability of the patient's gastrointestinal tract to process major nutrients, nutritional requirements, and fluid-electrolyte restrictions. We recommend an initial trial of simple polymeric diets in most patients with SIRS (Table 1). If these are poorly tolerated, specialized elemental diets are recommended. (See the chapter *Parenteral and Enteral Nutrition.*)

Feeding Protocol

A carefully designed feeding protocol is an important part of prevention and care of patients with SIRS. Aspiration of gastric residuals is performed every 4 hours for the first 24 hours and every 8 hours for the next 24 hours. We use 150 to 250 ml as an acceptable volume of aspirate. If the volume of aspirate exceeds this amount, enteral feeding should be temporarily discontinued for 4 hours and the gastric residual remeasured. The starting rate of infusion is 30 to 40 ml per hour, eventually reduced to 10 to 15 ml per hour, if intolerance to feeding is encountered.

Specialized Diets (Table 2)

Formulas containing increased amounts of branched-chain amino acids (BCAA) are recommended for patients with significant hepatic failure and intolerance of standard polymeric diets. As much as 50 percent of the total amino acid content of these formulas consists of BCAAs. The carbohydrate calories in these formulas are provided in the form of maltose-dextrin, whereas fats primarily come from medium-chain triglycerides and soy oil. The caloric density of these formulas is approximately 1.2 kcal per milliliter.

Renal failure is one of the later manifestations of SIRS. When it occurs, formulas containing crystalline essential amino acids as the sole source of protein are used. These formulas are lactose free, are hyperosmolar, and contain very little or no electrolytes. In theory, they minimize urea production by converting urea nitrogen into the nonessential amino acids. There is no evidence that any of these formulations are useful in chronic renal

Table 1 Simple Polymeric Diets*

Product	Concentration kcal/ml	Osmolality mOsm/kg	Carbohydrate		Fat		Protein	
			g/1,000 kcal	%kcal	g/1,000 kcal	%kcal	g/1,000 kcal	%kcal
Isocal HN	1.04	300	121	46	44	37	43	17
Ensure HN	1.06	470	141	53	35	30	44	17
Osmolite HN	1.04	300	141	53	37	30	44	17

*Incomplete listing.

Table 2 Elemental Diets*

Product	Concentration kcal/ml	Osmolality mOsm/kg	Carbohydrate		Fat		Protein	
			g/1,000 kcal	%kcal	g/1,000 kcal	%kcal	g/1,000 kcal	%kcal
Vivonex TEN	1.00	630	210	82	2.8	3	38	15
Alitra Q	1.00	5.75	165	66	15.5	13	52.5	21
Stresstein	1.21	910	142	57	23	21	58	23
Impact	1.00	375	132	53	28	25	56	22
Travasorb Hepatic	1.10	600	196	77.4	13	12	26.7	10.6
Hepatic-Aid	1.20	560	144	57.3	31	27.7	38	15
Travasorb Renal	1.35	590	200	81.1	13	12	1.7	6.9
Amin-Aid	2.00	700	187	74.8	24	21.2	10	4

*Incomplete listing.

failure, but they are reasonably effective in attempts to treat acute renal failure and avoid the need for dialysis. Once dialysis is instituted, a standard polymeric formula is recommended.

As noted, one of the important aspects of SIRS is the impaired functioning of both local and systemic components of the immune system. Enteral diets containing arginine, RNA, and omega-3 polyunsaturated fatty acids (PUFA) have been proposed to improve immune function. The immunomodulatory properties of arginine are related to its function as a lymphotrophic agent as well as its ability to stimulate pituitary growth hormone and insulin release. Lipids high in omega-3 PUFAs compete with omega-6 PUFAs crucial for the production of prostaglandins and leukotrienes. Omega-3 PUFAs also facilitate release of endothelium-derived relaxing factor, with resultant antithrombotic and antiatherosclerotic effects. A number of animal studies suggest that these diets are effective in improving immune function. There is no proof of the effectiveness of this diet in treating human patients with SIRS, but reduced rates of infections have been reported in burn patients who received omega-3 PUFA, arginine, histidine, and cysteine-enriched diets. We suggest that, owing to the grave nature of SIRS and the limited number of treatments available, immune-enhanced formulas are indicated in patients refractory to standard polymeric diets.

Several studies have evaluated the effects of glutamine-enriched diets in ICU patients. Glutamine is a primary fuel of the enterocyte, and its administration improves mucosal integrity in animal models of intestinal dysfunction. In a study of bone marrow transplant recipients, patients who received glutamine supplementation did not have the excessive expansion of extracellular fluids usually observed in individuals receiving standard amino acid diets. In addition, patients receiving glutamine diets had a shortened hospital stay and reduced infections. There is also evidence that patients receiving glutamine-enriched diets have lower rates of bacterial translocation rates, with a resultant decrease in the rate of bacterial infections. Glutamine-enriched diets (up to 40 g of glutamine per day) are recommended for selected patients with intestinal dysfunction and intolerance of standard polymeric diets.

A variety of dietary modifications are available for the treatment of patients with SIRS. The selection of a particular regimen for the individual patient presents a therapeutic challenge. Owing to the severity of SIRS, clinical judgment remains the most important factor in making this decision. As stated previously, the progression of symptoms in SIRS is often predictable. Appropriate nutrition should be used in conjunction with other therapies to halt the progression of the disease before it manifests itself as SIRS. Diets de-

signed to improve the immune status of patients are promising. Once SIRS has occurred, the appropriate diet should be based on the organ or organ system most severely compromised and the status of the gastrointestinal tract.

Complications and Monitoring of Enteral Feedings

A number of complications are commonly associated with enteral feedings, the most serious being pulmonary aspirations, contamination of equipment, tube blockage, food intolerance, and diarrhea. Most of these can be prevented if the following precautions are used. The tubes should be firmly taped to the bridge of the nose with minimal skin traction. Clear marking of the tube is important once the proper position has been established; this helps prevent mucosal destruction as a result of improper tube placement. Regular assessment of gastric residuals is important in reducing the incidence of aspirations. Assessments of gastric residuals should be performed in the first 24 to 48 hours after tube placement. Contamination of equipment can be controlled by aseptic techniques, which most importantly include the use of sterile gloves for feed changes. The tube should be flushed with at least 20 ml of sterile saline before and after each feeding to prevent both contamination and blockage. One should not immediately assume that if a patient develops diarrhea, it is necessarily due to the feeding. The precise cause should be sought and appropriate treatment implemented. The rate of feeding should be reduced if abdominal distention is observed, and if this does not resolve, discontinued.

SUGGESTED READING

Bone RC, Balk RA, Cerra FB, et al. Definitions for sepsis and organ failure and guidelines for the use of innovative therapies in sepsis. The ACCP/SCCM Consensus Conference Committee. American College of Chest Physicians/Society of Critical Care Medicine 1992; 101:1644–1655.

Cerra FB. Multiple organ failure syndrome. Dis Mon 1992; 38: 843–947.

Cipolle MO, Pasquale MO, Cerra FB. Secondary organ dysfunction. From clinical perspective to molecular mediators. Crit Care Clin 1993; 9:261–298.

Clevenger FW. Nutritional support in the patient with the systemic inflammatory response syndrome. Am J Surg 1993; 165 (2A Suppl):685–745.

Rombeau JL. Indications for and administration of enteral and parenteral nutrition in the critically ill. In: Carlson R, Geheb M, eds. Principles and practice of medical intensive care. Philadelphia: WB Saunders, 1993:1528–1551.

Rombeau JL, Rolandelli RH, Wilmore DW. Nutritional support. In: Wilmore DW, ed. Care of the surgical patient: American College of Surgeons. New York: Scientific American 1988; 10:1–39.

DIETARY-INDUCED SYMPTOMS

THEODORE M. BAYLESS, M.D.

Symptoms related to ingested foods can be as dramatic as the fatal food allergies seen in some children with a preexisting history of food allergy. At the other extreme, the relationship between eating a specific food and gastrointestinal symptoms can be very subtle as evidenced by the patient with undiagnosed celiac disease who has not recognized the correlation between eating wheat, rye or oats and his or her steatorrhea.

Although there are chapters in this edition on malabsorptive disorders, including carbohydrate intolerance, this chapter was added to put the symptoms of the patient who is complaining about diet-related symptoms into context with the physiologic and pathophysiologic responses to a meal.

PHYSIOLOGIC RESPONSES TO A MEAL

Motility

The physiologic postprandial events that occur as a subconscious painless process three times a day in healthy persons can result in uncomfortable symptoms in the 5 to 10 percent of the population who have functional bowel disease or organic intestinal disorders. As the antrum of the stomach is distended with a meal, the pyloric mechanism begins to triturate materials into the duodenum as ileal fluid begins to flow into the colon. The colon contents move distally, "pushing" contents which are now dehydrated into solid stool into the rectosigmoid. Those coordinated contractions move the feces into the rectum, producing the urge to defecate.

After the meal, propulsive activity occurs periodically in the small bowel, especially in the ileum. A digestive cycle, characterized by interdigestive migrating myoelectric complexes occurs about every 2 hours. Ileal propulsive waves were felt by three of six healthy controls. As will be discussed later, all 12 patients with irritable bowel syndrome (IBS) complained of cramping discomfort as individual prolonged propagated contractions (PPCs) occurred in the ileum. One could imagine that any degree of limitation to flow, as in acute inflammation with ulceration and edema or in partially obstructed Crohn's disease due to fibrosis and narrowing of the lumen, could produce more discomfort 1 or 2 hours after a solid meal.

Fluid Transport and Secretion

The colon serves both storage and dehydrating functions for the body. Approximately 1,000 to 1,500 ml of liquid contents enter the colon daily. In health, this volume is reduced by absorption to less than 150 ml.

Conditions which effect these fluid shifts can result in drier stools with constipation or in excessive fecal fluid content, diarrhea.

Dietary (exogenous) secretogogues, such as caffeine, can produce excessive net fluid and electrolyte accumulation in the small bowel of normal individuals. The mechanism for net fluid secretion with caffeine is by inhibition of phosphodiesterase and accumulation of cyclic adenosine monophosphate (AMP), a mediator of secretion in the intestine. This modest fluid excess is usually absorbed by the colon which can normally accommodate 2 liters per day and even 3 or 4 liters in the absence of bile salts. Of clinical importance, caffeine ingestion can cause diarrhea in a person with an ileostomy; someone with very rapid colonic transit, such as irritable bowel syndrome; or someone with altered colonic fluid absorption, as in a patient with collagenous colitis.

EXAGGERATED MOTOR RESPONSES TO A MEAL

Patients with the irritable bowel syndrome (IBS) exhibit exaggerated or prolonged electrical and motor responses to feeding both in the small bowel and the colon. Patients with diarrhea have shorter diurnal cycles in the small bowel (77 ± 10 minutes) compared to patients with IBS and constipation (118 ± 15 minutes) or to controls (113 ± 10 minutes). Patients with IBS also have more ileal propulsive waves and clusters of jejunal pressure activity. After a meal, patients with IBS exhibited the characteristic postprandial pattern of random irregular contractions.

Colonic motor activity, especially in the sigmoid seems to be exaggerated after a meal, especially a fatty meal. There are differences in electrical activity with a prolonged response in comparison to controls. The usual "gastro-colic" reflex is quicker and stronger, especially in patients with diarrhea or with left lower quadrant pain. Whitehead and Schuster have concluded that abnormal patterns of colonic motility and abdominal symptoms can be unmasked in IBS by various stimuli, including food, emotional stress, cholinergics and gastrointestinal peptides. There is also a high level of sensitivity of the small bowel in IBS to comparable stimuli. Phillips and co-workers have shown an impressive temporal relationship between dysmotility of the small intestine and abdominal symptoms in the IBS patient.

Intestinal distension, one of the physiologic responses to a meal, is intensified by the presence of excessive stool as with diarrhea or steatorrhea or by gas, as with carbohydrate malabsorption. It is important to remember that patients with IBS experience colonic contractions and pain with amounts of balloon distension that wouldn't effect "controls." Small bowel distension can also cause cramps and discomfort in IBS patients.

Therefore patients with IBS are likely to be more symptomatic with even modest amounts of intestinal gas.

This might occur after drinking large amounts of carbonated beverages, using an effervescent laxative, receiving an effervescent (air-contrast) upper GI series, undergoing an air contrast barium enema or eating cabbage, cole slaw or baked beans. IBS patients may experience pronounced gastrointestinal distress after ingesting small amounts of unabsorbed carbohydrates, such as 15 g of fructose (equivalent to a quarter pound of grapes). The combination of 25 g fructose and 5 g sorbitol (the sugars found in apple and pear juice) is also poorly tolerated by patients with functional bowel disease. These thresholds for carbohydrate malabsorption and symptom production in IBS patients, are definitely lower than in control subjects. Patients with constipation can be even more symptomatic after ingesting large amounts of potentially distending materials.

Recognizing that 10 to 12 percent of the population have the "tendency" to develop IBS is helpful when evaluating patients with inflammatory bowel disease or any other organic disorder. Some patients have IBS plus another disorder. Abdominal pain and bloating can occur in a patient with previous peptic ulcer surgery who has subtle fat and lactose malabsorption and underlying IBS. Lessening the bulky stools often makes management of the IBS easier. Another example of poorly tolerated left colon distension occurs in patients with both IBS and Crohn's disease who undergo ileal-right colon resection. The large fluid load, perhaps intensified by bile salt malabsorption, causes distension of the descending and sigmoid colon especially after a meal. The patient and sometimes the doctor are erroneously convinced that the Crohn's disease has activated in the left colon just a few weeks after a "negative" preoperative colonoscopy or barium enema.

SPECIFIC FOOD INTOLERANCES

Food Protein Allergies

Food allergy is a consideration when a specific food regularly precipitates symptoms in an individual (often a child) with a history of associated allergic reactions, such as asthma or atopic dermatitis. Clear examples of dietary protein allergy do exist, albeit rare compared to the frequency of IBS. Seafood, fruits, nuts, milk protein, and eggs are among the common foods incriminated. Fatal anaphylactic reactions, usually via pulmonary manifestations do occur but are preventable if the child carries an epinephrine syringe or if prompt medical attention is provided.

Gastroenterologists become skeptical about food "allergies" as described by patients with gastrointestinal complaints, especially IBS. Some of these intolerances are real and can be traced to carbohydrate malabsorption, such as lactose, fructose or sorbitol. Others are bothered by large, fatty or "rich" meals that stimulate the sigmoid colon causing pain or diarrhea within 30 minutes of starting the meal. Some patients are symptomatic one day but can eat the same food without symptoms another day. Careful questioning often reveals external psycho-social stresses or recent bouts of incomplete fecal evacuation as a non-dietary factor effecting meal or food tolerance.

Lactose Intolerance

Abdominal bloating and flatulence two to six hours after ingesting one or two glasses of milk or a large amount of frozen yogurt or ice cream, especially on an empty stomach, is the typical story obtained from about 75 percent of individuals with low intestinal lactase levels. This important topic is discussed in detail in the chapter *Carbohydrate Malabsorption*.

Based on our small population studies in the 1960s and 70s with Drs. Norton Rosensweig, Shi Shung Huang, and David Paige, we had predicted that 30 million Americans would be lactose intolerant as determined by a 50 gram lactose tolerance test (equal to 1 quart of milk). The pharmaceutical firms that market "lactase" now claim, that with the increased U.S. population, many of whom are from areas with a high prevalence of potential lactose intolerance, 50 million is a better estimate for the number of lactose-intolerant individuals. Again, it should be pointed out that those estimates are based on intolerance of 50 grams of lactose, equivalent to a quart of milk.

Opinions vary as to how many of these millions of people will be symptomatic with more physiologic amounts of milk. We predicted that 50 percent of lactose intolerant people could be symptomatic with one glass of milk (240 ml) on an empty stomach. Increasing the lactose load to two glasses (480 ml) could produce symptoms, usually flatulence or bloating in 75 percent. More recent studies with breath hydrogen testing still predict that at least 60 percent of those with lactose maldigestion will be symptomatic with a glass or glass and a half of milk. It is important to note that other workers disagree with this estimate of the frequency of potential milk intolerance. A recent review in the American Journal of Clinical Nutrition sponsored by the dairy industry, stated that very few people with lactose malabsorption would be seriously symptomatic with a glass of milk. Clinical experience teaches most experienced clinicians otherwise. It is true, however, that milk and lactose intolerance probably does not explain all of the symptoms for which millions of people are now buying lactase pills or drops or using lactose hydrolyzed milk.

Whether or not an individual with low intestinal lactase levels will be symptomatic depends upon: the amount of lactose; the dilution with other food; the rate of gastric emptying (slower with whole milk, with chocolate milk and with a meal); the levels of lactase in the duodenum and jejunum; and the irritability of the colon. Enzyme-specific activity is lowered by mucosal injury, such as celiac disease, giardiasis or bacterial overgrowth and perhaps alcoholism. Patients with co-existent IBS usually are more symptomatic with smaller sugar loads than "controls." Because we found that 15 of 20 known "milk intolerant" people who were fasting were symptomatic with 12 grams of lactose, we usually suggest that, as a test, a person who suspects they may be lactose intolerant try two glasses of skim milk (24 grams of lactose) on an empty stomach as a "tolerance test" after 2 to 3 days of avoiding dairy products. Skim milk and fasting are chosen because the lack of fat and other foods cause faster gastric emptying, less dilution of the lactose, and perhaps more symptoms, and thus provide a better "diagnostic" test.

The question arises as to how little lactose "should" bother a patient with lactose intolerance. Dr. Marshall Bedine and I could demonstrate an osmotic effect in the small bowel with 6 grams of lactose but not with 3 grams. However breath hydrogen testing is more sensitive and can detect as little as 1.5 to 2 grams of unabsorbed carbohydrate entering the colon. Some patients (many of whom are quite outspoken) feel they are intolerant of the milligram quantities of lactose in some foods and some medications. Most physicians haven't used double-blind placebo tablets to try to prove or disprove these "sensitivities" because many of these patients will continue to utilize rigid exclusion diets regardless of well-meaning medical advice. (Please see the chapter on fad diets.)

Fructose Intolerance

Fructose is transported by facilitated diffusion, not by active transport as is glucose. Dr. William Ravich and I showed that 70 percent of healthy lab personnel could not completely absorb 50 grams of a 20 percent solution of fructose (the amount of fructose in a pound of grapes) as judged by symptoms and breath hydrogen excretion. We recently confirmed this observation in first year medical students who ingested 50 grams of fructose as part of a physiology course laboratory experiment. Seventy percent of these presumably healthy students malabsorbed a portion of a 50 gram fructose load and were symptomatic, having cramps, flatulence or diarrhea. Patients with IBS are even more symptomatic with fructose or the potentiating combination of fructose and sorbitol.

One should suspect fructose intolerance as a cause of symptoms if a person is ingesting grapes, nuts, figs, dates, honey or apple or pear juice. Also many commercial fruit soft drinks, such as Fanta, as well as many popular cola drinks, contain 55 percent fructose solution as a sweetener. However since these beverages also contain glucose, the fructose absorption is enhanced and few symptoms occur on a fructose malabsorption basis. The carbonation and caffeine in soft drinks may be another source of dietary-induced symptoms.

Sorbitol Intolerance

Sorbitol, usually in "sugar-free" products or fruit juice can cause gastrointestinal symptoms. As discussed in the chapter *Carbohydrate Malabsorption,* sorbitol is a straight chain hexahydric alcohol which is only passively absorbed in the small bowel. Half of a group of healthy adults will be symptomatic with 10 grams of sorbitol while IBS patients are bothered by as little as 5 grams, especially if in combination with fructose, as in apple or pear juice. Other sources of sorbitol include peaches, pears, plums, sugarless gum, diet gum and mints. Treatment is to reduce or eliminate use of poorly absorbed carbohydrates in the symptomatic patient. However, some people build up a symptomatic tolerance to continued intake of sorbitol or xylitol. We also noted enhanced tolerance of platinit (a poorly absorbed synthetic carbohydrate) with prolonged intake.

Fiberophagia

Among the dietary trends that move back and forth across this continent, eating large amounts of dietary fiber is one of the more popular and self-sustaining. Symptoms that can be caused by newly started or excessive fiber intake include early satiety evoked by the delayed gastric emptying caused by soluble fibers as well as delayed small bowel transit. Some patients are quite symptomatic, especially in the first few days of excessive fiber intake.

An increase in breath hydrogen excretion can be detected 6 to 8 hours after a healthy person ingests eight slices of whole wheat bread. Presumably patients with co-existent IBS will be even more symptomatic with smaller quantities of fiber intake.

Gluten-containing breads can cause large volumes of colonic gas in healthy people. Thus it is not surprising that some patients with IBS and with Crohn's disease feel better on a gluten-free diet. For these reasons a "response" to a gluten-free diet is not equivalent to a diagnosis of celiac disease. The damaged small intestine, as in the infant with infectious diarrhea or the adult with tropical sprue will improve somewhat with a gluten-free diet. One should continue to insist on a flat distal duodenal or jejunal mucosal biopsy before considering the diagnosis of celiac disease. Celiac disease, discussed in a separate chapter, is one of the clearest examples of dietary-induced symptoms, although most patients have not recognized the relationship between grain ingestion and their symptoms.

Matzos, a form of unleavened bread eaten by Jewish people at Passover is probably another source of poorly-absorbed carbohydrate. Anecdotally, some patients report excessive gassiness during Passover. Perhaps this is another example of carbohydrate malabsorption.

Fatty Food Intolerances

Excessive fat intake will probably worsen the diarrhea of any patient with steatorrhea, regardless of cause. Lowering the fat intake is an important management step in the patient with a short bowel syndrome.

The colonic motor response to a fatty meal is a form of food intolerance that is not always appreciated by physicians. The exaggerated sigmoid colon contractions after a fatty meal, can be very painful to the patient with IBS and explaining the physiologic relationship helps the patient understand their symptoms and the relationship to large meals. Some patients with fatty food intolerance and irritable bowel syndrome have undergone cholecystectomy for probably asymptomatic gallstones only to return with postcholecystectomy diarrhea secondary to excessive bile acids and excessive fluid in the already irritable colon.

Dietary Secretagogues

The role of caffeine in producing excessive small bowel secretion is discussed in the physiology section of this chapter. As a therapeutic maneuver, decreasing caffeine intake may help the patients with non-specific watery diarrhea, collagenous colitis and, especially, the person with a high output ileostomy.

The author and a few acquaintances have noted severe intestinal cramps, pallor and sweating followed by diarrhea occurring about 30 minutes after ingesting foods containing even small amounts of garlic. The syndrome lasts about 20 minutes and the effect is usually enhanced by the ingestion of alcohol with the meal. The three physicians who have noted this intolerance were able to eat garlic until about age 25. Despite questioning hundreds of people, we have only found a few patients with this seemingly rare syndrome. Since garlic contains a number of potent amines and other chemicals, it is possible that one of these fractions (perhaps the one that acts as a laxative in cattle or as a vermifuge) is responsible for this unusual intolerance.

Gassy Patient

The chapters *Carbohydrate Malabsorption* and *Irritable Bowel Syndrome* provide clues that can be utilized in dealing with the patient with excessive flatulence and gassiness. Since one can produce IBS symptoms in almost anyone by constipating them with loperamide, rule number one in the gassy patient is to correct the altered bowel habits of their underlying IBS. Also, some psycho-social life stresses may exacerbate a "food intolerance" of previously-tolerated foods. If the alternating constipation and pellet-like stools of IBS continue, various dietary manipulations will be difficult, if not impossible, to evaluate.

COMMENTS

There are a modest number of people with potentially serious food protein allergies, sometimes manifested as extra-intestinal symptoms. Others, also small in number, are very symptomatic with one food substance such as garlic, or have the gluten-induced enteropathy of celiac disease. The key in many patients with persistent "food intolerances" despite your best efforts and perhaps that of your nutritionist, seems often to be the role of the irritable bowel syndrome in exaggerating physiologic responses to dietary stimuli. Patients are often convinced that what they eat causes symptoms. Sometimes they are right.

SUGGESTED READING

Alun-Jones A, McLaughlan P, Shorthouse M, et al. Food intolerance; a major factor in the pathogenesis of irritable bowel syndrome. Lancet 1982; ii:1115–1117.

Bayless TM. Coexistent irritable bowel syndrome and inflammatory bowel disease. In: Bayless TM, ed. Current Management of Inflammatory Bowel Disease, Toronto: BC Decker, 1989:59.

Bedine MS, Bayless TM. Intolerance of small amounts of lactose by individuals with low lactase levels. Gastroenterology 1973; 65: 735–743.

Friedman G. Diet and the irritable bowel syndrome. Gastroenterology Clin North Am 1991; 20:313.

Kellow JE, Phillips SF. Altered small bowel motility in irritable bowel syndrome is correlated with symptoms. Gastroenterology 1987; 91:1985–1993.

Levitt MD, Hirsh P, Fetzer CA, et al. H_2 excretion after ingestion of complex carbohydrates. Gastroenterology 1987; 92:383–389.

Rasmussen JJ, Gudman-Hoyer E. Functional bowel disease; malabsorption and abdominal distress after ingestion of fructose, sorbitol, and fructose-sorbitol mixtures. Gastroenterology 1989; 95:694–700.

Ravich WJ, Bayless TM. Carbohydrate absorption and malabsorption. Clinics in Gastroenterology 1983; 12:335–356.

Sampson HA, Mendelson L, Rosen J. Fatal and near-fatal anaphylactic reactions to food in children and adolescents. N Engl J Med 1992; 327:380–384.

Scrimshaw NS, Murray EB. The acceptability of milk and milk products in populations with a high prevalence of lactose intolerance. Am J Clin Nutr 1988; 48:1083–1159.

Snape J, Matarazzo SA, Cohen S. Effect of eating and gastrointestinal hormones on human colonic myoelectric and motor activity. Gastroenterology 1978; 75:373–378.

Wald A, Back C, Bayless TM. Effect of caffeine on the human small intestine. Gastroenterology 1976; 71:738–742.

GASTROINTESTINAL AND HEPATIC COMPLICATIONS OF BONE MARROW TRANSPLANTATION

TIMOTHY A. WOODWARD, M.D.
BERNARD LEVIN, M.D.

Bone marrow transplantation (BMT) has expanded into the 1990s as a major therapy for leukemia as well as solid malignancies (e.g., breast cancer), along with several nonmalignant disorders (aplastic anemia, congenital immunodeficiencies, homozygous hemoglobinopathies, and inborn errors of metabolism). However, serious and potentially fatal complications affecting almost all major organ systems may be encountered. This is particularly true of the gastrointestinal (GI) tract. Most GI problems in the setting of BMT have a characteristic chronology, allowing for a temporal classification (Table 1). Immediate enteric symptoms suggest toxicity engendered by the preparative regimen (chemoirradiation), whereas early and late complications are more likely due to graft-versus-host disease (GVHD) or infectious complications. Since infectious and immune-mediated complications often have similar presentations, an aggressive and prompt diagnostic and therapeutic approach is mandatory.

PREPARATIVE AND IMMEDIATE POST-TRANSPLANTATION COMPLICATIONS

The goal of preparative regimens in BMT is to achieve maximal malignant cell kill and sufficient immu-

Table 1 Temporal Classification of Gastrointestinal Complications of Bone Marrow Transplantation in Consecutive Post-Transplantation Periods

Immediate (days 0–25)*
  Hepatic veno-occlusive disease
  Intestinal chemoirradiation toxicity

Early (days 25-100)
  Acute hepatic GVHD
  Acute intestinal GVHD (enteritis)

Late (beyond day 100)
  Chronic hepatic GVHD
  Chronic enteric GVHD (esophageal)

Incessant and recurrent nausea and vomiting
  TPN-related hepatopathy
  Infection
    Early—bacterial and fungal
    Late—viral

*Day 0 = day of bone marrow transplantation.
GVHD = graft-versus-host disease; TPN = total parenteral nutrition.

nosuppression with minimal toxicity. Standard preparative regimens use cyclophosphamide and total body irradiation. Irradiation-free protocols are evolving, in particular busulfan and cyclophosphamide. Enterohepatic toxicity in all preparative programs usually develops within 3 weeks.

Intestinal Chemoirradiation Toxicity

Intestinal chemoirradiation toxicity manifests primarily in the small intestine and colon, with crampy abdominal pain, anorexia, and watery diarrhea occurring in the immediate post-transplant period. Symptoms generally resolve within 3 weeks unless GVHD and/or enteric infections supervene. Intestinal biopsies are not routinely done in the immediate post-preparative setting. Treatment is usually supportive, and total parenteral nutrition (TPN) is usually necessary for the 3 weeks required for the resolution of intestinal damage. Persistence of symptoms over 3 weeks should raise the suspicion of GVHD or enteric infections (Fig. 1).

Hepatic Veno-occlusive Disease

Hepatic veno-occlusive disease (VOD) evolves from microvascular damage to the small interhepatic venules, leading to venular obstruction together with damage to surrounding hepatocytes and sinusoids. Patients are considered to have VOD if they demonstrate two of the following three clinical criteria: jaundice, hepatomegaly, or unexplained weight gain within 14 days of bone marrow infusion. If only one feature is present or there are confounding events, (e.g., septicemia or pancreatitis), the diagnosis is uncertain. The incidence of VOD in BMT recipients is approximately 10 percent, with mortality rates varying between 30 and 40 percent.

Transjugular liver biopsy has been a major development in the diagnosis and management of VOD, particularly for distinguishing between VOD and GVHD or massive viral hepatitis (e.g., herpes or adenovirus groups). Adequate tissue is obtained in approximately 90 percent of liver biopsies. In addition, pressure gradients can be obtained. A hepatic wedge-free pressure gradient of greater than 10 mm Hg has an approximately 90 percent positive predictive value for a histologic diagnosis of VOD; the converse, i.e., the negative predictive value for less than 10 mm Hg, is 80 percent. The histologic appearance reveals occlusion of venular lumens by subendothelial reticulum or collagen fibers and atrophy of paracentral hepatocytes.

Newer preventive approaches and therapies can be added to the standard management of VOD (Table 2). Standard treatment entails maintaining intravascular blood volume as well as improving renal performance; this is accompanied by transfusion of red cells and infusion of colloid and albumin. Hemodialysis is occasionally necessary to control fluid accumulation and renal failure. Therapeutic paracentesis may be performed for refractory ascites, particularly when this is

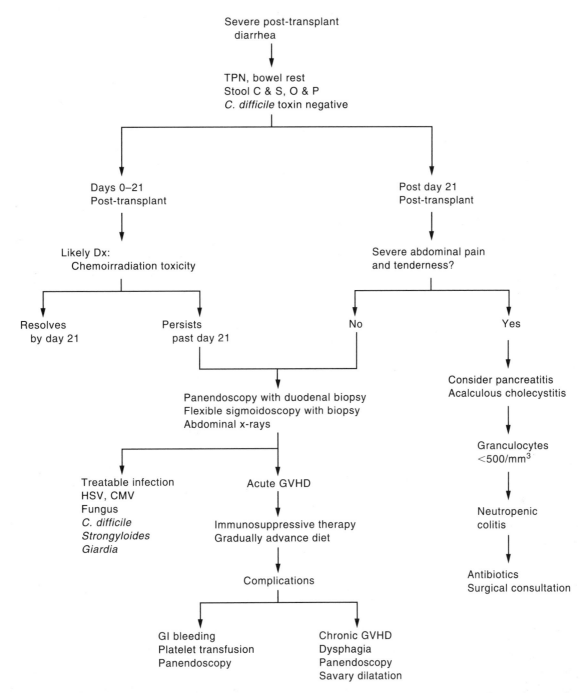

Figure 1 Algorithm for the management of severe diarrhea after bone marrow transplantation. C & S = culture and sensitivity; O & P = ova and parasites; Dx = diagnosis. (Modified from Gholson CF, LeMaistre CF, Levin B. Gastrointestinal problems after bone marrow transplantation. In: Bayless TM, ed. Current therapy in gastroenterology and liver disease. 3rd ed. Philadelphia: BC Decker, 1990:195; with permission.)

associated with dyspnea. Surgical measures are implemented only if the above therapies fail; in cases extending beyond 50 days after transplantation (when spontaneous resolution is rare), side-to-side portocaval shunts and orthotopic liver transplants have been employed. Transjugular intrahepatic portosystemic shunts (TIPSs) may present an alternative to surgical management of VOD in the future.

Table 2 New Modalities in Prevention and Treatment of Veno-occlusive Disease

Heparin
Prostaglandins of the E_1 group (PGE_1)
Recombinant tissue plasminogen factor (r-tPA)
TNF-alpha blockers (pentoxifylline, ciprofloxacin)
Ursodeoxycholic acid (UDCA)

Table 3 Clinical Stage of Acute Graft Versus Host Disease

Stage	Skin	Liver	Gut
+	Maculopapular rash <25% body surface	Bilirubin, 2–3 mg/dl	Diarrhea, 500–1,000 mg/day
+ +	Maculopapular rash 25%–50% body surface	Bilirubin, 3–6 mg/dl	Diarrhea 1,000–1,500 ml/day
+ + +	Generalized erythroderma	Bilirubin, 6–15 mg/dl	Diarrhea >1,500 ml/day
+ + + +	Desquamation and bullae	Bilirubin, >15 mg/dl	Pain or ileus

Modified from Hershko C, Gale RP. GVHD scoring system for predicting survival and specific mortality in bone marrow transplant recipients. In: Gale RP, Fox CF, eds. Biology of bone marrow transplantation. New York: Academic, 1980:59–67; with permission.

Several clinical studies have recently demonstrated a decrease in the incidence of VOD with either pentoxifylline (a rheoretic agent that diminishes the effect of mediators of inflammation, particularly TNF-alpha) or ursodiol (ursodeoxycholic acid, a hydrophilic bile acid used for the dissolution of gallstones). Prophylactic treatment with prostaglandins of the E_1 group (PGE_1) may reduce VOD, but caution is required because of side effects, (bullous skin lesions, edema, and postural hypotension), particularly in patients receiving cyclosporin. Tissue plasminogen activator (tPA) has been used to treat VOD, with results suggesting that it may reverse the natural history of even severe disease.

EARLY POST-TRANSPLANTATION COMPLICATIONS: ACUTE GRAFT VERSUS HOST DISEASE

The principal complication of BMT is still GVHD. Moderate to severe GVHD occurs in 35 to 60 percent of transplant patients and is the primary cause of death in 12 to 20 percent of all allogenic recipients. GVHD results from reactivity of engrafted immunocompetent lymphocytes against recipient tissue. Acute GVHD begins 20 to 80 days after transplantation. Chronic GVHD usually develops after 80 days and is generally preceded by acute GVHD, although it may arise de novo. Prognosis is related to clinical grade (Tables 3 and 4); more than 50 percent of patients with grades II to IV die of acute GVHD.

Graft Versus Host Disease Prophylaxis

Immunosuppressive prophylaxis is used to reduce the significant mortality associated with grades II to IV acute GVHD. Standard preventive regimens consist of two modalities: immunosuppression and T-cell depletion. Methotrexate, antithymocyte globulin, cyclosporine, and corticosteroids are used, either singly or in combination. Current data suggest that the combination of short-course methotrexate with cyclosporine reduces the incidence of severe acute GVHD to as little as 10 percent with donor-matched siblings.

Table 4 Clinical Grade of Acute Graft Versus Host Disease Severity

Grade	Degree of Organ Involvement
I	+ to + + skin rash, no gut involvement, no liver involvement, no decrease in clinical performance
II	+ to + + + skin rash; + gut involvement or + liver involvement (or both); mild decrease in clinical performance
III	+ + to + + + skin rash; + + to + + + gut involvement or + + to + + + liver involvement (or both); marked decrease in clinical performance.
IV	Similar to grade III but with + + to + + + + organ involvement and extreme decrease in clinical performance

Modified from Hershko C, Gale RP. GVHD scoring system for predicting survival and specific mortality in bone marrow transplant recipients. In: Gale RP, Fox CF, eds. Biology of bone marrow transplantation. New York: Academic, 1980:59–67; with permission.

T-cell depletion consists of removing T cells from the graft by either elutriation or anti–T cell monoclonal antibodies. Results have been mixed in several trials.

As with VOD, clinical trials have shown a decrease in the incidence of GVHD with pentoxifylline, and a reduction of grades II to IV GVHD from 68 percent in controls to 35 percent in those receiving the drug. Preliminary data from a multicenter study demonstrate the efficacy of monoclonal antibodies against the interleukin-2 (IL-2) receptor in decreasing GVHD; only 17 percent developed severe disease. Intestinal decontamination with nonabsorbable antibiotics and decontaminated food has also been shown to reduce the incidence of GVHD (see "Bacterial Infections" below).

Acute Enteric Graft Versus Host Disease

Acute enteric GVHD predominantly involves the terminal ileum and the right colon, presenting with nausea and vomiting, postprandial pain, and GI bleeding. Profuse diarrhea occurs and is often accompanied by passage of strands of intestinal epithelium. Protein loss is significant in the diarrheal fluid and is reflected in a decrease in serum total protein and albumin levels. Besides GVHD, residual effects of conditioning chemo-irradiation and/or enteric infection may also account for the clinical picture of enteropathy. In particular, certain viruses (cytomegalovirus [CMV], herpes simplex virus [HSV], coxsackievirus, rotavirus, and adenovirus) are major opportunistic agents associated with enteritis in this setting. Endoscopic biopsies can help distinguish between herpes virus enteritides and acute GVHD. Cytoplasmic inclusions may be seen in the biopsy specimen and help establish the diagnosis of CMV; acute GVHD is manifested histopathologically as crypt cell necrosis or drop-out, i.e., apoptosis.

Treatment is supportive and directed at specific clinical problems as they evolve. Initial management strategies entail bowel rest and TPN; investigations should be undertaken to exclude treatable pathogens causing pseudomembranous colitis or HSV enteritis. Caution should be employed with the use of antidiarrheal agents in order to avoid ileus, especially given the potential for neutropenic colitis, i.e., typhlitis, in this setting.

Abdominal pain in the early post-transplant period should raise suspicions of neutropenic colitis (with absolute neutrophil counts below 500 per cubic millimeter) and acalculous cholecystitis, especially after prolonged TPN when gallbladder stasis is thought to be the predisposing factor. Ultrasonography may suggest the diagnosis of acalculous cholecystitis by demonstrating an enlarged gallbladder with a thickened wall (greater than 6 mm), pericholecystic fluid, and tenderness to palpation with the ultrasound probe; treatment consists of surgery. Pancreatitis has been associated with BMT. Bezoars secondary to cellular debris and slough have been reported.

Most persistent GI bleeding is from diffuse esophagitis or gastroduodenal erosions, often fungal or viral in origin. A retrospective analysis demonstrated that the median time to a hemorrhagic event was 3 months, with bleeding complication being one of the major causes of death. Panendoscopy should be employed; if the results are negative, radionuclide bleeding scans should follow. Unfortunately, bleeding is usually diffuse, precluding successful endoscopic or angiographic intervention. Pneumatosis intestinalis may also affect recipients. Corticosteroid therapy, infection by gas-forming bacteria, and GVHD are believed to be predisposing factors. Treatment includes an elemental diet, antibiotics (specifically, intravenous [IV] metronidazole), and oxygen.

As outlined in Table 5, newer forms of treatment are emerging. Examples include ricin A-chain immunotoxins directed at T cells, as well as IL-2–receptor antagonists.

Acute Hepatic Graft Versus Host Disease

Cholestatic jaundice lasting longer than 21 days suggests GVHD. However, the differential diagnosis must include VOD, viral hepatitis (particularly hepatitis

Table 5 New Modalities in Prevention and Treatment of Graft Versus Host Disease

Prophylaxis
  Selective T-cell depletion (CD8, CD6)
  Fixed low number of T cells
  Specific elimination of alloreactive T cells
  GVL (graft-versus-leukemia) reactive lymphocyte returned to recipient
  Adoptive immunotherapy with donor LAK cells
  New immunosuppressors (rapamycine, FK506, deoxyspergualin, RS61443, Brequinar)
  Monoclonal antibodies (T-cell, p55, IL-2R)
  Anti-CD5 ricin A-chain immunotoxin

Treatment
  New immunosuppressors (e.g., FK 506, rapamycine)
  Monoclonal cell effector–specific antibodies (CD2, CD25, CD3, CD5, TCR alpha, beta Campath 1G)
  Monoclonal cytokine effector–specific antibodies (anti-TNF alpha)
  Anti-CD5 ricin A-chain immunotoxin
  Photopheresis UV-A + 8-MOP

Modified from Heuve P, Tiberghien P, Racadot E, et al. New modalities in the prevention and treatment of acute GVHD. In: Prevention and treatment of acute GVHD—new modalities. Bone Marrow Transplant 1993; 11 (Suppl):103–106.

B and C and CMV), and fungal infections (Fig. 2). Although jaundice may be severe, markedly elevated hepatocellular enzyme levels with prolongation of the prothrombin time and portosystemic encephalopathy are rare. Percutaneous liver biopsy with platelet counts less than 60,000 per cubic millimeter is unsafe. However, as mentioned, transjugular liver biopsy has somewhat lessened such concerns. Overall, a liver biopsy is probably not necessary if the patient presents with skin and intestinal manifestations of GVHD. In cases in which biopsy is warranted, histopathology reveals, after weeks to months of GVHD, extensive hepatocyte drop-out, sinusoidal fibrosis, and Kupffer-cell hyperplasia. Treatment consists primarily of immunosuppressive therapy, with milder cases slowly responding to cyclosporine, prednisone, or antithymocyte globulin. Most cases, unfortunately, evolve into chronic hepatic GVHD.

LATE POST-TRANSPLANTATION COMPLICATIONS: CHRONIC GRAFT VERSUS HOST DISEASE

Chronic GVHD develops 80 to 400 days after allogeneic BMT, and most cases follow previously diagnosed acute GVHD; 25 percent, however, arise de novo. Esophageal and hepatic involvement is common with chronic GVHD; death is usually due to systemic infection (particularly viral: CMV, HSV, and herpes zoster virus) secondary to profound impairment of the immune system.

Chronic Enteric Graft Versus Host Disease

The primary GI manifestation of chronic GVHD is esophageal disease. Chronic GVHD shares features of

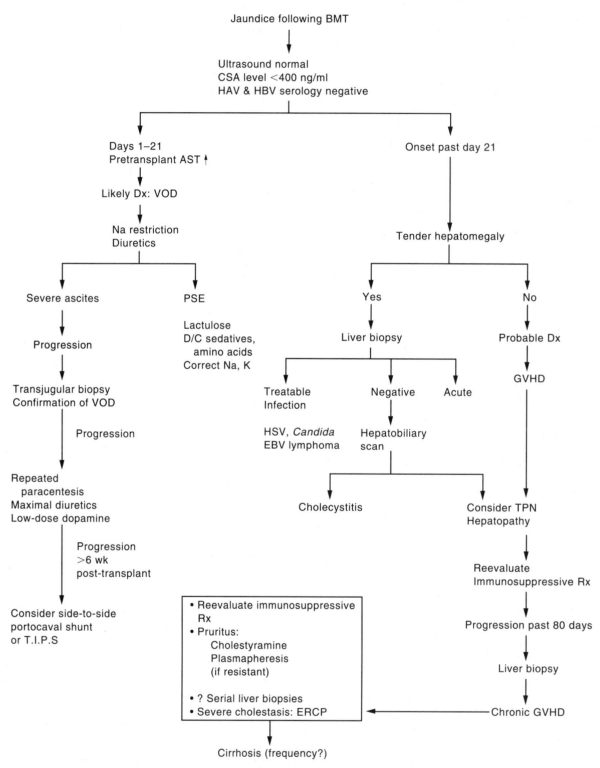

Figure 2 Algorithm for the management of jaundice after bone marrow transplantation. D/C = discontinue; Dx = diagnosis; EBV = Epstein-Barr virus; HAV = hepatitis A virus; HBV = hepatitis B virus; PSE = portosystemic encephalopathy. (Modified from Gholson CF, LeMaistre CF, Levin B. Gastrointestinal problems after bone marrow transplantation. In: Bayless TM, ed. Current therapy in gastroenterology and liver disease. 3rd ed. Philadelphia: BC Decker, 1990:197; with permission.)

various autoimmune disorders, e.g., scleroderma, and Sjögren's syndrome, both clinically and pathologically. Dysphagia, odynophagia, retrosternal pain, and weight loss are the usual presenting symptoms. Retrosternal pain is usually due to acid reflux onto denuded esophageal mucosa and responds to standard antireflux measures, including H_2-receptor antagonists. Caution should be employed with the latter in view of reports of drug-related myelosuppression in up to 5 percent of BMT patients treated with ranitidine. Endoscopy frequently reveals webs and strictures, usually in the proximal and middle esophagus. Biopsy is performed to exclude esophageal infection, specifically HSV and CMV. Particular histologic findings of chronic GVHD include lymphocytic and neutrophilic infiltrates with necrosis and desquamation of the squamous basal layer. Therapy includes Savary dilatation and treatment of any underlying infections. Recent trials also suggest a role for thalidomide (for an immunosuppressive effect of the drug, possibly similar to cyclosporine) in the treatment of chronic GVHD.

Chronic Hepatic Graft Versus Host Disease

Chronic liver disease is seen in almost all patients with chronic GVHD, manifesting usually as cholestasis with fluctuating jaundice. Progression to cirrhosis with portal hypertension is uncommon. Measures should be taken to exclude other potentially treatable diseases, such as chronic viral infections (in particular hepatitis B and C and CMV), infiltrative liver disease (tuberculosis), hepatic drug reactions (e.g., from trimethoprim-sulfamethexazole), and cholestasis secondary to drugs used to treat chronic GVHD (azathioprine and cyclosporine). Extrahepatic obstruction should be excluded by ultrasonography or endoscopic retrograde cholangiopancreatography (ERCP). Liver biopsies from patients with long-standing chronic GVHD reveal a marked reduction or complete absence of bile ducts. To circumvent subtle progression to cirrhosis in patients with clinically quiescent GVHD, serial liver biopsies may help guide immunosuppressive therapy.

GASTROINTESTINAL INFECTIONS POST-TRANSPLANT

The first 3 weeks after BMT represent the period in which infections from either bacterial or fungal organisms predominate until the initial neutropenia and other preparative toxicities resolve. Subsequent viral infections are common for up to 4 months and even longer after BMT owing to protracted restitution of immunocompetence.

Bacterial Infections

With the exception of *Clostridium difficile* enterocolitis, bacterial infections confined to the GI tract are uncommon. Septicemia due to invasion of gram-negative

flora through denuded mucosa is a persistent threat to neutropenic BMT recipients. Complete GI decontamination (accomplished with a regimen of tobramycin, 80 mg; vancomycin, 250 mg; polymyxin, 700,000 units; and nystatin, 3 million units all given orally, three times a day along with decontaminated food) with strict reverse isolation is the treatment of choice for the prevention of infections and GVHD in BMT recipients.

Typhlitis (neutropenic colitis) is a rare but well-recognized complication of BMT with an associated mortality rate of 50 to 100 percent. Suspicion should be alerted by the development of right lower abdominal pain in the setting of a decreased white blood cell count (less than 500 per cubic millimeter). As surgical intervention in the setting of BMT carries a very high perioperative mortality rate, treatment is conservative and includes bowel rest, IV fluids, and antibiotic coverage (a third-generation cephalosporin with an aminoglycoside plus the possible addition of metronidazole). Computed tomography (CT)-guided drainage has proved useful.

C. difficile enterocolitis may occur in the post-transplant period, presenting with fever, diarrhea, and abdominal pain. The sigmoidoscopic appearance may be atypical in neutropenic patients. Metronidazole, 500 mg every 8 hours, or oral vancomycin, 500 mg every 6 hours, is the treatment of choice. If ileus is present and the patient is not neutropenic, vancomycin can be given by enema, 1 g in 1 L of saline every 6 hours together with systemic vancomycin or metronidazole.

Fungal Infections

Infections with *Candida* species are a serious problem detected in up to 40 percent of BMT recipients at autopsy. The mortality rate for patients with systemic *Candida* infections in the early post-transplant period is 79 percent. The primary port of entry is through defects in the GI mucosa; the most important risk factors for the development of systemic *Candida* infection are increasing age and duration of neutropenia. Administration of recombinant G-CSF and/or GM-CSF may shorten the granulocytopenic period and thereby decrease the incidence of *Candida* infections. Fluconazole given prophylactically at 200 mg per day has proved safe and effective in decreasing the incidence of systemic candidiasis as well. *Aspergillus* and less susceptible *Candida* species may subsequently arise and cause infections, however. *Candida* esophagitis in neutropenic patients should be treated with IV amphotericin B, 0.3 mg per kilogram per day, although oral nystatin, 3 million units "swish and swallow," or clotrimazole, 100 mg troches every 8 hours, may suffice in non-neutropenic patients. The use of empiric amphotericin B in febrile patients not responding to empiric antibacterial agents has been successful.

Painful hepatomegaly suggests hepatic candidiasis. The characteristic bull's-eye lesions seen on CT or ultrasonography are evident only after neutropenia has resolved; therefore, liver biopsy may be necessary for early diagnosis.

Viral Infections

The esophagus and liver are frequent sites for viral infections in immunosuppressed patients after BMT. HSV reactivates in 60 to 80 percent of seropositive recipients; patients with higher pretransplant titers seem to be at an increased risk. Most HSV infections occur 1 month after BMT. Prophylaxis with oral and IV acyclovir, 500 mg per square meter every 8 hours for 7 days, is well established and also prevents varicella zoster.

The reactivation of CMV is a major cause of infection (in 50 percent of recipients) and death following BMT, usually 3 to 4 months after transplantation. CMV retinitis is rare in BMT recipients, in contrast to AIDS patients. Clinical disease is manifested by pneumonia, gastroenteritis, and hepatitis. Deep ulcerations may occur in the ileum or right colon, causing bleeding or perforation. Clinical data regarding the use of gancyclovir in the BMT setting have been equivocal; studies have shown that gancyclovir suppressed CMV infection without affecting the course of the disease. Fulminant hepatitis C after BMT has been reported.

Parasites

Giardia lamblia and coccidial organisms such as *Cryptosporidium*, *Microsporidium*, and *Isospora belli* are the most common parasites causing intestinal disease in immunodeficient patients, usually manifesting as nausea and vomiting, abdominal pain, malabsorption, and profuse watery diarrhea. In the BMT setting, *G. lamblia* has been associated with a protein-losing enteropathy in addition to chronic diarrhea and weight loss.

SUGGESTED READING

Bianco JA, Applebaum FR, Neumiunzitis, et al. Phase I–II trial of pentoxifylline for the prevention of transplant-related toxicities following bone marrow transplantation. Blood 1991; 78:1205–1211.

Careras E, Granenz A, Navasa M, et al. Transjugular liver biopsy in BMT. Bone Marrow Transplant 1993; 11:21–26.

Essell JH, Thompson JM, Herman GS, et al. Pilot trial of prophylactic ursodiol to decrease the incidence of veno-occlusive disease in allogeneic bone marrow transplant patients. Bone Marrow Transplant 1992; 10:367–372.

Henre P, Tiberghien P, Racadot E, et al. Prevention and treatment of acute GVHD–bone marrow transplantation: new modalities. Bone Marrow Transplant 1993; II(Suppl):103–106.

Korgnold R. Biology of graft vs. host disease. Am J Pediatr Hematol Oncol 1993; 15:18–27.

McDonald GB, Schulman HM, Sullivan KM, Spencer GD. Intestinal and hepatic complications of human bone marrow transplantation. Part I. Gastroenterology 1986; 90:460–477.

McDonald GB, Schulman HM, Sullivan KM, Spencer GD. Intestinal and hepatic complications of human bone marrow transplantation. Part II. Gastroenterology 1986; 90:770–784.

Schulman HM, Hinterberge W. Hepatic veno-occlusive disease – liver toxicity syndrome after bone marrow transplantation. Bone Marrow Transplant 1992; 10:192–214.

Vogelsang GB, Farmer ER, Hess AD, Altamonte V, et al. Thalidomide for the treatment of chronic graft versus host disease. N Engl J Med 1992; 326:1055–1058.

ACUTE INFECTIOUS DIARRHEA

RONALD E. MASON, M.D.
RALPH A. GIANNELLA, M.D.

Each year more than 5 million people die throughout the world from acute infectious diarrhea, and more than 80 percent are less than 1 year of age. Diarrhea caused by viruses, bacteria, or parasites, can be life threatening in the young, elderly, and malnourished. Before initiating specific therapy for acute infectious diarrhea, the clinician should exclude noninfectious causes of acute diarrheal syndromes such as divalent-cation exposure (Milk of Magnesia, magnesium sulfate), circulating secretagogues (e.g., VIP, carcinoid syndrome), laxative abuse, inflammatory bowel disease, carbohydrate malabsorption, and many others. Appropriate history taking and physical examination and prudent laboratory testing are essential to the diagnosis and management of acute infectious diarrhea.

This chapter focuses on the therapy for this disorder.

REHYDRATION

Prevention of dehydration, rehydration, and correction of electrolyte abnormalities should be the first consideration in the therapy for any patient with acute diarrhea, even though the exact cause cannot be immediately determined. The severity of volume depletion should be assessed with a detailed history and physical examination (Table 1). Determination of urinary output, stool frequency, orthostasis, pulse rates, absence of tears, depressed fontanelle (neonates); and decreased skin turgor are all important in assessing intravascular volume status.

Oral rehydration solutions (ORS) containing appropriate concentrations of glucose and sodium are adequate in many cases of mild to moderate dehydration in children or adults, and are as effective as intravenous (IV) therapy. Osmotically balanced, commercially available solutions are preferable to homemade ones (Table 2). Soft drinks, tea, and citrus juices contain little if any sodium chloride (even Gatorade contains only 24 mEq of sodium chloride per liter). Needless restriction of oral intake should be avoided. To avoid the possibility of hypernatremia in children, the American Academy of

Table 1   Dehydration: Signs and Symptoms and Treatment

Degree	Infant/Child	Adult	Treatment
Mild	Increased thirst Slightly dry mucous membranes	<5% weight loss Pale color Normal blood pressure	(ORS) 40–50 ml/kg over 4–6 hr

Moderate	Loss of skin turgor
	Dry mucous membranes
	Sunken eyes, lack of tears, depressed
	  fontanelle (infant)
	Decreased urine output
	5–9% body weight loss
		5–9% body weight weight loss
		Dry mucous membranes
		Orthostasis
		Decreased skin turgor, dusky skin
			(ORS) 100–150 ml/kg over 4–6 hr; if
			  tolerated, initiate maintenance phase
			  where intake equals losses

Severe	Cold extremities
	Hypotension
	Tachycardia
	Decreased or absent urine output
		>10% body weight loss
		Dry mucous membranes
		Hypotension
		Tachycardia
		Mottled skin
		Cold extremities
			IV fluids, D5NS starting at 10–20 ml/
			  kg/hr in adults; pediatric IV rates
			  should be obtained from text

ORS = oral rehydration solutions; D5NS = 5% dextrose in normal saline.

Table 2   Contents of Commonly Used Oral Rehydration Solutions

Product	CHO (g/L)	NA (mEq/L)	K (mEq/L)	Cl (mEq/L)	Base (mEq/L)	Osmolality (mOsm/L)
OTC						
WHO solution*†	20	90	20	80	30 (C)	310
Infalyte†	20	50	20	40	30 (B)	270
Lytren‡	20	50	25	45	30 (C)	290
Pedialyte‡	25	45	20	35	30 (C)	250
Rehydralyte‡	25	75	20	65	30 (C)	305
Resol‡	20	50	20	50	34 (C)	270
Ricelyte‡	30	50	25	45	34 (C)	200
Clear Liquids§						
Apple juice	120	3.5	28	30	0	730
Chicken broth	0	250	8	250	0	450
Cola	70–120	3	0.1	2	39 (B)	750
Gatorade	50	24	3	17	0	330
Jello	150–270	15–27	0.2	0	0	570–640
Tea	0	0	0	0	0	5

*Use for rehydration; all other solutions for maintenance therapy.
†Must be reconstituted with water.
‡Ready to use.
§Content may vary with specific brand.
CHO = carbohydrate; B = bicarbonate; C = citrate.
From Calligaro I. Treatment of acute diarrhea in children. Am Pharm 1992; NS32:29–34; with permission.

Pediatrics Committee on Nutrition recommends the administration of solutions containing 75 to 90 mEq of sodium per liter to rehydrate patients, and solutions containing 40 to 60 mEq of sodium per liter for maintenance therapy to replace ongoing losses and prevent recurrent dehydration. Solutions with higher sodium concentrations can be mixed with a solution with lower sodium content on a 1:1 ratio. Other experimental solutions containing food starches or glucose polymers may increase the absorption of fluid and electrolytes still further and may actually lessen the diarrheal fluid loss. These are not yet available.

Contraindications to ORS include severe dehydration, shock, glucose intolerance, and inability to tolerate oral solutions. Vomiting is not a contraindication in this setting; such patients should be given smaller amounts of ORS over short intervals.

Intravenous therapy is indicated when nausea or

vomiting precludes oral intake or when metabolic acidosis or shock is present. Total parenteral nutrition (TPN) may be indicated in severely nutritionally deficient patients in whom oral feeding has failed.

SYMPTOMATIC THERAPIES

Although most forms of acute infectious diarrheas are self-limited, many can benefit from symptomatic therapies. Many over-the-counter (OTC) as well as prescription medications are available. Anti-diarrheal agents are classified by their mechanism of action as antimotility agents, bulk-forming agents, adsorbents, and agents that alter intestinal secretion.

Antimotility Agents

Antimotility agents are in the opiate class of drugs and are very useful in providing symptomatic relief of acute diarrhea. Loperamide (Imodium) and diphenoxylate with atropine (Lomotil) are synthetic opiates, whereas codeine phosphate and paregoric are natural opiates. These drugs act on small intestinal smooth muscle by producing segmentation and inhibition of peristalsis, delaying gastrointestinal transit. They also stimulate water and electrolyte absorption; suppress gastric, pancreatic, and biliary secretions; and reduce stool volume. Their use in acute diarrhea associated with fever and dysentery has been controversial, but recent data document their safety and effectiveness in such situations.

Many of the opiate derivative antimotility agents have systemic side effects, including nausea, vomiting, constipation, and drowsiness. The recommended dosage of loperamide (liquid or capsule) for adults is 4 mg initially, then 2 mg after each diarrheal stool to a maximum of 16 mg a day.

Diphenoxylate-atropine also has side effects similar to those of loperamide, with the addition of anticholinergic effects (dry mucous membranes and skin, tachycardia, flushing, and urinary retention) related to the atropine. This drug should be used with caution in patients with heart disease, glaucoma, or prostatic hypertrophy. The initial dosage (2.5 mg per tablet or teaspoon) should be two tablets or 2 teaspoons up to four times a day. Codeine phosphate may be given in divided doses every 8 hours up to 180 mg per day. Paregoric liquid can be given to adults in dosages of 1 to 2 teaspoons four times a day.

Bulk-Forming Agents

Bulk-forming agents (polycarbophil, methylcellulose, and psyllium) absorb water, thereby providing bulk and increased form to stool. They are not systemically absorbed, are metabolically inactive, and are essentially free of systemic side effects. However, they are only marginally effective.

Anticholinergics

Anticholinergics (Bentyl, Donnagel) inhibit motility and are useful for episodes of abdominal cramping associated with diarrhea. They are not effective, however, for the control of diarrhea.

Adsorbents

Adsorbents include agents such as kaolin preparations, activated attapulgite, and activated charcoal. They theoretically adsorb toxins, viruses, and bacteria, thus preventing these substances from reaching the intestinal epithelia and exerting their effect. These agents also adsorb nutrients, enzymes, and other drugs.

Activated attapulgite is safe, is effective in reducing the number of stools, improves stool consistency, and can relieve cramps associated with diarrhea. It is a naturally occurring hydrous magnesium aluminum silicate with a large surface area capable of adsorbing eight times its weight in water. It is not systemically absorbed and has few side effects.

Antisecretory Agents

Bismuth preparations (Pepto-Bismol) can reduce the severity of virus-induced diarrhea, traveler's diarrhea, and others. A dose of 30 to 60 ml Pepto-Bismol every 30 minutes for eight doses is recommended.

ANTIMICROBIAL THERAPY (TABLES 3 AND 4)

The decision to use antibiotics for infectious diarrhea should be made carefully, because these are beneficial only in selected circumstances. Their use should be considered more strongly in very young, elderly, and immunosuppressed patients, since these groups have a higher morbidity and mortality rate from infectious diarrhea.

Empiric Antibiotic Therapy

Since most cases of acute infectious diarrhea are self-limited, antibiotics are not usually needed. However, in some situations (dysentery, evidence of systemic toxicity, immunocompromised patients, pregnant women), empiric therapy prior to isolation of a specific pathogen must be considered. Empiric use of antibiotics in these specific groups may improve the clinical outcome. The most common causes of bacterial enterocolitis in the United States are *Campylobacter, Salmonella,* and *Shigella* species. Trimethoprim-sulfamethoxazole (TMP-SMX) has been the mainstay of empiric therapy. New data suggest that ciprofloxacin and norfloxacin (quinolone antibiotics) are equal or superior to TMP-SMX for treatment of these infections in adults. They may also be beneficial in multiresistant strains of *Shigella* and *Salmonella*. Thus, the quinolones are now the drugs of choice for empiric antibiotic

Table 3 Antimicrobial Therapy for Acute Intestinal Infections

Organism	Indication	Adult Dosage	Pediatric Dosage	Comment
Salmonella	Asymptomatic carrier; exception: foodhandlers; daycare workers	None; Ampicillin or amoxicillin, 2–4 g/day × 6 wk; or TMP-SMX, 160–800 mg PO b.i.d. × 6 wk, or ciprofloxacin, 500 mg PO b.i.d.	None	? cholecystectomy if gallbladder disease present
	Gastroenteritis	Usually none	–	Confirm sensitivity in laboratory
	In severe cases, bacteremia or in patients at high risk; dissemination with localized suppuration (osteomyelitis)	Ciprofloxacin, 500 mg PO b.i.d., ampicillin or amoxicillin, 100 mg/kg/day IV or PO in 4 doses for 1–2 wk, or chloramphenicol, 100 mg/kg/day in 4 doses for 1–2 wk, or ceftriaxone, 1 g q 12hr for 2 wk	Ampicillin or amoxicillin, 100 mg/kg/day IV or PO in 4 doses for 1–2 wk, or ceftriaxone, 100–150 mg/kg/day q12hr for 2 wk	
Shigella	All isolates	TMP-SMX, 160–180 mg PO q12hr for 5 days, or ciprofloxacin, 500 mg PO b.i.d., or ampicillin, 500 mg q6hr for 5 days	TMP-SMX, 10 mg/kg/day of TMP, 50 mg/kg/day of SMX q12hr, or ampicillin, 50–100 mg/kg/day q6hr	Confirm sensitivity in laboratory
Campylobacter	Dysentery, severe infection	Erythromycin, 250–500 mg q.i.d. for 7 days, or ciprofloxacin, 500 mg b.i.d., or norfloxacin, 400 mg PO b.i.d.	Erythromycin, 10 mg/kg q6hr for 5–7 days	Eliminates organism from stool but not proved to diminish diarrhea; systemic infection may require parenteral therapy
Vibrio cholerae	All isolates	Tetracycline, 500 mg PO q6hr for 2 days, or TMP-SMX, 160–800 mg PO q12hr, or ciprofloxacin, 500 mg PO b.i.d.	TMP-SMX, 10 mg/kg/day of TMP, 50 mg/kg/day of SMX PO q6hr for 2–4 days	Tetracycline may discolor teeth in children
Noncholerae vibrios	Severe illness	Tetracycline, 250–500 mg PO q6hr, or furazolidone, 125 mg PO q6hr for 2–4 days	Furazolidone, 5 mg/kg/day PO q6hr for 2–4 days	
Yersinia	Severe or prolonged illness	Tetracycline, 250–500 mg PO q6hr for 7–10 days, or TMP-SMX, 160–800 mg IV, or ciprofloxacin, 500 mg PO b.i.d., or tobramycin, 3–5 mg/kg/day q8hr	Tobramycin, 6.0–7.5 mg/kg/day q6–8hr, or chloramphenicol, 50 mg/kg/day q6hr for 10 days	Diarrhea and mesenteric adenitis may subside spontaneously.
Escherichia coli	ETEC	TMP-SMX, 160–800 mg PO b.i.d. for 3–5 days, or ciprofloxacin, 500 mg PO b.i.d. for 3–5 days	TMP-SMX, 4 mg/kg/day of TMP, 20 mg/kg/day of SMX for 3 days	Diarrhea is self-limited; antibiotics may decrease duration
	EPEC	–	Neomycin, 30 mg/kg PO q8hr for 5 days	
	EIEC, EHEC	As for *Shigella*	None	
	EAEC	None	None	
Aeromonas and *Plesiomonas*	Dysentery, sepsis	TMP-SMX, 160–800 mg PO b.i.d., or ciprofloxacin, 500 mg PO b.i.d.	TMP-SMX, 4 mg/kg/day of TMP, 20 mg/kg/day of SMX	Cirrhotics may develop severe infection

ETEC = enterotoxigenic *E. coli*; EPEC = enteropathogenic *E. coli*; EIEC = enteroinvasive *E. coli*; EHEC = enterohemorrhagic *E. coli*; EAEC = enteroadherent *E. coli*; TMP-SMX = trimethoprim-sulfamethoxazole.

Table 4 Anti-Microbial Therapy of Sexually Transmitted Diseases of the Intestinal Tract

Organism	Indication	Dosage	Comment
Neisseria gonorrhoeae	Proctitis	Ceftriaxone, 250 mg IM and doxycycline, 100 mg PO b.i.d. × 7 days, or aqueous procaine penicillin G, 4.8 million units IM and 1 g of oral probenecid	Must treat sexual contacts
Chlamydia trachomatis	Proctitis, LGV	Tetracycline, 500 mg PO q.i.d. for 2–3 wk, or doxycycline, 100 mg PO b.i.d. for 2–3 wk	Severe disease may mimic Crohn's
Herpes simplex virus	Proctitis	Acyclovir, 400 mg PO 5 times a day for 10 days; IV acyclovir, 5 mg/kg q8hr for 5–7 days in severe disease	
Treponema pallidum	Proctitis, condyloma latum	Benzathine penicillin G, 2.4 million units IM (single injection)	Tetracycline and erythromycin can be used
Entamoeba histolytica	Diarrhea, dysentery	(Adults) metronidazole, 750 mg PO t.i.d. for 10 days, then iodoquinol, 650 mg PO t.i.d. for 20 days (Children) Metronidazole, 35–50 mg/kg/day in 3 divided doses for 10 days, then iodoquinol, 30 mg/kg/day in 3 divided doses for 20 days	Liver abscess or other extraintestinal amebic disease can occur
Giardia lamblia	Weight loss, diarrhea	(Adults) Metronidazole, 250 mg PO t.i.d. for 7 days, or quinacrine, 100 mg PO t.i.d. for 5–7 days, or furazolidone, 100 mg q.i.d. for 2–5 days (Children) Furazolidone, 6 mg/kg/day in 4 divided doses for 7 days, or metronidazole, 15 mg/kg/day in 3 divided doses for 7 days, or quinacrine, 6 mg/kg/day in 3 divided doses for 7 days	Metronidazole should be avoided in pregnant women, especially during first trimester Furazolidone is drug of choice in children

LGV = lymphogranuloma venereum.

therapy for infectious bacterial enterocolitis. There is concern over the use of quinolones in children because of their possible rheumatologic sequelae.

TREATMENT OF SPECIFIC INFECTIONS*

Salmonella

Salmonella infection results in a number of distinctive clinical syndromes: (1) self-limited gastroenteritis, which is the most common manifestation of nontyphoidal salmonellae; (2) enteric fever, characterized by remittent fever, headache, malaise, and anorexia (isolation of the *Salmonella* species from blood, bone marrow, or bile is usually required to make the diagnosis); (3) dissemination, with localized suppuration (abscess or osteomyelitis); and (4) the carrier state, i.e., carriage of *Salmonella* in stool for weeks to months after acute

*Editor's Note: Just a reminder; Since identifying a specific bacterial cause has therapeutic import in most settings, especially if there are polymorphonuclear white cells in the stool smear, appropriate stool cultures are important.

infection. The type of syndrome produced by *Salmonella* dictates the selection and duration of antibiotic therapy. Antibiotics should not be used to treat patients with mild uncomplicated gastroenteritis unless the illness appears to be evolving into a systemic process. Treatment with tetracycline, TMP-SMX, nonabsorbable oral aminoglycosides, and beta-lactam antibiotics does not influence the duration of symptoms, and prolongs fecal excretion of the organism. Antibiotic therapy should be given to patients with severe symptoms or suspected septicemia, patients at extremes of age, pregnant women, and patients with severe underlying illness or an immunocompromised state. Ciprofloxacin may shorten the duration of gastroenteritis symptoms and of excretion of the *Salmonella* organism. Thus, quinolones are the drugs of choice to treat severe *Salmonella* gastroenteritis in adults.

In cases of *Salmonella* bacteremia (enteric fever), antibiotic therapy with chloramphenicol, ampicillin, amoxicillin, or TMP-SMX for 10 to 14 days is indicated. Third-generation cephalosporins and the quinolone antibiotics are alternative choices. In particular, ciprofloxacin has been used for multiresistant *Salmonella* organisms (typhoid and nontyphoid). Corticosteroids as adjunctive therapy may be beneficial in severe cases of enteric fever (shock, altered mental status).

Dissemination with localized suppuration such as in osteomyelitis, endocarditis, or patients with AIDS and bacteremia should be treated for 4 to 6 weeks to prevent relapse.

Antibiotic treatment for *Salmonella* carriers remains controversial. The response to antibiotic therapy is variable. Cholecystectomy has been recommended in the past as therapy for chronic *Salmonella* carriers with concurrent cholelithiasis. In patients without gallbladder disease, ampicillin with probenecid or amoxicillin for 6 weeks is the treatment of choice for enteric carriers. When gallbladder disease is present, ciprofloxacin has been used with high success rates of eradicating the organism.

Shigella

Shigellae are divided into four serogroups: (1) *S. dysenteriae,* (2) *S. flexneri,* (3) *S. boydii,* and (4) *S. sonnei.* Sixty percent of cases in the United States are due to *S. sonnei,* and *S. flexneri* accounts for most of the remaining infections. Primarily a pediatric disease, *Shigella* symptoms include fever, abdominal pain, diarrhea, and dysentery. Hemolytic-uremic syndrome, disseminated intravascular coagulation, meningism, pneumonitis, and Reiter's syndrome can complicate the illness. Untreated, most symptoms resolve in 1 week. Antibiotic therapy shortens the duration of symptoms and carriage of the organism. Because of the increasing frequency of ampicillin resistance, the treatment of choice for shigellosis in both children and adults in the United States is TMP-SMX. However, there have been some reports of TMP-SMX resistance. Ciprofloxacin and norfloxacin have been dramatically effective in treating shigellosis (resistant strains). The safety and efficacy of these antibiotics in children is not known, and reports of drug-induced neurologic, dermatologic, and rheumatologic side effects have prohibited their use.

Campylobacter

Campylobacter species have been known to play a major role in diarrheal illnesses for the past 20 years. In the United States, *C. jejuni* is the most common species to cause infection. Other species are seen more often in immunocompromised hosts. Fever, headache, myalgia, cramping, abdominal pain, tenesmus, and diarrhea are common. Occasionally, bloody stools are seen.

Most patients have a self-limited illness and do not require antibiotics. Severe enteritis symptoms, enteritis persisting beyond 1 week, and evidence of systemic infection necessitate antibiotic therapy. Erythromycin is the drug of choice for *C. jejuni* infection, although it may not decrease the duration of illness. Quinolone antibiotics are also effective and may speed clinical recovery.

Yersinia

Yersinia enterocolitica is a rare infection in the United States, but in Northern Europe it is a common cause of diarrheal illness, especially in children.

Symptoms in children include fever, abdominal pain, and diarrhea that may be blood streaked. The illness usually resolves in 1 to 3 weeks, although chronic ileocolitis resembling Crohn's disease may occur. Older children may develop mesenteric adenitis presenting with fever, right lower quadrant abdominal pain, and leukocytosis—a syndrome resembling acute appendicitis. Adults may develop extraintestinal manifestations, including polyarthritis, Reiter's syndrome, erythema nodosum, and exudative pharyngitis.

In general, antibiotic therapy is not recommended, because this is usually a self-limited illness. Antibiotic therapy has not been shown to shorten its duration. Tetracycline, TMP-SMX, chloramphenicol, and aminoglycosides have all been used and recommended for septicemia or suspected septicemic illness.

Vibrio cholerae and Noncholerae Vibrios

Diarrhea with *V. cholerae* is very rare in the United States, although the organism may be endemic along the Gulf Coast. Untreated, symptomatic patients may experience stool rates of 1 liter per hour, dehydration, and death within 24 hours. Outbreaks occur in the warmer months and may be the result of eating inadequately cooked shellfish. Antibiotic therapy shortens the duration of diarrhea and reduces fluid loss. Tetracycline is the antibiotic of choice for both *V. cholerae* and noncholerae vibrio *(V. parahaemolyticus)* infections. Other effective agents include furazolidone (preferred in pregnant women and children), ampicillin, TMP-SMX, and doxycycline.

Aeromonas and Plesiomonas

Aeromonas hydrophila and *Plesiomonas shigelloides* have been associated with outbreaks of diarrhea after ingestion of contaminated water and shellfish. The clinical spectrum of disease ranges from mild diarrhea to dysentery, sepsis, and extraintestinal manifestations in patients with cirrhosis.

Antibiotic therapy is recommended for severe infections. Both organisms are sensitive to TMP-SMX and quinolones, as well as gentamicin, chloramphenicol, and third-generation cephalosporins.

Escherichia coli

Five forms of *E. coli* cause diarrheal illness: enterotoxigenic, enteropathogenic, enterohemorrhagic, enteroinvasive, and enteroadherent *E. coli.* These organisms may cause disease by several mechanisms, including elaboration of toxins and mucosal invasion.

Enterotoxigenic *E. coli* causes disease primarily in children in underdeveloped countries and is a major cause of traveler's diarrhea in adults. Disease is usually a self-limited syndrome of watery diarrhea caused by heat-labile and heat-stable enterotoxins. Oral rehydration is the mainstay of therapy. In adults TMP-SMX is recommended, with ciprofloxacin a good alternative. Antimotility agents provide symptomatic relief.

Enteropathogenic *E. coli* produces a diarrheal illness associated with fever and vomiting, primarily in neonates and infants. Management consists of correcting fluid loss and electrolyte imbalances. Oral nonabsorbable antibiotics (neomycin, colistin sulfate) and gentamicin have been used, but only in cases of severe illness.

Enteroinvasive *E. coli* causes an invasive dysenteric illness marked by fever, cramps, and watery diarrhea followed by passage of scanty stools containing blood and mucus. These organisms act similarly to *Shigella* species and can be treated in the same fashion.

Enterohemorrhagic *E. coli* represents distinct serotypes. Usually 0157:H7 causes an illness characterized by abdominal cramping, vomiting, and watery diarrhea, often followed by bloody diarrhea. The illness is usually self-limited. However, the young and elderly may develop potentially lethal complications of thrombotic thrombocytopenic purpura or hemolytic-uremic syndrome. Antibiotic therapy is recommended for severely ill patients, but its efficacy is debatable.*

Enteroadherent *E. coli* is characterized by its property of adherence to HEp-2 cell cultures. It causes mild diarrhea without dysentery. The disease is usually self-limiting and does not require antibiotic therapy.

VIRAL DIARRHEA

Specific viral causes of gastroenteritis have been recognized only for the past 20 to 25 years. Currently, at least five categories of viruses produce diarrheal illness in humans: rotavirus, Norwalk virus, enteric adenovirus, calicivirus, and other small round viruses. Astrovirus virus and enteric corona viruses are suspected of causing illness.

Rotavirus is the most common cause of viral diarrheal illness in children. It principally produces gastroenteritis in children between the ages of 6 and 24 months, most frequently during the winter. The syndrome is manifested by low-grade fever, large-volume watery diarrhea, vomiting, abdominal cramping, and (rarely) bloody diarrhea. The disease is usually self-limited and the mainstay of therapy is fluid and electrolyte replacement. Avoidance of milk products in adults and older children, and the use of dilute milk preparations in infants, is recommended to avoid aggravating the osmotic diarrhea that may be the result of rotavirus infection. Currently, no antiviral agent is available to treat rotavirus gastroenteritis.

---

*Editor's Note: This is the organism responsible for drastic falls in the stock prices of two famous (infamous) hamburger chains. A few patients were mistakenly subjected to colectomy in the belief that this was fulminant ulcerative colitis.

Norwalk virus is a significant cause of diarrhea in adults in developed countries. Symptoms include nausea, abdominal cramping, low-grade fever, myalgia, anorexia, headache, vomiting, and diarrhea, usually without bleeding. No effective antiviral agent is available, and fluid and electrolyte replacement and symptomatic treatment are the main cornerstones of therapy.

SEXUALLY TRANSMITTED DISEASES

An increasing number of enteric infections are now recognized as sexually transmitted diseases (STDs). Most are of bacterial and viral origin. However, protozoa and nematodes can now be included in the spectrum of STDs in which the human small intestine, large intestine, rectum, and anus may serve as reservoirs for distinct clinical illnesses. Homosexuals or bisexual males with multiple sexual partners appear to be at higher risk for such enteric infections, sometimes referred to collectively as the gay bowel syndrome. This term is somewhat a misnomer, as women who practice anal-receptive intercourse may acquire similar infections. Sexually transmitted infections are usually manifested as two distinct clinical syndromes: acute proctitis and a diarrheal syndrome. Acute proctitis is characterized by anal discharge or bleeding, anorectal pain, tenesmus, and dysenteric stools. The diarrheal syndrome is characterized by diarrhea, abdominal pain, and weight loss. Pathogens associated with acute proctitis include *Neisseria gonorrhoeae*, *C. trachomatis*, herpes simplex virus (HSV), and *Treponema pallidum*. Pathogens associated with the diarrheal syndrome include *Giardia lamblia*, *Entamoeba histolytica*, *Shigella*, and *Campylobacter* species.

Proctitis

Gonococcal proctitis may be asymptomatic or severe with rectal pain and discharge, hematochezia, constipation, or obstipation. Sigmoidoscopy reveals proctitis, and the diagnosis is confirmed by culture from rectal swabs. Recommended therapy consists of ceftriaxone, 250 mg intramuscularly in a single dose followed by doxycycline, 100 mg orally twice a day for 7 days. The traditionally preferred treatment is aqueous procaine penicillin G, 4.8 million units intramuscularly plus 1 g oral probenecid. Spectinomycin hydrochloride (TMP-SMX), kanamycin, tetracycline, and ampicillin have also been used.

Chlamydia proctitis is caused by *C. trachomatis*, the causative organism for lymphogranuloma venereum (LGV). A clinical syndrome of a mucopurulent discharge, tenesmus, and constipation may be seen. Rarely, chronic diarrhea and fistula formation mimicking Crohn's disease may occur. Sigmoidoscopy reveals proctitis, and the diagnosis may be made by a specific *Chlamydia* culture. The treatment of choice is tetracycline, 500 mg four times a day for 2 to 3 weeks. Alternative agents include doxycycline and erythromycin.

Herpes simplex proctitis is caused by HSV. Clinical disease includes anal pain, tenderness, tenesmus, discharge, and constipation. Typical small ulcers and vesicles are seen on sigmoidoscopy. For mild disease, acyclovir, 400 mg five times a day for 10 days, is effective. For more severe cases, IV acyclovir, 5 mg per kilogram every 8 hours for 5 to 7 days has been used. Topical acyclovir alone is less effective than oral or IV therapy.

Anorectal syphilis is caused by *T. pallidum*. Primary syphilis of the anorectum produces a chancre. Secondary syphilis produces flat, wartlike perianal and penile lesions called condyloma latum. Symptoms include tenesmus, mucoid discharge, and rectal pain. Diagnosis is confirmed by serologic testing or demonstration of the spirochete on dark-field microscopy of rectal biopsies. Treatment consists of a single dose of benzathine penicillin G, 2.4 million units in one injection. Oral tetracycline and erythromycin have also been effective.

Diarrheal Pathogens

E. histolytica and *G. lamblia* are the most common sexually transmitted parasitic diseases. *Enterobius vermicularis* and other helminths have been seen. *E. histolytica* is transmitted through oroanal intercourse. Patients may be asymptomatic or may have abdominal pain, blood-tinged diarrheal stools with fever, tenesmus, and malaise. Rarely, toxic megacolon and perforation can occur. Sigmoidoscopy may reveal erythema, edema, friable mucosa, and typical "hour-glass" trophozoite-ridden ulcers. Diagnosis is made by stool evaluation for ova and parasites. Treatment for proctitis or dysentery is oral metronidazole, 750 mg three times a day for 10 days followed by iodoquinol, 650 mg three times a day for 20

days. The chapter on intestinal parasites provides more details of therapy for amebiasis and giardiasis.

G. lamblia is also transmitted through oroanal intercourse. Symptoms include mild to severe cramps, bloating, anorexia, weight loss, and diarrhea. Diagnosis is made by identification of the organism from stool specimens or duodenal aspirate or biopsy. Metronidazole, 250 mg three times a day for 7 days, is effective. Quinacrine, furazolidone, and paromomycin can also be used.

Shigella and *Campylobacter* infections have already been discussed.

SUGGESTED READING

Anderson W, Mason RE. Diarrhea. In: Schwartz GR, et al, eds. Principles and practice of emergency medicine. 3rd ed. Philadelphia: WB Saunders, 1992:463–471.
Calligaro I. Treatment of acute diarrhea in children. Am Pharm 1992; NS32:29–34.
Levine GI. Sexually transmitted parasitic diseases. Primary Care 1991; 18:101–127.
Murphy GS, Ladaporn B. Ciprofloxacin and loperamide in the treatment of bacillary dysentery. Ann Intern Med 1993; 118: 582–586.
Pickering LK. Therapy for acute infectious diarrhea in children. J Pediatr 1991; 118:S118–S128.
Qadri SM. Infectious diarrhea. Postgrad Med 1990; 88:169–182.
Rubinoff MJ, Field M. Infectious diarrhea. Annu Rev Med 1991; 42:403–410.
Smith LE. Sexually transmitted diseases of the colon, rectum, and anus. Dis Colon Rectum 1990; 33:1048–1062.

TRAVELER'S DIARRHEA

CHARLES E. McQUEEN, M.D.
EDGAR C. BOEDEKER, M.D.

Traveler's diarrhea (TD) is a syndrome caused by ingestion of enteric pathogens, most of which can now be identified using specialized research and routine laboratory techniques. Such identification is not usually required to treat individual travelers safely and effectively. Breaks in sanitation in the chain of food preparation are thought to be the major contributors to the incidence of TD, but contamination of inadequately treated water supplies has been implicated in some areas. The degree of risk for acquiring illness can be semiquantitated according to the region of travel and susceptibility of the traveler. Travelers from developed regions of North America or Western Europe to developing regions of Africa, Asia, and Latin America

are at high risk (attack rates can exceed 50 percent), whereas travelers from developing to developed regions are at a lower risk for diarrheal disease (attack rates of 5 percent or less). A high prevalence of diarrheal illness in young children living at a destination predicts a high degree of risk for the adult traveler, perhaps reflecting immunologic naivety of the traveler and the children. This chapter describes our recommendations to adults for the prevention and treatment of TD.

DESCRIPTION

TD is a syndrome affecting travelers and characterized by the abrupt onset of three or more liquid stools in 24 hours or one or two liquid stools accompanied by abdominal cramps, vomiting, malaise, fever, or dysentery. The severity of illness ranges from being a mere nuisance to requiring hospitalization and parenteral therapy. Most cases are mild to moderate (typically four to five bowel movements per 24 hours) and without high fever or frankly bloody stools. TD was not implicated as either a primary cause of or a contributing factor to death in a retrospective study based on insurance claims of several hundred thousand Swiss travelers. Onset of diarrhea is usually 3 to 7 days after arrival in a developing country, but it may occur 7 to 10 days after return from travel, reflecting the incubation period for the pathogen. More than one episode may occur per trip, since different enteric pathogens may produce similar symptom complexes. Duration is less than 7 days (median, 3 to 4) in 90 percent of cases; fewer than 2 percent of cases persist longer than 30 days. Although not life-threatening, TD may cause significant disruption of schedules, decreased productivity, and general unpleasantness, particularly if toilet facilities are unavailable or not up to usual Western standards.

ETIOLOGY

Although some new etiologies undoubtedly remain to be discovered, the usual causes of traveler's diarrhea are no longer a mystery. TD is caused by pathogenic microorganisms, usually bacteria, which are transmitted through fecal contamination of food or beverages. When the best available laboratory techniques are used, a pathogen can be identified in up to 80 percent of cases. Even in the remaining 20 percent of cases, the favorable response to antibiotics indicates that most of these undiagnosed cases are also caused by bacteria. Noninfectious factors such as fatigue, anxiety, drugs, and special foods have been hypothesized to contribute to the illness, but are not well supported as causes of TD.

Escherichia coli pathogens are the agents most frequently isolated in surveys of TD, although *Campylobacter, Shigella, Salmonella,* and others have predominated in particular studies depending on the location, season, or circumstances of spread. Despite the technically difficult laboratory methods that are currently required for their identification, enterotoxigenic *E. coli* (ETEC) can be identified as the etiologic agent in at least 40 percent of cases of TD. Newly described enteroadhesive (enteroaggregative *E. coli*) varieties of *E. coli* have been suggested as less frequent causes of TD, accounting for some of the previously undefined cases. Bacterial pathogens that are consistently but less frequently isolated include *Salmonella, Shigella, Campylobacter,* Non-01 *Vibrios,* and *Aeromonas.* Parasites are infrequent causes, but *Giardia lamblia* should be considered if travel has been to an area where the risk of giardiasis is high (e.g., St. Petersburg), or if symptoms develop after the traveler returns home. Furthermore, *G. lamblia* and *Entamoeba histolytica* should be considered if diarrhea persists despite treatment with usual antimicrobials. Multiple pathogens can be identified in a significant percentage of travelers with diarrhea. This probably indicates the high degree of fecal contamination in the traveler's environment, rather than actual microbial synergy.

PREVENTION

Preventive measures fall into four major categories: (1) dietary discretion, (2) nonantimicrobial drugs, (3) prophylactic antimicrobials, and (4) vaccines (Table 1). Of these categories, we tend to rely almost entirely on the first. Prophylaxis with antimicrobial drugs, although of demonstrated short-term efficacy, *cannot* be recommended routinely. Currently recommended oral (or parenteral) vaccines for *Salmonella typhi* protect against typhoid fever, but do not provide protection against the multiple nontyphoid *Salmonella* serotypes which cause diarrhea, nor do they provide protection against ETEC, the most common etiology of TD. Although promising ETEC vaccines are in various stages of testing and development, none are available in the United States.

Dietary Discretion

Avoiding contaminated foods and beverages is prudent, inexpensive, and has the added advantage of preventing other food-borne illnesses such as hepatitis or food poisoning. Advising patients on dietary avoidance may seem complicated at first, since the list of foods that have been implicated in the transmission of TD is long. However, guidance can be simplified to a time-honored adage, a few specific pointers and a recommendation to follow common sense.

The adage "If you cannot boil it, cook it, or peel it, forget it," is sound advice. Untreated tap water and ice should be considered unsafe. Contrary to popular folklore, even undiluted whiskey does not have a high enough alcohol concentration to reliably eradicate bacteria that may contaminate the ice. Fresh vegetables and salads should be considered unsafe, especially in regions where fertilization with "night soil" (human waste) is practiced. Foods that have been cooked, allowed to stand, and then have been partially reheated pose a special hazard which may be difficult for the traveler to recognize. Perhaps for this reason, people are more likely to get TD from food served by street vendors than in private homes. Foods heated through to 68° C or greater (temperatures too hot to touch or eat without first cooling) can generally be considered safe.

Disappointingly few studies have shown clear benefit from attempts at dietary avoidance. Perhaps one reason for the paucity of data supporting dietary avoidance is that "mistakes" are often made by knowledgeable people who have limited choices, are hurried, or whose purpose for travel is to experience different cultures. One study revealed that 98 percent of informed travelers made at least one dietary "mistake" while vacationing. Interestingly, diarrheal illness was one of the commonest reasons for sick call during Operation Desert Shield, despite the widespread use of "MRE's" (meals ready to eat) prepared in the United States and bottled drinking water.

Carbonated beverages, bottled beer and wine, and well-cooked foods served hot are usually safe. Noncar-

Table 1 Prevention of Traveler's Diarrhea

Category	Agent	Recommendation	Comment
Dietary avoidance	Ice, tap water, vegetables, salads, street vendor foods, caffeinated beverages	Avoid	"Boil it, cook it, peel it, or forget it."
	Carbonated beverages, bottled beer and wines, well-cooked foods served hot, breads	Safe	Alcohol content in iced, mixed-drinks does not eradicate organisms. Non-carbonated bottled water may not be safe.
			Foods should be too hot to touch or taste when served. Breads with "wet" fillings or icings may not be safe.
	Iodine or chlorine water treatments combined with filtration	Useful	
Non-antimicrobials	Bismuth subsalicylate, 60 ml or 600 mg q.i.d.	Qualified recommendation	Avoid in patients on aspirin, with renal failure, or if elderly.
Antimicrobials	Fluoroquinolones: Ciprofloxacin 500 mg q.d. Norfloxacin 400 mg q.d. Trimethoprim-Sulfamethoxizole (160 mg/800 mg) q.d. Doxycycline 100 mg b.i.d. on day 1, then q.d.	Not recommended	Prophylactic antibiotics *not* recommended because of possible extreme risk. If elected, duration should not exceed 2 weeks, begin on day of travel and continue 2 days after return.
Vaccines	Not available for usual causative organisms		See text for recommendations re: hepatitis, cholera, and typhoid

bonated bottled water cannot always be relied upon. If tap water must be used, it should first be disinfected. Methods for disinfecting water include boiling or treating with iodine or chlorine. These methods may be as important for the elimination of enteric viruses, including those such as hepatitis A which do not usually cause diarrhea, as for bacterial pathogens commonly associated with TD. The method involves adding one tablet of iodine (tetraglycine hydroperiodide) to one quart of clear water (7 parts per million) or two tablets per quart if the water is cold or cloudy, indicating the presence of particulate matter. Similarly, chlorine tablets (calcium hypochlorite) can be added so that a level between 5 and 10 parts per million is reached (as determined by a portable colorimetric test kit). Both iodine and chlorine are effective in killing most bacteria or viruses, but iodine appears to be more effective against *Giardia* or *Amoeba*. A water purification kit that permits a glassful of water at a time to seep through an iodine resin is available in many sporting goods stores. Toxicity appears to be rare with these methods, but the chemicals do affect the taste of the water and they may be inconvenient. Water boiled 5 minutes at sea level is safe. If it is necessary to drink where the water may be unsafe and water purification systems are unavailable, drinking water obtained from the "hot" tap may provide a degree of protection if temperatures of 140° to 160° F are maintained, but this is clearly a less than optimal approach.*

*****Editor's Note:** At least one TD expert is known to carry a thermometer to test the temperature of the hot water in his hotel room.

Nonantimicrobial Drugs

Bismuth subsalicylate (BSS) (as Pepto-Bismol liquid, 60 ml four times daily, or two 300 mg tablets four times daily) taken throughout the period of travel reduces the incidence of TD by 40 to 60 percent. Although we do not unqualifiedly recommend BSS for prophylaxis, it is probably the safest, most effective nonantimicrobial drug for prophylaxis and is available without prescription in liquid or tablet form. There are several potential drawbacks to BSS. It turns stools black, the liquid form is bulky for the traveler to carry, and unfortunately, the minimal effective amount for prophylaxis is not known. Of more serious concern is the potential for salicylate intoxication particularly in patients who are elderly, have renal failure, or are on other medications containing salicylates. Neurologic side effects from bismuth intoxication are a theoretical problem and absorption may be increased if gastrointestinal disorders compromising mucosal integrity are present. Nevertheless, it seems unlikely that sufficient amounts of bismuth could be absorbed to reach neurotoxic levels if the subsalicylate form is taken for less than 3 weeks in otherwise normal individuals. But because of these uncertain risks and because effective treatment for TD (including BSS) can be made available, BSS was not recommended for prophylaxis at the most recent National Institutes of Health (NIH) Consensus Development Conference on TD. We feel, however, that the use of BSS, particularly in tablet form, can be an acceptable prophylactic measure to limit TD and that adverse reactions are unlikely to occur if care is taken not to administer this medicine concomitantly with other salicylates.

Antimotility agents, such as loperamide or diphenoxylate, should definitely not be given prophylactically, as these agents have been shown to increase the incidence of TD and may predispose to development of serious illness by inhibiting the normal protective action of peristalsis.

Other agents that should not be recommended because they are of unproven or minimal benefit include activated charcoal, kaolin, pectin, and lactobacillus preparations.

Antimicrobial Drugs

A growing list of antimicrobial drugs used for prophylaxis have been shown to decrease the incidence of TD by 70 to 90 percent. This list includes doxycycline, trimethoprim-sulfamethoxazole (TMP-SMX), erythromycin, amdinocillin, and various quinolones. Despite the efficacy of these drugs, we cannot recommend them for prophylaxis. Antimicrobial prophylaxis was discussed at length and rejected during the last NIH Consensus Development Conference on TD and a summary of the logic follows. On one hand, TD is usually a mild to moderate illness for which rapid, effective treatment can be made available in advance of travel. On the other hand, serious side effects from antibiotic therapy do occur (e.g., Stevens-Johnson syndrome, aplastic anemia, other idiosyncratic reactions, or antibiotic-induced colitis) and however rare, reach a statistical likelihood when one considers the number of travelers that would be at risk if antibiotics were given routinely. It is difficult to justify the risk of a potentially fatal illness for prophylaxis of an illness that is rarely fatal.

Some researchers have maintained that special classes of travelers could be identified for whom the risks of prophylaxis would be justified by the importance of their travel or by the possibility of occurrence of medical illnesses that would be worsened by dehydration. In general, however, we believe it is difficult to define categories of travelers for whom antibiotic prophylaxis is justified. The argument that special groups, such as businessmen on important trips, are more deserving of prophylaxis than the vacationer spending his own hard-earned money is difficult to support. Similarly, the wisdom of prescribing prophylactic antibiotics to those with pre-existing illness must be judged on a case by case basis. Nevertheless, since many travelers know of studies showing prophylactic efficacy of antibiotics and many define themselves as deserving prophylaxis, they may demand such protection from their physicians or else plan to obtain antibiotics in the countries to which they travel. In these situations, it is important for the physician to discourage prophylactic antibiotic use by carefully informing the patient of the extreme, if uncommon, risks of antibiotic therapy. Other less severe side effects, such as tetracycline-associated photosensitivity in the case of doxycycline, which occur with more predictable frequency, should also be mentioned. We should also emphasize to the patient that in the event of illness, rapidly effective therapy is available and will be provided. If the patient elects prophylactic antibiotics, he should be advised that such use should not be continued for more than 2 weeks.

Our major concern with regard to use of prophylactic antibiotics is increased risk to the individual patient. The possibility that prophylactic antibiotics taken by travelers could significantly contribute to an increase in resistant organisms in the environment should also be considered, but may not be a major concern. This is not to deny that antibiotic resistance is definitely increasing among enteropathogens isolated in developing countries where the use of antibiotics is widespread and often unrestricted. Nevertheless, antibiotic use by travelers has probably not been a major selective pressure in this developing resistance since it represents only a small proportion of antibiotic use in these countries. Moreover, it has been shown that the fecal flora of travelers quickly acquires the resistance pattern of the indigenous population of the developing countries, even though the travelers do not ingest antibiotics. Such emerging resistance is definitely a cause for concern, and may be expected to influence the effectiveness of antibiotics currently recommended for treatment.

Vaccines

Vaccines against two enteric pathogens, *Vibrio cholerae* and *Salmonella typhimurium,* are currently available, but neither is directed against organisms responsible for usual cases of TD. The present cholera vaccine, a killed preparation, gives short-lived (less than 6 months) protection against 01 vibrios, and this protection may be less for travelers from nonendemic areas than for residents of endemic areas. Despite the current (seventh) cholera pandemic which has spread through South America, the vaccine is not recommended for most travelers. It offers no protection against the emerging 0139 cholera strains newly epidemic in South Asia. According to World Health Organization (WHO) guidelines, no countries any longer require a certificate of cholera vaccination for entry.

The recommended typhoid vaccine is the orally administered live attenuated Ty21a strain marketed as Vivotif, Berna. This strain gives protection against *Salmonella typhi* similar to that achieved with killed bacterial preparations administered instramuscularly, but it is not associated with the severe systemic and local side effects (fever, nausea, vomiting, and muscle soreness) of the parenteral vaccine. These vaccines do not protect against non-typhoid salmonellae.

There is an ongoing effort to improve on available vaccines, as well as to develop effective vaccines against other enteric infections. Two new oral cholera vaccines, one a live-attenuated strain, and the other a killed whole cell product incorporating the B subunit of cholera toxin, may soon be available. One promising approach for immunization against other enteropathogens, involves engineering the oral attenuated *Salmonella* strain Ty21a as a carrier for antigens of other enteropathogens. Genetic material encoding for attachment factors or other immunogens present on the surface of pathogenic bacteria (such as *Shigella, Campylobacter* or ETEC) can be inserted into this short-lived, self-destructive strain which can then express these antigens. It is unlikely that such hybrid vaccines will be available for protection of travelers in the next 2 or 3 years. Closer to advanced development are killed, oral, whole cell vaccines for common phenotypes of ETEC and *Campylobacter* which are likely to be the first generation vaccines for TD.

A discussion of all currently available immunizations for traveler's diarrhea (including measles, meningitis, plague, polio, rabies, tetanus and diphtheria, and yellow fever) is beyond the scope of this chapter, but updated information can be found at intervals in publications such as the *Medical Letter.* Prophylaxis against hepatitis A in the form of immune serum globulin is recommended for travelers outside the usual tourist routes in areas where sanitation is poor. The recommended dose of immune serum globulin is 2 ml IM for stays less than 3 months or 5 ml for longer visits. Vaccination against hepatitis B is not generally recommended for travelers except to protect against transmission by sexual contact in endemic areas of Africa and southeast Asia.

TREATMENT

Treatment of TD (Table 2) falls into three major categories: (1) maintaining adequate hydration and replacement of electrolytes, (2) symptomatic treatment, and (3) specific antimicrobial therapy.

Maintenance of Hydration

The cornerstone for treatment of any diarrheal illness, including TD, is maintenance of adequate hydration and replacement of electrolytes. The tendency to stop oral fluids when diarrhea occurs is still distressingly common. Travelers should be advised that fluid replacement should be initiated at the onset of diarrhea and that volumes ingested should at least exceed stool losses and be sufficient to ensure the usual flow of urine. Fortunately, severe dehydration does not usually occur in the course of TD in adults. Therefore, in this setting, any acceptable source of fluids with some readily available, palatable source of salt (such as saltine crackers) will suffice. Commercial products such as Gatorade, although hypotonic, are usually adequate for adults. Resealable plastic bags containing a pinch of salt, a pinch of bicarbonate, and a tablespoon of sugar can be prepared in advance by the traveler to add to a liter of water when diarrhea begins. The World Health Organization and several commercial companies produce packets of an oral rehydration salts (ORS) powder that can be easily mixed with water and used in cases with more severe purging. These packets can be purchased in the United States, but they are also widely available in developing countries. Initially, ORS should be given to replace cumulative estimated diarrheal losses volume for volume; later, during the maintenance phase of diarrheal illness, ORS intake should be alternated with equal volumes of water to replace continued losses in the stool. It is rare that the oral route does not provide adequate rehydration in cases of TD. Because they may aggravate dehydration, alcoholic beverages as well as coffee and other caffeinated beverages are best proscribed if other acceptable fluids are available. See the chapter Dietary-Induced Symptoms for additional information on dietary "secretagogues."

Symptomatic Treatment

In mild to moderate cases of TD, treatment with synthetic opiates or BSS should provide adequate control of diarrhea and relief of symptoms.

The synthetic opiates, loperamide (Imodium) or diphenoxylate plus atropine sulfate (Lomotil) are rapidly effective at relieving cramps and decreasing frequency of stools. (See Table 2 for dosing recommendations.) There has been considerable debate concerning the advisability of using these preparations for treatment of TD, since in theory they may hinder the clearance of invasive pathogens. As stated previously these agents should not be used for prophylaxis, or in the presence of fever (greater than 101° F) or frankly bloody diarrhea indicating invasive pathogens. There is no evidence, however, that in the usual case of TD caused by ETEC or other noninvasive pathogens these agents worsen or prolong disease. Therefore, they can be recommended as reasonably safe and effective symptomatic therapy for uncomplicated TD, provided that their use is not continued beyond 36 hours. In choosing between the synthetic opiates, loperamide has the theoretical advantage of not crossing the blood-brain barrier and should therefore cause fewer central nervous system side effects. Neither loperamide or diphenoxylate should be used in children under 2 years old. A bottle containing 18 loperamide capsules can be purchased over the counter at local pharmacies for $6.99. A liquid over-the-counter formulation of loperamide is now available, indicating the general acceptance of this therapy for acute diarrhea.

As an alternative, for symptomatic relief in mild to moderate cases, BSS in liquid form (30 ml every 30 minutes for eight doses in adults) has also been shown to be effective (decreasing stools by 43 percent of non-treated levels). This is safe therapy but takes somewhat longer than the synthetic opiates (more than 4 hours, or not until the complete therapeutic dosage has been administered) to demonstrate its effects.

Antibiotic Therapy

For more severe cases, prompt antibiotic therapy is recommended. Although extensive laboratory studies have defined the causative agents of TD, it is impractical in the clinical setting to attempt to identify the causative organisms in uncomplicated cases of TD. Moreover ETEC, the most common agent of TD, are not identified

Table 2 Treatment of Traveler's Diarrhea in Adults

Category	Agent	Recommendation	Comment
Fluid and electrolyte replacement	Gatorade, clear sodas, flavored mineral water	Usually adequate	Increase intake to maintain usual urine output. Avoid caffeinated beverages, alcohol, and artificially sweetened beverages.
	Homemade solutions: pinch of salt, pinch of bicarbonate, 1 tbsp sugar per liter of water	Usually adequate	Economical. Packets can be prepared in advance.
	Oral rehydration solutions	Best	Parenteral fluids may be required if severe dehydration or intractible vomiting is present.
Symptom relief	Loperamide: 2 capsules, then 1 after each stool (not to exceed 8 capsules in 24 hours)	Preferred	Loperamide and diphenoxylate are both rapidly effective at relieving cramps and decreasing stool frequency, but loperamide avoids anticholinergic and CNS side effects. Neither drug should be used for more than 36 hours; avoid with temperature over 101°F or frankly bloody stools.
	Diphenoxylate with atropine: 2 tablets q.i.d., then taper to minimal maintenance dose	Alternate	
	Bismuth subsalicylate: 30 ml every 30 minutes for 8 doses	Alternate	Slower onset of action; turns stools black; watch for acetylsalicylic acid toxicity.
Antimicrobials	Ciprofloxacin: 500 mg b.i.d.	Preferred	Provide travelers with a 3-day supply to begin after 2 to 3 loose stools. Do not use in children, during pregnancy, or with history of reaction to nalidixic acid.
	Trimethoprim-sulfamethoxizole (160 mg/ 800 mg): 1 tablet b.i.d.	Alternate	Resistence is common. Does not cover *Campylobacter*. Do not use with history of sulfa allergy.
	Doxycycline: 100 mg b.i.d.	Alternate	Resistence is common. Sun sensitivity may be a problem. Antacids and sucralfate interfere with absorption.

by cultures for routine enteric pathogens. Antimicrobial therapy should be given empirically, based on our current knowledge of antibiotic sensitivity of the responsible pathogens and on empirical field trials. Such antimicrobial therapy appears to be safe and effective.

Several field studies have shown that the fluoroquinolone antibiotics (ciprofloxacin, norfloxacin, ofloxacin, fleroxacin) consistently decrease the duration of travel-related or domestically-acquired diarrhea from 3 or 4 days to 1 or 2 days. These drugs, which are related to the urinary tract antiseptic naladixic acid, work by inhibiting bacterial DNA synthesis by inhibiting bacterial DNA topoisomerases (gyrases). A number of considerations support fluoroquinolones as a first choice for empiric therapy of traveler's diarrhea. They are active in vitro against all known bacterial enteric pathogens at concentrations that are easily obtained in the serum and intestine after oral dosing. Effects on the normal anerobic flora are clinically insignificant. Pathogens disappear from stool cultures repeated 24 hours after the start of therapy, decreasing the potential for further spread of the pathogen. Fluoroquinolones have good activity against *Campylobacter* organisms. They do not convert *Salmonella* enteritis to the carrier state, which in the past complicated empiric therapy of enteric infections. Development of bacterial resistance to the fluoroquinolones is not plasmid mediated and occurs infrequently. Side effects are generally mild and occur at an acceptable frequency.

We recommend that patients obtain a supply of ciprofloxacin (provided no contraindications exist) sufficient to complete a 3 day course of treatment (500 mg orally twice a day). We advise patients to begin treatment after the third loose stool occurring in an 8-hour period, but caution them that nausea and vomiting without diarrhea are not indications for these drugs. Our reasons for choosing ciprofloxacin over other fluoroquinolones include greater firsthand experience with this drug, its availability in the United States, and its approval for treatment of enteric infections by the FDA, but there appear to be few data to recommend one quinolone over another. Six ciprofloxacin pills for a 3 day course costs the patient $20.80 at a local discount pharmacy. Unused drugs should be disposed of at the end of the trip. Efficacy appears to be enhanced if treatment is begun within 24 hours after the onset of symptoms. The addition of loperamide to the antibiotic regimen may further decrease the duration of diarrhea.

The quinolones should not be prescribed if there is a history of allergy to nalidixic acid. They also must not be given to children or pregnant patients because of the potential for damage to developing cartilage. Absorption is reduced by magnesium, aluminum or calcium antacids and by sucralfate and iron salts.

Trimethoprim-sulfamethoxizole (TMP-SMX) also decreases the duration of TD, and was the regimen of choice prior to the fluroquinolones (TMP-SMX, 160 mg/800 mg twice a day for 3 days). The appearance in many areas of drug-resistant pathogens and the occurrence of side effects now make this drug combination an alternate choice. Travelers taking this medication should be cautioned to seek medical attention for severe or persistent illness, which could indicate resistant organisms.

Doxycycline (100 mg twice a day) was effective treatment for TD and would be a good choice for patients with known reactions to fluroquinolones or TMP-SMX. Special cautions with regard to doxycycline include the likelihood of permanent staining of teeth, contraindicating its use in children; drug photosensitivity; fungal or bacterial overgrowth (e.g., candida vaginitis, candida esophagitis, pseudomembranous colitis); idiosyncratic reactions and interference with the absorption of antimalarials.

SUGGESTED READING

Consensus Development Panel. Traveler's diarrhea. JAMA 1985; 253:2700–2704.

DuPont HL, Ericsson CD. Prevention and treatment of traveler's diarrhea. N Engl J Med 1993; 328:1821–1827.

Sack RB. Travelers' diarrhea: microbiologic basis for prevention and treatment. Rev Infect Dis 1990; 12:S59–S63.

Steffen R. Epidemiologic studies of travelers' diarrhea, severe gastrointestinal infections, and cholera. Rev Infect Dis 1986; 8:Suppl 2:S122–S130.

Taylor DN, Sanchez JL, Candler W, et al. Treatment of travelers' diarrhea: ciprofloxacin plus loperamide compared with ciprofloxacin alone: a placebo-controlled, randomized trial. Ann Intern Med 1991; 114:731–734.

CLOSTRIDIUM DIFFICILE AND ANTIBIOTIC-ASSOCIATED COLITIS

JOHN G. BARTLETT, M.D.

Diarrhea is a relatively common complication of antimicrobial treatment. Most studies show the rates to be 2 to 5 percent for cephalosporins, 5 to 10 percent for ampicillin or amoxicillin, and 10 to 20 percent for clindamycin. These rates vary according to the definition of diarrhea, route of administration, and dosage.

Clostridium difficile is the major enteric pathogen implicated in patients with antibiotic-associated diarrhea. This organism causes a spectrum of clinical and pathologic changes ranging from the asymptomatic carrier state to life-threatening colitis. Risk factors for *C. difficile*–associated diarrhea or colitis include the following: First, exposure to an antibiotic, primarily an antibiotic that has an important impact on the colonic flora. Second, an age-associated risk with increased rates in the elderly. Third, approximately 3 percent of healthy adults harbor *C. difficile* and so presumably are susceptible if given appropriate antibiotics; others, especially in the setting of the hospital, acquire *C. difficile* from environmental sources, so that it is also recognized as a major nosocomial pathogen. Fourth, the organism must produce toxin, presumably toxin A, which is primarily responsible for clinical expression with diarrhea and colitis. The presumed mechanism is alteration of the fecal flora due to antibiotic exposure. This permits *C. difficile,* present as a component of the indigenous flora or acquired from an environmental source, to replicate in the relative microbial void. Replication of the vegetative forms of toxin-producing strains is associated with production of both toxins A and B. Toxin A appears to be primarily responsible for clinical expression; toxin B is responsible for the cytopathic effects noted with the standard tissue culture assay used for diagnosis. Almost all antibiotics have been implicated as inducing agents for this complication, although the major offenders are clindamycin, ampicillin or amoxicillin, and cephalosporins.

C. difficile causes a spectrum of changes ranging from the asymptomatic carrier state to life-threatening pseudomembranous colitis (PMC). In many cases, there is trivial or "nuisance" diarrhea, characterized by loose or watery stools, that resolves when the implicated antibiotic is simply discontinued. The frequency with which *C. difficile* toxin is found in patients with this type of complication after antibiotic exposure is 10 to 25 percent. With more advanced disease, there are often findings suggestive of inflammation or colitis with severe cramps, fecal leukocytes, systemic reaction with leukocytosis and fever, and evidence of colitis on endoscopy or computed tomographic (CT) scan. The frequency of *C. difficile* toxin in this setting when associated with antibiotic exposure is 40 to 80 percent. The most characteristic feature is PMC characterized by exudative plaquelike lesions that stud the colonic mucosa, as demonstrated by visual appearance on endoscopy or biopsy with histologic study. These lesions are usually found in association with the clinical features of colitis; anatomic changes are restricted to the colon (the small bowel is not involved), and fecal leukocytes are found in approximately 50 percent of cases. The frequency of *C. difficile* toxin in patients with antibiotic-associated PMC is 95 to 100 percent. PMC was commonly reported in the

1950s when it was ascribed to *Staphylococcus aureus,* and again in the 1970s when the most common inducing agent appeared to be clindamycin. PMC is infrequently encountered at present because early recognition and treatment prevents progression to this stage of disease, and because endoscopy, which is necessary to confirm the anatomic changes, is less frequently performed.

Most cases of antibiotic-associated diarrhea and many with colitis are associated with negative *C. difficile* toxin assays. Possible pathogens in this setting include *Salmonella,* enterotoxin-producing strains of *Clostridium perfringens, Candida albicans* (a controversial agent of antibiotic-associated diarrhea), and *S. aureus* (also controversial because many feel that the studies done in the 1950s implicating this organism were not convincing in retrospect). Most patients with negative *C. difficile* toxin assays have no alternative etiologic diagnosis.

DIAGNOSIS

C. difficile should be suspected in any patient with diarrhea as a complication of antibiotic exposure. This probability increases if the antibiotic was one of the "big three": clindamycin, cephalosporins, and amoxicillin/ampicillin. The probability of *C. difficile* is also greater if there is evidence of inflammation with fecal leukocytes, leukocytosis, fever, severe cramps, and/or tenesmus. Other clinical features highly suggestive of *C. difficile* include chronic or persistent diarrhea despite discontinuation of the implicated antibiotics, large losses of albumin with edema or even anasarca, and ileus or toxic megacolon. The finding of pseudomembranous lesions on endoscopy is virtually diagnostic of *C. difficile* in the setting of antibiotic exposure. In general, the more serious the illness, the more likely it is that *C. difficile* is involved.

Evaluation of patients who have antibiotic-associated diarrhea depends to a large extent on the diagnostic resources and the severity of illness. Most patients with this diagnosis have rather trivial complaints, and respond when the implicated antibiotic is simply discontinued or changed to an alternative agent that is less likely to cause this complication. Patients who have more serious illness undergo a diagnostic evaluation that may be divided into three categories: studies to determine the severity of the complications, studies of the anatomy of the lesion, and studies to determine whether *C. difficile* is responsible.

Patients who are severely ill with severe diarrhea often have complications reflecting dehydration, electrolyte abnormalities, and/or hypoalbuminemia. The diagnostic evaluation should include a complete blood count, serum electrolytes, and albumin levels. Ileus is suspected if the abdomen is distended or shows typical changes with auscultation. These patients should also undergo plain films of the abdomen and may require surgical consultation. Studies of the anatomy of the lesions traditionally require endoscopy to show colitis or PMC. Colonoscopy is often required since up to one-third of cases involve only the right side of the colon. CT is not the preferred diagnostic test for this condition but is often performed in the context of evaluation for intra-abdominal sepsis. Patients with *C. difficile*–associated colitis often show characteristic changes with a thick colonic mucosa, no involvement of the small bowel, and ascites fluid. The need to define the anatomy of the lesion is tempered greatly by the availability of diagnostic studies to detect *C. difficile* toxin, which is most important in terms of therapeutic choices.

Management strategies for patients with severe or moderately severe disease are based largely on the results of the *C. difficile* toxin assay. The standard test is the tissue culture assay to detect toxin B. This test is remarkably accurate if properly done, but results require 24 to 48 hours, and many laboratories do not perform tissue cultures, so that the specimen must be sent to reference laboratories that are sometimes at distant locations; this lengthens the time of reporting even further. In an effort to obtain a faster test that can be more easily incorporated into a diagnostic laboratory routine, there have been multiple alternative tests. The first such test in common use was the latex agglutination test originally designed to detect toxin A; subsequent studies showed that this actually detected an alternative protein produced by *C. difficile* and, perhaps not surprisingly, clinical trials have been disappointing. More recently, there have been multiple suppliers of reagents to perform enzyme immunoassays to detect toxin A, toxin B, or both. These tests provide results within 2 to 3 hours and show reasonable diagnostic accuracy, although many authors conclude that the tissue culture assay remains the "gold standard." For interpretation of *C. difficile* toxin assay results, it is crucial for the physician to know which of these diagnostic tests were made.

TREATMENT

The four components of treatment are supportive measures, avoidance of antiperistaltic agents, discontinuation of the implicated antimicrobial agent, and treatment directed against *C. difficile.*

Supportive measures include rehydration and correction of electrolyte imbalance. Rare patients may benefit from parenteral hyperalimentation. Antiperistaltic agents such as loperamide should be avoided, since these are known to promote the frequency and severity of *C. difficile*–associated diarrhea.

The inducing agent should be discontinued. If this is not possible, there should be a change to an alternative agent, preferably from the list of drugs that are unlikely to cause this disease: tetracyclines, sulfonamides, fluoroquinolones, metronidazole, parenteral aminoglycosides, and trimethoprim-sulfamethoxazole. As noted, drugs to avoid are clindamycin, ampicillin/amoxicillin, and cephalosporins.

The use of antimicrobial agents directed against *C. difficile* depends on the severity of symptoms and response to withdrawal of antibiotics. In many cases it is sufficient to simply discontinue the implicated agents. The major indications for treatment against *C. difficile* are persistent diarrhea, severe disease, and/or the necessity to continue antibiotics despite this complication. All are relative and require clinical judgment. The major deterrent to treatment with an antimicrobial agent is the possibility of a relapse, which is common, and of multiple relapses, which are uncommon but can be a major medical problem. Relapses are noted only with antibiotic treatment; they never occur when the disease resolves spontaneously or when it is managed with drugs other than antimicrobial agents. The major deterrent to treatment with vancomycin is its cost. The major deterrent to treatment with nonantibiotic agents such as cholestyramine or lactobacilli is the fact that they do not work very well. When specific treatment is indicated, the major options are metronidazole or vancomycin.

Metronidazole

Metronidazole is effective against nearly all strains of *C. difficile*. The drug is nearly completely absorbed in the small bowel, so that colonic levels are nil and it has minimal impact on the fecal flora. *C. difficile* is entirely restricted to the colonic lumen, so it is somewhat surprising that the drug works at all. Nevertheless, comparative trials seem to show benefits comparable with those observed with vancomycin. The only reason to prefer metronidazole is its cost, but the difference here is extraordinary. The wholesale price listing of metronidazole in the usual 10 day dosages is about $1.50 compared with $78 to $140 for vancomycin. The usual dosage of metronidazole is 250 mg three times daily or 500 mg twice daily for 7 to 14 days. The expected response is defervescence within 24 hours and a gradual reduction in diarrhea with normal bowel habits an average of 5 days after treatment. Post-treatment stool toxin assays should not be performed, since many patients with a good clinical response continue to show positive results for extended periods. The major side effects of metronidazole are gastrointestinal complications, primarily nausea and vomiting. The drug has been implicated in causing a disulfiram-like reaction in alcoholics, although I have never encountered a physician who witnessed this reaction despite the rather extensive use of this drug in diverse patient populations. Prolonged use of metronidazole has been complicated by a peripheral neuropathy that usually responds to drug withdrawal.*

Vancomycin

Vancomycin is the "gold standard" of treatment and is preferred for patients who are seriously ill. This agent is active in vitro against all strains of *C. difficile* and is not

_____

***Editor's Note:** Neuropathy is unusual at doses of 1,000 mg per day or less. One patient of mine who was taking 1,500 mg per day became ill after drinking three champagne cocktails.

absorbed when given orally, so that the levels within the colonic lumen are extremely high. The usual dose is 125 mg four times daily by mouth. Preparations include parvules of 125 mg and vials of 500 mg or 10 mg for intravenous (IV) use. The IV form is substantially less expensive than the parvules. My suggestion is to prescribe the 7 to 14 of 500 mg, each representing a 1 day supply. Some patients complain of bad taste or gastrointestinal intolerance, but most can take the drug with minimal difficulty. The anticipated response is defervescence within 24 hours and gradual resolution of diarrhea over an average of 4 to 5 days. Failure to respond is rare except in noncompliant patients, patients with ileus, or those with a concurrent disease process such as idiopathic inflammatory bowel disease.

Ileus

Ileus is a major therapeutic problem because the only treatment of patients with severe illness that has consistent results is oral therapy with vancomycin or metronidazole. IV metronidazole is often given in the hope that some will reach the colonic lumen via the inflamed bowel, although response is inconsistent. Alternative or additional strategies sometimes advocated are direct installation of vancomycin by a long tube from above, or by endoscopy or enema from below. Persistent symptoms in the face of ileus or toxic megacolon may require surgery, preferably with a cecostomy with preservation of the colon and direct installation of vancomycin.

Bacitracin

Bacitracin has gained modest interest as an alternative agent, but experience is limited, some strains of *C. difficile* are highly resistant, and the treatment is substantially more expensive than metronidazole. If used, the usual dose is 25,000 units four times daily by mouth for 7 to 14 days. The major reason to use bacitracin would be contraindications to metronidazole and vancomycin. This drug rarely solves the problems of failure to respond to vancomycin or multiple relapses with metronidazole or vancomycin.

Anion-Binding Resins

Cholestyramine and colestipol are anion exchange resins that bind both toxin A and toxin B of *C. difficile*. This is attractive, since it represents a nonantibiotic treatment of antibiotic-induced disease. However, clinical response rates are substantially less impressive than with vancomycin or metronidazole.

Relapses

The clinical pattern with relapse is highly stereotyped. Patients typically respond well to vancomycin or metronidazole and then have recurrence of diarrhea and cramps after these drugs have been discontinued, usually at 3 to 10 days. Patients usually know that it is the same problem, and toxin assays of stool are usually not necessary. Most patients who relapse respond to another course of the same drug or the alternative. However, a small subset of patients have multiple relapses. The record number of confirmed relapses in one patient in my experience is 26; the record duration of continuous treatment mandated by multiple relapses is 18 months, this being in a patient who could not tolerate metronidazole and paid an average of $1,030 per month for vancomycin.

The rate of relapses does not appear to be influenced by the selection of antibiotic for treatment (metronidazole, vancomycin, or bacitracin), the dosage of these drugs, or their duration. Therapeutic tactics that have been advocated for the patient with multiple relapses include the following:

1. Vancomycin combined with rifampin (600 mg per day) for 10 to 14 days.
2. Vancomycin or metronidazole for 10 to 14 days, followed by a 3 week course of cholestyramine (4 g packet three times daily), cholestyramine combined with lactobacilli (1 g as Lactinex four times daily), or low-dose, pulse vancomycin (125 mg by mouth every other day). The theoretical reason for this strategy is that the initial course of antibiotics is given to control the disease, and the 3 week course of nonantibiotic treatment (or low-dose vancomycin) is provided in an attempt to stabilize *C. difficile* for the 3 weeks required to re-establish the normal flora.
3. Tapering doses of vancomycin over a 6 week period.
4. Attempts to replenish the flora with colonic infusions of stool or a microbial cocktail. The use of stool from a healthy donor is problematic because it is mechanically difficult, is aesthetically displeasing, and, perhaps most important, may be associated with transmission of nasty viruses such as hepatitis virus or a retrovirus.

Epidemics

C. difficile is a nosocomial pathogen that may be epidemic or endemic in hospitals and nursing homes, i.e., in facilities where there is clustering of patients combined with high usage rates of antibiotics. Major epidemic sources of the organisms are patients with severe diarrhea, especially if incontinent, and epidemiologic studies in case-associated areas often show heavy contamination in toilet facilities and the hands of hospital personnel. Stool cultures often show that 20 to 30 percent of patients harbor *C. difficile*. Most of these patients do not have diarrhea, but they may represent a potential source of the continuing epidemic.

Standard practices to prevent epidemics or control minor outbreaks include (1) assiduous attention to enteric precautions; (2) assignment of patients, especially those with severe diarrhea or incontinence, to single rooms, preferably with bathroom facilities; and (3) antibiotic control to interrupt unnecessary use of clindamycin, ampicillin, or cephalosporins. A complete epidemiologic investigation requires stool cultures to identify carriers and typing of *C. difficile* isolates, using any of several typing methods currently available. These latter recommendations extend beyond the resources of most hospital laboratories, which generally do not offer *C. difficile* cultures, and the strain typing schemes are generally considered experimental. Some have suggested antibiotic treatment for all carriers of *C. difficile*, but it should be noted that neither metronidazole nor vancomycin predictably eradicates *C. difficile* from the colon owing to sporulation.

SUGGESTED READING

Barbut F, Kajzer C, Panas N, Petit JC. Comparison of three enzyme immunoassays, a cytotoxicity assay, and toxigenic culture for diagnosis of *Clostridium difficile*–associated diarrhea. J Clin Microbiol 1993; 31:963–967.

Bartlett JG. *Clostridium difficile:* clinical considerations. Rev Infect Dis 1990; 12:S243.

Bartlett JG. Treatment of *Clostridium difficile* colitis (editorial). Gastroenterology 1985; 89:1192–1195.

Fishman E, Kavuru M, Kulzman JE, et al. CT of pseudomembranous colitis: radiologic, clinical and pathologic correlation. Radiology 1991; 180:57–60.

Gerding DN. Diseases associated with *Clostridium difficile* infection. Ann Intern Med 1989; 110:255–257.

Leuong DYM, Kelly CP, Boguniewicz M, et al. Treatment with intravenously administered gamma globulin of chronic relapsing colitis induced by *Clostridium difficile* toxin. J Pediatr 1991; 118:633–637.

McFarland LV, Mulligan ME, Kwok RY, Stamm WE. Nosocomial acquisition of *Clostridium difficile* infection. N Engl J Med 1989; 320:204–210.

Schwan A, Sjolin S, Trottestam U, et al. Relapsing *Clostridium difficile* enterocolitis cured by rectal infusion of normal feces. Scand J Infect Dis 1984; 16:211.

Surawicz CM, McFarland LV, Elmer G, et al. Treatment of recurrent *Clostridium difficile* colitis with vancomycin and *Saccharomyces boulardii*. Am J Gastroenterol 1989; 84:1285–1287.

Tvede M, Rask-Madsen J. Bacteriotherapy for chronic relapsing *Clostridium difficile* diarrhoea in six patients. Lancet 1989; 6:1156.

Viscidi R, Willey S, Bartlett JG. Isolation rates and toxigenic potential of *Clostridium difficile* isolates from various patient populations. Gastroenterology 1981; 81:5–9.

INTESTINAL PARASITES

MARTIN S. WOLFE, M.D.

Intestinal parasites represent major disease problems worldwide, in both the developing and the developed world. Imported infections can be present in refugees and immigrants and in American travelers from the developing world. Domestic infection occurs in such situations as community water-borne outbreaks; hikers and campers who drink untreated stream water; children in and employees of day care centers; institutionalized individuals; male homosexuals; and persons eating raw or undercooked beef, pork, or fish. When a patient with one of these exposure histories presents with particular suggestive symptoms, the physician must consider intestinal parasites as the etiology before initiating a costly and time-consuming gastrointestinal (GI) evaluation. The proper performance of certain relatively simple and inexpensive laboratory procedures can frequently reveal an intestinal parasite as the cause of a perplexing symptom complex. Treatment, as described in this chapter, is usually straightforward, and results can be very satisfying to both patient and physician.

Most, but not all, of the drugs to be discussed are commercially available in the United States. Some are currently licensed for one indication but not for others. A few highly advantageous and superior drugs are not yet approved for use in the United States. Certain of these foreign-made drugs may be obtained from the Parasitic Disease Drug Service of the Centers for Disease Control in Atlanta, GA (tel. 404-639-3670).

Summaries of drug therapies for intestinal parasites can be found in *The Medical Letter on Drugs and Therapeutics* (see "Suggested Reading"). Relatively common side effects of important drugs discussed in this chapter are listed in Table 1. Consensus of safety of these drugs in pregnant women and young children is given in Table 2.

PROTOZOAN INFECTIONS (Tables 3 and 4)

Giardia lamblia

Giardia lamblia is the most commonly diagnosed intestinal protozoan in the United States. It is most frequently found in campers and hikers, travelers from and natives of the developing world, male homosexuals, and day care center children and staff. A number of large outbreaks have occurred as a result of faulty community water systems. Perhaps only 50 percent of infected children are symptomatic, whereas in my experience over 80 percent of adults have some related symptoms. Typical symptoms include foul diarrhea and flatulence, distention, weight loss, and fatigue. Most infected cases should be found positive after a series of stool specimens, usually three collected every other day. However, parasitic confirmation may be difficult in approximately 30 percent of those with *G. lamblia*. Some of these may be confirmed with duodenal aspiration or biopsy, but even these methods are not always helpful. Newer enzyme-linked immunosorbent assay (ELISA) methods of identifying *G. lamblia* antigen in the stool appear to be equal in sensitivity to well-performed stool examinations, but in my experience this test is rarely positive when stool tests performed in my laboratory are negative. Also, stool examinations are required to identify other potential pathogenic protozoa or helminths. In the recognition that it may not be possible in all cases to confirm infection, there is a definite role for empiric treatment in persons with an exposure history for and typical symptoms of *G. lamblia*, before disregarding the possibility of giardiasis.

The most commonly used drug for giardiasis is metronidazole in a 7 day course of 250 mg three times a day in adults and 5 mg per kilogram three times a day in children. This should cure close to 90 percent of those infected. In the absence of reinfection, treatment failure may represent drug resistance, among other possibilities. Side effects include metallic taste, dark urine, and occasional GI symptoms. Interestingly, metronidazole has never been approved in the United States for

Table 1 Common Adverse Effects of Antiparasitic Drugs

Bithionol (Bitin)	Photosensitivity skin reactions, vomiting, diarrhea, abdominal pain, urticaria
Diloxanide furoate (Furamide)	Flatulence, nausea
Furazolidone (Furoxone)	Nausea, vomiting, fever, rash
Iodoquinol (Yodoxin)	Rash, GI symptoms
Mebendazole (Vermox)	Occasional: diarrhea, abdominal pain
Metronidazole (Flagyl)	Metallic taste, nausea, dark urine
Niclosamide (Niclocide)	Occasional: nausea, abdominal pain
Paromomycin (Humatin)	GI symptoms
Praziquantel (Biltricide)	Sedation, dizziness, headache, abdominal discomfort
Quinacrine (Atabrine)	Diarrhea, headache, toxic psychosis
Thiabendazole (Mintezol)	Nausea, vomiting, dizziness
Trimethoprim-sulfamethoxazole (Bactrim, Septra)	GI symptoms, allergic skin reactions

From Wolfe MS. Infection caused by intestinal helminths. In: Kass EH, Platt R, eds. Current therapy in infectious disease. 3rd ed. Philadelphia: BC Decker, 1990:165, with permission.

Table 2 Use of Antiparasitic Drugs in Children and Pregnant Women

Drug	Toxicity in Pregnancy	Recommendation in Pregnancy	Recommendation in Young Children
Bithionol (Bitin)	Experience not extensive enough to recommend in pregnancy	Caution*	Use with caution* in children <8 yr
Furazolidone (Furoxone)	Safety has not been established	Caution*	Contraindicated in infants <1 mo of age
Iodoquinol (Yodoxin)	Safety has not been established	Best not to use	Long-term, high dosage must not be used
Mebendazole (Vermox)	Teratogenic and embryotoxic in rats	Caution*	Use with caution* in children <2 yr of age; has not been extensively studied
Metronidazole (Flagyl)	No adequate studies; a carcinogen in rodents	Caution*	No contraindication
Niclosamide (Nicloside)	Not absorbed; no known toxicity in fetus	Probably safe	Limited experience; use with caution* in children <2 yr of age
Paromomycin (Humatin)	Poorly absorbed	Considered safe	No contraindication
Praziquantel (Biltricide)	Increased abortion rate in rats; no adequate studies in pregnant women	Caution*	Safety in children <4 yr of age has not been established
Quinacrine (Atabrine)	Crosses placenta	Treatment of giardiasis should be postponed until after delivery	No contraindication
Thiabendazole (Mintezol)	No well-controlled studies done	Caution*	Safety and effectiveness not established in children <15 kg
Trimethoprim-sulfamethoxazole (Bactrim, Septra)	May interfere with folic acid metabolism	Caution*	Not recommended for infants <2 mo of age

*Caution: Use only for a strong clinical indication in the absence of a suitable alternative. Potential benefit should justify the potential risk to the fetus or young child.

From Wolfe MS. Infection caused by intestinal helminths. In: Kass EH, Platt R, eds. Current therapy in infectious disease. 3rd ed. Philadelphia: BC Decker, 1990:167, with permission.

Table 3 Drug Therapy for Intestinal Protozoan Parasites: Part 1

Parasite	Drug	Adult Dose†	Pediatric Dose*	Availability
Giardia lamblia	Metronidazole or	250 mg t.i.d. × 7 days	5 mg/kg t.i.d. × 7 days	Flagyl (tablets)
	Quinacrine HCL or	100 mg t.i.d. × 5 days	2 mg/kg t.i.d. × 5 days	Atabrine (tablets)
	Furazolidone	100 mg (tablet) q.i.d. × 7–10 days	1.25 mg/kg q.i.d. × 7 days (suspension)	Furoxone (tablets and suspension)
Dientamoeba fragilis	Paromomycin or	500 mg t.i.d. × 7 days	30 mg/kg/day in 3 divided doses × 7 days	Humatin (capsules)
	Iodoquinol or	650 mg t.i.d. × 20 days	40 mg/kg/day in 3 divided doses × 20 days	Yodoxin (tablets)
	Tetracycline	500 mg q.i.d. × 10 days	10 mg/kg/ q.i.d. × 10 days (max 2 g/day) above age 8 yr	
Balantidium coli	Iodoquinol or	As per D. fragilis	As per D. fragilis	
	Tetracycline	As per D. fragilis	As per D. fragilis	
Isospora belli	Trimethoprim-sulfamethoxazole (TMP-SMX)	160 mg TMP/800 mg SMX q.i.d. × 10 days, then b.i.d. × 3 wk	–	Bactrim (tablets) Septra (tablets)
Cryptosporidium	Spiramycin†	3 g/day in divided doses for 2–4 wk	–	Rovamycin (tablets)
Blastocystis hominis	Iodoquinol or	As per D. fragilis	As per D. fragilis	
	Metronidazole	As per G. lamblia	As per G. lamblia	

From Rakel RE. Conn's Current Therapy. Philadelphia: WB Saunders, 1993:520–525; with permission.
*All recommended drugs given by mouth.
†Not approved in the United States.

Table 4 Drug Therapy for Intestinal Protozoan Parasites: Part 2 (Amebiasis)

Parasite	Drug	Adult Dose†	Pediatric Dose*	Availability
Amebic dysentery	Metronidazole followed by:	750 mg t.i.d. × 10 days	45 mg/kg in 3 divided doses × 10 days	Flagyl (tablets or intravenous)
	Paromomycin	500 mg t.i.d. × 7 days	30 mg/kg in 3 divided doses × 7 days	Humatin (capsules)
	or			
	Iodoquinol	650 mg t.i.d. × 20 days	40 mg/kg in 3 divided doses x 20 days	Yodoxin (capsules)
Moderately severe non-dysenteric amebiasis	Metronidazole followed by:	500 mg t.i.d. × 10 days	30 mg/kg in 3 divided doses × 7 days	
	Paromomycin or iodoquinol as above			
Mildly symptomatic non-dysenteric amebiasis	Paromomycin	500 mg t.i.d. × 7 days	30 mg/kg in 3 divided doses × 7 days	
Asymptomatic cyst passer	Paromomycin			
	or	As above	As above	
	Iodoquinol			

From Rakel RE. Conn's Current Therapy. Philadelphia: WB Saunders, 1993:520–525; with permission.

giardiasis, but it remains a useful and essential drug. Careful observation and follow-up of treated patients have not revealed any carcinogenic or mutagenic effects of metronidazole. A number of related nitroimidazole drugs are available abroad but not in the United States. These include tinidazole and ornidazole, which have the advantage of a single treatment dose.

Quinacrine is the most effective anti-*Giardia* drug, therapy with which has frequently led to cure of patients who have failed on repeated or higher doses of metronidazole. The dosage is 100 mg (2 mg per kilogram for children) three times a day for 5 days. Tolerance is often poor in younger children, and placing the appropriate dose of the drug in a gelatin capsule may improve ingestion. Side effects include intestinal upset, headache, and yellow urine. Rarely, vomiting, diarrhea, cramps, fever, and skin rash may occur and necessitate cessation of the drug. A toxic psychosis, with either depression or excitation, occurs in about 1.5 percent of those taking quinacrine for giardiasis. These more troublesome side effects appear to be less likely when a 5 day, rather than the previous 7 day, course is used. Unfortunately, in 1993 the manufacturer became unable to obtain certain raw materials needed for production of quinacrine, and this drug is currently difficult if not impossible to obtain, both in the United States and abroad.

Furazolidone is the only anti-*Giardia* drug in the United States available as a suspension, making it particularly useful for young children. It is also available in tablet form. Cure rates of 75 to 90 percent have been reported. The adult dosage is 100 mg four times a day for 7 to 10 days; children should receive 1.25 mg per kilogram four times a day for 7 to 10 days. In my experience, side effects are not uncommon, including GI symptoms, fever, rash, urticaria, and (rarely) serum sickness. With the current unavailability of quinacrine, furazolidone should have increased use for those failing metronidazole therapy.

After treatment of giardiasis and other intestinal parasites, a series of stool examinations should be performed about 1 month later to assure parasitologic cure. When certain GI symptoms persist after treatment and parasites cannot be found, in addition to unconfirmed treatment failure, post-*Giardia* lactose intolerance and postmetronidazole intestinal candidiasis should be considered.

Entamoeba histolytica (Amebiasis)

Entamoeba histolytica has a worldwide distribution but is more prevalent in tropical areas, where invasive disease is frequent and symptoms tend to be more severe. Many of the cases identified in the United States are imported from more highly endemic areas by travelers and immigrants, but there is a low level of domestic endemicity.

Clinical features of amebiasis depend on the pathogenicity of the strain of *E. histolytica*. These are currently identifiable only with research techniques such as isoenzyme and polymerase chain reaction. The intensity of infection, bacterial flora, numerous host factors, and the site and extent of tissue damage also determine clinical features. The invasive amebiasis leading to dysentery or extraintestinal involvement occurs in only a few amebic infections. Most of those infected either have nondysenteric intestinal amebiasis with mild to moderate symptoms or are asymptomatic cyst passers. It is now believed that nonpathogenic strains, not necessarily requiring treatment, are predominant in asymptomatic cyst passers. However, more readily available and inexpensive strain typing techniques are necessary to confirm this in individual cases.

Acute amebic dysentery typically presents with severe abdominal cramps, chills, fever, prostration, and tenesmus. Stools are liquid and contain bloody mucus. In very severe fulminant disease, extensive colonic involvement may lead to massive destruction of the mucosa, hemorrhage, and perforation and peritonitis. It may be difficult to clinically differentiate acute amebic dysentery from inflammatory bowel disease, but it is essential to rule out an amebic etiology before treating with corticosteroids, as these drugs can exacerbate an acute amebic infection.

Treatment of acute amebic dysentery requires a potent, well-absorbed, tissue-active drug such as metronidazole. Most patients can tolerate oral treatment in a recommended course of 750 mg three times a day for 10 days (children, 45 mg per kilogram per day in three divided doses). Those unable to tolerate this drug orally should receive it intravenously. Emetine and dehydroemetine are older parenteral drugs that are now rarely used. After initial treatment with metronidazole, follow-up therapy should be with one of the poorly absorbed, primarily luminal-acting oral drugs, to eliminate all cysts and prevent possible relapse. These luminal-acting drugs include paromomycin (Humatin) in an adult dose of 500 mg three times a day for 7 days (children, 30 mg per kilogram per day in three divided doses); or iodoquinol (Yodoxin), 650 mg three times a day for 20 days (children, 40 mg per kilogram per day in three divided doses).

Amebic liver abscess presents with right upper quadrant pain and fever and is diagnosed by scanning or sonography and positive amebic serologic testing. Treatment is identical to that for acute amebic dysentery.

Moderate to mild, symptomatic, nondysenteric amebiasis may be treated relatively vigorously with metronidazole, 500 mg three times a day for 10 days (children, 30 mg per kilogram per day in three divided doses), followed by a luminal drug as above. Mildly symptomatic cases can often be treated with a course of a luminal drug alone; if this fails, more vigorous retreatment may be administered.

There are differences of opinion over the need to treat asymptomatic cyst passers. Research in male homosexuals who are asymptomatic cyst passers has shown that almost all infections are with nonpathogenic strains, suggesting that treatment, and certainly repeated treatment, may not be necessary in this population. Until more information on strains in other populations is available, it remains possible that some asymptomatic cyst passers can infect other people with differing host factors, or that long-term carriage of potentially pathogenic strains may lead to later active intestinal or hepatic disease. A luminal drug by itself, in doses cited above, is usually well tolerated and 80 to 90 percent effective in clearing asymptomatic infection. Metronidazole should not be used for this condition since it is so well absorbed that it is not effective against cysts in the bowel lumen.

Dientamoeba fragilis

Formerly considered an ameba, *Dientamoeba fragilis* is now recognized to be an ameba-like flagellate occurring only in a labile trophozoite form. This large bowel–dwelling, noninvasive, luminal parasite is associated with intermittent diarrhea, abdominal pain, distention, and gas. Preserved stool specimens and stained-slide examinations are usually required for diagnosis. Perhaps the most effective treatment is paromomycin, 500 mg three times a day for 7 days. Alternatives are iodoquinol (as for amebiasis) and tetracycline (500 mg four times a day for 10 days), but these are less effective.

Balantidium coli

This large ciliated protozoan is very rarely diagnosed in the United States. The drugs of choice are iodoquinol or tetracycline as for *D. fragilis*.

Isospora belli

This sporozoan parasite has a worldwide distribution and is rarely found in travelers. It is much more significant as an opportunistic infection in AIDS patients. Trimethoprim-sulfamethoxazole (TMP-SMX) has been found effective in a prolonged adult course of 160 mg TMP and 800 mg SMX four times a day for 10 days, then twice a day for 3 weeks.

Cryptosporidium

This coccidial parasite is a cause of highly lethal fulminant diarrhea in AIDS patients. It is also a common infection, usually water-borne or person-to-person, in otherwise healthy children and adults, in whom it causes a self-limited illness lasting 7 to 28 days. A satisfactory drug has not yet been identified. Experimental treatment with spiramycin (Rovamycine), octreotide, azithromycin, and paromomycin has led to improvement of diarrhea in some cases. Treatment is primarily directed toward the symptoms, including adequate fluid and nutritional support.

Microsporidiosis

An increasingly recognized cause of chronic diarrhea and weight loss in AIDS patients is microsporidiosis, particularly with *Enterocytozoan bienuesi*. Early cases were diagnosed by intestinal biopsy, examined under light microscopy and confirmed by electron microscopy. Recently, diagnosis has been found possible with direct fecal smears stained with a modified trichrome stain. At this time, no effective treatment is available. Partial remission has occurred with metronidazole and octreotide. Albendazole has been found to cause degenerative changes in the organism; it controls diarrhea and appears to be a useful palliative treatment.

Cyclospora-Like Bodies

Cyclospora are considered by many researchers to be coccidian parasites resembling a large species of *Cryptosporidium*. Outbreaks and individual cases in immunocompromised persons and normal travelers have been described. Symptoms include malaise, explosive watery diarrhea, cramps, and nausea that have lasted for up to 4 weeks with cycles of relapses and remissions. There is currently no published or anecdotal information on drug treatment of this infection.

Blastocystis hominis

This is a common parasite whose pathogenicity is debated. In asymptomatic persons harboring it, treatment need not be considered. In heavily infected symptomatic patients, I believe that there is usually an underlying unrecognized pathogenic protozoan causing symptoms, and I direct treatment toward the most likely clinically indicated causative parasite. Some workers have used iodoquinol and metronidazole for symptomatic *Blastocystis hominis* infections, but no drug has proved regularly effective, and no well-controlled studies have been reported.

Nonpathogenic Protozoa

A number of nonpathogenic amebae and flagellates are commonly found on stool examination. Although these are indicators of contamination, they should not be considered a cause of symptoms. If symptoms are present, further search should be made or empiric treatment given for a recognized or clinically suggested pathogenic parasite. These nonpathogens include *Entamoeba hartmanni, Entamoeba coli, Endolimax nana, Iodamoeba butschlii, Chilomastix mesnili,* and *Trichomonas hominis.*

HELMINTHIC INFECTIONS (Tables 5 to 7)

Ascaris lumbricoides (Roundworm)

Infections with this large roundworm are generally asymptomatic in the United States. A number of safe and highly effective drugs are available, but mebendazole (Vermox) in a regimen of 100 mg twice a day for 3 days in adults and children is the drug of choice.

Trichuris trichiura (Whipworm)

This parasite also does not usually cause symptoms and can be treated with a course of mebendazole as for *A. lumbricoides.*

Hookworm

In temperate areas, hookworm infection or an asymptomatic carrier state is much more common than heavier infections causing hookworm disease with anemia. Mebendazole, 100 mg twice daily for 3 days in adults and children, is the treatment of choice. If anemia is related to heavy infection, iron supplements must also be used.

Enterobius vermicularis (Pinworm)

This is a more common infection in middle-class American children than in children in the developing world. It is a major cause of perianal itching and restlessness in children, whose parents and siblings may also become infected. Single-dose treatment with 100 mg

Table 5 Drug Therapy for Intestinal Helminths: Part 1

Parasite	Drug	Adult Dose*	Pediatric Dose*	Availability
Ascaris lumbricoides	Mebendazole	100 mg b.i.d. × 3 days	Same as adult dose (>2 yr)	Vermox (tablets)
	or			
	Pyrantel pamoate	11 mg/kg single dose (max 1 g)	Same as adult dose (max 1 g)	Antiminth (suspension)
Trichuris trichiura	Mebendazole	As per *Ascaris*	As per *Ascaris*	
Hookworm	Mebendazole	As per *Ascaris*	As per *Ascaris*	
Necator americanus	or			
Ancylostoma duodenale	Pyrantel pamoate†	As per *Ascaris*	As per *Ascaris*	
Enterobius vermicularis	Mebendazole	100-mg single dose; repeat in 2 wk	Same as adult dose (>2 yr)	
	or			
	Pyrantel pamoate	11 mg/kg single dose; repeat in 2 wk	Same as adult dose	
Strongyloides stercoralis	Thiabendazole	25 mg/kg b.i.d. × 2 days (max 3 g/day)	Same as adult dose	Mintezol (suspension and tablets)
	or			
	Mebendazole†	As per *Ascaris*	As per *Ascaris*	
Trichostrongylus sp.	Thiabendazole†	As per *Strongyloides*	As per *Strongyloides*	
	or			
	Pyrantel pamoate†	As per *Ascaris*	As per *Ascaris*	
	or			
	Mebendazole†	As per *Ascaris*	As per *Ascaris*	

*All recommended drugs given by mouth.
†Considered an investigational drug for this purpose by the U.S. Food and Drug Administration.
From Wolfe MS. Infection caused by intestinal helminths. In: Kass EH, Platt R, eds. Current therapy in infectious disease. 3rd ed. Philadelphia: BC Decker, 1990:165; with permission.

Table 6 Drug Therapy for Intestinal Helminths: Part 2

Parasite	Drug	Adult Dose*	Pediatric Dose*	Availability
Tapeworms				
Taenia saginata	Niclosamide or	Single dose/4 tabs (2 g) chewed thoroughly	11–34 kg: single dose/2 tabs (1 g) >34 kg: single dose/3 tabs (1.5 g)	Niclocide (tablets)
Taenia solium	Paromomycin† or	1 g q 15 min × 4 doses	11 mg/kg q 15 min × 4 doses	Humatin (capsules)
Diphyllobothrium latum and *pacificum* *Dipylidium caninum*	Praziquantel†	15 to 20 mg/kg once	Same as adult dose	Biltricide
Hymenolepis nana	Niclosamide or	Single 2-g/dose × 6 days	As above for other tapeworms, single dose daily × 6 days	
	Praziquantel†	15 to 20 mg/kg once	Same as adult dose	
Schistosoma				
Schistosoma mansoni	Praziquantel or	40 mg/kg in 2 divided doses × 1 day	Same as adult dose	Biltricide (tablets)
	Oxamniquine	Caribbean and S. American strains: 15 mg/kg single dose African strains: 15 mg/kg b.i.d × 2 days	Same as adult dose	Vansil (tablets)
Schistosoma japonicum	Praziquantel	60 mg/kg in 3 divided doses × 1 day	Same as adult dose	
Schistosoma mekongi	Praziquantel	As per *S. japonicum*	As per *S. japonicum*	
Schistosoma intercalatum	Praziquantel	As per *S. mansoni*	As per *S. mansoni*	

*All recommended drugs given by mouth.
†Considered an investigational drug for this purpose by the U.S. Food and Drug Administration.
From Wolfe MS. Infection caused by intestinal helminths. In: Kass EH, Platt R, eds. Current therapy in infectious disease. 3rd ed. Philadelphia: BC Decker, 1990:165; with permission.

Table 7 Drug Therapy for Intestinal Helminths: Part 3

Parasite	Drug	Adult Dose*	Pediatric Dose*	Availability
Intestinal flukes				
Fasciolopsis buskii *Heterophyes heterophyes* *Metagonimus yokogawi*	Praziquantel†	25 mg/kg t.i.d. × 1 day	Same as adult dose	
Liver flukes				
Clonorchis sinensis *Opisthorchis viverrini*	Praziquantel	25 mg/kg t.i.d. × 1 day	Same as adult dose	
Fasciola hepatica	Bithionol† (capsule) or	30 to 50 mg/kg on alternate days × 10–15 doses	Same as adult dose	Parasitic Disease Drug Service, CDC, Atlanta, GA
	Praziquantel†	25 mg/kg t.i.d. × 1 day	Same as adult dose	
Paragonimus westermani	Praziquantel† or	25 mg/kg t.i.d. × 1 day	Same as adult dose	
	Bithionol†	As per *F. hepatica*	As per *F. hepatica*	

*All recommended drugs given by mouth.
†Considered an investigational drug for this purpose by the U.S. Food and Drug Administration.
From Wolfe MS. Infection caused by intestinal helminths. In: Kass EH, Platt R, eds. Current therapy in infectious disease. 3rd ed. Philadelphia: BC Decker, 1990:165; with permission.

mebendazole, repeated in 2 weeks, is highly effective and well tolerated, but reinfection may occur. It is acceptable practice to treat the entire family with the same regimen when at least one member is known to be infected. Pinworm eggs are uncommonly found in stool examinations, and a Scotch tape test is necessary to confirm the diagnosis.

Strongyloides stercoralis

This parasite has a unique autoinfection cycle that can allow self-perpetuating infection to continue for 30 to 40 years. The continued presence of this frequently unrecognized infection poses a potential threat of lethal dissemination by hyperinfection if an individual becomes immunosuppressed via human immunodeficiency virus

(HIV) infection or by treatment with cancer chemotherapy, radiation, or corticosteroids. Strongyloidiasis should be considered in anyone who has been in an endemic area and has otherwise unexplained eosinophilia with periodic diarrhea, urticaria, or creeping eruption on the buttocks or thighs, and possibly pulmonary complaints. Diagnosis can be confirmed by finding larvae in the stool or duodenal fluid. A positive serologic test for *Strongyloides* in the presence of the above signs and symptoms is also an indication for specific treatment. The only available drug for strongyloidiasis in the United States is thiabendazole (Mintezol) in a 2 day course of 50 mg per kilogram per day in two doses (maximum 3 g per day) for adults and children. Albendazole and ivermectin have shown a better effect against this parasite, but these drugs are not yet available in the United States. In disseminated strongyloidiasis, thiabendazole should be continued for at least 5 days in the above dosage.

Trichostrongylus sp.

This parasite resembles *Strongyloides stercoralis* in its symptoms and small bowel location, and is an uncommon cause of eosinophilia and intestinal problems in travelers. It is particularly common in Iran, Korea, and Indonesia. Thiabendazole, as used for strongyloidiasis in a 2 day course, is the treatment of choice.

Cestode (Tapeworm) Infections

Taenia saginata (the beef tapeworm), *Taenia solium* (the pork tapeworm), *Diphyllobothrium latum* (the fish tapeworm), and *Dipylidium caninum* are best treated with niclosamide (Niclocide) in a single 2 g dose (with reduced doses per weight for children). Praziquantel (Biltricide) and paromomycin (Humatin) are alternative drugs. *Hymenolepsis nana* (the dwarf tapeworm) and the much less common *Hymenolepsis diminuta* require a 6 day course of niclosamide in the above dosages.

Schistosomiasis

The most common form of intestinal schistosomiasis is infection with *Schistosoma mansoni*, common in tropical Africa and northeastern South America. Rare cases of *Schistosoma japonicum* from East Asia, *Schistosoma mekongi* in refugees from Southeast Asia, and *Schistosoma intercalatum* from Central Africa may also be seen. The treatment of choice for all these intestinal species, as well as for urinary schistosomiasis *(Schistosoma hematobium),* is with praziquantel in a single day course of 40 to 60 mg per kilogram per day in two divided doses for adults and children.

Intestinal Flukes

Fasciolopsis buskii, Heterophyes heterophyes, and *Metagonimus yokogawi* are very rare parasites in the United States. All can be treated with praziquantel, 75 mg per kilogram per day in three doses for 1 day for adults and children.

Liver Flukes

Clonorchis sinensis and *Opisthorchis viverrini* primarily infect the bile ducts, but diagnosis is usually made by finding eggs in the stool. These parasites are not uncommon in Southeast Asian refugees, who are generally asymptomatic. *Fasciola hepatica* can cause acute and chronic infections of the liver and the biliary tree. Eggs of *Paragonimus westermani* (the lung fluke) may be found in the stool. Praziquantel, in doses used for intestinal flukes, is the drug of choice for these flukes, except *Fasciola hepatica,* for which bithionol (an investigational drug available from CDC), 30 to 50 mg per kilogram on alternate days for 10 to 15 doses, is superior for both adults and children.

SUGGESTED READING

Campbell WC, Rew RS, eds. Chemotherapy of parasitic diseases. New York: Plenum, 1986. (Encyclopedic coverage of subject.)

Drugs for parasitic infections. Medical letter on drugs and therapeutics 1992; 34:17–26. (Particular parasites with drugs of choice and alternatives listed, with adult and pediatric doses, list of drugs with manufacturer, and adverse effects. Updated every 2 years.)

Gellin BG, Soave R. Coccidian infections in AIDS. Toxoplasmosis, cryptosporidiosis, and isosporiasis. Med Clin North Am 1992; 76:205–234. (Good description of attempts at drug treatment for cryptosporidiosis and isosporiasis.)

King CH, Mahmoud AAF. Drugs five years later: praziquantel. Ann Intern Med 1989; 110:290–296. (Describes advances in the knowledge of this very important anthelmintic drug in the 5 years since its introduction in the United States.)

Pawlowski ZS, ed. Intestinal helminthic infections. In: Bailliere's clinical tropical medicine and communicable diseases 2:No. 3, December 1987. (Deals with treatment of the most common intestinal helminthic infections as well as rare but clinically important infections.)

Sun T. Microsporidiosis in the acquired immunodeficiency syndrome. Infect Dis Newsletter 1993; 12:20–22. (Discusses drugs tried against microporidiosis.)

World Health Organization. WHO model prescribing information. Drugs used in parasitic diseases. Geneva: WHO, 1990. (A model whose objective is to provide source material for adaptation by national authorities to develop national drug formularies.)

WHIPPLE'S DISEASE*

WILLIAM O. DOBBINS III, M.D.

Whipple first described "intestinal lipodystrophy" in 1907 at an autopsy (at the Johns Hopkins Hospital) in a 36-year-old physician with features of a wasting disorder characterized by diarrhea, abdominal pain, arthralgia, and fever. Whipple's disease is a chronic, multisystem relapsing disorder that was uniformly fatal before the discovery that antibiotics were effective as treatment. Although fewer than 900 cases have been reported in the literature to date, recognition of this disorder and subsequent reporting have been on the rise for the past three decades. It primarily affects Caucasian males (8:1 male to female ratio) with a usual age at diagnosis of 40 to 49 years. The distribution initially appeared to be in North America and continental Europe, but is probably more widespread.

CLINICAL FEATURES

A bacterial cause for the disease was suspected by Whipple but not confirmed until 1961 when electron microscopy, also at Johns Hopkins, demonstrated the presence of rod-shaped bacteria in the foamy macrophages typical of the disease. These bacilli stain intensely with the periodic acid-Schiff (PAS) stain for glycoproteins and can be found in virtually any organ system, including heart, lung, brain, and gastrointestinal (GI) tract, but there is a marked predilection for the proximal small intestine. Dense infiltration with the bacteria-laden macrophages in the small intestine is associated with blunting and distention of the villi, dilated lipid-filled lacteals, and mesenteric lymphadenopathy. The finding of extracellular and intracellular Whipple's bacilli in intestinal tissue on small intestinal biopsy is diagnostic and differentiates the disorder from others characterized by intracellular PAS-positive bacilli, such as Mycobacterium avium-intracellulare in acquired immunodeficiency syndrome (AIDS) patients. These organisms, unlike Whipple's bacillus, are acid-fast staining. Indirect immunofluorescent staining of a bacillus of unique morphologic form suggests a single etiologic agent. Molecular genetic analysis of the bacterium have led to the identification of Tropheryma whippleii as the causative agent in this disease.

Patients typically present with a 5- to 10-year history of migratory polyarthralgias or nondeforming arthritis associated with fever, cough, abdominal pain, diarrhea, and malabsorption. Eventually, steatorrhea and severe weight loss may develop. Neurologic involvement is evident in 10 percent of cases and may manifest as personality changes, hypothalamic dysfunction, progressive dementia, visual disturbances, seizures, headache, meningitis, and peripheral neuropathy. Relapses have frequently been described especially in the central nervous system (CNS). Physical findings that are commonly present at diagnosis include generalized lymphadenopathy (50 to 55 percent), skin hyperpigmentation (40 to 54 percent), low-grade fever (30 to 50 percent), abdominal tenderness (50 percent), cardiac murmurs (30 percent), ill-defined abdominal mass (20 percent), ascites (10 percent), peripheral edema, splenomegaly, and glossitis. Hypotension is also common (70 percent) as a late finding. Abnormal laboratory findings include an elevated sedimentation rate, anemia of chronic disease (although iron deficiency and vitamin B_{12} malabsorption can occur), vitamin deficiencies, steatorrhea, low white blood cell count (usually due to decreased numbers of circulating T lymphocytes), and hypoalbuminemia.

There is strong evidence that an immune deficit may exist in individuals predisposed to develop Whipple's disease. In infected persons there is a decreased response of peripheral blood mononuclear cells to phytohemagglutinin (PHA) and concanavalin A (ConA) mitogens, both before and after treatment; impaired delayed cutaneous hypersensitivity, before and after treatment; and a 27 to 40 percent incidence of HLA-B27 antigen positivity. In this respect, the disease resembles other chronic disorders such as leprosy, chronic granulomatous disease, and AIDS in which a disorder of immune surveillance allows infection by usually nonpathogenic microbes.

Typical radiographic findings on upper GI series include flocculation, prominent duodenal and jejunal folds, luminal dilatation, and widening of the duodenal sweep from mesenteric nodal enlargement. The diagnosis is usually and most easily made by endoscopic small bowel biopsy, with the demonstration of an abundance of PAS-positive macrophages in the lamina propria and the presence of extracellular Whipple's bacilli by transmission electron microscopy. The characteristic organism may also be identified in other involved tissue.*

ANTIMICROBIAL THERAPY

Treatment with antimicrobial agents is universally effective in initial management of the disease. Choice of antibiotic is empiric. Chloramphenicol, tetracycline, trimethoprim-sulfamethoxazole (TMP-SMZ), penicillin, and streptomycin have been shown to be effective

---

*Editor's Note: Please see acknowledgment to Drs. Blades and Bonwell, who wrote on this topic in third edition.

---

*Editor's Note: With the development of PCR techniques to identify the organism and the immunofluorescent methods cited above, some of the "atypical" patients with CNS or ophthalmologic findings will be classifiable as Whipple's disease or some other illness. This is true of a man with oculomaticatory myorhythmia with the Whipple's organism in the brain and eye but not the gut. He was autopsied in 1931 before antibiotic usage.

in infected individuals or groups of patients. An appropriate antibiotic regimen results in alleviation of symptoms an average of 5 months after initiation of drug therapy, a normalization of the small bowel pattern on UGI series after 10 months, and histologic improvement an average of 14 months after therapy is begun. In patients exhibiting a curative response, clearance of extracellular and some intracellular organisms occurs. PAS-staining membranes may persist in macrophages of the lamina propria in asymptomatic individuals for years.

A retrospective study of 88 patients with Whipple's disease, compiled from a survey questionnaire sent to academic gastroenterology centers nationwide and from the medical literature by Keinath and colleagues reported tetracycline (49 of 88) alone as the most commonly employed antimicrobial regimen, followed by parenteral penicillin and streptomycin and oral tetracycline (15 of 88), or penicillin alone (eight of 88). In patients showing no evidence of clinical relapse, there was a mean follow-up of 8.2 years, with a range of 18 months to 27 years. Although the duration of therapy varied, the relapse rates for tetracycline and penicillin alone were 43 and 37 percent, respectively, suggesting that these are inadequate regimens especially when administered for less than 1 year. Eleven of these relapses occurred in the CNS, which underscores the need for an antimicrobial that effectively penetrates the blood-brain barrier in the absence of meningeal inflammation. In the same study, the only antibiotic treatment group in which there were no relapses consisted of three patients treated with oral TMP-SMZ.

In an article from the Mayo Clinic, Fleming and colleagues reported 29 patients with Whipple's disease that was diagnosed and managed at a single institution. The mean follow-up period was 6.4 years, with a range of 1 month to 26 years. Four patients whose condition was diagnosed before the recognition that antibiotics were effective therapy never received antibiotics. They all died within 9 months of diagnosis, which highlights the fatal nature of the disease when left untreated. Of the remaining 23 patients available to follow-up (two were lost to follow-up), 12 received tetracycline alone (1 g per day for an average of 16.6 months); eight received streptomycin, penicillin, or erythromycin for 7 to 14 days followed by tetracycline (1 g per day for 2 to 52 weeks); two received penicillin alone (5 days and 3 months, respectively); and one received penicillin and streptomycin for 3 weeks. The overall relapse rate was 9 percent, accounted for by one patient with a CNS relapse 2 years after cessation of therapy, and one with a clinical small bowel and pericardial relapse 12 months after cessation of therapy. Of interest, both patients had been treated with tetracycline alone for 9 and 18 months, respectively. The relapse rate in the group available for follow-up that received only tetracycline was 16.7 percent. It is important to note that of the 12 patients who received tetracycline alone and did not relapse, three received only 1 year of follow-up, and one died of a myocardial infarct 1 and 1/2 years after

therapy was completed. In addition, the two patients for whom follow-up was unavailable had received tetracycline alone.

In another report from Germany, von Herbay and Otto described 22 cases of Whipple's disease diagnosed at a single institution from 1965 to 1983. Follow-up was obtained for a median of 7.7 years (range 1 to 15 years). Follow-up was available for 2 years or more in 17 patients and 5 years or more in 11 patients. Sixteen of the 17 patients with adequate follow-up were treated with tetracycline for at least 2 years. The 17th individual received ampicillin and chloramphenicol intravenously. In those given tetracycline as primary therapy, there were four relapses, two in one patient. No CNS relapses were reported and all patients responded to further therapy. An overall relapse rate for tetracycline-treated patients was 25 percent, a figure at odds with these authors' conclusion that tetracycline for 2 years is a safe and effective long-term therapy.

Although the numbers are small, these studies represent the largest series of collected data on therapy for Whipple's disease. In view of the relapse data for single-agent treatment with either penicillin or tetracycline, initial therapy with either drug alone is inadequate. Neither agent effectively crosses the blood-brain barrier in the absence of meningeal inflammation. CNS relapse tends to be less responsive to subsequent therapy, and the long-term outcome is less favorable in CNS disease, with death occurring frequently. Because Whipple's disease is a multisystem disorder with symptoms and presumed infection for years before diagnosis, it is widely believed that this disorder involves the CNS at initial presentation in most patients. Therefore, initial therapy should always include an antimicrobial agent that penetrates uninflamed meninges, and a route of administration that ensures adequate cerebrospinal fluid levels. Of the antimicrobial agents used to date, parenteral penicillin, oral chloramphenicol, and oral TMP-SMZ all meet these requirements.

RECOMMENDED TREATMENT

Initial Therapy

Recommended therapy (Table 1) is based on a review of the collective experience in treating Whipple's disease. From these data, the ability to penetrate the bloodbrain barrier and the duration of initial therapy have been shown to be the most important considerations in antimicrobial management. The data supporting oral TMP-SMZ administered for 1 year or more as optimal therapy is sparse but convincing. However, there have been relapses in patients treated with this regimen. TMP-SMZ as a single oral agent has been successfully used to treat CNS relapse. Therefore, in individuals effectively able to absorb oral antibiotics, double-strength TMP-SMZ should be given twice daily for a minimum of 1 year. Owing to the excellent initial response and the paucity of experience with longer regimens, it is unclear whether therapy lasting longer

Table 1 Recommended Antimicrobial Regimens for Whipple's Disease

Antimicrobials	Route	Dosage	Duration
Initial Presentation			
TMP-SMZ	PO	1 DS tab 2×/day	1 yr
PCN G	IM	1.2 million U/day	10-14 days
STM	IM	1.0 g/day	10-14 days
followed by:			
TMP-SMZ	PO	1 DS tab 2×/day	1 yr
or:			
PCN VK	PO	250 mg 4×/day	1 yr
CHLORO	IV	250 mg 4×/day	10-14 days
followed by:			
TMP-SMZ	PO	1 DS tab 2×/day	1 yr
or:			
PCN VK	PO	250 mg 4×/day	1 yr
Relapse			
CHLORO	IV	250 mg 4×/day	2-4 wk
followed by:			
TMP-SMZ	PO	1 DS tab 2×/day	1 yr
or:			
PCN or	IV	20 million U/day	30 days
Cephtriaxone	IV	2g 2×/day	30 days
followed by:			
TMP-SMZ	PO	1 DS tab 2×/day	1 yr

TMP-SMZ = trimethoprim-sulfamethoxazole; PCN = penicillin; STM = streptomycin; CHLORO = chloramphenicol; DS = double strength.

than 1 year is of any clinical benefit. Folinic acid should be administered concurrently, particularly in malnourished patients, to prevent folic acid deficiency. Acceptable alternative antibiotic regimens include (1) intramuscular procaine penicillin G (1.2 million U) and intramuscular streptomycin (1 g) daily for 2 weeks, followed by 1 year of oral double-strength TMP-SMZ twice daily; (2) parenteral chloramphenicol (250 mg four times daily) for 2 weeks followed by oral double-strength TMP-SMZ twice daily. In the above regimens, penicillin VK (250 mg four times daily) or amoxicillin (250 mg three times daily) can be substituted for TMP-SMZ in sulfa-allergic patients.

With the institution of antimicrobial therapy, fever and diarrhea resolve quickly in 1 to 2 weeks. Resolution of arthralgias and cough follows, with subsequent weight gain. Malabsorption may persist for months. Fat-soluble vitamins and other nutritional deficits should be replaced as indicated. Since intracellular PAS-positive bacilli can persist indefinitely in patients otherwise completely recovered, it is not recommended to rebiopsy the small intestine or other involved tissue after appropriate therapy has been completed. If relapse is suspected, involved tissue should be biopsied and examined by electron microscopy for extracellular bacilli.*

---

*Editor's Note: Some pathologists believe that the usual PAS-positive bacterial material disappears with therapy, leaving only granular PAS-positive material in macrophages. We used repeat intestinal biopsies as some measure of the adequacy of treatment, but this may be fallacious, since some CNS relapses have presented with negative jejunal mucosal biopsies.

Relapse Therapy

Relapse can occur at any time after cessation of treatment. The duration of remission may bear a direct relationship to the length of initial therapy. Some patients treated with antimicrobial agents for only 3 to 4 weeks are completely free of disease 10 to 15 years later, but it is generally agreed that relapse is more likely to occur when an antimicrobial drug is administered for less than 1 year. In addition, CNS relapse is more likely to occur when initial therapy does not include an antimicrobial agent that effectively penetrates uninflamed meninges. CNS disease is the more serious form of relapse, since it responds less well to further therapy. When CNS disease is suspected, either initially or at the time of relapse, the cerebrospinal fluid should be examined for the presence of PAS-positive macrophages. Although progression of disease in the CNS can sometimes be halted, complete resolution of neurologic dysfunction is unusual. Typical features of CNS relapse include dementia, ataxia, hypothalamic dysfunction, ophthalmoplegia, and seizures. Treatment of CNS relapse should include 2 to 4 weeks of parenteral therapy, followed by 1 year or more of double-strength TMP-SMZ twice daily. The parenteral regimen should consist of either chloramphenicol, penicillin, or cephtriaxone in appropriate doses. In individuals for whom parenteral therapy may not be feasible, oral double-strength TMP-SMZ, three times daily for 2 weeks, then twice daily for at least 1 year, may be effective. Careful long-term follow-up should always be pursued. Despite appropriate therapy, relapse may occur in certain individuals.

Acknowledgment. Acknowledgment is made to Edmond W. Blades and John G. Banwell, who wrote on this topic in the third edition.

SUGGESTED READING

Adler CH, Galetta SL. Oculo-facial-skeletal myorhythmia in Whipple's disease: Treatment with ceftriaxone. Ann Intern Med 1990; 112:467–469.

Bayless TM. Whipple's disease. In: Gorbach SL, Bartlett JG, Blacklow NR, eds. Infectious diseases. Philadelphia: WB Saunders, 1992:649.

Dobbins WO III. Whipple's disease. Springfield, Ill: Charles C. Thomas, 1987.

Fleming JL, Wiesner RH, Shorter RG. Whipple's disease: clinical, biochemical, and histopathologic features and assessment of treatment in 29 patients. Mayo Clin Proc 1988; 63:539–551.

Keinath RD, Merrell DE, Vlietstra R, Dobbins WO. Antibiotic treatment and relapse in Whipple's disease: long-term follow-up of 88 patients. Gastroenterology 1985; 88:1867–1873.

Knox DL, Bayless TM, Pittman FE. Neurologic disease in patients with treated Whipple's disease. Medicine 1976; 55:467–476.

Relman DA, Schmidt TM, MacDermott RP, Falkow S. Identification of the uncultured bacillus of Whipple's disease. N Engl J Med 1992; 327:293–301.

Volpicelli NA, Salyer WR, Milligan FD, et al. The endoscopic appearance of the duodenum in Whipple's disease. Johns Hopkins Med J 1976; 138:19–23.

von Herbay A, Otto HF. Whipple's disease: a report of 22 patients. Klin Wochenschr 1988; 66:533–539.

PARENTERAL AND ENTERAL NUTRITION*

MARGARET MALONE, Ph.D., M.R.Pharm.S.
LYN HOWARD, M.B., F.R.C.P., F.A.C.P.

Over the centuries, many heroic attempts have been made to feed malnourished patients through enteral tubes or by vein infusion. However, these therapies did not become widely used until certain technical developments made such artificial feeding clinically feasible, more acceptable to patients, and safer. Tube enteral nutrition (EN) expanded once soft, small-bore, nasally inserted tubes and endoscopic gastrostomies were developed. Parenteral nutrition (PN) expanded once the technique of central vein catheterization and more complete intravenous (IV) nutrient solutions became available. Both therapies expanded from the "acute" care hospital setting to the more "chronic" care ambulatory setting, after this transfer was shown to be safe. Reimbursement mechanisms were established and home infusion services were developed to support and monitor these off-site patients. Table 1 provides an estimate of the total number of United States patients on EN and PN therapy in 1992 and the approximate number of dollars spent. This amounted to 18.5 million patients at an approximate cost of $8.5 billion: a little over 1 percent of the entire health care budget.

Like respiratory support, cardiac monitoring, or dialysis treatment, PN is often part of the management of high-acuity patients in an intensive care unit (ICU). In such patients, it is very difficult to demonstrate that specialized nutrition support (SNS) is cost effective.

***Editor's Note:** This is the chapter we've been seeking for those of us who serve as "pseudo"-nutritionists. It includes information for both medical and surgical conditions.

Table 1 Estimated Cost and Number of Persons Receiving Parenteral and Tube Enteral Nutrition in 1992

	No. of Persons (thousands)		Estimated Cost ($ millions)	
	Parenteral	Enteral	Parenteral	Enteral
Hospital	500	1,000	6,000	1,200
Home	42	148	636	287
Nursing home	1	160	6	410
Dialysis centers	3	<1	20	<1

Total persons = 1,854,000   Total cost = $8.56 billion

Hospital estimate based on Infusion Industry market data and on data from Anderson AF, Steinberg EP. JPEN 1986;10:3–8, with the dollars increased by 11.6% per year, the quoted growth rate. Nonhospital estimate based on Medicare data and North American HPEN Registry information, Oley Foundation, Albany, NY.

Many of these patients die despite high-intensity care. In fact, a study showed that patients requiring SNS had four times the average hospital stay and stayed 2.7 times longer than patients in the same diagnosis-related group who were not receiving SNS. Despite these unfavorable statistics, SNS is the cornerstone in many clinical situations to bringing patients through major surgery and other severe illness. An important challenge is to demonstrate clinical and cost benefit in well-designed prospective randomized controlled trials (PRCTs). In the present climate of health cost constraint, such trials must measure hard clinical end points such as mortality rate, length of hospital stay, and frequency of complications. It has been shown that a major complication such as wound dehiscence or pulmonary embolism increases the cost of a patient's hospital care by about $50,000. For SNS to be cost effective, it must not only reduce mortality rate, hospital stay, and complications but also induce these positive results without adding serious therapy-related complications such as pneumothorax from subclavian line placement or aspiration pneumonia from tube feeding. With this in mind, the section of this chapter that discusses indications for SNS emphasizes the findings of PRCTs and points out where an evaluable trial has not been done.

Before looking at how and when to provide SNS, it is important to consider the rationale for the use of nutritional therapy. There are perhaps three reasons for using SNS. The first is to support a patient through an illness associated with a prolonged inability to eat. A simple example is a young man with a ruptured appendix, peritonitis, and ileus. It may be weeks before his gastrointestinal (GI) tract tolerates a regular diet, but if he is adequately supported, complete recovery can be expected. Second, SNS may be used to treat established malnutrition and redress the complications of malnutrition such as impaired wound healing, compromised immunity, and delayed mobilization. The third rationale is the least established; it involves nutritional manipulations that can alter metabolic functioning and may therefore provide adjunctive treatment. An example is the use of branched-chain amino acids (BCAAs) in portal encephalopathy or early enteral feeding to prevent bacterial translocation and reduce the systemic hypercatabolic response.

To maintain realistic expectations of SNS, it is important to keep a rationale in mind. Most well-nourished patients can survive 10 days of marginal postoperative nutrition; hence, routine postoperative PN is likely to be associated with more harm than benefit and may be unwarranted. Likewise, patients with metastatic cancer are frequently cachectic, but currently available formulations apparently cannot reduce cytokine-induced wasting, so again SNS is likely to cause more harm than benefit.

After much ethical and legal processing, SNS has been deemed active treatment and not a comfort measure. This is appropriate, since SNS is invariably associated with some degree of discomfort. This means that a patient or the legal guardian must formally consent to SNS.

At least 20 percent of hospitalized patients show evidence of malnutrition. Many of these patients can benefit from SNS, but some cannot. In those who are terminally ill, wasting is often an inherent part of the disease course. Distinguishing between reversible and irreversible clinical situations requires knowledge and experience: knowledge of the remediable features of the primary pathologic process and experience with the benefits and hazards of SNS. Figure 1 is an algorithm to help clinicians determine where SNS is indicated, emphasizing the point at which it is essential to involve the patient and family in the decision. This algorithm does not address the question of withdrawing SNS. For a conscious patient, the physician makes this decision with the patient and family. For a patient who is unconscious or for other reasons unable to make medical decisions, withdrawal of SNS requires a written directive or the approval of a previously appointed health care proxy. For this reason, before initiating SNS, it is important to make sure the patient has written a living will and has appointed a health care proxy, and that the SNS stopping point is clearly addressed.

ASSESSMENT OF NUTRITIONAL STATUS

Evaluation of nutritional status is important in order to identify patients who are severely malnourished and also to predict those likely to be at risk for clinically significant nutritional impairment. However, difficulties arise because none of the measurements used in practice are indicators solely of nutritional status. Some of the common criteria used to monitor and assess nutritional status are described in Table 2. As a general guideline, any patient who is 25 percent below ideal body weight, shows evidence of significant muscle wasting, and has a serum albumin level of 2.8 g per deciliter or less is seriously malnourished.*

Most of these measures are static, i.e., they do not reflect functional status and rarely alter significantly during short-term SNS. For this reason, alternative methods of assessment continue to be evaluated. Tests of muscle function and respiratory function reserve may be useful in predicting clinically significant nutritional impairment. New technologies using dual energy x-ray absorption (DEXA) allow independent measurement of total body fat and the mineral compartment of the body. A combination of DEXA, in vivo neutron activation analysis measurements of nitrogen and chloride, and tritium dilution (injection of tritiated water) allows a complete assessment of the body compartments.

GENERAL NUTRITIONAL REQUIREMENTS

Fluid Requirements

Fluid requirements can be estimated as 35 to 40 ml per kilogram per day or 1,500 ml for the first 20 kg plus 20 ml per kilogram for body weight greater than 20 kg plus any additional abnormal fluid losses.

On average, most adults drink 1,000 to 1,500 ml of liquids per day. A commonly overlooked additional source of fluid is that which comes from solid food intake, which is around 1 liter per day, giving an actual fluid intake closer to 2,500 ml per day. In addition, the metabolism of ingested fuels produces another 500 ml of water.

Calorie Requirements

Although estimations of caloric requirements are based on measures of energy expenditure, there is evidence that in the stressed state the body cannot always effectively use a similar amount of exogenously supplied calories.

---

*Editor's Note: The pre- and postoperative nutritional support chapter that follows uses 15 percent below ideal body weight, and serum albumin less than 3.0 g, to define a patient "at risk."

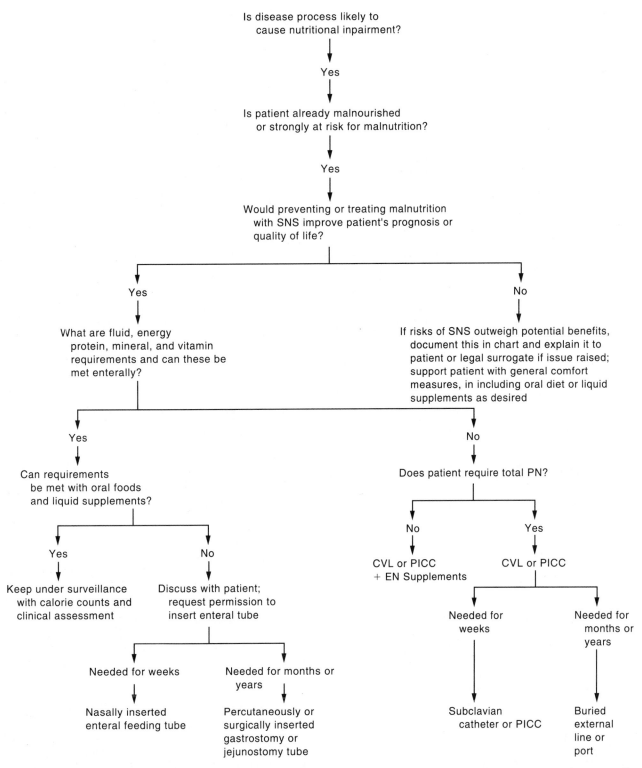

Figure 1 Algorithm for deciding whether specialized nutrition support (SNS) is indicated. CVI = central venous line; PICC = peripherally inserted central catheter. (From Howard L. Chapter 76. In: Isselbacher KJ, Braunwald E, Wilson JD, et al, eds. Harrison's principles of internal medicine, 13th ed McGraw-Hill, Inc. [in press]; with permission.)

Table 2 Assessment of Nutritional Status

Method of Assessment	Degree of Malnutrition		
	Normal	Moderate	Severe
Routine methods			
Ideal weight (IBW) (%)*	100	60–80	<60
Creatinine height index	100	60–80	<60
Triceps skinfold thickness	M 12.5	7.5–11.3	<7.5
(TSF, mm)	F 16.5	9.9–14.9	<9.9
Midarm muscle circumference	M 29.3	17.6–26.4	<17.6
(MAMC, cm)	F 28.5	17.1–25.7	<17.1
Serum albumin (g/dl)	3.5–5.0	2.1–3.0	<2.1
Serum prealbumin (mg/dl)	>20	10–15	<10
Serum transferrin (mg/dl)	200–400	100–150	<100
Retinol binding protein (mg/dl)	3–6	2–3	<2
Total lymphocyte count 10^6/l	1.8–3.0	0.8–1.2	<0.8
Delayed hypersensitivity index (DHI)†	2	1	0
Experimental Methods (Functional Tests)			
Prognostic nutritional index (PNI) %‡	<40	40–50	>50
Subjective global assessment (SGA)§	A	B	C
Grip strength/skeletal muscle function	82	65	50

*IBW (male) = 50 kg + 2.3 kg for each inch >60″; IBW (female) = 45.5 kg + 2.3 kg for each inch >60″.

†DHI quantitates the amount of induration elicited by skin testing with a common antigen such as *Candida*, PPD, or mumps. Induration grade 0 = <0.5 cm, 1 = 0.5 cm, 2 = 1.0 cm.

‡PNI % is a weighted combination = 158 − 16.6 × albumin (g/l) − 0.78 × TSF (mm) − 2 × transferrin (g/l) − 5.8 × DHI.

§SGA: clinical assessment based on weight change, dietary intake change, GI symptoms >2 weeks, functional capacity, disease and relation to nutritional status, physical findings.

In practice, for most purposes, general calorie requirements can be estimated using the values in Table 3. A second more tailored method of calculating resting energy expenditure (REE) is based on the Harris-Benedict equation, which takes into account additional patient variables:

$$REE\ Males = 66 + [13.7 \times wt\ (kg)] - [5 \times ht\ (cm)] - [6.8 \times age\ (yr)]$$
$$REE\ Females = 655 + [9.6 \times wt\ (kg)] + [1.7 \times ht\ (cm)] - [4.7 \times age\ (yr)]$$

The calculated REE is then modified on the basis of activity and stress factors that increase calorie requirements.

Energy requirement = REE × activity factor × injury factor
Activity factor: 1.2 (in bed), 1.3 (ambulatory)
Stress factor: 1.2 (minor operation), 1.35 (trauma), 1.6 (sepsis), 2.1 (burns)*

Where available, a more sophisticated approach may be adopted using indirect calorimetry, which estimates expenditure based on oxygen utilization and carbon dioxide production during metabolism:

Calorie expenditure = [(3.78 × VO_2 L/min] + [1.16 × VCO_2 L/min)] × 1440 min/day, where

*Editor's Note: A range of stress factors for surgical patients is given in Table 2 in the next chapter on surgical aspects of nutrition.

Table 3 General Calorie Requirements

Normal maintenance/elective surgery	25 kcal/kg/day
Trauma, acute pancreatitis, inflammatory bowel disease	30 kcal/kg/day
Sepsis, minor burns	35 kcal/kg/day
Major burns, severe trauma	40 kcal/kg/day

Table 4 Interpretation of Respiratory Quotient (RQ) Values

RQ	Interpretation	Recommended Action
0.7	Fat catabolism	Increase calories
0.8	Protein catabolism	Increase calories
0.9	Normal state	Maintain
1.0	Carbohydrate catabolism	Maintain
>1.0	Fat synthesis	Decrease calories

VO_2 = oxygen consumption and VCO_2 = carbon dioxide production

VO_2 is invalid in patients requiring mechanical ventilation who have chest tubes and/or when FIO_2 (fractional inspired oxygen) is greater than 50 percent. Values are also inaccurate when the nutritional regimen or the patient is unstable. Interpretation of respiratory quotient, RQ = VCO_2/VO_2, may be of value in assessing the impact of Nutrition Support as indicated in Table 4.

Protein Requirements

The adult daily requirements for protein in hospitalized patients are:

Maintenance	1.0 g/kg/day
Mild stress	1.2 g/kg/day
Moderate stress	1.5 g/kg/day
Severe stress	2.0 g/kg/day

Electrolyte Requirements

For the average patient with no abnormal losses, the daily electrolyte requirements for enteral and parenteral intake are outlined in Table 5. Modifications are necessary to take account of abnormal GI fluid losses (Table 6) and altered disease state and severity.

Micronutrient Requirements

There are commercially available multivitamins, multi–trace element preparations, and also EN formulations that follow the American Medical Association guidelines for daily maintenance requirements. In the case of enteral tube feeds, a minimum of 1,500 kcal should be given to provide sufficient micronutrients. Additional quantities of specific individual micronutrients may be needed to correct a particular deficiency or correct for abnormal losses. The daily micronutrient requirements, associated signs of depletion, and appropriate monitoring tests in adults are described in Table 7.

MANAGEMENT OF THE PATIENT REQUIRING NUTRITIONAL SUPPORT

The purposes of monitoring are (1) to ensure early recognition of metabolic, mechanical, and infectious problems; and (2) to follow the patient's progress in meeting the goal of therapy. As mentioned earlier, the assessment of nutritional depletion and repletion is difficult, and the clinician must often rely on broad clinical end points; e.g., a previously debilitated patient now being able to clear secretions, get out of bed, or be self-caring indicates improvement in strength and well-being.

The monitoring of patients who require SNS varies with their clinical status and the route of nutrient administration. A typical monitoring schedule is described in Table 8. While the adage "if the gut works, use it" holds up well, it is essential when using the enteral route to ensure that the prescribed amount of feed is being infused and that feeding is not constantly interrupted or discontinued, leading to inadequate intake.

COMPLICATIONS OF NUTRITIONAL SUPPORT

Complications are often classified as mechanical, metabolic, or infectious. Acute complications occurring in the first few days of therapy are usually metabolic because of fluid or electrolyte imbalance or associated with catheter insertion or enteral tube placement. Infectious complications can occur anytime, although line sepsis rarely accounts for fever within the first 48 to 72 hours. Later complications after 3 months of therapy are micronutrient deficiencies or physical damage to the catheter or feeding tube. Multiple-lumen catheters are associated with an increased risk of infection owing to more frequent connections and disconnections for intravenous access. Safe management requires strict adherence to aseptic techniques. Some complications associated with PN catheters can be resolved without removing the catheter (Table 9).

SNS teams have shown their cost effectiveness by

Table 5 Adult Electrolyte Requirements per 24 Hours

Electrolyte	Enteral (g)	Parenteral (mmol)
Sodium	1–3	50–120
Potassium	2–5	40–60
Magnesium	0.3	5–10
Phosphorus	0.8–1.2	20–45
Calcium	0.8–1.2	5–7.5
Chloride	2–5	150–180

Table 6 Enteric Fluid Volumes (L/day) and Their Sodium, Potassium, Chloride, and Bicarbonate Content (mmol/L).

	L/day	Na	K	Cl	HCO_3
Enteric secretions					
Saliva	1–2	10	30	10	30
Gastric juice	2	60	9	90	0
Pancreatic fluid	?	130	5	75	90
Bile	2–3	150	10	90	70
Small bowel	1	100	5	100	20
Colon	Variable	40	100	15	60

Enteric secretions are also rich in magnesium, calcium, zinc, and copper. Losses are increased by steatorrhea and diarrhea. Potassium losses are small except in secretions distal to the ileocecal valve. The regulation of Na-K exchange in the bowel is partially controlled by aldosterone's influence on the colon. Bicarbonate losses must be replaced as acetate or lactate in TPN solutions to avoid large alterations in the pH of the final solution.

Table 7 Vitamin and Micronutrient Requirements in Adults

Nutrient	Daily Requirement		Signs of Deficiency	Method of Assessment
	Enteral	Parenteral		
Iron (mg)	10	1–2	Hypochromic, microcytic anemia	Serum iron, ferritin, TIBC
Zinc (mg)	15 + 15–30 mg/l of diarrheal or ileostomy output	3–12	Growth retardation, Diarrhea, alopecia Hypogonadism, skin lesions, immune deficiencies, night blindness, taste, disturbances, and wound healing	Serum zinc, metallothionine 2 activity
Copper (mg)	2–3	0.3–0.5	Anemia, neutropenia, depigmentation of hair and skin, defective elastin synthesis—bone defects, CNS changes, hypotonia, hypothermia	Serum copper
Iodine (mg)	0.15	0.15	Hypothyroidism	Thyroid function tests
Manganese (mg)	2–5	2–5	Defective growth, bony anomalies, reproductive dysfunction, CNS abnormalities	Serum manganese
Chromium (mg)	0.015 + 20 μg for GI losses	0.015	Glucose intolerance, peripheral neuropathy, metabolic encephalopathy, cardiovascular disease	Serum chromium
Molybdenum (mg)	0.05–0.3	0.01–0.5	Headache, night blindness, cholestasis, lethargy, coma, abnormal purine and amino acid metabolism	Serum molybdenum
Selenium (mg)	0.05–0.2	0.05–0.1	Myalgia, muscle tenderness, red blood cell fragility, cardiomyopathy, weakness, hair loss	Serum selenium, RBC glutathione peroxidase activity
Ascorbic acid (mg)	60	100	Poor wound healing, capillary fragility, hemorrhage, aching joints, loose teeth, bleeding gums if teeth present	Serum vitamin C, WBC vitamin C
Thiamine (mg)	1.4	3.0	Beri-beri, cardiomyopathy, neuropathy, Wernicke-Korsakoff syndrome, fatigue, depression, encephalopathy	Transketolase activity
Riboflavin (mg)	1.6	3.6	Angular stomatitis, cheilosis, glossitis, nasolabial dermatitis, dry eyes, achlorhydria	Serum vitamin B_2
Niacin (mg)	18	40	Pellagra, dermatitis, diarrhea, dementia, glossitis, fissuring and swelling of tongue	NAD and NADP levels
Biotin (μg)	60	60	Dermatitis, alopecia, neuritis	Serum biotin
Pantothenic acid (mg)	5	15	Usually seen only with severe B complex deficiency	
Pyridoxine (mg)	2	4	Dermatitis, cheilosis, glossitis, anemia	
Folic acid (μg)	400	400	Megaloblastic, macrocytic anemia, glossitis	Serum and RBC folate
Cobalamin (μg)	3	5	Macrocytic anemia, neuropathy, dementia	Serum B_{12}
Vitamin A (IU)	1,000	3,300	Xerophthalmia, keratomalacia, night blindness	Serum vitamin A
Vitamin D (μg)	10	5	Rickets, osteomalacia, bone pain	Serum 25(OH) vitamin D
Vitamin E (mg)	8–10	10–15	Cardiomyopathy, hemolysis, megaloblastic anemia, edema, skin lesions	Serum vitamin E
Vitamin K (μg)	70–140	200	Clotting abnormalities	Prothrombin time

TIBC = total iron-binding capacity; NAD = nicotinamide-adenine dinucleotide; NADP = NAD phosphate.

Table 8 Monitoring Patients Receiving Nutritional Support

Assessment Parameter	Frequency
Clinical Well-being	
Vital signs	
Body weight	Daily
Fluid and nutrient intake	
Laboratory Data	
Urine glucose	Four times daily first 24 hr then daily
Blood glucose by capillary stick	
Serum glucose, Na, K, Cl, HCO₃, BUN	Daily until stable then twice weekly
Serum albumin, liver function tests, serum Ca, P, Mg, creatinine	Baseline then weekly
Hematology Data	
Hemoglobin, hematocrit, WBC + differential, prothrombin time, partial thromboplastin time	Baseline then weekly
Folate + vitamin B₁₂, Fe + transferrin	As indicated
Micronutrient assays	
Serum lipids	
Nitrogen balance	

Table 9 Catheter-Related Complications

Complication	Management
Thrombosis	*Urokinase lock*: 5,000 units urokinase dissolved in 2 ml saline, instilled into catheter, left in situ for 30–60 min, then withdrawn; if unsuccessful, may attempt urokinase infusion, 40,000 units/hr for 6 hr
	Streptokinase lock: 5,000 units/ml instilled to fill internal volume of catheter, dwell time 30 min then withdrawn
	Tissue plasminogen activator: used on an investigational basis in urokinase failures, 2 mg/2 ml with a 4 hr dwell time
Infection	*Antibiotic lock technique*: Limited studies have reported the efficacy of treating cather-related sepsis with a high concentration of an appropriate antibiotic, e.g., amikacin, 1.5 mg/ml; minocycline, 0.2 mg/ml; vancomycin, 1–5 mg/ml, left in situ for 12 hr
Occlusion	*With lipid*: Limited experience in clearing lipid-occluded catheters with 3 ml 70% ethanol, dwell time 1 hr
	With drugs/electrolytes: Where alteration of pH will improve the occluding agent's solubility, 1 ml 0.1 N hydrochloric acid or 8.4% sodium bicarbonate may be instilled, dwell time 1 hr

reducing the incidence of catheter-related sepsis, decreasing wastage of solutions, and encouraging EN rather than PN, whenever feasible.

INDICATIONS AND CONTRAINDICATIONS IN SPECIFIC CLINICAL CONDITIONS

Since SNS is an expensive therapy, particularly when administered parenterally, it is important to know where clinical benefit is likely to occur. In the following sections, various clinical conditions are reviewed and the important issues highlighted. Contraindications to EN are listed in Table 3 in the next (surgical nutrition) chapter.

Perioperative Nutrition

Clinical Issues:

1. What are the risks and benefits of pre- and/or postoperative nutrition, particularly in terms of morbidity and mortality?
2. What is the most effective route of nutrient administration?

A large cooperative Veterans Administration study and a meta-analysis of 18 smaller studies showed that preoperative nutrition is of benefit in severely malnourished patients only. Patients with mild to moderate malnutrition in the nutritionally supported treatment group showed no clear benefit and a greater incidence of complications than the control patients.

The duration of preoperative support has also been investigated in several PRCTs. Two to 3 days of IV

nutrition before surgery does not influence surgical outcome, and 5 to 7 days produces equivocal results, but in several studies 7 to 10 days of preoperative PN resulted in a significant reduction in postoperative complications and mortality in severely malnourished patients.

Postoperative SNS administered parenterally or enterally in critically ill patients has been demonstrated in PRCTs to reduce mortality, infectious complications, and length of ICU stay. A number of studies have indicated that early enteral feeding via a jejunostomy within the first 24 to 48 hours, even with small amounts, prevents bacterial translocation and reduces proinflammatory cytokine responses. These studies showed that jejunal feeding is tolerated even though the patient frequently has gastric atony and colonic ileus.

Inflammatory Bowel Disease*

Clinical Issues:

1. Does SNS have a primary role in treating inflammatory bowel disease (IBD) or is the role simply one of correcting secondary complications of malnutrition?
2. Does the route of administration make a difference?

IBD, particularly Crohn's disease, is often associated with severe hypoalbuminemia and weight loss.

---

*Editor's Note: A subsequent chapter on enteral feeding in Crohn's disease provides detailed information. The surgical chapter that follows also discusses IBD.

Anemia and vitamin and mineral deficiencies are also common.

Some new data suggest a possible role for a modified oral diet in the maintenance of disease remission. Several studies have compared steroid therapy with elemental diets and have found that steroids are somewhat more effective in inducing and maintaining a remission in Crohn's disease. However, in some clinical situations, particularly with children or in preoperative build-up, avoidance of steroids is preferred, and elemental diets may be more appropriate therapy, even though these usually involve a nasogastric tube.

Recent studies found no difference between elemental and polymeric diets. Several small studies have demonstrated no substantial benefit from the parenteral route. We interpret these data as tending to refute the hypothesis of food acting as an allergen in the pathogenesis of IBD. In fact, "bowel rest" is essentially bowel starvation, and depriving the gut of all substrates may be detrimental.

The possible value of soluble fiber in sustaining colonic short-chain fatty acid levels, the preferred fuel of the colonocyte; the role of glutamine as the preferred fuel for the enterocyte; and the anti-inflammatory role of omega-3 fatty acids, nucleotides, and arginine are all under investigation.

Pancreatitis

Clinical Issues:

1. Can the gut be used without exacerbating the pancreatitis?
2. Should SNS be a routine part of management?
3. Are there any contraindications to the use of IV fat as a calorie source?

Pancreatic secretion is stimulated by IV feeding and enteral nutrients that are delivered proximal to the ligament of Treitz. J-tube feeding appears to be well tolerated in up to 80 percent of patients with acute pancreatitis.

PN does not alter medical outcome in mild to moderate pancreatitis. In severe pancreatitis, malnutrition is associated with a poorer outcome, and hence SNS is probably justified.

In the absence of hyperlipidemia and impaired triglyceride clearance or thrombocytopenia, IV lipids can be administered without exacerbating pancreatitis, and provide a useful calorie source in a patient who may have impaired insulin secretion. Careful monitoring of acid-base balance is essential in patients with pancreatic fistulas or surgical drains, owing to loss of large amounts of bicarbonate in the pancreatic fluid.

Liver Disease

Clinical Issues:

1. Is there a role for BCAA-enriched formulas?

2. What are the constraints for SNS in a patient with acute or chronic liver dysfunction?

Malnutrition is common with advanced liver disease. Adequate protein intake may be constrained by the development of portal encephalopathy. Several studies have shown benefit from branched-chain (leucine, isoleucine, and valine) amino acid–enriched solutions in patients who cannot tolerate enough protein to achieve nitrogen balance. The rationale behind BCAA therapy is that patients with liver impairment have increased muscle breakdown for gluconeogenesis and reduced muscle and plasma BCAA levels, with a relative increase in aromatic amino acid (AAA) levels. This imbalance favors the transport of tryptophan, an aromatic amino acid, across the blood-brain barrier, leading to an increase in brain serotonin, which is a tryptophan breakdown product and a central nervous system (CNS) depressant. Since BCAA-enriched formulas are very expensive, they should be reserved for patients who cannot tolerate adequate protein intake (0.5 to 0.8 g per kilogram per day) without developing encephalopathy. These are only occasional liver failure patients.

In less severe liver disease, the protein intake should ideally be between 0.8 and 1 g per kilogram per day. The aim should be to meet the caloric requirement while keeping the serum glucose below 200 mg per deciliter. Fat emulsions must be used cautiously because of decreased lipid clearance. Sufficient fat must be provided to meet essential fatty acid requirements (5 percent of daily calories or 200 ml of 20 percent lipid emulsion twice weekly). A recent randomized study of alcoholic cirrhotic patients showed that the provision of a modest daily enteral oral supplement, on an outpatient basis, significantly reduced morbidity and hospitalization rates. This benefit appeared to relate primarily to a decrease in the incidence of infection.

Limited data suggest that aggressive post–liver transplant nutrition (1.5 g per kilogram per day of protein and 35 kcal per kilogram per day) is beneficial. Since many candidates for transplantation are malnourished, preoperative build-up is desirable. The ratio of plasma BCAA to AAA appears to be predictive of graft survival. To date, the benefit of post-transplant BCAA infusions has not been fully investigated. Infusion of BCAA increases the BCAA:AAA ratio, as would be expected, but no differences in outcome or encephalopathy have been demonstrated.*

Alterations in Liver Function Tests in Patients on Parenteral Nutrition

The incidence of abnormal liver function test results (raised alkaline phosphatase and transaminase levels) is reported to be 25 to 100 percent in patients on PN. Peak levels usually occur within 1 to 4 weeks of starting PN and then remain stable or decline despite continued therapy. A raised bilirubin level is less frequent (0 to 46

***Editor's Note:** There are three chapters on liver transplantation in this edition.

percent). Histologically, steatosis is more common in adults and cholestasis in children. Periportal fibrosis advancing to cirrhosis is a rare but serious complication of long-term PN that occurs more often in infants than in adults. Many etiologic factors have been proposed, including excessive administration of dextrose; lithocholic acid toxicity after bacterial overgrowth; bacterial translocation; and inadequate provision of sulfur-containing amino acids, to sustain normal levels, and of cytoplasmic antioxidants such as selenium and vitamin E. The presence of sodium bisulfite in the PN solutions may be an oxidant stress. Methods of reducing liver abnormalities have included the avoidance of overfeeding by accurate estimation of requirements, cyclic feeding with periods off the PN each 24 hours, maintenance of some enteral intake whenever possible to stimulate bile flow, and the use of oral antibiotics to reduce bacterial overgrowth.

Renal Disease

Clinical Issues:

1. Does SNS improve the outcome in acute renal failure (ARF)?
2. What is the role of essential amino acid solutions?
3. What is the role of SNS in the support of malnourished dialysis patients?
4. What is the place in therapy of novel methods of nutrient delivery during dialysis?

Acute Renal Failure

ARF in patients with major trauma is associated with a high mortality rate. Many of these patients have multiorgan failure that makes SNS very complex in terms of fluid and electrolyte monitoring. Early studies demonstrated an improved outcome in patients who received PN that supplied both essential amino acids and dextrose, compared with dextrose-only solutions. As a consequence, expensive specialized renal support solutions, rich in essential amino acids or their keto analogs, have been advocated. More recent randomized studies have shown no greater benefit of these special amino acid formulas compared with more standard amino acid solutions. In general, patients with ARF who are not on

dialysis require a reduced fluid and protein intake (0.5 to 0.6 g per kilogram per day of protein) with normal calorie requirements and generous micronutrients except for vitamin A, which accumulates.

Chronic Renal Failure Patients on Dialysis

A summary of nutritional requirements associated with different methods of dialysis is presented in Table 10.

Intradialytic Parenteral Nutrition (IDPN). IDPN is usually administered in the last 90 minutes of the hemodialysis treatment period. Limited data are available from a few studies that evaluated intradialytic infusion of calories, essential amino acids, and histidine along with a high protein–high calorie oral intake. These studies have shown improved appetite, serum protein levels, and body weight in malnourished patients. Problems may be experienced with postinfusion hypoglycemia when PN is abruptly halted at the end of dialysis. Glucose administration should not exceed the known maximal oxidation rate of 1.2 g per kilogram per dialysis treatment. Replacing some of the calories with lipid may limit glycemic problems, but hypertriglyceridemia should be avoided. Patients with end-stage renal disease have around 75 percent of normal lipid clearance. Lipid infusions should not be administered at more than 1 g per kilogram per hour and should be withheld if serum triglycerides are more than 300 mg per deciliter before dialysis. There are no studies comparing IDPN with improved enteral intake alone as might be achieved by cycled tube EN.

Peritoneal Dialysis. Amino acids are a good osmotic agent providing twice the osmotic load of glucose. The benefits of using some amino acids rather than just glucose in the peritoneal dialysis solution are the reduction in glucose load, reduced hypertriglyceridemia, and decreased protein loss with normalization of serum amino acids. Standard continuous ambulatory peritoneal dialysis (CAPD) solutions contain either a high glucose (4.25 percent, 486 mOsm) or a low glucose (1.5 percent, 347 mOsm) concentration. Amino acid CAPD solutions are glucose free and contain high amino acids (2.5 percent, 460 mOsm) or low amino acids (1.0 percent, 364 mOsm) with standard electrolyte concentrations. Acidosis may occur, possibly because of free

Table 10 Nutritional Requirements of Dialysis Patients

Type of Dialysis	Calorie Requirements	Protein Requirements	Comments
Hemodialysis	Intake and loss from hemodialysis fluid minimal	1–1.2 g/kg/day	Water-soluble vitamins lost in dialysate; iron required with erythropoietin; micronutrients (e.g., copper and zinc) lost in dialysate
Peritoneal	Patients absorb 60%–80% of dialysate glucose, average 8 kcal/kg/day	1.2–1.5 g/kg/day	Increased protein loss in peritonitis, water-soluble micronutrients lost in peritoneal dialysis fluid
Hemofiltration	Limited data available; 43% of infused glucose retained	Estimated losses around 11 g/day	

sulfur from methionine in the amino acid solutions. Small studies have used one amino acid exchange followed by three glucose exchanges per day, or alternating amino acid and glucose solutions. The peritoneal use of solutions containing lipid has so far been evaluated only in animal studies.

Lung Disease

Clinical Issues:

1. Is an increased REE associated with lung disease?
2. What is the optimal fuel source in patients with severe lung disease?

Patients with severe lung disease have a 15 to 20 percent increase in energy expenditure owing to the increased work of breathing. If this increased expenditure is not taken into account, patients with chronic lung disease gradually lose weight. Loss of any excess weight may be desirable, but if the weight loss impairs the respiratory muscle strength, ciliary clearance function, and immunocompetence, the patient is at greater risk for acute exacerbations. In patients who are being weaned off a ventilator, glucose should be given at no more than 5 mg per kilogram per minute and lipid at no more than 1 to 1.5 g per kilogram per 24 hours. The provision of excessive carbohydrate calories increases carbon dioxide production both by increasing metabolic rate and by stimulating lipogenesis. This may lead to worsening of the respiratory status. Lipids should not provide more than 40 percent of the nonprotein calories and should be discontinued if serum triglyceride levels are higher than 250 mg per liter. Controversy exists over the use of lipids with regard to impaired lung diffusion due to coating of red blood cells, deposition in the alveolar wall, and increased blood viscosity. The effect of lipids on the inflammatory response appears to be dose and rate related. Slow infusions (for more than 10 hours) are predominantly vasodilatory; fast infusions (for less than 5 hours) exhibit vasopressor and proinflammatory changes. Protein intake should be between 1.2 and 1.5 g per kilogram per day. A protein meal is known to enhance the ventilatory response to carbon dioxide. Electrolytes should be monitored closely, particularly potassium, phosphorus, calcium, and magnesium, as deficiency adversely affects respiratory muscle function.

Chronic pulmonary disease patients who are less than 90 percent of their ideal body weight demonstrate a greater 5 year mortality, independent of their pulmonary status. Since these patients have been shown to be hypermetabolic, the recommended calorie intake is 1.7 times the REE. Short-term studies over 3 months have demonstrated improved respiratory muscle function with improved nutritional intake.

Patients with cystic fibrosis (CF) are often undernourished because of malabsorption, anorexia, and increased expenditure (30 percent greater than normal) caused by the work of breathing and repeated infections.

Although prognosis is most related to the patient's pulmonary function, nutritional status is also important. Data from studies in children and adolescents suggest improvement in pulmonary function in the very young and stabilization of lung disease in older children, with better nutritional status achieved by using tube EN delivered through a gastrostomy. The psychological consequences of this aggressive approach have not been properly assessed. Also, most CF patients have reduced GI motility and are at risk for gastroesophageal reflux and aspiration. This should be assessed before a gastrostomy is inserted, since an antireflux procedure may also be needed.

Cancer

Clinical Issues:

1. Does SNS improve the outcome in cachectic cancer patients?
2. Does SNS in cancer patients increase lean body mass?
3. Does SNS improve patients' tolerance of cancer therapy?

One of the most striking forms of malnutrition is that seen in cancer cachexia. Most PRCTs designed to evaluate the risk-benefit ratio of SNS are too small to avoid a type II error, in which an important benefit is missed. From the limited data available, there appears to be no place for routine use of PN in patients with cancer. In fact there is a fourfold increase in the incidence of infection in cancer patients who receive PN, and a meta-analysis of available studies failed to demonstrate any clinical benefit in terms of survival, treatment tolerance, or tumor response. Despite this seeming lack of benefit, SNS may be justified for a finite period if normal intake is totally inadequate, such as during aggressive chemotherapy or in the severely malnourished cancer patient undergoing surgery.

Well-nourished bone marrow transplant recipients receiving prophylactic SNS before and during transplantation were shown to have significantly better late survival. EN appears to be as effective as PN where it is tolerated.

Human Immunodeficiency Virus–Positive Patients

Clinical Issues:

1. Does SNS early in the disease delay progression to symptomatic illness?
2. Does SNS late in the disease process alter survival or improve the quality of life?

The answers to these important clinical questions are not yet known. It is clear that from the moment of infection the virus is constantly replicating and that the immune status of the patient influences the disease-free interval. Thus, children who contracted human immu-

Table 11 Summary of Outcome on Home Parenteral and Enteral Nutrition

Diagnosis	No. of Pts	Average Age (yr)	Mortality* Rate on Rx	Time on Rx (% on >1 yr)	Comps per yr† Rx rel.	Dx rel.	Rehabilitation‡ C	P	M	Comments
Home Parenteral Nutrition										
Crohn's disease	480	35	5% p.a.	25	0.9	1.1	70	27	3	Usually justified
Ischemic bowel disease	274	60	10% p.a.	52	1.3	1.0	50	40	10	Usually justified
Motility disorder	264	45	10% p.a.	50	1.2	1.0	50	40	10	Usually justified
Radiation enteritis	123	57	15% p.a.	48	0.7	1.0	40	50	10	Usually justified
Congenital bowel defect	127	4	6% p.a.	44	2.0	1.0	65	25	10	Usually justified
Chronic adhesive obstructions	94	52	15% p.a.	40	1.5	1.3	30	65	5	Usually justified
Hyperemesis gravidarum	85	27	0% p.a.	Aver. dur. 8wk (2-30)	1.5	3.5	69	13	1	Usually justified
Cystic fibrosis	46	16	50% p.a.	50	0.8	3.7	20	60	20	Occasionally justified
Chronic pancreatitis	102	37	10% p.a.	20	1.2	2.5	60	30	10	Occasionally justified
AIDS	200	30	50% in 6 mo 20% survival rate >1 yr	5	1.4	3.2	6	64	30	Occasionally justified
Active cancer	1672	42	50% in 6 mo 25% survival rate > 1 yr	7	1.0	4.0	30	65	15	Justified in patients with treatable disease (e.g., in bone marrow transplant patients) or if the cancer is indolent; rarely justified in nontreatable metastatic bowel obstruction
Home Enteral Nutrition										
Active cancer	1296	60	50% in 6/12 30% SR >1 yr	5	0.4	2.8	20	60	20	Justified in patients with treatable disease or an obstructing cancer that can be bypassed by a feeding tube
Neurologic disorders of swallowing	918	65	40% first yr then levels off	30	0.3	1.0	10	20	70	Usually justified

*The cause of death in >95% of patients is the underlying illness or other causes unrelated to an HPEN complication.
†Refers only to those complications that result in rehospitalization.
‡Rehabilitation is designated as Complete (C), Partial (P), or Minimal (M), in relation to the patient's ability to sustain normal age-related activity. "Complete" means normal functioning; "partial" implies some limitation of activity; "minimal" indicates barely ambulatory or bedridden.
Data derived from North American HPEN Registry, 1985–1991.
Reproduced with permission from Oley Foundation, Albany, NY.

Table 12   Indications for Home Parenteral and
Enteral Nutrition

Home Parenteral Nutrition (HPN) is an appropriate therapy if the
patient meets all the following criteria:
1. The patient has severe bowel dysfunction that is expected to
   persist for a long time
2. The patient cannot be maintained by oral feeding or tube enteral
   nutrition alone
3. The therapy will restore, or sustain the patient at, a normal
   nutritional status
4. The therapy will restore, or sustain the patient at, a partial or
   complete level of rehabilitation
5. The patient has sufficient home support to manage HPN therapy
   comfortably and without undue hazard

Home Tube Enteral Nutrition (HEN) is an appropriate therapy if
the patient meets all the following conditions:
1. The patient cannot be maintained through dietary adjustment or
   oral supplements alone
2. The patient has severe bowel dysfunction that is expected to
   persist for a long time
3. The patient can experience sufficient nutritional benefit and
   rehabilitation so that the undertaking makes sense to the patient
   and family
4. The patient is medically stable and has sufficient home support
   to be managed on HEN therapy comfortably and without due
   hazard

nodeficiency virus (HIV) from Factor VIII have a longer disease-free interval than drug addicts, who are immunologically stressed by other diseases such as hepatitis. Nutritional status has a major influence on immune function. AIDS patients with HIV GI disease or an opportunistic GI infection often have fat and bile acid malabsorption, lactase deficiency, increased zinc and protein losses, and (in the presence of terminal ileal disease) vitamin B_{12} deficiency. General recommendations are that when nutritional intake meets more than two-thirds of the needs, only counseling is appropriate. If less than two-thirds of the required intake is being met, SNS may be indicated, preferably by the enteral route. There is no evidence that sterile supplements or elemental feeds are especially beneficial. Currently, data showing benefit from nutritional intervention are very limited, and large multicenter studies are needed to ensure best use of the available health care resources.

HOME PARENTERAL AND ENTERAL NUTRITION (HPEN)

A few patients require long-term SNS, which can be administered at home. Table 11 summarizes outcome data for 12 HPEN-treated disorders, and Table 12 presents the currently accepted indications for HPEN. Since HEN is about one-tenth the cost of HPN, it is the most desirable route where feasible. HPN complications result in an average rehospitalization rate of once a year, half of these admissions being due to suspected or confirmed sepsis. With greater HPN experience over the past 20 years, metabolic complications have decreased, particularly for patients managed by nutrition specialists from large teaching centers. Important issues currently facing long-term HPN patients are thrombosis of PN catheters, metabolic bone disorders, liver disease, and micronutrient deficiencies.

Psychosocial Issues

Patients requiring HPEN report feelings of anger and frustration, as well as altered body image. It is important to consider the impact of SNS on the quality as well as the quantity of life. Patients describe feelings of being unsupported in their home environment, particularly after the first 6 to 12 months when the assumption is often made that they are coping well. Support groups coordinated by the Oley Foundation offer a valuable contact point and reference source for HPEN patients, the parents of children requiring HPEN, and their physicians. In addition, self-help groups and support associations exist for specific disease states (e.g., CF, IBD, and pseudo-obstruction). These groups may have both local and national contact points.

SUGGESTED READING

De Meo MT, Van de Graaff W, Gottlieb K, et al. Nutrition in acute pulmonary disease. Nutr Rev 1992; 50:320–328.

Hill GL. Body composition research: implications for the practice of Clinical Nutrition. JPEN 1992; 16:197–218.

Lipman TO. Clinical trials of nutrition support in cancer. Hematol Oncol Clin North Am 1991; 5:91–102.

Quigley EMM, Marsh MN, Shaffer JL, Martin RS. Hepatobiliary complications of TPN. Gastroenterology 1993; 104:286–301.

White BJ, Madara EJ. The self help source book. 4th ed. Denville NJ: American Self-Help Clearinghouse, St Clare's Riverside Medical Center, 1991.

Wolfson M. Use of nutritional supplements in dialysis patients. Semin Dialysis 1992; 5:285–290.

Wolk R. Intraperitoneal nutrition. Hosp Pharm 1992; 27:893–905.

PRE- AND POSTOPERATIVE NUTRITIONAL SUPPORT

GREGORY M. TIAO, M.D.
JOSEF E. FISCHER, M.D.

The history of nutritional support dates as far back as nutrient enemas performed by ancient Egyptians. However, intravenous (IV) supplementation of high-calorie and protein nutrient mixtures has been practiced only over the past 25 years. While the initial research and clinical enthusiasm concentrated on parenteral nutrition, attention within the past decade has focused on the gut. What follows applies to either modality. Although the gut should be used preferentially, the nutritional needs of many patients will be met only by total parenteral nutrition (TPN), either alone or complementing enteral feedings.*

In the surgical setting, nutritional supplementation is often initiated as an attempt to decrease operative risk. We believe that the significance of nutritional support to operative procedures is of the same magnitude as antibiotics, fluid and blood transfusions, and critical care monitoring and allows us to perform more extensive procedures on sicker patients with expectations of better outcome.

NUTRITIONAL ASSESSMENT: IDENTIFYING THE PATIENT AT RISK

Nutritional assessment, a clinical term, attempts to estimate changes in body nutritional composition in order to predict the risk of a given treatment for a particular patient. Nutritional status is currently assessed by thorough history and physical examination, anthropometry, biochemical evaluation, immunocompetence, and functional capacity.

A history of recent weight loss, anorexia, or a disease process that interferes with oral intake should alert the clinician to the possibility of malnutrition. A physical examination that demonstrates muscle wasting, loose skin, and the edema of hypoproteinemia is confirmatory. Several studies have demonstrated that experienced clinicians can identify malnourished patients as accurately as multiple complex tests.

Anthropometry, i.e., structural measurements such as midarm muscle circumference and triceps skinfold thickness, is inaccurate and has very low sensitivity in predicting complications. In addition, biochemical abnormalities due to malnutrition are manifest long before demonstrable anthropometric changes occur.

Biochemical evaluation has focused on plasma protein concentrations, most notably albumin; low serum albumin correlates with rates of mortality and/or complications. More recent studies focusing on hepatic synthesis of short-turnover proteins such as transferrin, retinol binding protein, and prealbumin may be even more accurate, as these proteins with shorter half-lives measure smaller and more recent changes as compared with albumin.

Immunocompetence can be assessed by delayed cutaneous hypersensitivity or anergy. During the initial years of nutritional assessment, this was a widely used method, but unless these antigens are *injected,* they are without value for measuring operative risk. In studies by Christou and Tellado, anergy to cutaneous recall antigens was associated with high mortality and morbidity. This is associated, but not coincident, with severe malnutrition; moreover, as Christou emphasized, the defect is immunologic and not nutritional.

Functional capacity is a global measure of an individual's capacity for work and muscle endurance, with dysfunction classified in terms of duration and type. The type of dysfunction is categorized into working suboptimally, ambulatory, and bedridden. Hand dynamometry is a study of muscle function in which muscle strength is evaluated by either grip strength or as force-frequency characteristics and rate of recovery from fatigue after electrical stimulation of the ulnar nerve. Both functional capacity and hand dynamometry may reflect a functional counterpart of severe protein-calorie malnutrition.

The ultimate goal of nutritional assessment is to determine which specific patient is at risk for complications. Although the methods discussed above have shown statistical correlation, all can be nonspecifically affected by disease and other factors. As a result, clinical judgment is critical to the decision process. We believe, when all the studies are evaluated, that the patient at risk can be recognized in the following manner.

1. Recent (over 3 to 4 months) weight loss of more than 15 percent body weight, and/or body weight of less than 80 to 85 percent ideal body weight.
2. Serum albumin in a stable hydrated patient of less than 3.0 g per deciliter.

These two simple parameters will probably define the population at risk. Additional corroborative information includes

3. Anergy to injected skin recall antigens by the technique of Christou and Tellado.
4. True transferrin of less than 200 mg per deciliter.
5. A history of functional impairment (after Windsor and Hill).
6. Significant deficits in hand dynamometry.

INDICATIONS FOR NUTRITIONAL SUPPORT

In deciding whether a patient requires nutritional support in the preoperative period, the following factors

---

***Editor's Note:** This chapter supplements and complements the preceding chapter, *Parenteral and Enteral Nutrition.*

should be taken into consideration: (1) the premorbid state (healthy or otherwise), especially the nutritional status; (2) the age of the patient; (3) the duration of starvation; (4) the degree of anticipated insult; (5) the likelihood of resuming normal intake soon; (6) weight loss of 15 percent; (7) a serum albumin level less than 3.0 g per deciliter. Supporting values include transferrin of less than 200 mg per deciliter and anergy. These criteria indicate the type of patient in whom septic complications are likely to develop, and once developed may more often end in death, as compared with recovery from treatment in normal patients.

The indications and criteria listed above also apply to patients in the postoperative period. In a routine postoperative hospital course after intra-abdominal surgery, most patients can tolerate a 5 to 7 day fast without difficulty. If the hospital course is complicated and prevents nutritional intake beyond this time frame, nutritional intervention should be considered. The details of controlled trials of pre- and postoperative nutritional supplementation are given in the preceding chapter.

Specific situations in which nutritional intervention should be strongly considered and undertaken include the following.

Gastrointestinal-Cutaneous Fistulas. Patients with this type of fistula represent the classic indication for TPN. Gut failure is obvious and oral intake may increase fistula output. TPN increases spontaneous closure of fistula, and if spontaneous closure does not occur, the patient is better prepared for surgery. More recently, greater emphasis has been placed on the use of the gut. To do so effectively requires at least 4 feet of gut in continuity and access to it. Enteral nutrition here may not achieve targeted nutritional requirements and may require further supplementation with TPN.

Renal Failure. In patients whose need for dialysis is uncertain or those in nonoliguric renal failure, TPN containing essential amino acids and hypertonic dextrose is most useful. Dialysis may be delayed as hyperkalemia and accumulation of blood urea nitrogen are decreased by the dextrose and essential amino acid solution. Excessive fluid administration is limited by use of the hypertonic dextrose, which also minimizes free water produced internally by catabolism. Once dialysis is well established, some authors advocate use of a more complete solution, but the relative merits of a more complete solution as opposed to a solution limited to essential amino acids alone is not clear. Details on nutrition supplementation in renal failure are given in the preceding chapter and in Table 10 of that chapter.

Short Bowel Syndrome. There has been little alternative to long-term TPN in this syndrome. It is now common for these patients who otherwise would almost certainly have died to survive for more than 10 years on home TPN. Some of these patients exhibit sufficient hypertrophy of remaining small bowel to obviate or decrease the need for TPN, especially when combined with careful oral supplementation. Small bowel transplantation, as discussed in a separate chapter, may be

indicated for those who cannot be maintained on long-term home TPN. This option is also considered in the chapter *Short Bowel Syndrome.*

Hepatic Failure. Improved survival is also seen in patients with hepatic failure given aggressive TPN. Patients with liver disease are often malnourished secondary to excessive alcohol intake and decreased food intake. We use an amino acid solution enriched in branched-chain amino acids and deficient in aromatic amino acids that will increase tolerance to administered protein, and in meta-analysis has been shown to promote arousal from hepatic encephalopathy. Details are provided in the preceding chapter.

Inflammatory Bowel Disease. In patients with Crohn's disease, TPN and bowel rest can be useful; however, such therapy has never been subjected to randomized clinical trial. A recent long-term study analyzing the results of parenteral nutrition for acute exacerbations of Crohn's disease has revealed that after 15 months, only 15 percent of the patients had avoided operation. Chemically defined diets also promote remission in Crohn's disease and may be used primarily or as a bridge to full oral intake after remission induced by TPN. Ulcerative colitis does not generally respond to short-term TPN, nor is long-term TPN indicated, since sphincter-saving operations produce a long-term cure. However, we find that TPN is useful in preparation for the Soave procedure. In-hospital TPN, usually for less than 2 weeks, in conjunction with antibiotics allows rectal mucosa to heal, thereby facilitating rectal mucosectomy.

Table 1 Indications for Nutritional Support

Primary therapy
  Efficacy shown*
    Gastrointestinal-cutaneous fistulas
    Renal failure (acute tubular necrosis)
    Short bowel syndrome
    Acute burns
    Hepatic failure (acute decompensation superimposed on
      cirrhosis)
  Efficacy not shown
    Crohn's disease
    Anorexia nervosa

Supportive therapy
  Efficacy shown*
    Acute radiation enteritis
    Acute chemotherapy toxicity
    Prolonged ileus
    Weight loss preliminary to major operation
  Efficacy not shown
    Before cardiac surgery
    Prolonged respiratory support
    Large wound losses

Areas under intensive study
  Patients with cancer
  Patients with sepsis

*This indicates that randomized prospective trials or similar investigations have suggested that such nutritional intervention results in changed (improved) outcome.

Prolonged Ileus. Prolonged ileus after an abdominal procedure may necessitate a course of TPN until the ileus subsides.

Table 1 lists indications for which nutritional support has proved efficacious, either as primary therapy in which nutrition has been shown to influence the disease process, or supportive therapy in which adequate nutritional support has been reached but no change in the disease process has occurred. Cancer and sepsis are two areas in which the role of nutritional support is under intensive study.

Each clinician must determine the criteria relevant to a given patient. Older patients do not tolerate starvation as well as younger patients, and critically ill patients should receive supplementation more quickly than the less severely stressed.

NUTRITIONAL REQUIREMENTS

Protein

Of the three major food groups (protein, fats, and carbohydrates), protein is the most important, being the effector of all organic functions. The balance between protein synthesis and degradation is critical. Protein synthesis is energy requiring, whereas breakdown yields only one-fourth of the energy in energy-rich phosphate that synthesis requires; the remainder is expended as heat. Clearly, use of protein for energy is wasteful. Moreover, there is no body store for protein (for example, as glycogen is for carbohydrate); thus, every protein broken down for gluconeogenesis removes a functional protein.

One can approach protein requirements by assuming that after some 4 to 5 days on a calorically adequate, protein-free diet, nitrogen excretion is minimal and represents true requirements. Thus, for an adult on a calorically adequate, protein free diet, there is daily loss of 37 mg nitrogen per kilogram in the urine, 12 mg per kilogram in feces, 5 mg per kilogram to the integumentary system, and 2 to 3 mg per kilogram to evaporation, making a total of 56 to 57 mg per kilogram per day or, in terms of whole protein, 0.34 g per kilogram per day. With various corrections and allowances for low-value biologic protein, the average normal requirement is 0.8 g of protein per kilogram per day or 56 to 60 g per day for a 70 kilogram adult. Stress increases the requirement to a maximum of 1.5-2.5 g per kilogram per day, with the lower figure probably being preferred.

Calories

Energy Requirements

The body can use three sources for energy: protein, carbohydrate, and fat. Amino acids contribute 15 percent of normal energy expenditure; the remaining 85 percent is derived from carbohydrate and fat, primarily from fat utilization. Caloric requirements can be estimated by indirect calorimetry (using oxygen consumption to determine caloric needs) or the Harris-Benedict equation given in the preceding chapter. The result of the Harris-Benedict equation is basal energy expenditure. This is multiplied by a stress factor that can be derived from Table 2 to yield resting energy expenditure (REE), which defines the caloric needs per 24 hours of an individual patient in a given state of stress.

In the past it was common for patients to receive 3,500 to 4,000 calories per day. This oversupplementation can result in excessive lipid deposition, carbon dioxide retention, immunosuppression, hepatic steatosis, and carbohydrate intolerance. "More" is not necessarily better. At present, mean caloric supplementation is closer to 1,800 to 2,000 calories per day; an increase to 2,500 calories per day, as required in stress states, is quite rare.

Each method of determining caloric needs requires some correction. One should add 15 percent to metabolic cart measurements for activity. For example, if a patient's caloric requirements were 1,500 calories based on either indirect calorimetry or the Harris-Benedict equation, we would supplement with an extra 225 calories to account for activity; thus, the patient would receive 1,775 calories per day.

Calorie-Nitrogen Ratio

The energy required for protein synthesis has been estimated as a ratio of 100 to 150:1 (i.e., 100 to 150 nonprotein calories per gram of nitrogen) in normal adult patients. This ratio changes with the disease state; in sepsis, a lower ratio is thought appropriate, whereas in uremia a ratio as high as 300 to 400:1 has been advocated. The key is to maintain adequate nitrogen amounts and to vary the caloric intake to maximize protein synthesis.

Carbohydrates

Glucose is the preferred carbohydrate source in traditional TPN and is the "gold standard" for protein sparing. A minimum of 400 calories per 24 hours, and up to 1,800 calories in the resting fasting state, minimizes protein breakdown. In addition, red blood cells must use glucose and white blood cells, and the central nervous system "prefers" glucose.

Fat

In normal resting starvation, fat provides the bulk of the body's calories. Lipolysis is encouraged by stress.

Table 2 Stress Factors in Injury and Infection

Clinical State	Stress Factor
Postoperative (uncomplicated)	1.1
Multiple fractures	1.1–1.3
Severe infection	1.3–1.6
>20% third-degree burn	1.5–2.1

Also, when fat emulsions are given to supply 4 percent of caloric needs, essential fatty acid requirements are met. Optimal visceral protein synthesis results when 20 to 25 percent of the nonprotein calories is administered as fat emulsion.

Vitamins and Trace Elements

Vitamins and trace elements should be supplemented when giving parenteral nutrition. Most authorities advocate two to five times the requirement for water-soluble vitamins (no toxicity) and minimal daily requirements for fat-soluble vitamins (see Table 7 in preceding chapter).

Deficiencies in zinc, copper, magnesium, selenium, and chromium have been reported in patients on parenteral nutrition. Zinc is the element most frequently reported deficient and results in impaired wound healing, altered white blood cell function, skin lesions, and decreased taste acuity.

MECHANISM OF DELIVERY

Two routes are possible: the enteral route using either the stomach or small intestine, and the parenteral route. If the gastrointestinal (GI) tract can be used, the enteral route is preferred. Recent clinical and experimental evidence suggests that enteral nutrition is physiologically superior to parenteral nutrition. The reasons for this may include protection and improvement in hepatic function, in that it mimics the normal ingress of nutrients so that the liver can store, process, and release nutrients; and probable maintenance of gut mucosal integrity, particularly in burns and hemorrhagic shock. When mucosal integrity is not protected, an increase in bacterial translocation or their products may occur. The benefits of enteral feedings may be achieved when only a portion of needs is administered enterally, with the remainder given by the IV route. The most recent estimates suggest that as little as 20 percent of calories by the GI tract may be effective.

Enteral nutrition is not, however, necessarily "safer" than parenteral nutrition. Deaths with enteral nutrition are generally due to aspiration when gastric motility suddenly changes with sepsis. One death from aspiration is equivalent to the mortality rate over 2 to 3 years of a well-operated parenteral nutrition program, despite the danger of catheter sepsis (which in well-operated units should be less than 3 percent).

Enteral nutrition can be administered into either the stomach or the small intestine. From the standpoint of safety, but not physiology, it is safer to give diets in the small intestine either by passing a tube via the mouth, nostril, or gastrostomy into the duodenum, or by a small catheter jejunostomy. Patients should be infused constantly, with the bolus technique reserved for special situations. To prevent reflux and aspiration, patients should be maintained at a 30-degree angle, and gastric tube feedings should generally cease by 11 PM, when only

Table 3 Contraindications to Enteral Feeding

Inability to establish enteral access safely
Intestinal obstruction
High-output fistula
Ischemic bowel
Known intolerance to enteral feeding
  Malabsorption
  Acute exacerbation of inflammatory bowel disease
Bowel length <4 feet
Patient refusal

skeletal nursing shifts are present. Because there can be a rapid change in gastric or intestinal motility with the onset of sepsis, aspiration may result. Thus, it is often safer (though not necessarily more physiologic) to deliver diets into the small intestine. In initiating gastric feedings, osmolarity is first advanced and then volume. If administration is made into the small bowel, volume should be increased first and then osmolarity. Most patients do not tolerate small bowel administration of osmolar concentrations greater than 500 to 600 mOsm.

Tube feedings should be initiated at 20 to 40 ml per hour of near iso-osmolar feedings, and advanced 20 ml per hour per day to the targeted rate. Gastric residuals should be checked every 4 hours. If the residual is greater than 50 percent, feeding should be held. If, after 4 hours, less than half the original aspirate remains, tube feeds should be resumed at a rate 20 to 40 ml per hour less than the original rate. Enteric intolerance will be manifested with nausea, vomiting, crampy abdominal pain, and distention as well as large residuals.

In general, where possible, enteral nutrition is the preferred route of administration of nutritional support; however, enteral nutrition often is not possible in the surgical patient. Table 3 lists contraindications to enteral nutrition. In these patients, parenteral nutrition is the only alternative route. A central venous catheter dedicated to TPN will reduce the incidence of catheter-related sepsis. Safe TPN requires an organization of nurses, physicians, and pharmacists and an enforced protocol. For most patients, a 15 percent dextrose formula with 5 percent amino acids is appropriate, with 20 to 25 percent of nonprotein calories as a lipid emulsion. This standard formula is initiated at a rate of 40 ml per hour. Serial monitoring of electrolytes, blood urea nitrogen (BUN), and serum and urine glucose levels should be obtained, especially in critically ill patients. Once tolerance is achieved, TPN is increased at a rate of 20 ml per hour per day until the targeted caloric needs are met. When GI tract function improves, enteral nutrition should be instituted and TPN weaned at a rate of 20 ml per hour per day until 40 ml per hour is reached, at which time TPN can be stopped. Weaning at a faster rate may result in rebound hypoglycemia.

ADEQUACY OF SUPPORT

Once the decision has been made to give a patient nutritional support, he or she should be monitored to ensure the adequacy of support and to prevent metabolic complications. Weekly transferrin, prealbumin, and retinol binding protein measurements provide an objective evaluation of efficacy. Those who do not improve with initial treatment undergo bedside indirect calorimetry and 24 hour urinary nitrogen excretion studies. Critically ill patients are monitored more aggressively, with indirect calorimetry and nitrogen excretion studies used as a part of the initial evaluation. Once stability of parenteral nutrition is reached in patients who are not critically ill, routine monitoring including complete blood count, electrolytes, BUN, creatinine, liver function status, prothrombin time and partial thromboplastin time, calcium, magnesium, and phosphate can be obtained twice weekly.

COMPLICATIONS

Metabolic complications are common with parenteral supplementation and can also occur with enteral support. Strict monitoring of input and output, daily weights, serial serum and urine glucose, serial electrolytes, liver function tests, and plasma triglycerides will help avoid the more common metabolic abnormalities.

Enteral Complications

The most common enteral nutrition complications arise from improper placement of the feeding catheter, resulting in aspiration. Proper tube placement should be confirmed by radiography before any feeding catheter is used. Perforation is rare but can occur, especially when feeding tubes utilizing rigid stylets to aid in tube placement are used. Another very common complication of enteral feeding results from solute overload. Inappropriately rapid administration of hyperosmolar solutions results in diarrhea, dehydration, electrolyte imbalance, and hyperglycemia, as well as electrolyte loss in diarrhea, with hyperosmolar nonketotic coma the possible result. All these problems can be avoided if care is taken when administering support. Aspiration can be minimized if all tube positions are radiologically confirmed, the head-up position of 30 degrees is used, and there is judicious advancing of enteral formulas as described above. Dehydration can be prevented by carefully advancing osmolarity and (after excluding other causes of diarrhea) using Kaopectate and opiate-like medications to prevent excessive diarrhea.

Parenteral Complications

Parenteral complications may be grouped into three categories: technical, metabolic, and septic.

Technical Complications

These relate to catheter placement and include pneumothorax, arterial lacerations, hemothorax, mediastinal hematoma, brachial plexus injury, hydrothorax, thoracic duct injury, and air or catheter embolism. Indwelling catheters may also erode into adjacent structures. Subclavian thrombosis commonly occurs, and if sepsis complicates the thrombosis, may be the source of septic thrombi.

Metabolic Complications

Plasma electrolyte abnormalities and disorders in glucose metabolism are common and may be minimized by careful monitoring with appropriate supplementation. Essential fatty acid, vitamin, and trace metal deficiencies can be avoided by daily supplementation. Liver function derangements may occur in any patient regardless of TPN composition, and manifest with abnormalities in aspartate aminotransferase, alanine aminotransferase, gamma-glutamyl transferase, and alkaline phosphatase. Hepatic steatosis also can occur, most commonly from excessive glucose administration. The specific cause of this dysfunction is unclear. Elevated serum bilirubin rarely occurs as a metabolic complication and usually means sepsis. As discussed in the preceding chapter, liver failure, although uncommon, can occur with prolonged TPN.

Septic Complications

Catheter sepsis is potentially the most lethal complication in patients receiving TPN. Bacterial sepsis is directly related to catheter care and can be reduced to the current minimum of less than 1 percent by careful attention to detail and avoidance of multiuse catheters. Fungemia, a far more serious complication, is thought to result from *Candida* entry via the GI tract. Oral nystatin may prevent candidal colonization but is not universally effective.

SPECIAL FORMULATIONS

Enteral and parenteral nutrition formulas can be balanced and nutritionally complete, or can be tailored to a specific disease. Of the many tailored formulas, efficacy has been established in a few, the most widely accepted being those designed for patients with hepatic and renal failure.

Of patients with liver failure, an estimated 50 percent develop grade 2 or worse encephalopathy if attempts are made to provide adequate dietary protein; however, limiting protein can have serious metabolic implications. These patients will benefit from formulas high in branched-chain amino acids and low in aromatic amino acids. The electrolyte formulation is also altered for these patients in response to their electrolyte abnormalities as a result of liver failure.

Patients with renal failure but not yet on dialysis have poor tolerance of both protein and fluid loads. Thus, renal formulas provide small amounts of high biologic quality amino acids and high concentrations of dextrose to limit both protein and fluid infusion. Once the patients progress to dialysis, the restrictions defined above can be diminished.

COMMENTS

The field of nutritional support has evolved from an initial period of enthusiastic, uncritical acceptance to a more critical review with demands for efficacy. The definition of nutritional needs in specific disease states has now begun. Nutritional supplementation in some patients who are malnourished will improve their outcome after surgery. We, as clinicians, must appropriately choose those who may benefit from such intervention.

SUGGESTED READING

Buzby GP, et al (Veterans Affairs Total Parenteral Nutrition Cooperative Study Group). Perioperative total parenteral nutrition in surgical patients. N Engl J Med 1991; 325:525–532.

Christou NV, Tellado JM. In vitro polymorphonuclear neutrophil function in surgical patients does not correlate with anergy but with "activating" processes such as sepsis or trauma. Surgery 1989; 106:718.

Fischer JE, ed. Total parenteral nutrition. 2nd ed. Boston: Little, Brown, 1991.

Fischer JE. Metabolism in surgical patients. In: Sabiston DC, ed. Textbook of surgery. 14th ed. Philadelphia: WB Saunders, 1991:103.

Rombeau JL, Caldwell MD, eds. Enteral nutrition (Vol 1); Parenteral nutrition (Vol 2). Philadelphia: WB Saunders, 1990.

Windsor JA, Hill GL. Weight loss with physiologic impairment: a basic indicator of surgical risk. Ann Surg 1988; 207:290.

CROHN'S DISEASE: ENTERAL FEEDING

COLM O'MORAIN, Ph.D.
AIDEEN McGUINNESS, B.Sc.

There is as yet no definitive treatment for Crohns disease since its etiology remains unknown. However, diet has been implicated in both the development of the disease and its treatment. Nutritional support is often required in the course of the disease because of the associated prevalence of malnutrition, owing to a combination of malabsorption, reduced food intake, protein exudates into the gut, drug-nutrient interactions, and increased nutrient requirements.

ELEMENTAL DIET

An elemental diet provides all nutrients in their simplest forms: protein as amino acids, carbohydrate as glucose or maltodextrins, and fat as short-chain triglycerides. The use of an elemental diet to treat exacerbations of Crohn's disease has proved as effective as steroids, the standard treatment, in six controlled studies to date (Table 1).

In a controlled study by O'Morain and colleagues, 21 hospitalized patients with acute Crohn's disease were randomized to receive as sole treatment either an elemental diet (Vivonex) or prednisolone, 0.75 mg per kilogram of body weight for 4 weeks. Assessment at 4 weeks and again at 12 weeks showed that patients given the elemental diet improved as much as those on steroids

Table 1 Controlled Trials Comparing Elemental Diet with Steroids in the Treatment of Active Crohn's Disease

Study	No. of Patients	Duration (wk)	Outcome (%) Diet	Outcome (%) Steroids
O'Morain (1984)	21	4	81	80
Saverymuttu (1985)	32	1.5	94	100
Seidman (1989)	18	3	78	68
Sanderson (1987)	17	6	88	86
Hunt (1989)	29	4	100	100
Okada (1990)	20	6	> > >	

Steroid dosage is 0.5–0.75 mg/kg/day in each study.

by the defined criteria. At a follow-up examination 3 months later, those in the steroid group were taking 10 to 20 mg prednisolone daily, while those in the elemental diet group required no specific treatment. At 3 months, the serum albumin level, which is a reliable laboratory index of activity, was significantly higher in the elemental diet–treated group.

In Teahon and colleagues' long-term study of 113 patients treated with an elemental diet (Vivonex—96 orally, 17 via a nasogastric tube), 85 percent obtained clinical remission. Twenty-four of these had continued their previous maintenance dose of steroids, while 72 were treated with elemental diet alone. The chances of obtaining remission were not related to disease site, severity, or duration. Of the 17 patients defined as treatment failures, seven had been unable to tolerate the diet. In terms of long-term maintenance of remission in the same group of patients, there was a 22 percent relapse rate within 6 months, with a 38 percent probability of still being in remission at 3 years. Those with ileal disease only tended to fare better: no early relapse, with a 3 year remission rate of 54 percent. A further comparison of long-term outcome of diet versus steroid-induced remission showed no significant difference in the relapse rates between the two groups at 1, 3, and 5 years.

ELEMENTAL VERSUS POLYMERIC DIET

Elemental diets have been compared with polymeric diets and produced conflicting results in four recent controlled trials (Table 2). The results from three imply that elemental diet is equivalent to or preferable to polymeric diet. The patient numbers in the fourth study are quite small, and although the number of remissions are similar according to the modified simple index, only a few in each group had normal laboratory indices at that stage. It is also notable that in some of the patients with apparently active disease, no activity was demonstrable by indium-leukocyte scanning.

In a controlled trial of oligopeptide diet versus steroids plus sulfasalazine in 104 Crohn's disease patients, the drug treatment group fared significantly better in obtaining remission (78 percent versus 53 percent). However, the feed used, Peptisorb, has as its protein sources hydrolyzed lactalbumin, meat protein, and soybean, so it is possible that these may have a greater antigenicity than some other feeds. The analysis was made on an "intention-to-treat" basis and there was a significantly higher dropout owing to poor compliance with the feed.

Because of its characteristics, an elemental diet reduces pancreatic, biliary, and intestinal secretions; is non antigenic; and therefore may be more beneficial than a polymeric diet in active Crohn's disease.

TOTAL PARENTERAL NUTRITION

Total parenteral nutrition (TPN) has been used as a primary treatment in the hope of improving the patient's nutritional status and of alleviating the acute attack by resting the bowel. In a controlled randomized trial of 51 patients with active Crohn's disease, there was no significant difference in the number of remissions achieved after 21 days of treatment with TPN, polymeric enteral feed, or peripheral parenteral nutrition with oral diet (71, 58, and 60 percent, respectively). At 1 year, the probability of being in remission for each group was 42, 55, and 56 percent, respectively. The authors and an accompanying editorial concluded that bowel rest was not a major factor in achieving or maintaining remission. Considering the complications and extra expense that may be associated with TPN, it is now widely agreed that the enteral route of feeding is preferable in most groups of patients.

PRACTICAL USE OF AN ELEMENTAL DIET

The use of an elemental diet (Table 3) incorporates a team approach. The dietitian, nurse, and physician must all work closely and the patient must be fully cooperative. We use the elemental diet as our primary mode of treatment for exacerbations of Crohn's disease. In our experience, patients are often ill enough to require hospitalization, which allows complete supervision and guidance during the initiation of the diet. Patients who have used the diet in the past may be started on an outpatient basis, with an "open door" arrangement should problems occur, and weekly follow-up otherwise.

After treatment is fully discussed with the patient, the elemental feed (E028 Extra) is introduced as a chilled flavored drink in increasing osmolarity over 3 to 4 days. A few patients may experience some side effects as a result of the feed's high osmolarity, in which case the concentration is increased more gradually. We find the first few days the most difficult for patient compliance; as symptoms usually improve rapidly, patients are then more positive toward the treatment. Since palatability has been a problem with many feeds available, we find the use of a fine-bore nasogastric tube for feeding beneficial in some patients. However, recent developments in the manufacture of the elemental feed have

Table 2 Comparison of Recent Controlled Trials of Elemental versus Polymeric Diets in Active Crohn's Disease

	Giaffer (1990)	*Raouf (1991)*	*Rigaud (1991)*	*Park (1991)*
Design	Random	Random	Random (2 centers)	Random double-blind
Elemental feed	Vivonex	Elemental 028	Vivonex	Elemental 028
Polymeric feed	Fortison	Triosorbon	Nutrison Realmentyl	Enteral 400
Patient location	Inpatient then outpatient	Inpatient then outpatient	Inpatients (NG tube)	Inpatients (NG tube)
Duration	28 days	21 days	28–42 days	28 days
Concurrent medications	Withdrawn	Unchanged	Steroids, <20 mg/day	None
No. of Patients	30	24	30	14
Results				
Elemental	12/16	9/13	10/15	2/7
Polymeric	5/14	8/11	11/15	5/7

NG = nasogastric.

Table 3 Factors to Improve Compliance With Elemental Diet

Gradual introduction
Chilled feed
Nasoenteric feeding tube
Team approach

Table 4 Patients Suitable for Elemental Diet

Initial presentation of Crohn's disease
Exacerbations of Crohn's disease
Fistulas
Steroid dependency
Growth failure in children with Crohn's disease

vastly improved palatability, and as a result tolerance and compliance.

The elemental feed is increased to cover estimated protein requirements, and caloric intake is further supplemented to requirements with glucose polymers, minerals, and hard candies. Black tea or coffee and water are also permitted. All sources of dietary protein or fat are excluded.

Indices of disease activity, including erythrocyte sedimentation rate, C-reactive protein, serum albumin, hemoglobin, body weight, and anthropometric assessments are measured weekly to monitor progress. If clinically improved, patients are generally allowed home on the diet between days 4 and 7, with weekly follow-up. Those who show no improvement in clinical or laboratory assessment within 7 to 10 days may be assigned to alternative treatments as clinically indicated.

The ideal duration of treatment required for elemental diet has not yet been established. After 10 days the clinical symptoms have generally subsided, but intestinal inflammation may persist at this stage, and laboratory indices may not yet have returned to normal. We generally encourage patients to continue the diet for 3 to 4 weeks. They are then gradually reintroduced to a low-residue diet and can return within 2 to 3 weeks to a normal, well-balanced intake with nutritional supplements as appropriate. Extra caution is required with strictures. Some patients may continue to avoid particular foodstuffs that they find provoke symptoms. Although a procedure of staged food reintroduction with identification of specific food intolerances is advocated by some workers in England, we have tried this and not found it to carry any advantages.

Conditions in which an elemental diet is useful are listed in Table 4.

Fistulas

Elemental diets have proved particularly effective in the management of Crohn's fistulas since the elemental diet is absorbed in the proximal intestine, thus allowing the affected area to heal. However, the duration of treatment is generally longer for fistulas; we have successfully treated one such patient with elemental diet at home for 6 months.

Crohn's Disease in Childhood

Some centers in Canada have used intermittent elemental diet therapy to combat growth failure in children with Crohn's disease, and noted positive results.

In a controlled study of eight children with growth failure resultant from Crohn's disease who were treated for a period of 1 month every 4 months with elemental diet (Vivonex, nocturnally via a nasogastric tube, with flavored elemental feed during the daytime), lean body mass was significantly increased, while disease activity and steroid requirement decreased. Because of their adverse effects on growth, daily steroid use should be avoided in children if possible.

Steroid Dependency

The elemental diet has also proved beneficial in groups of patients who are steroid dependent. The elemental diet in these patients in our experience facilitates the tapering of steroid dosage. As a tertiary referral center, we also tend to see a proportion of patients who have previously used steroids but suffered side effects, and we are therefore keen to try alternative modes of treatment.

EFFECT OF AN ELEMENTAL DIET

How an elemental diet can be beneficial in Crohn's disease is as yet uncertain. Since its component nutrients are absorbed in the proximal intestine, it may have its effect by allowing a medical bypass of the diseased distal bowel; it has little residue, with reduced stimulation of motility or secretions.*

Nutritional Factors

As previously stated, malnutrition is often present with Crohn's disease, so nutritional therapy is indicated. Although the improvement in nutritional status is beneficial to the patient, this does not usually occur until after the clinical improvement has already taken place, so the elemental diet must therefore have a more fundamental effect.

Medical Bypass

The elemental diet is almost completely absorbed in the proximal intestine, leaving only endogenous matter to enter the remainder of the intestine. This bypass may

---

*Editor's Note: This is a key question: Why do elemental diets (and other alterations in luminal contents) result in such a rapid improvement? Dr. O'Morain's article and table in Gastroenterology Clinics in 1990 was excellent.

allow the diseased section of the gut to rest and inflammation to subside.

Flora Alterations

An elemental diet may benefit patients by inducing a positive change in bowel flora. We have not found any difference in amount or type of fecal flora before and after treatment with elemental diet, although this is a very inaccurate mode of assessment. In a controlled study, two groups of patients received TPN and steroids, with sulfasalazine and metronidazole where indicated. One group also randomly received whole-gut lavage with 18 L saline over 2 hours, followed by 4 g 5-aminosalicylic acid on two occasions in the first week. The lavage group were found to have a significantly more rapid fall in Crohn's disease activity and circulating endotoxin, plus a shorter duration of hospital stay. It is thus possible that an elemental diet may induce an improvement by a reduction in circulating endotoxin.

Mucosal Permeability

It may be that an abnormality of mucosal permeability in Crohn's disease allows microbial or dietary antigens access to the mucosa, resulting in the observed alteration in immune function, and possibly causing the chronic inflammation seen. In a study of intestinal permeability as assessed by polyethylene glycol 400 (PEG 400), chromium-labeled ethylenediaminetetraacetate (^{51}Cr EDTA), and lactulose-rhamnose, a significant increase in urinary excretion of these probes occurred in Crohn's disease patients, indicating increased permeation. Another study involving the use of an elemental diet as treatment showed a significant decrease in urinary excretion of EDTA and lactulose-rhamnose; the authors concluded that the elemental diet decreased intestinal permeability. Conflicting results have been reported in studies of the intestinal permeability of relatives of Crohn's patients depending on the probe used, reflecting the different permeation pathways used by each probe.

A reduction in protein exudation into the gut has also been reported after 8 days' treatment with elemental diet.

Amino Acids

The presence of amino acids rather than whole protein may confer a lower antigenicity on the elemental diet compared with polymeric feeds. Glutamine and arginine are two amino acids recently discovered to be essential in stressed states, instead of nonessential, as was previously assumed. Glutamine has been shown to be a major fuel of the small intestine, as well as having an effect on enterocyte function and the stimulation of trophic gut hormones. Steroids have been shown to stimulate the release of glutamine from muscle and to increase intestinal glutamine utilization. In stressed states, body stores of glutamine may be rapidly depleted. Arginine has proved to have beneficial effects on the immune system distinct from its nutritional benefits. As yet, these two novel substrates are not contained in commercial polymeric or parenteral nutritional products, whereas they are present in elemental feeds.

COMMENTS

Elemental diets are useful in inducing remission in active Crohn's disease and are free from the side effects noted with other treatments. More research is necessary to discover their mode of action and optimal duration of treatment, and to learn possible ways of maintaining long-term remission in Crohn's disease.

SUGGESTED READING

Giaffer MH, et al. Lancet 1990; 1:816–819.

Hunt JB, et al. Gastroenterology 1989; 96:A224.

Okada M, et al. Hepatogastroenterology 1990; 37:72–80.

O'Morain CA. Crohn's disease: treatment and pathogenesis. Boca Raton, FL: C.R.C. Press, 1987.

O'Morain CA, et al. Br Med J 1984; 288:1859–1860.

Park RHR, et al. Eur J Gastrol Hepatol 1991; 3:483.

Raouf AH, et al. Gut 1991; 32:702–707.

Rigaud D, et al. Gut 1991; 32:1492–1497.

Sanderson IR, et al. Arch Dis Child 1987; 61:123–127.

Saverymuttu S, et al. Gut 1985; 26:994–998.

Seidman EG, et al. Gastroenterol Clin North Am 1989; 17:124–155.

Teahon K, et al. Gut 1990; 31:1133–1137.

METABOLIC BONE DISEASE

BESS DAWSON-HUGHES, M.D.

Osteoporosis and osteomalacia occur with increased frequency in patients with a variety of gastrointestinal (GI) disorders. Metabolic bone disease may result from (1) nutritional deficiency of calcium and vitamin D; (2) failure of fat emulsification and digestion, seen in circumstances of pancreatic insufficiency or partial gastrectomy (inadequate gastric mixing); (3) decreased intestinal transit time from structural disease in the small bowel—intestinal bypass surgery, blind loops, fistulas, bacterial overgrowth, and so forth; or (4) altered vitamin D status caused by fat malabsorption. Thus, patients with a wide variety of GI disorders may have increased intake requirements of calcium and vitamin D. Adrenal corticosteroid therapy is also an important deleterious factor in many patients.

The symptoms of osteoporosis and early osteomalacia are limited to those associated with fractures (Table 1). With early osteomalacia, cortical bone loss predominates, whereas with osteoporosis, trabecular bone loss usually predominates. As vitamin D deficiency progresses, the classic picture of osteomalacia develops: bone pain and tenderness and muscle weakness. Biochemical features of osteoporosis and osteomalacia are given in Table 1.

The fat-soluble vitamin D is supplied by ultraviolet-stimulated production in skin and by absorption from the diet. Skin production is highly variable and depends not only on the extent and duration of skin exposure but also on the degree of skin pigmentation, sun-screen use, and latitude. For example, at a latitude of 42°N (e.g., Boston), essentially no conversion of 7-dehydrocholesterol to vitamin D_3 occurs in skin after as much as 3 hours of sun exposure during the months of November to March. Dietary vitamin D as cholecalciferol (D_3) or ergocalciferol (D_2) is absorbed in the distal ileum by a process that requires the presence of bile salts. These compounds are sequentially hydroxylated, first in the liver to form 25-hydroxy vitamin D [25(OH)D] and then in the kidney to form 1,25-dihydroxy vitamin D [$1,25(OH)_2D$]. It is the latter compound that is metabolically active in stimulating the active transport of calcium across the intestinal mucosa. Each of these metabolites is available for oral administration. Selected pharmacologic properties of these compounds are given in Table 2.

Prevention and treatment of metabolic bone disease are most effective in patients whose general nutritional status (e.g., protein, calories, phosphorus, magnesium) is good. Patients with GI disease may also have concurrent bone disease of other causes such as advanced renal disease or primary hyperparathyroidism. Under these circumstances, specialized therapeutic approaches with calcitriol or dihydrotachysterol or surgery may be required. Specific treatment with calcium, vitamin D, and estrogen for metabolic bone diseases resulting from GI disorders is the focus of this chapter.

CALCIUM

In all patients with GI disorders who are at risk for or already have bone disease, adequate calcium intake is

Table 1 Selected Features of Metabolic Bone Disease

	Osteoporosis	Osteomalacia	
		Early	Established
Clinical			
Bone fractures	+	+	+/−
Bone pain	−	−	+
Muscle weakness	−	−	+
Biochemical			
Calcium, phosphorus	nl	nl	↓
Alkaline phosphatase	nl	↑	↑ ↑
Parathyroid hormone	↓ -nl- ↑	nl- ↑	↑
25(OH)D, ng/ml	nl	<30	<30
$1,25(OH)_2D$, pg/ml	↓ -nl	↓ -nl- ↑	↓ -nl- ↑
Bone mineral density			
Cortical sites	↓ -nl	↓	↓
Trabecular sites	↓	↓	↓

Table 2 Pharmacologic Properties of Vitamin D Metabolites

Metabolite	Time to Peak Serum Concentration	Onset of Hypercalcemic Action	Duration of Action
Ergocalciferol or cholecalciferol	–	12–14hr*	Up to 6 mo
Calcidiol [25(OH)D]	4 hr	12–24 hr	15–20 days†
Calcitriol [$1,25(OH)_2D$]‡	2 hr	2–6 hr	1–2 days

*Therapeutic effect may take 10 to 14 days.
†Increased two to three times in renal failure.
‡Not recommended for patients with gastrointestinal disorders but included here for comparison.

essential. A total intake of 1,000 to 1,500 mg of elemental calcium daily is recommended. Food sources are preferred, although some supplements are often needed. In general, most of the widely used calcium supplements are equally well absorbed and may be taken throughout the day. When calcium carbonate is being used, however, it should be taken with meals, since calcium from this preparation is not as well absorbed in the fasting state by people with hypo- or achlorhydria. In addition, the daily quota of a calcium supplement should be taken in split dosages of 500 mg or less. When taken in smaller doses, net absorption of calcium is greater and the risk of acid rebound, seen in patients with peptic ulcer disease, is reduced.

VITAMIN D

Several principles should be considered before the form and dosage of vitamin D therapy are selected for a specific patient. These include (1) the pathophysiology of the underlying GI disorder, (2) the severity of the bone disease, and (3) other medications.

Early or Impending Vitamin D Deficiency

Patients at risk for developing bone disease on the basis of a wide variety of GI disorders, and those who have had a spontaneous fracture, should undergo an initial evaluation, including an assessment of cortical (e.g., two-thirds distal radius) and trabecular (lumbar spine, os calcis) bone mineral density and measurement of serum alkaline phosphatase, parathyroid hormone, and 25(OH)D concentrations. Although a wide normal range is frequently given, it is desirable to maintain the serum concentration of 25(OH)D above 30 ng per milliliter. On a hospital diet, the 25(OH)D concentration can increase by up to 1 ng per milliliter daily. Thus, a blood sample taken on admission provides the best index of vitamin D status. If the 25(OH)D concentration is less than 30 ng per milliliter (more likely to occur in winter at high latitudes), the patient should be given 400 IU (10 μg) of vitamin D daily. It is useful to categorize patients according to their response to this therapy.

Normal Responders

On 400 IU of vitamin D daily, the serum 25(OH)D concentration is expected to normalize over the ensuing several weeks and plateau in the range of 30 to 55 ng per milliliter. In contrast, the 1,25(OH)$_2$D concentration may rise out of the normal range, sometimes reaching 100 to 150 pg per milliliter after 5 to 10 days of therapy. In general, patients with the lowest 25(OH)D concentrations before treatment have the greatest increment in 1,25(OH)$_2$D on vitamin D supplementation. Normalization of the 25(OH)D concentration on 400 IU of vitamin D daily indicates that the vitamin D deficiency resulted from inadequate intake or mildly impaired absorption. To monitor therapy, patients should have serum 25(OH)D concentration measured annually, in the winter, and the dosage of vitamin D should be adjusted as needed to maintain the 25(OH)D concentration in the desired range of 30 to 55 ng per milliliter. Parent vitamin D is appropriate therapy for these patients, since they have demonstrated the capacity for absorption and 25-hydroxylation. Monitoring of patients at risk for metabolic bone disease should be continued on a long-term basis, since the time before the appearance of symptomatic bone disease often exceeds 10 years.

Finally, patients with low bone density, with or without fractures, and normal 25(OH)D concentrations should be treated with calcium supplementation and, where appropriate, estrogen replacement (see below).

Abnormal Responders

In patients who do not achieve a serum 25(OH)D concentration in the range of 30 to 55 ng per milliliter after several weeks of treatment with 400 IU of vitamin D daily, malabsorption of vitamin D should be suspected. To evaluate this, a calcidiol [25(OH)D] loading test is recommended. This is performed by administering 10 μg per kilogram of calcidiol orally in the morning after an overnight fast, and measuring the serum 25(OH)D concentration just before and 4 and 8 hours after the dose. The calcidiol, dissolved in propylene glycol, should be given with a light breakfast; the patient can have normal meals thereafter. An increment of 70 to 150 ng per milliliter above the baseline 25(OH)D concentration occurs in normal individuals. The peak concentration usually occurs at 4 hours but may be seen at 8 hours after the dose. The test offers the advantages of repleting body stores of vitamin D and giving an indication of the presence and degree of malabsorption so that the oral therapeutic dose can be more accurately estimated. Although there may be a slight increase in serum calcium, e.g., from 9.5 to 9.7 mg per deciliter, there is no risk of hypercalcemia after this test. With the results of the loading test, the therapy required to normalize the serum 25(OH)D concentration can be estimated.

The metabolite calcidiol is preferred therapy for patients with vitamin D malabsorption because it is better absorbed (more water soluble) than the parent compound. In addition, normal absorption data needed to assess the degree of vitamin D malabsorption are available (given above), and the onset of action is rapid (Table 2). Calcidiol should be given orally in an amount that will maintain the serum 25(OH)D concentration in the range of 30 to 55 ng per milliliter. For patients with moderately impaired calcidiol absorption, I treat initially with 20 to 40 μg of calcidiol per day. Serum calcium and 25(OH)D concentrations should be measured monthly until the correct dose is determined; thereafter, the serum 25(OH)D concentration can be checked every 6 months. It should be recognized that the absorption of calcidiol will vary with the severity of malabsorption in a given patient. Thus, during periods of increased fat malabsorption, whether due to worsening GI disease or to noncompliance with medications, the serum 25(OH)D concentration must be followed more frequently. In diseases such as sprue, there may be little correlation between fecal fat levels and vitamin D malabsorption. Thus, one cannot assume that because fat malabsorption is minimal, the probability of vitamin D deficiency is minimal. Finally, for patients with advanced liver disease who may have substantial reduction in 25-hydroxylase activity, calcidiol therapy is preferred.

ESTABLISHED OSTEOMALACIA

In patients with symptoms and biochemical features of established osteomalacia (Table 1), a calcidiol loading test as described above is recommended. This gives an indication of the presence and degree of malabsorption and provides a loading dose of 25(OH)D. Normal absorbers should be treated with 20,000 to 50,000 IU of parent vitamin D daily, and malabsorbers with 40 to 80 µg of calcidiol. Treatment should be adjusted, as needed, to maintain the 25(OH)D concentration in the high-normal range. Intake of calcium and phosphorus should be increased to 1,500 to 2,000 mg daily, as needed, to achieve and maintain normal serum concentrations. This therapy will result in increased urinary calcium excretion. To prevent calcium oxalate stone formation, urine oxalate excretion must be normal and urine calcium excretion no higher than 300 mg daily. Therapy should be continued until the serum alkaline phosphatase decreases to the upper limit of the normal range, indicating that excess osteoid has been mineralized. This takes months in cases of severe osteomalacia. At this point, calcium intake should be lowered to prevent overshoot hypercalciuria and risk of formation of kidney stones. The serum concentration of parathyroid hormone often takes months to years to normalize.

Bone mineral deficits in osteomalacia resulting from the associated secondary hyperparathyroidism have been estimated at 20 to 40 percent for cortical and 30 percent for trabecular bone. With treatment, recovery of the trabecular bone deficit in the ilium has been good (80 percent), whereas recovery of cortical losses (in the ilium and radius) has been no more than 10 to 15 percent. This underscores the importance of early recognition and prevention of vitamin D deficiency.

DRUG-DRUG INTERACTIONS

Several drugs interact with the various vitamin D metabolites. Large amounts of aluminum hydroxide, present in some antacids, may precipitate bile acids and thus decrease vitamin D absorption. Concurrent use of magnesium-containing antacids and vitamin D therapy may result in hypermagnesemia. Cholestyramine binds endogenously formed 25(OH)D as it undergoes enterohepatic circulation, and also binds ingested cal-

cidiol. Anticonvulsants, rifampin, and primidone accelerate metabolism of 25(OH)D by hepatic microsomal enzyme induction and thereby increase the requirement for vitamin D. Isoniazid interferes with the activity of the 25-hydroxylase and 1-α-hydroxylase enzymes.

Glucocorticoid therapy is sometimes required in patients with GI disorders. This has several effects on calcium and bone metabolism, the most important of which are inhibition of bone formation and suppression of gonadal hormone levels. In addition, glucocorticoids reduce calcium absorption and increase renal loss of calcium. The latter may result in secondary hyperparathyroidism and an associated increase in bone resorption. Many patients on glucocorticoid therapy develop osteoporosis characterized by rapid loss of trabecular bone and fractures typically of the vertebrae, ribs, and hips.* A minimum of 1,500 mg of calcium per day, sufficient vitamin D to maintain a high normal serum 25(OH)D concentration, and hormone replacement therapy are recommended for postmenopausal women. Although variably effective, this therapy does not cause hypercalcemia.

ESTROGEN

General guidelines for the use of estrogen in the treatment of osteoporosis also apply to patients with GI disorders. Estrogen therapy is most effective in preventing bone loss when administered to women within 5 to 10 years after menopause (whether natural or surgical). Estrogen therapy is generally appropriate for those with (1) early menopause, (2) low or low-normal bone density, or (3) several risk factors (e.g., immobilization and other inactivity, smoking, excess caffeine and alcohol use, positive family history) when confirmatory bone mineral density measurements are unavailable. To reduce the risk of endometrial cancer, progesterone should also be given. One effective regimen is equine conjugated estrogens, 0.625 mg orally on days 1 to 25, and medroxyprogesterone, 10 mg daily on days 15 to 25 of each month. Another is to take estrogen and medroxyprogesterone, 2.5 mg daily. Both may result in withdrawal bleeding. The beneficial effect of estrogen appears to be complemented by an adequate calcium intake and physical activity.

Estrogen therapy is associated with numerous side effects, including hypertension and deep-vein thrombophlebitis. An association with breast cancer risk with long-term use, although not established, remains an area of concern and active investigation. For in-depth descriptions of possible side effects of estrogen and progesterone, see the *Physicians' Desk Reference*.

---

*Editor's Note: In a study of prevention of corticosteroid osteoporosis, 1,25-dihydroxy vitamin D (calcitriol, 0.5 to 1.0 µg daily) and calcium (1,000 mg per day), with or without salmon calcitonin (400 IU per day intranasally), prevented bone loss in the lumbar spine in patients on long-term steroid therapy.

SUGGESTED READING

Lukert BP, Raisz LG. Glucocorticoid-induced osteoporosis: pathogenesis and management. Ann Intern Med 1990; 112:352–364.
Parfitt AM, Rao DS, Stanciu J, et al. Irreversible bone loss in osteomalacia. J Clin Invest 1985; 76:2403–2412.

Riggs BL, Melton LJ III. The prevention and treatment of osteoporosis. N Engl J Med 1992; 327:620–627.
Sambrook P, Birmingham J, Kelly P, et al. Prevention of corticosteroid osteoporosis. A comparison of calcium, calcitriol, and calcitonin. N Engl J Med 1993; 328:1747–1752.

FOOD FADS AND ALTERNATIVES

VICTOR HERBERT, M.D., J.D.
TRACY STOPLER KASDAN, M.S., R.D.

"For every complicated problem there is a simple solution—and it is wrong."

(H.L. Mencken)

Food faddism is an unusual pattern of food behavior enthusiastically adopted by its adherents. It is commonly expressed by (1) beliefs that particular foods or food substances can cure diseases, (2) elimination of certain foods from the diet, and/or (3) emphasis on "natural" foods.

There are three kinds of alternatives: genuine, questionable, and blatantly fraudulent. Genuine alternatives are those that successfully answer the three basic questions of efficacy and safety:

1. Is a remedy better than placebo or than doing nothing?
2. Is it as safe as placebo or as doing nothing?
3. If there is any question about safety, does the potential benefit exceed the potential harm?

Quackery is promotion for profit of questionable medical (including nutritional) schemes or remedies. This definition distinguishes folk practices and neighborly advice from practices done for financial gain.

Questionable alternatives are those that have not successfully answered the three basic questions. Questionable alternatives represented as genuine and used to make a profit are fraudulent since, by legal definition, the two requisite elements of civil fraud are deception and profit. For criminal fraud, a third element is required—scienter. Scienter means the culprit is deliberately deceiving, and knows or should know that his or her representations of efficacy and safety are unsupported by anything other than "best cases."

*Editor's Note: Gastroenterologists are asked nutrition-related questions almost daily. Here are some facts and some strong opinions.

"Best cases" are not evidence of either efficacy or safety because on investigation they invariably prove to be "cures that are not." These fake "cures" fall into six categories:

1. The disorder is self-limiting, and will go away with no treatment. Eighty percent of all symptoms with which patients present go away within a day to a month with no treatment. This is why quacks have eighty percent satisfied customers.
2. The patient was "cured" of a disease he or she never had.
3. The cure or remission was induced by genuine therapy but the quack remedy also given was credited.
4. The disease was progressing silently but was erroneously believed to be cured.
5. The patient is dead but fraudulently represented as cured.
6. The patient had a spontaneous remission publicized as a success, but the proponents failed to keep score and publicize all the failures before and after each "success." The difference between promoters of quack remedies and promoters of legitimate remedies is that only the latter keep score.

Faddists and quacks urge everyone to distrust large food companies, government regulators, and scientific health professionals. This negative philosophy is essential because without it, consumers would have no reason to buy health food industry products or to consult "alternative" practitioners.

Fundamental to nutrition scams is the use of buzzwords which, although in fact are deceptive and misleading, evoke Pavlovian approbation. Among such words are "alternative," "natural," "organic," "supplement," and "antioxidant." They make great advertising copy, but poor common sense and poor science. The fact is that if it is sensational about nutrition, it is not true; and if it is true, it is not sensational.

MISLEADING CLAIMS

Nutrition faddism and quackery are promoted with four basic fallacies:

1. Our food supply is nutritionally inadequate because our soils are depleted and important nutrients are removed by food processing. These claims encourage the purchase of "organic," "natural," and "health" foods.
2. Most health problems result from faulty diet and can be treated with "nutritional" methods. These types of claims are used to market hundreds of "food supplements," "health foods," and quack dietary methods.
3. Americans are in danger of being poisoned by food additives and pesticides residues. This claim is used to promote the sale of "organic" and "natural" foods.
4. Personal experience is the best way to tell whether something is effective. This claim encourages people to disregard scientific studies and rely on testimonial evidence.

Because of their charisma, glibness, charm, and simple "sound-bite" solutions to complex problems, the gurus of questionable nutrition practices are confidence men and women par excellence. They are the favorite guests of talk show hosts, and the favorite sources used by newspapers and magazines for nutrition information and advice. Their books, with sound-bite titles offering simple (and fraudulent) solutions to complex problems, are almost invariably best sellers, illustrating the maxim that scams sell and science doesn't.

Responsible health professionals, encountering these gurus on talk shows or elsewhere, invariably make the mistake of appealing to their consciences. This is fatal, because they don't have consciences. Typically, the responsible professional will say, "But you would have to agree that what you say has never been proven either effective or safe." To which the guru, with no conscience, replies, "It certainly is effective and safe, and I have a thousand patients that prove it." End of argument — guru wins.

It is impossible to get patients to understand they have been misled without recognizing oneself, and helping the patient to recognize, that a majority of the gurus of questionable nutrition practices are in fact sociopath-psychopaths, as delineated in the American Psychiatric Association: DSM III (*Diagnostic and Statistical Manual III*). Key characteristics of these gurus include deceitfulness, manipulative skills, ability to lie with no sense of guilt or feelings of remorse, and the attitude that the suckers who are dumb enough to believe them deserve to be taken.

Caveat. As psychiatrist Stephen Barrett points out, "Many quacks are true believers, who are delusional and lie in the service of their delusions." Thus, while they are guilty of the *civil* offense of fraud, which requires only the two legal elements of deception and profit, they may lack the third legal element, *scienter* (legalese for "they consciously know, or should know, they are lying"), which is required for *criminal* fraud.

FAD DIETS

"Vegetarianism"

Vegetarianism has been popular in many parts of the world throughout history. We put the word in quotes because it means different things to different people. Adherents range from those who eliminate only red meat to those who limit their diets to a single food. Some objective definitions help to clarify various vegetarian practices:

Vegans, or strict vegetarians, consume no animal products (meat, fish, poultry, eggs and egg products), dairy (including, but not limited to, milk and cheese), but eat only food from plant sources such as grains, legumes, fruits, vegetables, nuts, and seeds. They constitute about 2 percent of American vegetarians.

Ovolactovegetarians avoid all meat but include in their diet egg and dairy products along with all foods from plant sources. Groups that advocate avoidance of animal slaughter generally subscribe to this practice.

Lactovegetarians eliminate only meat and eggs not dairy products. This form of vegetarianism is practiced by groups such as Hare Krishnas, some Yoga groups, and Trappist monks.

Semi- or partial vegetarians usually refuse red meat but may eat chicken and/or fish along with ovolactovegetarian fare and small amounts of meat.

Classifying the degree of vegetarianism solely on the consumption or exclusion of animal food does not take into account the additional diet modifications practiced by many vegetarian adults. For example, some vegans eat only raw plant food. One group, fruitarians, limits diet to fruits, nuts, seeds, olive oil, honey, and, in some cases, whole grains. Some individuals devise their own eclectic variations. Other variables frequently associated with vegetarianism include the use of "organically grown" (i.e., without artificial fertilizers or pesticides) or natural foods, avoidances of refined sugar and processed foods, use of megadoses of vitamin supplements, and inclusion of certain foods in the misguided belief that they have special health-promoting or disease-preventing properties.

Because of the many variations on the theme of vegetarianism, generalizations about the adequacy of vegetarian diets are difficult. Some vegetarian diets are well balanced and healthful, others are too restrictive, and still others are borderline. Each must be evaluated on its own merits.

Many individuals and groups have practiced vegetarianism on a long-term basis and demonstrate excellent health. As with other nutritionally sound diets, those traditional vegetarian diets that are characterized by moderation, variety, and balance pose fewer risks than do those that involve extensive food avoidance or excesses. Dietary restrictions are most hazardous to those whose well-being is already stressed, such as those who are ill or recovering from disease, cancer patients, pregnant or lactating women, and infants and growing children.

Semivegetarians, who eliminate red meat but include fish and/or fowl in their diets, are at no greater risk than omnivores for malnutrition. Red meat is higher in saturated fats than many other foods so eating excessive amounts is not prudent. Red meat is nutrient dense, so modest amounts (3 ounce portions) are a dietary plus.

Similarly, lacto- and ovolactovegetarians have adequate sources of essential nutrients in their eggs and milk, which provide generous amounts of high-quality protein. Care must be taken, however, to assure enough absorbable iron in the diet, since dairy products are poor sources of it and the iron in plant foods averages only 3 percent absorbability as compared to the average 15 percent absorbability of iron in meat, fish, and poultry.

For those who eliminate all animal products from their diets, careful planning is necessary to ensure a good balance of essential amino acids, sufficient calories, and adequate sources of vitamins D, B_{12}, riboflavin, calcium, iron, and zinc. Details of such planning are in the chapter "Vegetarianism" in *The Mount Sinai School of Medicine Complete Book of Nutrition* (see Suggested Reading), and in the looseleaf *Diet Manual Including a Vegetarian Meal Plan,* published by the Seventh-Day Adventist Dietetic Association, PO Box 75, Loma Linda, California 92354.

Zen Macrobiotic Diets

The Zen macrobiotic diet consists of ten sequential vegetarian diet stages, each more restrictive and therefore more dangerous than its predecessor. Followers of such diets believe that sequentially eliminating more and more specified foods from the diet as one progresses through the ten stages will result in a happy, harmonious life. As the individual progresses through the stages, desserts, fruits and salads, animal foods, soup, and vegetables are eliminated one by one and replaced by increased amounts of cereal grains. All dietary stages also encourage food restriction. This continues until, at the highest level, only brown rice and small amounts of water or herbal tea are consumed. The lower level diets can meet nutritional needs, but strict adherence to the higher-level diets has resulted in serious malnutrition and even death. When a young woman eating such a diet died of undernutrition in New Jersey, a grand jury indictment was brought against her guru.

Infants of parents who use the Zen macrobiotic diet are typically fed a food mixture called *kokoh,* which is made up of ground seeds, brown rice, beans, wheat, oats, and water. Kokoh is deficient in several vitamins and minerals, including calcium, iron, and vitamin B_{12}. Since Zen followers frequently refuse nutrient supplementation, extreme growth retardation and death have been reported in infants on this diet.

Reducing Diets (Food Plans)

Until the first law of thermodynamics is repealed, there will be only one way to lose weight—consume less calories than one burns. This can be done responsibly or irresponsibly.

Gurus of irresponsible weight loss regimens point out that their diets "work," i.e., people lose weight on them. Of course they "work." Anyone will lose weight on any diet whose bottom line is that one eats each day less calories than one burns. Their regimens are irresponsible because they are unsafe.

For example, several people who sued a popular diet guru, claiming that his high-fat weight loss diets gave them heart attacks, have won six-figure judgments. Typically, when a nutrition guru settles out of court a suit by a victim, a condition of the settlement is that the victim not disclose either the size of the settlement or that the guru did harm. The same is true when supplement profiteers settle out of court suits by their victims for the harms done by the supplements.

Responsible weight loss involves following a food plan incorporating the 3-5-7 of good nutrition: 3 basic words, 5 basic food groups, and 7 dietary guidelines. Reducing diets are irresponsible in direct proportion to the degree in which they deviate from the 3-5-7 of good nutrition. To determine whether any reducing diet is responsible or irresponsible, one simply determines how closely they follow the 3-5-7, or how widely they deviate therefrom.

The 3 basic words are moderation, variety and balance. Moderation means not eating either too much or too little of any one food or nutrient. Variety means consuming as wide a variety as one can afford from each of the five basic food groups, as well as within each of the groups. Balance is both the balance achieved by following the rules of moderation and variety, and the balance of calories in versus calories out. For weight loss and to sustain muscle tone, this requires adequate exercise to ensure that energy intake is a little less than energy output.

The five basic food groups were incorporated by the U.S. Departments of Agriculture and of Health and Human Services in a food guide pyramid (Fig 1). There is also a sixth, "other" group, consisting of fats and oils, sweets, salty snacks, alcohol, other caloric beverages, and condiments. This sixth group, whose main function is to enhance palatability, is meant to be consumed in modest amounts, so as not to take the place (especially in a weight loss regimen) of adequate quantities of the five basic food groups.

Note in Figure 1 that the number of servings from each of the five food groups that one should consume each day depends on one's genetic blueprint. For example, if a person is among the approximately 12 percent of Americans with a gene for enhanced iron absorption, he or she should eat more portions from the plant origin groups (average iron absorption 3 percent) than from the animal origin groups (average iron

Food Guide Pyramid
A Guide to Daily Food Choices

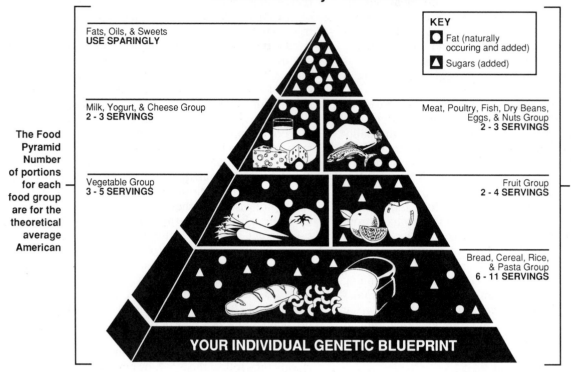

KEY
◯ Fat (naturally occuring and added)
▲ Sugars (added)

Fats, Oils, & Sweets
USE SPARINGLY

Milk, Yogurt, & Cheese Group
2 - 3 SERVINGS

Meat, Poultry, Fish, Dry Beans, Eggs, & Nuts Group
2 - 3 SERVINGS

The Food Pyramid Number of portions for each food group are for the theoretical average American

Vegetable Group
3 - 5 SERVINGS

Fruit Group
2 - 4 SERVINGS

Number of portions from each food group may need to be increased or decreased by each individual according to his or her Genetic Blueprint.

Bread, Cereal, Rice, & Pasta Group
6 - 11 SERVINGS

YOUR INDIVIDUAL GENETIC BLUEPRINT

Figure 1   The U.S. food guide pyramid, modified to take genetic variability into account. (Copyright 1992, Victor Herbert.)

absorption 15 percent). Additionally, one should avoid alcohol and supplements of vitamin C each of which enhances iron absorption.

The seven U.S. dietary guidelines are: (1) eat a variety of foods, (2) maintain healthy weight, (3) choose a diet low in fat, saturated fat, and cholesterol, (4) choose a diet with plenty of vegetables, fruits, and grain products, (5) use sugars only in moderation, (6) use salt and sodium only in moderation, and (7) if you drink alcoholic beverages, do so in moderation.

ALTERNATIVE DIETARY PATTERNS

When not modified by the appropriate adjective (genuine, questionable, or fraudulent), the term "alternative dietary pattern," like the term "alternative health care," is misleading. Since unsound dietary patterns are not true alternatives to sound ones, the term "unscientific" or "dubious" dietary pattern is more appropriate. Most so-called alternative dietary patterns are in fact either of questionable safety or downright fraudulent.

Health Foods

The term "health food" was created by the health food industry to label what they sell. Strictly speaking, therefore, grains, fruits, vegetables, and supplements are not "health foods" if sold in a grocery in a section not labeled "health foods," but are if sold in a section so labeled or in a health food store.

All food is health food in moderation. Any food is junk food in excess. No food in moderation is junk food. Any food in excess is junk food.

Promoters of "health foods" as healthier foods appear unfamiliar with the realities of toxicants naturally occurring in foods, such as aflatoxin in some "health food" peanut butters. Nor do they appear aware of food-borne disease, such as that due to bacteria in unpasteurized milk and cheese. They seem to be as unaware of the health value of many food additives as they are of the harms from megadoses of vitamins and minerals.

The public needs more responsible books and television shows on nutrition science and fewer "nutrition guru" shows and books. The public must learn that if the book or guru promotes pills, powders, and potions instead of food, they can't be trusted. In fact, even the "harmless" daily vitamin-mineral supplement may not be fully trustworthy, although to question it today, when about half of all Americans take such a supplement, is like questioning motherhood. Nothing is perfect; 100 percent safety is impossible to provide.

"Organic" and "Natural" Foods

Organic means containing a carbon skeleton. Natural means unprocessed. "Organic" suggests safer and more nutritious foods than conventionally grown foods. "Natural" foods are produced and marketed with a minimum of processing and without the use of additives or artificial ingredients.

Supplements

The Random House Dictionary definition of the word "supplement" is "something added to complete a thing, supply a deficiency, or reinforce or extend a whole." The vitamins, minerals, herbs, and other substances sold to the American public by the supplement industry are in fact not supplements, since the average American diet is complete, has no deficiencies, and needs no reinforcement or extension. Claims for, and

problems resulting from, supplements are listed in Table 1.

Deception by omission (which the law calls fraudulent concealment) is the stock in trade of the supplement industry. One example is that they inform the public of the 6 percent of the population who may be helped by supplements containing iron and/or vitamin C because they are in negative iron balance (fertile and pregnant women, infants, and children at the onset of puberty). They conceal from the public that twice as many (12 percent, mainly males) are in positive iron balance and can only be harmed by the very same supplements.

The consensus of the November 1 through 3, 1993 Food and Drug Administration (FDA) Public Conference on Antioxidant Vitamins and Cancer and Cardio-

Table 1 Popular Supplements: Help or Harm?

Supplement	Claims	Problems From Excess	Good Sources
Fiber	Lowers cholesterol Lowers risk of colon cancer Lowers weight Helps glucose control	GI obstruction Decreased absorption of calcium, zinc, and iron	Whole grains, fruits and vegetables
Omega-3-fatty acids	Lowers cholesterol Lowers blood pressure Lowers risk for heart disease	Vitamin A toxicity Increased serum cholesterol Increased bleeding problems	Fish oil (bluefish, mackerel, salmon, herring); linseed, canola walnut oils; purslane, spinach, some lettuces; some nuts
Vitamin A	Reduces wrinkles Reduces acne Treats epithelial-origin cancers	Liver damage Birth defects Skin irritation	Liver; fish oil; fortified milk
Beta carotene (precursor to Vitamin A)	Reduces risk for cancer and heart disease	Turns skin yellow Worsens liver damage from alcohol	Dark green, orange, yellow fruits and vegetables
Vitamin C	Enhances iron absorption Reduces cold symptoms via antihistaminic effect	Enhances iron absorption Oxalate kidney stones Diarrhea	Citrus fruits (and juices); sweet (and white) potato; broccoli; cabbage
Vitamin E	Reduces aging of skin Reduces risk for heart disease and cancer Enhances immunity	Enhancing immunity makes worse immune endocrine (e.g., diabetes, thyroid) and autoimmune (e.g., lupus, etc.) disorders	Poultry and seafood; seeds and nuts; cooked greens; wheat germ and fortified cereals; eggs
Iron	Provides energy	Iron overload promotes diabetes, liver disease, heart disorders; Reduced zinc absorption	Meat, fish and poultry are all 15 percent absorbable; vegetables are 3 percent absorbable
Lecithin	Lowers blood cholesterol Cures arthritis Reduces memory loss Reduces skin problems Reduces gallstones Reduces nervous disorders Aids in weight loss	Excessive sweating Appetite loss GI distress Excessive salivation Depression Nervous system disorders	Soybeans; egg yolk; legumes; whole grains Note: The body makes all the lecithin it needs. Supplements are pure scam.
Niacin	Doses large enough to lower cholesterol act by damaging liver enzymes, not by vitamin action	Hot flushes Itchy skin Liver dysfunction GI upset	Poultry; seafood; nuts; potatoes; whole grains
Selenium	Reduces the risk of cancer	Large amounts produce severe toxicity and promote cancer Diarrhea Hair and nail loss	Poultry; egg yolk; seafood; whole grains; mushrooms; onions

vascular Disease was that labeling and advertising should be for consumer education, should be consistent with scientific evidence about which there was substantial agreement in the scientific community, and should be neither deceptive nor misleading (as, for example, by presenting only the upside and leaving out the downside).

The nutrition scientists at the Conference agreed that vitamins C, E, and beta carotene are mischaracterized by describing them solely as "antioxidant" (fighter against harmful free radicals), since they are in fact *redox* agents, antioxidant in some circumstances (often so in the physiologic quantities found in food), and *pro-oxidant* (producing billions of harmful free radicals) in other circumstances (often so in the pharmacologic quantities found in supplements).

Vitamin C is a special case, since, in the presence of iron, it is violently pro-oxidant, and, for genetic reasons, about 10 percent of American whites and perhaps as many as 30 percent of American blacks have a positive iron balance and too much body iron.

People with positive iron balance can be harmed by vitamin C supplements because vitamin C can enhance iron absorption, and can release toxic amounts of iron from the increased body iron stores of people in positive iron balance in quantities so great that they exceed the capacity of iron-binding proteins to bind them, resulting in the generation of billions of harmful free radicals which promote cardiovascular disease, cancer, and death.

Representing these vitamins as "antioxidant" in either labeling or advertising is a consumer deception, since it tells the consumer only the upside and omits the downside. At the conference we recommended that, to protect the public, the FDA and Federal Trade Commission should forbid using the word antioxidant to describe the preceding vitamins in labeling or advertising, and that every advertisement and label for vitamin C supplements should include the following:

> NOTICE: Do not take this product until your blood iron status has been determined. Six percent of Americans are in negative iron balance, and this product may help them. Twelve percent of Americans are in positive iron balance and this product may hurt them.

We further recommended that all labeling and advertising for vitamin C supplements should also bear the following:

> "NOTICE TO HEALTH PROFESSIONALS: Iron status is determined by measuring serum ferritin and, if it is high, also measuring serum iron. Alternatively, it is measured by determining percent saturation of the serum iron binding capacity."

Scientific evidence presented at the FDA conference indicated that the anticardiovascular disease and anticancer actions of beta carotene very likely have to do with chemical properties of beta carotene entirely distinct from antioxidant properties. In addition, the pro-oxidant effects of beta carotene, and its many other properties totally unrelated to antioxidant action, were delineated by James Allen Olson, one of the world's leading authorities on vitamin A and beta carotene. Also at the FDA conference, Max K. Horwitt, the world's foremost authority on vitamin E, submitted a letter stating (emphases ours):

> "Any toxicity of vitamin E has, so far, not proved to be a problem but I remain cautious. *Very high levels of antioxidants in blood and tissues may make them pro-oxidants.* A number of reports have shown that the tocopherols can inhibit platelet adhesion and aggregation. . . . *My position on health claims on labels is that they should be absent or stated very conservatively.*"

The study of 30,000 Chinese published in the September 15, 1993 *Journal of the National Cancer Institute,* widely misrepresented as showing that supplements of vitamin E and beta carotene protected against cancer, in fact merely showed that when one corrected vitamin E and beta carotene *deficiencies,* rampant in that Chinese population but almost unknown among Americans, the frequency of esophageal and gastric cancer was reduced.

It has been known for many years that a number of nutrient deficiencies can promote certain gastrointestinal cancers, and correcting those deficiencies reduces the frequencies of those cancers. Our 1992-3 studies in the north of China, where vitamin B_{12} deficiency and folic acid deficiency are rampant, showed that providing the missing vitamin B_{12} and folic acid reduced the frequency of esophageal cancer, and even partially reversed esophageal dysplasia, the intermediate lesion between normality and cancer. (That part of the dysplasia consisting of cells already DNA damaged to become committed cancer cells is not reversed; the *uncommitted* cells reverse to normal.)

Our work suggests that, where vitamin C appears to act against cancer, it may be acting in its role of preserving folic acid against oxidative destruction. It may be the folic acid that suppresses the development of cancer, by methylating DNA. Since methylation of DNA "switches off" cell proliferation, for 3 decades our laboratory has been trying to methylate malignancy DNA to "switch it off".

SUGGESTED READING

Barrett S and The Editors of Consumer Reports. Health schemes, scams, and frauds. New York: Consumer Reports Books, 1990.

Butler KA. A consumer's guide to "alternative medicine": A close look at homeopathy, acupuncture, faith healing and other unconventional treatment, Buffalo: Prometheus Books, 1992:130.

Hare RD. Without conscience: The disturbing world of the psychopaths among us. New York, London, Toronto, Sydney, Tokyo and Singapore: Pocket Books, 1993.

Herbert V. Everyone should be tested for iron disorders. J Am Diet Assoc 1992; 92:1502–1509.

Herbert V. Does mega-C do more good than harm, or more harm than good? Nutr Today 1993; 28(1):28–32.

Herbert V. Vitamin pushers and food quacks. In: Barrett S, Jarvis W, eds. The health robbers: A close look at quackery in America. Buffalo: Prometheus Books, 1993:23.

Herbert V, Barrett S. Fads, frauds, and quackery. In: Shils ME, Olson JA, Shike M, eds. Modern nutrition in health and disease. 8th ed, Vol 2. Baltimore: Lea & Febiger, 1994:1526.

Herbert V, Subak-Sharpe G, eds. The Mount Sinai School of Medicine complete book of nutrition. New York: St. Martin's Press, 1990.

Simopoulos AP, Herbert V, Jacobson B. Genetic nutrition: Designing a diet based on your family medical history. New York: Macmillan, 1993.

Tyler VE. The honest herbal: A sensible guide to the use of herbs and related remedies. 3rd ed. New York, London, & Norwood (Australia): Pharmaceutical Products Press, 1993.

SMALL INTESTINE

SMALL BOWEL ENDOSCOPY

GARTH GEORGE, M.D.
JAMIE S. BARKIN, M.D., F.A.C.G., F.A.C.P.

The small intestine beyond the duodenal third portion and extending to the ileum has been unknown territory for the gastrointestinal (GI) endoscopist. Fortunately, the past few years have been an escalating period of innovation for small bowel instruments, which have enabled endoscopists to examine and provide therapy for these areas. In this chapter, we outline the available methods that have expanded our diagnostic and therapeutic capabilities.

METHODS

Several enteroscopes and different techniques have been used to visualize the small bowel. These are classified as (1) push enteroscopy, (2) pull enteroscopy, and (3) intraoperative enteroscopy.

Push Enteroscopy

Enteroscopy was performed initially in the early 1970s with a standard, orally passed pediatric or adult colonoscope, which could be advanced to approximately 20 to 50 cm beyond the ligament of Treitz, into the proximal jejunum. Since then, new classes of very flexible enteroscopes have been developed. Initially, the Olympus SIF-10, a 165 cm flexible enteroscope, attained easy passage up to 60 cm beyond the ligament of Treitz. However, further advancement was not possible secondary to "looping" of the instrument in the stomach. The SIF-10L, approximately 200 cm in length, was developed along with the use of a stiffening overtube; the latter enables further passage. The technique of using an overtube with an enteroscope entails (1) passing the enteroscope beyond the second portion of the duodenum, where it is fixed and then straightened along the lesser curvature of the stomach; and (2) pushing the overtube already loaded onto the enteroscope, into the second portion of the duodenum, under fluoroscopic guidance. The scope is then advanced without looping in the stomach. This enteroscope has an outer diameter of 11.3 mm, a biopsy channel of 2.8 mm, and excellent tip deflection with a field of view of 120 degrees. Therefore, biopsy, cautery, and polypectomy can be easily performed with this instrument.

Subsequently, newer prototypes have been developed, including the SIF-10.5L with a larger outer diameter, and the newest fiberoptic enteroscope, the SIF-3000, which is 2,995 mm long and has a working length of 2,675 mm. We have shown that this latest prototype attains a median distance of 150 cm past the ligament of Treitz at its maximal insertion, allowing farther visualization than with previous enteroscopes. Video enteroscopes such as the SIF-100L generally seem to be easier to pass than fiberoptic instruments owing to their greater flexibility, reaching approximately 108 cm beyond the ligament of Treitz.

Sonde Enteroscopy

The technique of passage of the sonde-type enteroscopes, including the SIF-SW and SSIF-VII, involves nasal placement. These scopes are approximately 9 feet long, with only up-down controls, and depend on intestinal peristalsis to permit their endoluminal passage. Once the enteroscope is pushed into the stomach, a gastroscope is passed orally. The sonde scope is grasped and carried to the distal duodenum, facilitating its passage; the small bowel is visualized only upon withdrawal. The advantage of these enteroscopes is that they may permit examination of the entire small intestine. However, their disadvantages include the long duration of the procedure (an average of 6 hours); incomplete visualization, especially areas of lost visualization upon withdrawal, precluding examination; and more important, the lack of therapeutic potential, as there is no biopsy or therapeutic channel owing to its small size. Fortunately, the findings on sonde enteroscopy correlate well with lesions found at intraoperative enteroscopy (IOE).

Intraoperative Enteroscopy

In patients with occult bleeding who are to undergo diagnostic laparotomy, IOE is mandatory. This allows for visualization of the entire small bowel as well as the marking of lesions that ordinarily would not be found with external visualization of the small bowel. IOE is performed by the endoscopist, who orally passes a colonoscope at the time of surgery, through the pylorus, into the duodenum, to beyond the ligament of Treitz. Once beyond the ligament of Treitz, the surgeon helps to advance the scope through the bowel to its maximal insertion. During the insertion, the surgeon views the bowel from its serosal surface while the endoscopist views its mucosal surface. After maximal insertion is achieved, the surgeon pleats the small bowel over the endoscope so that when the procedure is completed, the bowel looks like a "slinky." Before IOE, the bowel must be freed of any adhesions and the ileocecal valve area must be cross-clamped to prevent colonic dilation. A colonoscope is best used, as it rarely loops in the stomach and reaches the area of the ligament of Treitz relatively easily. This "ultimate" endoscopic, small bowel procedure, makes possible localization of occult causes of bleeding in up to 40 percent of patients, as well as surgical removal of bleeding lesions.

The advantages of IOE include complete endoscopic visualization of the small bowel. This could be frustrated by (1) extensive neoplasia involving the gut and mesentery or (2) dense adhesions from previous operations, both of which may limit full endoscopic insertion. Unfortunately, while this procedure is successful in locating the source of bleeding, it is often tedious, is difficult to perform, and requires general anesthesia and laparotomy. In addition, prolonged postprocedure ileus is not unusual. Lewis and Waye have shown that small bowel enteroscopy using the sonde-type enteroscope and IOE appear to be comparable in terms of depth of insertion and ability to detect small bowel vascular ectasias.

DIAGNOSIS AND THERAPY

The advent of small bowel enteroscopies (SBEs) has allowed visual examination of the proximal to middle small bowel during push enteroscopy, and the entire small bowel during sonde and intraoperative enteroscopy. Apart from diagnosis, the advantages of push and intraoperative enteroscopy are their therapeutic benefits. They make possible coagulation of bleeding lesions, using bicap and heater probe, removal of polyps, and the obtaining of multiple directed biopsies of lesions and mucosa. However, push enteroscopy is limited by its depth of insertion, which involves visualizing the proximal third of the small bowel. The advantage of sonde enteroscopy is thus its greater length of visualization.

INDICATIONS AND FINDINGS

The most common indications for SBE are occult bleeding in approximately 75 percent of cases and suspected small bowel disease or localized lesions in the remaining 25 percent. Occult bleeding is defined as either ongoing bleeding evidenced by heme-positive stool, need for hematemics or transfusion, or patients who have intermittent documented bleeding of clinical significance in which standard work-up has been unrevealing. Patients with these bleeding patterns should undergo endoscopy and colonoscopy and x-ray examination of the small bowel before enteroscopy. Lesions are found in approximately 40 percent of patients with occult bleeding; half of these are proximal to the ligament of Treitz and are overlooked. Among the most common gastric lesions are linear erosions where the hiatal hernia passes through the diaphragm. The other major indication for SBE is abnormal small bowel seen by x-ray or suspicion of small bowel mucosal disease. SBE allows us to obtain directed small bowel biopsies and cultures and has become the accepted method. Therefore, biopsy technique is important, as it permits routine acquisition of adequate tissue. Specimens are obtained perpendicular to the intestinal folds, with only one per passage of biopsy forceps. This technique allows adequate specimens that are not crushed to be collected, and obtaining six specimens obviates the need to orient the specimens before placing them in formalin. This permits maximal interpretation by the pathologist and appropriate orientation by chance.

Small Bowel Lesions

A variety of small bowel lesions may result in occult bleeding (Table 1).

Vascular Lesions

Arteriovenous malformations (AVMs) are the most common lesions in patients with occult bleeding. The push enteroscopy technique enables visualization and coagulation of these lesions. Unfortunately, long-term therapy is a problem, as the patients may rebleed. In our ongoing study, we showed that after long-term therapy with norethindrone (Ortho-Novum), 1/50 mg twice daily in 30 patients with AVMs, there was no recurrence of GI blood loss in patients followed for longer than 2 months. Blue rubber bleb nevus syndrome, in which patients have AVM-like lesions on the skin and in the small bowel, frequently leads to significant GI hemorrhage. These endoluminal lesions can be treated with coagulation via the enteroscope.

The small bowel can be affected by vasculitides (e.g., polyarteritis, Henoch-Schönlein purpura), which can be visualized and biopsied at enteroscopy. It is unknown whether coagulation of these lesions has a therapeutic role.

Tumors

The small intestine is not a common area of the GI tract for tumor occurrence, probably because of rapid transit time and the proficient immune system. The duodenum, "centimeter for centimeter," is the most frequent site of carcinoma compared with the jejunum or

Table 1 Small Bowel Diseases Identified by Endoscopy

Vascular lesions
    Arteriovenous malformations
    Polyarteritis nodosa

Tumors
    Leiomyomas
    Leiomyosarcomas
    Adenocarcinomas
    Malignant lymphoma
    Lipomas
    Carcinoid
    Ileal angiosarcoma
    Leukemic ulcer

Diverticulosis
    Meckel's jejunal

Benign ulcers
    Nonspecific
    Non–steroid-induced (jejunal)
    Tuberculous (ileal)

Hereditary conditions
    Peutz-Jeghers syndrome
    Blue rubber bleb nevus

Mucosal disorders
    Malabsorption

ileum. However, a variety of benign and malignant tumors are found in patients with occult bleeding distal to the ligament of Treitz, which have been overlooked by small intestinal series. These patients may present with vague abdominal discomfort, nausea and/or emesis, and occult GI blood loss. Pathologically, these lesions include leiomyomas and ulcerated leiomyomas, adenocarcinomas, melanomas, and carcinoids. In addition to obtaining tissue diagnosis, the push enteroscope, with the benefit of fluoroscopy, allows the surgeon to localize these lesions accurately.

Benign Ulcers

Nonspecific and non–steroid-induced ulcers can be localized and therapy administered with injection sclerotherapy or coagulation probes using the prototype enteroscopes. If bleeding cannot be controlled, fluoroscopy can help determine good site localization to assist the operating surgeons, as these lesions can be notoriously difficult to detect by gross examinations. If lesions cannot be located at the time of laparotomy, IOE can be used for definitive localization.

Chronic ulcerative jejunoileitis is a condition in which enterocyte destruction outstrips the mitotic capacity of the stem cell, with histologic features of mucosal atrophy along with crypt hyperplasia, villous atrophy, and an inflammatory cell infiltrate. It is thought to be associated with celiac sprue. Clinically, these patients fail to respond to gluten withdrawal and may be harbingers of T-cell small intestinal lymphoma. These lesions are usually in the jejunum and are easily reached

by the enteroscope where the mucosa appears consistent with sprue but with ulcerations. Therefore, if localized lymphomatous infiltrates are found, surgical excision is mandatory.

Diverticulosis

Although jejunal diverticula are not as common a source of blood loss as colonic diverticula, they may bleed and have been shown to be actively bleeding during enteroscopy. Therefore, in patients with occult bleeding who have jejunal diverticula, it is not unreasonable to evaluate surgical therapy. The second manifestation of jejunal diverticula is bacterial overgrowth. Enteroscopy can also be used to obtain organisms via aspiration in cases of suspected bacterial overgrowth.

Currently, push enteroscopy is unable to diagnose Meckel's diverticulum because of its location in the distal ileum. However, diagnosis has been made by IOE and should be attainable by sonde enteroscope. Unfortunately, there is no therapeutic role for this instrument if areas of active bleeding are identified.

Hereditary Conditions

Peutz-Jeghers syndrome is manifested by GI polyposis and mucocutaneous pigmentation. Its complications are due to the large number of intestinal polyps and include bleeding, obstruction, and intussusception. Traditionally, surgical management has been used to relieve these complications, at which time palpable polyps are removed by multiple enterotomies, and patients may require surgery every 2 to 3 years because of associated risks of GI malignancy. Present-day enteroscopy has the ability to (1) endoscopically remove smaller polyps; (2) provide an accurate assessment of the extent of disease; (3) decrease the number of enterotomies, thus saving viable small intestine; and (4) treat bleeding lesions.

Mucosal Disorders

We and others have shown biopsy specimens obtained by push enteroscopy in patients with suspected malabsorption to be adequate for diagnostic purposes in 76 to 100 percent of cases. All the spruelike disorders are easily diagnosed, along with infective diseases of the small intestine. Classically, the endoscopic findings of celiac sprue are loss of duodenal folds due to atrophy of the bowel. However, early in the process, scalloping of the valvulae conniventes, especially on their luminal edge, is seen on close inspection.

COMMENTS

We foresee future adaptations of enteroscopic instruments that will enable access to the distal ileum by push enteroscopy with its current, therapeutic advantage, and/or development of a sonde enteroscope with therapeutic capabilities. Enteroscopy is becoming a routine endoscopic procedure.*

SUGGESTED READING

Lau WY. Intra-operative enteroscopy—indications and limitations. Gastrointest Endosc 1990; 36:268–271.

Lewis BS, Waye JD. Total small bowel enteroscopy. Gastrointest Endosc 1987; 33:435–438.
Rosen S, Barkin JS. Enteroscopy. In: Barkin JS, O'Phelan CA, eds. Advanced therapeutic endoscopy. New York: Raven Press, 1990: 163–168.
Wenger J, Barkin JS. Endoscopic morphology of the small bowel. In: Haubrich WS, Schaffner F, eds. Bockus gastroenterology. 5th ed. Philadelphia (in press).

---

*Editor's Note: The mythical "trip through the GI tract with gun and camera" is now complete.

NSAID-INDUCED INJURY TO THE SMALL AND LARGE INTESTINES

INGVAR BJARNASON, M.D., M.Sc., M.R.C.Path.
ANDREW MacPHERSON, M.A., Ph.D., M.R.C.P.

Many drugs have intestinal side effects, either as a consequence of their action on intestinal motility (e.g., opiates, tricyclic antidepressants) or in terms of a direct effect on mucosal integrity or function (e.g., neomycin can cause blunting of intestinal villous structure with steatorrhea, and colchicine may cause hemorrhagic gastroenteritis through inhibition of intestinal cell division). It is important to understand the intestinal side effects of these medications in order to eliminate the offending drug, or in the case of purgative abuse to be aware of the possible diagnosis. Relatively few drugs require specific treatment for intestinal side effects generated by therapeutic doses. One example is the effect of folate in counteracting the antimetabolite effects of methotrexate. In this respect the nonsteroidal anti-inflammatory drugs (NSAIDs) are in a unique position. Although they are highly successful, and the frequency of long-term use attests to their therapeutic usefulness in rheumatoid arthritis and other arthropathies, they can cause adverse effects in the digestive system.

NSAIDs cause damage throughout the gastrointestinal (GI) tract and there is great awareness of their effect on the stomach and duodenum, because of potentially catastrophic ulcer perforations or hemorrhage. The adverse effects on the small intestine are common in long-term NSAID users, but frequently are clinically occult. The approach to possible prevention and treatment of NSAID-related problems distal to the duodenum varies greatly, depending on the subspeciality of each physician and local referral habits. Hence, a general practitioner giving short courses of NSAIDs may not perceive a problem, while the rheumatologist is often puzzled by the fact that many patients with intestinal bleeding and iron deficiency anemia have normal gastroscopy and colonoscopy findings. In specialist gastroenterology practice, a subgroup of rheumatoid patients may be referred with long-standing severe iron deficiency or hypoalbuminemia without apparent cause after conventional investigation. This is a difficult patient group, many of whom have had repeated courses of oral iron and some of whom have even had intravenous iron infusions, which are said to carry the risk of a flare-up of the rheumatoid disease itself. In these patients, NSAID enteropathy is almost always the cause. Treatment of the enteropathy depends largely on the duration of symptoms and their functional consequences, as well as on the severity of the laboratory findings.

No fully randomized placebo controlled trial on the effectiveness of drug treatment of NSAID enteropathy has been published. Such studies are unlikely to appear in the near future because the pharmaceutical industry does not yet see this as a profitable investment area.

TREATMENT OF NSAID ENTEROPATHY

Our initial objective is to reduce the inflammation as quickly and effectively as possible. The obvious approach is to stop the NSAID, but this is often impractical because patients usually have severe rheumatoid arthritis requiring NSAIDs for control of joint pain. Moreover, once NSAID enteropathy is established, it may take up to 18 months to clear after discontinuation of these agents. If we are concerned about the particular NSAID an individual patient is taking, we now tend to try nabumetone (see below) in a large dose, 1.0 g twice daily. However, as with other agents, we have some reservations about its efficacy in pain relief.

Metronidazole

Oral metronidazole (200 mg four times daily in England*) is the first drug that we use in these patients, as it reduces both inflammation and blood loss. Its mode of action is uncertain. It has some effects on the immune system, but these are probably too mild to account for its action. It is more likely that it acts through its antimicrobial activity on the anaerobic intestinal flora, which indeed may be the main neutrophil chemoattractant in NSAID enteropathy. It is suggested that if one can reduce neutrophil activation and migration, there will be a concomitant reduction in tissue damage assessed by blood and protein loss.

Patients are advised to swallow, not chew, the tablets and to abstain from alcohol because of the occasional disulfiram-like reaction. We continue this therapy empirically for 6 weeks, after which time there is usually evidence of reduced inflammation and bleeding (demonstrated by the use of radioisotope traces). Side effects are infrequent, but we have limited the length of treatment to 6 months because metronidazole is associated with neuropathy when given on a long-term basis. Nevertheless, it may be necessary, particularly in patients with hypoalbuminemia, to continue the course, in which case they are warned to look out for symptoms of neuropathy. After the course of metronidazole, there are a number of possible strategies to keep the inflammation under control. The choice of drug depends on the medical history of the patients.

Misoprostol

If patients have a history of gastroduodenal complications of NSAIDs, we give oral misoprostol, a minimum of 200 μg twice a day and up to 200 μg four times a day if they take a NSAID more frequently. It may be important to take the two drugs together, although we know of no study to justify this. It has been shown that misoprostol reduces inflammation in the small intestine, but in a double-blind, placebo-controlled trial it was not significantly better than placebo. This was thought to be due to the small size of the trial. Misoprostol's action in the small intestine is unknown. One possibility is that the inflammation is reduced by virtue of its action in increasing intestinal blood flow, cell proliferation, and mucus secretion. If it is well tolerated, we continue misoprostol indefinitely. However, diarrhea may be a problem in up to 15 percent of patients (depending on how diarrhea is defined), in which case we have stopped treatment, perhaps reintroducing misoprostol later.

Sulfasalazine

We treat most patients, however, with oral sulfasalazine, 1.0 g three times a day. This has been shown to

reduce both inflammation and blood loss caused by NSAIDs in the small intestine, and there is an additional advantage over other forms of treatment in that sulfasalazine clearly has a disease-modifying action on the arthritis itself. We start patients on 500 mg twice daily for 1 week and gradually build up the dose to 1.0 g three times a day. While nausea and headache is minimized, up to one-quarter of patients still experience side effects that necessitate discontinuing treatment. These side effects usually occur early and tend to be a nuisance rather than serious or life-threatening. We have occasionally seen serious complications from sulfasalazine, including pancytopenia and hemolytic anaemia, but these are rare compared with those noted with other disease-modifying drugs (e.g., gold, penicillamine). It is recommended that patients have regular biochemical and hematologic screening during the first 3 months of treatment and every few months thereafter.

Mesalamine

Because of the intolerance problem with sulfasalazine, we have tried research patients on an early-release 5-amino salicylic acid (ASA) preparation, mesalamine (Pentasa), 500 mg three times a day. Nausea and headache are not a problem because these symptoms are due to the sulfapyridine moiety of sulfasalazine. There have been consistent decreases in intestinal inflammation after 6 weeks of treatment, similar to those seen with sulfasalazine, but there is presumably no joint disease-modifying action, as this theoretically resides within the sulfapyridine part of the sulfasalazine molecule or the entire molecule. No major side effects of mesalamine are reported, but there has been recent concern about the possible nephrotoxicity of certain 5-ASA preparations. As with sulfasalazine, we continue the drug for as long as the patients require NSAIDs.

Monitoring Therapy

It is easy to document reduced intestinal inflammation and blood loss in a research setting, but this is expensive. It is also notoriously difficult to carry out an indium-111 leukocyte and chromium-51 (^{51}Cr) labeled red blood cell study on an outpatient basis, as it involves a 5 day fecal collection and daily blood sampling. A conventional ^{51}Cr protein loss study is even more demanding and requires daily blood sampling and a 10 day fecal stool collection. A compromise must therefore be made. The main parameter of use to assess a favorable response is the serum albumin level in patients treated for hypoalbuminemia, but this leaves a major complication in the assessment of iron deficiency in patients with rheumatoid arthritis. Here the conventional indices for assessing responses to treatment change independently of iron deficiency because of the anemia of chronic disease. Also, iron status is dependent on food intake and absorption as well as blood loss. We therefore use a "rule of thumb" that hemoglobin levels below 10.0 g per deciliter in patients with rheumatoid arthritis are usually due to iron deficiency. Sequential hemoglobin estimations below this level may reflect the lack of effectiveness of treatment. Generally, albumin levels tend to increase over the first 4 weeks of metronidazole therapy, but it is rare to see them normalize if the initial albumin level was below 20 g per liter. The improvements in hemoglobin levels are less obvious and occur over months rather than weeks.

Medication Choices

The precise choice of drug to use after metronidazole is always difficult to justify because of the limited studies of their effectiveness. In general, we prefer to use sulfasalazine because of its disease-modifying action on the rheumatoid process itself. When side effects limit its use, we give misoprostol, which is usually well tolerated. Pentasa (mesalamine), a 5-ASA preparation that releases part of the dose in the small intestine, is currently used only for research purposes in our unit.

Prophylaxis

The idea of preventing NSAID-induced enteropathy is interesting but not necessarily sound. Patients are usually asymptomatic from the enteropathy, and treatment is only occasionally required. However, there has been no attempt to prevent the intestinal inflammation in humans, possibly because such studies are demanding and require untreated patients to be studied before treatment is started and after 6 months, a formidable task in the hospital setting. One of the most interesting possibilities for prevention, as yet untested, is the prescription of pro-NSAIDs. These drugs are inert until converted to an active NSAID in the liver after absorption. The strongest candidate for a relatively safe pro-NSAID at this time is nabumetone (Relafen), which has the additional advantage that its active metabolite is not excreted in bile. Most, if not all, other NSAIDs have a biliary secretion component that may be important in the pathogenesis of the intestinal inflammation. Although we place many patients on nabumetone, we still fear that the systemic effects of NSAIDs are sufficient to perpetuate the enteropathy, and in relation to the small intestine there are no data to show that it is any better than the other NSAIDs.

Ulcerations and Strictures

Another complication of NSAID enteropathy consists of intestinal ulcers and strictures. The strictures may be unique, multiple (three to 70), thin (2 to 4 mm), concentric, septate-like narrowings causing symptoms of intermittent subacute small intestinal obstruction. The type of surgery is straightforward: the ulcers and fibrous strictures require resection with end-to-end anastomosis; the diaphragms may need only stricturoplasty.

Table 1 Summary of Adverse Effects of Ingested NSAIDs on Large Intestine

Type of Damage	Drug Involved
"Normal" Colon	
Colitis	Fenemates
	Ibuprofen
	Naproxen
	Piroxicam
	Aspirin
Eosinophilic colitis	Naproxen
Pseudomembraneous colitis	Diclofenac
Collagenous colitis	Indomethacin
	Fenbrufen
Colonic ulcers*	Various
Perforation and bleeding†	Various
Pre-existing disease	
Complications of diverticular disease (perforation, fistulas, bleeding)	Various
Relapse of inflammatory bowel disease	Various

Most of the reports of adverse effects of NSAIDs on the normal large bowel are in the form of case reports, but the effects of NSAIDS on pre-existing disease are rather more common than their effect on the "normal" colon.
*Not always possible to distinguish from a colitis.
†Some cases may represent small intestinal bleeding.

TREATMENT OF NSAID-INDUCED COLONIC DISEASE

Table 1 lists some of the complications of NSAIDs in the large intestine. In general, these side effects are sufficiently rare to warrant case report publications. Treatment is simply supportive, consisting of discontinuing the drugs when possible and treating the condition whether or not it was associated with NSAIDs. Two aspects merit consideration, however.

First, NSAIDs may cause a colitis, which is most noticeable after treatment with fenemates (mefenamic and flufenamic acid). The clinical setting is one of unexplained diarrhea after months of NSAID treatment, which becomes bloody when the patient continues to take the fenemate. Treatment is simply to change to another NSAID, as the adverse reaction is presumably not due to the common action of NSAIDs in inhibiting cyclooxygenase. Second, there is increasing evidence that NSAIDs are associated with an aggressive form of diverticulitis (fistulas and perforations). In the setting of severe diverticulitis, it may be prudent to stop the NSAID temporarily and switch to a non-NSAID analgesic. Clinicians must be aware of this complication of NSAID ingestion and refrain from prescribing NSAIDs for mild or nonspecific abdominal pain.

SUGGESTED READING

Bjarnason I, Hayllar J, Macpherson A, Russell A. Side effects of nonsteroidal antiinflammatory drugs on the small and large intestines in man. Gastroenterology 1993; 104:1832–1847.
Bjarnason I, Hayllar J, Smethurst P, et al. Metronidazole reduces

inflammation and blood loss in NSAID enteropathy. Gut 1992; 33:1204–1208.

Bjarnason I, Hopkinson N, Zanelli G, et al. The treatment of non-steroidal anti-inflammatory drug induced enteropathy. Gut 1990; 31:777–780.

Bjarnason I, Zanelli G, Smith T, et al. Nonsteroidal antiinflammatory drug induced intestinal inflammation in humans. Gastroenterology 1987; 93:480–489.

CELIAC SPRUE AND RELATED PROBLEMS

PAUL J. CICLITIRA, M.D., Ph.D., F.R.C.P.

Celiac disease may be defined as a condition in which there is an abnormal jejunal mucosa that improves morphologically when gluten is removed. The condition, commonly called celiac sprue or gluten-sensitive enteropathy, was previously called nontropical sprue, celiac syndrome, idiopathic steatorrhea, or primary malabsorption. Dermatitis herpetiformis is a related condition in which there is an itchy, blistering skin eruption frequently affecting the knees, elbows, buttocks, and back. The diagnosis of dermatitis herpetiformis includes the finding of granular IgA at the dermoepidermal junction of uninvolved skin.

DIAGNOSIS

There are a variety of screening tests for celiac disease. Those most favored include the detection of antiendomysium, reticulin, or gliadin serum antibodies. Definitive diagnosis requires a jejunal or small intestinal biopsy, which should be taken with a Watson or Crosby peroral suction biopsy capsule. The current practice is for duodenal biopsies to be routinely taken through an endoscope. However, many other conditions may cause duodenitis that results in histologic appearances similar to those observed in celiac disease. Should there be any doubt about the correct diagnosis, either further biopsies of the small intestine distal to the first part of the duodenum should be obtained at upper gastrointestinal endoscopy, or a peroral suction biopsy of the jejunum should be undertaken.

The characteristic histologic changes in a small intestinal biopsy are villous atrophy, crypt hyperplasia, a chronic inflammatory cell infiltrate of the lamina propria, lymphocytic infiltration of the epithelium, and a decrease in the epithelial surface-cell height. Confusion can occur when these changes are only mild, particularly when only one endoscopic duodenal biopsy is histologically assessed and when this has been cut obliquely. Because several other conditions, including giardiasis and tropical sprue, produce histologic changes in small intestinal villous morphology, additional biopsies should be obtained if the diagnosis is in doubt. A follow-up biopsy should be obtained 4 to 6 months after starting treatment with a gluten-free diet, at which time there should have been an improvement in the small intestinal morphology. If the diagnosis is still in doubt, it is mandatory to take an additional jejunal biopsy after a formal gluten challenge. The patient should receive at least 40 g of gluten per day for a minimum of 2 weeks, and in the case of children, 6 weeks. If the patient experiences severe symptoms on gluten challenge, the date of the biopsy may be brought forward. The development of symptoms on gluten challenge without evidence of an abnormal small intestinal biopsy result, is insufficient to make the diagnosis, since some patients with the irritable bowel syndrome have an exacerbation of their symptoms associated with gluten ingestion.

TREATMENT

Patients with celiac disease should be treated with a gluten-free diet, avoiding all products containing wheat, rye, barley, and oats. Because the toxicity of oats is debated, some physicians permit oats to be taken, but it is my practice to exclude them strictly. Foods containing partial hydrolysates of gluten proteins, such as beer, which contains alcohol-soluble barley prolamins, should be strictly excluded from the diet. It has been known for some years that patients with celiac disease have a 10 to 15 percent chance of developing a small intestinal T-cell lymphoma. It was recently shown that this incidence is decreased on a gluten-free diet but not on a gluten-reduced diet. Patients with celiac disease must therefore be advised to take a strict gluten-free diet. In addition, those who have a normal or reduced gluten intake frequently develop nutritional deficiencies, particularly of iron and folic acid. The latter is important in women of child-bearing age, as low folate levels at conception are associated with an increased risk of neural tube defects in the fetus.

Most patients improve rapidly on a gluten-free diet; some improve well on a partial gluten-free diet. It is not customary to discuss this with the patients because it might give them a false sense of security. A small minority of patients with untreated celiac disease can become very ill and require treatment with a short course of oral or parenteral steroids (see below).

Adolescent patients often stop their diet in the mistaken belief that they have "grown out of" their celiac disease. This myth is perpetuated by gastroenterology textbooks published during the 1950s that propounded this idea. It is a particular problem in some European countries where patients with celiac disease are returned to a normal diet at this age. Adolescent patients with a confirmed diagnosis must be maintained on a strict gluten-free diet, or permanent growth retardation will result. Should the diagnosis be in any doubt, a gluten challenge and repeat jejunal biopsy should be undertaken. The patients often remain well, even if they return to a normal diet, perhaps because of the increased levels of circulating sex hormones associated with puberty. It should not be forgotten that puberty is a stressful time and adolescents fear that celiac disease may make them different from their peers. The problem can usually be overcome by introducing them, through their local celiac association, to others of the same age and background who have come to terms with a gluten-free diet.

Reproductive Problems

There is usually a delay in the menarche, typically of 1 year, in an untreated celiac girl. Amenorrhea lasting more than 3 months, unrelated to pregnancy, occurs in one-third of women of child-bearing age. The average age at menopause in untreated celiac patients is 45, compared with 53 in those on a gluten-free diet. Many celiac patients appear relatively infertile but eventually conceive; the mean time for celiac patients to conceive is 19 months on a normal diet and 12 months on a gluten-free diet. Infertile celiac patients frequently become pregnant shortly after starting a gluten-free diet. Spontaneous abortion is more common in untreated celiac patients (18 percent of pregnancies compared with 9 percent in those on a gluten-free diet). Recurrent abortions may be a presenting feature. Given these problems associated with pregnancy, unless there is a pressing urgency in view of the age of the patient, those female patients with untreated celiac disease should be given a strict gluten-free diet before intensive investigation for infertility.

Male patients with untreated celiac disease may experience some reduction in potency. Fertility and normal sperm counts are restored by a gluten-free diet even after some years of oligospermia. Low levels of plasma testosterone, free testosterone, and plasma 5-dihydrotestosterone are reported, and the plasma luteinizing hormone level is frequently raised. This may, in part, explain the commonly observed delay in puberty and development of secondary sex characteristics in untreated male patients. These abnormalities usually resolve after treatment with a strict gluten-free diet, although improvement may take up to 2 years.

Gluten-Free Diet

A gluten-free diet is low in roughage and therefore frequently induces troublesome constipation. This usually responds to the addition of regular dietary rice bran and a proprietary preparation of ispaghula husks.

Patients may supplement their diet with commercial gluten-free products, which are available on prescription in many European countries. Many gluten-free flours and bread mixes are based on purified wheat starch from which most gluten proteins have been removed. Most patients with celiac disease can tolerate these products well, with an improvement both in symptoms and in the morphology of their small intestinal villous architecture. However, a few celiac sufferers are unable to tolerate these products. These individuals should be advised to take a strict gluten-free diet in which the only commercial gluten-free products ingested are not based on wheat starch. Most gluten-free products available in North America avoid the use of wheat starch; in Europe the converse is true. The marked gluten sensitivity of a small minority of celiac patients was reported after the finding that ingestion once a week of a Communion wafer based on wheat flour was sufficient to cause symptoms of growth retardation in a child affected with the condition. The symptoms resolved when the patient stopped taking Communion wafers. Gluten-free Communion wafers are available, although these are not currently accepted by some church authorities, leading to upsetting decisions for the patients.

Specific dietary deficiencies can occur in celiac disease and should be corrected. These include iron, folic acid, calcium, and, very rarely, vitamin B_{12} deficiency.

Patients who fail to adhere strictly to a gluten-free diet may have continued ill health and recurring symptoms that can usually be traced to dietary lapses, either deliberate or accidental. Difficulty may arise when a food is taken that is thought to be gluten free but in fact contains gluten. An unusual cause of failure to respond to a strict gluten-free diet is the development of a small intestinal lymphoma, jejunal ulceration, or the unmasking of a concurrent complicating condition such as chronic pancreatitis. Rarely, a patient on treatment may deteriorate and die unaccountably.

In one report, 70 percent of celiac patients on a gluten-free diet quickly returned to normal health, with improvement within 2 weeks. The remaining 30 percent could be divided into three groups. Patients in the first group experienced progressive deterioration, which was halted in some cases by corticosteroids but which continued to death in others. Those in the second group were found to have an associated pancreatic lesion, and those in the third group were found not to adhere strictly to the diet, but even when this was corrected their minor abdominal symptoms and diarrhea persisted. It is important not to forget these observations, since it cannot always be assumed that dietary failure is an explanation for ill health.

Steroids

Celiac disease can be controlled by systemic corticosteroids, with rapid cessation of diarrhea, weight gain, and improvement in fat absorption. However, within a few days of stopping treatment, there is usually a deterioration. Steroids are indicated for the treatment of celiac crises that involve severe diarrhea, dehydration, weight loss, acidosis, hypocalcemia, and hypoproteinemia. They have also been used to treat gliadin shock, an anaphylactic reaction that rarely occurs in treated patients subject to gluten challenge.

There is rarely a need to use steroids. Steroids are most commonly given to complement a strict gluten-free diet when the serum albumin level is markedly depressed. They may be used in an attempt to bring the associated protein-losing enteropathy under control. The use of azathioprine as a steroid-sparing agent, at a dose of 1.5 mg per kilogram, has been reported. There is a theoretical potential for the use of more specific immunotherapy in the form of cyclosporin A for nonresponsive, life-threatening disease, although the role of these agents in clinical practice remains to be established. In my experience, this agent may exacerbate rather than alleviate symptoms.

The dosage of steroids used varies according to clinical requirements. If a patient requires intravenous (IV) fluid replacement because of vomiting, diarrhea, or surgery, IV hydrocortisone should be given, 100 mg every 6 hours. Individuals who are eating normally but exhibiting a crisis should be given 40 to 60 mg prednisolone daily. The normal dosage of prednisolone for gluten-sensitive enteropathy that has not responded adequately to a strict gluten-free diet is 5 to 20 mg a day. It should be feasible within a matter of weeks to reduce a high dose. Should this prove impossible without a recurrence of symptoms, clinicians must be alert to the possibility of either inadequate dietary compliance or complications such as lymphoma or ulcerative jejunitis.

TREATMENT OF COMPLICATIONS

Carbohydrate Intolerance

Many patients with gluten-sensitive enteropathy have lactose or sucrose intolerance at the time of diagnosis. Only a few patients continue to be troubled with disaccharidase deficiencies after treatment; these develop diarrhea and abdominal pain with lactose or sucrose. These conditions may be diagnosed either by enzyme assays of the mucosa from part of a repeat jejunal biopsy or by the appropriate sugar permeability study. If concomitant disaccharidase deficiency is diagnosed, the relevant disaccharide should be excluded from the gluten-free diet. Many of the currently available gluten-free products are lactose free.

Bacterial Overgrowth

A minority of treated celiac patients suffer from small intestinal bacterial overgrowth, which can be diagnosed by an abnormal breath hydrogen test, a bile acid breath test, an abnormal urinary indican excretion test, or an abnormally high small intestinal aspirate bacteriologic count. Should bacterial overgrowth persist, patients may be given antibiotics such as oxytetracycline, 250 mg four times a day, rotated every 2 weeks with another agent such as co-trimoxazole (80 mg trimethoprim and 4 mg sulfamethoxazole), one tablet twice a day. A 10 day course of metronidazole, 200 mg three times a day, is frequently helpful in small bowel bacterial overgrowth; its potential side effects preclude long-term therapy.

Neurologic Complications

Neurologic complications may occur rarely. These include Korsakov's syndrome and an unusual encephalitis, the precise etiology of which is unknown. Patients are normally given a 5 day course of high-dose vitamin supplementation, usually injectable Parentrovite, for both of these conditions, and maintained on a strict gluten-free diet. No other specific therapy is indicated and most patients recover.

Associated Diseases

Numerous disease associations can occur with celiac disease and are listed in Table 1. These include a variety of autoimmune disorders associated with the extended genetic haplotype HLA-B8, DR3, DQ2, frequently present in celiac disease. If a patient with celiac disease becomes unwell, investigations should be undertaken to exclude other autoimmune disorders, and a detailed family history sought.

The prevalence of diabetes mellitus in celiac disease has been reported as 4 to 10 percent. Diarrhea may be a symptom of both disorders. Diagnosis and insulin therapy are standard, but the dietary treatment of the patient's gluten sensitivity will necessarily be complicated by the need for sugar balance. The services of a competent dietitian are essential.

Thyroid disease affects 4 to 6 percent of patients with celiac disease, either as thyrotoxicosis or as hypothyroidism. Symptoms of unexplained weight loss or general lassitude should prompt the institution of thyroid function tests and appropriate treatment.

Celiac patients have a higher incidence of certain liver disorders, including chronic active hepatitis, primary cirrhosis, and sclerosing cholangitis. Diagnosis of these conditions should be followed with the appropriate therapy. Chronic fibrosing alveolitis and other interstitial lung disease, including idiopathic pulmonary hemosiderosis, have been reported in association with celiac disease. These conditions should be sought, particularly if celiac patients experience any respiratory problems. There is a known association of celiac disease with inflammatory bowel disease, especially ulcerative proctocolitis. Patients with this complication can be improved with a gluten-free diet and also with either oral salazopyrine or mesalazine and corticosteroid enemas.

Table 1 Conditions Associated with Celiac Disease

Disease	Approximate Reported Incidence (%)
First-degree relative of celiac patients	10
Dermatitis herpetiformis	80–100
IgA deficiency	20
Hyposplenism	100
Aphthous ulceration	5
Cow's milk protein intolerance	10
Small intestinal T-cell lymphoma	15
Thyroid disease	6
Diabetes mellitus	10
Cutaneous vasculitis	U
Fibrosing alveolitis	U
Sjögren's syndrome	U
Polyarteritis	U
Addison's disease	U
Systemic lupus erythematosus	U
Ulcerative colitis	U
Rheumatoid arthritis	U
Idiopathic pulmonary hemosiderosis	U
Glomerulonephritis	U
Schizophrenia	U
Sarcoidosis	U
Histocompatibility antigens HLA-B8, DR3, DQ2 (Northern European population)	98

U = incidence unknown.

DERMATITIS HERPETIFORMIS

Skin disorders in celiac disease are common, including psoriasis, eczema, and pustular dermatitis. Atopic eczema in patients with celiac disease may respond to a gluten-free diet. A number of rare skin disorders have been reported in association with celiac disease, including cutaneous amyloid, cutaneous vasculitis, nodular prurigo, acquired ichthyosis, epidermal necrolysis, pityriasis rubra pilaris, and mycosis fungoides. All should be given the appropriate specific therapy.

Dermatitis herpetiformis complicates 2 to 5 percent of cases of gluten-sensitive enteropathy. All cases of dermatitis herpetiformis exhibit a degree of gluten-sensitive enteropathy, although the precise relationship to celiac disease remains unclear. In some families multiply affected with celiac disease, some members are reported to have dermatitis herpetiformis. This skin condition is characterized by a symmetric, itchy, papular, vesicular eruption, usually affecting the elbows, knees, buttocks, sacrum, face, neck, and trunk and occasionally the mouth. The predominant symptoms are itching and burning, which may be so severe as to cause pain. Because of the severe irritation, patients more commonly present with excoriated papules, often on a background of raised erythematous plaques.

The condition was observed in 1940 to respond to sulfapyridine and subsequently to dapsone, which has become the first-line treatment, at a dose of 50 to 100 mg a day. Patients should also be advised to take a strict gluten-free diet, as this results in a significant improvement after 6 to 12 months and permits a reduction in the dose of, or elimination of the need for, dapsone. Months or years are normally needed for the full benefit of a gluten-free diet to be obtained. For this reason, many patients are unwilling to accept the diet. However, it is worth explaining to them that continuation of a strict gluten-free diet will eventually allow them to reduce and subsequently discontinue dapsone therapy, with its possible side effects.

A few individuals are unable to tolerate dapsone because of its side effects, which include a dose-dependent hemolytic anemia, methemoglobinemia, and headache. These patients can alternatively be treated with sulfapyridine, 500 mg three times a day.

ULCERATIVE JEJUNITIS AND LYMPHOMA

Controversy has surrounded the association between lymphoma and celiac disease with respect to the nature of the tumor, the enteropathic process, and the relationship between dietary exposure to gluten and the chances of developing a lymphoma. A common pattern is the return of symptoms of diarrhea, associated with both weight loss and lassitude in a patient with established celiac disease. The diagnostic dilemma with such a return of symptoms in a previously well-controlled patient with adult celiac disease is to distinguish dietary lapses from the development of lymphoma or the possibility of ulcerative ileojejunitis. The latter should be considered as a stage in the potential development of the complicating lymphoma. Manifestations such as fever, lymphadenopathy, hepatomegaly or splenomegaly, or abdominal masses or ascites may help solve the diagnostic conundrum, but these suggest more advanced disease. Rather than having an insidious presentation, acute small intestinal perforation or obstruction, or less commonly gastrointestinal hemorrhage, may present as an acute emergency.

Early diagnosis of lymphoma frequently requires an exploratory laparotomy. Standard small intestinal diagnostic maneuvers, including jejunal biopsy and small bowel barium studies, are likely to have a low yield, even when the lymphoma is suspected, because of the associated subtotal villous atrophy. The histologic appearance of peripheral lymph nodes, the liver or bone marrow may be diagnostic, and lymphangiography, ultrasonography, computed tomography scanning, or nuclear magnetic resonance scanning to detect lymphodenopathy may be positive, although these investigations cannot exclude the diagnosis of early lymphoma. Whether enteroscopy will help in such patients is considered in a separate chapter.

Blood tests are unhelpful. Hypoalbuminemia and a high erythrocyte sedimentation rate may occur, although these tests do not offer any specificity for the diagnosis. Laparotomy therefore becomes an early diagnostic tool at which time resection of suspicious areas of intestine, including full-thickness biopsy of a normal area together with lymph node and liver biopsies, should all be undertaken. Debate continues over whether a splenectomy should be performed.

Patients with celiac disease and ulcerative jejunitis should be advised to continue with a gluten-free diet. However, if they remain ill with severe lassitude or any other problems, they should be referred for surgical resection of the affected area of the small intestine. This frequently results in resolution of the symptoms. Should frank lymphoma be present either in the intestine or elsewhere, the patient should be referred to an oncologist for appropriate chemotherapy.

SUGGESTED READING

Branksi D, Rozen P, Kagnoff MF, eds. Gluten-sensitive enteropathy. Frontiers of gastrointestinal research. Vol 19. London: Karger, 1992.

Ciclitira PJ. Coeliac disease & related disorders and the malignant complications of coeliac disease. In Bouchier I, Hodgson H, eds. gastroenterology: clinical science and practice. London: Bailliere Tindall, WB Saunders, 1993 (in press).

Hagman B, ed. The gluten-free gourmet: living without wheat. New York: Henry Holt, 1990.

Marsh MN. Coeliac disease. Blackwell Scientific Publications, 1992.

APPENDIX

Information about gluten-free products:

Celiac Disease Foundation, PO Box 1265, Studio City, CA 95614-0265

The Canadian Celiac Association, National Office, 6519B Mississauga Road, Mississauga, Ontario, L5N 1A6 (Tel: 416 567-7195)

The UK Coeliac Society, PO Box 220, High Wycombe, Bucks, HP11 2HY, England

Suppliers of gluten-free products:

United States:

Alpineaire Foods, PO Box 926, Nevada City, CA 95959 (Tel: 916 272-1971)

Anglo-Dietetics Ltd, 641 Lancaster Pike, Frazer, PA 19335

Arrowhead Mills, PO Box 2059, Hereford, TX 79045 (Tel: 806 364-0730)

Bickford Flavors, 19007 St Clair Avenue, Cleveland, OH 44117-1001 (Tel: 800 283-8322)

Celiac Cooks, PO Box 728CD, Ramsay, NJ 07446 (Tel: 800 934-0987)

Chicago Dietetics Supply Inc, 405 Shawmut Avenue, La Grange, IL 60525

Cooks Flavoring Co, 3319 Pacific Avenue, Tacoma, WA 98408 (Tel: 206 727-1361)

Cybros Inc, PO Box 851, Waukesha, WI 53187-0851 (Tel: 800 876-2253)

Desoles Nutritional Foods, 2120 Jericho Turnpike, Garden City Park, NY (Tel: 516 742-1818)

Dietary Specialties Inc, PO Box 227, Rochester, NY 14601 (Tel: 800 544-0099)

El Molino Mills, 345 N Baldwin Park Blvd, City of Industry, CA 91746

Ener-G-Foods Inc, PO Box 24723, Seattle, WA 98124-0723 (Tel: 800 331-5222)

Fantastic Foods, 1250 N McDowell Blvd, Petaluma, CA 94954 (Tel: 707 778-7801)

Foodcare Inc, PO Box 40, 205 South Main, Seymour, IL 61875 (Tel: 217 687-5115)

Food for Life Baking Co Inc, 2991 East Doherty Street, Corona, CA 91719 (Tel: 714 279-5090)

G & I Kosher Bakery, 76-10 Main Street, Flushing, NY 11367 (Tel: 718 261-1167)

The Gluten-Free Pantry, PO Box 881, Glastonbury, CT 06033 (Tel: 203 633-3826)

Legumes Plus Inc, PO Box 383, Fairfield, WA 99012 (Tel: 800 845-1349)

Life Force Nutritional Products Inc, PO Box 1317, San Marcos, CA 92069-1317 (Tel: 818 952-4433)

Lundberg Family Farms, PO Box 369, Richvale, CA 95974-0369 (Tel: 916 882-4551)

Mallard Pond Farms, 746 Mallard Pond Drive, Boulder, CO 80303 (Tel: 800 533-2676)

Mrs Leepers Pasta, 11035 Technology Place, Suite 300, San Diego, CA 92127 (Tel: 619 673-0073)

Moore Natural Foods, 5209 SE International Way, Milwaukie, OR 97222 (Tel: 503 654-3215)

Omega Nutrition, 1720 Labounty Road, Ferndale, WA 98248 (Tel: 604 322-3862)

Original Rice-Crust Pizza, PO Box 3608, Chico, CA 95927 (Tel: 800 521-6727)

Pacific Rice Products, PO Box 2060, Woodland, CA 95695 (Tel: 916 662-5056)

Pamela's Products, 136 Utah Avenue, South San Francisco, CA 94080 (Tel: 415 952-4546)

Quinoa Corporation, PO Box 1039, Torrance, CA 90505

The Really Great Food Company, PO Box 319, Malverne, NY 11565 (Tel: 516 593-5587)

Red Mill Farms Inc, 290 South 5th Street, Brooklyn, NY 11211 (Tel: 718 384-2150)

Miss Roben's, 5500 Huntington Parkway, Bethesda, MD 20814 (Tel: 718 384-2150)

Shelton's Poultry, 204 North Loranne Avenue, Pomona, CA 91767 (Tel: 714 623-4361)

Shiloh Farm, PO Box 97, Sulpher Spring, AK 72768

Snackcracks, PO Box 3608, Chico, CA 95927 (Tel: 800 521-6727)

Sterk's Bakery Ltd, MPO Box 2703, Niagara Falls, NY 14302

Tad Enterprises, 9356 Pleasant, Tinley Park, IL 60477 (Tel: 708 429-2101)

Trillium Health Products, 655 South Orcas Street, Seattle, WA 98108 (Tel: 800 800-8455)

Vans International Foods, 1751 W Torrance Blvd, Unit K, Torrance, CA 90501 (Tel: 213 320-8611)

Vita Wheat Baked Products Inc, 11839 Hilton Road, Frendale, MI 48220

Walnut Acres, Penns Creek, PA 17862

White Oaks Farm, 13 Lake Street, Sherborn, MA 01770 (Tel: 508 653-5953)

Canada:

Carol's Gluten-Free Products, Mt Brydges, Ontario (Tel: 519 264-1028)

DE-RO-MA 1983, Food Intolerance Centre, Laval, PQ (Tel: 800 363-3438)

El Peto Products Ltd, Kitchener, Ontario (Tel: 800 387-4064)

Kingsmill Foods Ltd, Toronto, Ontario (Tel: 416 755-1124)

Liv-n-well Distributor's Ltd, Richmond, BC (Tel: 604 270-8474)

Mt Baked Products, London, Ontario (Tel: 519 672-3104)

Nelson David of Canada, St Boniface, MB (Tel: 204 237-9161)

Pastariso Products Inc, 55 Ironside Crescent, Units 6 & 7, Scarborough, Ontario, M1X 1N3 (Tel: 416 321-9090)

Speciality Food Shop, Head Office, 2 Carlton Suite 1310, Toronto, Ontario, M5B 1J3 (Tel: 416 593-5997; Fax: 416 593-6362)

Speciality Food Shop, Radio Centre Plaza, Lower Level Mall, 875 Main Street West, Hamilton, Ontario, L85 4P9 (Tel: 800 268-7010)

Sterk's Bakery Ltd, 3866 23rd Street, Vineland, Ontario, L0R 2C0 (Tel: 416 562-3086)

England:

Cantassium, 225-229 Putney Bridge Road, London, SW15 2PY (Tel: 081 874-1130) (Trufree Products)

Cow & Gate Ltd, Trowbridge, Wilts, BA14 8YX (Tel: 0225-768381) (Glutenex Biscuits)

Farley Health Products, Nottingham, NG2 3AA (Tel: 0602-507431) (Farley's Gluten-free Biscuits)

Food Watch, Butts Pond Industrial Estate, Sturminster Newton, Dorset, DT10 1AZ (Tel: 0258-73356)

General Designs Ltd, PO Box 38E, Worcester Park, Surrey, KT4 7LX (Tel: 081 337-9366) (Ener-G and Pastariso Products)
Grove Fruit Products, Milton Hill, Abingdon, Oxon, OX14 4DP
Kallo Foods Limited, Sunbury on Thames, TW16 7JS (Tel: 081 890-8324) (Kallo Products)
Larkhall Laboratories Ltd, 225 Putney Bridge Road, London, SW15 2PY
The Mustard Shop, 3 Bridewell Alley, Norwich, NR2 1AQ (Genuine Mustard, coded GDSF)

Nutricia Dietary Products Ltd, 494-496 Honeypot Lane, Stanmore, Middlesex, HA7 1JH (Tel: 081 951-5155; Fax: 44 81 951-5623) (GF Dietary, Glutafin, Loprofin, Rite Diet Products)
Scientific Hospital Supplies Ltd, 100 Wavertree Boulevard, Wavertree Technology Park, Liverpool, L7 9PQ (Tel: 051 228-1991) (Juvela Products)
Ultrapharm Ltd, PO Box 18, Henley on Thames, Oxon, RG9 1AW (Tel: 0491-578016) (Aproten, Arnott's Rice Cookies, Schar, Ultra products)

CARBOHYDRATE MALABSORPTION

RICHARD J. GRAND, M.D.
ROBERT K. MONTGOMERY, Ph.D.
HANS A. BÜLLER, M.D.

GENERAL CONCEPTS

Carbohydrate digestion reduces complex nutrients into smaller components suitable for absorption. Starch digestion is accomplished in two phases: an initial intraluminal phase mediated by salivary and pancreatic amylase, and a mucosal phase characterized by surface digestion at the intestinal microvillus membrane. Disaccharides undergo surface hydrolysis followed by uptake of monosaccharides by microvillus membrane carriers.

Carbohydrate Intake

In infants, carbohydrates account for 35 to 55 percent of daily calories ingested, and these are mainly in the form of lactose. As weaning foods are introduced, carbohydrate intake varies and approaches the composition commonly found in adults. The average adult ingests 300 g of carbohydrates per day in approximately the following distribution: 52 percent of daily calories as starch (mainly cereals and potatoes), 37 percent as sucrose, 5 percent as lactose (mainly in milk), and 3 percent as fructose (in fruit and honey). Glycogen, glucose, and maltose are minor constituents of the diet, and cellulose accounts for approximately 4 g of carbohydrates per day.

Digestion

Salivary amylase initiates starch hydrolysis in the mouth, and this process accounts for not more than 30 percent of total starch hydrolysis. As salivary amylase is

Supported in part by National Institutes of Health Research Grant DK 32658; Grant P30 DK 34928 to the Center for Gastroenterology Research on Absorptive and Secretory Processes, New England Medical Center Hospitals, Boston, MA; a grant from Nutricia, Zoetermeer, The Netherlands; and a NATO Collaborative Research Grant.

inactivated by an acid pH, no significant hydrolysis of carbohydrates occurs in the stomach. The intraluminal phase of starch digestion depends on pancreatic amylase to complete hydrolysis, yielding oligosaccharides of varying lengths. This process is extremely rapid; 75 percent is completed in the proximal 2½ feet of jejunum within 10 minutes after passage into the small intestine.

The mucosal phase is characterized by surface digestion of oligosaccharides released by amylase. It also includes hydrolysis of the disaccharides maltose, sucrose, and lactose by specific disaccharidases: maltase-glucoamylase, sucrase, and lactase. The rates of maltose and sucrose hydrolysis are rapid as they are readily cleaved, and the released monosaccharides rapidly absorbed. Lactose digestion is slower, and hydrolysis is the rate-limiting step for the overall process of absorption. The final uptake of monosaccharides is accomplished by the sodium-dependent glucose carrier.

Colonic Salvage

When carbohydrates are not absorbed by the small bowel, they are passed rapidly to the colon as a consequence of the osmolarity of the intraluminal oligosaccharides. In the colon, they are converted to short-chain fatty acids and hydrogen gas by the bacterial flora, producing acetate, butyrate, and propionate. The short-chain fatty acids are absorbed by the colonic mucosa, and this route salvages malabsorbed carbohydrates for energy use. This is a mechanism by which the adult colon salvages carbohydrate, especially from wheat starch, and the newborn colon salvages lactose. This fermentative process not only conserves nutritionally important carbohydrate, but also serves as the basis for the breath hydrogen test (discussed below).

SYMPTOMS AND SIGNS OF CARBOHYDRATE MALABSORPTION

In considering clinical symptoms induced by the ingestion of carbohydrates, the term *carbohydrate intolerance* is often applied. This is characterized by abdominal pain, cramps or distention, nausea, flatulence, and diarrhea or vomiting. The abdominal pain may be crampy in nature and may be periumbilical or lower quadrant. Borborygmi may be audible on physical examination and to the patient. Carbohydrate intolerance generally produces abnormal stools, which are usually bulky, frothy, and watery. In severe cases, mostly in infants, acidosis and dehydration may be a problem. Vomiting after lactose ingestion is often seen in adolescents.

Several factors account for the variability of symptoms produced by carbohydrate ingestion in people who are intolerant. This pathophysiology is of particular importance in those with lactose intolerance accompanying low lactase activity, but similar mechanisms apply to people with sucrose intolerance or other sugar intolerances, and those with intraluminal phase defects in carbohydrate digestion. Important factors include the osmolarity and fat content of the food in which the sugar is ingested, the rate of gastric emptying, sensitivity to intestinal distention produced by the osmotic load of unhydrolyzed carbohydrate in the upper small bowel, the rate of intestinal transit, and the response of the colon to the carbohydrate load. In general, the higher the osmolarity of gastric contents and the higher the fat content of the diet containing the specific sugar involved, the slower the gastric emptying and the lesser the symptoms induced by sugar. Different individuals appear to have more or less sensitivity to abdominal distention and complain differently when ingested carbohydrates stimulate an influx of water into the lumen of the small intestine, or when the production of gas leads to distention of the colon.* Patients with greater tolerance report fewer symptoms. These subjective responses are difficult to quantify. Intestinal transit is also influenced by the quality of the diet and individual motility patterns. Accordingly, some lactose- or sucrose-intolerant people experience very rapid movement of sugar to the cecum, while others have slower motility. Fecal flora are known to adapt to digested carbohydrate. Thus, if carbohydrates are provided slowly over a long period in many "intolerant" people, the flora may adapt to the load, and symptoms produced by gas and acid in the colon may be reduced or eliminated. This mechanism of lactose tolerance in people with low lactase levels accounts for the discrepancy between "lactase deficiency" and lactose intolerance.†

The term *carbohydrate malabsorption* is generally reserved for patients for whom the intestinal malabsorption of sugar or complex carbohydrates has been investigated using an appropriate test of absorption (e.g., lactose or sucrose absorption test) or malabsorption (lactose or sucrose breath hydrogen test, or breath hydrogen production after the ingestion of complex carbohydrate). Carbohydrate malabsorption may be due to pancreatic insufficiency with impairment of the

intraluminal phase of starch digestion, or to disaccharidase deficiency characterized by an absence or very low levels of specific microvillus membrane enzymes.

CONFIRMATORY TESTS

The diagnosis of carbohydrate malabsorption is based on the combination of clinical findings and results of appropriate tests. The presence of low fecal pH or reducing substances indicates carbohydrate malabsorption, but these tests are valid only when carbohydrate has been ingested, intestinal transit time is rapid, stools are collected fresh, and assays are performed immediately and when bacterial metabolism of colonic carbohydrate is incomplete. In general, carbohydrate malabsorption is best confirmed by means of more specific tests, especially as sucrose is a nonreducing sugar and requires special techniques for detection in stool.

The capacity for sugar absorption can be measured using a lactose or sucrose (tolerance) absorption test. In adults, it has a sensitivity of 75 percent and a specificity of 96 percent. However, in children as well as in adults, oral tolerance tests are cumbersome, invasive, and time-consuming and have largely been replaced by the breath hydrogen test.

This test really measures carbohydrate nonabsorption, rather than carbohydrate hydrolysis and monosaccharide uptake. Its sensitivity and specificity are superior to those for absorption tests, and it is simple and noninvasive. The breath hydrogen test can be performed in people of all ages. The dose is customarily 2 g of carbohydrate per kilogram body weight (maximum, 50 g in adults). Breath hydrogen is sampled before ingestion of sugar, and at 30 minute intervals after ingestion of sugar for 3 hours. We customarily use a value of Δ 10 parts per million as normal, comparing samples obtained after carbohydrate ingestion to the baseline value. Values between Δ 10 and 20 parts per million may be indeterminate unless accompanied by symptoms, but values over Δ 20 parts per million are representative of carbohydrate malabsorption. False-positive test results are seen with inadequate pretest fasting or when the patient has smoked recently, and false-negative results are obtained when patients have recently used antibiotics or are nonhydrogen producers (approximately 1 to 5 percent of the population). In children under 5 years of age, an abnormal lactose breath hydrogen test result always signifies abnormal intestinal mucosa or bacterial overgrowth, both of which require further definition by appropriate diagnostic tests. A normal breath hydrogen test does not rule out an intestinal mucosal lesion and cannot be used to avoid an intestinal biopsy. The glucose breath hydrogen test can be used for the diagnosis of bacterial overgrowth syndromes.

The assay of disaccharidase activity in small bowel biopsy samples establishes the presence of disaccharidase deficiency and has been used to define populations at risk for low lactase levels. However, when low lactase activity accompanies intestinal injury, the lesion may be

---

*Editor's Note: Since intestinal distention is not well tolerated by patients with irritable bowel syndrome (IBS), it is not surprising that IBS patients are often among those most "sensitive" to unabsorbed carbohydrates.

†Editor's Note: In the past, we usually reserved the term *lactose intolerance* for those symptomatic with some quantity of lactose, commonly 50 g in adults.

focal or patchy; consequently, intestinal biopsy samples may not yield an abnormal result. Clinical and biochemical data must always be compared to obtain the correct diagnosis.

APPROACH TO THE PATIENT

Patients who have symptoms and signs of carbohydrate malabsorption should be evaluated in a systematic fashion (Table 1). The clinical findings may not immediately suggest a diagnosis of carbohydrate malabsorption, as many patients with this diagnosis actually have a clinical pattern more like that seen in irritable bowel syndrome (IBS). Secondary causes of carbohydrate malabsorption must be sought and appropriate confirmatory tests obtained. When considering lactose malabsorption, especially in infants and young children, the possibility of milk protein allergy must be ruled out.

It is important to remember that lactose malabsorption may occur in patients with other disorders (e.g., IBS); thus, a lactose breath hydrogen test for elimination of lactose from the diet should, in some people's minds, be part of the evaluation of patients suspected of having IBS.

Intraluminal Phase Defects

Pancreatic amylase deficiency is seen with hereditary diseases of the exocrine pancreas, particularly cystic fibrosis and Shwachman's syndrome, and with pancreatic insufficiency due to alcohol, and bacterial overgrowth. Most patients with cystic fibrosis have absent or low levels of amylase activity, but their symptoms are usually more attributable to fat than to carbohydrate maldigestion. Shwachman's syndrome, consisting of exocrine pancreatic insufficiency and hematologic and skeletal abnormalities, is the second most common cause of hereditary pancreatic insufficiency in children. Amylase activity is low or absent in such infants and they have diarrhea and malabsorption. Low amylase levels in adults with pancreatic insufficiency are well described, and bacterial overgrowth may produce intraluminal fermentation. Amylase deficiency is generally successfully treated by the administration of pancreatic supplements, achieving virtually complete carbohydrate digestion. There is a chapter on the treatment of pancreatic insufficiency. Bacterial overgrowth syndrome is treated with appropriate antibiotics.

Mucosal Phase Defects

Lactose Malabsorption

Lactose malabsorption occurs in three clinical settings: (1) racial/ethnic lactose malabsorption, (2) developmental lactase deficiency, and (3) congenital lactase deficiency.

Racial/ethnic lactose malabsorption is the most common form of genetically determined reductions of

Table 1 Disorders of Carbohydrate Absorption

Intraluminal phase defects
  Primary
    Cystic fibrosis
    Shwachman's syndrome
  Secondary
    Pancreatic insufficiency due to alcohol
    Bacterial overgrowth

Mucosal phase defects
  Primary
    Lactose
      Racial/ethnic
      Developmental
      Congenital
    Sucrose
      Sucrase isomaltase deficiency
    Glucose-galactose malabsorption
  Secondary
    Bacterial overgorwth
    Mucosal injury
      Infectious enteritis
      Giardiasis
      Celiac sprue
      Drug-induced enteritis
      Inflammatory bowel disease
      Radiation enteritis
    Acquired glucose malabsorption

lactase activity. This clinical finding has been termed *lactase deficiency*, although this term is really a misnomer, as most of the world's populations develop low intestinal lactase levels during mid-childhood (approximately age 5). This finding is most prominent in Asian, African, and indigenous populations (Table 2). Peoples of Scandinavian or Caucasian genetic background have acquired a high degree of lactose tolerance as adults, with preservation of intestinal lactase activity. In the United States, it is customary to expect normal lactase activity in all children until 5 years of age. Lactose intolerance detected in children before this age usually indicates an underlying mucosal lesion or bacterial overgrowth syndrome.

There is no evidence that lactase deficiency or lactose malabsorption is a normal part of the aging process. Thus, in the mixed population of Caucasian extraction, the normal aging process does not lead to lactase deficiency. However, alterations in motility secondary to other disorders, or intestinal injury, may produce lactose intolerance.

Developmental lactose malabsorption is a consequence of gestational age. During fetal development, lactase activity rises late in gestation, so that 28 to 32 week premature infants have reduced lactase activity. If they are otherwise healthy, the colon can salvage unabsorbed carbohydrate so that these infants are not nutritionally compromised and do not have diarrhea.

Primary lactase deficiency is characterized by the absence of lactase activity in the small intestine, normal histologic appearance, and normal levels of other disaccharidases. This is a very rare syndrome associated with diarrhea from birth in affected infants.

Table 2 Distribution of Lactase Phenotypes in Selected Populations

United States		Europe		
Population	Low Lactase (%)	Country	Population	Low Lactase (%)
Northern European	7	Sweden	Swedes	1
Whites	22	Netherlands	Dutch	0
African Americans	65	Austria	Austrians	20
American Indians	95	France	French	32
Vietnamese	100		Southern Franch	44
		Italy	Northern Italians	50
			Southern Italians	72
			Sicilians	71

Data from Montgomery R, Buller HA, Rings EHHM, et al. Lactose intolerance and regulation of small intestine lactase activity. In: Berdanier CD, Hargrove JL, eds. Nutrition and gene expression. Boca Raton: CRC Press, 1992: 23–53; with permission.

Treatment. The treatment of lactose malabsorption includes four general principles: (1) reduction or restriction of dietary lactose, (2) substitution of alternative nutrient sources to avoid reduction in energy and protein intake, (3) regulation of calcium intake, and (4) use of a commercially available enzyme substitute. When lactose restriction is necessary, the patient must be instructed to read labels of commercially prepared foods, because hidden lactose may be difficult to identify. Table 3 summarizes the lactose content of selected foods. Complete restriction of lactose-containing foods should be necessary only for a limited period to ascertain the specificity of the diagnosis. As some patients can tolerate graded increases in lactose intake, small quantities of lactose may subsequently be reintroduced into the diet, careful attention being paid to associated symptoms. Because of its high sugar and fat content, ice cream may be a good way to introduce lactose into the diet. Calcium is supplemented in the form of calcium carbonate; "Tums" is popular and effective. Standard preparations contain 500 mg of calcium carbonate, equivalent to 200 mg of elemental calcium, which is 20 percent of the USRDA (U.S. recommended daily allowance) for adults. In infants and young children, liquid calcium gluconate is readily tolerated and available. When complete lactose restriction is recommended, the RDA for calcium should be provided as a supplement.

Commercially available "lactase" preparations are actually bacterial or yeast beta-galactosidases. When added to lactose-containing food or when ingested with meals containing lactose, these are effective in reducing symptoms and breath hydrogen values in many lactose-intolerant subjects. However, these products are not capable of completely hydrolyzing all dietary lactose, and the results achieved in individual patients are variable. Some of the commercial "lactase" preparations are listed in Table 4. LactAid liquid may be added to milk (14 drops per quart), which is then refrigerated overnight before use. The resulting hydrolysis of lactose (which is approximately 90 percent effective) produces a sweeter taste than milk containing lactose. Lactrase capsules may

Table 3 Lactose Content of Selected Foods

Product	Unit	Lactose (approx. g/unit)
Milk	1 cup (244 g)	11
Low-fat milk, 2% fat	1 cup (244 g)	9–13
Skim milk	1 cup (244 g)	12–14
Nonfat dry milk, instant	1-½ cup (91 g)	46
Whipped cream topping	1 tbs (3 g)	0.4
Light cream	1 tbs (15 g)	0.6
Cheese		
Cheddar	1 oz (28 g)	0.4–0.6
Cream	1 oz (28 g)	0.8
Parmesan, grated	1 oz (28 g)	0.8
Cheese, pasteurized, processed		
American	1 oz (28 g)	0.5
Swiss	1 oz (28 g)	0.4–0.6
Cottage cheese	1 cup (210 g)	5–6
Ice cream		
Vanilla, regular	1 cup (133 g)	9
Sherbet, orange	1 cup (193 g)	4
Ice, orange	100 g	0

Modified from Hyams JS. Carbohydrate malabsorption. In: Bayless T, ed. Current therapy in gastroenterology and liver disease. 3rd ed. Philadelphia: BC Decker, 1990:266.

Table 4 Some Commercial "Lactase" Substitutes

Name	Dose Form	Supplier
LactAid	Liquid/tablets	LactAid, Inc.
Lactrase	Capsules	Kremers-Urban
LactAce	Capsules	Nature's Way Products, Inc.
DairyEase	Tablets	Glenbrook Laboratories
Lactrol	Caplets	Advanced Nutritional Technology

be taken orally with lactose-containing foods, as can the other products listed in Table 4, but the individual dosage required and responses to individual products must be tested in each patient. It should be noted that "acidophilus milk" is not sufficiently lactose depleted. Live culture yogurt, which contains endogenous beta-galactosidase, is a useful alternative source for calcium and calories and may be well tolerated by some lactose-intolerant patients. However, yogurts that contain milk products added back after fermentation, such as most frozen yogurts, may produce symptoms. While consumption of yogurt alone by low-lactose individuals reduces symptoms, consumption of yogurt together with additional lactose does not do so.

Sucrose Malabsorption

Sucrase isomaltase deficiency is an uncommon autosomal recessive disorder. Sucrose intolerance presents at different ages. In infants, symptoms may appear when sucrose is introduced into the diet; in younger children, chronic diarrhea may occur alternating with constipation and confusing the diagnosis. Occasionally, the first manifestations appear in adulthood with complaints of carbohydrate malabsorption, or may mimic IBS. The diagnosis is most easily achieved by means of the sucrose breath hydrogen test. Treatment is accomplished by restriction of dietary sucrose. Some studies that describe provision of exogenous sucrase activity using viable yeast cells *(Saccharomyces cerevisiae)* may assist in sucrose tolerance.

Glucose Galactose Malabsorption

This is a rare disorder detected in neonates who develop diarrhea with ascitic stools and who have fecal-reducing substances present after the first feeding of glucose water. The diagnosis in these patients can be confirmed with a flat glucose and a normal fructose tolerance test. The diagnosis can be confirmed in vitro by measurement of glucose transport in small bowel biopsy or by intraluminal perfusion.

Fructose Malabsorption

Fructose malabsorption (Table 5) is uncommon. However, the ingestion of large amounts of fructose (particularly in the form of fruit juices) by infants and young children may lead to diarrhea and symptoms of carbohydrate malabsorption because of an ingested load of fructose in excess of the capacity of the small intestine to absorb the sugar. Fruit juice ingestion by infants and young children may produce the syndrome of "chronic nonspecific diarrhea" or "toddler's diarrhea" and can be rapidly reversed by reducing dietary fructose.

The sugar alcohol of fructose (sorbitol) (Table 6) is not well tolerated by most people. It is poorly absorbed in the small intestine and its transport to the colon may be associated with symptoms of carbohydrate malabsorption. Sorbitol can be found in "dietary" products such as chewing gums and "low-sugar" fruits and fruit juices. In the appropriate clinical setting, a search for sorbitol-containing foods in the diet and elimination of offending substances may lead to resolution of symptoms.

Table 5 Fructose Content of Foods

Figs*	30.9†
Dates*	23.9†
Prunes*	15.0†
Grapes*	8.0†
Soft drinks containing high-fructose syrup	37.5‡

*Dried.
†Per 100 g edible portion.
‡Per 18–19 oz of soda.
From Ravich WJ, Bayless TM, et al. Fructose: incomplete intestinal absorption in humans. Gastroenterology 1983; 84:26; with permission.

Table 6 Sorbitol Content of "Sugar-Free" Products and Various Foods

"Sugar-free" gum	1.3–2.2 g/piece
"Sugar-free" mints	1.7–2.0 g/piece
Pears	4.6*
Prunes	2.4*
Peaches	1.0*
Apple juice	0.5*
Pear juice	2.0*

*Grams of sorbitol per 100 g dry matter or 100 g juice. Dry weight equals 15% of fresh weight.
From Hyams JS. Sorbitol intolerance: an unappreciated cause of functional gastrointestinal complaints. Gastroenterology 1983; 84:30; and Hyams JS, et al. Carbohydrate malabsorption following fruit juice ingestion in young children. Pediatrics 1988; 82:64; with permission.

Secondary Carbohydrate Malabsorption

Bacterial overgrowth or stasis syndromes may be associated with increased fermentation of dietary carbohydrates in the small bowel. Clinical symptoms of carbohydrate intolerance are often found. The diagnosis may be suspected when a very early peak of breath hydrogen is detected during a carbohydrate challenge.

Carbohydrate malabsorption frequently occurs after mucosal injury of the gastrointestinal tract, causing villus flattening or damage to the intestinal epithelium. Disorders that often produce this lesion are listed in Table 1. When the mucosa is damaged, lactase is usually the first affected disaccharidase, presumably because of its distal location on the villus. Treatment of the primary disorder is mandatory for the return of lactase activity, which often lags behind the return of normal intestinal structure. Prolonged lactose intolerance, which may persist for months after healing starts, is unique to this disaccharidase, and its biochemical basis is unexplained.

Secondary sucrase isomaltase deficiency is usually of less clinical significance than lactase deficiency. Enzyme activity is not totally lost and usually does not reach the low levels of primary sucrase isomaltase deficiency; thus, patients tend to tolerate some sucrose intake. Maltase-glucoamylase deficiency is related to the severity of the mucosal lesion and is usually of minimal clinical significance in most patients.

The principles of treatment for carbohydrate malabsorption in patients with secondary disorders are identical to those for the primary disorders in addition to therapy for the underlying problem.

MISCELLANEOUS OBSERVATIONS

Patients demonstrating symptoms compatible with a diagnosis of carbohydrate malabsorption, but for whom specific testing fails to reveal an abnormality, may have symptoms related to starch ingestion. A careful dietary history should be obtained and appropriate breath hydrogen testing performed. The custom of eating extremely-high-fiber foods may predispose some people to symptomatic carbohydrate malabsorption. Flatulence associated with ingestion of a variety of beans and other vegetables considered to be gas producing may be somewhat relieved by the use of a new commercial product, Beano.

Patients whose main complaints are increased flatulence may or may not have carbohydrate malabsorption, but this possibility should be ruled out by appropriate testing. Swallowed air also may lead to flatulence, but air swallowing is more often accompanied by excessive belching. The ingestion of large quantities of air may be due to psychogenic factors, to crying in infants, to gum chewing, or to the consumption of carbonated drinks. Appropriate dietary recommendations may lead to resolution of symptoms.*

---

*Editor's Note: Since unabsorbed carbohydrates are the main source of short-chain fatty acids, a major energy source for the left colon, it is possible that in the future we may want to feed some poorly absorbed carbohydrates to patients with ulcerative colitis. This might supplement short-chain fatty acid enemas.

SUGGESTED READING

Büller HA, Grand RJ. Lactose intolerance. In: Creger WP, Coggins CH, Hancock EW, eds. Annual review of medicine: selected topics in the clinical sciences. Vol 41. Palo Alto: Annual Reviews, 1990:141–148.

Corazza GR, Strocchi A, Rossi R, et al. Sorbitol malabsorption in normal volunteers and in patients with coeliac disease. Gut 1988; 29:44–48.

Escher JC, de Koning ND, van Engen CGJ, et al. Molecular basis of lactase levels in adult humans. J Clin Invest 1991; 89:480–483.

Harms HK, Bertele-Harms RM, Bruer-Kleis D. Enzyme-substitution therapy with the yeast Saccharomyces cerevisiae in congenital sucrase-isomaltase deficiency. N Engl J Med 1987; 316:1306–1309.

Hoekstra JH, van Kempen AAMW, Kneepkens CMF. Apple juice malabsorption: fructose or sorbitol? J Pediatr Gastroenterol Nutr 1993; 16:39–42.

Mobassaleh M, Montgomery RK, Biller JA, Grand RJ. Development of carbohydrate absorption in the fetus and newborn. Pediatrics 1985; 75(Suppl):160–166.

Montgomery R, Büller HA, Rings EHHM, et al. Lactose intolerance and regulation of small intestine lactase activity. In: Berdanier CD, Hargrove JL, eds. Nutrition and gene expression. Boca Raton: CRC Press, 1992: 23–53.

Rosado JL, Solomons NW, Lisker R, et al. Enzyme replacement therapy for primary adult lactase deficiency. Effective reduction of lactose malabsorption and milk intolerance by direct addition of beta-galactosidase to milk at mealtime. Gastroenterology 1984; 87:1072–1082.

INTESTINAL PSEUDO-OBSTRUCTION AND OTHER NEUROMUSCULAR DISORDERS

MICHAEL CAMILLERI, M.D.

Motility disorders resulting from abnormal neuromuscular function in the digestive tract are increasingly being recognized because of greater awareness on the part of clinicians and improved diagnostic methods. New therapeutic approaches have provided an added incentive to diagnose these disorders.

These disorders typically present with stasis of content within the regions affected. Esophageal involvement results in dysphagia or odynophagia; hypotensive or hypocontractile lower esophageal sphincter function results in gastroesophageal reflux disease, a frequent complication of progressive systemic sclerosis. Gastroparesis and chronic intestinal pseudo-obstruction produce nausea, vomiting, bloating, distention, early satiety, and diffuse abdominal pain. In the more severe expression of these disorders, the clinical picture may simulate obstruction, but no mechanical factor (e.g., stricture) can be identified radiologically. Colonic inertia results in intractable constipation, despite the usual treatments such as bulk, osmotic, or stimulant laxatives.

In general, these disorders are difficult to treat, and a caring sympathetic attitude goes a long way to reassure the patient of the physician's commitment to provide relief despite the adversities encountered.

PRELIMINARY CONSIDERATIONS IN PLANNING THERAPY

There are four questions to be considered in the first approach to the patient. First, is there an acute or

Table 1 Examples of Categories of Chronic Intestinal Pseudo-obstruction

	Myopathic	*Neuropathic*
Infiltrative	Progressive systemic sclerosis (PSS)	Early PSS
	Amyloidosis	Amyloidosis
Familial	Familial visceral myopathies (autosomal dominant/ recessive)	Familial visceral neuropathies
General neurologic diseases	Myotonic and other dystrophies	Diabetes
		Porphyria
		Brainstem tumor
		Multiple sclerosis
		Spinal cord transection
Infectious		Chagas' disease
		Cytomegalovirus
Drug-induced		Tricyclic anti-depressants
		Narcotic bowel syndrome
Neoplastic		Paraneoplastic (bronchial small cell carcinoma)

From Camilleri M. Medical treatment of chronic intestinal pseudo-obstruction. Pract Gastroenterol 1991; 15:10–22; with permission.

chronic problem? Second, is the disease due to a neuropathy or a myopathy? Third, what is the patient's state of hydration and nutrition? Finally, which regions of the digestive tract are affected?

Identification of neuropathic or myopathic pathophysiology starts with the clinician's search for an underlying endocrine, metabolic, or collagen vascular disease such as hypothyroidism, hyperparathyroidism, or progressive systemic sclerosis (Table 1). The presence of pupillary, autonomic, cranial, or peripheral nerve abnormalities suggests that a neurologic disorder may be affecting the extrinsic neural control of the gut. A careful history of concomitant medication use may identify the factor causing or aggravating the motility disorder. Mechanical obstruction should be excluded by barium radiography or endoscopy. Endoscopy is particularly useful in the esophagus or stomach, where dilatation is rarely needed but may be therapeutic. Colonoscopy helps to rule out mechanical obstruction. Transit measurements (usually by radiopaque markers in the colon or by scintigraphy in other regions) quantitate the degree of stasis. Multilumen manometry or solid-state transducers mounted on a tube currently provide the best nonoperative methods to document the underlying pathophysiologic process. Normal amplitude but incoordinated contractions suggest a neuropathic process; low-amplitude pressure profiles suggest a myopathic process. Mechanical obstruction of the intestine may be suspected if there are characteristic, nonpropagated, prolonged phasic contractions in the upper small bowel. Laparotomy merely to obtain a full-thickness biopsy is avoided in order to reduce the risk of subsequent adhesive obstructions.*

TREATMENT

Acute Intestinal Pseudo-Obstruction

Three general approaches should be instituted when this acute intestinal pseudo-obstruction is diagnosed: correction of potential etiologic factors, decompression, and prokinetic medications. This involves restoration of normal circulating potassium and calcium levels, and withdrawal of medications such as anticholinergics, alpha$_2$-adrenergic agonists, or calcium channel blockers. Decompression of the upper digestive tract is achieved by a nasogastric or nasojejunal tube. There is no evidence that longer tubes decompress more efficiently. Colonic decompression is performed initially by colonoscopy; there is no definite guideline to determine when decompression should be carried out. However, the consensus is that the risk of ischemic injury and perforation of the colon appears to increase when its diameter exceeds 15 cm. Hence, decompression is indicated when this diameter is reached or when sequential radiographs show progressive dilatation that is likely to reach that dimension. At the time of colonoscopy, a soft-tipped, Teflon-coated guidewire is inserted into the proximal colon, and a colonic decompression tube with multiple sideholes is introduced along the guidewire. The tube's position is then checked by fluoroscopy or abdominal radiography and any kinks in the tube are removed.

There is anecdotal evidence, usually based on single case reports, that prokinetic medications accelerate the resolution of acute intestinal pseudo-obstruction (Table 2). Thus, intravenous cisapride (10 to 20 mg every 8 hours), neostigmine (0.5 mg every 4 to 8 hours), and erythromycin (200 mg every 8 hours) may be useful adjuncts to decompression or a wait-and-see policy.

Chronic Intestinal Pseudo-Obstruction

The principal methods of management are (1) correction of hydration, electrolyte depletion, and nutritional deficiencies; (2) prokinetic agents; (3) suppression of bacterial overgrowth; (4) decompression; and (5) consideration of surgical treatment (Table 3).

Correction of Dehydration and Electrolyte Depletion

This is particularly important during acute exacerbations of chronic pseudo-obstruction syndromes. Nutritional support is tailored according to the severity of the deficiencies and of the motility disorder. Trace element and dietary deficiencies may complicate small

---

***Editor's Note:** Also, some patients with scleroderma have had a prolonged period of pseudo-obstruction after surgery, sometimes lasting weeks.

Table 2 Medications Available for Gastric and Small Intestinal Motility Disorders

Drug	Usual Dose	Clinical Efficacy	
		Acute	Chronic
Stasis			
Metoclopramide	10–20 mg t.i.d.	+	−
Bethanechol	10–25 mg t.i.d.	±	−
Erythromycin	125–500 mg t.i.d.	+	−
Cisapride	10–20 mg t.i.d.	+	±
SC octreotide	50 μg h.s.	±	?
Accelerated transit			
Codeine	30–60 mg q.i.d.	+	+
Loperamide	2–4 mg q.i.d.	+	+
Diphenoxylate	5 mg q.i.d.	+	+
Clonidine	0.1–0.2 mg q.d.	+	+
SC octreotide	50–500 μg t.i.d.	+	±

+ = yes; − = no; ± = equivocal; SC = subcutaneous;
Adapted from Prather CM, Camilleri M. Medical management of small bowel motilities disorders and chronic intestinal pseudo-obstruction. Pract Gastroenterol 1992; 16:25–37; with permission.

Table 3 Principles of Medical Treatment of Chronic Intestinal Pseudo-Obstruction

Correction of dehydration and electrolyte depeletion
Nutrition: oral, enteral, or parenteral
Stimulation of propulsion
Treatment of complications, e.g., bacterial overgrowth
Decompression
Consideration of surgical treatment

From Camilleri M. Medical treatment of chronic intestinal pseudo-obstruction. Pract Gastroenterol 1991; 15:10–22; with permission.

bowel motility disorders and require correction. Dietary measures include the use of low-fiber, polypeptide, or hydrolyzed protein supplements as well as provision of recommended intakes of iron, folate, calcium, and vitamins D, K, and B_{12}. In patients with more severe symptoms, these supplements may have to be delivered by a feeding tube inserted into the small bowel. A 48 to 72 hour trial of nasojejunal feeding at up to 80 ml per hour is first performed. In my experience, percutaneous endoscopic jejunostomy tubes are associated with more practical problems than direct jejunostomy tubes inserted at minilaparotomy. Hence, I choose to place operatively any tubes that I anticipate will be needed for more than 3 months. An added advantage of this approach is that it also allows for a full-thickness biopsy of small intestine to be taken for histologic examination.

In the most severe small bowel motility disorders, usually those with hollow visceral myopathy or extensive involvement with progressive systemic sclerosis, parenteral nutrition is often necessary, although many patients continue to tolerate some oral feeding.

Prokinetic Agents

These agents are being increasingly used for neuromuscular motility disorders. There is very little evidence that they are effective for myopathic processes, but they should be used, provided they are not associated with adverse effects.

The time-honored but generally ineffective agents bethanechol (cholinergic agonist), neostigmine (cholinesterase inhibitor), and metoclopramide (peripheral cholinomimetic, partial 5-HT$_4$ agonist and dopamine D$_2$ antagonist) have been replaced by a new generation of agents that have less side effects and greater efficacy (see Table 2).

Cisapride, a substituted benzamide with peripheral cholinomimetic and 5-HT$_4$ agonist actions but no central or hormonal side effects, is probably the best prokinetic agent available at the present time. It stimulates transit at all levels of the digestive tract and has an excellent side effect profile. Although its use is associated with tachyphylaxis, there is documented efficacy in both double-blind, medium-term trials (4 to 8 weeks) and prolonged open treatment trials (1 year). Clinical experience suggests that, despite tachyphylaxis, a 2 to 3 week "drug holiday" may restore its efficacy. Cisapride may induce abdominal cramping or increased bowel movements, but these rarely necessitate cessation of the drug. It was recently approved by the Food and Drug Administration for use in patients with reflux esophagitis. The usual dosage is 10 to 20 mg three times a day and every bedtime.

The dopamine D$_2$ antagonist domperidone does not cross the blood-brain barrier (unlike metoclopramide), but its clinical efficacy appears limited to mild motility disorders.

Erythromycin, a macrolide antibiotic that stimulates motilin and probably cholinergic receptors, has been shown to induce dumping of solids from the stomach, to stimulate gastric emptying in a variety of gastric motility disorders, and to have some efficacy in a small trial in chronic intestinal pseudo-obstruction. Tachyphylaxis and gastrointestinal (GI) upset preclude its use beyond 10 to 15 days. It is best used as a GI motor stimulant for acute exacerbations of chronic motility disorders, typically when the patient requires hospitalization for correction of hydration and electrolyte depletion. The usual dosage is 3 mg per kilogram by infusion every 8 hours; when the patient can tolerate oral feedings, oral erythromycin, 200 mg three times a day, is given 30 minutes before meals. After about 1 week's treatment with erythromycin, an alternative prokinetic (e.g., cisapride) is administered.*

Octreotide, a synthetic cyclized somatostatin analog, induces pressure profiles that resemble interdigestive motor complexes in the small intestine and has been proposed as a potential treatment for patients with small bowel scleroderma. The initial report in the literature requires confirmation; specifically, its effects on the more advanced and more commonly encountered myopathic stage of small bowel scleroderma require careful evaluation. The usual dosage is 50 µg subcutaneously at bedtime. Higher doses may aggravate steatorrhea by inhibiting pancreatic exocrine function; chronic use may also result in gallstone formation.

Chronic constipation in these neuromuscular disorders often requires combination approaches with bulk formers, osmotic laxatives (e.g., lactulose, 30 ml twice a day), and stimulant laxatives (e.g., bisacodyl) or prokinetic agents (e.g., cisapride). Judicious use of enemas (soap and water or Fleets) is also indicated to induce one bowel movement per week.

Suppression of Bacterial Overgrowth

Broad-spectrum antibiotics (e.g., doxycycline, metronidazole, ciprofloxacin) provide symptomatic relief, particularly in patients who have fat malabsorption associated with bacterial overgrowth.

Decompression

Decompression is rarely necessary for chronic pseudo-obstruction. Venting enterostomy creates an effective means to relieve gaseous distention and bloating, and significantly reduces the frequency of nasogastric intubations or hospitalizations for acute exacerbations in patients with severe pseudo-obstruction requiring central parenteral nutrition.

Surgical Treatment

Surgery should be considered whenever the motility disorder is localized or the portion of gut affected is resectable. In clinical practice, the three situations most commonly amenable to surgical therapy are (1) colectomy with ileoproctostomy for severe, intractable, idiopathic constipation when pelvic floor function is normal; (2) duodenojejunostomy for megaduodenum; and (3)

completion gastrectomy for patients with post–gastric surgery stasis syndrome. A word of caution is warranted, since motility disorders are often more generalized than is apparent from patient symptoms, and this may lead to "recurrence" postoperatively. Surgical treatment is also mandatory when a complication such as perforation, stricture, internal herniation, or volvulus is demonstrated in patients with a known underlying motility disorder. Surgical relief may significantly affect the patient's symptoms and tolerance of oral nutrition. Intestinal pacing and small bowel transplantation remain experimental procedures at present but may become viable options in the future.

ESOPHAGEAL DYSFUNCTIONS IN NEUROMUSCULAR DISEASES

Two issues require special comment. Several neurologic disorders (e.g., brainstem strokes, amyotrophic lateral sclerosis) result in pharyngeal and upper esophageal dysfunction causing transfer dysphagia. Rehabilitation by a swallowing education program is not always successful, and percutaneous endoscopic gastrostomy is a useful alternative to overcome tracheal aspiration and nutritional depletion that result from transfer dysphagia.

Reflux disease in progressive systemic sclerosis requires an aggressive, multifaceted approach with antacid regimens, including histamine H_2-receptor antagonists, proton-pump inhibitors (e.g., omeprazole, 20 mg twice a day), and possible addition of a prokinetic agent (e.g., cisapride, 10 to 20 mg three times a day) to enhance esophageal clearance. Reflux strictures may require endoscopic dilatation. Surgical correction of reflux by fundoplication should be approached cautiously, since a tight wrap may result in intractable dysphagia.

Editor's Note: The dramatic reports of intestinal pseudo-obstruction in association with small cell carcinoma of the lung (Sodhi N, et al. Dig Dis Sci 1989; 34:1937–1942) should be kept in mind. These patients had enteric plexus autoantibodies (Lennon VA, et al. Gastroenterology 1991; 100:137–142).

SUGGESTED READING

Camilleri M. Disorders of gastrointestinal motility in neurologic diseases. Mayo Clin Proc 1990; 65:825–846.
Camilleri M. A guide to the treatment of GI motility disorders. Drug Ther 1991; 21:15–28.
Camilleri M. The current role of erythromycin in the clinical management of gastric emptying disorders (editorial). Am J Gastroenterol 1993; 88:169–171.
Camilleri M, Phillips SF. Acute and chronic intestinal pseudo-obstruction. Adv Intern Med 1990; 36:287–306.
Krishnamurthy S, Schuffler MD. Pathology of neuromuscular disorders of the small intestine and colon. Gastroenterology 1987; 93:610–639.
Schuffler MD. Chronic intestinal pseudo-obstruction syndromes. Med Clin North Am 1981; 65:1331–1358.
Soudah HC, Hasler WL, Owyang C. Effect of octreotide on intestinal motility and bacterial overgrowth in scleroderma. N Engl J Med 1991; 325:1461–1467.

****Editor's Note:** There are some reports of smaller doses of erythromycin (50 mg) working in the small bowel, while larger doses are more effective in the stomach. Dr. Marvin Schuster describes using ½ tsp of EryPed 200 syrup. He also mentions that low doses (70 mg) have some effect on the stomach.

SHORT BOWEL SYNDROME

A. J. RATE , F.R.C.S.
MILES IRVING , M.D., F.R.C.S.

Intestinal failure may be defined as the reduction of functioning gut mass below the minimal amount necessary for adequate digestion and absorption of nutrients. One of the major causes of this is the short bowel syndrome (SBS).*

In adults, small bowel function remains satisfactory if over 2 m of healthy small bowel remains. If less than 60 to 80 cm of healthy small bowel is left, adequate function is unlikely unless parenteral fluid or nutrients are given. Function may improve spontaneously as adaptation of the residual bowel occurs.

ETIOLOGY

The causes of SBS are many. In children, the principal causes follow surgery for congenital abnormalities (e.g., atresia, volvulus, or gastroschisis). In adults, SBS is caused by the surgical treatment of Crohn's disease, mesenteric infarction, and a host of less common problems (Table 1). By far the most common cause of SBS is Crohn's disease, so surgery for this condition should be conservative, with resections limited. The use of stricturoplasty to avoid resection should be encouraged.

Factors that influence the degree of physiologic and metabolic disturbance are as follows:

1. *Extent of resection.* The more small bowel resected, the greater is the effect.
2. *Site of resection.* Jejunal resections are tolerated better than ileal resections. The ileum can adapt to perform jejunal function, whereas the jejunum is unable to absorb vitamin B_{12} and bile salts, which have specific active transport sites in the ileum. Motility in the ileum is also slower than in the jejunum, allowing more time for absorption.
3. *Presence of ileocecal valve.* This structure slows intestinal transit and reduces bacterial colonization of the ileum from the colon.
4. *Presence of stomach or colon.* The postgastrectomy syndrome is characterized by diarrhea and occasionally malabsorption. An intact colon can adapt to absorb extra fluid and electrolytes. However, unabsorbed bile salts have a choleretic effect on the colon, causing accentuation of diarrhea and fluid-electrolyte loss.

---

*Editor's Note: Professor Irving and his group direct the largest home TPN service in Great Britain. They are also beginning to evaluate the results of small bowel transplantation in patients with chronic intestinal failure.

Table 1 Causes of Short Bowel Syndrome in Adults

Crohn's disease
Mesenteric infarction (secondary to arterial or venous thrombosis or embolism)
Radiation enteritis
Intestinal volvulus
Trauma
Internal hernias
Multiple fistulas
Small bowel tumors
Morbid obesity (bypass surgery)

5. *Age of patient.* Younger patients usually adapt better (both physically and mentally) to SBS than older patients.
6. *Presence of disease in residual bowel.* This may limit the absorptive and adaptive potential in the residual bowel.

PATHOPHYSIOLOGY

SBS is usually "acquired" suddenly, after massive surgical resection of the small bowel. The pathophysiologic changes that occur result from the sudden loss of absorptive area and the associated reduced intestinal transit time. Maldigestion of food is uncommon, whereas malabsorption of fats, carbohydrates, and proteins is present in various degrees of severity. Carbohydrate absorption is usually less affected than protein or fat absorption; by 6 weeks, it has normally returned to adequate levels in most patients. Protein absorption recovers at a slower rate and is also often at a satisfactory level. However, fat absorption is most severely affected; only a proportion of ingested fat is absorbed after adaptation. The enterohepatic circulation of bile salts is impaired and cannot be fully compensated for by the increased hepatic synthesis of bile salts that occurs in SBS. Other nutrients that may also be malabsorbed in SBS include vitamins (e.g., fat-soluble and B_{12}), trace minerals, and electrolytes (e.g., calcium or magnesium). Lactose intolerance may also be noted, with worsening of the diarrhea after lactose ingestion.

Other pathophysiologic processes occurring in SBS include the following:

1. *Gastric hypersecretion.* Increased gastric acid production is sometimes associated with hypergastrinemia. This is probably due to loss of inhibitory hormones normally produced by the small bowel. The decreased intraluminal pH further impairs lipid digestion, inactivates pancreatic enzymes, and stimulates peristalsis. Within 1 year, this state has usually resolved.
2. *Gallstone formation.* After ileal resections, the reduction in bile salt reabsorption leads to a lithogenic state favouring cholesterol stone formation.
3. *Renal calculus formation.* Renal stones are very

common in SBS. Dehydration reduces the glomerular filtration rate, which leads to production of concentrated urine. This favors stone formation. Oxalate absorption in the presence of an intact colon is high, again conducive to stone formation.

4. *Nephropathy.* In SBS, acid-base and electrolyte imbalance (hyponatremia, hypokalemia, and metabolic acidosis) may all impair renal function.
5. *Liver disease.* Elevation of liver enzymes and serum bilirubin levels is common. This may lead to clinical liver disease, cirrhosis, or even hepatic failure. Bacterial overgrowth in SBS may contribute to this failure.
6. *Metabolic bone disease.* Hypocalcemia, hypomagnesemia, and malabsorption of vitamin D can all lead to osteomalacia and pathologic fractures.
7. *Pancreatic function.* Exocrine function can diminish as a result of reduced levels of secretin and cholecystokinin, normally produced by the small bowel.
8. *Intestinal motility.* Ileogastric reflexes are disturbed and the local enteric control of coordinate peristalsis is affected. This, along with loss of intestinal length, leads to reduced transit times for enteric contents.

ADAPTATION

After resection, adaptation occurs in the residual bowel. Most is seen in the first 6 months, but changes have been shown to continue into the third year after resection. The changes include cellular hyperplasia, villous enlargement, intestinal lengthening and dilatation, altered motility, increased absorptive ability, and increased activity of brush border enzymes. Factors thought responsible for these changes are usually divided as follows:

1. **Luminal:**
   a. *Alimentary secretions.* Pancreaticobiliary secretions cause mucosal hypertrophy. Gastroduodenal secretions may have a role in producing epidermal growth factor, which increases crypt cell production in both the small and large intestine.
   b. *Ingested nutrients.* Sugars, proteins, and fatty acids have direct effects on the intestine to stimulate enzyme production and are trophic to the intestinal villi. These effects are very important in the adaptation process; hence, early introduction of enteral feeding, as soon as the clinical situation allows, is a major stimulus for intestinal adaptation to proceed.
2. **Humoral:** Hormones (e.g., enteroglucagon) are thought to stimulate mucosal growth in SBS.

Adaptation in motility occurs with a tendency toward increased transit time. The mechanisms for this are uncertain but are thought to result from a failure to initiate coordinated peristalsis and from diminished peristaltic contractions. As a result of the adaptation processes, a patient with SBS may have different digestive and absorptive capabilities and therefore require either little or up to total nutritional support. This may range from requiring no dietary restriction to enteral supplements, to electrolyte infusions, to a varying number of days of intravenous (IV) feeding, or to being totally dependent on home parenteral nutrition (HPN). The situation does not remain static: patients may require different degrees of support at different times, as further adaptation continues or as disease progresses.

MANAGEMENT

After massive small bowel resection, the immediate risks to the patient are dehydration and electrolyte imbalance. Patients require IV fluids to keep apace with ongoing losses (diarrhea, stomal or fistula fluid) as well as daily maintenance needs. Assessment of the balance is made by clinical examination; fluid-balance charts (especially monitoring urinary output), supplemented by biochemical analysis of urine and serum electrolytes; and electrolyte analysis of other losses (stomal or fistula fluid). Without this IV therapy, patients quickly become dehydrated, develop hyponatremia, hypokalemia, and oliguria and progress to hypovolemic shock. Acute renal failure will follow, which if sustained will be irreversible and lead to death. During this early period of treatment, total parenteral nutrition (TPN) is usually begun. This is necessary in the short term while intestinal recovery and adaptation occur, but it may also be needed as definitive treatment.

Enteral feeding is introduced as soon as the clinical condition allows. Isotonic sugar-electrolyte solutions are used to maximize absorption. The type and content of enteral feeding thought best for adaptation has undergone many changes. Low-fat diets and changes in the medium- and long-chain triglyceride content have all been advocated. Low-fat diets are less palatable, and now that the fat content is thought to be unimportant, patients should be encouraged to eat what they like.

The most important management of the diarrhea associated with SBS is fluid replacement. IV fluids and enteral sugar-electrolytes are used. When possible, we use a commercially produced oral preparation (Diarolyte). In 1 L of water of this preparation there is 50 mmol of sodium, 20 mmol of potassium, 40 mmol of chloride, 30 mmol of bicarbonate ions, and 111 mmol of glucose. Antidiarrheal agents, such as loperamide (2 mg capsules) first and then codeine, are added in increasing dosages tailored to the response. Cholestyramine (4 g three times a day) can also be used if bile salt malabsorption is thought to be a problem, although this drug is rather unpleasant to take. Gastric secretion can be decreased by using H_2 blockers (cimetidine or ranitidine). Our own preference is for the newer proton-pump inhibitors (omeprazole). The dose is tailored so that the stomal or fistula fluid pH is greater than 6.0. These agents have been shown to reduce the volume of stomal output in SBS. Stomal output can also be increased if patients attempt to quench their thirst by lemonade or fizzy drinks, because of their osmotically active contents. Somatostatin and its analogs (e.g., octreotide) can also be used to reduce diarrhea or stomal output in SBS. A dose of 50 mcg three times daily, intravenously or subcutaneously, is started. In patients who do not respond to the antidiarrheal measures described above, this can be increased to 100 mcg three times daily. The effects appear to have the greatest impact in those patients with the greatest absorptive defect. Absorption is improved, and therefore diarrhea lessened, by slowing intestinal transit. Gastric acid and pancreatic fluid secretion also are both suppressed. This may allow patients to have shorter periods of diarrhea and decreased volumes of parenteral fluids. The antisecretory effects of octreotide appear to be maintained with long-term use. Unfortunately, subcutaneous injections of this drug may be painful, and patients often prefer to do without rather than face repeated injections. Some also develop increasing steatorrhea.

NUTRITION

As mentioned, nutrition should be instituted early in the treatment of SBS. It has been shown that prompt introduction of TPN in SBS prevents early weight loss, achieves a positive nitrogen balance, and improves survival. It is infused via a cuffed central venous catheter, tunneled to the anterior chest wall, at a site accessible for the patient in case training for HPN is necessary. Our preferred method is to insert a silicone, Dacron-cuffed catheter (e.g., Broviac) into the cephalic vein in the deltopectoral groove. This is advanced under radiologic screening to lie in the superior vena cava.

Complications of central venous catheterization and TPN are well known but can be reduced in specialized units with well-motivated medical and nursing staff to acceptable levels. Our current figures for catheter-related complications are one septic episode (line or exit site) per 111 months of HPN, one mechanical occlusion every 148 months of HPN, and one episode of any catheter complication every 5 to 6 months of HPN. The experience in the U.S. program is given in the chapter on parenteral and enteral nutrition.

As adaptation occurs, the total dependence on TPN may subside, with the result that it is possible to reduce the number of days on TPN until IV nutrition or electrolyte infusions are not needed at all. This process can take several years to occur as adaptation develops. Our usual regimen for TPN is a standard glucose-based feed providing 2,000 kcal and 9 g of nitrogen daily. Trace minerals and vitamins are also given, and extra fluid and electrolytes to allow for other losses that occur. Fat solutions are given to avoid fatty acid deficiencies. We infuse 500 ml of a 10 percent fat solution (e.g., Intralipid) twice weekly.

Monitoring of patients is by clinical examination supplemented by biochemical analysis of blood and urine, as described in the earlier chapter on parenteral and enteral nutrition. Weekly 24 hour collections of urine are performed in the early stages to measure sodium and potassium excretion. This often shows evidence of deficiency or overload of these electrolytes before changes occur in serum electrolyte levels.

Home Parenteral Nutrition

HPN is an expensive treatment with well-recognized although largely preventable complications (catheter sepsis and occlusion, metabolic disorders). Therefore, alternative methods to treat SBS that could reduce these risks seem sensible. Most of these involve surgery.*

SURGERY

Surgical intervention is usually responsible for producing SBS by treating the primary condition. This mainly occurs in the context of an immediately life-threatening situation. However, in some situations, careful surgical decisions can limit the severity of the resultant SBS, or can make nursing and patient care easier. Surgical strategy to improve the outcome is primarily directed toward avoidance of any unnecessary resection. When the blood supply to the bowel ends is precarious, exteriorization of the bowel ends producing stomas is much safer than an anastomosis. A stoma is easier to manage than a fistula, which may occur if there is an anastomotic leak. A jejunocolic anastomosis may lead to intolerable diarrhea, whereas a high-output jejunostomy may be more satisfactory for both patient and nurses to manage. If possible, surgeons should perform stricturoplasty in preference to resection in Crohn's disease. Preservation of the ileocecal valve is recommended.

Surgery after this period is directed toward ways of minimizing the effects of SBS, or efforts to return the patient to a normal dietary intake. This is considered after a period of time to allow adaptation to occur. Methods available, which have had varying levels of experience and success, are discussed in the following paragraphs.

Intestinal Lengthening Procedures

Bianchi in 1980 described a technique whereby the small bowel mesentery was divided longitudinally to produce two leaves, which each supplied one-half of the bowel. This bowel was divided with a GIA stapler to produce two side-by-side tubes equal in length but smaller in diameter than the original bowel. This

---

*Editor's Note: As discussed below, the use of glutamine and growth hormone as described by Wilmore and colleagues at the Massachusetts General Hospital may provide a method to wean some patients off home TPN (see the O'Dwyer reference).

technique has been used with some success but is technically difficult, and complications of obstruction and anastomotic leakage have been reported.

Interpositional Loops

Reversed intestinal loops have been used in the "dumping" syndrome to slow intestinal transit and gastric emptying. This technique has been tried in SBS with varying degrees of success. The length of bowel used as the loop is critical, since long loop lengths are associated with intestinal obstruction, often necessitating dismantling the loop. Other disadvantages of these loops are that with time they can lead to bacterial overgrowth, causing further malabsorption, and that in the long term the loops fail to act as a reverse loop. Colonic interpositional loops have also been tried, again with some success. In general, because of limited experience and well-known complications, loop surgery has not yet made a great impact on surgery for SBS.

Recirculating Loops

An isoperistaltic loop is produced to overcome the problem of intestinal obstruction. However, lack of experience currently prevents evaluation of this technique. The problems of stasis, bacterial overgrowth, and the increased number of anastomoses make this a risky procedure. With all loop surgery, there is the added danger of losing the loop with ischemia because of the surgical difficulty. This obviously makes the length of bowel remaining even shorter.

Artificial Sphincters

Since the presence of an intact ileocecal valve affects the severity of SBS, several techniques have been described to re-create a sphincter. At present few human data are available, but animal studies suggest that in creating the valve or sphincter, the benefits may outweigh the risks.

SMALL BOWEL TRANSPLANTATION

There has been a resurgence of interest in small bowel transplantation (SBT) in the past decade. The technique of transplantation was developed in the late 1950s. The three major problems of graft rejection, graft-versus-host reaction, and sepsis are now better understood and managed. The major advances have been with the use of immunosuppressive agents such as FK506, monoclonal antibodies, and improved perioperative care (including TPN). With these advances, SBT is likely to be the preferred surgical option for many patients with SBS in the not too distant future. This approach is discussed in detail in a separate chapter.

THE FUTURE

Apart from the exciting progress being made in small bowel transplantation, other new methods emerging for treatment of SBS include the following:

1. *Growing intestinal mucosa* on serosal patches in vivo to increase the surface area of the bowel.
2. *Electric pacing of the intestine,* which may produce slowing of intestinal transit, or even reverse the direction of peristalsis to allow increased time for absorption of intestinal contents.
3. *Glutamine infusions* or enteral supplements, which may produce mucosal growth to help reduce parenteral intake. Glutamine, which is abundant in normal diets, has not been formulated in parenteral nutrition until recently. Along with the use of growth hormone and high-fiber diets, it may allow intestinal adaptation to occur up to a point at which normal dietary intake is possible again.

Editor's Note: Professor Irving and others, such as the transplant groups at Pittsburgh, Toronto, and Omaha, will be providing guidelines to help us select patients with chronic intestinal failure who would be suitable candidates for small bowel transplantation when home TPN or external feeding is not effective.

SUGGESTED READING

Allard JP, Jeejeebhoy KN. Nutritional support and therapy in the short bowel syndrome. Gastroenterol Clin North Am 1989; 18:589–601.

Cuschieri A, Giles GR, Moossa AR. Short gut syndrome. In: Wright J, ed. Essential surgical practice. 2nd ed. 1988:1145–1148.

Devine RM, Kelly KA. Surgical therapy of the short bowel syndrome. Gastroenterol Clin North Am 1989; 18:603–618.

Purdum PP, Kirby DF. Short bowel syndrome: a review of the role of nutrition support. JPEN 1991; 15:93–101.

O'Dwyer ST, Smith BJ, Wilmore DW, et al. Maintenance of small bowel mucosa with glutamine-enriched parenteral nutrition. JPEN 1989; 13:579–585.

SMALL BOWEL TRANSPLANTATION

JAMES C. REYNOLDS, M.D.
PHILIP PUTNAM, M.D.

Small bowel transplantation (SBT) is the latest achievement in visceral organ transplantation, following successes in heart, lung, pancreas, liver, and kidney replacement over the past two decades. With advances in the operative approaches and transplant immunology, transplantation has become a practical therapeutic option for patients with permanent dysfunction of these organs.

Successful SBT was first reported in a multivisceral transplantation procedure. Grant et al. reported the first isolated intestinal transplant with graft survival exceeding 1 year in 1990. Although advances during the past 5 years have promoted an increase in the number of patients undergoing SBT and in the number of centers participating in the development of this new technology, the impact of SBT as a therapeutic option for the many disorders that result in dependence on total parenteral nutrition (TPN) continues to evolve.

Prolonged use of TPN may lead to chronic liver disease and even liver failure, particularly in patients with the "short gut syndrome". Initial experience with SBT suggested that graft survival was enhanced by simultaneous replacement of the liver along with the small intestine. Therefore, SBT appeared to be particularly suitable for patients with short gut syndrome and liver failure. Subsequent success with isolated SBT has made that initial impression seem less universal, thereby fostering investigation into other disease entities that might be amenable to transplantation before the development of end-stage liver disease (ESLD).

The broader application of this surgical therapy to other small intestinal diseases remains to be clarified. There is reason to hope that transplantation may be an alternative therapy for severe disorders of the small intestine including Crohn's disease, celiac sprue or vasculitis-induced intestinal dysfunction, as well as congenital small intestinal disorders such as hollow visceral myopathy, chronic neuropathic intestinal pseudo-obstruction, or microvillous inclusion disease.

INDICATIONS AND CONTRAINDICATIONS

Currently, transplantation of the small intestine is made available only to those patients with major loss and/or dysfunction of the small intestine who cannot sustain an adequate nutritional balance by oral intake. These patients suffer from the wide variety of disorders (Table 1). At present, identification of optimal candidates for SBT from within these groups is hampered by

Table 1 Indications for Small Bowel Transplantation

In Children:
Short gut syndrome due to:
  Gastroschisis
  Malrotation
  Necrotizing enterocolitis
  Volvulus intussception
Microvillous atrophy
Pseudo-obstruction

In Adults:
Short gut syndrome due to:
  Ischemic bowel injury
  Mesenteric thrombosis
  Traumatic bowel injury
    Motor vehicle accident
    Surgical trauma
    Gunshot wound
  Polyposis syndromes
    Gardner's syndrome
    Peutz-Jeghers syndrome
    Desmoid tumor
Immune mediated bowel diseases
  Advanced Crohn's disease
  Refractory celiac sprue
  Ulcerative jejunitis
  Vasculitis

limited experience, concerns over graft survival, as well as practical and financial factors.

Among this large group of potential transplant candidates, two cohorts of patients have been identified who appear to be ideal candidates. As noted above, this includes patients with short gut syndrome who have developed ESLD as a consequence of TPN. Such patients receive the same potent immunosuppressant medications required to prevent rejection as they would after liver transplantation. Furthermore, the transplantation of the two organs may lead to an increased rate of survival of the grafted small intestine.

The second patient population are those for whom TPN is becoming an increasingly dangerous and impractical option. These patients are severely limited by recurrent episodes of bacterial sepsis and/or difficult central venous access. These complications arise from difficulties maintaining intravenous lines and from thrombosis of central veins. Because transplantation itself is not feasible if all central venous sites have become dysfunctional, the decision regarding SBT must include consideration of this factor.

Patients who are not dependent on TPN are not currently considered for SBT because of the risk of transplantation and immunosuppressant drugs. At the same time, patients with severe Crohn's disease, celiac sprue, or vasculitis-induced bowel injury, may be among the first to undergo SBT before the use of TPN has caused ESLD. These patients are already receiving immunosuppressant agents, including corticosteroids, azathioprine (Imuran), cyclosporine or FK-506.

SBT is contraindicated in patients over the age of 60, with incurable cancer, active infection, or psychiatric disorder which influence patient compliance.

CURRENT EXPERIENCE

Published experience with human transplantation has occurred in Europe, Canada, and the United States. The report of the first long-term graft and patient survival by Grant and colleagues has been followed by reports from a consortium in Europe and from Pittsburgh. The longest survival in the world is from Deltz Krell, who had a small bowel transplant from a living donor. Of 15 transplanted patients in the European series, four achieved long-term survival and independence from TPN. All patients are on prednisone and cyclosporine and most also receive Imuran or OKT-3. There were three deaths. The initial Pittsburgh experience involved nine patients, but has increased to more than 50 adults and children.

Current actuarial survival of patients undergoing small bowel transplantation is 80 percent at 3 months, 72 percent at 1 year, but only 59 percent after 2 years. Graft losses have become increasingly frequent after 18 months of survival. The initial success of the University of Pittsburgh small bowel program is related to the vast experience gained through animal research and by the transplantation of other organs, as well as the availability of FK-506, an immunosuppressant drug which is 50 times more potent than cyclosporine. Methods to reduce the chronic graft infection and infectious complications that limit long-term survival are under intense investigation.

The technical factors which provide for the optimal retrieval of donor graft through an en-bloc liver–small bowel resection have been described. Skillful resection reduces cold ischemic injury and optimizes the preservation of intestinal epithelium and neural structures.

DIFFERENCES BETWEEN TRANSPLANTATION OF SMALL BOWEL AND OF OTHER ORGANS

Factors which limit the success of SBT are different from those which initially restricted the transplantation of other solid organs. Lung, heart, and liver transplantations were primarily limited by technically difficult anastomosis and the practical limitations of performing orthotopic transplantation. Considerable technical difficulties are encountered when orthotopic transplantation is performed including the need to maintain normal physiology and hemodynamic stability during the removal and replacement of a vital organ, and the need to perform many vascular and other anatomical anastomosis rapidly and precisely. Each anastomosis has a potential to stenose from scar formation, to leak, or to become occluded by thrombosis.

Although it is an orthotopic procedure, the technical demands of SBT are considerably less. The original organ is usually absent, which substantially reduces the magnitude of the surgical procedure. Furthermore, SBT primarily involves creation of "routine" intestinal anastomoses and vascular anastomoses that are less technically challenging than those performed in heart, lung, or liver transplantation.

Despite the reduced technical demands, successful SBT depends on recovery of small intestinal function. For TPN to be discontinued the transplanted intestine must be able to support the patient's nutritional status from enterally-administered nutrients, which requires intact (or at least, compensated) secretion, digestion, absorption, and motility. Failure of any component will markedly influence the success of refeeding.

Several important changes, each with the potential to prevent recovery of function, occur as a consequence of removal of the intestine from the donor or while the specimen is in preservative solution during transport. For example, all extrinsic innervation (both sympathetic and parasympathetic) is divided during removal of the intestine from the donor. Normally, these neurons from the central nervous system provide a neuromodulatory influence on the intrinsic (enteric) nervous system and the hormone-secreting cells of the intramucosal neuroendocrine system. These intrinsic neuroendocrine systems play an essential role in the control of gastrointestinal motility. With the loss of extrinsic modulation during SBT, motility remains independent of extrinsic neural innervation. Our observation suggests that nerve regrowth in patients with failed grafts months after transplantation and reinnervation does not occur.

Post-transplant intestinal motility also may be altered by the loss of continuity between the smooth muscle syncytium (including the enteric nervous system) of the native gastroduodenal segment and the donor intestine as a result of the proximal anastomosis. Recovery of the coordinated motility, as evidenced by the propagation of Phase III of the migrating motor complex has *not* been seen in patients studied in our institution to date.

The lymphatic system also is disrupted by transplantation. Intestinal lymphatics are not in continuity with the recipient's lymphatic system immediately after transplant, potentially interfering with normal fat transport and lymphocyte movement, but this problem appears to be transient and to have little overt clinical consequence. Connections apparently are re-established within weeks to months of transplantation.

Another important function of the small intestine that may be altered by transplantation involves the mucosal defense system. Transplantation and rejection alter the integrity of epithelial cell adhesions and may lead to both increased bacterial transudation and impaired absorption. In addition to nonspecific factors such as mucus, motility, and epithelial adhesion, mucosal defense depends on immunologically-active cells which protect the body from invasion by micro-organisms and from potentially damaging substances in the lumen of the intestine. The small intestine is one of the largest lymphoid organs of the body. Fully 25 percent of its gross weight is made up of immunoactive cells. When this system breaks down, bacteria, yeast, and other toxins may invade the bloodstream leading to sepsis and even death. This breakdown may occur not only in the newly transplanted organ, but whenever the transplanted organ is damaged by rejection which occurs despite improved immunosuppressant medications.

The large number of donor immune regulatory cells that are contained within the intestine at the time of transplantation allows for the potential development of graft versus host disease (GVHD). During GVHD, immunocompetent (donor) lymphocytes and dendritic cells leave the small intestine and circulate throughout the recipient, where they can cause damage to a variety of organs. Fortunately, these invading immune cells tend to be destroyed by the host immune system, or disabled by immunosuppressant medications. Because of this, severe GVHD after SBT is unusual. However, this process may be intense, and one death in our early experience was due to GVHD.

The development of SBT has necessitated the clarification of specific histologic criteria for rejection. Unfortunately, biopsy alone may not provide a reliable means of detecting rejection. While cyclosporin with prednisone may provide adequate immunosuppression for liver transplantation, this regimen has not been as successful in SBT. FK-506 in combination with other immunosuppressants appears to provide more effective prevention of rejection and GVHD.

Finally, it is important to note that ethical considerations that have surrounded the transplantation of other organs (e.g., liver transplantation in an alcoholic patient) are not common for small intestinal diseases.

FUTURE DIRECTIONS

Improvements in SBT will require advances in our understanding of the role of preservation solutions to maintain normal neural and muscular function of the gut during the cold schemic injury which occurs while the organ is in transit to the recipient. Better understanding of factors which lead to the indefinite survival of small bowel grafts is needed. Recent observations that the graft and host become chimeric in multiple organs other than the graft may provide the key to graft survival. Pharmacological agents must be developed to limit rejection and GVHD with fewer side effects. The role of techniques such as irradiation of the donated bowel to further disable immunocompetent donor cells need to be established. In addition, the development of immunosuppressant medications which will permit the host immune system to engraft into the donor small intestine and replace the mucosal defense system is essential.

Improvements in surgical technique may allow "split donor grafts" to become possible in many patients, since shorter lengths of bowel can provide not only complete nutritional needs but also may result in less severe GVHD.

Other surgical advances are possible. Recently, a portion of donor colon has been included in our transplant procedure to combat excessive fluid and electrolyte losses which accompany the creation of an ileostomy in patients without adequate native colon. Current data are insufficient to comment on the effectiveness of this procedure, though initial observations are encouraging.

In addition, improvements in SBT have already begun to allow patients with whole gut malfunction (e.g., hollow viscus myopathy, chronic gastrointestinal pseudo-obstruction, total aganglionosis), who are not only TPN dependent but also unable to tolerate oral intake because of gastric dysfunction, the possibility of multi-visceral transplantation with resumption of oral intake. Several patients have received multivisceral transplants, including stomach, duodenum, small intestine, liver, and pancreas with impressive early success.

Small intestinal transplantation has progressed considerably over the past 5 years. Much effort will be required to bring its level of acceptance to that currently enjoyed by more established solid organ transplantation, but these continued advances may soon provide a practical solution so that SBT can be made available to intestinally-disadvantaged patients who desperately desire a more normal lifestyle.*

SUGGESTED READING

Abu-Elmagd K, Fung JJ, Reyes J, et al. Management of intestinal transplantation in humans. Transplant Proc 1992; 24:1243–1244.

Casavilla A, Selby R, Abu-Elmagd K, et al. Logistics and technique for combined hepatic-intestinal retrieval. Ann Surg 1992; 216:605–609.

Langrehr JM, Hoffman RA, Demitris AJ, et al. Evidence that indefinite survival of small bowel allografts achieved by a brief course of cyclosporine or FK506 is not due to systemic hyporesponsiveness. Transplantation 1992; 54:505–510.

Quigley EMM, Spanta A, Rose SG, et al. Long-term effects of jejunoileal autotransplantation on myoelectrical activity in canine small intestine. Dig Dis Sci 1990; 35:1505–1517.

Schmid T, Oberhuber G, Korozski G, et al. Histologic pattern of small bowel allograft rejection in the rat: Mucosal biopsies do not provide sufficient information. Gastroenterology 1989; 96:1529–1532.

Starzl TE, Rowe MI, Todo S. Transplantation of multiple abdominal viscera. JAMA 1989; 261:1449–1457.

Starzl TE, Todo S, Tzakis A, Murase N. Multivisceral and intestinal transplantation. Transplant Proc 1992; 24:1217–1223.

Todo S, Tzakis A, Abu-Elmagd K, et al. Intestinal transplantation in composite visceral grafts or alone. Ann Surgery 1992; 216:223–233.

Tzakis A, Todo S, Reyes J, et al. Clinical intestinal transplantation: Focus on complications. Transplant Proc 1992; 24:1238–1240.

Watson AJ, Lear PA, Montgomery A, et al. Water, electrolyte, glucose, and glycerine absorption in rat small intestinal transplants. Gastroenterology 1988; 94:863–869.

---

*Editor's Note: As feasibility of SBT improves we will face the interesting dilemma of deciding which patients with "small bowel insufficiency" on home TPN should be offered SBT. A number of people could be kept on home TPN for the price of one transplant. The author of this chapter gives some good guidelines, especially for those who can't stay on TPN because of infections or vascular problems.

HYPERLIPIDEMIAS

WILLIAM G.M. HARDISON, M.D.

Over the past 30 years there has been a growing awareness that our society's leading cause of death and morbidity, cardiovascular disease, is potentially preventable. This has led to the development of a variety of drugs effective in lowering elevated blood lipid levels, thought to be a major cause of cardiovascular disease. However, these drugs are expensive. Furthermore, as physicians learn more and more about hyperlipidemias, the definition of "desirable" levels becomes more stringent, so that a progressively larger segment of the population falls within the defined high-risk category. These latter two facts promise to clash head-on with the need to prioritize health expenditures to reduce the proportion of the gross domestic product devoted to health care in the United States.

The development of simple and convenient ways of obtaining a blood lipid profile has made mass screening practical. The relationship between cardiovascular events and high blood lipid levels, as well as the prevalence of cardiovascular disease, makes such screening desirable. The potent drugs now available for treating hyperlipidemias make screening essential. Such screening measures have shown that up to one-third of the U.S. adult population merit some form of intervention. In those aged 65 or over, a growing segment of our population, the situation is similar. It has been estimated that, on the basis of total cholesterol levels, 46 percent deserve a lipoprotein profile and 36 percent are eligible for some form of intervention, according to the National Cholesterol Education Program (NCEP) guidelines. Of those, 12 to 15 percent will require some form of drug therapy to reach "target" lipid levels; this percentage, of course, depends on the chosen target. The cost of screening and indicated treatment has been estimated to be somewhere between $1.6 and $16.8 billion in 1995, depending on the assumed efficacy of diet and the drug regimen selected. Recommendations leading to this level of intervention will have to be scrutinized closely by bodies responsible for slowing the growth of health expenditures. Progressively, the difficult question will not simply be *how* to treat but how to treat most cost effectively and, more important, *whom* to treat. The answers will not be found in this chapter but will unfold, perhaps painfully, as diseases and conditions compete for the limited health dollar.

One other consideration has surfaced to complicate these already complex issues. Lowering of cholesterol may be associated with its own risks. This was apparent in the early trials with clofibrate. Although this drug

lowered the coronary death rate, it did not decrease overall mortality. The "excess" deaths in the group with successful cholesterol lowering were statistically significant, although no reasonable hypothesis was devised to explain them. The same trend (not significant) was noted in the Helsinki primary prevention trial with gemfibrozil. Since then, meta-analyses have confirmed the excess of noncoronary deaths in the group of patients in whom cholesterol had been successfully lowered. This phenomenon has been referred to as the U-shaped total mortality curve. Currently, this is an area of intense controversy, some believing that the data are related to unidentified confounding variables, and others believing that the data warrant at least temporary restriction of primary prevention to only those patients at the highest risk for coronary heart disease.*

WHOM TO TREAT

As considered and enlightened as all the bodies have been in drawing up recommendations for lipid screening and treatment, much controversy still exists, and we are apt to see modifications of these recommendations over the next few years or more. The recommendations in this chapter reflect those generally accepted today for screening and treatment. Discussion of available therapies emphasizes cost, toxicity, and efficacy rather than mechanisms of action. Rarer forms of hyperlipidemias are properly managed by experts in metabolic disease and are not discussed in detail. Thresholds for treatment are based on those values obtained with the standard lipid profile: total cholesterol (TC), triglycerides (TG), low-density lipoprotein cholesterol (LDL-C) and high-density lipoprotein cholesterol (HDL-C). Because of biologic and technical variances, it is recommended that decisions be based on two or three separate assays taken several weeks apart. Although the form of HDL and the level of the recently identified small lipoprotein Lp[a] may have prognostic import, they have not yet been integrated into the profile on which recommendations for treatment are based.

In treating hyperlipidemias to prevent coronary morbidity and mortality, it is important to distinguish between primary and secondary prevention. In secondary prevention, one is dealing with a population that has already manifested coronary heart disease (CHD); in primary prevention, one is dealing with a population that is at risk but has yet to manifest CHD. All agree that aggressive control of hyperlipidemia is appropriate in secondary prevention. Disagreement exists about the threshold for aggressive treatment in primary prevention.

In general, treatment can be subdivided into "hy-

Supported by the V.A. Research Service and Grant #DK23446 from the National Institute of Diabetes and Digestive and Kidney Diseases.

*Editor's Note: Have we been wrong to tell patients with ileal resections and quite low cholesterol levels not to worry about the low values? The EKBOM and ADAMI studies from Uppsala, Sweden, did find excessive cardiovascular deaths with inflammatory bowel disease. Is there a link?

gienic" measures and drug therapy. Table 1 summarizes current recommendations that combine recommendations formulated in 1988 by the NCEP with those resulting from a 1992 National Institutes of Health (NIH) Consensus Panel Statement. In devising these recommendations, the NCEP recognizes LDL-C as a factor increasing the risk of coronary events and HDL-C as a factor decreasing that risk. The recommendations also consider TG as a risk factor, although at present it is not clear that this is a truly independent risk factor in nondiabetic individuals. Two-stage screening is recommended: first, TC is measured; if this is sufficiently high, lipoprotein analysis is performed. The 1988 guidelines were fairly simple: a lipoprotein profile is obtained if TC of 240 or more (units of mg per deciliter) or if TC of 200 to 239 and either CHD or two risk factors (Table 2) exist. The 1992 conference extended these indications to include patients with established CHD, TC of 200 or more, or TC less than 200 but with HDL-C of 35 or less plus any risk factor. It is clear that the 1992 recommendations include measurement of HDL-C in all patients screened, provided that accuracy of measurement, appropriate counseling, and follow-up can be assured. Since only measurement of TG in addition is necessary

to derive a lipoprotein profile, it is likely that such a profile will in practice become the initial screening assay in adults. The 1992 recommendations also include performing a lipoprotein profile in the presence of those diseases known to be associated with high TG levels and with CHD (e.g., diabetes, central obesity, peripheral vascular disease, and hypertension). As of 1992, treatment is recommended only after a lipoprotein profile has been obtained. It is likely that in the near future the desirable LDL-C limit in patients with two or more CHD risk factors may be set even lower (≤ 100 mg per deciliter or less), and even initial screening will be based on lipoprotein profile.

HOW TO TREAT

Hygienic Measures

Hygienic measures include not only diet and activity modification, but, even more important, treatment of conditions that increase the risk of coronary artery disease (CAD) directly (hypertension, smoking, diabetes mellitus) or that alter the lipid profile in such a way that CAD risk is increased. Table 3 lists the latter conditions. All these conditions must be dealt with in addition to any other hypolipidemic therapy used.

Diet therapy has great appeal: it promotes normalization of weight, is free of harmful side effects, and ostensibly costs little. The problems lie in implementation. It is difficult to alter behavior, and measures designed to promote compliance (education, supervision, and encouragement) can be costly. In one recent study, a reduction in fat content to 20 percent of total calories was feasible, but the cost of instruction and support was estimated at $551 per participant over 1 year. However, the more modest reductions in fat content in the NCEP/American Heart Association step 1 and step 2 diets should be easier to achieve. The assistance of a dietitian is essential in implementing diet therapy. As an adjunct to diet therapy, the patient, if sedentary, must undertake regular aerobic exercise. The amount must depend on the general medical condition of the patient, but a minimum of 30 minutes of brisk walking at least three times a week is necessary. Exercise not only facilitates weight loss but also independently elevates HDL-C.

Table 1 Treatment Recommendations

LDL-C (mg/dl)	TG (mg/dl)	HDL-C (mg/dl)	Treatment
≥ 160			Hygienic measures; if target not reached, drug therapy if LDL-C ≥ 190 or two risk factors present
130–159			Hygienic therapy; consider drug therapy if CHD or multiple risk factors present
< 130	250–500	≥ 35	Hygienic therapy for elevated TG; no drug therapy
< 130	≤ 250	< 35	Hygienic therapy for HDL-C; no drug therapy
< 130	250–500	< 35	Hygienic therapy; if target not reached, consider drug therapy if CHD or multiple risk factors present
	> 500		Hygienic therapy; if target not reached, drug therapy to prevent pancreatitis; drug therapy initially if history of pancreatitis

CHD = coronary heart disease.

Table 2 Risk Factors for CHD (Other Than Preexistent CHD)

Male gender or postmenopausal female
Smoking
Central obesity (≥ 30% overweight)
Hypertension
Family history of CHD
Diabetes mellitus
History of occlusive vascular disease
LDL-C ≥ 160 mg/dl
HDL-C < 35 mg/dl

Table 3 Conditions that Produce Dyslipidemias

Conditions That Increase LDL-C	Conditions That Decrease HDL-C	Conditions That Increase TG
Diabetes mellitus	Diabetes mellitus	Diabetes mellitus
Nephrotic syndrome	Hypertriglyceridemia	Renal insufficiency
Cholestasis	Obesity	Obesity
Hypothyroidism	Cigarette smoking	Alcohol intake
Progestins	Progestins	Estrogens
Anabolic steroids	Beta blockers	Beta blockers
	Lack of exercise	Lack of exercise
	Anabolic steroids	

Much recent research has gone into the type of fatty acid that is most beneficial in diets designed to lower blood lipid levels. "The more unsaturated the better" is no longer a valid concept. It has been shown that, although substitution of polyunsaturates for saturates lowers LDL-C, polyunsaturates do not possess any independent cholesterol-lowering properties and can lower HDL-C. It has recently been shown that the saturates with the greatest potential for raising serum cholesterol are palmitic (16:0), myristic (14:0), and possibly lauric (12:0) acids. On the other hand, the saturate stearic acid (18:0) and its monounsaturate oleic acid do not raise cholesterol or reduce HDL-C. This has led to a recommendation that polyunsaturates not comprise over 10 percent of dietary calories. Fish oils, although lowering TG, have no effect on LDL-C and tend to lower HDL-C. They are not currently recommended as part of a cholesterol reduction diet. *Trans*-unsaturated fatty acids (hydrogenated vegetable oil) behave as the cholesterol-elevating saturated fats. The essential features of the cholesterol-lowering diets are shown in Table 4. Total calories are adjusted to promote weight reduction in the obese. A step 1 diet should be pursued for a minimum of 3 months. If the lipoprotein values have not then reached the target level, the patient should be placed on the step 2 diet. If after 3 more months lipoprotein values are still not at target levels, the use of drugs can be considered.

A few special considerations are relevant in prescribing weight reduction diets for the elderly. Severe reduction in dairy products may deprive these patients of a necessary source of calcium, so that the diet may have to be supplemented with calcium. Constipation may be a problem, so that adequate fiber in the diet must be ensured or a stool-bulking agent may be necessary.

Drug Therapy

Hygienic therapy is considered benign intervention that brings a variety of benefits and no liabilities. It is therefore recommended for both primary and secondary prevention in the young and old. Drug therapy is not so benign: each drug carries some toxicity and considerable cost. Added to this is the previously mentioned U-shaped curve of death rate versus LDL-C level. These

considerations have led a number of experts to express major reservations, at least for the present, about the use of cholesterol-lowering drugs for primary prevention except in the highest-risk groups such as those with LDL-C levels of 160 mg per deciliter or more with two or more risk factors for CHD. When considering drug therapy in older patients, one must take into account the generally reduced toxic-therapeutic dose ratios of most drugs as well as the patient's overall functional condition.

Niacin (Nicotinic Acid)

Niacin is by far the most cost-effective lipid-lowering agent available, but it unfortunately is plagued by side effects. The agent reduces TG, reduces LDL-C, and raises HDL-C, all worthwhile goals. At high dosage, LDL-C levels may be lowered as much as 40 percent and HDL-C levels elevated as much as 20 to 35 percent. Side effects, however, limit its use. It produces flushing in almost all patients; it may precipitate diabetes mellitus in those with impaired glucose tolerance; and it may increase uric acid, produce gastrointestinal (GI) side effects, and exacerbate peptic ulcer disease. It is therefore not recommended for patients with diabetes mellitus, a history of gout, or peptic ulcer. It can also produce abnormal liver test results; these generally resolve with continued therapy, but may progress and rarely eventuate in hepatic necrosis. This latter complication has been reported especially with a slow-release form of niacin designed to minimize the flushing that follows a dose. Because of the high cost and augmented toxicity of the slow-release form, it should be avoided. Since the flushing is prostaglandin mediated, it may be mitigated by low-dose aspirin (e.g., ¼ to ½ tablet) taken with each dose of niacin. Untoward side effects can also be minimized by starting with a low dose (e.g., 100 mg three times a day) and increasing the dose slowly over 2 to 3 weeks to a final dose of 1500 mg per day. It should be given with meals to minimize GI side effects. A lipoprotein profile should be repeated at that point. If target values are not reached, the dose may be cautiously increased to a total of 3 to 5 g per day if tolerated. Since liver abnormalities are dose related, liver enzymes must be observed closely. As effective and cheap as the drug is, its side effects are such that only two-thirds or fewer of patients started on the drug will remain on it. Continuous dosing is important because discontinuation, even for several days, will lead to renewed symptoms of flushing and itching if the full dose is immediately reinstituted. Niacin has been shown to reduce the risk of CHD in large controlled trials and even to cause partial regression of atherosclerotic lesions.

Bile Acid–Binding Resins (Cholestyramine and Colestipol)

These agents lower LDL-C levels by an average of 10 to 20 percent at full dosage. They have little effect on HDL-C (perhaps a 5 percent increase over 4 months of

Table 4 Diet Therapy of Elevated LDL-C*

	Stage 1 Diet	Stage 2 Diet
Total fatty acids	≤ 30	≤ 30
Saturated fatty acids	≤ 10	≤ 7
Polyunsaturated fatty acids		≤ 10
Monounsaturated fatty acids	10–15	10–15
Carbohydrates	50–60	50–60
Protein	10–20	10–20
Cholesterol	≤ 300 mg/day	≤ 200 mg/day
Total calories	To achieve and maintain desirable weight	

*Figures in % of total calories

therapy). They are the most expensive drugs in terms of both monthly cost and per 1 percent reduction in LDL-C. These are safe drugs in that there are no serious side effects. However, symptoms of abdominal bloating and constipation are frequent and limit the number of patients willing to continue therapy for long periods. The only hazard is that these resins bind certain drugs in the intestine and alter their systemic availability (e.g., digoxin, tetracycline and certain other antibiotics, warfarin, thyroxine, propranolol, and phenobarbital). Resins can also elevate TG, especially in patients with some degree of hypertriglyceridemia to begin with. TG levels should therefore be monitored. The resins can be started at a relatively low dose (4 to 5 g twice daily) and lipoproteins measured after 4 to 6 weeks. If target values are not reached, the dose may be doubled. Other medications the patient may be using should be taken 1 to 2 hours after or 4 to 5 hours before resin is taken. Mild laxatives or stool softeners may be necessary to alleviate constipation. Resins have been shown in large controlled trials to reduce the risk of CHD.

Fibric Acid Derivatives

The only one used extensively in the United States currently is gemfibrozil, which is not a potent agent for reduction of LDL-C. However, it is effective in lowering TG and it also increases HDL-C. With the usual dose of 600 mg twice daily, expected reductions of LDL-C range from 0 to 15 percent and of TG 35 percent, and increases of HDL-C range from 5 to 15 percent. It is especially effective in hypertriglyceridemic patients. Unlike niacin and bile acid–binding resins, gemfibrozil is not associated with unpleasant side effects except for occasional GI distress, and it is well accepted by patients. Its cost is substantially higher than that of niacin but less than that of the resins, calculated in terms of both monthly drug cost and overall cost per 1 percent reduction in serum cholesterol. The relative cost of this agent will probably fall significantly when its patent expires in 1993. Gemfibrozil may occasionally produce hepatotoxicity and a myositis characterized by muscle cramping and elevated creatine kinase. It is known to potentiate the effect of warfarin. In some hypertriglyceridemic patients, it may paradoxically increase LDL-C, and this needs to be monitored. Finally, the fibrates increase cholesterol saturation in bile and may increase the likelihood of cholelithiasis, cholecystitis, and cholecystectomy with their attendant morbidity and mortality risks. It should not be used in patients with cholelithiasis or a history of cholecystitis. Gemfibrozil has been shown in a large controlled trial to reduce the risk of CHD, especially in the group with low HDL-C levels in addition to high TG and LDL-C.

HMGCo-A Reductase Inhibitors

Three agents are now available: lovastatin, simvastatin, and pravastatin. Lovastatin, which has been used for 5 years, is the agent I have most experience with.

These are potent agents for lowering LDL-C and are accompanied by few side effects. Some reduction of VLDL-C also occurs. At a dose of 20 mg twice daily, one may expect a 25 to 35 percent decrease in LDL-C, a 20 percent fall in TG, and possibly a small (5 to 10 percent) rise in HDL-C. The fall in LDL-C is dose dependent from 10 mg to about 80 mg per day, so that the dose may be adjusted according to need. A starting dose of 20 mg once daily is appropriate. Lovastatin is the only agent for which the relative cost has been calculated. The cost of the drug itself is similar to that of gemfibrozil, although in terms of per 1 percent reduction in LCL-C, it is the next cheapest drug to niacin. The patent on lovastatin does not expire until 1997, but competition from other HMGCo-A reductase inhibitors on the market may lower prices a little. Lovastatin may cause minor elevations of transaminase levels, which should be monitored over the first few months of therapy. Serious liver disease is extremely rare. Myopathy and, rarely, rhabdomyolysis may occur. This latter complication occurs most often when niacin, clofibrate, or cyclosporine are used with lovastatin. Although HMGCo-A reductase inhibitors have not been subjected to controlled studies to document that they reduce the risk of CHD, their potent lipid-lowering effects indicate that they almost surely do.

Probucol is the latest addition to the armamentarium of cholesterol-lowering drugs. Although approved for lowering LDL-C, it is relatively weak in this regard. At 500 mg twice daily, it is less effective than either bile acid–binding resins or HMGCo-A reductase inhibitors in lowering LDL-C. In addition, it lowers HDL-C. This does not conform with present concepts of drugs that should be effective in treating hyperlipidemias. Probucol's major appeal is that it may affect favorably those factors responsible for genesis of the atherosclerotic lesion. Oxidative modification of LDL particles is thought to promote atherogenesis by stimulating cholesterol accumulation in macrophages, with resultant death and release of chemotactic agents and lymphokines. Probucol is the first agent that disrupts this chain of events by its antioxidant and free radical scavenging properties. Animal studies suggest that it can retard the development of atherosclerotic lesions and actually accelerate reabsorption of xanthomatous deposits in animal models and in humans. Although HDL-C is lowered, probucol may selectively reduce a form of HDL not directly responsible for reverse cholesterol transport. Probucol has not yet been shown in large trials to lower the risk of CHD. Currently, there is great interest in these and similar agents, and one may expect more information soon on their place in the treatment of patients at risk for CHD.

SPECIAL CONSIDERATIONS

Age

It makes no sense to treat an elderly person for hyperlipidemia if prognosis is measured in months to a few years or if disease has severely impaired the quality of life. Likewise, it makes no sense to withhold treatment in an otherwise healthy and vigorous patient 70 years old simply because of age. Physicians agree that quality of life and expected longevity weigh heavily in any therapeutic decision for the elderly, and treatment for hyperlipidemia is no exception. If the decision is to treat, however, certain considerations must be kept in mind. I have already mentioned the dangers of insufficient calcium intake and of constipation. Deprived of customary diet, an elderly person may simply not consume enough to ensure adequate nutrition. Compromises must be made. Also, the elderly generally tolerate drugs less well than younger persons, so that toxicity must be carefully monitored. If these considerations are kept in mind, advanced age, in the absence of debilitating or life-threatening disease, should be no contraindication to therapy. Although the proportion of the elderly cohort dying of CHD is less than that in some younger cohorts, the absolute death rate from CHD is higher because the total death rate is higher.

Severe Hypercholesterolemia Unresponsive to Diet and Drug Therapy

Removal of the ileum reduces both of these effects, the hepatic free cholesterol pool falls, LDL receptors become up-regulated, and the hepatic uptake of plasma LDL-C increases. It has been shown that hypercholesterolemic patients subjected to surgical bypass of the distal third of the small bowel have fewer combined nonfatal myocardial infarctions and deaths from CHD than a control group over a 10 year period. They also have lower total and LDL cholesterol levels. However, no studies have been performed comparing the efficacy of such surgery with the newer antihyperlipidemic drugs. Until this is done, the place of surgery in the treatment of hyperlipidemia cannot be established.

For patients with no functional hepatic LDL receptors, those with homozygous familial hypercholesterolemia, liver transplantation has been effective therapy. Such patients are an obvious early target group for gene therapy if and when it becomes available. Such therapy would certainly be preferable to liver transplant.

SUGGESTED READING

Brett AS. Treating hypercholesterolemia. How should practicing physicians interpret the published data for patients? N Engl J Med 1989; 321:676–680.

Denke MA, Grundy SM. Hypercholesterolemia in elderly persons: resolving the treatment dilemma. Ann Intern Med 1990; 112: 780–792.

Goldman L, Gordon DJ, Rifkind BM, et al. Cost and health implications of cholesterol lowering. Circulation 1992; 85: 1960–1968.

Grundy SM, Getz G. Dietary influences on serum lipids and lipoproteins. J Lipid Res 1990; 31:1149–1172.

Jacobs D, Blackburn H, Higgins M, et al. Report of the conference on low blood cholesterol: mortality associations. Circulation 1992; 86:1046–1060.

Schulman KA, Kinosian B, Jacobson TA, et al. Reducing high blood cholesterol level with drugs. Cost-effectiveness of pharmacologic management. JAMA 1990; 264:3025–3033.

DIABETIC DIARRHEA

UMA SUNDARAM, M.D.
HENRY J. BINDER, M.D.

Diabetic diarrhea is the appelation usually applied to the patient with insulin-dependent diabetes mellitus who has profuse watery, nonbloody diarrhea without evidence of nutrient malabsorption and with normal intestinal histopathology. It is assumed, but certainly not established, that diabetic diarrhea is a result of autonomic neuropathy. Such patients frequently, but not always, have peripheral neuropathy and/or other evidence of autonomic neuropathy. Since therapy for diabetic diarrhea is less than perfect at best and since other diarrheal disorders associated with diabetes have specific treatment, a discussion of the therapy for diabetic diarrhea must first emphasize the differential diagnosis of diarrhea in the patient with diabetes so that appropriate management can be employed.

In general, the clinician can place a diabetic patient with diarrhea in one of four categories: (1) diabetic diarrhea (as defined above); (2) diarrhea associated with diabetes (e.g., stasis syndrome leading to bacterial overgrowth and resulting in diarrhea); (3) concomitant presentation of diarrhea and diabetes (e.g., islet cell tumors); and (4) diarrhea *not* related to the diabetes. In this last situation, care must be taken to review carefully the patient's history to identify other causes of diarrhea. This is especially necessary for hospitalized patients, many of whom have iatrogenic diarrhea (e.g., medications, enteral feedings, antacids).*

Diarrhea is not uncommon in patient with diabetes. Its incidence ranged from 10 percent to as high as 22 percent in one survey. Diabetic diarrhea is typically found in patients who have had diabetes for more than 10 years. These patients invariably have peripheral

---

*****Editor's Note:** Clinically, I have used the presence or absence of steatorrhea as a branching point in the differential diagnosis. A 3 day stool collection that reveals high volume but no increased fat is most typical of "diabetic diarrhea." Steatorrhea leads one to consider other mechanisms.

neuropathy. Diabetic diarrhea is more common in men than in women; tends to be episodic, lasting from a few days to weeks; and is often nocturnal.*

DIARRHEAL CONDITIONS ASSOCIATED WITH DIABETES

Celiac Sprue

Although the exact pathophysiology of diabetic diarrhea is yet to be established, several other associated conditions may, at least in part, cause diarrhea in diabetes. For example, celiac sprue has been reported in several studies to be more common in diabetics than in the general population. When this diagnosis is made in diabetic diarrhea, treatment must be that for celiac sprue, i.e., a gluten-free diet. Satisfactory control of diabetes in these patients may be difficult to achieve until the malabsorption of nutrients associated with celiac sprue is corrected.

The diagnosis is made by the combination of a characteristic "flat" jejunal biopsy and both clinical and histologic improvement after institution of a gluten-free diet for 4 to 6 weeks. An empiric trial of a gluten-free diet is *not* recommended as treatment of diarrhea in diabetics, not only because of the difficulty in complying with such a restrictive diet, but also because there may be other causes of diarrhea in diabetics as discussed below.

Exocrine Pancreatic Insufficiency

A deficiency of pancreatic enzymes may also be found in insulin-dependent diabetics. This may be due to the elevated levels of glucagon found in these patients, or to structural damage to the pancreas. Regardless of the cause, if the pancreatic exocrine deficiency is severe enough, steatorrhea may result. If pancreatic malabsorption is diagnosed, pancreatic enzyme replacement should be initiated. However, pancreatic enzymes are not useful in patients without steatorrhea. Conversely, somatostatin, an inhibitor of pancreatic secretion, has been used in some studies as treatment for diabetic diarrhea with limited success.

Bile Acid Malabsorption

Bile acid malabsorption in the small intestine has been proposed as a cause of diarrhea in some diabetics on the basis of enhanced fecal excretion of bile acids and a decreased bile acid pool in these patients. The pathophysiologic basis for this bile salt wasting is not known. Furthermore, this hypothesis cannot be generalized to all diabetics with diarrhea because less than 15 percent have enhanced fecal bile acid loss. Also, treatment with cholestyramine, the standard therapy for

bile acid diarrhea, produces variable results, at best, in diabetic patients with diarrhea.†

Diabetic Neuropathy

Visceral autonomic neuropathy is common in diabetics and may play a role in the pathogenesis of diarrhea in diabetics. This neuropathy may contribute to diarrhea in one of three ways: intestinal dysmotility, altered fluid and electrolyte transport in the intestine, and anal sphincter incontinence.

While neuropathy of the gut may result in intestinal dysmotility, it is not clear whether an alteration in motility in fact causes diabetic diarrhea. There is no correlation between either enhanced or reduced transit time as a result of altered motility and the presence of diarrhea in these patients. Indeed, small bowel transit times have been reported to be shortened, lengthened, or unchanged in diabetic diarrhea in different studies. Morphologic studies of the intestine demonstrate degenerative changes of the vagal and sympathetic nervous system, albeit not uniformly. Degenerative changes of the enteric nervous system have been observed even less consistently. Further, enteric neuropathy does not correlate with the presence of diarrhea in diabetics. Thus, whether or how the variable changes in intestinal innervation and the consequent effect on intestinal motility cause diarrhea in diabetes is controversial.

There is, however, some experimental evidence to suggest that the loss of autonomic innervation of the intestine in diabetes may affect fluid and electrolyte transport in the intestine and lead to diarrhea. Stimulation of intestinal alpha$_2$-adrenergic receptors enhances intestinal fluid and electrolyte absorption in experimental animals. Second, diabetes induced by streptozotocin causes adrenergic neuropathy and a decrease in fluid and electrolyte absorption in in vitro studies. This abnormality can be reversed by the alpha$_2$-receptor agonist clonidine. These observations are considered the scientific basis for the earlier anecdotal observation that clonidine reduced stool output in some patients with diabetic diarrhea. Thus, it has been postulated that autonomic neuropathy causes denervation of enterocytes, resulting in reduced adrenergic drive, and that pharmacologic doses of clonidine are required to enhance fluid absorption in the diabetic patient. Generally, up to 1 mg clonidine a day is necessary to reduce diarrhea. Despite these relatively high doses, this agent often does not cause hypotension and does not exacerbate the postural hypotension that is common in diabetics with neuropathy. Clonidine therapy is also discussed in the chapter on secretory diarrhea.

Finally, it is important to keep in mind that changes in both motor function and electrolyte transport may be

---

*Editor's Note: The article by Valdovinos and colleagues from the Mayo Clinic (cited in the Suggested Reading list) is an excellent approach to patients with diabetes and chronic diarrhea.

†Editor's Note: Excessive bile acid loss occurs in various "rapid-transit" diarrheas, such as that caused by magnesium sulfate. If present, in a diabetic with diarrhea, a trial of cholestyramine plus large doses of loperamide or deodorized tincture of opium would seem reasonable if other causes of diarrhea have been eliminated, i.e., excessive caffeine or lactose intake.

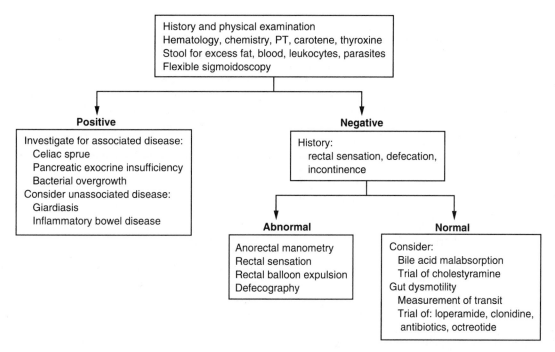

Figure 1 Algorithm for the management of patients with diabetes and chronic diarrhea. PT = prothrombin time. (From Valdovinos MA, Camilleri M, Zimmerman BR. Chronic diarrhea in diabetes mellitus: mechanisms and an approach to diagnosis and treatment. Mayo Clin Proc 1993; 68:698; with permission.)

involved in diarrhea resulting from diabetic neuropathy—a situation that most likely occurs in idiopathic "diabetic diarrhea." Some categories of diarrhea resulting from diabetic neuropathy, including fecal incontinence, are more fully discussed below as well as in the chapters on constipation and incontinence. An algorithm for approaching the patient with chronic diarrhea is presented in Figure 1.

Stasis Syndrome

Even though intestinal motility abnormalities ranging from rapid to normal to delayed transit have been described in diabetes, it is reasonable to consider bacterial overgrowth in diabetics with diarrhea as a consequence of stasis syndrome. Small intestinal bacterial overgrowth has been demonstrated by the presence of abnormal ^{14}C-glycocholate breath tests in these patients. Bacterial overgrowth can lead to diarrhea and/or steatorrhea. Bacterial deconjugation of bile salts leads to luminal deficiency of the conjugated bile acids necessary for fat digestion and absorption, resulting in steatorrhea.

Indirect evidence for bacterial overgrowth as one cause of diarrhea in diabetes is the finding that in some diabetics broad-spectrum antibiotics temporarily alleviate diarrhea. The bacterial cultures from the small intestine in diabetics with diarrhea demonstrate polymicrobial flora that usually contain *Escherichia coli* and *Bacteroides*. Fortunately, a wide variety of antibiotics are effective in the eradication of these bacteria. A 2 week course of a broad-spectrum antibiotic such as tetracycline or ampicillin, 1 g a day, is generally sufficient.

Alternatively, one may consider metronidazole.

Despite some supportive evidence, it must be remembered that bacterial overgrowth in diabetics is not a universal finding. In one study, it was found in less than 20 percent of diabetics with diarrhea. Furthermore, since antibiotics do not alter the neurogenic basis for intestinal stasis, bacterial overgrowth will recur in these patients. Unfortunately, no treatment is available to address the underlying motor abnormality.

Diabetic Diarrhea

The exact pathophysiology of idiopathic diabetic diarrhea is yet to be elucidated. However, as previously discussed, it is likely that diabetic neuropathy, by altering intestinal motility and/or fluid and electrolyte transport, may lead to diarrhea. The clinician who has excluded (1) diarrhea not associated with diabetes; (2) diarrhea that is associated with diabetes; and (3) concurrent presentation of both is left with this diagnosis of exclusion: idiopathic diabetic diarrhea. Since the pathophysiology of this condition is not known, it is not surprising that there is no adequate treatment. Any one of the above other situations may subsequently become apparent.

Treatment of diabetic diarrhea must be undertaken on a case-by-case, trial-and-error basis. Often, more than one treatment modality may be necessary. For example, it is reasonable to start these patients on clonidine; if response is limited, synthetic opiates (e.g., loperamide) should be given, but often there is limited response to these also. Alternatively, patients can be given a trial of broad-spectrum antibiotics for 2 weeks and, if not responsive, clonidine and/or opiates considered. Use of pancreatic enzymes to treat diabetic diarrhea should be restricted to those patients who have steatorrhea (greater than 7 g fecal fat excretion per day). While pancreatic enzymes have limited utility even in patients with steatorrhea, they have no role in the typical diabetic who has diarrhea without steatorrhea. Somatostatin should be reserved as a last option because it is expensive, inconvenient, and frequently of little benefit. Finally, it cannot be emphasized enough that the cause may be iatrogenic. Thus, repeated careful history taking and review of the medical records is crucial. It is important to make sure that these patients are not excessively indulging in sugarless dietary items (e.g., candy, gum). These substances are often used by diabetic patients, are rich in nonabsorbable sorbitol as sweetener, and may lead to osmotic diarrhea.*

Fecal Incontinence

The neuropathy of diabetes may also affect the innervation of the anal sphincter, and fecal incontinence is found in about one-third of patients with diabetes. However, fecal incontinence may or may not coexist with diabetic diarrhea. In one survey, 20 percent of patients with diabetes reported incontinence, but only half of these reported diarrhea. Incontinence and diarrhea occur at approximately the same time: about 10 to 12 years after the onset of diabetes. Contrary to the popular misconception, incontinence is not necessarily nocturnal in diabetics. Only three of 16 patients reported nocturnal fecal incontinence in one study. Some patients may describe incontinence as diarrhea. Thus, a careful history is necessary to distinguish between these two entities. Anorectal motility is helpful to establish anal sphincter dysfunction. A 24 hour stool collection of less than 250 g should suggest such a diagnosis. Biofeedback to control anal incontinence is invariably of little benefit in these patients. Attempts to "firm up" the stool with bulking agents such as Metamucil and anticholinergics are of limited use but should be made.†

CONCOMITANT PRESENTATION OF DIARRHEA AND DIABETES

The coexistence of diarrhea and diabetes may be noted in patients with islet cell tumors of the pancreas.

For example, diarrhea and diabetes may be found in 20% of patients with glucagonoma. However, since diabetes is a relatively common disease and diarrhea may be found in up to 20 percent of patients with diabetes, it is not cost effective to screen every diabetic with diarrhea for this *very rare* islet cell tumor. Other signs and symptoms of glucagonoma such as weight loss, glossitis, and the characteristic rash found in this disease should heighten the suspicion of the clinician for this diagnosis. Glucagonoma is diagnosed when a high level of glucagon is found in plasma. Islet cell tumors are discussed in a chapter in the section of the book devoted to pancreatic diseases.

Diabetes of short duration, absence of neuropathy, and diarrhea may be found in patients with somatostatinoma. Again, this is an extremely rare condition, and not all diabetics with diarrhea need be screened for this tumor, the presence of which is usually established by high levels of somatostatin in the serum. The chapter on endocrine tumors also discusses somatostatinoma.

SUGGESTED READING

Fedorak RN, Field M, Chang EB. Treatment of diabetic diarrhea with clonidine. Ann Intern Med 1985; 102:197–199.

Feldman M, Schiller LR. Disorders of gastrointestinal motility associated with diabetes mellitus. Ann Intern Med 1983; 98: 378–384.

Koletzko S, et al. Prevalence of coeliac disease in diabetic children and adolescents. Eur J Pediatr 1988; 148:113–117.

Ogbonnaya KI, Arem R. Diabetic diarrhea. Arch Intern Med 1990; 150:262–267.

Schiller LR, et al. Pathogenesis of fecal incontinence in diabetes mellitus. N Engl J Med 1982; 307:1666–1671.

Valdovinos MA, Camilleri M, Zimmerman BR. Chronic diarrhea in diabetes mellitus: mechanisms and an approach to diagnosis and treatment. Mayo Clin Proc 1993; 68:691–702.*

Wald A. Diabetic diarrhea and fecal incontinence. Practical Gastroenterol 1993; 4:20–28.

Whalen GE, Soergel KH, Geenen JE. Diabetic diarrhea. Gastroenterology 1969; 56:1021–1032.

*Editor's Note: A very useful article with a rational approach to the patient with chronic diarrhea and diabetes.

---

*Editor's Note: This is an important consideration in *any* patient with excessive gas or diarrhea, not just those with diabetes. The chapter *Carbohydrate Malabsorption* provides more details.

†Editor's Note: A detailed discussion of incontinence in diabetes is presented in the chapter *Fecal Incontinence.*

CROHN'S DISEASE OF THE SMALL BOWEL

LLOYD R. SUTHERLAND, M.D.C.M., M.Sc., F.R.C.P.C., F.A.C.P.

The management of patients with Crohn's disease of the small intestine remains a challenge for physicians. Because patients cannot be cured of this disease, physicians not only must treat the acute or active episode but also need to consider that the natural history of the disease suggests that recurrence is only a matter of time. Differing strategies may be required for the management of the acute episode, while other options, including perhaps doing nothing, may be more appropriate for maintaining disease remission.

THERAPEUTIC ALTERNATIVES

A variety of therapies have been suggested as effective for active small bowel Crohn's disease, including pharmacologic therapy, nutritional intervention, and surgery. The reader is directed to the chapters *Crohn's Disease: Enteral Feeding* and *Crohn's Disease: Surgical Management* for detailed reviews of the nutritional and surgical approaches to this disease. I will comment only on nutrition and surgery as compared with pharmacologic intervention.

PREFERRED APPROACH

General Principles

I believe it is appropriate to emphasize to patients that Crohn's disease is a lifelong disorder and that their lives will be characterized by relapses and recurrences. In the initial interviews, I generally point out that for most patients with Crohn's disease, the "good times" (remission) outnumber the "bad times" (recurrence). Since this is a lifelong disease, patients should be empowered through education (e.g., discussion, pamphlets) to assist in its management.

A healthy lifestyle is important. Patients should be encouraged to take all things in moderation, to enjoy an active social and physical life, and not to let the disease overwhelm their lives. I believe that ample rest, recreation, and opportunities for socialization should be sought, but that patients should try to maintain as normal a lifestyle as possible. I always refer patients to the Crohn's and Colitis Foundation of America (444 Park Avenue S, New York, NY, 10016, 1-800-343-3637) or Crohn's and Colitis Foundation of Canada (301-21 St. Clair Ave E, Toronto, ON, M4T 1L9) and provide them with the appropriate pamphlets.

My patients consult a dietitian familiar with Crohn's disease, who reviews the basic principles of nutrition, conducts a thorough analysis of current intake, and offers suggestions for improving nutrition. The goal is a healthy, balanced nutritious diet with adequate calories and fiber. Occasionally, the elements of a lactose-free or low-residue diet can also be introduced. Patients with Crohn's disease who smoke should be actively discouraged from doing so and offered support while withdrawing from nicotine. There is growing literature that implicates smoking as a risk factor not only for the development of Crohn's disease but also for continuing disease activity. Crohn's disease patients who smoke report more relapses and resections than those who do not smoke.

Advice about the use of oral contraceptives is often sought. Although a few of my patients report that use of the contraceptive was associated with worsening of disease, there is no convincing evidence to support restricting this medication. With the exception of early case reports of a colonic (perhaps ischemic) lesion that regressed in women taking oral contraceptives, the current literature does not support the concept that oral contraceptive use is a cause of continuing disease activity.*

Symptomatic Therapy

In addition to the specific anti-inflammatory, antibiotic, and immunosuppressant agents used in the therapy for Crohn's disease, patients often need medications directed toward specific symptoms. Diarrhea is a common complaint that may persist after induction of remission. Antidiarrheal agents such as loperamide or diphenoxylate are often helpful; I tend to prefer loperamide because of its longer half-life. For a few patients, codeine, 30 mg two or three times daily, may be required. For patients with severe diarrhea, I initiate therapy with 4 to 6 mg twice daily rather than giving it after each bowel motion; patients can then adjust the dose downward if necessary. In certain situations, the diarrhea is related to loss of bile salt receptors in the terminal ileum secondary either to disease or to resection. Cholestyramine, one scoop (4 g) or one packet in apple sauce, binds bile salts and reduces the diarrhea.

A request for analgesics should always be considered carefully and sympathetically by the physician. However, one should be cautious, because the patient has a lifelong disease and potentially may require long-term analgesics. Crohn's patients are just as susceptible to the addictive potential of the more potent analgesics as the general population, and this risk should always be discussed frankly with them. I usually begin with acetaminophen, 500 mg every 4 to 6 hours. If this does not suffice, I advance to acetaminophen-codeine combinations, which not only provide relief for pain but

---

*Editor's Note: Because severe colitis and high-dose adrenocortical steroid therapy may be associated with hypercoagulability, I discourage oral contraceptive use in that subset of patients.

also help control diarrhea. I rarely resort to anileridine (Leritine) or other potent narcotics for long-term pain control. For some patients, referral for relaxation therapy or training in meditation techniques may also help. It is a good idea to identify one physician, either the gastroenterologist or primary care physician, who will take responsibility for providing all analgesic prescriptions.

SPECIFIC THERAPY

Active Disease

Currently available pharmacologic therapies for the treatment of active small bowel Crohn's disease are listed in Table 1. These include the 5-aminosalicylates, corticosteroids, antibiotics, and immunosuppressants. All have been assessed in a variety of clinical trials of varying quality and sample size. In reviewing the literature, a useful rule of thumb is that trials that include less than 100 patients may not provide sufficient information on which to base therapeutic decisions.*

5-Aminosalicylates

A variety of delivery systems have been developed to deliver and release 5-aminosalicylate (5-ASA) in the small and large intestine. The first of these systems was sulfasalazine, which consists of a molecule of 5-ASA linked by a diazo bond to sulfapyridine. Bacteria in the large intestine split the bond and released the 5-ASA into the colon. In theory, sulfasalazine would be of little benefit to patients with small bowel disease, but it is possible that in patients who either have resection of the ileocecal valve or strictures or enteroenteric fistulas, sufficient bacteria may be present to break the bond and release the 5-ASA.†

Two newer 5-ASA delivery systems have been developed to release 5-ASA specifically into the small intestine. Pentasa contains microspheres of 5-ASA in methylcellulose and begins release of 5-ASA in the duodenum and upper small intestine. Salofalk, Mesasal, Claversal, and Rowasa are essentially the same and represent a pellet of 5-ASA wrapped with a pH-sensitive resin that in theory dissolves at pH > 6 and therefore is

Table 1 Specific Drug Therapies for Active Small Bowel Crohn's Disease

5-Aminosalicylates
  Sulfasalazine
  Asacol
  Pentasa
  Claversal/Mesasal/Salofalk
Corticosteroids
Antibiotics
  Metronidazole
Immunosuppressants
  Azathioprine
  Mercaptopurine

released in the terminal ileum. Asacol, another pH-sensitive preparation, is coated with another resin that dissolves at pH greater than 7 is thought to be more appropriate for inflammatory bowel disease of the large intestine. However, articles suggesting usefulness in maintaining remissions in patients with ileitis may point to some role in treating active small bowel Crohn's disease. The newer 5-ASA preparations have fewer side effects than sulfasalazine. Many of the problems associated with sulfasalazine are thought to be related to the sulfapyridine carrier.

Few large trials have assessed the use of 5-ASA for small bowel Crohn's disease. I use 5-ASA for active small bowel Crohn's disease in patients with mildly active disease or for those who are concerned about the side effects of corticosteroids. The medication is expensive, often costing over $100.00 (Canadian) per month of therapy. As the onset of action is relatively slow, patients should be cautioned that 5-ASA takes time to have an effect. In a small comparative study with corticosteroids, patients who received steroids had a prompter response, but by 6 weeks there were no differences in remission between the two groups. There are no comparative data to favor one preparation over the other, and I use either Pentasa, 1 g four times daily, or Salofalk, Mesasal, Claversal, or Rowasa, 1 g three times daily. My opinion is that although 5-ASA may have a limited role in the treatment of active disease, it will have its greatest impact in the maintenance of remission once that has been achieved (see below); however, this remains to be proved.

Corticosteroids

There is almost universal agreement amongst gastroenterologists that corticosteroids are the mainstay of therapy for patients with moderate to severely active small bowel Crohn's disease. Several multicenter trials in North America (prednisone) and Europe (methylprednisolone) have documented the superior efficacy of steroid therapy compared with placebo, sulfasalazine, and various nutritional approaches. Unfortunately, prolonged use of corticosteroids carries the potential for a variety of side effects. The benefits and risks should be discussed with the patient. Side effects can conveniently

---

*Editor's Note: Lest we forget, not all the therapeutic questions confronting the clinician have yet been asked (much less answered) by large clinical trials. When they have, this may be a thinner book.

†Editor's Note: Three types of evidence suggest that in fact sulfasalazine may have anti-inflammatory actions. First, Azad, Kahn, and Truelove showed that sulfasalazine enemas were as effective for proctitis as 1 g 5-ASA enemas. Second, Stenson and colleagues demonstrated effects of the sulfasalazine molecule on steps in prostaglandin metabolism not accomplished by 5-ASA. Third, and perhaps least objective, a number of pragmatic clinicians, championed by Franz Goldstein, have thought that some of their patients with small bowel Crohn's disease benefited from sulfasalazine used with or without prednisone.

be divided into those that are related to the total cumulative dose (metabolic bone disease, cataracts) and those that are not (increased susceptibility to infection, diabetes mellitus, hypertension).

There is little agreement among gastroenterologists about dosage and duration of treatment. When steroids are indicated, I usually initiate therapy with between 40 and 50 mg prednisone taken once a day. There is no evidence that higher doses increase the effectiveness of therapy. By taking the medication in the morning, patients tend to report less disturbance of nighttime sleep. I taper the prednisone by 5 mg a week until the 15 mg a day level is reached, and then reduce the steroid by 2.5 mg a week. I have not been impressed with alternate-day steroids, although my colleagues in pediatrics continue to use this method. French investigators have demonstrated that colonoscopy has no role to play in determining how quickly therapy is to be tapered. There is no evidence that continuing steroid therapy reduces the probability of recurrence after clinical remission is induced.

Frequently, Crohn's disease patients are severely ill and require hospitalization. In this situation I prescribe intravenous corticosteroids until the disease begins to settle down: hydrocortisone sodium succinate (Solu-Cortef), 100 mg every 6 or 8 hours. Although others have recommended using adrenocorticotropic hormone (ACTH), extrapolating from the ulcerative colitis trial of ACTH versus Solu-Cortef, rather than other forms of steroids, I do not. If fistulas or strictures are suspected, the use of antibiotics in addition to steroids should be considered (see below).

Is combination therapy (5-ASA and corticosteroid) ever warranted? Many physicians, including myself, use combinations for patients with active disease, but there is little evidence in the literature on which to base such a decision. One trial demonstrated that combination therapy proved beneficial compared with sulfasalazine alone, but another suggested that the combination was less effective than corticosteroid therapy by itself. Further trials are needed.

Antibiotics

Only one antibiotic, metronidazole, has been shown in clinical trials to warrant consideration for the treatment of small bowel Crohn's disease. On the basis of the current literature, it is difficult to be a strong proponent of its use, but in patients with ileocecal disease it may be considered a second- or third-line therapy. Metronidazole does, however, appear to provide effective therapy for patients with perianal disease, although this has never been documented by a clinical trial. One trial could not demonstrate significant differences between 750 and 1,500 mg a day given in divided doses. I tend to use 1 g a day for up to 16 weeks. Patients should be cautioned about peripheral neuropathy (generally related to total cumulative dosage) and avoidance of alcohol. Triple antibiotic therapy should be considered

for patients who present with a tender, painful abdominal mass that may be an abscess.

Immunosuppressants

In my opinion, the use of immunosuppressants such as azathioprine, 6-mercaptopurine and cyclosporin A should be restricted to patients with (1) extensive small bowel disease or multiple resections who have failed to enter remission after a course of steroids, (2) toxic side effects from corticosteroids, or (3) a clinical relapse as steroids are tapered. I stress the importance of *extensive* disease, because I believe that a patient who is not doing well and has only 20 to 30 cm of terminal ileal disease should be offered the option of surgery before immunosuppressants.

Although there is a body of literature that supports the use of azathioprine or 6-mercaptopurine, not all clinical trials have demonstrated efficacy. Both physician and patient should understand that it may take up to 6 months for a clinical response to become apparent. In general, immunosuppressant therapy should not be given as monotherapy; it is introduced while the patient is still on corticosteroids (20 mg daily). I generally begin therapy with 50 mg per day of 6-mercaptopurine along with weekly complete blood counts for the first month. If the white blood cell count remains above 5,000, the dosage may be slowly increased during the second month to 100 mg daily. Once the dose is stabilized, blood counts can be reduced to once a month. Despite the impressive list of side effects for immunosuppressants, which should be related to the patient, reports from large centers suggest that, aside from pancreatitis, most patients tolerate the medication reasonably well. After 2 to 3 months of therapy and if the patient is in remission, the corticosteroids can be withdrawn. The optimal duration of therapy cannot be determined, as most patients who respond to immunosuppressants and are then withdrawn from therapy relapse within a relatively short time.

Recently, there has been interest in the use of cyclosporin A for Crohn's disease. I am not one of the proponents of its general use. The original international study (Denmark, Italy, Canada) demonstrated efficacy only when the drug was given as adjunct therapy for patients already on corticosteroids. A large Canadian trial found it had no effect on mild to moderately active disease. Cyclosporin is expensive, has significant renal toxicity, and, when given in high doses, is associated with an increased risk of opportunistic infection.

Unproven Therapies

In an open study, methotrexate has been suggested as an effective, relatively rapid-acting agent for patients with active disease. A North American double-blind trial is currently under way. Budesonide, one of the new generation of corticosteroids, has a 90 percent first-pass hepatic metabolism, suggesting an opportunity for a corticosteroid with local effects and without the usual side effects. Dose finding and comparative studies are currently under way.

Fistulizing Disease

Enteroenteric fistulas are common in patients with small bowel disease. Extensive fistula formation may be an indication for immunosuppressants, since they have been described as particularly effective in this situation. This has not been confirmed by a specific clinical trial. Fistulas may involve other abdominal organs and can present as an abdominal mass with abscess formation. Such patients should be started on triple antibiotics (metronidazole, ampicillin, and gentamicin), and steroids should be instituted after 48 hours.*

Stricturing Disease

Crohn's disease has a tendency toward fibrous strictures as part of the healing process of inflammation. When patients present with obstruction, the clinical challenge is to separate active inflammation from a fixed fibrostenotic lesion that will not respond to medical therapy. Helpful clues that point to the latter include the absence of other systemic complaints (fevers, chills, anorexia, malaise) and precipitants of obstruction such as nuts or popcorn. A brief trial of steroids may be indicated to relieve the inflammatory component of the stricture. Referral to a surgeon for resection or stricturoplasty is indicated.

Indications for Surgery

From the perspective of the gastroenterologist, the indications for surgery in Crohn's disease may be divided into (1) those that are relatively acute, such as obstruction related to stricture, intra-abdominal or perianal abscess, and massive bleeding; and (2) those that fall into the category of intractable disease. There is no readily agreed definition of intractable disease; in effect, each patient defines the limit of his or her tolerance of medical therapy and gastrointestinal symptoms. It is my feeling that patients who actively participate in the discussion of surgery accept their procedures better than those who feel that surgery was imposed on them.

MAINTENANCE OF REMISSION

A salient feature of Crohn's disease is its propensity for relapse. In fact, if a patient has had only one episode of Crohn's disease in the remote past, the diagnosis should be re-evaluated; the patient may have had an infectious ileitis such as *Campylobacter* or *Yersinia* infection. Patients enter a clinical remission via either a

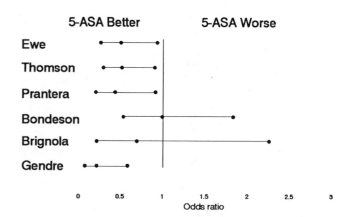

Figure 1 Odds ratios along with Cl_{95} for several studies that have examined the efficacy of 5-aminosalicylate (5-ASA) therapy for maintenance of remission. Values of less than 1 imply a beneficial effect for 5-ASA.

medical or a surgical approach. Endoscopic studies demonstrate that disease recurs rapidly after resection, and that at least aphthous ulceration within the neoterminal ileum is seen in most patients within 6 months after surgery. Belgian colleagues suggest that the endoscopic appearance of the neoterminal ileum can predict the risk of clinical recurrence. To be effective, therapy should be introduced as soon as possible after surgery.

There is no evidence to suggest that the use of corticosteroids will maintain remission. Until recently, it was thought that 5-ASA did not confer the same remission-sustaining properties they demonstrated in ulcerative colitis. This conclusion may be erroneous, since the early studies in the 1970s had small sample sizes and heterogeneous populations. These studies assessed sulfasalazine, which requires bacterial action to release 5-ASA. Over the last 5 years an increasing number of studies using a variety of 5-ASA delivery systems have suggested that pharmacologic therapy can alter clinical recurrence. Although not as dramatic as in ulcerative colitis, the risk of recurrence may be reduced by 30 to 40 percent (Fig. 1). Many studies suggest that early introduction of 5-ASA (within 3 months of surgery) may identify a group of patients who will benefit from prophylactic therapy. Details of patient selection and appropriate dosage should be defined. As gastroenterologists, we tend to see maintenance therapy in the context of peptic ulcer disease as prescribing 50 percent of active disease therapy. In the future, the concept of continuous full-dose therapy may have to be emphasized for patients with Crohn's disease.†

FUTURE THERAPIES

Therapy for Crohn's disease is changing with the introduction of newer medications along with continued

---

*Editor's Note: Although our experience is uncontrolled, we use an abdominal computed tomographic scan to evaluate new abdominal masses before instituting steroid therapy. If an abscess is found, percutaneous or surgical drainage is usually requested.

---

†Editor's Note: Although I have advocated maintenance therapy with alternate-day prednisone, sulfasalazine, and/or azathioprine, none of my observations are controlled.

evaluation of nutritional interventions. The observation that patients with AIDS and Crohn's disease reported improvement in their Crohn's disease as their HIV infection progressed has led to the concept of selective modulation of T-cell function. Further advances in therapy can be expected.

SUGGESTED READING

Archambault A, Feagan B, Fedorak R, et al. The Canadian Crohn's Relapse Prevention Trial (CCRPT) (abstract). Gastroenterology 1992; 102:A591.

Brynskov J, Freund L, Rasmussen SN, et al. A placebo-controlled, double-blind, randomized trial of cyclosporine therapy in active chronic Crohn's disease. N Engl J Med 1989; 321:845.

International Mesalazine Study Group. Coated oral 5-aminosalicylic acid versus placebo in maintaining remission of inactive Crohn's disease. Aliment Pharmacol Ther 1990; 4:55.

Landi B, Anh TN, Cortot A, et al. Endoscopic monitoring of Crohn's disease treatment: a prospective, randomized clinical trial. Gastroenterology 1992; 102:1647.

Malchow H, Ewe K, Brandes JW, et al. European Cooperative Crohn's Disease Study (ECCDS): results of drug treatment. Gastroenterology 1984; 86:249.

Martin F, Sutherland LR, Beck IT, et al. Oral 5-ASA versus prednisone in short term treatment of Crohn's disease: a multicentre controlled trial. Can J Gastroenterol 1990; 4:452.

Present DH. 6-Mercaptopurine and other immunosuppressive agents in the treatment of Crohn's disease and ulcerative colitis. Gastroenterol Clin North Am 1989; 18:73.

Rasmussen SN, Lauritsen K, Tage-Jensen U, et al. 5-Aminosalicylic acid in the treatment of Crohn's disease. A 16 week double-blind, placebo-controlled, multicenter study with Pentasa. Scand J Gastroentol 1987; 22:877.

Rijk MC, Van Hogezand RA, Van Lier HJJ, et al. Sulphasalazine and prednisone compared with sulphasalazine for treating active Crohn's disease. Ann Intern Med 1991; 114:445.

Singleton JW, Summers RW, Kern F, et al. A trial of sulfasalazine as adjunctive therapy in Crohn's disease. Gastroenterology 1979; 77:887.

Summers RW, Switz DM, Sessions JT Jr, et al. National Co-operative Crohn's Disease Study: results of drug treatment. Gastroenterology 1979; 77:847.

Sutherland L, Singleton J, Sessions J, et al. Double blind, placebo controlled trial of metronidazole in Crohn's disease. Gut 1991; 32:1071.

Tremaine WJ. Maintenance of remission in Crohn's disease: is 5-aminosalicylic acid the answer? Gastroenterology 1992; 103:694.

CROHN'S DISEASE IN CHILDREN AND TEENAGERS: SPECIAL PROBLEMS

GEORGE D. FERRY, M.D.

Prednisone and sulfasalazine continue to be the drugs most often used in children with Crohn's disease, but experience is growing with a number of alternative medications. The new 5-aminosalicylic acid (5-ASA) derivatives for oral and rectal use, along with immunosuppressive drugs, give physicians some choice in tailoring treatment to specific disease sites and complications. The therapeutic goal for an acute flare-up of Crohn's disease is to control inflammation and reduce symptoms as quickly as possible. Although there is often a reluctance to use prednisone in children because of suppression of growth, this and other side effects must be weighed against a slow or inadequate response to other drugs. Physicians caring for children and adolescents must adjust drug doses carefully by weight and clinical response, watch growth carefully, and deal with changing emotional and developmental problems and parental concerns over a broad age range.

MILD TO MODERATE ILEITIS AND ILEOCOLITIS

Seventy percent of patients with Crohn's disease have inflammation in the ileum or ileum and colon. Children most often present with abdominal pain, diarrhea, weight loss, and/or fever. The severity may vary depending on the location and extent of disease. A transient decrease in height velocity is also common, and occasional patients present with growth failure.

My usual treatment for mild to moderate ileitis or ileocolitis is prednisone, 0.5 to 1.0 mg per kilogram per day up to 40 mg daily (Table 1). Symptoms often improve within 1 to 2 weeks, at which time the dose of prednisone can be tapered by 2.5 to 5 mg per week, depending on the clinical response. With the first episode of Crohn's disease, I try to wean patients off prednisone by 10 to 12 weeks. If symptoms recur as the dose is lowered, I wean more slowly and often switch to an every-other-day schedule when the dose is approximately 20 mg per day. This can be accomplished by continuing to taper the alternate-day dose every 1 to 2 weeks, or by switching from 20 mg daily to 40 mg every other day and continuing to taper the dose as above. Side effects, including acne, cushingoid appearance, and mood changes, are common in spite of tapering doses of prednisone. Adolescents are particularly distressed with these side effects, and I try to decrease the dose as rapidly as the clinical response allows. In the short term, these doses of prednisone have

Table 1 Medical Treatment of Ileitis and Ileocolitis

Prednisone	
Moderate disease	0.5–1 mg/kg/day (30–40 mg/day)
Severe disease	2 mg/kg/day (60 mg/day)
Tapering dose*	2.5–5 mg/wk
Maintenance†	0.25–0.5 mg/kg q.o.d.
Sulfasalazine	
Treatment	60–75 mg/kg/day up to 4.0 g/day
Maintenance	30–40 mg/kg/day up to 2.0 g/day
Metronidazole	15 mg/kg/day up to 750 mg/day
Azathioprine	2.0 mg/kg/day up to 150 mg/day
6-Mercaptopurine	1.5 mg/kg/day up to 150 mg/day
Cyclosporine	
Oral	7 mg/kg/day
IV	4 mg/kg/day
Mesalazine	Up to 2.4 g/day
Olsalazine	30–40 mg/kg/day up to 2–3 g/day

*After 2–4 weeks and an adequate clinical response.
†Average doses for alternate-day prednisone: 20 mg q.o.d. for children over 40 kg; 15 mg q.o.d. for 20–40 kg; 10 mg or less for children <20 kg.

no negative effect on growth and may actually stimulate a short growth spurt from increased intake and decreased inflammation. Switching to alternate-day prednisone, 10 to 20 mg every other day, often controls inflammation and helps maintain growth.

As I taper prednisone, I often begin a maintenance dose of sulfasalazine, 30 to 40 mg per kilogram per day up to 2.0 g per day. I divide the dose into two or three doses per day so that school age children do not have to take medication at school. Although some question remains about the benefit of maintenance therapy, I generally continue sulfasalazine for at least 1 to 2 years, especially for Crohn's colitis. In very mild ileitis or ileocolitis without complications, I have used sulfasalazine as the initial treatment in doses of 60 to 75 mg per kilogram per day, up to 4.0 g daily. I add prednisone if symptoms increase or there is no improvement within 4 to 6 weeks. Sulfasalazine may inhibit absorption of folic acid and I suggest that patients take 1 mg of folic acid per day.

Side effects of sulfasalazine are common, and 15 percent of children have to discontinue the drug because of headache, rash, or neutropenia. In cases in which I feel maintenance therapy to be essential (e.g., continued mild symptoms, growth failure) I use mesalazine (Asacol), 1.2 to 2.4 g per day, or prednisone, 10 to 20 mg every other day. Mesalazine releases 5-ASA in the distal small bowel and colon and appears to be well tolerated in patients who cannot take sulfasalazine. Although my experience is limited in Crohn's disease, I have used this drug successfully in children with ulcerative colitis.

Careful follow-up of clinical status, abnormal laboratory findings, nutritional status, and growth is essential. Initial follow-up visits are scheduled for 2 to 4 weeks, then monthly for two or three visits, depending on the clinical status. More frequent visits give children and their parents ample opportunity to ask questions about the disease. This also allows the medical and nursing staff to discuss the chronic nature of inflammatory bowel disease and to stress the importance of compliance. For

adolescents, I provide extra time alone to establish rapport and to offer support and understanding about the difficulty in coping with a chronic illness. I also offer literature from the Crohn's and Colitis Foundation of America (CCFA) and ask patients and families to view one of the video tapes that discusses coping with Crohn's disease and colitis. Once a patient is in remission, I arrange a follow-up visit every 6 months to monitor clinical status and growth and to give support to the patient and family. Any abnormal laboratory findings are followed until normal, especially the sedimentation rate. I have not found the Crohn's Disease Activity Index (CDAI) useful in children, but I am evaluating a pediatric index (PCDAI) that uses clinical, laboratory (hematocrit, sedimentation rate, albumin), and growth parameters to assess activity.

MODERATE TO SEVERE ILEOCOLITIS

For more severe disease associated with fever, bloody diarrhea, cramping pain, weight loss, and anemia, or other systemic signs of illness, I start prednisone, 2 mg per kilogram up to 60 mg per day. If there is vomiting, abdominal tenderness with guarding or rebound, severe pain, suspected abscess, or fistula, patients are hospitalized for intravenous (IV) corticosteroids, fluids, and bowel rest. As symptoms improve over the first few days, I initiate oral feedings. With continued anorexia, the presence of a fistula, or partial obstruction, I offer an elemental diet, even if this requires the introduction of a nasogastric tube. If tube feedings are not tolerated, I place a central venous catheter and start total parenteral nutrition (TPN). Once patients have responded, I switch to an equivalent dose of oral prednisone and taper slowly as for mild to moderate cases.

STEROID-DEPENDENT PATIENTS

Some children with large and small bowel involvement respond initially to prednisone, but each time the dose is lowered they have a relapse or a significant increase in symptoms. Sulfasalazine and other 5-ASA drugs may not prevent relapse, and other approaches are indicated. After the second relapse or increase in symptoms, I try to switch to alternate-day prednisone. A dose of 15 to 20 mg per kilogram every other day is generally well tolerated and effective in many children. If this is unsuccessful, I add 6-mercaptopurine (6-MP), 1.5 mg per kilogram per day, or azathioprine, 2.0 mg per kilogram per day. Once I start an immunosuppressive agent, I discontinue sulfasalazine. I do not decrease the dose of prednisone for 4 to 6 weeks, since I do not anticipate a real effect from immunosuppressive drugs before this time. I tend to be slower in reducing prednisone in these circumstances and may make a change every 2 weeks rather than once a week, depending on the severity of the disease. Often it is necessary to continue immunosuppressive drugs for 1 or 2 years or more, and I have had some patients on these drugs for 6 to 8 years. I monitor blood counts very closely, starting at 2 and 4 weeks, then monthly for the first year, and then every 3 to 6 months. If there is a decrease in the white blood cell count, I decrease the medication or stop it if the count does not improve. The long-term use of immunosuppressive drugs appears to be safe, but patients and parents are warned that an increased risk of cancer has been suggested, albeit minimal. Any potential for late complications must be weighed against steroid dependence and significant side effects from daily prednisone.*

COLITIS

Mild left-sided colitis and pancolitis, either Crohn's disease or ulcerative colitis, are generally treated with sulfasalazine, 60 to 75 mg per kilogram per day, up to 4.0 g daily. With significant rectal or rectosigmoid disease, I often add 5-ASA enemas or hydrocortisone enemas, twice daily for the first week, then once daily for 1 to 2 weeks or until a good clinical response is documented. Most patients are unwilling to use enemas for an extended period; many children complain of increased pain, diarrhea, or bleeding with enemas and will not tolerate their use. For more severe cases of colitis, with anorexia, anemia, severe pain, and more frequent bloody stools, I give prednisone as described for ileocolitis. I add sulfasalazine as I begin to taper the prednisone.

Localized proctitis is rare in my practice, but hydrocortisone enemas or foam, 5-ASA enemas, or suppositories have all been effective in some patients. In others, the inflammation is resistant and tends to relapse frequently. Most children find oral medication preferable to enemas or suppositories, and in some cases of proctitis sulfasalazine has been effective.†

Symptomatic treatment with loperamide or other drugs to decrease intestinal activity may provide some relief from pain and constant trips to the bathroom. I have not seen complications with these medications in patients with mild to moderate disease, but am cautious in more severe disease because of the potential for ileus and megacolon.

In fulminant colitis, with persistent bloody diarrhea, a requirement for blood transfusions, and no response to prednisone over 2 weeks, I begin IV cyclosporine, 4 mg per kilogram per day, divided into two doses or infused continuously.‡ I adjust this dose to maintain cyclosporine trough levels between 200 and 300 µg per deciliter. If there is no response within 7 to 10 days or if the patient deteriorates, a total colectomy is recommended. My experience with total colectomy and an ileal J-pouch anastomosis for fulminant ulcerative colitis has been excellent in terms of continence and patient satisfaction. Fulminant colitis has been uncommon in Crohn's disease and indeterminant colitis. In these cases I see mostly chronic, unremitting disease, for which 6-MP or azathioprine may be effective in inducing remission and lowering the requirement for prednisone.

COMPLICATIONS

Strictures are common in Crohn's disease, and resection or stricturoplasty is indicated if symptoms persist in spite of treatment with corticosteroids or other medications to control inflammation. It is important to recognize when narrowed bowel is due to scar formation, so that side effects from excessive use of corticosteroids can be avoided. Resection of a short stenotic section of involved bowel gives good results, but I am now gaining experience with stricturoplasty, which allows correction of obstruction without resection.§

Fistula and abscess formation are also common in Crohn's disease and require both medical and surgical treatment. One to 2 weeks of IV broad-spectrum antibiotics, corticosteroids, and bowel rest may help decrease inflammation. Depending on the location of the fistula or abscess, I start one of the elemental diets within the first week if possible. If symptoms persist, or if patients have some degree of obstruction or very severe disease, I leave the bowel at rest and use TPN. If symptoms subside and the abscess decreases in size on computed tomography (CT) or ultrasonography, I may choose resection or continued observation. A few such abscesses have disappeared on x-ray examination and patients have remained asymptomatic. I have successfully drained a number of abscesses with ultrasound-directed needle aspiration and placement of a small drain. Many of these patients recover clinically and are reluctant to consider resection of the diseased segment.¶

---

*Editor's Note: Pediatric gastroenterologists are increasingly willing to give azathioprine or 6-MP to teenagers with chronic unresponsive disease or those who are steroid dependent. The response rate of 70 percent seems to be similar in both adolescents and adults. It would be helpful if there were a central registry for such patients so that data on possible complications, such as infertility, could be put into perspective with data on other patients who have not received these agents. This might be a reasonable challenge for the CCFA.

†Editor's Note: As stated, proctitis that remains localized to the rectum or sigmoid is unusual in teenagers. It is not uncommon to see seemingly localized disease extend within months or a year to left-sided colitis or even pan-colitis. I usually avoid giving a firm prognosis to young people with seemingly localized disease.

‡Editor's Note: IV cyclosporine therapy has provided prompt responses (6 or 7 days) in some young people with fulminant colitis of short duration, but the results seem to be less consistent than in adults, where a 60 to 70 percent response rate is expected.

§Editor's Note: Patients with jejunoileitis don't usually come to surgery for treatment of obstruction before 10 to 12 years of disease.

¶Editor's Note: It is gratifying to note the increasing willingness of physicians to treat transmurally aggressive ileal disease with bowel rest, antibiotics, and even at times steroids. We find CT scans very helpful in evaluating right lower quadrant abdominal masses. Drainage of obvious abscesses still seems prudent before starting steroids.

UPPER INTESTINAL DISEASE

I am performing upper endoscopy more often in children with ileitis or Crohn's disease of the colon and upper intestinal symptoms. Gastric, duodenal, and esophageal erosions and microscopic inflammation are common. Ranitidine or omeprazole do not appear to provide much relief from symptoms, and I have used a moderate dose of prednisone in some cases.*

NUTRITIONAL SUPPORT

In any patient with weight loss, a decrease in linear growth, anemia, low serum albumin levels, or other signs of undernutrition, I evaluate general eating habits and ask for a 4 day diet record. Laboratory evaluation includes a complete blood count, serum albumin, blood urea nitrogen, electrolytes, calcium, and phosphate. Every effort is made to improve intake, focusing on specific deficiencies and general energy and protein intake (Table 2). Nutritional supplements with high caloric density and high protein are often helpful (Table 3), but in my experience many children and adolescents will not take more than 8 to 10 ounces a day. Carnation Instant Breakfast, which provides 250 kcal per 8 ounces, is a good substitute for some of the ready-mixed products, as it is quite palatable, has a variety of flavors, and is less expensive than many prepared supplements. For lactose intolerance, a lactose-free supplement is necessary.

Vitamin, iron, and mineral supplementation is often required, and needs should be assessed by the diet record and appropriate blood tests. Zinc and magnesium

Table 2 Energy and Protein Requirements in Crohn's Disease

Acute undernutrition: normal height for age, weight for height less than 5th percentile
Use 4 day diet record as baseline for increasing calories and protein
Use RDA for age to calculate appropriate caloric intake; adjust for level of activity and intestinal losses due to diarrhea
With low serum albumin, increase protein intake to 2.0–3.0 g/kg/ day for young children, 1.5 g/kg/day for older children (may increase more if significant fecal losses)

Chronic undernutrition: height less than 5th percentile, weight for height less than 5th percentile
Calculate height age
Use RDA for height age as goal for appropriate intake
Increase gradually to 140%–150% of RDA as needed to improve nutrition
Increase protein intake to 1.5 g/kg/day for older children (may increase more if significant fecal losses)

Mild chronic undernutrition or steroid effect: height less than 5th percentile, weight for height normal
Calculate height age
Use RDA for height age as goal for appropriate intake (if height is low owing to chronic steroid use, increasing intake may not be desirable)
Maintain normal protein intake

*__Editor's Note:__ Omeprazole seems to be somewhat helpful if combined with anti-inflammatory medications. Heretical as it may seem, I think sulfasalazine has some local effect in the esophagus, stomach, and duodenum (after all, it does work as an enema for proctitis).

Table 3 Commonly Used Nutritional Supplements

Type	Product (kcal/ml)	Protein Source (g/dl)	Carbohydrate (g/dl)	Fat g/dl (% MCT)	Osmolality (mOsm/kg water)
Complete oral or tube feeding	Instant breakfast: 1/ml	Cow's milk: 6	15*	4	
	Ensure†: 1	Casein, soy: 3.5	13.7	3.5	470
	Ensure Plus: 1.5	Casein, soy: 5.5	20	5.3	690
	Sustacal: 1	Casein, soy: 6.1	14	2.3	620
	Sustacal HC: 1.5	Casein: 6.1	19	5.8	650
	Nutren 1: 1	Casein: 4	12.7	3.8 (24)	300
	Nutren 1.5: 1.5	Casein: 6	17	6.8 (50)	410
	Nutren 2: 2	Casein: 8	19.6	10.6 (73)	710
	Pediasure†‡: 1	Casein: 3	11	5	310
Complete tube feeding	Osmolite: 1	Casein, soy: 3.7	14.5	3.8 (50)	300
	Osmolite HN: 1	Casein, soy: 4.4	14	3.7 (50)	300
	Isocal: 1	Casein, soy: 3.4	13.3	4.4 (20)	300
	Isocal HCN: 2	Casein: 7.5	20	10.2 (40)	690
	Jevity§: 1	Casein: 4.4	15.5	3.7 (50)	300
Complete elemental	Peptamen: 1	Hydrolyzed whey: 4	12.7	3.9 (54)	270
	Vivonex: 1	Free amino acids: 3.8	20.5	0.28	630
	Tolerex¶: 1	Free amino acids: 2.0	22.6	0.14	550
	Vital HN: 1	Hydrolyzed whey, meat, soy: 4.2	18.5	0.1 (45)	500

*Diluted with milk, contains lactose.
†Available with fiber.
‡For ages 1–6 years.
§Has fiber.
¶Less protein may be appropriate for children.

are often included in vitamin supplements, and iron can be given separately for anemia due to blood loss.

In children who are significantly underweight (less than the 5th percentile weight for height), intake may need to reach 140 percent of the recommended daily allowance (RDA), or more, to reach a normal weight and height. Using a 4 day diet record as a start, and the RDA for height age as the goal, caloric intake can be increased in a stepwise fashion as tolerated. In patients unable to maintain an adequate intake owing to a poor response to medications, or complications of Crohn's disease, I use nasogastric tube feedings of complete or elemental formulas. A nighttime drip providing 500 to 1000 kcal per night is often enough to supplement oral intake adequately. For patients with minimal oral intake or in cases in which bowel rest is indicated, a 24 hour infusion is used. Patients with significant weight loss and/or low serum albumin levels are at risk for complications of malnutrition, and rapid nutritional intervention is indicated. A trial of enteral feedings should begin as soon as the clinical course allows. In chronic undernutrition, long-term goals are essential to help patients gain weight and catch up linear growth.

In severely ill patients who cannot be fed or who fail nasogastric feedings, peripheral or central IV nutrition is necessary. Indications for IV nutrition include persistent vomiting, ongoing fecal losses of blood and proteins, obstruction, or fistula or abscess that may require eventual surgery.

PERIANAL DISEASE

This is a particularly difficult disease medically, and for children and adolescents it adds a severe emotional burden that requires extra patience and understanding from physicians, nurses, and family. Treatment is often unsatisfactory, and many different medical therapies, nutritional approaches, or forms of surgery may be needed. The interest in using newer drugs is especially strong because of the frequent poor response.

I generally give metronidazole, 15 mg per kilogram per day, up to 250 to 500 mg three times daily. If there is active bowel disease or severe inflammation with draining fistulas, I also give moderate doses of prednisone. If there is no response, or perianal disease remains active, I switch to 6-MP and prednisone.

Although some patients respond to this combination, many continue to have active disease, and I have occasionally used oral cyclosporine, 7 mg per kilogram per day. If this is successful, I try to wean patients off this regimen within 3 months and maintain them on a combination of alternate day-prednisone and 6-MP.

GROWTH DELAY

In a few children, Crohn's disease is diagnosed as a result of a significant decrease in growth velocity and a subsequent fall in height percentiles. This is a challenging complication that requires dual goals of both decreasing active inflammation and providing adequate nutritional support. It is important to assess growth potential by using bone age and the Tanner stage of pubertal development. Boys over 14 and girls over 13 with no delay in bone age may have limited growth potential. Tanner stage III also suggests limited growth potential, but there is significant variation in response. In my experience, alternate-day prednisone, often with a maintenance dose of sulfasalazine, has been effective in improving growth in many patients. Occasionally I have used nighttime nasogastric tube feedings to boost caloric intake and improve growth.

SUGGESTED READING

Fonkalsrud EW, Loar N. Long-term results after colectomy and endorectal ileal pullthrough procedure in children. Ann Surg 1991; 215:57–62.

Hyams JS, Ferry GD, Mandel FS, et al. Development and validation of a pediatric Crohn's disease activity index. J Pediatr Gastroenterol Nutr 1991; 12:439–447.

Jackson WD, Grand RJ. Crohn's disease. In: Walker WA, Durie PR, Hamilton JR, et al, eds. Pediatric gastrointestinal disease. Philadelphia: BC Decker, 1991:592–608.

Markowitz J, Rosa K, Grancher K, et al. Long-term 6-mercaptopurine treatment in adolescents with Crohn's disease. Gastroenterology 1990; 99:1341–1351.

Motil KJ, Grand RJ. Ulcerative colitis and Crohn's disease in children. In: Kirsner JB, Shorter RG, eds. Inflammatory bowel disease. 3rd ed. Philadelphia: Lea & Febiger, 1988:227.

Palder SB, Shandling B, Bilik R, et al. Perianal complication of pediatric Crohn's disease. J Pediatr Surg 1991; 26:513–515.

Whitington PF, Barnes HV, Bayless TM. Medical management of Crohn's disease in adolescents. Gastroenterology 1977; 72: 1338–1344.

CROHN'S DISEASE: SURGICAL MANAGEMENT

JOE J. TJANDRA, M.D.
VICTOR W. FAZIO, M.D.

Crohn's disease is a diffuse, chronic, and transmural inflammatory condition that can involve any part of the gastrointestinal (GI) tract. It most commonly affects the terminal ileum but often extends to or is limited to the large bowel. Perianal involvement occurs in 20 to 90 percent of patients, depending on the diagnostic criteria and the reporting centers. In general, severe perianal disease is more common in patients with Crohn's colitis than in those with exclusively small bowel involvement.

Crohn's disease is commonly manifested as discontinuous and patchy inflammation with active disease, and stenotic skip areas may be found with grossly normal bowel in between. Aphthous ulceration is generally believed to be the first macroscopically recognizable sign of Crohn's disease. Symptoms relate to the ulcerated mucosa, to strictures, to intra-abdominal and/or perianal sepsis, and to a variety of extraintestinal manifestations.

SURGICAL MANAGEMENT

Crohn's disease is not curable by either medical or surgical treatment. The surgical procedure must have a specific and limited objective: to deal with the immediate effects of the disease, prevent certain complications, restore health, and permit withdrawal of steroids or immunosuppressive agents. The need for surgery is related to the duration of the disease and the anatomic site of involvement within the GI tract. Thus, most patients with Crohn's disease will undergo surgery during the course of their illness: 50 percent within 5 years of the diagnosis of small bowel disease and 66 percent within 10 years. Patients with ileocolic disease have the greatest need, and those with disease confined to the colon or rectum appear to have a somewhat lesser need for surgery. The anatomic pattern of disease also has an important bearing on the indications for surgery.

PREOPERATIVE PREPARATION

Anemia and fluid and electrolyte abnormalities are corrected before elective surgery. Significant nutritional depletion, if present, may require parenteral nutrition. The extent of Crohn's disease is determined by contrast study and colonoscopy as far as possible. Perioperative steroid coverage is used for patients who have been on steroids in the preceding 6 months. Perioperative antibiotics are used prophylactically for 48 hours but may be prolonged in highly contaminated cases. An appropriate bowel preparation is used. When there is severe obstruction, a more prolonged preparation without catharsis is used and a period of nasogastric decompression may be necessary. In patients in whom a stoma is a possibility (suspected abscess, perforation), preoperative marking of the stoma site is made.

SMALL BOWEL CROHN'S DISEASE

Indications for Surgery

Surgery is usually performed to treat complications rather than for failure to thrive or failed medical therapy. However, even among "experts," views differ regarding the management of specific cases. Common indications for surgery are shown in Table 1. Given a patient who has an adequate length of small bowel and who requires long-term (more than 3 to 6 months) steroids in dosages greater than 15 mg prednisone per day, we usually recommend surgery, either resection or stricturoplasty (SXPL) (see later).

Operative Strategy

Resection

For most patients with small bowel disease, bowel resection and anastomosis is the procedure of choice, especially in the presence of acute inflammatory phlegmon, overt perforation, fistula, long strictures (greater than 30 cm), and multiple strictures within a short segment. In most cases, a conservative margin of 2 to 5 cm of bowel is adequate. Lymphadenectomy of enlarged mesenteric lymph nodes is performed only if it does not compromise the vascular supply of the remaining bowel. There is no evidence that more radical margins result in fewer recurrences. Frozen section to ensure disease-free margins is probably unnecessary. Anastomosis can safely be made in segments of bowel with aphthous ulceration, provided that there is no severe overt disease such as ulceration or strictures. Anastomoses in bowel with microscopic evidence of Crohn's disease heal as well as those in normal bowel. Results are also similar in terms

Table 1 Primary Indications for Surgery

Indication	Ileitis/Ileocolitis	Colitis
Obstruction	+ + +	+
Perforative	+ + +	+ + +
Fistula		
Phlegmon/abscess		
Persistent hemorrhage	+ +	+ +
Chronic ill health (including severe disease, poor response to medical therapy, growth retardation)	+	+ + +
Perianal disease	+	+ + +
Toxic colitis/megacolon	N/A	+ +

+ + + = most common; + = least common.

of postoperative complications and recurrence rates between patients who have had a side-to-end and those with an end-to-end anastomosis. Our own preferred technique is the side-to-side anastomosis because of its larger lumen.

Stricturoplasty

With repeated bowel resections, there is the potential of ultimately leaving a functionally insufficient length of small bowel. It is now recognized that Crohn's disease is a chronic, relapsing, panintestinal disease and that microscopic and histochemical evidence of Crohn's disease may be present in grossly normal-appearing bowel. Thus, the philosophy for surgical treatment of small bowel Crohn's disease has swung in the direction of conservatism. The rationale of SXPL is that it increases the diameter of the bowel and relieves the obstruction without sacrificing any small bowel. The principles and nomenclature of the operation are analogous to those of pyloroplasty. For strictures shorter than 10 cm, a Heineke-Mikulicz SXPL is performed. Strictures longer than 10 cm are best dealt with by Finney SXPL. For long strictures that are close together, Finney SXPL will result in long bypass segments where stasis can be a problem. In these circumstances, it is often better to reconstruct the posterior wall in a Finney fashion but to close the anterior enterotomy in a Heineke-Mikulicz manner. A very long isolated stricture (greater than 30 cm) is often best dealt with by resection. Only short strictures of the duodenum are suitable for SXPL. We do not perform SXPL on colonic strictures because preservation of length of large bowel is not so critical and the healing can be less predictable.

A number of studies have attested to the safety and efficacy of SXPL in the treatment of selected strictures of the small bowel and an anastomosis (small bowel, ileocolic, or ileorectal). In our experience of 452 SXPLs in 116 patients, there has been no mortality. Septic complications occurred in 6 percent and were similar to those with resection. Obstructive symptoms were relieved in 99 percent of patients. Symptoms recurred in 24 percent of patients after a median follow-up of 3 years; all of them had new strictures or perforative disease elsewhere.* The rate of symptomatic restricture of the SXPL sites was 2.8 percent after a median interval of 3 years.

Several factors have been examined for association with septic complications after SXPL. These include the presence of perforative components distant from the SXPL sites, steroid dosage, synchronous resection, previous bowel resection, the number of SXPLs, the length of stricture, and a serum albumin level less than

30 g per liter. Only the last of these factors has been found to be associated with an increased incidence of septic sequelae.

Selection of appropriate patients, attention to perioperative care, and techniques of SXPL are important factors for a good outcome. There are certain situations in which SXPL should be particularly considered:

1. Diffuse Crohn's disease with symptomatic strictures, especially if there is dilatation of proximal bowel.
2. Previous extensive (longer than 100 cm) resection of small bowel.
3. Recurrence of symptoms within 12 months of previous resection.
4. Evidence of short bowel syndrome.
5. The presence of fibrotic strictures.

There are circumstances, however, in which SXPL is contraindicated:

1. Overt perforation.
2. Fistula or inflammatory phlegmon at the operative site.
3. Multiple strictures within a short segment.
4. Excessive tension at the SXPL closure site.
5. A serum albumin level less than 20 g per liter.

Bypass Surgery

Diversion of the fecal stream around the segment of bowel involved with Crohn's disease while leaving that segment in place was recommended in the past. However, there is often bacterial overgrowth in the bypassed segment. Patients will also have a persistent inflammatory process in the bypassed bowel segment, with the potential for abscess, bleeding, or perforation. Many have persistent debilitating extraintestinal manifestations. In addition, about one-third of all adenocarcinomas reported have been in the bypassed segment. Thus, bypass surgery is now rarely performed, except for gastroduodenal Crohn's disease. Occasionally, if the patient is particularly ill or if the surgeon feels that the situation is technically formidable, unilateral exclusion bypass can be carried out. The bypassed segment is resected several months later.†

Special Problems

Abscess

In the presence of a localized abscess, including a psoas retroperitoneal abscess, a preliminary computed tomography (CT)-guided drainage of the abscess, fol-

---

*Editor's Note: The recurrence of symptoms in one-fourth of the patients was due to "new strictures" or "perforative disease elsewhere." At present we have no medical therapy that prevents fibrosis and scarring, but we do have long-term medication programs that can suppress disease activity and probably lessen morbidity. We need a controlled trial of medical therapy after stricturoplasty.

---

†Editor's Note: As more attention is focused on dysplasia and carcinoma in Crohn's disease, it is clear that there is dysplasia in the small bowel near the cancers. Since these loops (and retained rectal stumps) are rarely accessible to surveillance, the advice to remove bypassed segments is usually reasonable.

lowed by definitive resection and anastomosis several weeks later, is helpful. This downstages the degree of sepsis, provides guidance to deep-seated abscesses such as a psoas abscess, and allows primary bowel anastomosis. If an occult abscess is encountered during a planned laparotomy, the site is drained and quarantined with omental interposition, and bowel resection is then performed. In most cases, a primary anastomosis is still possible. In very ill patients with significant sepsis, a diverting ileostomy may be prudent.

Fistula

Enterocutaneous fistulas that arise within the first week after surgery are probably due to technical problems rather than residual Crohn's disease. These are best treated by early laparotomy, exteriorization of fistula, or a proximal stoma. Those arising after the first week are usually managed by nonoperative means, including total parenteral nutrition (TPN). Those arising from recurrence of Crohn's disease are usually treated by resection. Patients who have had multiple recurrences (potential short bowel syndrome) and who have a low-output "pouchable" fistula are also best treated nonoperatively initially. In extreme cases, home parenteral nutrition may be indicated. There is a separate chapter on parenteral nutrition.

Enteroenteric fistulas are not always symptomatic and do not always demand surgical treatment. Ileoileal and ileosigmoid fistulas are treated by resection and anastomosis of the primary fistulizing disease, which is usually in the distal ileal segment. Secondary sites often are not involved by Crohn's disease and can usually be managed by wedge excision of the fistula and closure of the enterotomy. In cases of ileosigmoid fistula, endoscopic examination of the sigmoid colon is helpful to determine whether it contains Crohn's disease. In some of these cases, there is a significant phlegmonous reaction at the parasigmoid tissues that necessitates formal sigmoid resection and anastomosis.

Ileoduodenal fistula is usually a manifestation of Crohn's disease of the terminal ileum. Many have had previous ileocolic resection for Crohn's disease. Recurrent disease at an ileocolic anastomosis predisposes to fistulization to the underlying second and third parts of the duodenum. Attention to technical detail may prevent this rare complication. In most cases, ileocecal resection, without mobilization of the ascending colon, keeps the anastomosis in the right lower quadrant. If the disease recurs or if the ascending colon must be resected, consideration should be given to resection of the proximal transverse colon so that the anastomosis is on the left side of the abdomen. Surgery is indicated if symptoms are not controlled by nonoperative means or if there is significant obstruction or sepsis. The ileal disease is excised. Debridement of the edges of the duodenum and primary closure is possible in some patients, but larger duodenal defects are best dealt with by side-to-side duodenojejunal anastomosis.

Ileostomy fistula is managed by resection and neoileostomy, unless the fistula is superficial to the skin level and easily pouchable. Relocation of the stoma may be required if the original aperture in the abdominal wall harbors residual sepsis.

Ileovesical fistula can occur. Removal of the fistulizing ileal segment is necessary. The bladder defect is closed if possible and separated from the abdominal cavity by omental interposition. Foley catheter drainage of the bladder is maintained for 7 to 10 days postoperatively.*

Obstructive Uropathy

Obstructive uropathy is often the result of retroperitoneal inflammation and fibrosis, and compression by ileocecal or colonic phlegmon. Resection of the enteric disease alone is often adequate, and ureterolysis is rarely necessary.

GASTRODUODENAL CROHN'S DISEASE

Gastroduodenal Crohn's disease is unusual. Duodenal Crohn's disease is more common, affecting around 2 percent of patients with Crohn's disease. Operative intervention is required in at least one-third of patients. The most common indication for surgery is obstruction (70 percent); others include pain, unresponsiveness to medical therapy, and severe hemorrhage. If the diagnosis of Crohn's disease is certain preoperatively, gastrojejunostomy with truncal vagotomy is the preferred surgical option. Because of concerns with postvagotomy diarrhea, particularly in patients who have had previous ileocecal resection, other authors have advocated gastrojejunostomy with highly selective vagotomy. Simple bypass without vagotomy is associated with a high incidence of marginal ulceration. Gastrectomy is also associated with significantly higher morbidity than non-Crohn's cases.

CROHN'S DISEASE OF COLON AND RECTUM

In general, few patients with extensive Crohn's colitis secure long-term remission with medical treatment, and most require surgery. The probability of surgical treatment for primary Crohn's colitis has been estimated as 35 percent ± 7 percent at 5 years and 39 percent ± 7 percent at 10 years for recent-onset disease, rising to 72 percent ± 6 percent at 6 years from the first admission to the hospital.

---

*Editor's Note: There is a small but vocal group of gastroenterologists who point out the usually benign nature of ileovesical fistula *without* ascending urinary tract infection. Some urge no therapy; others stress the use of 6-mercaptopurine (6-MP). Since most of the patients I see have the fistula at the site of an obstructed ileal segment, most are urged to undergo ileal resection and fistula take-down.

The indications for surgery are somewhat different in Crohn's colitis from those in ileocolic or ileal disease (see Table 1). A greater proportion of patients undergo surgery for intractability or anorectal disease. Less commonly, the indication may arise more acutely owing to fulminant disease (phlegmon, abscess, fistula, bleeding, toxic megacolon, perforation). Most commonly the need for surgery becomes apparent gradually over months or years from increasing inability to maintain the patient in a reasonable condition during times of exacerbation, despite increasing doses of steroids.*

Surgical Options

In our experience, the most common operation performed was proctocolectomy in one or more stages (76 percent), followed by abdominal colectomy with or without anastomosis (21 percent). Much less commonly, ileostomy alone or bypass (3 percent) was performed.

Proctocolectomy and Ileostomy

Proctocolectomy and ileostomy is most appropriate in the presence of extensive Crohn's colitis, especially if there is serious anorectal disease. This can be performed as a one-stage procedure in the elective setting, with a mortality rate of less than 2 percent. The procedure also appears to carry the lowest clinical recurrence rate, averaging around 20 percent. Goligher suggested that although there is a linear increase in recurrence during the first 10 years after proctocolectomy, it tends to plateau at the 20 percent range thereafter. However, this operation is associated with significant morbidity, notably unhealed perineal wounds (10 to 30 percent), small bowel obstruction, and ileostomy complications.†

When there is fulminant colitis or severe malnutrition or perineal sepsis, it is preferable to perform a staged procedure after initial abdominal colectomy with or without anastomosis, completed by proctectomy at a second stage. Less commonly, a diverting loop ileostomy is constructed initially for severe rectal and suppurative perianal disease, followed by second-stage proctocolectomy.

Perineal proctectomy is completed by the endoanal technique with intersphincteric dissection between the internal and external anal sphincters. This minimizes perineal wound problems. Others have advocated transecting the rectum at the level of the levators, leaving a small anorectal stump and avoiding a perineal wound altogether. We find that even in these circumstances, drainage from the anus still occurs and perirectal fistulas may persist.

Abdominal (Subtotal) Colectomy

Abdominal (subtotal) colectomy is often performed in acute situations, as previously discussed. It is also considered when the rectum is compliant and relatively spared of disease, there is a lack of significant perianal sepsis or fistulas, and there is no extensive ileal disease. This technique is also an acceptable alternative when the diagnosis of Crohn's disease versus ulcerative colitis is uncertain. One-stage primary ileorectal anastomosis is usually performed unless there is toxic colitis, associated intra-abdominal sepsis, significant malnutrition, or significant rectal or perianal disease. In such circumstances, an initial ileostomy and Hartmann's closure of the rectum is performed, followed, if appropriate, about 6 to 12 months later by a secondary ileorectal anastomosis. It is desirable to conserve the entire rectum and even the distal sigmoid, if the extent of the disease makes that possible, to provide a good reservoir capacity for stool. In our own experience with 118 patients with an ileorectal anastomosis, there were no operative deaths. Anastomotic leaks occurred in 3 percent of patients. After a mean follow-up of 9.5 years, 61 percent retained a functioning ileorectal anastomosis, and less than half of these patients had recurrent disease that required nonoperative treatment with medications. The functions in some of these patients are not always satisfactory, but this situation may be preferable to a stoma for some patients. Twenty-three percent of the 118 patients ultimately required proctectomy and the remainder required proximal diversion. In patients with an excluded rectal stump, careful surveillance is important because of the risk of development of rectal carcinoma. Certainly, the presence of persistent and significant anorectal disease despite fecal diversion is a predictor of probably poor function with reanastomosis. If reanastomosis is not intended, we recommend removal of the rectal stump within 1 to 2 years after abdominal colectomy, unless the patient is elderly and frail.

Segmental Colectomy

Although segmental resection is the accepted treatment of choice for ileocolitis, the management of symptomatic and isolated segmental colitis is less clear. This condition is uncommon, occurring in 6 to 20 percent of patients. It could be in the form of segmental resection with colocolic or colorectal anastomosis, or an abdominoperineal resection of the rectum with end-colostomy, depending on the site of the lesion. In some patients, this has been done when the preoperative diagnosis was diverticulitis. The recurrence rate after segmental resection is high, being up to 60 percent at 5 years. However, this may be of value in elderly patients if the

---

*Editor's Note: This is the Crohn's colitis seen by physicians who do not use azathioprine or 6-MP. Those of us who do use immunomodulators for chronic unresponsive disease or for those dependent on steroids (13 percent of my Crohn's disease patients) rarely send patients to surgery for intractable but uncomplicated colitis. Whether we are creating a pool of people who will later develop dysplasia and cancer must also be considered.

†Editor's Note: It is commonly stated that if the ileum is grossly normal, there is only a 20 percent chance of recurrence in the ileostomy. The lack of contact with colonic contents may also play a role in this relatively low recurrence rate.

water-absorbing capacity of the right colon and the function of the ileocecal valve can be preserved.

TOXIC COLITIS/MEGACOLON

This occurs less commonly in Crohn's colitis than in ulcerative colitis. Histologic distinction between ulcerative colitis and Crohn's colitis can be confusing in the presence of fulminant colitis, especially if there is only mild inflammatory involvement of the rectum. The most satisfactory surgical treatment in an emergency is subtotal colectomy with end-ileostomy and Hartmann's closure of the rectum. This allows for removal of a majority of diseased bowel and establishment of a firm histologic diagnosis, and it does not preclude subsequent sphincter-sparing restorative procedures.

RECURRENCE AFTER SURGERY

The definitions of recurrent disease and indications for reoperation are variable and are different in different reports. This accounts for a wide variation in the reported rates of recurrence. In general, recurrence rates vary with the length of follow-up and the sites of disease. If recurrence is defined as a return of symptoms, including pain, fever, diarrhea, and weight loss, approximately 20 percent of patients experience recurrence by 2 years, 30 percent by 3 years, and 50 percent by 5 years. By contrast, endoscopic evidence of asymptomatic recurrent disease is apparent in 73 percent of patients 3 months after ileocolic resection. The anatomic pattern of disease also has an important impact on remission-free intervals. At 14 years after the initial operation, the cumulative risk of recurrence for patients with ileocolic disease was 50 percent ± 9.6 percent, whereas for terminal ileal disease alone it was 38 percent ± 6 percent, and for large bowel disease alone only 32 percent ± 7 percent. In a study, the number of sites involved by Crohn's disease is an important variable in the intra-abdominal recurrence rate. The annualized risk of recurrence was 1.6 percent for patients with single-site involvement and 4 percent for those with multiple-site involvement. Overall, when followed at 5 years, approximately one-quarter of patients with either small bowel resection or SXPL require treatment (operative and nonoperative) of recurrent disease at the sites of previous surgery or at new sites. While a bigger resection is not necessarily better in small bowel Crohn's disease, and the overall rates of reoperation for stricture at the sites of SXPL and resection are similar, this is not the case with Crohn's colitis. Thus, proctocolectomy and end-ileostomy has a lower recurrence rate than subtotal colectomy and ileorectal anastomosis, which in turn has a lower recurrence rate than segmental colectomy.

There is a predilection of recurrence for specific sites after certain surgical procedures. The most common site of recurrence after proctocolectomy and ileostomy is in the terminal ileum immediately proximal to the ileostomy; after ileorectal anastomosis, it is in the rectum or ileum; after ileocolic anastomosis, it is in the preanastomotic ileum; and after segmental colectomy, it is in the remaining large bowel. Late recurrences (after more than 10 years) are more often successfully managed nonoperatively than those that occur early. Trials evaluating adjuvant steroids, sulfasalazine, and azathioprine as prophylaxis against recurrences have been performed. There does not appear to be any benefit thus far.*

SPECIAL CIRCUMSTANCES

Proximal Diversion

Proximal diversion of the fecal stream may often improve the anorectal disease, at least temporarily. Its use as a staged procedure in preparation for later resection has been referred to earlier. With currently available perioperative care, this is becoming less necessary. With proximal diversion, the patient's general status is often improved and steroid dosage may be tapered before proctectomy is performed. It also decreases local sepsis and may improve subsequent perineal healing. However, of patients in whom a defunctioning ileostomy is performed as an elective surgical treatment of Crohn's colitis, less than 15 percent go on to reestablishment of intestinal continuity with a good result. Proximal diversion may have an adjunctive role in surgical repair of a perirectal fistula, but even this is not always necessary.

Proximal Resection in Anorectal Disease

Removal of proximal bowel disease leads to remission of anorectal disease in 30 to 50 percent of patients. Relief in this respect may be temporary (12 to 24 months). If the proximal disease is gross and is contiguous with anorectal disease, complete removal of all active disease in the area, even at the cost of the anal sphincters, is desirable.

Pouch Procedures

Pouch procedures, including the continent ileostomy and ileal pouch–anal anastomosis, are contraindicated in patients with known Crohn's disease because of the high risk of recurrence in and proximal to the ileal pouch, which could result in the loss of much precious small bowel. In our experience, when restorative proctocolectomy has been performed for patients with indeterminate colitis or with "ulcerative colitis" that subsequently proved to be Crohn's disease, a good functional outcome is still achieved in 65 percent of cases

---

*Editor's Note: Trials continue, with small bowel released 5-ASA looking promising, e.g., ASACOL, Pentasa, Salofalk. A preliminary short-term study of metronidazole seemed to lessen the severity of recurrence. A trial of 6-MP is under way.

at 3 year follow-up. The presence of any clinical features suggestive of Crohn's disease preoperatively, e.g., perianal disease, is associated with a high incidence of pouch sepsis and a poor outcome. By contrast, complication and pouch failure rates are very similar in patients with true indeterminate colitis and in those with typical ulcerative colitis. In very special circumstances, after a thorough discussion and the obtaining of informed consent, one may consider the staged conversion of a Brooke ileostomy to a continent ileostomy in selected patients who, after several recurrence-free years, desire an attempt at restoration of continence.

Balloon Dilatation

Balloon catheters passed by the radiologist or through an endoscope have been introduced into the strictured area and then inflated to dilate the stricture. The procedure appears to be relatively painless and safe in expert hands. Perforation has occurred and the long-term benefit is not clear. The technique should be regarded as experimental and be restricted to short strictures, such as in ileorectal anastomosis, in the pyloric canal, and in medically debilitated patients.*

Crohn's Disease and Adenocarcinoma

Adenocarcinoma of the small and large bowel affected by Crohn's disease is being reported with increasing frequency. Adenocarcinoma of the small bowel is difficult to diagnose preoperatively and carries a poor prognosis. It tends to affect more distal small bowel than in patients with non-Crohn's adenocarcinoma of the small bowel. Although the observed

---

*Editor's Note: Two excellent series on dilatation of colon and ileocolonic strictures in Crohn's disease, from Sweden and from Belgium, have taught us that strictures that are dilated 7 or 8 years after resection tend to stay open, while those in areas of actual disease tend to recur.

incidence is much higher, fewer than 100 cases have been reported in the literature to date. At least one-third of these have occurred in excluded small bowel segments. The relative risk of small bowel cancer in Crohn's patients probably exceeds 100, although this estimate is highly imprecise. Resection provides the only cure, although in many patients the cancer is advanced at surgery and is amenable only to palliative bypass.

The incidence of adenocarcinoma of the large bowel is much lower than that associated with ulcerative colitis. Patients with Crohn's colitis of more than 7 years' duration have an increased risk of up to twentyfold. Cancer has developed insidiously in bypassed segments of colon and defunctionalized rectal stumps because of difficulty with periodic surveillance.†

SUGGESTED READING

Becker JM. Surgical management of inflammatory bowel disease. Curr Opin Gastroenterol 1993; 9:600–615.
Fazio VW, Tjandra JJ. Stricturoplasty for Crohn's disease with multiple long strictures. Dis Colon Rectum 1993; 36:71–72.
Fazio VW, Tjandra JJ, Lavery IC, et al. Long-term follow-up of stricturoplasty in Crohn's disease. Dis Colon Rectum 1993; 36: 355–361.
Sayfan J, Wilson DA, Allan A, et al. Recurrence after stricturoplasty or resection for Crohn's disease. Br J Surg 1989; 76:335–338.
Schoetz DJ. Gastroduodenal Crohn's disease. Perspect Colon Rectal Surg 1992; 5:145–154.
Schrock TR. Surgery for Crohn's colitis. Curr Manage Inflamm Bowel Dis 1989; 1:290–294.
Tjandra JJ, Fazio VW. Crohn's disease: the benefits of minimal surgery. Can J Gastroenterol 1993; 7:254–257.

---

†Editor's Note: There is a chapter, also from the Cleveland Clinic, on neoplasia in inflammatory bowel disease. One major problem with Crohn's colitis is determining when the ulcers started, especially in people diagnosed after age 50. Sentiment seems to be building for some type of surveillance program in patients with long-standing extensive Crohn's colitis, especially if the illness started in childhood or adolescence.

ENTEROCUTANEOUS FISTULA

ADRIAN J. GREENSTEIN, M.D.

The management of enterocutaneous fistulas has improved dramatically over the past three decades, with significant advances in medical and surgical therapy. Both mortality and morbidity rates have been affected. Advances in overall management have resulted in increased spontaneous closure rates, lower operation rates, and fewer deaths. Mortality has been reduced from the 20 to 60 percent range to 5 to 20 percent by the use of parenteral nutrition, administration of newer antibiotics, and improved intensive care. Fluid and electrolyte imbalance and malnutrition, major causes of death in earlier years, are now successfully managed in almost all patients. Despite better imaging techniques, better management, better antibiotics, percutaneous drainage of complicating abscesses, and improved surgical techniques, the old enemies—sepsis and septic shock—remain the major cause of the residual mortality.

ETIOLOGY

Enterocutaneous fistulas may be divided into spontaneous and postoperative (post-traumatic) groups. The latter group is much more common and may follow surgery or penetrating trauma. Although some reports suggest approximately equal incidences originating from the upper (stomach, duodenum, and gastroduodenal anastomosis); middle (jejunum, and ileum); and lower (ileocolonic) gastrointestinal (GI) tract, the precise incidence at any one institution will be determined by the local distribution of disease. Thus, hospitals specializing in trauma, gastric or pancreatic diseases, inflammatory bowel disease, and oncologic surgery each deal with different incidences of the various types of external fistula.

MANAGEMENT

Anastomotic Leaks

Anastomotic leaks are the most lethal of enterocutaneous fistulas, are often difficult to diagnose before obvious leakage through the wound or drain site occurs, and usually (but not always) require surgical intervention, especially if located high in the GI tract and of high volume.

Gastroduodenocutaneous Leaks

During the era when peptic ulcer surgery was common, anastomotic leaks occurred occasionally, usually after Billroth I gastrectomy. Ischemia of the gastric stump, distal obstruction, tension at the suture line in high gastrectomy, and tumor at the line of resection in cases of gastric carcinoma all predispose to this complication. Duodenal stump leakage is more common and follows Billroth II gastrectomy with an overall incidence of 1 to 5 percent. Poor surgical technique, the difficult duodenal stump, and sepsis due to perforation of the original peptic ulcer are underlying causes. The development of acute gastroduodenocutaneous fistulas can be avoided or minimized by meticulous surgical technique, including insertion of a duodenostomy or gastrostomy when necessary.

Once the gastro- duodeno- or gastroduodenocutaneous fistula is established, one is faced with a serious management problem. The output is usually high, sepsis of the surrounding tissues is inevitable, and immediate therapy is mandatory. If a Jackson-Pratt or Penrose drain was inserted at the original surgery, it should be replaced by a high-flow sump drain and the patient placed on continuous suction drainage to prevent digestion of the skin and subcutaneous tissues. Appropriate antibiotic coverage should be started immediately. Accurate fluid and electrolyte replacement, milliliter for milliliter, of the precise electrolyte content of the aspirated fluid is essential, preferably in an intensive care unit. If there is an associated wound abscess, this should be surgically drained. Once the patient is stable, diagnostic fistulography should establish the site of origin of the fistula. Most duodenal stump leaks close within 3 to 4 weeks with continuous aspiration, provided that adequate high-calorie nutritional support is given by a central venous line, and that sepsis is controlled by antibiotics and adequate drainage. Surgical resection of an anastomotic leak site may be necessary. In the rare duodenal stump leak that fails to heal, one should suspect underlying Crohn's disease, persistent abscess, tumor, or distal obstruction at the gastroenterostomy. A Roux-en-Y duodenojejunostomy may be the best surgical solution in the intractible case.

Jejunal, Ileal, and Ileocolonic Leaks

Jejunoileal leaks are uncommon, as the blood supply of the small bowel is excellent, but most occur during attempts to carry out an anastomosis in the presence of dilated, edematous, obstructed, and unprepared bowel with associated sepsis. In these circumstances, a diverting ileostomy is safe and effective, although a second major intra-abdominal procedure is necessary. Jejunal contents will drain through the wound or drain site, and immediate surgery is generally advisable, especially if the site is lower in the ileum. A proximal diverting loop ileostomy, or resection and exteriorization of the original suture line with enterostomy, including drainage of the infected intestinal fluid and irrigation of the entire peritoneal cavity, is the minimal procedure. Enteroenterostomy may be carried out 3 or more months later when the patient has fully recovered and all sepsis is controlled. In some cases in which the severity of the original fistula does not preclude immediate reanastomosis, a concomitant proximal diverting loop ileostomy may be performed. This can be closed several months later without formal laparotomy through the ileostomy site.

Distal Colonic Leaks

If the output is low and the fistula small, conservative management with adequate drainage, control of infection, intravenous (IV) feeding or elemental diet, and early return to oral feedings may be tried. If this approach is unsuccessful, or the disruption is large, re-exploration with disconnection of the suture line, proximal colostomy, and closure of the distal stump should be undertaken. Colocolostomy can be performed after several months.

Chronic Fistulas

Spontaneous Enterocutaneous Fistulas

Spontaneous fistulas are rare; almost all external fistulas occur after abdominal surgery or penetrating trauma. When fistulas occur spontaneously, it is usually in the umbilical region, and occasionally in the linea alba above or below the umbilicus.

Umbilical fistulas may be of congenital or acquired origin. The draining umbilicus may be studied by fistulography, and the presence of a Meckel's diverticulum established by technetium 99m pertechnetate scan. Umbilical fistulas of congenital origin occur when the omphalomesenteric duct fails to obliterate and remains patent. Only 6 percent of patent vitellointestinal ducts have a patent ileocutaneous tract, while 10 percent have a solid cord that may predispose to internal herniation and obstruction; approximately 80 percent have a Meckel's diverticulum. If the former type has a large diameter, a fecal fistula may develop early in life or even in the neonatal period. If this is small, intestinal obstruction may produce an ileoumbilical fistula. Treatment is simple: exploratory laparotomy with transection of the patent omphalomesenteric duct and ligation on either side, preferably with resection of the intervening segment. If obstruction is present, the cause must be treated. In some cases a large or small omphalocele with pouting intestinal mucosa may be the clue to an underlying patent omphalomesenteric duct; in other instances (approximately 20 percent), herniation of small bowel through the umbilicus may be found. In these cases, complete excision of the umbilicus with disinvagination of the small bowel and resection of the segment, if necessary, should be carried out. If a segment of duct is present, it should be amputated from the ileum, and the bowel closed transversely.

Spontaneous acquired enteroumbilical fistula is usually secondary to Crohn's disease and originates most frequently from the underlying colon, but ileoumbilical fistulas, usually from the terminal ileum, also occur. These fistulas are rare, occurring in approximately 0.2 percent of patients with Crohn's disease. Although elemental diet, 6-mercaptopurine (6-MP), and azathioprine (Imuran) have been tried with limited success, long-term cure can best be achieved by resection of the underlying diseased segment with reanastomosis. I recently resected a spontaneous Crohn's ileocutaneous fistula through a large umbilical hernia, which had been treated for several years unsuccessfully with a combination of steroids and 6-MP, by means of wide excision of the entire umbilicus, infected tissue, and underlying diseased ileum en bloc. Reanastomosis was successfully accomplished by ileoileostomy at the primary operation.

Spontaneous external fistula, usually in the midline secondary to diverticulitis, occurs but is rare. Resection of the segment of diseased colon, with or without immediate reanastomosis, and with or without proximal diverting ostomy, is the preferred surgical treatment.

Spontaneous external fistulas secondary to underlying intestinal malignancy are exceedingly rare today, being due to neglect or late diagnosis, and are generally incurable. Complete resection, including the involved abdominal wall, gives the best palliation.

Postoperative Enterocutaneous Fistulas

Postoperative external fistulas are relatively common and usually develop through a previous incision or drain tract. Approximately 25 percent of all external fistulas are due to Crohn's disease. Simple incision and drainage of an intra-abdominal abscess in Crohn's disease without concomitant diversion will result in an enterocutaneous fistula in a high percentage of patients because the feeding focus remains in situ. External fistulas usually originate in the distal ileum or colon and rarely cause the skin excoriation and discomfort of high small bowel fistulas. They usually discharge pus or mucus intermittently and require one or several dressing changes daily. Although they may be tolerated for long periods, they seldom heal spontaneously, and persistent underlying disease, either primary or recurrent, is indicated. In the presence of Crohn's disease, simple appendectomy, or exploratory laparotomy without resection of an unrecognized perforated segment of small bowel, will result in a fecal fistula. If the disease was missed by the limited exposure of a McBurney incision, this fistula may be the presenting manifestation of this disease. A widespread misconception among physicians, including well-trained surgeons and gynecologists, is that if Crohn's disease is inadvertently encountered at emergency exploratory laparotomy, the abdomen should be closed. This may be appropriate for acute terminal ileitis or Crohn's disease of the nonperforating variety of recent duration. However, a laparotomy without resection is likely to lead to an intra-abdominal abscess, with or without fistula formation in the perforating forms: a prescription for disaster, when sealed fistulous tracts to the mesentery or adjacent bowel are opened up.

Reports of closure of such fistulas with prolonged IV alimentation, oral elemental diet, 6-MP, or metronidazole are not sanguine about the long-term outlook, as most fistulas recur after medical therapy is discontinued. Most patients ultimately need resection of diseased bowel together with the fistulous tract, and do well thereafter. Complex fistulas may occur in Crohn's disease, including multiple enterocutaneous tracts, multiple communicating intestinal fistulas, ileovesicocutaneous fistulas, ileosigmoidocutaneous fistulas, jejunocolocutaneous fistulas, and numerous other varieties. I have seen as many as five concomitant jejunocolic fistulas, and five ileoileal fistulas with concomitant ileocutaneous fistulas. It is at times fortunate that all the fistulas can arise from a short segment of ileum. The key to management is simultaneous closure or resection of all these complex fistulas. Preoperative imaging of the extent of disease and fistulization can be helpful.

Fistulas originating at a suture line heal in the same way as other suture line fistulas in the absence of actual overt disease at the anastomosis, distal obstruction, foreign body, or carcinoma.

Duodenocutaneous fistulas, particularly in Crohn's disease, should be treated by closure, preferably in two layers, with onlay of a jejunal patch.

Peri-Ileostomy Fistulas

Peri-ileostomy fistulas are a particularly unpleasant form of external fistula having the problem of persistent drainage from an ileocutaneous fistula combined with the difficulty of maintaining the seal of an appliance. The latter problem may produce severe skin excoriation. When such fistulas are preceded by a parastomal abscess, or when multiple fistulas are present, the skin surface is usually grossly irregular, and transposition of the stoma to the left lower quadrant of the abdomen may be necessary after resection of the diseased segment of ileum proximal to the stoma. This may be done through a formal laparotomy incision, or by the direct stoma-to-stoma technique.

Carcinomas in Crohn's disease have presented as ileocutaneous or ileovesical fistulas, particularly when occurring in bypassed loops of bowel. In such cases, palliative resection should be attempted, but no cures have been reported and death usually ensues within a few months to a year.

High-Output Jejunal Fistulas

High-output fistulas, especially with sepsis, loss of fascial tissues of the anterior abdominal wall, and excoriation of the skin by intestinal fluid, remain a most difficult management problem. Special skin care is necessary, often requiring the skills of a stomatherapist. Nutritional support is essential, as healing may take a long time. The key is to reduce output to a minimum. This is accomplished by making the patient NPO and giving parenteral nutrition for both adequate caloric intake and reduction in output of bile and pancreatic fluids.

In recent years, a number of publications have evaluated the use of somatostatin and octreotide, a long acting analog, in patients with fistulas. Somatostatin acts by decreasing gastric, pancreatic, and jejunal secretion via secretory inhibition of a number of secretagogues, including enteroglucagon, gastrin, secretin, VIP, glucagon, and pancreatic polypeptide. Somatostatin and its analog have been found useful as an adjunct to standard treatment. In some studies, rapid reduction in fistula output was noted, and in a review of ten separate studies a closure rate of approximately 80 percent in 175 patients at a mean of 7.2 days was found. Use of somatostatin should substantially reduce hospital stay if further studies confirm these early results. In many patients, fistulas take a month or longer to heal. A multi-institutional, prospective randomized controlled study is urgently required to determine the true value of somatostatin for enterocutaneous fistulas, although initial reports seem promising. These drugs have also been used for pancreaticocutaneous fistulas, also with a remarkable immediate reduction in pancreatic output, and reported rapid closure of fistulas, but also without a randomized controlled trial.

Perianal Fistulas and Abscesses

Anorectal abscesses and fistulas are a common complication of Crohn's disease, being least frequent in ileal disease (approximately 20 percent), most frequent in distal colonic disease (approximately 60 percent), and of intermediate incidence in the ileocolonic form of disease (45 percent). These perianal lesions may precede the onset of the intestinal disease by as long as 20 years. They are particularly troublesome and painful, but the extensive excavation of some perianal fistulas and abscesses results from reluctance to treat these lesions actively for fear of aggravating the local condition. This problem should be seen less often now with early local drainage and fistulotomy, and with use of the Parks internal sphincterectomy. This latter procedure partially resects and divides the internal sphincter, removes the area of local fibrosis, and allows the abscess to drain internally. Although in many instances complete healing will not be achieved, especially if the active intestinal disease is not controlled, this conservative form of treatment leads to a satisfactory clinical result in most patients.

Occasionally, severe perianal disease is associated with severe distal Crohn's colitis, fecal incontinence, and/or anorectal stricture with obstruction. Total proctocolectomy and ileostomy is the only solution to this intractable problem. Fecal diversion alone does not result in healing of extensive perianal disease. Rarely, a perianal fistula originates in the upper rectum or a loop of ileum with perirectal tracking of the fistula. Correction of the proximal disease with ileal resection is the solution to this unusual high fistula of ileal origin. Proctocolectomy may be necessary for high rectal fistulas if the perianal abscess and fistulas are incapacitating or track to the buttocks or hip joints, and if the colonic disease is extensive and severe. Fecal diversion may play a useful adjunctive role in the surgical management of perianal Crohn's disease, but it is of extremely limited value as definitive therapy, especially in patients with concomitant rectal involvement, in whom the long-term success rates are less than 20 percent.

COMMENTS

Enterocutaneous fistulas no longer present the specter of a high mortality rate or an intractable long-term problem. Although many acute fistulas respond to medical therapy, judicious surgical intervention usually resolves the problem in the remainder. Chronic fistulas usually require surgical management, with a high success rate and a low mortality rate, utilizing our armamentarium of excellent anesthesia, preoperative mechanical bowel preparation with appropriate antibiotics, intestinal resection rather than bypass, and advanced postoperative care in an intensive care unit when necessary.

SUGGESTED READING

Bury KD, Stephens RD, Randall HT. Use of a chemically refined liquid elemental diet for nutritional management of fistulas of the alimentary tract. Am J Surg 1971; 121:174–183.

Fazio VW, Church JM, Jagelman DG, et al. Colocutaneous fistulas complicating diverticulitis. Dis Colon Rectum 1987; 30:89–94.

Fischer JE, Foster GS, Abel AN, et al. Hyperalimentation as primary therapy for inflammatory bowel disease. Am J Surg 1973; 125: 165–175.

Greenstein AJ, Dicker A, Meyers S, Aufses AH Jr. Periileostomy fistulae in Crohn's disease. Ann Surg 1983; 197:179–182.

Greenstein AJ, Kark AE, Dreiling DA. Crohn's disease of the colon. I. Fistula in Crohn's disease of the colon, classification presenting features and management in 63 patients. Am J Gastroenterol 1974; 62:419–427.

Greenstein AJ, Sachar DB, Tzakis A, et al. The course of enterovesical fistulae in Crohn's disease. Am J Surg 1984; 147:788–792.

Grosman I, Simon D. Potential gastrointestinal uses of somatostatin and its synthetic analogue octreotide. Am J Gastroenterol 1990; 85:1061–1072.

Hiley PC, Cohen N, Present DH. Spontaneous umbilical fistula in granulomatous (Crohn's) disease of the bowel. Gastroenterology 1971; 60:103–107.

MESENTERIC ISCHEMIA

PETER HUGH MacDONALD, M.D., F.R.C.S.C.

IVAN T. BECK, M.D., Ph.D., F.R.C.P.C., F.A.C.P., F.A.C.G.

Ischemic bowel disease occurs when blood flow to any part of the intestine is suddenly or chronically diminished or fully interrupted. This may be caused by inadequate systemic blood flow or local vascular abnormalities. Because of the frequency of inadequate vascular supply in the elderly, ischemic bowel disease occurs most often in older patients. It may also be seen in younger patients with vascular abnormalities such as vasculitis, collagen diseases, or diabetes or in those who are taking vasoconstrictor drugs. The approach to therapy depends on the type of vessel involved. Thus, to provide appropriate treatment, it is necessary to acquire a thorough understanding of the pathophysiology of the different ischemic syndromes. Accordingly, in this chapter we provide a short review on the classification and pathophysiology of intestinal ischemia.

GENERAL CONCEPTS

Classification of Intestinal Ischemia

The extent of intestinal ischemia and the pathologic consequence depends on the size and location of the occluded or hypoperfused vessels. The clinical presentation is also different, depending on the acuteness or chronicity of the vascular occlusion. Because certain acute events may change to a chronic condition, a clear-cut classification of ischemic bowel disease is very difficult. From a clinical and pathologic point of view, we find it useful to classify ischemic bowel disease according to the size of the vessels that are hypoperfused or occluded. This is because the clinical picture, investigation, and therapy in patients with mesenteric artery or vein occlusion are often different from those in patients in whom the cause of the disease is occlusion or hypoperfusion of the intramural vessels (Fig. 1). As the classification of syndromes in this Figure 1 is based on the pathophysiologic mechanisms, we will discuss therapy based on this classification.

In our experience, ischemic colitis is more common than acute mesenteric ischemia. Overall, acute ischemia is much more common than chronic forms of the disease. Also, ischemia of arterial origin is far more frequent than that of venous disease. It is now recognized that many reported cases of mesenteric vein thrombosis were in fact incorrectly diagnosed cases of nonocclusive ischemia, and it is now believed that the true incidence of mesenteric vein thrombosis is quite low.

Pathophysiology of Intestinal Ischemia

Vascular Anatomy

The anatomy of the splanchnic circulation is complex and extremely variable. The finer details are really important only to the invasive radiologist, whereas the clinician need only be concerned with some of the more constant and important features. The blood flow to the splanchnic organs is derived from three main arterial trunks: the celiac, superior mesenteric, and inferior mesenteric arteries. The celiac artery supplies blood to the foregut (stomach and duodenum), the superior mesenteric artery to the midgut (duodenum to transverse colon), and the inferior mesenteric artery to the hindgut (transverse colon to rectum). Each arterial trunk supplies blood flow to a section of the gastrointestinal (GI) tract through a vast arcade network, a system that is generally protective against ischemia. In the event of an arterial obstruction distal to the main arterial trunk, GI blood flow can usually be maintained through collateral vessels. As shown in Figure 2, additional vascular protection is obtained from anastomotic connections between the three arterial systems.

Communication between the celiac system and the superior mesenteric system generally occurs via the superior pancreaticoduodenal and inferior pancreaticoduodenal arteries. The superior mesenteric and inferior mesenteric systems are joined by the arc of Riolan and the marginal artery of Drummond, vessels that

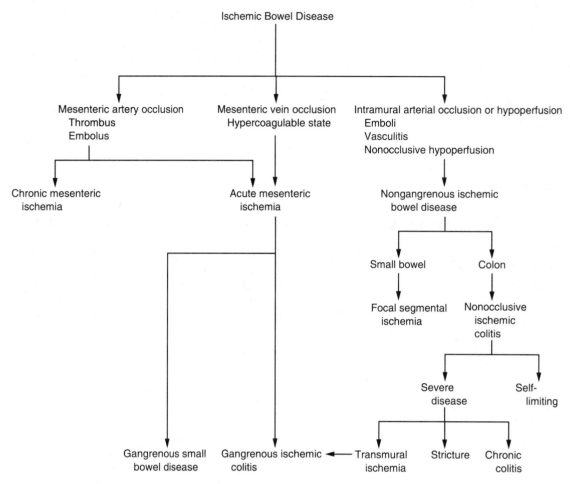

Figure 1 Classification of intestinal ischemia.

connect the middle colic artery (a branch of the superior mesenteric artery) and the left colic artery (a branch of the inferior mesenteric artery). In addition, communication exists between the inferior mesenteric artery and branches of the internal iliac arteries via the rectum. The caliber of these anastomotic connections varies considerably, depending on the existence of vascular disease, but it is important to realize that in chronic states of vascular insufficiency, blood flow to an individual system can be maintained through these anastomotic connections even when an arterial trunk is completely obstructed. It is not uncommon to find one or even two arterial trunks completely occluded in the asymptomatic patient. In fact, there are reports of occlusion of all three trunks in patients who are still maintaining their splanchnic circulation. However, in up to 30 percent of people, the anastomotic connections between the superior and inferior mesenteric arteries, via the arc of Riolan and the marginal artery of Drummond, can be weak or nonexistent, making the area of the splenic flexure particularly vulnerable to acute ischemia or failure of a surgical anastomosis. Another area of relatively poor collateral circulation is at the rectosigmoid junction, where the anastomotic connection be-

tween the most inferior sigmoid artery and the superior rectal artery (critical point of Sudeck) is often weak. These areas of poor collateral circulation are often referred to as the *watershed areas*.

Physiology of Splanchnic Blood Flow

Splanchnic blood flow varies in the fasting and nonfasting state, but on average it receives approximately 30 percent of the cardiac output. Blood flow through the celiac and superior mesenteric trunks is about equal (approximately 700 ml per minute in adults) and is twice that which flows through the inferior mesenteric trunk. In comparison with other tissue layers of the gut, the mucosa has the highest metabolic rate and thus receives about 70 percent of the splanchnic blood flow. Per unit tissue, the small bowel receives the most blood, followed by the colon and then the stomach.

Much has been written on the control of GI blood flow and many factors are involved. It is not the intent of this chapter to review the intricacies of physiologic control, but rather to highlight some important points. Vascular resistance is proportional to $1/r^4$ (where r = the radius of the vessel). Thus, the smaller the

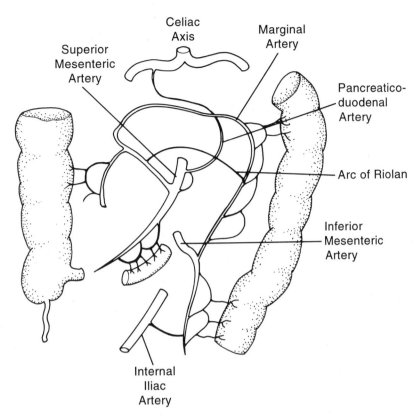

Figure 2 Splanchnic circulation.

artery, the greater is its ability to effect vascular resistance. Most blood flow control occurs at the arteriolar level, the so-called resistance vessels. Very little control of blood flow occurs at the level of the large arterial trunks. In fact, the diameter of these large arterial trunks can be compromised by 75 percent before blood flow is reduced. Additional control of blood flow occurs at the level of the precapillary sphincter. In the fasting state, only one-fifth of capillary beds are open, leaving a tremendous reserve to meet increased metabolic demands.

Among the most important control mechanisms of splanchnic blood flow are the sympathetic nervous system, humoral factors, and local factors. The sympathetic nervous system through alpha-adrenergic receptors plays an important role in maintaining basal vascular tone and in mediating vasoconstriction. Beta-adrenergic activity appears to mediate vasodilation, and it appears that the antrum of the stomach may be particularly rich in these beta receptors. Humoral factors involved in the regulation of GI blood flow include catecholamines, the renin-angiotensin system, and vasopressin. These humoral systems may play a particularly important role in shock states, and in some patients may play a role in the pathogenesis of nonocclusive ischemia. Local factors appear to be mainly involved in the matching of tissue blood flow to the metabolic demand. An increased metabolic rate may produce decreased Po_2, increased Pco_2, and an increased level of adenosine, each of which can mediate a hyperemic response. Finally, many inves-

tigators have now identified an important contribution by endothelin and endothelium-derived relaxing factor (nitric oxide) in the local control of intestinal blood flow.

The integration of these control systems, and their alteration by factors such as vascular disease, motor activity, intraluminal pressure, and pharmaceutical agents, remain poorly understood. The key to our understanding and successful treatment of intestinal ischemia lies in a better knowledge of this physiology.

Pathophysiology of Intestinal Ischemia

Intestinal ischemia occurs when the metabolic demand of the tissue supersedes the oxygen delivery. Obviously, many factors may be involved in this oxygen need/demand mismatch. These include the general hemodynamic state, the degree of atherosclerosis, the extent of collateral circulation, neurogenic/humoral/local control mechanisms of vascular resistance, and abnormal products of cellular metabolism before and after reperfusion of an ischemic segment.

Of all the intestinal wall tissue layers, the mucosa is the most metabolically active. Mechanisms that bring about redistribution of intramural blood flow have been identified. In general, they function to protect the mucosa against ischemia, but despite these mechanisms, the mucosal layer is the first tissue layer to demonstrate signs of ischemia. Changes at the cellular level begin at the tip of the villi. With ongoing ischemia, ultrastructural changes begin within 10 minutes and cellular damage is extensive by 30 minutes. Sloughing of the villus tips is followed by edema, submucosal hemorrhage, and eventual transmural necrosis.

The intestinal response to ischemia is first characterized by a hypermotility state. It is this intense motor activity that results in the patient experiencing severe pain, even though the ischemic damage may be limited to the mucosa at this stage. As the ischemia progresses, motor activity ceases and the gut mucosal permeability increases, leading to an increase in bacterial translocation. With transmural extension of the ischemia, visceral and parietal inflammation develop, resulting in peritonitis.

An important factor often responsible for or aggravating intestinal ischemia is the phenomenon of vasospasm. It has been well demonstrated that both occlusive and nonocclusive forms of arterial ischemia can result in prolonged vasospasm even after the occlusion has been removed or the perfusion pressure restored. This vasospasm may persist for several hours, resulting in prolonged ischemia. The mechanism responsible for this vasospasm is not clearly defined. To date, many of the interventional techniques used to treat mesenteric ischemia have been directed at counteracting this vasospasm.

A second factor that may be responsible for accentuating ischemic damage is reperfusion injury. In the laboratory, reperfusion has been shown to cause more cellular damage than is brought about during the actual ischemic period. Parks and Granger showed in an animal model that the injury after 1 hour of ischemia and 3 hours of reperfusion is more severe than that observed after 4 hours of continuous ischemia. The mechanism responsible for this reperfusion injury appears to be related to the release of harmful reactive oxygen metabolites, which are thought to be released from adhering polymorphonuclear leukocytes. It is not known what role ischemia reperfusion injury plays in humans with occlusive and nonocclusive disease.

ACUTE SUPERIOR MESENTERIC ISCHEMIA

Presentation and Diagnosis

The key to diagnosis lies in a high index of suspicion. Patients with advanced ischemia are usually not a challenge to diagnose, presenting with diffuse peritonitis, shock, and severe metabolic derangements. Often, these patients cannot be salvaged, and the mortality rate is reported to be between 70 and 90 percent. The patient with early ischemia is far more challenging to diagnose and stands to benefit most from a correct diagnosis.

The typical patient with mesenteric ischemia is usually over 50 years of age and often has a history of cardiac and peripheral vascular disease. In the early stage of ischemia the patient complains of severe abdominal pain in the absence of peritoneal findings; hence, the standard expression, "pain out of proportion to the physical findings." Other nonspecific symptoms

such as nausea, vomiting, and altered bowel habit may be present but are not particularly helpful in the diagnosis.

Laboratory Findings

Many studies have attempted to identify a biochemical marker of early ischemia. Creatine kinase, alkaline phosphatase, lactate dehydrogenase, diamine oxidase, and inorganic phosphate are among the biochemical markers that have been examined. Although all of these eventually become altered with intestinal ischemia, no single marker reliably identifies early ischemia, and thus in the clinical setting they are not particularly useful.

Management

General Concepts

If a diagnosis of mesenteric ischemia is being considered, the subsequent investigation and management must proceed in an efficient and aggressive fashion if morbidity and mortality are to be reduced. Initial management of all patients consists of resuscitation, the degree of which varies widely with the degree and extent of ischemia. Patients with early ischemia require very little resuscitation, whereas those with infarcted intestine may require admission to a critical care unit for invasive monitoring. Insertion of a Swan-Ganz catheter with central pressure monitoring can be very useful in resuscitating the shocked patient with underlying cardiac disease. It must be kept in mind that in patients with extensive and advanced infarction, complete "stability" may never be obtained, and thus investigation and treatment should proceed without extensive delay. However, ongoing patient "instability" is no doubt an ominous sign. As a general rule, vasopressors to support blood pressure should be avoided as they may further increase the degree of intestinal ischemia. The role of antibiotics is not clear-cut. Our policy is to administer broad-spectrum antibiotic coverage as soon as possible to patients presenting with peritonitis. In those without peritonitis, antibiotics are used in the perioperative period should surgery be required.

Clearly, several intra-abdominal disease processes can present in a fashion identical to that of mesenteric ischemia. Thus, initial investigation is aimed at ruling out other causes of abdominal pain and peritonitis. An upright and supine plain film of the abdomen should be obtained in all patients. Although these films may support a diagnosis of ischemia, as indicated by bowel wall thickening and "thumbprinting," their main purpose is to rule out visceral perforation or bowel obstruction. In many centers, computed tomography (CT) is being used as a first-line investigation in patients with abdominal pain. Several markers of intestinal ischemia have now been described by radiologists with expertise in CT scans, including bowel wall thickening, mucosal edema, pneumotosis, and mesenteric and portal vein gas. By means of large injections of peripheral venous contrast material, mesenteric arterial and venous occlusion can now also be identified in some patients. Of course, many of these findings are not specific, and thus we do not currently advocate the CT scan as a diagnostic test for intestinal ischemia. However, in certain situations, a high index of suspicion that a disease process other than ischemia is involved will necessitate its use. For example, it is sometimes difficult to differentiate acute pancreatitis from abdominal ischemia. Both can present with hyperamylasemia and/or peritonitis. This is one situation in which an abdominal CT scan may be useful to rule out retroperitoneal inflammation.

Ultrasonography combined with Doppler assessment of blood flow in the splanchnic arterial and venous system is now being used in some centers to screen for mesenteric ischemia. Our personal experience with this technique is limited, and the exact role this technique will play is not clearly defined. There is experimental evidence from a rabbit model of ischemia that magnetic resonance imaging (MRI) may also be of significant use in the diagnosis of mesenteric ischemia. Certainly, both arterial and venous abnormalities as well as the extent of the collateral circulation can be identified in some patients through MRI technology, but further clinical experience is required before this technique can be completely evaluated.

Angiography remains the "gold standard" in the diagnosis of mesenteric ischemia and, as will be discussed, may play a significant role in the treatment of such patients. We believe that all patients with suspected mesenteric intestinal ischemia should undergo angiography to confirm the diagnosis and assist treatment planning. This approach should include those patients presenting with peritonitis. Often, there is a tendency to take patients with peritonitis straight to the operating room without performing angiography. These patients need to be treated in an expedient fashion, but the short delay involved in obtaining an angiogram may prove beneficial. Not only will it identify patients who may require embolectomy or vascular reconstruction, but it will also provide a means to treat vasospasm in the perioperative period. Such a treatment policy has two implications. First, for management to be effective, an invasive radiologist must be available at all times and a system must be in place that allows the angiography suite to function with a short lead time. Second, the physician must realize that an appreciable number of negative angiographic results should be expected with this low angiography threshold.

The treatment algorithm we recommend is outlined in Figure 3. Essentially, patients are divided into two groups: those with peritonitis and those without. Although all patients with peritonitis require laparotomy, the exact treatment plan for both groups of patients is dictated by the angiographic findings, which fall into four major categories, as outlined below.

Thrombotic Occlusion. This finding is usually identified with an aortic flush of contrast dye, but it is sometimes difficult to differentiate from a proximal arterial embolus. The other pitfall is that this finding sometimes represents a chronic obstruction not neces-sarily related to the patient's current symptoms and findings. Most of these patients require arterial reconstruction, although the final treatment plan will be based on the exact vascular anatomy and degree of collateral circulation. Patients with peritonitis may also require a bowel resection. Perioperative papaverine infusion in these patients may be useful; however, depending on the site of vascular obstruction, it may not be possible to secure a catheter for infusion.

Major Embolus. Major emboli are usually in the proximal portion of the superior mesenteric artery. Most of these patients should be referred to surgery for consideration of embolectomy regardless of the presence or lack of peritoneal findings. Papaverine infusion in the perioperative period should be used to reduce vasospasm-induced ischemia.

Minor Embolus. These emboli are limited to the branches of the superior mesenteric artery or to that portion of the vessel distal to the origin of the ileocolic artery. Unless peritoneal signs are present, these patients should be managed with papaverine infusion and observation.

Vasospasm (Nonocclusive Ischemia). Vasospasm may occur in response to a mechanical arterial obstruction, but when it is the sole finding it is diagnostic of nonocclusive ischemia. The recommended management is papaverine infusion.

Papaverine Infusion

Papaverine has been recommended as a mainstay of medical therapy for mesenteric ischemia. Although we support its use, it must be stressed that its efficacy has not been absolutely proved by the proper clinical trials.

Papaverine is a smooth muscle relaxant. Administered systemically, it nonspecifically dilates the vascular tree. However, since it is almost completely metabolized by a single pass through the liver, selective administration into the mesenteric circulation produces very few systemic effects. This allows vasodilatation in the mesenteric circulation to occur without a drop in systemic blood pressure. Typically, papaverine is infused into the mesenteric circulation (usually the superior mesenteric artery) after angiography-guided selective catheterization of an arterial trunk. Papaverine is dissolved in normal saline to a concentration of 1 mg per milliliter, although a higher concentration can be used. Heparin should not be added to the solution, as it will crystallize. The infusion is started at 30 mg per hour and may be increased to 60 mg per hour. In most cases the papaverine infusion is maintained for 24 hours. The catheter is then flushed with normal saline for 30 minutes and angiography is then repeated. If vasospasm persists, the cycle should be repeated every 24 hours for a maximum of 5 days. During the papaverine infusion, the patient's systemic vital signs must be monitored. A sudden drop in blood pressure usually suggests that the catheter has slipped out of the mesenteric circulation into the aorta. Repeat angiography at the bedside can be performed to confirm this. Generally, papaverine infu-

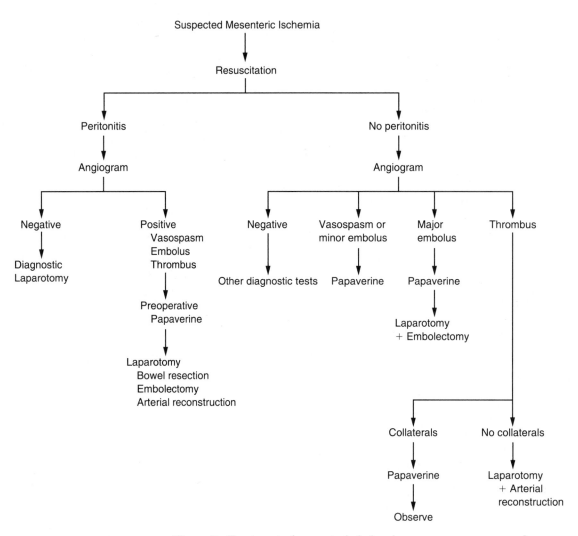

Figure 3 Treatment of mesenteric ischemia.

sion is quite safe, and major complications are usually related to the initial passage of the arterial catheter. Complications include injury to the femoral artery, dislodgment of atherosclerotic plaques with embolic accidents in the lower extremities, and the formation of a false aneurysm after the catheter is removed.

Surgical Management

The role of surgery is to evaluate the viability of ischemic bowel, resect if necessary, and if possible alleviate or bypass a vascular obstruction. If possible, the vascular surgery should be performed first so that its effect on intestinal viability can be assessed.

One of the most difficult decisions the surgeon has to make is to determine whether the bowel injury is reversible or not. Subjective criteria such as bowel wall color, the presence of peristalsis, and the presence of palpable mesenteric pulses are often used. Unfortunately, these criteria can lead to an inaccurate assessment in over 50 percent of cases. This has led surgeons to adopt a second-look approach, with which only the most obviously infarcted gut is resected and any questionable bowel is left in situ. A second look within 24 hours is then used to decide on the need for further resection. More recently, several objective measurements have been employed to assess bowel viability, including fluorescence staining, laser Doppler flowimetry, surface oximetry, and intramural pH measurements. At present, no single technology has been widely adopted, but as these techniques are further refined they may eventually play a valuable role in the assessment of intestinal viability.

A second difficult situation for the surgeon is the management of patients with near-total intestinal infarction. Even with resection, the mortality rate in this group of patients is very high, and survivors are often dependent on total parenteral nutrition (TPN) indefinitely. In elderly patients with other underlying medical problems, many surgeons choose to close without resection. The approach in a younger patient with a catastrophic vascular accident tends to be more aggressive, particularly with increasing advances in bowel transplantation.

CHRONIC MESENTERIC ISCHEMIA

Owing to the vast collateral arterial network of the gut, chronic mesenteric ischemia is relatively uncommon. In almost all patients, the cause is related to atherosclerosis. Classically, it is written that these patients present with a similar symptom complex, namely, postprandial abdominal pain, "fear of eating," and weight loss. Unfortunately, most patients do not present with these classic symptoms, and as with other ischemic syndromes the physician must maintain a high index of suspicion. The diagnosis is made with angiography and the treatment is surgical. Because the symptoms of chronic mesenteric ischemia in the elderly often closely resemble those of functional dyspepsia, it can be difficult to decide whether arteriography with its inherent dangers is indicated. Thus, the disease may run a prolonged course before diagnosis and effective treatment is employed.

Many surgical procedures have been described for the treatment of chronic mesenteric ischemia, of which aortovisceral bypass and endarterectomy are employed most commonly. More recently, balloon angioplasty has been used, but early results suggest that the recurrence rate may be high.

NONGANGRENOUS ISCHEMIC BOWEL DISEASE

Etiology

Contrary to mesenteric ischemia, in which occlusion of major vessels is the cause of the disease, the ischemia in nongangrenous ischemic bowel disease is caused by hypoperfusion and occasionally secondary occlusion of intramural vessels and the gut wall microcirculation. Many factors may precipitate this disorder. Most often, hypoperfusion is caused by vascular disorders, such as collagen disease, vasculitis, and atherosclerosis or by increased viscosity of the blood in polycythemia vera. Sudden acute hypotension due to hemorrhage, acute myocardial infarct, congestive heart failure, and vasoconstricting drugs may also precipitate local ischemia in patients with already impaired local circulation. Because the disease involves the vessels of the bowel wall, localization is always segmental, and thus there is usually an adequate collateral circulation. As a result, the ischemia-induced necrosis is rarely transmural and peritonitis is a rare complication. Nongangrenous ischemic bowel disease may involve the small bowel as "focal segmental ischemia" or the colon as "nongangrenous ischemic colitis."

Focal Segmental Ischemia

The clinical course of this condition is variable and depends on the severity of the infarct. Limited necrosis may heal completely. Ongoing repeated injury may cause chronic enteritis almost indistinguishable from Crohn's disease. In other patients the necrotic ulcer may lead to late stricture formation, or may become transmural and cause peritonitis. The diagnosis is always difficult, as the symptoms may be those of chronic recurrent abdominal pain, bowel obstruction, or frank peritonitis. Unless there is complete spontaneous resolution, the treatment is surgical and the diagnosis is often made only on the resected specimen.

Nongangrenous Ischemic Colitis

Pathogenesis

Ischemic colitis was first described by Boley and co-workers in 1963. The disease was classified by Marston and colleagues in 1966 into three major forms: gangrenous, stricturing, and transient colitis. Since that time, it has become clear that there are only two major forms: gangrenous and nongangrenous ischemic colitis (see Fig. 1). These two forms are in fact two different diseases, with different etiologies and clinical courses, and require entirely different approaches to their management. Gangrenous ischemic colitis is caused by obstruction of the mesenteric vessels and was discussed in the section on acute mesenteric ischemia. Occasionally, transmural gangrene may develop when nongangrenous ischemic colitis slowly progresses to transmural necrosis. The recognition and management of this complication of nongangrenous ischemic colitis are discussed in this section.

Nonocclusive ischemia of the small bowel is rare, but there appears to be a predilection of the colon for local vascular hypoperfusion. The relative frequency of colonic involvement may be explained by the following factors: in comparison with the small intestine, the colon receives less blood, has a less well developed collateral circulation, has a different neuroendocrine control, and an ongoing motor activity that may predispose it to a temporary decrease in blood flow. Not only is the colonic blood flow quantitively smaller than that of the small intestine, but it also has fewer vascular collaterals and has susceptible "watershed areas." Recent evidence in our laboratory demonstrated that in the colon of the dog, unlike the small intestine, the major local vasoconstrictory substance is angiotensin, and the vessels of the colon respond more vigorously to hypotension than do those of the small intestine. Also, elevated intramural pressure during increased motility in patients with constipation, diverticular disease, and cancer of the colon may lead to diminished gut wall blood flow. Similarly, distention with air during colonoscopy or barium enema may temporarily reduce blood flow to the colon.

Under specific conditions, nonocclusive ischemic colitis can also occur in the young (Table 1). This sometimes has iatrogenic causes such as contraceptive medication or nonsteroid anti-inflammatory agents.

Clinical Presentation

The clinical presentation is characterized by a sudden onset of severe crampy abdominal pain, diarrhea, hematochezia, and occasionally melena. On physical examination, the abdomen may be distended. There

Table 1 Causes of Nonocclusive Ischemic Colitis

Acute diminution of colonic intramural blood flow
  Small vessel obstruction
    Collagen vascular disease
    Vasculitis, diabetes
    Oral contraceptives
  Nonocclusive hypoperfusion
    Hemorrhage
    Congestive heart failure, myocardial infarction, arrhythmias
    Sepsis
    Vasoconstricting agents: digitalis, vasopressin, ergot, NSAIDs
    Increased viscosity: polycythemia, sickle cell disease,
      thrombocytosis

Increased demand on marginal blood flow
  Increased motility
    Mass lesion, stricture
    Constipation
  Increased intraluminal pressure
    Bowel obstruction
    Colonoscopy
    Barium enema

are bowel sounds and no signs of peritoneal involvement. The patient may have one of the associated diseases such as hypotension, ischemic heart disease, or polycythemia or one of the iatrogenic causes such as oral contraceptives or digitalis (see Table 1). Occasionally, the specific event that precipitated the attack cannot be determined, especially in the elderly. The early clinical presentation is so similar to that of acute infectious colitis, ulcerative colitis, Crohn's colitis, and pseudomembranous colitis that the differentiation can be established only by excluding infection (including *Clostridium difficile*) and by demonstrating the classic radiographic or colonoscopic findings of ischemic colitis. Investigation must be carried out within 24 to 48 hours of the onset of the disease, as the typical findings tend to disappear rapidly. Because large vessels are never involved, angiography has no place in the diagnosis of nongangrenous ischemic colitis. The first radiologic examination should be an abdominal survey film, which may demonstrate "thumbprinting" in air-filled segments of the colon. Thumbprinting is caused by intramural hemorrhage but can be mimicked by severe mucosal and submucosal edema. Typically, colonic involvement is segmental. Although any part of the colon may be affected, the "watershed" areas of the splenic flexure and the rectosigmoid junction are most commonly involved. Thumbprinting can be better demonstrated by barium enema, and the submucosal hemorrhage by colonoscopy. Because distention of the colon with air may compress intramural blood vessels and decrease blood flow, barium enema and colonoscopy must be carried out carefully with minimal air insufflation. Colonoscopy is preferable to barium enema because early inspection and biopsy can differentiate between the thumbprinting caused by submucosal hemorrhage and that caused by severe edema due to inflammatory bowel disease (IBD) or colitis of other etiology. After 24 to 48 hours, the hemorrhage resolves and the mucosa becomes necrotic. If colonoscopy is performed at this stage, the endoscopist

may have great difficulty in differentiating the necrosis and ulceration caused by ischemic colitis from that caused by Crohn's disease or pseudomembraneous enterocolitis. The pathologist reviewing biopsies taken a few days after the onset of the disease may have similar difficulties. Not infrequently, only time will tell whether the patient has IBD or ischemia. One cannot help but wonder what proportion of late-onset IBD or Crohn's disease in young women on contraceptive medication is actually due to ischemia.

As shown in Figure 1, the disease can progress in four ways. Mild disease may resolve spontaneously. The symptoms and physical findings subside within 24 to 48 hours and complete resolution should occur within 2 to 3 weeks. In some patients the disease does not resolve and they may suffer from ongoing or recurrent chronic colitis, indistinguishable from IBD. Since the pathologic response of colonic tissue to chronic injury is restricted to a very few factors, such as infiltration with leukocytes, crypt abscess, hemorrhage, necrosis, ulceration, and regeneration of crypts, the pathologist may have difficulty in differentiating ongoing ischemic colitis from Crohn's colitis. Hemosiderin, a sign of previous bleeding, is often considered a typical manifestation of ischemic colitis. Unfortunately, this finding is not restricted to ischemic disease; it can be seen in any type of colitis, including IBD, in which hemorrhage has occurred in the past. Furthermore, ischemia may be one of the etiologic factors involved in Crohn's disease.

Chronic disease may resolve, relapse, or progress to deeper intramural necrosis. If the necrosis stops in the submucosa or muscularis, the patient may exhibit toxic symptoms such as chills, fever, severe bloody diarrhea, abdominal distention, diminished bowel sounds, leukocytosis, anemia, elevated platelet count, and electrolyte disturbances. If it does not progress further, intramural necrosis will heal with stricture. In some instances, the necrosis results in toxic megacolon, and if the intramural necrosis becomes transmural, acute peritonitis may ensue. This usually occurs slowly and may take several days to develop. This progression must be detected early by careful follow-up.

Treatment

Appropriate treatment depends on an accurate diagnosis. Infectious causes, bacterial and amebic dysentery, and all other infectious enteropathies must be excluded. Exclusion of IBD at the early stage is less important, but other local precipitating causes of ischemia such as diverticulitis or cancer must be detected and appropriately treated. As to the immediate management of patients, we prefer to consider treatment under the following three categories: (1) nonspecific medical supportive therapy, (2) specific medical treatment, and (3) surgical therapy.

Nonspecific Medical Supportive Therapy. While investigation of the cause is progressing, fluid and electrolyte balance must be carefully maintained. Intake by mouth is restricted according to the severity of disease. The need for nutritional support depends on the patient's overall nutritional status. Well-nourished patients can be maintained for a few days without specific support, except for what they receive in intravenous solutions. Very rarely, severely undernourished patients may have to be started on TPN at an early stage. Bleeding is rarely sufficient to require blood transfusion, but if severe anemia is present, it may be necessary to transfuse an elderly patient who has atherosclerosis, angina, or a myocardial infarct. This requires careful balancing of the cardiac and hematologic state to ensure that one does not overload an already precariously maintained circulation. Usually, patients with acute colitis request medication to relieve symptoms, but the use of analgesics and antispasmodic or antidiarrheal agents is contraindicated because these drugs may lead to an inert bowel and possibly a toxic megacolon.

Depending on the progression of the disease and the patient's response to feeding, a low-residue diet may be slowly started. In chronic ischemic colitis, enteric feeding may be required. It is our experience that diarrhea and abdominal pain may become worse on enteric nutrition in some patients. Dilution of the solution, constant slow administration over 24 hours, or the use of an iso-osmotic product may overcome this problem.

Patients must be carefully followed to detect deterioration. There is no good experimental evidence to support the value of antibiotics, but in a patient who shows signs of deterioration one should start antibiotics, using triple therapy (metronidazole, amoxicillin, and an aminoglycoside) or a beta lactam. If there is further progression and patients develop increasing peritoneal signs, surgery may become necessary, even if they appear to be a poor surgical risk. One of the major errors is to delay surgery to the point where a patient who was previously a poor risk has become so sick that successful surgery becomes impossible.

Specific Medical Treatment

Colitis. Specific therapy for colitis is not needed in mild self-limiting disease. The value of therapy for chronic ongoing disease is questionable. No experimental data are available to assess the effectiveness of drugs used in IBD for the treatment of chronic ischemic colitis. If one considers how difficult it is to ascertain by prospective double-blind studies the success of medical therapy (sulfasalazine [Azulfadine], 5-aminosalicylic acid [5-ASA], steroids, metronidazole, or immuno suppressive agents) in IBD, because of the lower incidence of ischemic colitis, there is little likelihood that controlled studies will ever be available for this disease. Taking this limitation into consideration, we believe that in long-standing progressive disease a trial with sulfasalazine or 5-ASA by oral and/or (depending on the location of the disease) rectal administration may be justified. If patients do not respond, a trial with steroids may be attempted, although it is difficult to predict the outcome. No experience exists with metronidazole and immunosuppressive agents.

One may question whether vasodilators, (e.g., pa- paverine, angiotensin converting enzyme [ACE] inhibitors) may be useful in the management of this disease. Once the symptoms have developed and the patient is seen by the physician, the intramural ischemic injury has already occurred. There is no evidence to indicate either that vasodilators may be useful in reverting the pathologic findings and thus facilitating recovery, or that these agents may prevent recurrence or progression to chronic disease.

Precipitating Disease. Another type of specific therapy is directed toward the condition that precipitated the ischemic attack. Treatment of heart disease, change of digitalis to other medication (e.g., ACE inhibitors), discontinuation of estrogens, management of diabetes, recognition and treatment of vasculitis and polycythemia, for example, may prevent recurrences in the future but may not necessarily alter the outcome of already established chronic disease.

Surgical Therapy

Acute Colitis. Uncontrollable hemorrhage is rare, but if it occurs, resection may be necessary. As already discussed, transmural necrosis and toxic megacolon leading to peritoneal signs require immediate surgical intervention.

Late Complications. About one-third of patients with severe ischemic colitis develop strictures, usually within 6 months after the onset of the disease. Patients present with obstructive symptoms, and barium enema and colonoscopy demonstrate an area of narrowing. If colonoscopic dilatation fails and symptoms persist, surgical resection or stricturoplasty may be necessary.

COMMENTS

Within the last decade, the morbidity and mortality rates of ischemic bowel disease decreased considerably. Recent advances, better radiologic and surgical techniques, new methods in measuring tissue blood flow, advances in intensive care medicine, and appropriate nutritional support have already improved the outcome of these diseases. Further research to obtain a better understanding of the physiology of the regulation of blood flow should lead to an even better approach to these patients.

SUGGESTED READING

Boley SJ, Brandt LJ, guest eds. Intestinal ischemia. Surg Clin North Am 1992; 72:1.

Carratu R, Parisi P, Agozzino A. Segmental ischemic colitis associated with nonsteroidal antiinflammatory drugs. J Clin Gastroenterol 1993; 16:31–34.

Kvietys PR, Barrowman JA, Granger DN. Pathophysiology of the splanchnic circulation. Vols 1 & 2. Boca Raton, FL: CRC Press, 1987.

MacDonald PH, Dinda PK, Beck IT. The role of angiotensin in the intestinal vascular response to hypotension in a canine model. Gastroenterology 1992; 103:57–64.

SECRETORY DIARRHEA

JUDY H. CHO, M.D.
EUGENE B. CHANG, M.D.

Active secretion of water and electrolytes is a major component of most diarrheal diseases, including those caused by infection, inflammation, and circulating secretagogues. These conditions can be acute self-limited processes or chronic lifelong disorders. When active secretion is the major component of the disease, the diarrhea is typically profuse and watery (often more than 1,000 g per day). Although typically referred to as "secretory diarrheas," these disorders arise from impaired absorption of water and electrolytes as well as increased secretion. The diagnosis of secretory diarrhea is suggested when the concentration of stool $(Na^+ + K^+) \times 2$ approximately equals total stool or blood osmolality. In addition, in most cases of secretory diarrheas, the diarrhea continues despite fasting for 24 to 48 hours.

The focus of this chapter is on general considerations in the treatment of secretory diarrheas as well as the use of more specific agents for chronic diarrheas. Infectious diarrheas make up a large percentage of diagnosed secretory diarrheas, and specific antibiotic treatments for individual disorders are discussed in other chapters. Specific therapies associated with bile acid– and fatty acid–induced diarrheas are also discussed in other chapters. In inflammatory bowel disease (IBD), the local production of inflammatory mediators that both increase secretion and decrease absorption of intestinal water and electrolytes contributes significantly to the diarrhea observed with acute flare-ups. The main treatment of secretory diarrhea associated with IBD is therefore directed toward decreasing the underlying inflammatory process. This chapter focuses on the general medical management of secretory diarrheas, including hormone-related secretory diarrheas resulting from VIPomas and the carcinoid syndrome.

FLUID AND ELECTROLYTE REPLACEMENT

Initial considerations in the treatment of patients with secretory diarrheas should include replacement of lost fluid and electrolytes. Typically, patients presenting with secretory diarrheas exhibit dehydration, hypokalemia, and metabolic acidosis, although metabolic alkalosis is seen in some cases of secretory diarrhea. Since hypokalemia results from intestinal losses, it should be corrected promptly with potassium replacement as total body volume is being replaced, taking advantage of the avid urinary potassium retention. However, the presence of high urinary $[K^+]$ in the setting of diarrhea resulting from laxative abuse should suggest the possibility of concomitant diuretic abuse. The severity of initial presentation determines whether oral or intravenous replacement should be attempted. The concentration of sodium and potassium in replacement solutions is not critical in the absence of renal insufficiency. When renal insufficiency does exist, the concentrations of sodium and potassium replacement need to be lowered. In short bowel syndrome, the concentration of sodium in replacement solutions often needs to be higher.

The principle behind oral rehydration therapy is that while absorption of sodium by some carriers is impaired in secretory diarrheas, absorption via Na-glucose and Na–amino acid cotransporters is intact. Therefore, glucose-based oral rehydration solutions improve fluid and electrolyte balance by increasing intestinal absorption. As intestinal secretion and absorption are separate processes, oral rehydration therapy may temporarily worsen diarrhea. The present World Health Organization (WHO) formulation contains 3.5 g of sodium chloride, 1.5 g of potassium chloride, 2.9 g of trisodium citrate dihydrate, and 20 g of glucose per liter of water. More recently, rice-based oral rehydration solutions containing glucose polymers have been shown to not only increase absorption, but also decrease stool volume output and provide greater caloric intake without increasing osmolality.

PHARMACOLOGIC AGENTS USED IN THE TREATMENT OF SECRETORY DIARRHEAS

Pharmacologic agents used to treat secretory diarrheas can be divided into those accepted agents commonly in use and experimental or unproved agents (Table 1). Currently used pharmacologic agents act by (1) increasing contact time between luminal contents and the intestine, thereby increasing absorption; (2) increasing the absorption efficiency of enterocytes directly; and (3) interrupting cellular signal transduction events (secondary messengers) that lead to intestinal secretion.

Accepted Agents Commonly in Use

Opiates

Opiates are a mainstay of treatment of mild to moderate secretory diarrheas. They increase smooth muscle tone throughout the gastrointestinal (GI) tract and decrease peristaltic contractions. Consequently, there is a decrease in gastric emptying time as well as an increase in transit time. The resultant increased contact time between intestinal contents and mucosa produces increased absorption. In addition, naturally occurring opiates and some synthetic opiates (e.g., loperamide) increase the absorptive efficiency of enterocytes and possess antisecretory properties.

Synthetic opioids such as diphenoxylate (Lomotil), 2.5 mg diphenoxylate plus 25 μg atropine per tablet, and loperamide (Imodium), 2 mg loperamide per tablet, have much more potent GI effects than morphine, and

Table 1 Pharmacologic Agents Used in the Treatment of Secretory Diarrheas

Medication	Indication	Side Effects	Comments
Agents Commonly in Use			
Opiates	First-line therapy for mild to moderate diarrheas	Abdominal discomfort, constipation, toxic megacolon, nausea, vomiting, CNS (drowsiness, respiratory depression); Lomotil has anticholinergic side effects	Minimal or no risk of physical dependence; loperamide (Imodium) does not cross BBB and does not have CNS side effects
Octreotide	Severe diarrhea not responsive to other therapy; major indications: VIPomas, carcinoid syndrome, diabetic diarrhea, AIDS enteropathy	Increased incidence of gallstones, mild abdominal pain/nausea that resolves with continued therapy, malabsorption from pancreatic insufficiency, mild hypo/hyperglycemia	Use limited by cost and subcutaneous administration
Alpha$_2$-agonists	Major use is in treatment of diabetic diarrhea; also used in short bowel syndrome	Orthostatic hypotension, drowsiness	Taper dose when discontinuing therapy
Corticosteroids	Inflammatory diarrheas, VIPomas unresponsive to octreotide alone	Standard glucocorticoid side effects	Use in secretory diarrheas limited by side effects
Prostaglandin synthetase inhibitors	Inflammatory diarrheas	Generally mild and reversible	Decrease AA metabolites, which are potent secretagogues
Experimental or Unproved Agents			
Calcium channel blockers	Reported use in chronic infectious diarrheas	Cardiovascular	Often not useful as a single agent
Trifluorperazine and chlorpromazine	Reported use in cholera, VIPomas	Retinopathy, movement disorders, blood dyscrasias, abnormal liver function tests	Monitor side effects carefully

AA = arachidonic acid; AIDS = acquired immunodeficiency syndrome; BBB = blood-brain barrier; CNS = central nervous system.

also have much fewer central nervous system (CNS) effects than morphine and thus a smaller abuse potential. The recommended maximal dose of both Imodium and Lomotil is eight tablets a day or 16 mg loperamide and 20 mg diphenoxylate a day, although 32 mg Imodium has been used without untoward effects. For acute symptoms, two tablets of Imodium are given, followed by an additional tablet with each loose stool. Two tablets of Lomotil four times a day can be given acutely for initial control and the dose tapered subsequently.

At large doses, diphenoxylate does possess some CNS effects, while loperamide does not cross the blood-brain barrier; thus, even in large doses, the latter appears to have few CNS side effects. The potential for abuse with diphenoxylate has been reduced by combining it with atropine in commercial preparations (Lomotil), so that unpleasant anticholinergic side effects will result if high doses are used. Other side effects of synthetic opiates include abdominal discomfort, nausea, intractable constipation, and, in some cases, toxic megacolon.

Octreotide

Octreotide (Sandostatin) is a synthetic octapeptide that is a long-acting somatostatin analog. Like somatostatin, octreotide suppresses secretion of gastroenteropancreatic peptide hormones such as VIP and serotonin. Thus, a major use of octreotide has been in the treatment of severe diarrhea associated with metastatic carcinoid syndrome and VIPomas. Octreotide also inhibits VIP, serotonin, and prostaglandin E_1-induced anion secretion in both small and large intestine and has been shown to stimulate sodium chloride (NaCl) absorption in animal studies. Therefore, octreotide has also been used to treat a broad array of non–hormone-related secretory diarrheas. Acquired immunodeficiency syndrome (AIDS)-related secretory diarrhea unassociated with identifiable pathogens occurs commonly, and in nonrandomized trials octreotide has been reported to decrease stool output effectively. The effectiveness of octreotide in AIDS-associated secretory diarrheas where a specific pathogen has been identified has also been reported. Carcinomas of the medullary thyroid elaborate calcitonin, an intestinal secretagogue. Although the treatment of choice is surgical removal, cases of metastatic medullary thyroid carcinoma with severe secretory diarrhea may respond to octreotide therapy. However, in our experience, diarrhea resulting from medullary thyroid carcinoma represents one of the few predominantly secretory diarrheas not responsive to octreotide therapy. Secretory diarrheas associated with intestinal graft-versus-host disease that do not initially respond to prednisone therapy have been reported to improve with octreotide therapy. Other reported uses of octreotide in the treatment of diarrheas include therapy for intestinal amyloidosis, short bowel syndrome, chemotherapy-induced diarrheas, villous adenoma–associated secretory diarrheas, and Zollinger-Ellison syndrome.

The use of octreotide is limited to cases of severe diarrhea refractory to other treatments because of its high cost and also because it is presently available only in injectable form. The initial dosage is 50 μg subcutaneously two to four times a day up to a recommended maximal daily dose of 1500 μg per day in divided doses two to four times a day, although there is little experience with daily doses above 750 μg. The half-life of octreotide ranges from 90 to 120 minutes, and peak concentrations are attained approximately 1 hour after administration.

Side effects of octreotide include the development of nausea and mild abdominal cramping, which usually resolve on continued therapy; and pain at the injection site, which can be minimized by injecting slowly and warming the solution before injection. Mild hypo- or hyperglycemia can result from alterations in secretion of the counter-regulatory hormones insulin, glucagon, and growth hormone. Some patients report lighter stools than usual, and a few (less than 2 percent) develop fat malabsorption from decreased pancreatic enzyme secretion, which often abates with time, presumably owing to subsequent adaptation. Because octreotide inhibits gallbladder emptying, it has been associated with the development of gallbladder sludge and gallstones. No recommendations are available currently on the advisability of preventive therapy for patients requiring long-term octreotide.

Alpha₂-Agonists

Noradrenergic innervation of the intestinal mucosa is known to promote absorption. Since patients with refractory diabetic diarrhea invariably have autonomic neuropathy, concomitant noradrenergic denervation in the intestine may contribute significantly to the secretory diarrhea seen in these patients. In addition, alpha₂-agonists increase intestinal transit time, thereby increasing contact time for absorption. Clonidine, an alpha₂-agonist, has been used successfully to treat diabetic diarrhea, as discussed in the chapter on diabetic diarrhea. Dosage is started at 0.1 mg per day and increased slowly. The maximal effective dose is 1.0 to 1.2 mg per day in divided doses, although lesser amounts of 0.4 to 0.6 mg per day in divided doses are usually needed. Transdermal preparations of clonidine applied weekly can also be used and provide more stable therapeutic levels. Clonidine has also been used to treat diarrhea associated with short bowel syndrome in combination with opiates, and for alcohol withdrawal.

A major limitation to the use of clonidine has been cardiovascular toxicity, especially the development of orthostatic hypotension. Newer formulations of alpha₂-agonists should decrease these problems in the future. When discontinuing clonidine, the dose should be tapered slowly over 4 to 5 days to avoid withdrawal symptoms of rebound hypertension, headache, nausea, and vomiting.

Corticosteroids

In addition to their anti-inflammatory actions, corticosteroids alleviate diarrhea by increasing electrolyte absorption. This effect is mediated by corticosteroid-induced increased expression of absorptive carrier proteins. Improved absorption may contribute to the early improvement in diarrhea seen in acute flare-ups of IBD treated with corticosteroids. Although side effects limit their use in most cases of secretory diarrhea, corticosteroids have been used to treat VIPoma-associated diarrhea refractory to octreotide alone.

Prostaglandin Synthetase Inhibitors

Mucosal production of arachidonic acid (AA) metabolites in inflammatory disorders such as IBD or infectious diarrheas contributes to acute exacerbations of diarrhea, as a number of inflammatory mediators are potent secretagogues. Therefore, prostaglandin synthetase inhibitors such as 5-acetylsalicylic acid (5-ASA) derivatives should be useful in the treatment of inflammatory diarrheas. While the beneficial effect of 5-ASA derivatives in the treatment of IBD is primarily through preventing and decreasing inflammation, antisecretory effects may play a significant role in the early improvement in diarrhea seen in the treatment of acute flares.

Bismuth subsalicylate (Pepto-Bismol) is used primarily for prophylaxis and treatment of acute infectious diarrheas. Its beneficial effects are mediated through both antimicrobial effects and anti-inflammatory actions of the salicylate moiety. Long-term use of bismuth compounds has been associated with the development of encephalopathy. This is a rare complication with currently available preparations, but long-term bismuth usage should be avoided and drug-free intervals introduced.

Adsorbent Agents

Adsorbent agents such as psillium husk, methylcellulose, and calcium polycarbophil avidly absorb intraluminal water, resulting in firmer stool consistency and a decreased number of stools. However, they do not affect the total amount of fluid or electrolytes excreted and may actually increase stool volume. Therefore, they are not used to treat diarrheas resulting primarily from increased secretion. An exception to this is the use of the adsorbents cholestyramine or colestipol, anion exchange resins that bind bile salts, to treat bile salt–induced secretory diarrheas.

Experimental or Unproved Agents

Calcium Channel Blockers

Since one of the intracellular mediators of intestinal secretion is calcium, calcium channel blockers, which decrease intracellular calcium, could be useful in the treatment of secretory diarrheas. In fact, one of the well-known side effects of verapamil is constipation. Although not established therapy, verapamil has been used to treat chronic infectious diarrheas. However, it is often not useful as a single agent.

Neuroleptics

Neuroleptic agents such as trifluoroperazine and chlorpromazine act to decrease intestinal secretion by binding to the calcium-calmodulin complex and inactivating it. Their use has been reported for the treatment of VIPomas and cholera. Significant side effects are common and include development of retinopathy, movement disorders, blood dyscrasias, and abnormal liver function test results, which must be monitored carefully.

Berberine

Berberine is a plant alkaloid that has been used as an antidiarrheal agent in Asia for years. Animal studies suggest that it inhibits secretion and increases absorption. In addition, it may have an antimicrobial action in infectious diarrheas. Extensive experimental trials are lacking at this point, and it remains an experimental agent.

Leukotriene Synthesis Inhibitors

An alternative mechanism for decreasing mucosal production of AA metabolites is via inhibition of the leukotriene pathway. Specific inhibitors of this pathway such as MK-886, an inhibitor of 5-lipoxygenase activating protein (FLAP), are under development and study.*

SPECIAL CONSIDERATIONS

VIPomas

The major mediator of the pancreatic cholera syndrome of watery diarrhea and hypokalemia is VIP. Since the profuse diarrhea is inadequately controlled with traditional agents such as opioids, the mainstay of initial management is currently octreotide. Octreotide suppresses secretion of VIP and decreases intestinal secretion. Whether it affects tumor size has

---

*Editor's Note: Zilenton, a 5-lipoxygenase inhibitor, is being tested in patients with ulcerative colitis.

been somewhat controversial. Enough cases have been documented to suggest that octreotide does exert a beneficial effect on tumor growth rate, but this beneficial effect is temporary and unpredictable in individual patients.

The dosage of octreotide required to attain control of the diarrhea varies greatly, ranging from 150 to 750 µg per day in divided doses; however, doses over 450 µg per day are usually not required. After initial control of the diarrhea is attained, precise localization of the VIPoma and surgical excision should be attempted, as 50 percent of all VIPomas are benign. The tumor most often originates in the pancreas, but other sites include the stomach and upper duodenum. Bronchogenic carcinoma, ganglioneuroma, or ganglioneuroblastoma can also secrete VIP and cause this syndrome.

When surgical excision is not possible, debulking of large tumors may be helpful if symptoms are poorly controlled by medical management. The number of these cases is decreasing with the advent of octreotide. Some patients initially controlled with octreotide subsequently relapse and require higher doses or the addition of corticosteroid therapy. Prednisone, 40 mg per day, can be used for initial management, with the dose tapered as control of symptoms is maintained. 5-Fluorouracil and streptozotocin have resulted in objective improvement in metastatic disease.

Carcinoid Syndrome

The carcinoid syndrome consists of watery diarrhea, flushing, right-sided endocardial fibrosis, and bronchospasm resulting from excessive production of serotonin and/or other bioactive amines. Almost all cases of carcinoid syndrome involve metastatic disease; however, since the tumor is very slow-growing, long-term medical management of symptomatic secretory diarrhea is often required. Octreotide is the mainstay of medical management; as with VIPomas, it acts by decreasing hormonal secretion as well as through more general effects on intestinal secretion and absorption. Improvement of symptoms is observed in 92 percent of patients started on octreotide, and 66 percent exhibit biochemical evidence of diminished serotonin release, such as a decrease in urinary 5-hydroxyindoleacetic acid levels. As with VIPomas, octreotide exerts a beneficial, if temporary, effect on tumor growth.

Initial control of symptoms is usually achieved with doses between 100 and 600 µg per day. As with VIPomas, patients may relapse after achieving initial control and require higher doses. The median daily maintenance dose is 450 µg per day. In addition to producing symptomatic relief of diarrhea, octreotide improves the flushing associated with the carcinoid syndrome. Cyproheptadine, 4 to 12 mg three times a day, has also been used to treat diarrhea associated with the carcinoid syndrome, but this agent rarely improves the symptoms of flushing.

SUGGESTED READING

Cello JP, Grendell JH, Basuk P, et al. Effect of octreotide on refractory AIDS-associated diarrhea. Ann Intern Med 1991; 115:705–710.

Ely P, Dunitz J, Rogosheske J, Weisdorf D. Use of a somatostatin analogue, octreotide acetate, in the management of acute gastrointestinal graft-versus-host disease. Am J Med 1991; 90:707–710.

Gaginella TS, O'Dorisio TM, Fassler JE, Mekhijian HS. Treatment of endocrine and nonendocrine secretory diarrheal states with sandostatin. Metabolism 1990; 39:172–175.

Gorbach SL. Bismuth therapy in gastrointestinal diseases. Gastroenterology 1990; 99:863–875.

Kvols LK. Therapy of the malignant carcinoid syndrome. Endocrinol Metab Clin North Am 1989; 18:557–568.

O'Dorisio TM, Mekhjian HS, Gaginella TS. Medical therapy of VIPomas. Endocrinol Metab Clin North Am 1989; 18:545–555.

Proceedings, Sandostatin, State of the Art. Metabolism 1992; 41(9 Suppl 2).

Smith MB, Chang EB. Antidiarrheals and cathartics. In: Wolfe MM, ed. Gastrointestinal pharmacotherapy. Philadelphia: WB Saunders, 1993:139–156.

Zheng BY, U KM, Lu RB, et al. Absorption of glucose polymers from rice in oral rehydration solutions by rat small intestine. Gastroenterology 1993; 104:81–85.

COLON AND RECTUM

ACUTE APPENDICITIS

DAVID A. APPEL, M.D.
GORDON L. TELFORD, M.D.
ROBERT E. CONDON, M.D., M.S.

Acute appendicitis is one of the most common causes of an acute abdominal emergency and accounts for approximately 1 percent of all surgical operations. The disease is rare in infants but becomes increasingly more prevalent in the teens and early adulthood, reaching a maximal incidence between 10 and 30 years. After age 30 the incidence declines but the disease can occur at any age.

The most widely accepted theory of the pathogenesis is that appendicitis results from obstruction of the lumen followed by bacterial overgrowth and infection. The lumen becomes obstructed by hyperplasia of lymphoid follicles, or by a fecalith, foreign body, stricture, tumor, or other pathologic condition. Mucus builds up behind the obstruction and bacterial overgrowth ensues. Pressure within the lumen gradually rises and lymphatic drainage ceases. This results in further edema formation which eventually interrupts both venous drainage and arterial inflow. The appendix becomes gangrenous and eventually perforates if left untreated. The obstruction hypothesis has been challenged.

CLINICAL FEATURES

The diagnosis of acute appendicitis is based upon a thorough history and physical exam supplemented with appropriate laboratory and radiologic exams. Typically, the history begins with crampy abdominal pain that is often poorly localized in the epigastrium or peri-umbilical area and is accompanied by anorexia and nausea. Vomiting, if it occurs, appears next. Anorexia is such a common finding that if it does not exist the diagnosis of appendicitis should be questioned. As the appendix becomes more inflamed it begins to irritate the adjacent parietal peritoneum and perceived pain shifts to the right lower quadrant (RLQ) and becomes localized.

Focal peritoneal signs, including point tenderness, involuntary guarding, percussion tenderness and rebound tenderness may now be elicited on examination of the RLQ and at McBurney's point ("between an inch and a half and two inches from the anterior spinous process of the ilium on a straight line drawn from the process to the umbilicus"). Rovsing's sign, pain in the RLQ when palpation pressure is exerted in the left lower quadrant, is another way of demonstrating referred rebound tenderness and is sometimes helpful in making the diagnosis.

Muscle guarding, or voluntary resistance to palpation, roughly parallels the peritoneal inflammatory process. As the disease progresses voluntary guarding is replaced by reflex involuntary rigidity, a classic sign of intense peritoneal inflammation. An occasionally helpful sign is the psoas sign—pain noted upon passive extension of the right hip. A positive psoas sign is said to indicate irritation of the psoas muscle by an inflamed retrocecal appendix.

A low grade fever is another clinical feature. A temperature above 38° C may indicate complicated appendicitis involving perforation or abscess formation. Occasionally a mass may be palpated on examination of the RLQ. Generally this is a late finding and can represent abscess formation in the case of a ruptured appendix, or simply a phlegmon, an inflammatory mass of omentum and loops of bowel adherent to the inflamed appendix.

Appropriate laboratory studies include a complete blood count with differential and a urinalysis. The white blood cell count and white cell differential are usually abnormal in appendicitis, but the degree of abnormality does not correlate with the extent of inflammation. Up to one third of patients may have a normal total leukocyte count in the presence of acute appendicitis. The white cell differential, however, shows a shift to the left in most patients. Less than 4 percent of patients with acute appendicitis have both a normal differential count and a normal total leukocyte count.

Posteroanterior and lateral chest x-rays should be obtained. The chest x-ray is generally normal in acute appendicitis, but the examination is performed to rule out pneumonia which can produce abdominal pain and mimic appendicitis, especially in children.

Radiographic examination of the abdomen does not show any pathognomonic signs in early appendicitis. The only exception is the occasional finding of an appendiceal fecalith. In late, complicated disease there may be scoliosis to the right, absence of the right psoas shadow, absence of small bowel gas in the RLQ, or interruption of the preperitoneal fat line in the flank.

In patients with an atypical history or physical findings, further diagnostic studies might include abdominal ultrasonography, barium enema, or computed tomography (CT). Ultrasound of the RLQ may reveal an enlarged, inflamed appendix and can be very useful in evaluating the pelvic organs of the female. Barium enema can be performed on those patients in whom the diagnosis remains unclear. Positive findings include non-filling or partial filling of the appendix, often associated with extrinsic pressure defects in the cecum ("reverse 3 sign"). A CT scan is especially useful for those patients with a mass palpable on examination. An abscess, if present, can be managed at this time with percutaneous catheter drainage under CT guidance.

PREOPERATIVE MANAGEMENT

All patients with suspected appendicitis should be admitted to the hospital and surgical consultation obtained. Serial examinations should be performed by a single examiner in those patients in whom the diagnosis is unclear. Once the diagnosis of acute appendicitis is made, rapid preparation for operation is required. Intravenous fluid resuscitation is undertaken with lactated Ringers solution or normal saline to restore urine output to 50 ml per hour. In a healthy adult this should only take one to two hours but, in the very young and very old, resuscitation may require a longer time. No person should be subjected to operation who has not been adequately fluid resuscitated.

Antibiotics are given in the immediate preoperative period, usually at induction of anesthesia, for uncomplicated appendicitis. For simple appendicitis a single dose of a broad spectrum antibiotic (usually a second generation cephalosporin) is adequate. The chosen drug should cover gram negative enteric bacilli and anaerobes. If perforated appendicitis is suspected a drug with a broader range of antimicrobial coverage may be selected and be administered for a longer period.

SURGICAL TECHNIQUE

Once fluid resuscitation is complete the patient is taken to the operating room and anesthetized. The abdomen is palpated for evidence of a RLQ mass which might indicate phlegmon or abscess. A transverse incision is made in the RLQ. If a mass is present the incision should be made transversely over the most prominent aspect of the mass. The muscles are split along their fibers and the peritoneum is entered. Peritoneal fluid is cultured. The appendix is located by following the anterior cecal taenia to the appendiceal base. The inflamed appendix is then coaxed into the wound. Occasionally, as in a retrocecal appendix, the right colon may need to be mobilized in order to locate the appendix. The mesoappendix is divided serially between absorbable sutures. With the appendix freely mobilized the base is clamped, ligated, and divided. The appendiceal stump is not inverted routinely. If inversion is performed, it is done with a Z-stitch instead of a purse string and the stump is not ligated. The peritoneum and muscles are closed in layers and the skin closed primarily.

If a normal appendix is found, it should be removed to prevent future diagnostic confusion. A systematic exploration of the abdomen is undertaken to evaluate for other causes of the clinical signs and symptoms. The cecum and terminal ileum are examined for evidence of regional enteritis (Crohn's disease), infectious ileitis, or malignant disease. Next, the terminal three feet of ileum is examined for Meckel's diverticulitis. The intraabdominal colon, gallbladder, duodenum, and stomach should be palpated. If enlarged lymph nodes are present in the mesentery, the diagnosis may be mesenteric adenitis and a representative node should be excised and sent for culture and histology. Finally, the pelvic organs of the female are inspected either visually or by palpation. This allows for evaluation and surgical management of ovarian tumor, ectopic pregnancy, or tubo-ovarian abscess. Exploration should not cease until the cause of the illness has been located or the surgeon is certain that no treatable lesion is present in the abdominal cavity.

Laparoscopy is becoming increasingly popular in the diagnosis and treatment of suspected appendicitis. The one clear advantage of the laparoscopic method is the avoidance of an appendectomy scar. Virtually the entire abdomen can be examined with the laparoscope, avoiding a larger abdominal incision. When the diagnosis is uncertain, laparoscopy is an efficient diagnostic tool. If appendicitis is identified, the uncomplicated inflamed appendix can be easily removed via the laparoscope. A recent prospective randomized study comparing laparoscopic versus open appendectomy found no significant differences postoperatively for pain score, analgesic requirements, hospital stay, or recovery time. The laparoscopic procedure takes longer and is considerably more expensive, however.

POSTOPERATIVE TREATMENT

A nasogastric tube is rarely required in patients with uncomplicated disease. Patients with uncomplicated appendicitis usually require 24 to 36 hours of intravenous hydration postoperatively until bowel function returns. The diet is then advanced. Discharge is usually on the second or third postoperative day. A single dose of antibiotic may be given immediately postoperatively, but longer antibiotic therapy is not necessary unless perforated or gangrenous appendicitis was present.

COMPLICATED APPENDICITIS

Complicated appendicitis is synonymous with gangrenous and perforated appendicitis. The untreated inflamed appendix becomes gangrenous and may perforate with time. Accumulated pus then spills into the peritoneum. Most often the omentum and surrounding bowel wall off the area and an abscess or phlegmon forms. On examination, a tender mass may be felt in the RLQ. The patient's temperature generally increases and the white blood cell count may be elevated. In general, complicated appendicitis or an appendiceal abscess should be managed by appendectomy or abscess drainage. In some patients, however, appendicitis evolves in a more desultory fashion, culminating in an abscess but without much systemic reaction. Such patients may be treated initially with intravenous hydration, nasogastric decompression, and intravenous antibiotics. Fever should resolve in 24 to 36 hours and the abdominal mass and pain should subside over the next 5 to 7 days. The patient then should return in 6 weeks for an interval appendectomy. Those patients failing nonoperative management should, obviously, undergo operation as soon as such an outcome is suspected.

Operative management of complicated appendicitis depends on the findings. If there is diffuse peritonitis, the appendix is removed and the abdomen irrigated with generous volumes of saline. Drains are not placed. Postoperatively, patients are treated with broad spectrum antibiotics providing aerobe-anaerobe coverage for 5 to 10 days. Prolonged ileus and a need for nasogastric decompression can be expected. Intravenous antibiotics are continued postoperatively and switched to the oral route when the diet resumes. Operative wounds are left open at the skin level to prevent wound infection. After appropriate granulation tissue has formed the skin can be closed secondarily with paper tape.

If an abscess has formed, simple drainage is performed. This can be done operatively or percutaneously with ultrasound or CT guidance if the abscess has been detected preoperatively. Closed suction drains are placed into the abscess cavity and left in place until drainage becomes minimal (< 50 ml per day) and the patient has no fever. Approximately 6 weeks later the patient is returned to the operating room for an interval appendectomy.

APPENDICITIS IN PREGNANCY

Appendicitis occurs once in every 2,000 pregnancies and is the most common extrauterine condition requiring an abdominal operation during pregnancy. Appendicitis occurs more frequently during the first two trimesters. During this period symptoms do not differ much from those of a nonpregnant woman. During the last trimester the situation is altered by displacement and lateral rotation of the cecum and appendix by the enlarging uterus. Consequently, pain is felt in the right flank or right upper quadrant, which can confuse the diagnosis and may delay therapy.

Treatment consists of urgent appendectomy once the diagnosis is made. If rupture has not occurred, operation generally does not disturb the pregnancy. Premature labor occurs in about half of the women who develop appendicitis during the third trimester. The prognosis for the infant is directly related to birth weight. In complicated appendicitis with peritonitis, fetal loss occurs much more often and is related not only to prematurity but also sepsis.

INCIDENTAL APPENDECTOMY

Incidental appendectomy involves removal of the non-inflamed appendix during an abdominal operation performed for other reasons. Advocates of the procedure argue that it prevents the future development of appendicitis and does so with little or no added morbidity, operative time, or cost. In most cases, the procedure is performed on women undergoing hysterectomy or cholecystectomy who are more than 30 years of age. Their future risk of developing appendicitis is minimal and incidental appendectomy affords them no measurable benefit. Analysis of the risk-benefit balance in relation to the age specific incidence of appendicitis indicates that incidental appendectomy is appropriately done only in children under 10 years of age. The procedure requires that the patient needs an abdominal operation for another reason, and such situations are rare in the young child.

COMPLICATIONS

Postoperative complications occur in approximately 5 percent of uncomplicated appendicitis cases and in more than 30 percent of complicated cases. The most frequent complications are wound infection, intraabdominal abscess, fecal fistula, and intestinal obstruction. Wound infection is the most common complication and is treated by opening the skin and subcutaneous tissues. The wound is then allowed to heal by secondary intention.

Intraabdominal abscesses occur in up to 20 percent of patients with gangrenous or perforating appendicitis. The abscess causes recurrent fever, malaise, and anorexia beginning in the early postoperative period. A CT scan is very useful in diagnosing and treating an intraabdominal abscess. All abscesses must be drained, either percutaneously or surgically.

Fecal fistulas are manifested by feculent wound drainage. They often close spontaneously and may not require further surgical management.

SUGGESTED READING

Condon, RE. Incidental appendectomy is rarely indicated. In Simmons RL and Udekwu, AO, eds: Debates in Clinical Surgery. Chicago: Year Book Medical Publishers, 1990:91.
Condon RE, Telford GL. Appendicitis. In: Sabiston DC, ed., Textbook of Surgery. Philadelphia: WB Saunders Company, 1991.
Doherty GM, Lewis FR Jr. Appendicitis: continuing diagnostic challenge. Emerg Med Clin North Am 1989; 7:537–553.

Tate JJT, Dawson JW, Chung SCS, et al. Laparoscopic versus open appendectomy: prospective randomized trial. Lancet 1993; 342: 633–637.
Warren JL, Penberthy LT, Addiss DG, et al. Appendectomy incidental to cholecystectomy among elderly medicare beneficiaries. Surg Gynecol Obstet 1993; 177:288–294.

CONSTIPATION

ARND SCHULTE-BOCKHOLT, M.D.
TIMOTHY R. KOCH, M.D.

DEFINITION AND EPIDEMIOLOGY

Constipation remains difficult to define within the general population. Patients who complain of constipation may describe infrequent defecation, pain or straining with defecation, passage of firm or small-volume material, increased difficulty initiating evacuation, or a feeling of incomplete evacuation. Bowel frequency has been used as an objective criterion, and a range between three and 21 bowel movements weekly is thought to be normal defecation frequency. We define chronic constipation as a disorder lasting 6 months or longer in which individuals have two or fewer bowel movements per week. We consider a diagnosis of acute constipation in those individuals who have recently (less than 6 months previously) had either decreased frequency of bowel movements or increased difficulty initiating evacuation.

Constipation is one of the most common digestive disorders. It affects nearly 5 million people in the United States, corresponding to a prevalence rate of 2 percent, and 2.5 million people consult a physician yearly because of constipation. The occurrence of constipation increases with advancing age, rising exponentially in prevalence after the age of 65. This disorder is three times more common in women than in men. Constipation affects nonwhites more frequently than whites and is noted in people with low income or lack of formal education, indicating that environmental factors play a role in the development of constipation.

In the United States, laxatives are prescribed for more than 3 million people yearly, and 15 percent of women and 2 percent of men use laxatives on a regular basis. An estimated $250 million is spent yearly on laxatives purchased without a prescription, and the total amount spent on laxatives, including prescriptions, is at least $450 million yearly. These numbers are similar to those reported in European studies, and it has been noted that laxative use, as expected, increases with patient age.

Table 1 Causes of Constipation

Nerve disorders	Smooth muscle disorders
Hirschsprung's disease	Scleroderma
Central nervous system diseases	Amyloidosis
Heavy metal poisoning (e.g. lead/mercury)	Metabolic/endocrine disorders
	Hypothyroidism
Mechanical obstruction	Diabetes mellitus with autonomic neuropathy
Neoplasia and strictures	Uremia
Rectocele	Hypercalcemia/hypokalemia
Rectal prolapse	
Endometriosis	Idiopathic constipation
	Outlet obstruction
Medication induced	Slow transit/colonic inertia
Opiate analgesics	Normal transit/irritable bowel syndrome
Anticholinergic agents	
Calcium channel antagonists	
Calcium-containing supplements	
Aluminum-containing antacids	
Vinca alkaloids	
Polystyrene binding resins	

COMMON CAUSES

Constipation is a symptom that may be present in many underlying disorders. Therefore, before beginning medical treatment, it is important to consider known treatable causes of constipation (Table 1). In general, we are more aggressive in excluding known causes of constipation in patients presenting with acute constipation (lasting less than 6 months). In more than 50 percent of individuals seen for a complaint of constipation, it is not possible to find a specific cause. These patients are classified as having idiopathic constipation.

AGENTS USED FOR TREATMENT OF CONSTIPATION

Five major groups of agents have been used in the medical treatment of constipation (Table 2).

Bulk Agents

Bulk agents include soluble and insoluble fiber supplements. Fiber and fiber supplements are a diverse group of nonstarch carbohydrates that are not digestible by humans. Cellulose and lignin are fibrous and insoluble and have their greatest effect on fecal bulk. Noncellulose polysaccharides include hemicellulose, pectin, gums, algal polysaccharides such as guar, and the synthetic resin polycarbophil. These substances are viscous and soluble, have a high water-binding capacity, and appear to influence colonic motility. Most soluble fibers are digested by bacteria and may contribute to a laxative action by increasing osmotic pressure of stool and increasing fecal mass. Colonic bacterial fermentation of soluble fibers may also produce metabolites that directly influence fluid transport and motility. However, water-soluble fiber supplements may slow nutrient absorption and decrease transit through the upper gastrointestinal (GI) tract.

Colonic gas formation is a common side effect, but often subsides after a week owing to adaptation of intestinal flora. Patients with GI stenosis or intestinal pseudo-obstruction should avoid fiber. Cellulose may bind cardiac glycosides and other drugs; therefore, ingestion of drugs and laxatives should be separated in time as much as possible. Intestinal obstruction and bezoar formation are unusual complications from the use of fiber supplements. Allergic reactions have also been described, especially with plant gums, but fiber supplements generally have the fewest side effects among laxatives.

Osmotic Agents

Osmotic agents increase the water content of fecal material, an effect that may be beneficial in patients with constipation, since studies of colonic motility have suggested that transit of liquid fecal material in the human colon is more rapid than transit of solid material. Magnesium salts such as sulfate or citrate of magnesia have been extensively used and are relatively safe if used as directed. They are contraindicated for long-term use in patients with congestive heart failure or renal insufficiency. Patients receiving these agents for long-term use should periodically undergo screening of the serum magnesium level. Sodium phosphate is another salt often used as an osmotic laxative; it is more pleasant tasting than magnesium salts, but phosphate and sodium accumulation can occur in patients with diminished renal function.

In patients with renal insufficiency, poorly absorbed mono- or disaccharides or alcohol derivatives (e.g., lactulose, sorbitol, or glycerol) may be beneficial in treatment of constipation. These substances increase osmotic pressure in the colon and are metabolized by

Table 2 Agents used in Treatment of Constipation

Group	Comments
1. Bulk/fiber	Least side effects but may cause obstruction
a. Soluble:	Fermentation increases flatus
psyllium, guar, pectin	
b. Insoluble/inorganic:	Not fermented
cellulose, polycarbophil salts	
2. Osmotic	May impair fluid and electrolyte balance
a. Salts:	Inexpensive
magnesium salts,	Magnesium accumulation if renal insufficiency
sodium phosphate	Phosphate accumulation if renal insufficiency
b. Sugars or sugar alcohols:	Increases flatus
Lactulose, lactose, mannitol,	Expensive
sorbitol, glycerol,	
polyethylene glycol solutions	
3. Stimulants/irritants	Tachyphylaxis occurs
Bisacodyl and phenolpthalein (diphenols),	Active only if bile salts and bacteria present
cascara/senna/aloe/casanthranol	Require bacterial cleavage
(anthraquinones),	
Castor oil (ricinoleic acid),	Not routinely used, poor taste
Docusate salts,	Poorly effective
Chenocholic acid	Expensive
4. Prokinetic agents	Abdominal cramping; avoid in outlet obstruction
Cisapride	
Bethanecol chloride	
Neostigmine bromide	May induce cholinergic crisis
Naloxone hydrochloride	Requires parenteral delivery
5. Enema and suppository	
Sodium phosphates, glycerol, sorbitol,	Self-administered enema may produce
lactulose, mineral oil, bisacodyl, CO_2-	perforation
producing suppository	

colonic bacteria to increase intraluminal bacterial mass. Sorbitol 70 percent syrup and glycerol are less expensive alternatives to lactulose. Most patients receive benefit from 30 ml of these substances once or twice daily, although the therapeutic dose has to be determined empirically; 1 to 3 days may be required before a laxative effect begins. Common side effects include gas formation due to fermentation by colonic bacteria.

Polyethyleneglycol (PEG: MW3350 daltons) electrolyte solutions are nonabsorbable polyalcohols in a saline isotonic solution containing 60 g PEG per liter. These solutions are commonly used in preparation for colonoscopy, since there is no net ion absorption or loss and dehydration does not occur because of their isotonicity. In patients with constipation, PEG solutions have been given at a dose of 3 to 4 L to obtain colonic cleansing once or twice weekly. Alternatively, these patients have been treated with 250 to 500 ml of PEG solution daily. A relative disadvantage of PEG solutions is their high price.

Stimulant Laxatives

Irritant or stimulant laxatives include anthraquinone compounds such as the extracts of senna, aloe, cascara, or rhubarb and diphenylmethane derivatives, including phenolphthalein and bisacodyl. These substances have a prokinetic action, increase intestinal secretion, and diminish intestinal absorption. The active ingredients in the anthraquinone group are glycoside derivatives of danthron. Danthron itself has been withdrawn from the market because of its association with hepatic and intestinal tumors. Anthraquinones are nonabsorbable, and the active component, rheinanthrone, is formed by bacterial cleavage. By contrast, bisacodyl and phenolphthalein are absorbed by the small intestine, undergo glucuronidation in the liver, and are then excreted into the bile. Glucuronidated derivatives are not absorbable and will pass into the colon, where deconjugation by bacteria forms the active diphenol compound. These substances have a laxative effect only if bile flow is not obstructed and bacteria are present in the colon. Owing to the enterohepatic circulation, their laxative effect is delayed until 6 to 10 hours after ingestion.

The dosage of anthraquinones for constipation is variable, because most commercial preparations are not standardized. The adult dose for the proprietary preparation cascara sagrada (casanthranol) is 30 mg per day; the usual dose of bisacodyl is 10 to 15 mg per day, and of phenolphthalein 30 to 200 mg per day.

Stimulant laxatives, especially if used for acute constipation, cause abdominal cramping and tenesmus in 10 percent of patients. Melanosis coli is a reversible black-brown discoloration of the colonic mucosa that begins abruptly at the ileocecal valve and may progress distally to the dentate line. It is found frequently in patients who chronically use stimulant laxatives, especially anthraquinones. However, there is no present evidence that melanosis coli has a pathophysiologic

importance. Stimulant agents generally should not be prescribed for longer than 2 weeks. It is presently unclear whether long-term use of these substances can damage the enteric nerve system. It is well known that patients using these substances on a long-term basis may require increasing doses. Unfortunately, older patients may develop fecal incontinence while using stimulant laxatives. Allergic reactions, including Stevens-Johnson syndrome, have been described in patients receiving stimulant laxatives.

There is a group of stimulant and irritant laxatives that we do not use in our clinical practice. Castor oil, obtained from the bean of the castor plant *Ricinus communis,* has been used since the time of the ancient Egyptians. It contains ricinoleic acid, has a terrible taste, and affects both secretion and motility. Castor oil causes cramping abdominal pain by a prokinetic effect on the small bowel. Bile acids, such as cholic acid (0.25 g three times daily) or chenodeoxycholic acid (0.25 to 0.5 g three times daily), reduce net absorption of water and electrolytes. These substances are quite expensive for use as a first-line drug in treatment of constipation. We do not use mineral oil because reflux of this material can cause lipid pneumonia. Available studies have shown minimal benefit from wetting agents or surfactants, such as docusate salts, in treatment of constipation. These docusate salts may cause increased absorption of other drugs being given concurrently.

Prokinetic Agents

Prokinetic agents or drugs that function as neurotransmitter agonists have potential use in patients with slow transit constipation, but may increase abdominal symptoms in those with constipation related to an outlet obstruction. Bethanechol chloride is a muscarinic-cholinergic agonist that increases phasic contractions in human colon at a dose of 10 to 50 mg three times daily. Neostigmine bromide is an anticholinesterase agent that is rarely used because of the possible initiation of a cholinergic crisis. A newly available prokinetic agent, cisapride, releases acetylcholine at the level of the nerve plexus and induces phasic colonic contractions. It may function as a serotonin[4]-receptor agonist to stimulate GI motility. It is a promising drug for treatment of patients with mild to moderate slow transit constipation. A frequently used dosage is 10 to 20 mg up to three times daily. Cramping abdominal pain and chest pain due to its prokinetic effects on the stomach and esophagus have been noted.

The opiate antagonist naloxone hydrochloride has been used for idiopathic slow transit constipation. Its use has been limited by the necessity of parenteral administration and high cost.

Suppositories and Enemas

The final group of agents frequently used to treat constipation are suppositories and enemas. Bisacodyl, a known stimulant laxative, is commonly used in suppository form (10 mg) or in enema form (10 mg per 30 ml). After rectal administration, it initiates defecation within 15 to 60 minutes. Some patients note cramping abdominal pain, and a burning sensation in the rectum associated with mild proctitis has been observed.*

Sorbitol, glycerol, and lactulose are commercially available in both suppository and enema form. These compounds function as rectal irritants (by dehydration of exposed mucosa), and rectal discomfort or a burning sensation has been reported. Carbon dioxide–producing suppositories (a mixture of sodium bicarbonate and potassium bitartrate) distend the rectum with CO_2 and stimulate colorectal contractions. This mechanism may be beneficial in patients with chronic constipation and secondarily diminished rectal sensation of distention. We do not routinely advise patients to use enemas at home owing to the possibility of perforation of the anal canal or rectum by the enema tip.

UNPROVED THERAPY

There is little scientific evidence to support the widespread belief that increased water consumption, physical exercise, or abdominal massage is beneficial as primary therapy in patients with chronic constipation. It has been shown that water consumption has to be increased to more than 4 L daily before stool consistency is affected. This is due to the large resorptive capacity of the small and large intestine.

Psychotherapy may be helpful in coping with the irritable bowel syndrome (IBS) but has not been shown to have an effect on intestinal transit. Erythromycin has been used as a prokinetic agent in treatment of small bowel pseudo-obstruction, but it does not affect colonic motility.

COMBINATION THERAPY AND HERBAL PREPARATIONS

We recommend that physicians use only one or two preparations from each main group of agents in treating constipation. This permits improved awareness of specific effects and potential side effects of different agents. There is no evidence that combinations of laxatives have an advantage over preparations containing a single ingredient. We discourage our patients from using herbal tea preparations and other "natural" laxative preparations because the substances in these preparations are poorly defined pharmacologically, are not consistent in the amount of drug that is present, and may contain hepatotoxic alkaloids.

---

*Editor's Note: The acute proctitis occurring with bisacodyl or with hypertonic phosphate enemas (Fleet's) should be kept in mind when they are used in preparation for sigmoidoscopy.

MANAGEMENT

Standard Evaluation and Treatment

Figure 1 presents our algorithm for the laboratory investigation and treatment at the initial presentation of a patient with constipation. In the first visit, we complete a history and physical examination, including a rectal examination. Our goal is to try to differentiate among complaints of acute constipation (less than 6 months), progressive symptoms, and chronic constipation (more than 6 months).

In patients with acute constipation or progressive symptoms (especially those who are over 40 years old), metabolic or endocrine disorders associated with constipation should be excluded by examining serum potassium, calcium, glucose, creatinine, and thyroid stimulating hormone levels. We also perform proctosigmoidoscopy and barium colon x-ray examination to exclude mechanical obstruction due to neoplasms, diverticular strictures, or endometriosis. If this laboratory evaluation provides a specific diagnosis, we treat the underlying disease. If no specific diagnosis is made, we recommend a high-fiber intake as described below.

In patients with chronic constipation, we initially recommend a high-fiber intake. The average American diet is estimated to include 15 to 20 g of fiber daily. To utilize fiber in the therapy for constipation, we recommend 30 to 50 g of total fiber intake daily. Specifically, patients can take bran (8 g fiber per 30 g serving); shredded wheat (3 g fiber per 30 g serving); corn meal (5 g fiber per 120 g serving); brown rice (5.5 g fiber per 120 g serving); whole wheat or rye bread (2 g fiber per 30 g serving); brown, Navy, or red beans (8 g fiber per 120 g serving); corn, broccoli, or peas (4 g fiber per 120 g serving); prunes (5.5 g fiber per 120 g serving); and an apple or pear (5 g fiber per medium fruit).

Since most individuals seem unable on a daily basis to reach 30 to 50 g of total fiber intake, they will require fiber supplements, which are best taken with a meal and adequate fluid intake. Among commonly used supplements, psyllium obtained from *Plantago* seed should be taken in a dose of 3 to 4 g of fiber in at least 250 ml of fluid such as fruit juice (as a taste corrector) up to three times daily. Patients who continue to have excessive flatulence may benefit by substituting a polycarbophil salt, 1 g up to four times daily.

When we instruct patients on a high-fiber intake, we also discuss the initiation of the gastrocolonic response. In most individuals, gastric distention can increase phasic contractions of the rectosigmoid region. Because of the normal circadian rhythm of colonic motility, this response may be more pronounced in the morning. We recommend that patients eat a warm meal or drink a warm fluid after arising in the morning.

In patients with chronic constipation who have not improved with a high-fiber intake, we perform the above-described laboratory evaluation; if this provides a specific diagnosis, we treat the underlying disease.

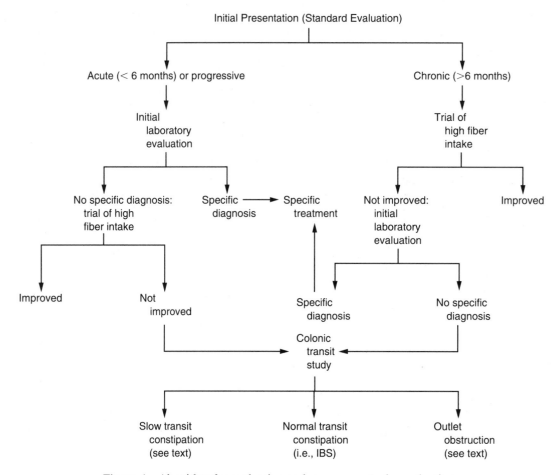

Figure 1 Algorithm for evaluation and management of constipation.

Failure of Standard Treatment

In patients with constipation whose laboratory results are normal and who have not improved with a high-fiber intake, we proceed to a colonic transit study. These patients by definition have idiopathic constipation, and this test is performed to determine the subtype of constipation. Because of improved patient compliance and ease of interpretation, we use the Hinton method for examination of colonic transit. After fecal disimpaction (if appropriate), the patient ingests a single gelatin capsule containing 20 nonabsorbable markers (Sitzmarks). During the study, the patient refrains from all laxatives, suppositories, enemas, and constipation-associated medications. An abdominal flat plate x-ray film is taken at 5 days. In multiple published studies, normal individuals pass at least 80 percent, or 16 of 20 markers, at 5 days. If the study is abnormal, markers may be retained in the rectosigmoid region (consistent with a diagnosis of outlet obstruction) or more diffusely throughout the colon (consistent with slow transit constipation).

In patients with outlet obstruction, we routinely advise a low-residue diet. As supplemental therapy, the regular use of glycerol or CO_2-producing suppositories (two to three mornings a week) may be beneficial in maintaining rectal evacuation. Also, in patients with continued abdominal symptoms, we recommend addition of an osmotic agent such as citrate of magnesia, 30 to 120 ml at bedtime, or sorbitol 70 percent syrup, 30 to 60 ml at bedtime. Some patients prefer to use citrate of magnesia intermittently (120 to 240 ml twice weekly). A more complete discussion of the evaluation and treatment of patients with outlet obstruction is offered in the chapter *Chronic Constipation: Matching Type to Treatment*.

In patients with normal transit constipation (probable IBS), the main goal is usually relief of chronic abdominal pain. We first try to determine whether pain is relieved after colonic cleansing with either citrate of magnesia, 120 to 240 ml, or PEG solution, 2 to 4 L. If pain relief is satisfactory, we begin the stepwise management approach described above for patients with outlet obstruction. Unfortunately, most individuals have continued abdominal pain after colonic cleansing. The evaluation and treatment of patients with IBS is discussed in a separate chapter.

In patients with slow transit constipation, we routinely advise a low-residue diet. A few patients with slow transit constipation obtain relief from abdominal pain by colonic cleansing but cannot maintain colonic evacuation. These patients may obtain long-term improvement of symptoms by chronic use of a polymeric liquid diet, or an alternative treatment, a trial of a prokinetic agent such as cisapride, 10 to 20 mg up to three times daily, may be warranted. The evaluation and treatment of patients with slow transit constipation is discussed in the chapter on chronic constipation.

Laxative and Enema Dependency

After evacuation of the colon by means of a stimulant laxative or enema, it may be several days before a spontaneous bowel movement occurs. Patients may assume that they are constipated, and a vicious cycle develops in which they become dependent on the daily use of a laxative or enema to produce defecation. Secondary hyperaldosteronism, steatorrhea, hypoalbuminemia, and osteomalacia have been described as additional problems that can develop in laxative dependency.

In patients with dependency, our initial goals are to determine whether there is a treatable cause of constipation and whether there is objective evidence of colorectal dysmotility. We complete the laboratory investigation described above and initiate proper treatment if a specific diagnosis is made. Next, if the patient has an impaction, we obtain colonic cleansing with either osmotic laxatives or prolonged use of a polymeric liquid diet. After disimpaction and in patients with no evidence of a fecal impaction, a colonic transit study is performed (described above) while the patient maintains a regular diet and avoids laxatives and enemas.

Patients with slow transit constipation or outlet obstruction are treated as described above. In most patients who have normal transit constipation, we initially convert them from use of stimulant laxatives or enemas to osmotic agents or suppositories, and we discuss initiation of the gastrocolonic response as described above. It is very important at this stage to reassure patients that there is no evidence for abnormal movement of solid material through the colon or rectum, and to discuss the possible side effects of continued use of stimulant laxatives or enemas. As a next step, we try to slowly increase fiber intake up to 30 to 50 g fiber daily while tapering the intake of osmotic agents or suppositories. Laxative dependency has not been well studied, but in 50 percent of cases it appears possible to discontinue stimulant laxatives after introducing a high-fiber diet. In many cases, it is possible to convert patients' stimulant laxative use to suppository use. In some patients, the believed need for routine use of stimulant laxatives and enemas cannot be overcome, and we then consider a psychiatric evaluation. In general, these patients have a great obsession about their bowel movements.

Pregnancy

Patients presenting with constipation during pregnancy should initially receive a trial of 30 to 50 g of daily fiber intake. If this is not effective, lactulose or sorbitol may be used safely. Studies examining the possible side effects of stimulant laxatives during pregnancy have been contradictory. Both the sennosides and bisacodyl have been examined for their embryonic and fetotoxic influences, and it is presently not clear whether they can be safely used in pregnancy. It has been suggested that castor oil can initiate uterine contractions and should not be used. Both bisacodyl and sennosides appear in breast milk in the postpartum period, but the concentrations are so low that no side effects should be expected in breast-feeding babies. We do not recommend the regular use of enemas. Either bisacodyl or CO_2-producing suppositories should be safe in inducing rectal evacuation.

Spinal Cord Injury

Spinal cord injuries interrupt both afferent and efferent innervation of the anal sphincter. Constipation, like urinary bladder retention, commonly occurs shortly after the injury (so-called spinal shock). In a bowel rehabilitation program, it is recommended that patients have 30 to 50 g daily of fiber intake and take daily advantage of the normal gastrocolonic response that occurs 20 minutes after breakfast. When beginning this bowel program, the spinal injury patient also has to initiate defecation by learning to apply digital rectal stimulation in combination with either a bisacodyl or glycerol suppository or a CO_2-producing suppository, to induce rectal distention. Before beginning digital stimulation, feces present in the lower rectum should be removed digitally. A well-lubricated gloved finger should be inserted 2 to 3 cm into the rectum. A gentle circular motion toward the sacrum will relax the external anal sphincter, and stimulation of the autonomic nerves in the S2-S3 segment will initiate a rectal peristaltic reflex. After 1 to 2 minutes of digital stimulation, the suppository should be inserted as high above the sphincter as possible and held in place for 15 seconds. After waiting 20 minutes, digital stimulation is repeated for periods of 3 minutes every 5 to 10 minutes until defecation occurs. During this time, the patient should attempt to use Valsalva's maneuver, if possible. Alternatively, the patient can lean forward to increase intra-abdominal pressure. If defecation is not achieved within 30 minutes, a second suppository may be inserted and the above sequence repeated.

It is important to obtain regular evacuation of the rectum at least once every 3 days, because a stool-filled colon in these patients can induce bladder spasms with urinary incontinence and autonomic hyperreflexia in patients with T4-T6 or higher lesions. The symptoms of autonomic hyperreflexia are a rise in blood pressure, headache, and profuse sweating above the lesion. If routine evacuation is not obtained in these patients, fecal impaction can cause diarrhea by leakage of fecal fluid around a rectal impaction.

Cancer Chemotherapy

Chemotherapy, especially with vinblastine or vincristine, is associated with the development of constipation. The vinca alkaloids can damage afferent and efferent rectal innervation and potentially damage the enteric nervous system. Stimulant laxatives therefore may not be effective, and osmotic laxatives such as lactulose, sorbitol, or PEG solution are alternatives. Magnesium laxatives and sodium phosphate should be avoided owing to possible magnesium retention or water and electrolyte depletion. Enemas or suppositories should not be used in view of the possible development of anal or rectal injury with resultant bleeding or infection. Fiber supplements may be helpful in patients complaining of difficulty initiating defecation or passage of hard feces.

SUGGESTED READING

Andorsky R, Goldner F. Colonic lavage solution (PEG) as a treatment for chronic constipation: a double-blind, placebo controlled study. Am J Gastroenterol 1991; 85:261–265.

Drossman DA, Thompson WG. The irritable bowel syndrome: review and a graduated multicomponent treatment approach. Ann Intern Med 1992; 116:1009–1016.

Hepner G, Hofman AF. Cholic acid therapy for constipation. Mayo Clin Proc 1973; 48:356–358.

Krevsky B, Maurer AH, Malmud LS, Fisher RS. Cisapride accelerates colonic transit in constipated patients with colonic inertia. Am J Gastroenterol 1989; 84:882–887.

Lederle FA, Busch DL, Mattox KM, et al. Cost-effective treatment of constipation in the elderly: a randomized double-blind comparison of sorbitol and lactulose. Am J Med 1990; 89:597–601.

Müller-Lissner S. Effect of wheat bran on weight of stool and gastrointestinal transit time: a meta-analysis. Br Med J 1988; 296:615–617.

Snape WJ Jr, Carlson GM, Cohen S. Human colonic myoelectric activity in response to Prostigmin and the gastrointestinal hormones. Dig Dis Sci 1977; 22:881–887.

Staumont G, Frexinos J, Fioramonti J, Bueno L. Sennosides and human colonic motility. Pharmacology 1988; 36 (Suppl 1):49–56.

CONSTIPATION IN CHILDREN

JONATHAN A. FLICK, M.D.

DIAGNOSTIC CONSIDERATIONS

Constipation is a frequent complaint of childhood that accounts for a significant portion of subspecialty consultations in pediatric gastroenterology. It should be recognized that normal stool frequency, size, and consistency are variable during infancy and childhood, and change with development. Most breast- or bottle-fed infants defecate with each feeding. Older children normally pass between three bowel movements per day and one every other day. Failure to evacuate on a regular basis leads to chronic stool retention and overflow incontinence, or encopresis. Encopresis is a hallmark of chronic childhood constipation and is often the symptom for which medical attention is first sought.

A differential diagnosis of childhood constipation is listed in Table 1. The two most important diagnostic considerations are functional constipation (known also as acquired megacolon or psychogenic constipation) and Hirschsprung's disease (congenital megacolon or aganglionosis). These entities are discussed in more detail below. Additional etiologies include local mechanical factors such as acquired fissures, strictures of congenital or acquired origin, and anterior displacement of the anus. The latter, a developmental anomaly, may be suspected by the finding on physical examination of an anus located less than one-half the distance posterior from the scrotum to the coccyx (or less than one-third

Table 1 Differential Diagnosis of Constipation in Childhood

Idiopathic ("functional")

Local mechanical factors
  Fissures
  Strictures
  Tumors
  Anterior anal displacement

Systemic/metabolic disorders
  Hypothyroidism
  Diabetes mellitus
  Hypokalemia
  Hypocalcemia
  Cystic fibrosis
  Malabsorption
  Intestinal pseudo-obstruction

Drugs
  Antacids (calcium, aluminum-containing)
  Anticholinergics
  Anticonvulsants
  Iron
  Opiates
  Laxative abuse
  Lead intoxication

Neurogenic disorders
  Hirschsprung's disease
  Neurofibromatosis
  Myelodysplasia
  Spinal cord injury
  Cerebral palsy
  Mental motor retardation
  Infant botulism

Psychiatric
  Anorexia nervosa
  Attention-deficit hyperactivity disorder

Table 2 Differentiating Features Between Hirschsprung's Disease and Functional Constipation

Feature	Hirschsprung's Disease	Functional Constipation
Delayed passage of meconium	>95%	Rare
Symptoms as newborn	Almost always	Unusual
Late onset (>3 yr)	Rare	Common
Encopresis	Rare	Common
Failure to thrive	Common	Rare
Obstructive symptoms	Common	Rare
Anal sphincter tone	Increased	Decreased
Rectal ampulla	Narrowed	Enlarged
Stool in ampulla	Rare	Common
Stool caliber	Narrow	Large
Male predominance	Yes	Yes

the vagina-coccyx distance in girls). Malabsorption syndromes of childhood, including cystic fibrosis and celiac disease, may present with constipation rather than the more expected diarrhea. As in adults, a variety of drugs have been associated with childhood constipation. Children with cerebral palsy or mental motor retardation frequently suffer from chronic constipation that may be multifactorial in cause, including neuromuscular dysfunction, dietary habits, and drug (i.e., anticonvulsant) therapy.

Hirschsprung's disease occurs in one in 5,000 live births and accounts for up to 25 percent of cases of neonatal obstruction. Delay in passage of meconium beyond the first 24 hours after birth is seen in up to 95 percent of affected infants. Although 80 percent of cases are recognized by 1 year of age, there is sometimes a delay in diagnosis until later in childhood or adulthood. Hirschsprung's disease should therefore be considered in any child with chronic constipation beginning in early infancy. Table 2 compares several differentiating features between Hirschsprung's disease and chronic functional constipation.

THERAPEUTIC APPROACH

Acute Constipation

Acute constipation in childhood is most often a self-limited condition precipitated by a variety of factors, including systemic illness, change in diet, and travel. The otherwise well infant who continues to feed well and is without vomiting, abdominal distention, or colic should be managed expectantly. In this regard, it should be noted that an occasional breast-fed infant may pass stools once weekly or less often. However, if excessive irritability, poor feeding, significant abdominal distention, or other obstructive symptoms prompt treatment, several options are available. Gentle rectal stimulation by careful insertion of a well-lubricated rectal thermometer may suffice. Alternatively, a small glycerin suppository or enema (Babylax) may be employed. Repeated rectal manipulation, however, should be avoided. In

older children suffering from an acute episode of constipation, milk of magnesia (1 to 2 tbsp), senna (e.g., Senokot granules, ½ to 1 tsp, or Senokot syrup, 1 to 2 tsp) or, for those old enough to swallow pills, bisacodyl (5 mg) may be given.

Chronic Constipation in Infants

As discussed earlier, it is important to exclude Hirschsprung's disease in chronically constipated infants. Features suggestive of Hirschsprung's disease should prompt appropriate diagnostic studies, which might include anorectal manometry, rectal suction biopsy, and/or barium enema examination. Consultation with a pediatric gastroenterologist or pediatric surgeon should be obtained.

When Hirschsprung's disease and other organic causes have been excluded, the indications for treatment include pain with bowel movements, anal fissures, poor feeding, vomiting, and other obstructive symptoms. In general, dietary treatment of the chronically constipated infant is preferred to chronic rectal stimulation. Prune juice, 2 ounces diluted with 2 ounces of water once or twice daily, may suffice. Alternatives include dark corn syrup and malt soup extract (Maltsupex). Either may be administered as 1 to 2 tsp in 4 ounces of formula or water, once or twice daily. For infants aged 6 months or older, a laxative fruit (prunes, plums) should be added to the diet. Mineral oil preparations should not be used in children under 1 year of age.

Chronic Constipation in Toddlers and Older Children

A successful treatment program begins with an explanation to the child and parents of underlying pathophysiologic mechanisms. It is important that the family, as well as teachers and other caretakers, recognize that encopresis is a result of chronic fecal retention, rectal distention, and diminished sensory feedback, rather than simply the child's lack of motivation to attend to a defecatory urge. It is also stressed that a successful treatment program will take several months to accomplish, during which time therapy as described below must be consistently administered on a daily basis.

"Clean-Out"

Medical therapy is divided into initial "clean-out" and subsequent maintenance phases (Table 3). "Clean-out" can usually be accomplished with a series of hypertonic phosphate enemas, one daily for 3 to 4 days, or until the rectum is essentially clear of fecal residue. Most school-age and older children may safely receive standard-sized (4.5 ounce) enemas; pediatric (2.25 ounce) enemas may be given to younger patients. Because hyperphosphatemia and hypocalcemic tetany have been reported with prolonged retention of hypertonic phosphate enema fluid, enemas should be discontinued if evacuation does not occur within 24 hours. In this case, isotonic saline enemas may be used. The

Table 3 Therapy for Chronic Constipation in Toddlers and Older Children

Initial "clean-out"	Hypertonic phosphate enemas, one daily for 3–4 days (alternatives: high-dose mineral oil, magnesium citrate, colonic lavage solution, manual disimpaction)
Maintenance therapy	Medical: emulsified mineral oil preparation, 2 tbsp twice daily (titrate) (alternatives: lactulose, cathartic agents, every-other-day enemas) Dietary: high-fiber diet Behavioral: toilet-sitting routine (maintain proper posture), calendar reward system

effectiveness of the "clean-out" may be enhanced by oral administration of mineral oil preparations (see below) for several days before enema use. If the retained fecal mass is particularly hard, a mineral oil enema (60 to 120 ml) may be given as the first of the series.

Alternatives to enemas for initial colonic cleansing include high-dose mineral oil by mouth (15 to 30 ml per year of age per day, maximum 240 ml), oral magnesium citrate (one ounce per year of age, maximum 10 ounces), polyethylene glycol–electrolyte lavage solutions, and manual disimpaction. The latter two modalities should be reserved for cases of fecal impaction refractory to enemas. Colonic lavage solutions may be given at a rate of 40 ml per kilogram per hr (maximum 2 L per hour) until the rectal discharge is clear. This may require 24 or more hours to accomplish, using volumes far greater than those employed for adult colonoscopy preparation. Since few children will drink such large volumes, delivery of the solution via nasogastric tube is most frequently required, usually in an inpatient setting. Simultaneous administration of oral clear liquids or intravenous fluids is necessary to prevent dehydration. Manual disimpaction is a frightening and uncomfortable procedure for a child and should rarely be necessary. When it is required, performance under sedation or general anesthesia is recommended.

Continued soiling after the initial series of enemas should alert the physician to possible inadequate colonic cleansing, best assessed by repeat rectal examination. Additional enemas should be given as needed. In contrast, a successful "clean-out" results in prompt cessation of encopresis. However, because of chronic rectal distention, altered rectal compliance, and increased sensory threshold, most constipated children still do not have a normal defecatory urge after even successful "clean-out." Maintenance therapy is therefore instituted to effect regular evacuation and prevent fecal reaccumulation in the still-dilated rectal ampulla.

Maintenance

Maintenance therapy has medical, dietary, and behavioral components. The traditional therapeutic agent is light mineral oil, given in large doses. This has the advantages of being effective and inexpensive, but it has some objectionable qualities with regard to taste, consistency, and leakage from the rectum. Emulsified mineral oil preparations (Agoral, Kondremul, or Milkinol) are therefore preferred. An initial dose of two tbsp twice daily may be increased every several days as necessary until the child is passing soft stools on a daily basis. Oil leakage from the rectum may indicate too high a dose but is more often an overflow phenomenon secondary to an inadequate initial "clean-out" or formation of a new impaction. Because these agents act as lipid solvents, they should not be administered with meals, to minimize the small risk of interference with fat-soluble vitamin absorption. A more genuine concern is that of oil aspiration leading to lipid pneumonia; the use of mineral oil preparations is therefore contraindicated in children under the age of 1 year and those with gastroesophageal reflux or an impaired gag reflex.

Habit Training

Several alternatives to the above-outlined approach have been described. With so-called habit training, children attempt a bowel movement daily for 10 minutes after a meal. If no stool is produced on 2 consecutive days, an enema is given. This technique has been reported to be effective, but compliance with long-term enema administration may be poor. Lactulose syrup may be useful, especially in children who refuse mineral oil. An initial dose of 0.5 g per kilogram body weight per day may be increased every several days to a maximum of 1 g per kilogram twice daily. The effectiveness of cathartic agents and stimulant laxatives is limited by the excessive abdominal cramping they may induce. In addition, their long-term use may lead to a cathartic colon. Limited experience suggests that the prokinetic agent cisapride, 0.2 mg per kilogram three times daily, may be useful in some children with chronic constipation.

Dietary Management

Like adults, constipated children may benefit from a high-fiber diet. A child's acceptance of substituting bran-containing for processed cereals, whole-wheat for white bread, and so forth, is probably most determined by the family's overall dietary habits. Popcorn is a good source of fiber that most children will readily consume. Fiber supplements in liquid suspension form are usually rejected. Specific dietary restrictions are not routinely indicated.

Behavioral Management

A regular toilet-sitting routine should be instituted whereby the child sits for 10 minutes twice daily. This is best done after mealtimes, to capitalize on the gastrocolic reflex. It is important that the child sit well back on the toilet seat and be provided with adequate foot support to raise the knees above the level of the hips, to facilitate descent of the rectal sling.

Because of the rectal sensory deficit present in this disorder, there is little value in punishing the child for episodes of soiling. More helpful is positive reinforcement of first compliance with a toilet-sitting program, and later, successful defecation. Many children respond favorably to a calendar system with paste-on stars applied to days on which these goals are achieved.

Biofeedback training has been used in children with functional constipation and encopresis. Overall, it appears to be of equivalent efficacy to standard mineral oil therapy. It may be of particular value in children with abnormal defecation dynamics as determined by anorectal manometry. Children must be of sufficient age to cooperate with the procedure. A considerable commitment of time is required of the physician and child enrolled in such a program.

Referral of chronically constipated children for psychological evaluation is not routinely indicated. Although behavioral abnormalities are present in some children, these are usually secondary to the social consequences of fecal soiling and often resolve with successful medical management. Furthermore, the results of psychotherapy as sole treatment for functional constipation and encopresis have not been encouraging. Psychiatric evaluation may, however, be indicated for the occasional encopretic child without stool retention, because a high incidence of behavioral disorders has been found in these youngsters. Counseling may also be helpful for children who refuse medications or toilet sitting.

RESULTS OF THERAPY

Functional constipation with encopresis has a generally good prognosis, although therapy may be required for many months or even longer. Relapses are not uncommon and may require a repeated course of enemas and increased doses of mineral oil preparations. When the child is having bowel movements every day or two and is no longer soiling, medication may be slowly tapered over several months.

SUGGESTED READING

Blisard KS, Kleinman R. Hirschsprung's disease: a clinical and pathologic overview. Hum Pathol 1986; 17:1189–1191.

Clayden GS. Management of chronic constipation. Arch Dis Child 1992; 67:340–344.

Hatch TF. Encopresis and constipation in children. Pediatr Clin North Am 1988; 35:257–280.

Ingebo KB, Heyman MB. Polyethylene glycol–electrolyte solution for intestinal clearance in children with refractory encopresis. Am J Dis Child 1988; 142:340–342.

Loening-Baucke V. Persistence of chronic constipation in children after biofeedback treatment. Dig Dis Sci 1991; 36:153–160.

Lowery S, Srour JW, Whitehead WE, Schuster MM. Habit training as treatment of encopresis secondary to chronic constipation. J Pediatr Gastroenterol Nutr 1985; 4:397–401.

Nolan T, Debelle G, Oberklaid F, Coffey C. Randomized trial of laxatives in treatment of childhood encopresis. Lancet 1991; 338:523–527.

Staiano A, Cucchiara S, Andreotti MR, et al. Effect of cisapride on chronic idiopathic constipation in children. Dig Dis Sci 1991; 36:733–736.

Wald A, Chandra R, Gabel S, Chiponis D. Evaluation of biofeedback in childhood constipation. J Pediatr Gastroenterol Nutr 1987; 6:554–558.

CHRONIC CONSTIPATION: MATCHING TYPE TO TREATMENT

JOHN H. PEMBERTON, M.D.

Constipation is a complex condition with multiple dietary, physiologic, anatomic, and psychosocial causes. Its manifestations vary from mild to incapacitating. Constipation is a subjective complaint that may reflect various diseases and mechanisms; the term encompasses infrequent defecation as well as difficulty with defecation.*

Although most patients are treated medically with success or improvement, some appear refractory to such maneuvers. Patients with constipation are rarely referred to the surgeon, and then usually only as a last resort. However, when patients *are* referred, advances in evaluation have helped to define the indications for surgery and the likelihood of success. The aim of this

---

*Editor's Note: Although there is overlap with other chapters, I have tried to give each author an opportunity to "state his case" in the management of these often uncomfortable and unhappy patients. Please read on because the discussion of classification, surgical treatment, and biofeedback for constipation is unique.

chapter is to examine current approaches to evacuation management in patients with severe chronic constipation. The chapters on constipation, constipation in children, and incontinence provide additional relevant information and some similar tables.

DEFINITIONS

It is important that treatment decisions be based on etiology. Causes of constipation may be labeled broadly as "extracolonic" (Table 1) or "colonic," the latter being divided into problems of colonic dysmotility or of disordered defecation (Table 2). Although such an extensive classification of extracolonic causes is intimidating, it is important to have it at hand. (There are some differences from the table in the chapter on constipation.)

"Colonic constipation" may be caused by structural (e.g., volvulus, stricture, megacolon) or functional abnormalities. Functional constipation refers to that which is chronic (lifelong), severe, and lifestyle altering, and that which is present in patients with a normal-sized colon. The major causes of such functionally significant chronic severe constipation in adults are either slow transit constipation, disordered defecation, or a combination of the two. An overall approach to patients with constipation is illustrated in Figure 1.

SELECTED CLINICAL FEATURES AND MANAGEMENT

Extracolonic constipation and structural disorders are discussed in the other chapters on constipation.

Idiopathic Megarectum and Megacolon

Idiopathic megarectum and megacolon are diagnosed by barium enema; if the lumen of the colon at the sacral promontory is 6 cm or more, a diagnosis of megacolon is substantiated. A lateral view of the pelvis must be performed to rule out a narrow distal segment of aganglionosis (which occurs in Hirschsprung's disease). Unlike Hirschsprung's disease, which occurs predominantly in men, the distribution of idiopathic megacolon is equal among the sexes and the colon has normal ganglia. The cause is controversial, but megabowel may be an acquired condition related to refusal to defecate during toilet training. There is also the possibility that some patients have a congenital abnormality.

Adult patients with idiopathic megacolon are divided into two main groups: those who develop symptoms in childhood, and those who present sporadically later in life with constipation and abdominal pain but no soiling. In addition to contrast enema evaluation, colon transit time and pelvic floor studies should be performed.

Patients with idiopathic megacolon who have prolonged colon transit time and normal pelvic floor

Table 1 Extracolonic Causes of Chronic Constipation

Faulty Diet and Habits
  Inadequate bulk (fiber)
  Excessive ingestion of foods that harden stools (e.g., cheese)
  Lack of exercise
  Ignoring the call to stool

Pharmacologic
  Analgesics
  Antacids
  Anticholinergics
  Anticonvulsants
  Antidepressants
  Antiparkinsonian agents
  Diuretics
  Ganglionic blockers
  Monoamine oxidase inhibitors
  Iron
  Laxative abuse
  Arsenic, lead, mercury, phosphorus poisoning
  Opiates
  Phenothiazines

Metabolic and Endocrine
  Amyloidosis
  Diabetes mellitus
  Hypothyroidism
  Hypercalcemia
  Hypokalemia
  Hyperparathyroidism
  Hypopituitarism
  Pheochromocytoma
  Pregnancy
  Porphyria
  Uremia

Psychiatric
  Depression
  Psychoses
  Anorexia nervosa

Neurologic
  Spinal
    Neoplasm
    Lumbosacral cord trauma
    Paraplegia
    Multiple sclerosis
    Tabes dorsalis
    Shy-Drager syndrome
    Meningocele
  Cerebral
    Neoplasm
    Parkinson's disease
    Stroke
  Iatrogenic
    Immobilization
    Resection of nervi erigentes
  Peripheral
    Ganglioneuromatosis (von Recklinghausen's disease)
    Autonomic neuropathy

function are candidates for surgical treatment if medical measures do not relieve the constipation. Optimal medical management consists of developing a regular habit of attempted defecation each day, regular and continuing use of laxatives (magnesium sulfate or lactulose), and sporadic use of enemas or suppositories. Surgical management consists of subtotal colectomy with ileorectal anastomosis; the rationale is that liquid stool will be expelled efficiently by normal pelvic floor motions. If a megarectum is present, however, the Duhamel operation is an appropriate alternative. If megabowel is present (megacolon plus megarectum) and the patient is young, ileoanal anastomosis is useful.

Table 2 Causes of Chronic Severe "Colonic" Constipation

Colonic motor disturbance
    Slow transit
    Constipation-predominant irritable bowel syndrome

Defecation dysfunction
    Anismus
    Descending perineum syndrome
    Hirschsprung's disease
    Disturbed rectal sensation
    Occult rectal prolapse
    Procidentia (complete prolapse)
    Rectocele

Colonic Constipation

Slow Transit Constipation

Patients with slow transit constipation (STC) are defined by the abnormally slow transit of radiopaque markers through the colon. In my practice, a transit time greater than 72 hours is consistent with STC. Patients with STC should subsequently undergo a pelvic floor evaluation to prove normal function, because difficulty with defecation may contribute to STC.

Several recent studies have reviewed the surgical management of severe chronic constipation. I evaluated 277 patients with long-standing intractable constipation. Patients underwent colonic transit studies, anorectal manometry, electromyography (EMG), scintigraphic balloon topography, scintigraphic evacuation, balloon expulsion, and defecography. The diagnostic tests categorized patients as having STC (n = 29), pelvic floor dysfunction (PFD) (n = 37), combined STC and PFD (n = 14), and normal transit constipation (NTC) (n = 197). Thus, even among a tertiary referral popula-

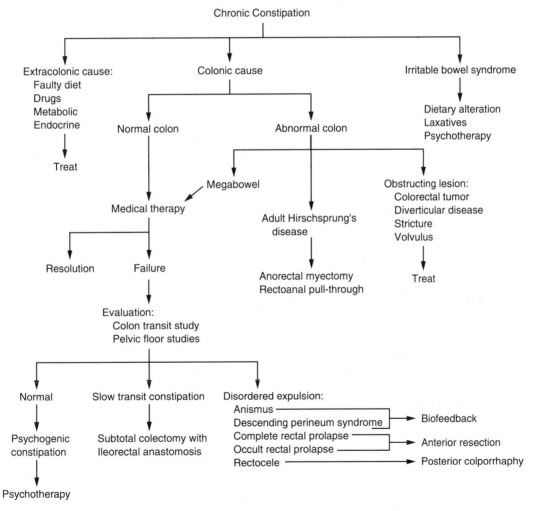

Figure 1 Algorithm for an approach to the patient with constipation.

tion of severely constipated patients, only 30 percent had a quantifiably definable abnormality of colonic or pelvic floor function. The patients with NTC received further symptomatic care; whether NTC is the same as, or a variant of, irritable bowel syndrome (IBS) is controversial. The patients with PFD underwent aggressive pelvic floor retraining with biofeedback. Abdominal colectomy with ileorectostomy was offered to patients with STC and to those with combined STC and PFD who successfully completed pelvic floor retraining initially. There was no operative mortality; 11 percent of patients developed small bowel obstruction. One patient with an ileosigmoidostomy (upon further evaluation) developed recurrent constipation and required revision to an ileorectal anastomosis. At a mean of 20 months' follow-up, the mean daily stool frequency was four, with no incontinence or need for laxatives or stool-bulking agents. These results confirm that an aggressive evaluation strategy identifies the small subset of patients with STC who may achieve prolonged relief from constipation after abdominal colectomy and ileorectal anastomosis. Table 3 compiles several series describing the results of surgery for constipation. The heterogeneous results reflect the heterogeneous nature of the patients operated on; patients in most of these series were not evaluated preoperatively with transit or pelvic floor studies.

Unfortunately, some patients develop a megarectum with impaired rectal sensation and recurrent severe constipation after ileorectostomy. For these patients, if aggressive medical therapy fails, proctocolectomy with permanent ileostomy or ileoanal anastomosis are the available surgical alternatives. Although the reported experience is limited, the results of proctocolectomy and ileoanal anastomosis for constipation have been encouraging.

Failure to Relieve Constipation. Failure to relieve constipation over time after ileorectal anastomosis is usually caused by unrecognized PFD or whole gut dysmotility (pseudo-obstruction of the small bowel). Whether small bowel manometry and/or scintigraphic gastric emptying and small bowel transit studies should be administered *routinely* preoperatively in patients considered for colectomy is controversial. In a patient complaining of postprandial nausea, bloating, belching, or upper abdominal distress, the threshold for performing small bowel manometry or scintigraphic transit studies should be low. Subtotal colectomy and ileorectal anastomosis may not, however, be contraindicated in some patients with whole gut pseudo-obstruction. In addition, such testing might better identify patients who may experience a poor result postoperatively.

It is clear from the results of surgery for STC that patient selection is key. Selection is improved by more clearly delineating subgroups of patients with "colonic" constipation and, to this end, objective tests of small bowel, colon, and pelvic floor function are mandatory.*

Normal Transit Constipation

Constipation-Predominant Irritable Bowel Syndrome. Unlike patients with STC, patients with NTC have relatively normal colon transit, periods of diarrhea alternating with constipation, an impressive degree of left lower quadrant pain, and diverticular and sigmoid muscular hypertrophy. The challenge in these patients is to identify them properly and thus not remove the colon; the results of surgery for NTC and IBS are nearly always unsatisfactory. Appropriate dietary habits and psychological management strategies are much more valuable.

Disordered Defecation

Pelvic Floor Dysfunction (Anismus)

The physiologic abnormality in this condition is failure of the striated muscles of the pelvic floor to relax upon straining to defecate. Failure of relaxation precludes descent of the pelvic floor and straightening of the anorectal angle. In some patients with anismus, not only does the puborectal muscle fail to relax, but it may actually increase its firing rate. Such paradoxical firing, however, sometimes occurs in healthy controls.

The clinical findings include inability to initiate defecation, incomplete evacuation, a history of manual disimpaction, laxative and enema abuse, leakage, rectal pain, and the assumption of contorted postures for defecation. On examination, patients often cannot push the perineum downward, and the puborectal muscle remains prominent posteriorly in the upper anal canal on digital examination. These patients may even contract the external anal sphincter and puborectal muscle against the examining finger while straining to defecate. Importantly, transit through the colon may be impaired in patients with anismus; sometimes (rarely), improvement in anismus leads to improved colon transit.

Surgical approaches to anismus have included partial division of the puborectal muscle and anorectal myectomy. These attempts nearly always fail and are not recommended for the management of patients with pelvic floor dysfunction. I prefer newer approaches aimed at retraining the muscles of the pelvic floor to relax during defecation straining.

Techniques of Pelvic Floor Retraining. Biofeedback is now a well-established (but still controversial) form of treatment for obstructed defecation, and several techniques have produced promising results. One is an ambulatory approach using a three microballoon system. Among 16 patients studied, seven could expel a 50 ml rectal balloon before biofeedback compared with nine patients afterward. After six weeks of training, nine of 16 patients no longer exhibited paradoxical sphincter contraction during defecation. At 12 months' follow-up, these nine patients had no symptomatic recurrence of outlet obstruction.

Another technique uses EMG recording of the external sphincter for pelvic retraining. Among 15 patients with anismus, after a mean of 3 weeks of outpatient training, 13 were able to expel a rectal balloon

Table 3 Results of Colectomy for Constipation

Author	No.	Operation Performed	Success (%)
Sunderland et al (1992)	18	Ileorectostomy	16 (89)
Pemberton et al (1991)	38	Ileorectostomy (IS-L)	36 (95)
Wexner et al (1991)	16	Ileorectostomy	15 (94)
Beck et al (1989)	14	Ileorectostomy	14 (100)
Yoshioka and Keighley (1989)	40	Ileorectostomy (34) Cecorectostomy (5) Ileosigmoidostomy (1)	23 (58)
Akervall et al (1988)	12	Ileorectostomy (12)	8 (67)
Kamm, Hawley, and Lennard-Jones (1988)	44	Cecorectostomy (11) Ileorectostomy (33)	22 (50)
Vasileusky et al (1988)	51	Ileosigmoidostomy (46) Ileorectostomy (5)	40 (78)
Leon, Krishnamurthy, and Schuffler (1987)	13	Ileorectostomy	10 (77)
Roe, Bartolo, and Mortenson (1986)	7	Ileorectostomy	5 (71)
Keighley and Shoulder (1984)	10	Ileorectostomy	9 (90)
Preston et al (1984)	16	Ileorectostomy (8) Cecorectostomy (8)	14 (88)
Belliveau (1982)	29	Ileosigmoidostomy (20) Ileorectostomy (9)	15 (75) 7 (78)
Lane and Todd (1977)	14	Cecorectostomy (5) Ileorectostomy (3) Left hemicolectomy (2) Ileosigmoidostomy (1) Sigmoid colostomy (3)	4 (80) 1 (33) 1 (50) 1 (100) 1 (33)

compared with two patients before biofeedback. Biofeedback also led to less perianal pain at defecation, less difficulty with defecation, and reduced time spent straining at stool. Stool frequency also increased from a mean of five per week to seven per week. The clinical improvement was not associated with anorectal manometric changes, but defecography in six patients showed less paradoxical sphincter contraction during straining.

Another series of 18 patients with paradoxical puborectal contraction and chronic constipation used an EMG-based biofeedback training program. Mean stool frequency increased from 4.6 laxative-induced evacuations per week to 7.3 spontaneous evacuations per week following biofeedback.

Other series using surface EMG and behavioral relaxation techniques for retraining pelvic floor muscles confirm these results. Of nine patients with constipation from pelvic floor obstruction, all experienced reestablishment of normal defecation after treatment, although three required repeat training episodes. Similarly, 13 of 15 patients with paradoxical external sphincter contraction improved after using anal EMG probes. Interestingly, in several studies, EMG and manometric findings consistent with paradoxical sphincter contraction resolved in most patients.

I have used pelvic floor retraining in ten patients with PFD; seven successfully achieved spontaneous bowel movements. One patient failed because of psychological problems and the other two failed because there was accompanying STC. Pelvic floor retraining at Mayo Clinic is a multimodality approach aimed at teaching patients to defecate effectively. Dietary ma-

nipulation, stool bulkers, biofeedback techniques using an anal electrode, balloon pull-through, and defecation simulation are all employed. Finally, psychological counseling is usually indicated and is quite helpful.

Patients with abnormal colonic transit *and* disordered expulsion have a combined disorder. If no anatomic defect is found, pelvic floor retraining with biofeedback techniques is indicated primarily. If retraining is successful and the patient can be taught to evacuate efficiently, the colon transit study is repeated. In a few patients, transit returns to normal. In others, transit remains prolonged; in such patients, colectomy and ileorectal anastomosis may be indicated if symptoms are disabling. Pelvic floor retraining thus appears to be a useful treatment for patients with obstructed defecation, but only comparative trials will show which technique is best.

Hirschsprung's Disease

Congenital aganglionosis is an extremely rare cause of *adult constipation*. Nonetheless, it does occur and should be suspected when symptoms have been present since birth and barium enema shows a widened rectal vault above the level of the anorectal ring. Absence of the rectoanal inhibitory response and ganglion cells confirm the diagnosis. The biggest problem in diagnosing Hirschsprung's disease definitively is the wide variation in the density of ganglion cells at the level of the anorectal junction in perfectly healthy people.

Once the condition is diagnosed, surgery is indicated. The surgical goal is to bypass or excise completely the aganglionic segment. The Swenson, Duhamel, and Soave operations have been devised for this purpose.

Rectocele

Patients with functionally significant rectoceles on defecating proctography undergo operative repairs only after medical options have been exhausted. A functionally significant rectocele is one that fills preferentially during defecating proctography. Rectoceles within 7 to 8 cm of the sphincter (low) are best treated by transanal repair. Midlevel rectoceles are best treated with obliterative sutures. Patients who have high rectoceles should be repaired transvaginally via a posterior colporrhaphy, because a rectal approach provides inadequate exposure.

Descending Perineum Syndrome

The cause of profound perineal descent is probably injury of the sacral nerves and/or pudendal nerves and damage to the pelvic floor and external anal sphincter muscles during childbirth, and/or chronic straining at stool. An abnormal degree of perineal descent occurs in a high percentage of patients with constipation and chronic straining at stool; conversely, most patients with perineal descent give a history of excessive straining to achieve a bowel movement. Fecal incontinence may occur later in the natural history of perineal descent. At my institution, patients with profound perineal descent and obstructed defecation undergo pelvic floor retraining with, frankly, fair to poor results. If perineal descent occurs with occult intussusception, anterior resection may cure the prolapse, but the perineal descent, with its symptoms, invariably persists.

Rectal Prolapse

Anterior mucosal prolapse, internal rectal intussusception, solitary rectal ulcer syndrome, and abnormal perineal descent are frequently seen in patients with obstructed defecation. Patients presenting with anterior mucosal prolapse and perineal descent have a 30 percent chance of becoming incontinent over the subsequent 5 years and a 20 percent risk of developing complete rectal prolapse. A high proportion of patients with complete rectal prolapse suffer from chronic constipation, but a role for this symptom in the genesis of rectal prolapse has not been established convincingly. Moreover, a cause-and-effect relationship between pelvic floor weakness and rectal prolapse has never been proved.

It seems likely that without repair of a rectal prolapse, incontinence will develop, as repeated traction on the pudendal nerves during prolapse and descent of the perineum leads to permanent neurapraxia. Repeated dilatation of the anus by the intussusceptum also damages the anal sphincter muscles. Complete rectal prolapse is the condition for which operative treatment is most clearly indicated. Two approaches give satisfactory results.

In frail or debilitated patients, a perineal approach results in fewer systemic complications, while still having an acceptable chance of success. The procedures of Delorme and Altemeier both yield reasonable results.

Most patients are best served by an abdominal approach, whereby the rectum is completely mobilized and either resected or fixed to the sacrum. Performance of a concurrent sigmoid resection is controversial, but is advised if the anastomosis is performed in the peritonealized portion of the completely mobilized rectum. Sigmoid resection enhances fixation and reduces the frequency of postoperative constipation.

Approximately half of the 50 percent of patients with full-thickness rectal prolapse who are incontinent preoperatively continue to be so postoperatively. It remains an unfortunate fact that not one of the procedures used for treating rectal prolapse deals with any of the potential underlying factors; indeed, constipation is a common preoperative symptom that often becomes more frequent after rectopexy. This is probably the reason that rectopexy alone fails to alleviate the symptoms of obstructed defecation associated with occult rectal prolapse.

The management of occult rectal prolapse remains a challenging problem. Bowel retraining, with avoidance of straining, and biofeedback techniques have been used with some success in some patients. Bulk laxatives are unhelpful. The role of surgical procedures is controversial and we do not operate on such patients.

COMMENTS

Because our understanding of constipation is imperfect, treatment rationales are likewise imperfect. Conservative nonsurgical measures are indicated for the great majority of patients with constipation. There is little doubt, however, that more aggressive measures are indicated in a distinct and increasingly definable minority of such patients. Importantly, rational management strategies depend upon classifying patients objectively. Clearly, advances in the management of constipation will be made only by classifying, treating, and then following patients closely over time.

SUGGESTED READING

Bartolo DC. Pelvic floor disorders: incontinence, constipation, and obstructed defecation. In: Schrock TR, ed. Perspectives in colon and rectal surgery. St. Louis: Quality Medical Publishing, 1988:1.

Duthie GS, Bartolo DCC. Abdominal rectopexy for rectal prolapse: a comparison of techniques. Br J Surg 1992; 79:107–113.

Fleshman JW, Dreznik Z, Meyer K, et al. Outpatient protocol for biofeedback therapy of pelvic floor outlet obstruction. Dis Colon Rectum 1992; 35:1–7.

Pemberton JH, Rath DM, Ilstrup DM. Evaluation and surgical management of severe chronic constipation. Ann Surg 1991; 214:403–413.

Phillips SF, Pemberton JH. Megacolon: congenital and acquired. In: Sleisenger MH, Fordtran JS, eds. Gastrointestinal disease. Philadelphia: WB Saunders, 1993:888–897.

Read NW, Timms JW, Barfield LJ, et al. Impairment of defecation in young women with severe constipation. Gastroenterology 1986; 90:53.

Schlinkert RT, Beart RW Jr, Wolff BG, Pemberton JH. Anterior resection for complete rectal prolapse. Dis Colon Rectum 1985; 28:409–412.

Turnball GK, Ritvo PG. Anal sphincter biofeedback relaxation treatment for women with intractable constipation syndrome. Dis Colon Rectum 1992; 35:530–536.

Wexner SD, Daniel N, Jagelman DG. Colectomy for constipation: physiologic investigation is the key to success. Dis Colon Rectum 1991; 34:851–856.

HERNIA

J. LAWRENCE FITZPATRICK, M.D.
ANTHONY L. IMBEMBO, M.D.

A hernia develops secondary to a weakness in an investing musculofascial layer with resultant protrusion of normally contained contents through that point of weakness. The abdomen is the most common site for hernia development due to the generation of positive intra-abdominal pressure. Two factors contribute to the formation of a hernia. Any condition causing a chronic increase in intra-abdominal pressure may be contributory. Examples include obstructing lesions of the genitourinary or gastrointestinal tract, obesity, ascites, chronic peritoneal dialysis, pregnancy, or chronic cough. The second requisite for hernia formation is weakness in the investing layer. Points of relative weakness usually occur either at the edge of a fascial or muscular band, or at a point of penetration of the abdominal wall by structures such as the spermatic cord or femoral vessels. The essential component of any hernia repair is restoration of the integrity of the investing layer. When possible, treatable causes of increased intra-abdominal pressure should be addressed as well, in order to decrease the risk of recurrence.

Untreated hernias almost invariably enlarge. This is usually due to gradual attenuation of the surrounding fascia along with actual enlargement of the defect. As a result, an increasingly greater volume of intra-abdominal contents can protrude through the defect. This presents two problems. The fascial edges become weaker and separate further so that attempts at primary closure become increasingly difficult. Secondly, in some cases, the volume of the peritoneal cavity decreases as visceral herniation increases. This may be associated with loss of abdominal domain, thereby precluding successful reduction.

The entrapment of abdominal viscera within a hernia sac constitutes incarceration. When this involves omentum or preperitoneal fat alone, the symptoms are those of pain and local irritation. However, incarceration of intestine usually results in nausea, vomiting, abdominal distention, and obstruction. An incarcerated hernia is initially managed with attempted manual reduction. Gentle pressure is applied after the patient has been moderately sedated. If manual reduction is unsuccessful, emergent surgical exploration, reduction, and repair are indicated. Incarceration is more likely to occur with herniation through a small fascial defect. Manual reduction should be attempted only when it is certain that strangulation has not occurred.

Strangulation occurs when the blood supply to the hernia contents is compromised, usually by the fascial ring. Venous compromise is more common than arterial obstruction. Impaired perfusion may ultimately lead to ischemic necrosis, or perforation, developments which markedly increase overall morbidity and mortality. Usually, compromised bowel may be explored and resected through the fascial hernia defect; however, formal laparotomy is required in some patients. Strangulation should be suggested by increasing tenderness over an irreducible mass, nausea, vomiting, fever, leukocytosis, or radiologic studies consistent with bowel obstruction. The ultimate goal is to repair hernias electively, thereby precluding the potential for incarceration and strangulation.

DIAPHRAGMATIC HERNIA

Paraesophageal Hernia

The most common paraphrenic hernia is the sliding hiatus hernia. Unlike almost all other hernias, this lesion does not incarcerate. Sliding hiatus hernia is of concern only because of its frequent association with gastroesophageal reflux and its complications. In contrast, surgical correction is almost always indicated for a paraesophageal hernia. With a true paraesophageal hernia, the anatomic gastroesophageal junction is located in its normal position, 5 to 6 cm below the diaphragm. Instead, the stomach flips or turns in such a way that the greater curvature slips into the mediastinum adjacent to the esophagus through the abnormally widened esophageal hiatus. On occasion, a paraesophageal hernia has a sliding component, as well. Paraesophageal hernia may cause a variety of clinical problems. The mucosa within the herniated stomach may exhibit venous congestion or frank ulceration with resultant gastrointestinal bleeding. Dysphagia secondary to esophageal compression or dyspnea due to pulmonary compromise may both occur. Many patients experience severe pain after meals due to distention of the herniated stomach. The most feared problem, however, is incarceration and strangulation. Perforation may then follow, either in the abdomen or the mediastinum. This catastrophic occurrence is associated with a high mortality rate and significant reconstructive problems.

Repair of a paraesophageal hernia usually is accomplished via an abdominal approach. The stomach is reduced into the abdomen and the diaphragmatic crura narrowed posterior to the esophagus to prevent recurrence. The stomach is usually sutured to the undersurface of the diaphragm, as well. If there is an associated sliding component, an anti-reflux procedure may be added, usually a Nissen fundoplication. A gastrostomy may help to fix the stomach to the anterior abdominal wall, thereby reducing the low recurrence rate still further.

There is a separate chapter on antireflux surgery.

Congenital Diaphragmatic Hernia

Bochdalek and Morgagni hernias are congenital diaphragmatic hernias, usually diagnosed in infancy but occasionally identified later in life.

The foramen of Bochdalek hernia is due to incomplete fusion of the pleuroperitoneal fold with the developing body wall (anteromedial anlage). The defect is usually located far laterally on the left, but occasionally involves the right hemidiaphragm. As a result, there is in utero herniation of abdominal viscera into the developing thoracic cavity. When this occurs on the left, the stomach, spleen, splenic flexure, and small bowel may all herniate. On the right, the liver mass usually obstructs some of the defect, resulting in a lesser degree of herniation. This hernia usually presents in the immediate neonatal period. The infant has a scaphoid abdomen and abdominal viscera are present in the left chest. It is the severe respiratory distress of these infants which prompts evaluation. Urgent or emergent repair is required, usually performed through the abdomen. The diaphragmatic hernia is usually repairable by unfolding the diaphragm and attaching it to the chest wall. Occasionally, prosthetic material is necessary. The most important determinant of infant survival is the developmental status of the left lung with its potential for persistent fetal circulation causing respiratory failure. Delayed diagnosis results when respiratory distress is not present at birth. The child may feed poorly or evidence intermittent gastrointestinal obstruction. Decreased breath sounds in the left chest may be noted and the diagnosis should be confirmed by radiologic study. Elective repair is indicated. Due to their stable respiratory status, these children generally do quite well.

The other congenital diaphragmatic hernia occurs through the foramen of Morgagni. This defect is located in the midportion of the diaphragm anteriorly. Failure of the developing diaphragm to fuse with the fascia arising from the posterior sternum is responsible. The defect may remain asymptomatic due to obstruction by the subjacent left lobe of the liver. Evaluation is prompted by symptoms of obstruction or poor feeding. Radiologic studies show herniated abdominal viscera in the lower

anterior mediastinum. Hernia contents may include a segment of small bowel, transverse colon, or omentum. Repair is accomplished using an abdominal approach. The prognosis is good and recurrence is rare.

ABDOMINAL WALL HERNIA

The investing musculofascial layers of the abdominal cavity comprise a barrel-like support system. These layers slide upon each other, often in a scissor-like fashion, thereby enhancing overall strength. Points of relative weakness occur wherever the supporting structure is penetrated, such as at the deep inguinal ring by the spermatic cord. Relative weakness is also present at points of attachment and at the limits of the fascial expanse. It is at these various locations that hernias typically occur.

Umbilical Hernia

Umbilical hernia can present at any age. In infants, umbilical hernias occur because of failure of the midline abdominal fascia to fuse completely at the umbilicus. At the end of the first trimester, the exteriorized mid-gut returns to the abdominal cavity, but the umbilical arteries and vein, as well as the urachus continue to traverse the abdominal wall at this site. This results in a point of relative weakness at the superior aspect of the umbilicus. Umbilical hernias occur in as many as 10 percent of African-American children, but to a much lesser extent in white infants. The resulting bulge varies in size and is most apparent when the child is crying or straining at stool.

Unlike most other hernias, the mere presence of an umbilical hernia does not mandate surgical repair. Approximately 90 percent of these defects will obliterate spontaneously, usually by the second year of age. Spontaneous resolution is most apt to occur if the defect is less than 1 cm in diameter. Any hernia whose contents are incarcerated must be repaired; however, this is rarely a problem in infants. If the hernia persists after 2 years of age, particularly if it is enlarging or the fascial defect is greater than 1 to 1.5 cm in size, it is not reasonable to expect spontaneous closure. Repair should be performed before the child reaches school age. An infraumbilical incision is used with the child under general anesthesia. The usual technique consists of transverse closure of the fascia. Results are usually excellent with little cosmetic deformity.

In adults, umbilical hernias comprise a different spectrum of disease. The hernia usually develops as a consequence of increased intra-abdominal pressure, most commonly due to pregnancy, ascites, or obesity. Commonly, the adult umbilical hernia contains only omentum or preperitoneal fat. However, abdominal viscera can herniate making incarceration and strangulation possible. For this reason, and the likelihood of continued enlargement, umbilical hernias in adults are almost always repaired. The approach is similar to that used for infants. However, repair of a chronic defect may be more complicated due to attenuation of the surrounding fascia. As a result, prosthetic reinforcement of the repair may be necessary.

The presence of an umbilical hernia in a patient with ascites presents special problems. There is a significant possibility of erosion of the attenuated skin overlying the defect. Such erosion may result in evisceration and/or peritonitis. Every effort should be made to control the ascites. This will facilitate subsequent repair and decrease the risk of recurrence. Mortality rates of up to 20 percent have been reported for emergency repair of a ruptured umbilical hernia in a patient with ascites due to cirrhosis.

Epigastric Hernia

Epigastric hernias occur through the linea alba anywhere between the xiphoid and the umbilicus. The fibers of the linea alba decussate in an oblique manner making for points of relative weakness. It is preperitoneal fat or omentum which usually protrudes through the defect. These defects are typically small and may be multiple. Symptoms are usually noted in the fourth or fifth decade. Findings consists of small reducible bulges, often with localized pain and tenderness. Incarceration is unusual. The defects may be difficult to appreciate and, in some instances, are only identified at local exploration for evaluation of chronic pain. In a patient with persistent superficial epigastric pain and an otherwise negative evaluation, epigastric hernia must be considered. These hernias should be repaired under general anesthesia. The entire linea alba should be opened vertically so that multiple defects can be repaired simultaneously. Otherwise, a recurrence rate as high as 10 percent may be expected due to failure to identify all defects.

A separate, but related problem is rectus diastasis, a diffuse widening of the linea alba. The normal width of the linea alba varies from 2 to 3 mm to 2 cm. When the linea alba is so widened that there is a protrusion through it, diastasis is present. Since this is a generalized attenuation rather than a well-defined defect, diastasis is not associated with symptoms or risk of incarceration. Repair usually is not required and when performed is done primarily for cosmetic reasons.

Incisional Hernia

The terms ventral and incisional hernia are used interchangeably to refer to a defect in a previous abdominal wound. These most often occur in laparotomy incisions, but may also develop at drain sites or stab wounds. These hernias are, by definition, of the acquired type. Their formation is usually due to a combination of factors including both technical problems of wound closure and underlying conditions which compromise wound healing, such as advanced age, malnutrition, ascites or underlying malignancy. Chronic elevation of intra-abdominal pressure may also contribute to inci-

sional hernia formation. Significant elevation of intra-abdominal pressure may occur secondary to obesity, chronic obstructive pulmonary disease with cough, or obstructive uropathy. A wound infection at the fascial level significantly impairs healing diminishing the long-term strength of the fascial closure. Diabetes and corticosteroid therapy both predispose to incisional hernia formation. Technical errors include improper placement of sutures, apposition of inadequate attenuated fascia, or closure of fascia under tension.

In the immediate postoperative period, fascial dehiscence is heralded by leakage of serosanguinous intraperitoneal fluid from the wound. Evisceration may follow in some cases. Immediate repair, if permitted by the patient's condition, is indicated to prevent evisceration. More commonly, incisional hernia appears much later as a progressively enlarging bulge within a previous incision. Symptoms may include local pain or an irreducible mass. Small defects are more likely to result in incarceration and strangulation. In general, these hernias should be repaired to prevent the latter complications and because progressive enlargement only increases the difficulty of repair. In extreme cases, very large hernia sacs may be associated with loss of abdominal domain for the herniated viscera. Correction is usually accomplished under general anesthesia. When the defect is small, repair with native tissue is almost always possible. With a large defect due to complete breakdown of the wound or chronic attenuation of the fascia, prosthetic material may be needed to bridge the defect. Depending on the size of the defect and the type of repair required, recurrence rates may be high, reflecting, in a large part, the underlying problems which contributed to hernia formation initially. In patients who are not considered to be reasonable candidates for repair, use of supportive binders may produce symptomatic improvement.

Incisional hernias most often develop in mid-line incisions. It is generally felt that transverse abdominal incisions are under less tension, therefore resulting in a lesser incidence of hernia formation.

Lumbar Hernia

These rare hernias are of two distinct types. The superior lumbar hernia begins at the tip of the twelfth rib at the point where the neurovascular bundle penetrates the fascia, thereby producing a site of potential weakness. The inferior lumbar hernia occurs superior to the iliac crest, just anterior to the paravertebral muscles. It is not clear whether lumbar hernias are due to progression of a congenital weakness or to attenuation of normal fascia in response to progressive increase in intra-abdominal pressure. Lumbar hernias may manifest as vague discomfort or progressive swelling. In the evaluation of lumbar hernia, a renal cause for pain must be ruled out. These hernias rarely cause gastrointestinal symptoms, but may become quite large over time, particularly in obese patients.

Asymptomatic lumbar hernias do not require repair,

as there is no risk of incarceration or strangulation. This is fortunate because repair often presents a major technical challenge. The fascia inferior and posterior to either defect is well-anchored and cannot be advanced readily. As a result, any repair is under significant tension. Prosthetic material or complex rotation of adjacent fascia is required for all but the smallest lumbar hernias. Recurrence rates may be as high as 5 percent.

Spigelian Hernia

The Spigelian hernia is probably discussed far more often than it is encountered. It is a small defect occurring in the semilunar line, just outside the lateral margin of the rectus sheath. The semilunar line is an aponeurotic strip extending from the ninth costal cartilage to the pelvis. The Spigelian hernia develops at the point where the inferior epigastric vessels penetrate this structure, thereby creating a fascial defect. This hernia is usually located a few centimeters inferior and lateral to the umbilicus. Spigelian hernia can occur in all age groups, but most frequently is seen in the young active population. It may present after strenuous exercise. The initial manifestation is often very localized, severe pain, without an apparent cause. The defect is quite small with only a minimal hernia sac, which may be contained within the muscular layer (intramural). While ultrasound and computed tomography (CT) have been proposed for diagnosis, they are rarely helpful. A high index of suspicion is essential for diagnosis. Once other causes of intra-abdominal or abdominal wall pain have been ruled out, persistent symptoms mandate local exploration. The incision is made over the point of tenderness. Repair consists of reduction of the hernia sac and ligation of the inferior epigastric vessels at the point where they penetrate the fascia. The fascial defect can be closed primarily in almost all instances. Long-term results are excellent.

Obturator Hernia

This rare hernia typically causes small bowel obstruction. It occurs in the obturator space where the neurovascular bundle pierces the pelvic fascia. The space is bounded by the pubic ramus superiorly and the ligamentous attachments of the obturator muscles posteriorly and laterally. A taut unyielding defect results. Should a loop of bowel manage to traverse this fibrous opening, there is a high likelihood of incarceration and strangulation. Obturator hernias occur much more frequently in women, with a ratio of 6:1. They are commonly encountered in middle-aged women after multiple pregnancies, suggesting that progressive relaxation of the pelvic fascia may contribute to formation of the defect.

Clinical examination rarely suggests an obturator hernia. Small bowel obstruction is the usual presentation. On occasion, the hernia may cause pressure on the obturator nerve resulting in pain along the medial aspect of the thigh. This pain may be intensified by extension of the hip and improved by flexion (Howship-Romberg

sign). There may also be sensory deficits in the anterior and medial thigh. A CT scan may demonstrate the hernia. If this diagnosis is suspected, urgent laparotomy is required to prevent strangulation. Quite often the diagnosis of obturator hernia is made only at the time of laparotomy performed for bowel obstruction of uncertain etiology. Once identified at laparotomy, the hernia contents are reduced and bowel resection performed, if indicated. The hernia sac is excised and the defect approximated with simple sutures. Due to the tendinous nature of the defect, tension on the repair is not unusual. Prosthetic material may be used to reinforce the repair as long as there is no bowel compromise. In the presence of contamination, a rotational flap consisting of fascia or peritoneum may be employed to cover the defect. Due to the associated bowel obstruction and strangulation, morbidity and mortality rates of obturator hernia approach 10 percent. While perineal and inguinal approaches have been described, the transabdominal approach seems to be the best option.

GROIN HERNIAS

Femoral Hernia

A femoral hernia results from attenuation of the transversalis fascia surrounding the femoral canal. This defect is located medial to the femoral vein and may be identified clinically as a bulge presenting just beneath the inguinal ligament. The incidence of femoral hernia is much higher in older women than in either males or nulliparous females. This suggests that stretching and relaxation of the fascia is responsible for the eventual formation of the hernia defect.

Due to the high incidence of associated incarceration or strangulation, femoral hernias should be repaired upon identification. Particularly in obese patients, the femoral hernia may be identified only at the time of laparotomy for small bowel obstruction. As for the obturator hernia, the hernia contents are then reduced and the fascial defect closed transabdominally. When diagnosed pre-operatively, even in the face of incarceration, the defect is exposed using a preperitoneal inguinal approach. The sac can usually be reduced by this means. Repair of the defect consists of reinforcement of the posterior inguinal wall with obliteration of the femoral canal medial to the vessels. This is usually accomplished with native fascia. However, particularly in the older woman with markedly attenuated fascia, the use of prosthetic material to either plug the femoral defect or reconstruct the posterior inguinal wall is helpful.

Indirect Inguinal Hernia

This hernia is felt to be a congenital defect secondary to the incomplete obliteration of the processus vaginalis during fetal development. By definition, an indirect inguinal hernia arises lateral to the inferior epigastric vessels and presents through the deep inguinal ring. Since the right testicle descends later than the left, the indirect hernia is more frequent in infants on the right. There is a 10 to 30 percent incidence of bilaterality in infant males, supporting the concept of bilateral inguinal exploration at the time of repair, particularly if the visible hernia is on the left. The indirect inguinal hernia usually presents with a visible bulge, frequently extending into the scrotum. Identification of the hernia is an indication for repair, as incarcerated hernia is the leading cause of bowel obstruction in infants and young children.

In infants and young children, the initial step in repair is isolation of the spermatic cord or round ligament. The hernia sac is freed from the cord to the level of the deep inguinal ring where the contents are reduced and the sac ligated. In females the round ligament is excised, allowing for complete closure of the deep inguinal ring. In males, several sutures may be required to tighten the ring around the spermatic cord. Care must be taken to not compromise the arterial supply or venous drainage of the testicle.

In adults, the basic pathophysiology of indirect inguinal hernia is the same. However, the deep inguinal ring is often enlarged significantly, and, in fact, may extend medially to involve much of the inguinal floor. Therefore, after reduction and closure of the sac, the integrity of the posterior wall of the inguinal canal must be assessed. If the floor is attenuated, fascial reinforcement is indicated. Long-term results are good with accepted recurrence rates being less than 5 percent. Recurrences are most often due to failure to recognize a direct or femoral component, or to inadequate closure of the deep inguinal ring.

Direct Inguinal Hernia

This hernia is due to attenuation of the inguinal floor medial to the inferior epigastric vessels. It is felt to be an acquired defect and is usually seen in older individuals. Repair involves reduction of the hernia contents and reconstruction of the posterior inguinal floor. In many instances this may be accomplished by rotation of substantial adjacent fascia. However, this can result in a repair under tension. A relaxing incision in the anterior rectus sheath may facilitate rotation. When native tissue is markedly attenuated, as is often the case with large hernias, prosthetic material may be necessary for successful repair. Long-term recurrence rates for direct inguinal hernia repair are as high as 25 percent.

TECHNICAL INNOVATIONS

The surgical approach to repair of most hernias has remained constant for many years. However, the last decade has seen increasing acceptance of prosthetic materials for repair. These are used to accomplish a "tension free" repair by bridging the fascial defect, generally resulting in less postoperative discomfort. Decreased tension is thought to result in lower recurrence rates. The placement of prosthetic material usually prolongs the procedure, however. In addition, its use may increase the risk of infection, a complication which necessitates mesh removal and almost certain hernia recurrence. In general, there appears to be a trend towards more liberal use of prosthetic material for primary repair, as well as much more frequent use for repair of recurrences. In the latter instance, the native fascia may be much less mobile than normal due to previous scarring.

Laparoscopic Herniorrhaphy

The explosion of laparoscopic-assisted surgery within the past several years has spawned new approaches to inguinal and femoral hernia repair. The approach is not readily applicable to upper or central abdominal wall defects because of their size and difficulty with exposure. Laparoscopic repair is a technique in evolution and results need to be evaluated carefully over the next several years, especially as techniques are refined further. An earlier chapter, *Laparoscopic Surgical Procedures: Present and Future*, presents additional useful information.

Laparoscopic-assisted repair approaches the site of weakness transabdominally. A patch of prosthetic material is laparoscopically placed to cover the defect from within. Therefore, a proposed advantage of the laparoscopic approach is creation of a tension-free repair. There is certainly less postoperative pain and earlier return to normal activity is standard, often in 10 days. Bilateral hernias may be repaired through the same small incisions. Among the potential disadvantages of laparoscopic-assisted repair is the need for general anesthesia. Conventional repair can be done under local anesthesia with or without supplemental sedation. Laparoscopy also requires entry into the peritoneal cavity with potential for bowel injury and subsequent adhesion formation.

The approach continues to evolve, progressing from an initial prosthetic plug technique, to intraperitoneal dissection, and most recently to a preperitoneal approach. There is still a significant learning curve with this approach, as for all laparoscopic procedures. Finally, and perhaps most importantly, the long-term durability of these repairs has not been established. Most early reports provide, at most, 2 year follow-up. Recent reports suggest recurrence rates of less than 5 percent for primary mesh repairs utilizing conventional techniques. This is the standard against which laparoscopic repair will have to be compared. The final verdict requires much longer follow-up and systematic evaluation before the precise role for laparoscopic-assisted hernia repair can be defined.

SUGGESTED READING

Madden JL. Abdominal Wall Hernias: An Atlas of Anatomy and Repair. Philadelphia: WB Saunders, 1989.
Nyhus LM and Condon RE, eds. Hernia. 3rd ed. Philadelphia: JB Lippincott, 1989.
Skandalakis JE, Gray SW, Mansberger AR Jr, et al. Hernia: Surgical Anatomy and Technique. New York: McGraw-Hill, 1989.

LEFT-SIDED ULCERATIVE COLITIS AND ULCERATIVE PROCTITIS

PHILIP B. MINER, Jr., M.D.

Patients with left-sided ulcerative colitis or ulcerative proctitis represent a significant proportion of those seen with inflammatory bowel disease (IBD). Seventy percent of patients with ulcerative colitis have disease limited to the left side. The advent of flexible sigmoidoscopy has (1) allowed us to identify this group more efficiently, (2) improved our understanding of the natural history, and (3) permitted us to evaluate the efficacy of new modes of therapy, including topical medications. Complementing these basic diagnostic understandings, recent analysis of the anorectal physiology of IBD has improved our ability to manage and treat this often frustrating disease. One of the most important symptoms in patients who have left-sided ulcerative colitis is tenesmus (spasm of the rectum related to inflammation in the distal colon). The traditional approach to tenesmus is to decrease rectal inflammation. Improved understanding of anorectal physiology allows intervention in other important ways. The unique metabolic regulation of the left colon dependent on short-chain fatty acids, a chief energy source for colonocytes of the left colon, may explain the value of short-chain fatty acids in treating distal colitis. As we become more familiar with the physiology of inflammation, the nutrient requirements of the left colon compared with the right colon, and the characteristics of the distal colon that cause symptoms of diarrhea, we will have new tools with which to treat these diseases.

BASIC CONCEPTS

Easy access to office-based flexible sigmoidoscopy by the family practitioner or internist has made the diagnosis of left-sided ulcerative colitis far easier. In a patient presenting with bloody diarrhea of more than 2 weeks' duration associated with symptoms of tenesmus and bloody, mucoid stools, the clinician should perform flexible sigmoidoscopy. If possible, the flexible sigmoidoscope should be passed beyond the line of demarcation of the disease in order to evaluate the extent of mucosal inflammation and the inflammatory characteristics of the mucosa such as edema, erythema, granularity, and ulceration. The pattern of inflammation with areas spared of disease may suggest either a disease of infectious origin or perhaps Crohn's disease. Biopsies are useful at the line of demarcation, in the area of active disease, and above the line of demarcation of disease, but for practical purposes the extent of disease should be determined by visual recognition and not microscopic changes.

In patients with left-sided ulcerative colitis or ulcerative proctitis, the apparent paradox of diarrhea as well as constipation often occurs. This is due to the disturbed anorectal physiology that occurs with inflammation of the distal colon. In left-sided ulcerative colitis or ulcerative proctitis, the rectal tone is increased and the rectum is far more sensitive to volume distention. These changes are present even in the absence of active inflammation. Rectal reactivity and spasm induce diarrhea while impairing proximal colonic motility. This arrested stool movement permits desiccation of stool with the failure of delivery of stool into the inflamed rectum. An understanding of this concept is important for management of patients, as avoiding constipation is a critical issue in left-sided ulcerative colitis. The frequent observation that symptoms of irritable bowel syndrome (IBS) occur in conjunction with inflammatory disease may be linked to the high number of mast cells at the line of demarcation and in the proximal mucosa in left-sided disease. It has been shown that 70 percent of patients with IBS have increased numbers of mucosal mast cells, and 60 percent of those with IBD have increased mast cells at the line of demarcation of the disease. Increased mucosal mast cells may explain the symptoms of abdominal pain, urgency, and occasional incontinence associated with anorectal dysfunction.

In a separate study of patients with increased gastrointestinal mast cells, we demonstrated similar rectal reactivity to low volume balloon distention with increased rectal tone to the changes in ulcerative colitis patients. This observation is practical with regard to management, as antihistamines often modulate the spasm and reactivity in the rectum and can be used as adjunctive therapy for managing symptoms in patients with left-sided ulcerative colitis. The strategy of using antihistamines for retention of enemas or decreasing the feeling of tenesmus has been useful in patients with active distal inflammation. It is also important to avoid using antimotility agents, which may increase the level of constipation in patients with limited ulcerative colitis. Occasionally, stool softeners are required to make sure that hard stool located above the area of inflammation does not complicate the illness. Dietary intake of sugars can have important ramifications in these patients, since disaccharide malabsorption can lead to an increase in abdominal pain and gas. Avoidance of simple sugars, including lactose, is a useful dietary adjunct for improving symptoms.*

---

*Editor's Note: Since short-chain fatty acids, a preferred nutrient for the left colonocytes, are derived from unabsorbed carbohydrates, perhaps we will want to feed some well-tolerated, poorly absorbed carbohydrates.

SPECIFIC TREATMENT FOR COLONIC INFLAMMATION

Sulfasalazine

Traditional treatment of IBD with sulfasalazine remains an important part of the management of left-sided ulcerative colitis and ulcerative proctitis. This inexpensive and effective drug continues to be useful in long-term management despite the emergence of new mesalamine derivatives. Sulfasalazine has a long history of safety and efficacy, although there is a significant complication rate, with headaches and nausea in approximately 20 percent of patients. In the mid-1970s, studies were conducted to distinguish between the effects of sulfapyridine and those of 5-aminosalicylic acid (5-ASA) (mesalamine); it was determined that mesalamine was effective when given in the form of enemas for left-sided disease. This has led to the emergence of numerous new mesalamine formulations; it is emphasized that although many new such formulations are available, sulfasalazine was the first mesalamine-based compound. It can be used in many patients as the only drug, or can modify the cost of the new mesalamine drugs by being used in conjunction with the newer agents to decrease the total cost of management. A bacterial azoreductase breaks the bond in sulfasalazine between sulfapyridine and 5-aminosalicylate.

New Salicylates

Local Therapy (Table 1)

The efficacy of mesalamine was first demonstrated via direct application of mesalamine by enemas in patients with left-sided ulcerative colitis. Mesalamine enemas (Rowasa) proved more effective than glucocorticoid enemas in managing not only symptoms but also endoscopic and histologic appearance. The formulation of effective mesalamine enemas has been a major step in the improvement of symptoms, since the response is extremely rapid and highly effective. The low toxicity and rapid onset of action will keep these enemas at the forefront of management of left-sided disease; they have been effective in as proximal a location as the splenic flexure. In addition to the enemas, local therapy may be given in the form of mesalamine suppositories, which are effective in left-sided disease and have the advantage of greater mucosal adherence and less extensive distribution. Using frequent flexible sigmoidoscopy, I have noticed that the last area of improvement after oral drugs and enemas is the rectosigmoid junction. The suppositories can apply medication to this area more effectively than the enemas. A patient with a reactive rectum must evacuate the enema either proximally into the sigmoid or descending colon or out of the rectum. Suppositories can be used to decrease the inflammation in the rectum and rectosigmoid junction to allow the enemas to be retained in a more efficient fashion. This is an important management caveat. Rectal evacuation of the enema explains why it can be effective to the splenic flexure and why there may be a delay in the therapeutic response, which can be adjudicated by suppository therapy. Although topical medication can be used for long-term management, the value of enema therapy needs to be reconciled with costs and patient preferences as new oral drugs emerge.*

Oral Preparations

The observation that sulfasalazine improved patients with ulcerative colitis led to the inevitable studies to determine whether the sulfapyridine or 5-ASA component was effective in treating the inflamed colonic mucosa. Once it was understood that 5-ASA was as effective as sulfasalazine in treating ulcerative colitis, efforts were made to develop methods for delivering mesalamine to the colon (Table 2). Sulfasalazine is split by a bacterial azoreductase present in the colonic microbiologic flora; this breaks the bond between sulfapyridine and 5-ASA. The strategy of using bacterial azoreductase enzymes was used in the development of

---

*Editor's Note: Conventional wisdom held that 5-ASA suppositories work best for distal disease less than 15 cm in area, but the author's experience says otherwise. He is recommending suppositories in the morning and enemas in the evening.

Table 1   Rectal Preparations

Product	Preparation
RoWASA*/Salofalk/ Claversal (Reid-Rowell, US) (Interfalk, Canada) (SmithKline, International)	Enemas (4 g/60 ml buffered suspension pH 4.5)* Suppository (0.5 g/1 g)*
Pentasa (Marion, US) (Ferring, Denmark)	Enema (1, 2, 4, g/dl) Buffered suspension pH 4.8
4-ASA	Enema (2 g Na-4-ASA — requires reconstitution)

*Available in the United States.
From Hanauer SB. Ulcerative proctitis and left-sided colitis. In: Bayless TM, ed. Current therapy in gastroenterology and liver disease. 3rd ed. Philadelphia: BC Decker, 1990:336.

Table 2 New Salicylates (Oral)

Product	Preparation	Dose	Delivery
Pentasa* (Marion, U.S.) (Ferring, Denmark)	Mesalamine encapsulated in ethylcellulose microgranules	250 mg	Time/pH release 30%–55% urinary recovery
Asacol* (Norwich-Eaton, U.S.) (Tillots, U.K.)	Mesalamine coated with Eudragit-S	400 mg	Release at pH > 7 20%–35% urinary recovery
Claversal/Salofalk (SmithKline/Falk)	Mesalamine in sodium/glycine buffer coated with Eudragit-L	250–500 mg	Release at pH > 6 25%–45% urinary recovery
RoWASA (Reid-Rowell)	Mesalamine in enteric-coated compress, coated with coteric opadry	250–500 mg	Release at pH > 4.5 ≈ 60% urinary recovery
	Mesalamine in enteric-coated tablet coated with Eudragit-L100	250–500 mg	Release at pH > 5 ≈ 30% urinary recovery
4-ASA (Reed and Carnrick)	Enteric coated with Eudragit compound	500 mg	Time/pH release
Dipentum* (Pharmacia)	Olsalazine (azodisalicylate)	250 mg	Two molecules of 5-ASA released into colon ≈ 25% 5-ASA urinary recovery
Balsalazide (Brorek)	4-aminobenzoyl-β-alanine-5-ASA	500 mg	Inert carrier delivers 5-ASA into colon

*Available in the United States.

From Hanauer SB. Ulcerative proctitis and left-sided colitis. In: Bayless TM, ed. Current therapy in gastroenterology and liver disease. 3rd ed. Philadelphia: BC Decker, 1990:336.

olsalazine (Dipentum), which combined two 5-ASA molecules that could be separated by bacterial diazoreductase. Although this drug is very effective for ulcerative colitis, it has the disadvantage of inducing diarrhea in 15 to 20 percent of patients through activation of small bowel fluid secretion. In patients with constipation and distal disease, this observation can be used to treat both colonic inflammation and the constipation due to impaired colonic function with dehydration of stool in the proximal colon.

Other medications are being developed that combine mesalamine with an inert carrier, which should obviate the complications of sulfapyridine and the small intestinal secretion by olsalazine. These are not currently available in the United States, although there is extensive experience with Balsalazide outside this country. Another delivery strategy encapsulates a large amount of drug with an Eudragit coating that dissolves with change in pH in the terminal ileum or cecum. Asacol uses this strategy to release the contents of the 400 mg capsule into the cecum. This is an effective way of delivering medication to the colon; however, the renal excretion of mesalamine indicates that there is probably some release proximal to the ileocecal valve, and a few patients report seeing undissolved capsules in their stools. Microencapsulation with ethylcellulose was a strategy used to develop Pentasa. With this method, there is gradual release of 5-ASA throughout the small bowel and colon from a semipermeable ethylcellulose membrane. This form of release also delivers mesalamine to the colon, but the urinary secretion of mesalamine indicates small bowel release as well. Although this is uncertain at present, release in the small bowel may be beneficial in Crohn's disease.

One of the principal advantages of the mesalamine derivatives is their relative safety compared with sulfasalazine. In contrast to the 20 percent incidence of side effects seen in patients on sulfasalazine, the side effects associated with mesalamine derivatives are a fraction of that number. The wide array of drug release profiles allows flexibility in dosing and tailoring medication release profiles to disease distribution for long-term therapy. Even in male patients without obvious disease or toxicity, sulfasalazine induces sperm changes. Male infertility can be corrected by removal of the sulfapyridine moiety. Males should discontinue sulfasalazine and initiate mesalamine or olsalazine if they wish to father children. The oral drugs provide a convenient dosage form for patients and are effective in over 70 percent of those with left-sided ulcerative colitis.*

Glucocorticoids

Glucocorticoids, whether topical or systemic, have played an important role in long-term management of IBD. As with mesalamine, local application of glucocorticoids rapidly improves the disease through direct contact with the mucosa with active drug, and limits the side effects. Although it was thought for many years that glucocorticoids would be rapidly absorbed by the inflamed colon, it is the mucosa in remission that rapidly absorbs glucocorticoid enemas, in contrast to limited absorption by actively inflamed mucosa. Glucocorticoids improve tenesmus and can be used as adjunct therapy with 5-ASA drugs either rectally or orally. Glucocorti-

---

***Editor's Note:** The 70 percent response to Asacol was in patients with mild to moderate colitis and at a dosage of 4.8 g per day. Only 25 percent went into remission with olsalazine; 50 percent responded to 3 g.

coids as foam or topical cream preparations may be utilized for distal disease. As with mesalamine, enema administration extends further into the colon for use in more proximal disease. Newer glucocorticoids such as budesonide are rapidly metabolized by the liver and thus have high first-pass clearance, which limits their systemic toxicity. Although none of the new-generation glucocorticoids have been approved for use in the United States, this major advance in glucocorticoid formulation should allow local high-dose glucocorticoid therapy with limited side effects.

Immunomodulators

Immunosuppressants such as 6-mercaptopurine and azathioprine should be cautiously administered to patients with left-sided disease, in view of their potential toxicity. Approximately 50 percent of patients with left-sided disease respond, but there is a lag period of 60 to 90 days between administration and the onset of action. There is a relative prednisone-sparing effect with sufficient immunosuppressant to improve long-term symptoms.

Emerging New Therapies

A variety of new medications are being used for the treatment of distal proctitis, proctosigmoiditis, and left-sided disease. These include methotrexate (which acts as an interleukin-1 antagonist), interleukin-1 antagonists, 5-lipoxygenase inhibitors (Zileuton), hydroxychloriquine, and short-chain fatty acid enemas. Of these, only short-chain fatty acids are unique for left-sided disease. There is emerging recognition that the left and right sides of the colon use different metabolic substrates to support mucosal integrity. If these agents are confirmed as important, they may be useful adjunctive therapy for improving resistant left-sided disease in limited colitis or pancolitis.*

MANAGEMENT DECISIONS

Management focuses on evaluation of the extent of colonic mucosal involvement and the state of the mucosa proximal to the line of demarcation. If there is considerable uninvolved colon with the possible exception of a cecal patch, the disease should be considered to be left-sided colitis. If a line of demarcation can be established and an infectious etiology excluded, the first line of treatment depends on the extent of mucosal involvement. If more than 25 cm of the colon is involved, mesalamine enemas or local glucocorticoid enemas are most useful. The superior efficacy of mesalamine enemas compared with glucocorticoid enemas suggests that mesalamine should be a first course of treatment

---

*Editor's Note: The combination of short-chain fatty acids as a source of nutrients with 5-ASA, an anti-inflammatory agent, may prove useful in patients with resistant distal disease.

unless there is known sensitivity to mesalamine drugs. Disease extending less than 25 cm is effectively covered by mesalamine suppositories. Even though suppositories contain only 500 mg of drug, mucosal adherence and limited migration improve their efficacy in the rectum and distal sigmoid. If disease extends to the splenic flexure, oral adjunct therapy with mesalamine-based drugs, including azulfidine, olsalazine, or the newer-release mesalamine preparations (Asacol, Pentasa) in doses of 1 to 4 g, should often help suppress the disease. As specific symptoms are elucidated, the most disconcerting symptom should be identified and treated. Tenesmus should be treated with topical therapy. The low-volume suppository or glucocorticoid cream treatment is desirable, since medication-induced tenesmus and rectal spasm are volume related. When rigid sigmoidoscopy was the only way to visualize the mucosa, the important caveat for rectal management was that the physician not be deceived by an improvement in the rectum due to local therapy. With the use of flexible sigmoidoscopy, this does not appear to be a problem, since this procedure goes well beyond the direct contact area of local treatment and can move up to the line of demarcation. I have found local therapy to be the most effective management for these patients.

RECURRENT DISEASE

Therapy for recurrent episodes of colitis is an interesting topic requiring special assessment. I recently reported my approach to the problem of recurrence, which I believe is often associated with a systemic or enteric infection. The hypothesis that best explains the activation of the colitis by infection is as follows: before the infectious episode, colonic inflammation was controlled by medication that suppressed the immune system sufficiently to allow mucosal recovery. The tenuous balance between controlled homeostatic inflammation (normal) and the pathobiologic inflammation that induces mucosal disease is disrupted by the stimulation of the immune system, which has been activated to protect the body against a nonintestinal infection. Generally, activation of colonic symptoms occurs within 1 week of resolution of the systemic infection, such as an upper respiratory illness. Colonic infection with *Clostridium difficile* or other enteric infectious agents also appears to be important. I approach management of a recurrent episode by careful evaluation for treatable infection while aggressively re-establishing topical treatment and stressing the importance of compliance with drugs. Maintenance therapy is discussed below.

REFRACTORY DISEASE

If the patient is refractory to treatment, re-evaluation is essential to eliminate extension of colitis or undiagnosed disease. Possible unrecognized problems include concurrent infection, solitary rectal ulcer syndrome due to the prolapse of mucosa down into the anal canal, ischemic changes, coexistent IBS, drug-induced colitis, and mesalamine sensitivity. Each of these problems may mimic active IBD. We have recently begun to recognize an emerging group of patients with typical left-sided colitis that undergoes a gradual transition from active mucosal inflammation to a refractory disease with deep ulcerations and small areas of spared mucosa while under conventional management. Although this disease looks like Crohn's disease after the transition, transmural changes or changes consistent with Crohn's disease cannot be verified on biopsy. I believe this emerging group of patients with indeterminant colitis may be a subset of IBD with mucosal changes related to the unique metabolism of the left side of the colon. The partial repression of the disease occurs as a response to medications, and the escape from control that occurs is related to differences in the mucosal metabolism of short-chain fatty acids.

A common problem with long-term local treatment is failure to retain the enema or rapid proximal migration of the enema, leaving the distal colon inadequately treated. Although suppositories are helpful, it is also important to consider the possibility of decreasing reactivity of the rectum with antihistamines or anticholinergic agents. When this strategy is attempted, it is important to avoid constipation above the area of active inflammation.

LONG-TERM MANAGEMENT

Two principal issues are part of long-term management. The first is colonic surveillance for dysplasia and cancer. Cancer in the left side of the colon, although delayed, is an important risk. Intermittent flexible sigmoidoscopy to the line of demarcation of the disease should be performed with biopsies for dysplasia.*

The second principal issue is maintenance therapy. It has been shown that maintenance therapy with 1 g

---

*Editor's Note: Although I usually perform one colonoscopy at 8 to 10 years to determine the extent of microscopic disease, there is no evidence that this is necessary. Reliance on the extent of gross disease may be sufficient.

mesalamine enemas is successful in left-sided colitis. It was possible to maintain patients in remission over the entire period, and yet when the medication was decreased, they had the same flare pattern as the controls admitted to the study 1 year previously. Anecdotal experience suggests that enemas can be used every other day or every third day for long-term management. A large study, currently being evaluated, should determine whether intermittent therapy with 4 g enemas would be successful in maintaining remission. Oral therapy is an alternative, with a mesalamine dose equivalent to 2 g sulfasalazine. In patients with limited disease, I often discontinue all therapy 6 to 10 months after successful induction of remission after the first attack, to assess the possibility that the patient might be free of symptoms without medication.

Editor's Note: We ask contributors to give us their approach. This chapter does just that and provides many "new" ideas for the clinician.

SUGGESTED READING

Biddle WL, Greenberger NJ, Swan JT, et al. 5-Aminosalicylic acid enemas: effective agent in maintaining remission in left-sided ulcerative colitis. Gastroenterology 1988; 94:1075–1079.

Danielsson A, Lofberg R, Persson T, et al. A steroid enema, budesonide, lacking systemic effects for the treatment of distal ulcerative colitis or proctitis. Scand J Gastroenterol 1992; 27:9–12.

Hermens DJ, Miner PB Jr. Exacerbation of ulcerative colitis. Gastroenterology 1991; 101:254–262.

Miner PB Jr, Biddle WL. Maintaining remission in distal ulcerative colitis and ulcerative proctitis. Can J Gastroenterol 1990; 4:476–480.

Petitjean O, Wendling JL, Tod M, et al. Pharmacokinetics and absolute rectal bioavailability of hydrocortisone acetate in distal colitis. Aliment Pharmacol Ther 1992; 6:351–357.

Rao SSC, Read NW, Brown C, et al. Studies on the mechanism of bowel disturbance in ulcerative colitis. Gastroenterology 1987; 93:934–940.

Rao SSC, Read NW, Davison PA, et al. Anorectal sensitivity and responses to rectal distention in patients with ulcerative colitis. Gastroenterology 1987; 93:1270–1275.

Scheppach W, Sommer H, Kirchner T, et al. Effect of butyrate enemas on the colonic mucosa in distal ulcerative colitis. Gastroenterology 1992; 103:51–56.

Sutherland LR, May GR, Shaffer EA. Sulfasalazine revisited: a meta-analysis of 5-aminosalicylic acid in the treatment of ulcerative colitis. Ann Intern Med 1993; 118:540–549.

ULCERATIVE COLITIS

DANIEL H. PRESENT, M.D.

Ulcerative colitis is a complex illness. Current knowledge indicates that there are underlying genetic factors that predispose to its development. This is suggested by the increased incidence noted in first-degree relatives and in the Jewish population, concordance in monozygotic twins, and the association with a distinctive serum antineutrophilic cytoplasmic antibody in ulcerative colitis patients as well as their first-degree relatives. Finally, there is a selective reduction in colonic glycoproteins in patients and families as well as monozygotically unaffected twins. It has been suggested that the disease may be triggered by multiple factors, including superimposed infections (*Salmonella,* viral) and the taking of nonsteroidal anti-inflammatory agents. Attacks may even occur in a seasonal pattern. Discontinuation of cigarette smoking appears to be a major factor in either initiation or worsening of the inflammatory process. Once the condition is under way, multiple alterations in patients' immune response have been noted with subsequent enhancement of cytokine release and alterations of the lipoxygenase and cyclooxygenase pathways.

Although many drugs are available to treat active ulcerative colitis, there is no standard management for this complex clinical condition, and artful individualization is required for most patients. Current therapeutic approaches are directed toward manipulation of the nonspecific inflammatory pathways as well as the more specific initial immune response.

VARIABLES AFFECTING MANAGEMENT

Management with available agents varies according to several factors, the most important being the extent of involvement and severity of disease. Other potential differences include whether this is an initial attack, a recurrent flare-up, or chronic refractory activity.

Extent of Disease

Almost by definition, ulcerative colitis involves the rectum, which is the most active segment in most patients, even in those in whom involvement is extensive. The clinician should carefully note the extent of the inflammatory process, i.e., proctitis (involvement up to 10 to 15 cm), proctosigmoiditis (activity up to 30 to 40 cm), left-sided colitis (up to the splenic flexure), extensive (to the hepatic flexure), or universal (to the cecum).

When disease is only distal (proctitis and proctosigmoiditis), the involved segment often must be treated more intensively, and a major error in management of extensive ulcerative colitis is failure to use topical in addition to oral or parenteral medications. The institu-tion of concurrent rectal therapy will help more quickly alleviate symptoms such as diarrhea, bleeding, and tenesmus. For example, high-dose oral steroids may effectively treat refractory distal proctosigmoiditis, but when steroid doses are decreased exacerbation is common if concomitant rectal therapy has not been instituted and maintained. An accurate measurement of extent is important in terms of potential development of fulminant disease (rarely seen in limited proctitis and proctosigmoiditis) and increased cancer risk (also not seen in proctitis and proctosigmoiditis), but of highest risk in universal disease that has been present for 8 or more years.

There have been infrequent reports of "skip" areas in ulcerative colitis, especially in the right colon. The significance of these skip areas is uncertain, but they may serve to predict those patients in whom the disease process will extend in the future.

Proctitis and proctosigmoiditis have been reported to extend in 10 to 30 percent of patients, and endoscopic re-evaluation may be required with the passage of time. Barium enemas are not accurate in describing the extent and should mainly be used to evaluate strictures and scarring of the colon and the presence of small bowel inflammation that may suggest Crohn's disease. Colonoscopic biopsies demonstrating microscopic activity when the colon appears grossly normal are of little to no value in guiding the choice of therapy. For example, if the gross extent of the disease is 30 cm and biopsies show universal disease, distal topical therapy is often all that is required for symptomatic clinical relief. It is uncertain whether the proximal positive biopsy findings are forerunners of extension and therefore an indication for oral preventive therapy.

Activity of Disease

Ulcerative colitis disease is usually defined in terms of symptoms that are correlated with endoscopic findings. Mild disease is associated with four or fewer loose bowel movements daily with occasional blood and associated with abdominal cramps, blood, and infrequently tenesmus. Systemic symptoms are not present. Endoscopy shows erythema, edema, and mild friability of the mucosa. In moderate disease, there are movements ranging from four to eight daily with urgency, a nocturnal pattern, blood in the stool, abdominal discomfort, and some systemic symptoms such as weight loss, mild anemia, and low-grade fever of less than 100°F. Blood chemistries are usually unremarkable, and endoscopy shows spontaneous bleeding and friability, increased mucoid material in the lumen, and scattered ulcerations. Severe attacks are classically described by the passage of six or more bloody stools daily accompanied by systemic symptoms such as fevers of 100°F or greater, weight loss, tachycardia, anemia with a hemoglobin count of 10 g per deciliter or less, and hypoalbuminemia. Endoscopy demonstrates all of the above-noted findings seen in moderate disease plus large amounts of blood in the lumen and large areas of ulcerated denuded mucosa. Plain abdominal x-ray films often demonstrate a column of air in the descending and transverse colon, or even a full-blown toxic megacolon.

I believe that treatment should be primarily directed at symptoms and not at endoscopic findings. The latter should be used as guidance for the duration of specific therapy (Table 1).

DIET AND NONSPECIFIC THERAPEUTIC MEDICATIONS

Although patients and families initially focus on dietary alterations in an attempt to manage ulcerative colitis, there is unfortunately little to be gained from dietary therapy. Thus far, no one specific diet or elimination of potential irritants has been successful, other than producing a mild improvement in bowel symptoms.

If diarrhea is a major symptom, bulk such as raw fruits and vegetables should be eliminated. However, in distal proctitis and proctosigmoiditis in which proximal constipation is common, extra bulk in the diet may be required or the addition of psyllium compounds that may be useful in relieving the constipation. Gas-producing foods such as beans or cabbage and stimulants, or laxatives such as caffeine or dietary (sorbitol-containing gum) are best avoided when cramps and/or diarrhea are prominent. Milk is often inappropriately withheld from patients with ulcerative colitis. Since lactase deficiency is not observed in most patients, lactose intolerance should be documented before complete exclusion is advised, especially in young children. Elemental diets and predigested supplements have never been shown to play any role in suppressing inflammation in ulcerative colitis, as contrasted with Crohn's disease, and are indicated only if there is significant nutritional depletion and a normal diet cannot be tolerated. In fact, total parenteral nutrition (TPN) has shown no efficacy in several controlled trials in the management of severe ulcerative colitis. TPN should not be used as primary therapy but only to improve the nutritional status in depleted patients before surgery or while waiting for acute therapy (such as cyclosporine) to become active.

Emotional factors have not been shown to be etiologic and rarely worsen already active disease. Psychotherapy rarely if ever alters the clinical course and is best used as supportive therapy unless the patient has an underlying separate psychiatric disorder. Family therapy and mutual support groups (as sponsored by the Crohn's and Colitis Foundation of America) are valuable in the long-term adjustments to this chronic illness. A major benefit is a concerned and caring physician who will be available to answer questions and personal concerns, especially in the early phases of the illness and at the time of hospitalization or complications.

SYMPTOMATIC DRUG THERAPY

It is not unique to observe patients with ulcerative colitis who are taking a variety of medications (5-aminosalicylic [5-ASA] agents, steroids, immunosuppressives), whose main symptom is diarrhea, and who are not receiving an antidiarrheal agent. Choices include diphenoxylate, 2.5 to 5 mg; loperamide, 2 to 4 mg; deodorized tincture of opium, 5 to 15 drops; and codeine, 15 to 30 mg, all given up to four times daily. Individuals vary as to which of these agents is most effective. All are best given 15 to 30 minutes before meals and before sleep. Addiction is rare and the only major concern regarding these symptomatic agents is that during a severe, systemic attack there is the potential of triggering a toxic megacolon. This complication occurs infrequently, but antidiarrheals are best avoided with severe disease. However, when the activity is controlled, they can be reinstituted.

Irritable bowel syndrome (IBS) is a common gastrointestinal (GI) disorder and the astute clinician will observe symptoms of IBS superimposed on the symptoms of the active colitis in about 15 percent of patients. The use of anticholinergics such as dicyclomine, 10 to 20 mg before meals and sleep, bulking agents, and occasional antidepressants such as amytriptaline, 10 to 20 mg at sleep, may be valuable for symptomatic relief when IBS symptoms are present. Excessive bowel movements after an otherwise successful ileoanal anastomosis may occasionally be the result of a superimposed IBS and will require symptomatic medications.

SPECIFIC DRUG THERAPY

Salicylates (5-ASA Compounds)

Sulfasalazine

Sulfasalazine (Azulfidine) was the original, and is still the foundation and most commonly used drug in the treatment of ulcerative colitis. The drug consists of 5-aminosalicylic acid bound by an azo bond to sulfapyridine. About 20 percent of the parent compound is absorbed in the small intestine and excreted predominantly unmodified in bile. Colonic bacteria are responsible for azo bond reduction, thereby releasing 5-ASA and sulfapyridine. The latter is absorbed from the colon and acetylated by the liver (slow acetylation results in an increased incidence of sulfapyridine side effects). If given orally alone or uncoated, 5-ASA is rapidly absorbed in the jejunum, whereas when azo-bonded 5-ASA is released by bacteria, colonic absorption is limited, and the active moiety is thus distributed throughout the colon. 5-ASA is acetylated by colonic epithelium and excreted primarily in the stool.

The mechanism of action is uncertain and various proposals have been put forward, including inhibition of: the lipoxygenase and cyclooxygenase pathways, free

Table 1 Drug Therapy for Active Ulcerative Colitis

Mild Acute Relapsing		Moderate Acute Relapsing		Severe Acute Relapsing	
Proctitis-proctosigmoiditis	Left-sided, universal	Proctitis-proctosigmoiditis	Left-sided, universal	Proctitis-proctosigmoiditis	Left-sided, universal
Symptomatic (bulk, antidiarrheals)	Symptomatic (antidiarrheals)	Symptomatic (antidiarrheals, bulk)	Symptomatic (antidiarrheals)	Symptomatic (antidiarrheals)	No antidiarrheals
Rectal steroids (? rectal 5-ASA)	Rectal steroids	Rectal steroids (? double-dose) (? plus rectal 5-ASA)	Rectal steroids, Oral steroids	Double-dose rectal steroids (? + rectal 5-ASA)	Rectal steroids × 2
? Oral 5-ASA	Oral 5-ASA	Oral 5-ASA in increasing doses	Maintenance of oral 5-ASA	Increased oral 5-ASA Oral steroids (? systemic ACTH or Solu-Cortef)	Maintenance oral 5-ASA, IV steroids, IV antibiotics, IV cyclosporine (if no response to steroids)

ACTH = adrenocorticotropic hormone.

radical scavengers, platelet activating factor, macrophage, neutrophil and mast cell function, and of production of cytokines as well as alterations in humoral immunity.

Approximately 75 to 80 percent of patients with mild to moderate ulcerative colitis are reported to be responsive to sulfasalazine, usually within 2 to 3 weeks. Some patients may require several months to show complete response. The drug should be started at 500 mg twice daily, with gradual increase over 1 to 2 weeks. Most patients respond to 3 g, but if activity persists the dose can be increased to 4 g daily or rarely higher, since most patients do not tolerate doses over 4 g. The drug is best given with meals to minimize side effects. Enteric-coated sulfasalazine is valuable and should be substituted if GI side effects are seen soon after initiation.

Of equal importance is the fact that sulfasalazine, in addition to quieting active ulcerative colitis, is effective in maintaining remission, with a three to four times lower relapse rate compared with placebo for 1 year's duration. Preventive dose-ranging studies have shown that 4 g is more effective than 2 g, which in turn is more effective than 1 g; however, the higher doses result in increased side effects. The ideal preventive dose is approximately 2 to 3 g daily for most patients. The need for frequent administration during the day often results in poor patient compliance. There are few more difficult tasks in clinical medicine than convincing teenagers or young adults who have been in clinical remission that they must remain on this drug for prevention. However, the effort is worth the rewards in terms of preventing exacerbations and possible extension of disease.

Adverse effects occur in about 20 percent of patients taking sulfasalazine, and approximately half of these will have to stop the drug. The most common side effects are related to sulfapyridine blood concentration and depend on the administered dose and the acetylator status. These include nausea and vomiting, anorexia, abdominal pain, heartburn, and occasionally diarrhea. As noted, slow increase in dosage and taking the coated preparation with meals result in increased tolerance. Other important side effects include impaired male fertility secondary to oligospermia, morphologic sperm abnormalities, and abnormal motility. All are reversible within 6 to 8 weeks of stopping the drug. Severe side effects include idiosyncratic rash (ranging from mild to Stevens-Johnson syndrome), fever, agranulocytosis, liver dysfunction (cholestasis, hepatitis, massive liver necrosis), and lupus-like phenomenon with Raynaud's syndrome and pericarditis. Pulmonary eosinophilic pneumonias, fatal fibrosing alveolitis, and severe depression have also been noted. Neutropenia may occur, making concurrent use of 6-mercaptopurine or azathioprine more difficult. Megaloblastic anemia and hemolysis have been reported. Although folate deficiency can occur, routine supplementation is not required since the deficiency is usually not clinically significant.* Initial reports recommending the use of folic acid to prevent the development of dysplasia or carcinoma have not been confirmed by subsequent studies. Uniquely, there have been reports of sulfasalazine producing exacerbation of colitis. This adverse effect appears to be related to the 5-ASA moiety as it has been observed with the newer 5-ASA analogs that do not contain sulfapyridine.

New Salicylates

Since many of the adverse effects of sulfasalazine are due to the sulfapyridine moiety, and since 5-ASA has been shown to be the active agent, there has been recent rapid development of newer 5-ASA formulations. Slow desensitization to sulfasalazine, which is effective in 80

*****Editor's Note:** I agree with the author: overt folate deficiency, as measured by red cell folate levels, is unusual with sulfasalazine therapy.

to 90 percent of allergic patients, has been abandoned in favor of these newer formulations. Alternative delivery systems either substitute a new carrier molecule for the sulfapyridine or coat the 5-ASA, protecting it from absorption in the jejunum and allowing subsequent release in the distal small intestine or colon where it can exert its effect.

Olsalazine (azodisalicylate, Dipentum) consists of two molecules of 5-ASA linked by the same azo bond as in sulfasalazine. It also requires reduction by colonic bacteria and is well tolerated in many patients who are sensitive or intolerant to the sulfapyridine component of sulfasalazine. It shows efficacy equal to that of sulfasalazine in mild attacks as well as in maintenance of remission. Therapeutic doses for active disease range from 1 to 3 g daily; the greatest effectiveness is seen with 3 g, whereas the preventive dose (which is FDA approved) is usually 1 g given as 500 mg twice daily. The major toxicity of this agent is diarrhea resulting from small bowel secretion of fluid; this is dose related and more common in patients with extensive colitis. Diarrhea can be diminished if the dose is increased gradually and given with meals. Diarrhea tends to improve with time, but in about 10 percent of patients the drug must be stopped because of this side effect.

Balsalazide (Colazide) links 5-ASA by an azo bond to 4-aminobenzoyl-β-alanine and is cleaved similarly to olsalazine and sulfasalazine, releasing the 5-ASA into the colon. Recent prevention studies suggest that higher oral doses are well tolerated and are more effective in maintenance of remission than lower doses of balsalazide. The major side effects of this agent are GI (abdominal discomfort, heartburn, and diarrhea). The maximal tolerable doses giving the greatest efficacy are yet to be determined.

Coated 5-ASA, also called mesalazine, contains no other compounds but is released at different sites in the small intestine, depending on the coating. Asacol is coated with Eudragit S, which dissolves at lumenal pH 7 (approximately at the terminal ileum and/or right colon). Claversal (Salofalk) is coated with Eudragit L and dissolves at a pH greater than 6. Studies have demonstrated that Asacol is effective in active mild to moderate ulcerative colitis and also in maintaining remission in ulcerative colitis patients. Of interest is the demonstrated efficacy of higher-dose Asacol (4.8 g daily, which is equal to about 10 g sulfasalazine) in over 60 percent of patients with mild to moderate ulcerative colitis, whereas 2.4 g is effective in 50 percent of patients and 1.6 g daily is no better than placebo. The drug is well tolerated and toxicity is similar to that seen with placebo. The standard dose of Asacol used by most clinicians to treat ulcerative colitis is 800 mg three times daily. This dose was approved by the FDA. Thus far, no one has determined the ideal time to give this medication in relation to meals. It has been shown that if Asacol is taken with food, the coated capsule may remain in the stomach for many hours and be released much later in the intestine.

With all the 5-ASA compounds, idiosyncratic allergy

to 5-ASA can be seen in the form of pericarditis, pleuritis, pancreatitis, and nephrotic syndrome. Nephrotoxicity is a potential long-term problem, as it has been noted in animals ingesting high doses of 5-ASA. My long-term experience indicates that sulfasalazine is safe during pregnancy and nursing, and preliminary data from Canada suggest that there are no complications with Asacol in pregnancy, but further evidence is awaited.

Pentasa is a sustained-release preparation that contains granules of 5-ASA coated with ethylcellulose. Release occurs with time and increased pH. Efficacy has been observed (and FDA approved) in active ulcerative colitis as well as in maintenance of remission. The response rate is once again similar to the above-mentioned preparations. Doses of 2 to 4 g daily are effective.

Despite the numerous new agents developed, none has so far proved more effective than the standard sulfasalazine. The advantage of the newer agents appears to be that of less toxicity in avoiding the sulfapyridine molecule; a major disadvantage is increased cost. Long-term data are required for accurate comparison of each of the new formulations in active disease and to establish the best dosage. It remains to be determined whether higher doses will give increased efficacy without increased toxicity. At this stage of our knowledge, perhaps more important than which formulation is given is the need to convince the patient to stay on medication for maintenance of remission.

Topical 5-ASA

Since the demonstration that 5-ASA was the active ingredient in sulfasalazine, topical 5-ASA has been used for distal disease. Initially, 5-ASA enemas (Rowasa) of 4 g daily were shown to be more effective than cortisone enemas containing 100 mg daily. In addition, 5-ASA enemas of 1 to 4 g daily have clearly proved more effective than placebo for mild to moderate disease. Clinical response is noted in about 70 to 75 percent of patients and does not appear to be dose related. Of greater importance may be the amount of fluid administered with the active ingredient. It is stated that 100-ml enemas will reach the splenic flexure in most patients, but U.S. preparations are produced as 60 ml, which may have less extensive distribution. Refractory patients may require 5-ASA enema therapy for several months to induce clinical remission, and relapse is high when the enema is discontinued in this group of patients. Prevention should be attempted, and enemas taken every other day or every third night are successful in most patients. 5-ASA suppositories (Rowasa) in doses of 200 mg, 1 g daily, are also effective for distal rectal activity, and if continued are more effective than placebo in maintaining remission. The optimal dose is yet to be determined. The toxicity of topical 5-ASA is similar to that seen with placebo and is usually idiosyncratic, in addition to occasional local irritation and pruritus.

There are no prospective studies determining the

best initial topical therapy of choice for active distal ulcerative colitis. Both 5-ASA and steroid enemas have been used initially with success, but it is important to remember that only the 5-ASA compounds are preventive. The short- and long-term role of oral 5-ASA in the treatment of proctitis and proctosigmoiditis is uncertain.

Corticosteroids

In the mid-1950s, steroids were shown to be more effective than placebo for ulcerative colitis, and they have become the treatment of choice for moderate to severe disease.

The mechanism of action is uncertain, with multiple anti-inflammatory and immune effects. Inhibition of bound arachidonic acid and decreased activity of by-products of the lipoxygenase and cyclooxygenase pathways are noted, as well as impaired neutrophil chemotaxis and phagocytosis, inhibition of cytokine production, and decreased capillary permeability.

In the 1960s, prednisone (the most frequently used corticosteroid) proved more effective at doses of 40 to 60 mg daily than at 20 mg daily. The 60 mg doses were associated with increased toxicity, and it was concluded that most patients with active disease should be given 40 to 45 mg daily, with tapering after a good response. Although the literature suggests that a once-daily dose is as effective as multiple doses, the studies are limited to few patients and short periods. My experience is that multiple doses are more effective if the patient is very active but result in increased side effects. For moderate to severe attacks, it is suggested that steroids be initiated in dosages three to four times daily, with a decrease to 1 to 2 times daily after a response has occurred. Overall, the response rate to oral steroids is greater than 75 percent. Tapering after response is usually in 5 mg decrements every 5 to 7 days, but this can be varied depending on the degree of clinical response and the severity of side effects. Relapse, when it occurs, is usually seen at dosages between 10 and 20 mg daily. There is no evidence that steroids are effective in maintaining remission, and therefore 5-ASA products are added (or maintained) once remission has been obtained. Steroids should then be discontinued.

For patients with severe disease, admission to the hospital is indicated with administration of intravenous (IV) steroids: hydrocortisone (Solu-Cortef), 300 mg daily, or methylprednisolone, 48 to 60 mg daily. There are no controlled trials to confirm my impression that continuous infusion is more effective than pulse administration. However, personal experience suggests that about 25 to 30 percent of all refractory patients on pulse IV steroids improve when switched to continuous infusion. In one controlled trial, adrenocorticotropic hormone (ACTH), 120 units by continuous daily infusion, was shown to be more effective than 300 mg hydrocortisone only in patients who had not been receiving previous steroids. It is suggested that ACTH

be used in this situation.* It is incorrect to switch a patient who is refractory to IV hydrocortisone to ACTH in the hope of further response. The response rate to IV steroids in active colitis is better than 60 percent.

Toxicity with steroids is extensive and can result in long-term irreversible effects. Toxic effects include emotional disturbances (occasionally psychosis), a cushingoid habitus, hyperglycemia, hypertension, electrolyte disturbances with hypokalemia and metabolic alkalosis, myopathy, and increased intraocular pressure. Other long-term complications include osteoporosis, aseptic necrosis of the hip, cataracts, growth retardation in children, and impaired immunity resulting in increased infections. Steroids must be used promptly when indicated but rapidly decreased and discontinued when not needed. If exacerbation occurs when lowering the dosage or if long-term steroid use is required, consideration must be given to other therapeutic tools such as immunosuppressive agents or surgery. Steroids can be safely given in pregnancy, in which the risk to mother and child of increased bowel inflammation far outweighs any potential side effects to the fetus.

Topical Steroids

Studies starting in the late 1950s were convincing that topical steroids were about four to five times more effective than placebo in the treatment of distal colitis. A response rate of over 70 percent is usually noted within 2 weeks. Some unresponsive patients with extensive disease seem to benefit from being given two enemas at the same time at night. Many patients cannot tolerate enema preparations when the disease is active, and for these Cortifoam, which is also more effective than placebo, should be used initially. Administration of the more tolerable foam preparation twice daily for 1 week usually quiets the rectal segment sufficiently for higher-reaching enema preparations to be administered and retained. The combination of topical and oral steroids is highly effective initial therapy for moderate to severe ulcerative colitis.

Because systemic absorption with potential toxicity is noted with prolonged use of rectal steroids, several newer steroid preparations with decreased absorption or less systemic availability have been developed. These include prednisolone-metasulphobenzoate, which is poorly absorbed and comparable in efficacy with prednisolone enemas or low-dose oral steroids. This preparation is not available in the United States. Tixocortol pivalate, with replacement at the 21-hydroxylate area with a thiol group esterified to pivalic acid, is inactivated by red blood cells and first-pass metabolism through the liver. This agent therefore does not suppress the hypothalamic-pituitary-adrenal axis. Large multicenter

***Editor's Note:** The use of ACTH, which is not popular with some who question the comparability of groups in the oft-cited paper, should be limited to 10 to 14 days' usage because of instances of bilateral and renal hemorrhage after several weeks of therapy.

trials have shown equal effectiveness with hydrocortisone enemas in short-term studies of 3 weeks, but approval and release of tixocortol pivalate has not occurred in the United States. Beclomethasone dipropionate, a rapidly metabolized steroid, has shown conflicting results compared with conventional topical steroids in distal disease. Fluticasone, a fluorinated steroid that is subject to first-pass metabolism, has also shown conflicting results, and further trials are ongoing.

Budesonide, a nonhalogenated glucocorticoid with potent anti-inflammatory activity, has proved more effective than placebo and prednisolone enemas in several studies. Dose-response studies suggest that a 2 mg dose is an attractive alternative to prednisolone enemas, in that minimal suppression is seen on the hypothalamic-pituitary-adrenal axis. The results of controlled trials will soon be available in the United States.

Immunosuppressive Agents

Recognition of the importance of immune system abnormalities in pathogenesis has resulted in increasing and better-defined indications for the use of immunosuppressives for ulcerative colitis.

Azathioprine/6-Mercaptopurine

Azathioprine is well absorbed and converted to 6-mercaptopurine in vivo, with subsequent impairment of purine synthesis. The exact mechanism of action is uncertain, especially in the low dosages used in inflammatory bowel disease (IBD). The first successful therapeutic report occurred in the early 1960s with subsequent uncontrolled literature showing a response rate of 80 percent (84 of 105 patients). In addition to the clinical response, healing of pyoderma gangrenosum was also noted. There are several controlled trials of the use of these agents in ulcerative colitis, with a demonstrated efficacy equal to that of sulfasalazine as well as significant steroid-sparing action. Since the drug takes a mean time of over 3 months for response, its use is limited in acute ulcerative colitis, in which steroids and 5-ASA agents are the drugs of choice.

The major indication is for patients with chronic refractory colitis or steroid-dependent disease and for those with significant early steroid toxicity (e.g., psychosis, aseptic necrosis of the hip, uncontrollable diabetes). Uncontrolled trials have been carried out with 6-mercaptopurine (6-MP) in which the clinical response and toxicity have been similar to those seen with azathioprine. Both drugs are to all intents and purposes similar and equally effective. 6-Mercaptopurine should be initiated in a dose of 50 to 75 mg daily; azathioprine at 75 to 100 mg daily. The dosage can be increased until leukopenia is observed, but most patients respond to 75 mg 6-MP (or 100 mg azathioprine). If they do not respond clinically with decreased requirements of steroids in 3 to 4 months, the dosage should be maximized to leukopenia and should not be considered ineffective until after at least 6 to 8 months of therapy. There is not always a correlation of clinical response and endoscopic findings after therapy with 6-MP and azathioprine, in that it is not unique to have a clinical remission with mild scattered inflammatory changes persisting on colonoscopy. In uncontrolled trials and in a recent double-blind withdrawal trial, 6-MP and azathioprine have proved preventive of relapse in ulcerative colitis. Approximately three-quarters of patients remain in remission once this has been obtained with these agents. Relapse on these agents, when it occurs, is often mild and responds to increasing doses of immunosuppressives or 5-ASA agents or a short course of topical or oral steroids. Surgery can be prevented with 6-MP or azathioprine in more than two-thirds of refractory cases.

Acute toxicity consists of allergic reactions such as rash, fever, and joint pains in about 2 percent; pancreatitis in 3 to 4 percent; and (rarely) hepatitis. Bone marrow depression is dose related and can be avoided with close monitoring of the white blood cell count during the first 1 to 2 months. Almost all acute toxicity and allergic reactions occur in the first 3 to 4 weeks of taking these agents and disappear if the drug is stopped. Although there has been great fear of long-term immunosuppression leading to superinfections and neoplasia or lymphoma, no association or increased risk has so far been noted in the more than 25 years of using these agents for IBD. Long-term studies in transplant patients and recent studies in IBD patients have shown no increase in fetal abnormalities in women or men taking 6-MP or azathioprine at the time of conception. Some clinicians have maintained these agents throughout pregnancy with no untoward side effects noted so far.

These agents should be initiated if ulcerative colitis patients do not go into remission or cannot discontinue systemic steroids after two attempts. I believe steroid use of 3 to 6 months' duration is an indication for the institution of 6-MP or azathioprine.*

Cyclosporine

Cyclosporine, a fungally derived immunosuppressive that inhibits the production of interleukin-2 as well as subsequent production of cytokines, has proved effective in ulcerative colitis as well as Crohn's disease. In uncontrolled studies and as recently confirmed in a controlled trial, continuous IV cyclosporine is effective when administered in a dose of 4 mg per kilogram daily to patients with severely active ulcerative colitis who have failed 10 or more days of IV steroids. In this group in whom colectomy was indicated, response was seen in 82 percent in 6 to 7 days, so that patients could leave the hospital well controlled on oral steroids (45 to 60 mg prednisone daily) and cyclosporine (6 to 8 mg per kilogram per day). The long-term response has been

---

*Editor's Note: As a personal approach, I use azathioprine as described except for patients with over 8 to 10 years' duration of colitis because of an unproved (and perhaps unfounded) concern about colon neoplasia. I favor colectomy for these latter patients. Connell et al (Abstract, Gastroenterology April 1994) cite 20 years' experience that shows no increase in colon cancer with azathioprine therapy.

satisfactory, and approximately 60 percent of the original study group of 46 patients have gone into complete clinical and endoscopic remission and been able to discontinue both steroids and cyclosporine. They are currently being maintained predominantly on 5-ASA compounds, with some patients taking 6-MP. A recent controlled trial of cyclosporine enemas has failed to confirm the efficacy in distal disease that was seen in several smaller uncontrolled series.

Cyclosporine has a high potential for toxicity, including hypertension, renal injury (which is dose related), hepatotoxicity, neurologic toxicity (tremors, paresthesias, and seizures), and long-term neoplasia. However, in series in which the drug was monitored carefully and used in the short term (less than 1 year), toxicity was not excessive. The clinician should obtain experience with this drug before using it extensively for ulcerative colitis.

Other Immunosuppressive Agents

Other immunosuppressives have yet to undergo extensive studies in patients with ulcerative colitis. In an uncontrolled study, intramuscular methotrexate, 25 mg once weekly, showed a response rate of greater than 70 percent. However, maintenance of response and significant steroid sparing have not been seen with lowering of the dose or switching to oral administration. A new potent immunosuppressive, FK506, has so far not been used extensively in ulcerative colitis. Dihydroxychloroquin (Plaquenil), a drug that inhibits lysosomal processing of antigens, was effective in a small uncontrolled series. A larger controlled trial using a dosage of 400 mg daily for 6 weeks was not more effective than placebo, but a new study, using higher doses for longer periods, is currently under way.

Other Agents

Space limits the discussion of a variety of agents that have been tried or are currently being studied in the management of ulcerative colitis, including topical lidocaine, acetarsol, sucralfate, short-chain fatty acids, and clonidine. Recently, a promising lipoxygenase inhibitor (Zileuton) has proved effective in those ulcerative colitis patients not taking sulfasalazine. Further studies using higher doses of this potentially promising drug are almost complete. Studies of omega$_3$ fatty acids, as found in fish oils, have produced modest clinical improvements in ulcerative colitis patients.* So far, there is no evidence that broad-spectrum antibiotics or metronidazole are effective therapy for ulcerative colitis, whether it be for moderate to severe disease or distal disease, or whether administered topically, orally, or intravenously.

*Editor's Note: Short-chain fatty acid enemas provide an energy source for the left colon cells and may prove useful in unresponsive patients. Zileuton provides an opportunity to see the effect of blocking one step in the inflammatory cascade. Other such products are also being considered.

FULMINANT COLITIS AND TOXIC MEGACOLON

Fulminant colitis is one of the severe complications of ulcerative colitis. Colectomy occurs in about 25 percent of patients and is required in almost 50 percent of patients if the entire colon is involved at the time of the acute attack. The typical clinical picture of severe colitis, described earlier, requires careful monitoring by both gastroenterologist and surgeon and must be treated intensively with all available modalities if recovery and remission are to be obtained. Certain therapies should always be initiated, including rapid admission to the hospital, the patient being given no food or fluid by mouth, and IV fluid, electrolyte, and blood replacement. Continuous IV steroids should be administered in the form of hydrocortisone, 300 mg daily; methylprednisolone (Solu-Medrol), 48 to 60 mg daily; or ACTH, 120 units daily (if no previous steroids have been given) over a 24 hour period. Rectal hydrocortisone enemas, 100 mg, should be administered twice daily; if these cannot be retained, Cortifoam should be given twice daily. Although the use of antibiotics is controversial, in view of the potential of minute sealed-off perforations, broad-spectrum IV coverage using an aminoglycoside, ampicillin, and metronidazole should be undertaken. There is no indication to start short-term 5-ASA orally or rectally if the patient has not been receiving these agents, but they should be maintained (when feedings are restarted) in those already taking them. There is no indication for 6-MP or azathioprine, because they take too long to be effective. There is no controlled evidence nor any indication for the use of TPN in these patients, and after they have stabilized (24 to 48 hours), oral feedings are allowed as tolerated. If the patient fails to respond to this regimen in 1 week, cyclosporine should be initiated, 4 mg per kilogram per day by continuous IV infusion. Failure to show any response to cyclosporine in 7 days or deterioration is an indication for surgery.

If toxic megacolon complicates fulminant colitis, all the above therapies should be continued plus cessation of oral feedings; passage of a long, small intestinal tube with suction drainage; and use of a rolling technique in which patients lie on the abdomen for 10 to 15 minutes every 2 hours while awake. This allows for passage of gas and easier decompression of the dilated colon.

SURGERY

Indications for surgery in ulcerative colitis can be specific or occasionally less well defined. Free perforation and unstoppable hemorrhage are fortunately rare but are clear indications for urgent colectomy. The finding of either cancer or confirmed high-grade dysplasia is an indication for surgery no matter what current therapy is being employed. Therapy for low-grade dysplasia is more controversial, but multifocal low-grade dysplasia found at a single endoscopy, or repeat low-grade dysplasia on sequential endoscopies, is an indication for colectomy. There is a separate chapter on this subject.

In fulminant colitis and toxic megacolon the indications for surgery are not clear-cut, but patients should be treated as outlined above, and if there is no response after adequate medication has been initiated or if there is a rapid decline after therapy (fever, hypotension), acute colectomy is indicated. In patients with chronically active disease, surgery is not indicated until there has been a trial of 6-MP or azathioprine. This requires that the treating physician not take too long to institute

Table 2 Drug Therapy for Chronic Refractory Ulcerative Colitis

Proctitis-proctosigmoiditis	Left-sided, Universal
Symptomatic (bulk and/or antidiarrheals)	Antidiarrheals
Double enemas (steroid × 2 or steroid + 5-ASA)	Steroids + 5-ASA enema
Maximize oral 5-ASA	Maximize oral 5-ASA
6-MP/azathioprine	6-MP/azathioprine
Course of IV steroids	Course of IV steroids
Surgery vs experimental agents	Surgery (especially if disease >8 yr)

6-MP = 6-mercaptopurine.

immunosuppressives, because steroid toxicity may destroy patients' health and so deplete them that there is no time for the immunosuppressives to be effective. Drug therapy for refractory patients should be maximized before colectomy (Table 2).

SUGGESTED READING

Biddle WL, et al. 5-Aminosalicylic acid enemas: effective agent in maintaining remission in left-sided ulcerative colitis. Gastroenterology 1988; 94:1075.
Habal FM, Hui G, Greenberg GR. Oral 5-aminosalicylic acid for inflammatory bowel disease in pregnancy. Gastroenterology 1993; 105 (in press).
Janowitz HD. Systemic corticosteroid therapy of ulcerative colitis. Gastroenterology 1985; 89:1189.
Lichtiger S, Present DH. Preliminary report: cyclosporine in treatment of severe active ulcerative colitis. Lancet 1990; 336:16.
Peppercorn MA. Sulfasalazine: pharmacology, clinical use, toxicity and related new drug development. Ann Intern Med 1984; 3:337.
Present DH. 6-Mercaptopurine and other immunosuppressive agents in the treatment of Crohn's disease and ulcerative colitis. Gastroenterol Clin North Am 1989; 18:57.
Sheppach W, Sommer H, Kirchner T, et al. Effect of butyrate enemas on the colonic mucosa in distal ulcerative colitis. Gastroenterology 1992; 103:51–56.
Truelove SC, Witts LJ. Cortisone in ulcerative colitis. Final report on a therapeutic trial. Br Med J 1955; 2:1041.

CROHN'S COLITIS

MARK A. PEPPERCORN, M.D.

Although Crohn's disease may involve any portion of the gastrointestinal (GI) tract, approximately one-third of patients have disease limited to the small intestine, about one-half have ileal and colonic involvement, and the remaining one-fifth have colitis only. Of those with colonic disease, the rectum or rectosigmoid is spared in approximately 50 percent. One-third of patients have perianal lesions and up to one-fifth may have associated manifestations of skin, joint, and liver disease.

The clinical course of this idiopathic disorder, which involves the bowel in a transmural fashion, is one of unpredictable spontaneous exacerbations characterized by episodes of crampy abdominal pain and diarrhea, with or without bleeding. Microperforations often present with an acute picture of localized peritonitis resembling appendicitis or diverticulitis. Fistula to surrounding organs such as the bladder lead to complications that may dominate the clinical picture, while progressive segmental fibrosis may lead to episodes of partial colonic obstruction. Recently, it has been appreciated that colon

cancer may be as much of a long-term risk for patients with Crohn's colitis as for those with ulcerative colitis.

The diagnosis of Crohn's colitis today is usually established endoscopically with findings of focal ulcerations surrounded by edematous mucosa. Colonic biopsies show focal acute and chronic inflammation and may reveal granulomas in up to one-third of patients. Barium x-ray examinations characteristically show segmental disease with skip areas and asymmetric involvement of the bowel wall. Crohn's colitis needs to be distinguished from acute forms of colitis (bacterial, amebic, viral, ischemic) by appropriate investigations; from the other major cause of chronic colitis, ulcerative colitis, which involves only the mucosa of the colon in a continuous fashion beginning in the rectum; and from both diverticulitis and obstructing or perforating colon cancer.

THERAPEUTIC ALTERNATIVES

Drugs are the principal form of therapy for acute exacerbations of Crohn's colitis and may also be useful in sustaining remissions. For many years, sulfasalazine has been the mainstay for such patients, and now a variety of oral and topical aminosalicylates based on the structure of sulfasalazine can be used for those intolerant of, allergic to, or unresponsive to sulfasalazine.

Standard oral corticosteroids such as prednisone

and methylprednisolone and topical hydrocortisone, used alone or in combination with sulfasalazine, have proved effective for outpatients with exacerbations of Crohn's colitis, while parenteral forms including hydrocortisone, methylprednisolone, and prednisolone as well as adrenocorticotropic hormone have been used for severe and fulminant disease. There are now emerging topical and oral preparations of rapidly metabolized steroids that may be as effective with regard to anti-inflammatory activity but with less toxicity.

There has been increasing interest in the use of antibiotics for active Crohn's disease. Metronidazole has become an established agent to treat both Crohn's colitis and perianal Crohn's disease. Ciprofloxacin appears to be useful for perianal disease and may, along with other broad-spectrum antibiotics, have a primary role in the treatment of active ileal and colonic disease. Moreover, antituberculous agents look promising for both active and remitted disease in selected patients.

The therapy for Crohn's colitis has been greatly influenced in the past decade by increasing acceptance of the immunomodulators 6-mercaptopurine (6-MP) and azathioprine, which appear effective both in active disease and in sustaining remissions of Crohn's colitis. For patients intolerant of or refractory to these agents, there have been promising results from trials with cyclosporine and methotrexate, and in very preliminary studies of anti-CD4 monoclonal antibodies as well as alpha-interferon.

Other innovative modalities that may be of benefit in a given refractory patient include T-cell apheresis, immunoglobulin infusions, oxygen-derived free radical scavengers, and, for those with severe perineal disease, hyperbaric oxygen.

Finally, in patients with well-established symptoms, one should not forget the role of antidiarrheal drugs such as loperamide, diphenoxylate with atropine, and codeine as well as cholestyramine for those with nonstenosing ileal disease and ileal resection, and anticholinergic agents such as hyoscyamine, propantheline, and dicyclomine.

In addition to drug therapy, nutritional treatment with modification of the diet and use of enteral and parenteral feedings as primary therapy should be considered in selected patients. Behavior modification and psychotherapy, with and without the use of psychotropic agents, may be important for certain individuals. Finally, surgery may be necessary for patients with Crohn's colitis who are refractory to medical therapy or who suffer an irreversible complication of the disease.

PREFERRED APPROACHES TO THE USE OF SPECIFIC DRUGS

Sulfasalazine

Since its introduction into clinical medicine over 50 years ago, sulfasalazine has been a mainstay of treatment for both ulcerative colitis and Crohn's disease. Controlled trials have shown the effectiveness of the drug in active Crohn's ileocolitis and colitis. Although many physicians who use the drug are convinced that it also works in a subset of patients with ileitis alone, most controlled trials have not shown efficacy in this patient group. Similarly, although controlled trials have not shown sulfasalazine to be effective in maintaining remission in Crohn's colitis, in contrast to its accepted role as prophylaxis in remitted ulcerative colitis, many clinicians keep patients with Crohn's colitis on the drug indefinitely once they have achieved remission.

Sulfasalazine has been my therapy of choice for any patient with mild to moderate symptoms of Crohn's colitis. I begin at an initial dose of 500 mg orally twice daily, with advancement over several days to 1 g orally three to four times daily. Since sulfasalazine may interfere with dietary folate absorption, I add folic acid, 1 mg per day. Clinical improvement usually occurs within 3 to 4 weeks, at which time the dose can be tapered to 2 or 3 g per day and maintained for an additional 3 to 6 months. The response to therapy is judged almost exclusively on clinical grounds, including the signs and symptoms of abdominal pain, diarrhea, and bleeding as well as improvement in laboratory parameters, including hematocrit, white blood cell (WBC) count, sedimentation rate, and albumin. There is not a good correlation between endoscopic appearance and clinical response, so follow-up with endoscopy is generally not indicated.

If the patient achieves remission and prefers not to be on long-term treatment, the drug can be stopped. For those who wish to continue therapy despite the lack of clear evidence of long-term benefit, maintenance therapy with 2 g sulfasalazine is continued. Some, however, believe that higher doses (3 to 4 g per day) are needed to improve the long-term prophylactic effect. In patients who relapse quickly but respond to reinstitution of therapy, indefinite long-term use of sulfasalazine should be considered.

Sulfasalazine's usefulness is limited by a high incidence of intolerance and allergic reactions. Nausea, anorexia, and headache can be overcome by lowering the dosage, and dyspepsia may be decreased by using an enteric-coated form. Mild neutropenia and mild degrees of hemolysis may also be reversed by lowering the dosage. The complete blood count (CBC) should be monitored frequently at first and then periodically on chronic therapy. Minor allergic reactions such as rash and fever may be overcome in up to 75 percent of patients by a process of gradual desensitization. More serious side effects such as agranulocytosis, severe hemolysis, hepatitis, pancreatitis, pneumonitis, neuropathy, alteration of sperm count and sperm morphology, and exacerbation of colitis necessitate discontinuing the drug. Sulfasalazine can be used safely during pregnancy and nursing.

Sulfasalazine consists of sulfapyridine linked to 5-aminosalicylic acid (5-ASA) via an azo bond. The drug is partially absorbed from the proximal GI tract, and a portion of the absorbed drug is excreted unchanged in the urine. The remaining absorbed portion returns unchanged to the small intestine via the bile, where, together with the unabsorbed portion, it traverses the intestine until it encounters the bacterial flora primarily in the distal ileum and colon. The azo bond is broken by the action of the intestinal bacteria with release of sulfapyridine and 5-ASA. The sulfa portion is largely absorbed, metabolized by the liver, and excreted in the urine. The 5-ASA metabolite, in contrast, stays largely in contact with the colon and is excreted in the feces. These observations suggested that sulfasalazine might be serving as a prodrug delivering an active component (5-ASA) to distal disease sites. This hypothesis, coupled with observations that most of the drug's toxicity related to the sulfa portion, led to the development of a new group of agents, the aminosalicylates.

Aminosalicylates

Controlled trials of topical 5-ASA in both suppository and enema form (known as mesalamine in the United States and mesalazine in Europe) have clearly established its effectiveness in ulcerative proctitis and distal ulcerative colitis. Only a few patients with distal Crohn's colitis or Crohn's proctitis have been treated with topical 5-ASA in an organized fashion, although there has been the impression that the agent does not work as well in distal Crohn's disease as it does in distal ulcerative colitis. Nonetheless, I have used 5-ASA enemas in patients with Crohn's disease isolated to the rectum or the left colon with success, beginning with one enema every night and then tapering to every other night or every third night, similar to its usage in distal ulcerative colitis. The topical preparations available in the United States include Rowasa enemas and suppositories. Neither has been approved by the Federal Drug Administration (FDA) for use in Crohn's disease.

Several formulations of oral 5-ASA agents have been developed and studied. These include olsalazine (Dipentum), which links 5-ASA to itself via an azo bond; balsalazide (Colazide), which links 5-ASA to an inert polymer, also via an azo bond; and slow or delayed release forms of mesalamine, which encapsulate 5-ASA in ethylcellulous microspheres (Pentasa) or coat it with an acrylic resin (Eudragit) that dissolves at pH greater than 6 or 7 (Asacol, Claversal, Rowasa).

The oral agents have proved effective in active and remitted ulcerative colitis. Studies of the use of these oral 5-ASA drugs in Crohn's disease have been limited. In the largest and most promising study, 310 patients with mildly or moderately active Crohn's disease involving the small and large bowel were randomized to Pentasa at doses of 1, 2, or 4 g per day or to placebo over a 16 week period. In the trial, 64 percent of the patients on the 4 g dose improved, with 43 percent achieving full remission. These contrasted with a 36 percent overall improvement rate in those on placebo, with only a 11 percent remission rate. The 1 and 2 g per day dose results were comparable with those seen on placebo. Neither the disease site nor previous medication usage affected the outcome.

Although the slow-release and delayed-release oral 5-ASA agents may have an advantage over sulfasalazine in small bowel Crohn's disease, it is unlikely that they will be any more effective than sulfasalazine in Crohn's colitis. The oral 5-ASA agents should be considered for patients with Crohn's colitis who are intolerant of or allergic to sulfasalazine. As suggested by the Pentasa study, the dosage may have to be pushed to the higher range (e.g., Asacol, 4.8 g; Dipentum, 3.0 g) to realize an effect in active disease. Currently, Dipentum, Asacol, and Pentasa are available in the United States but have received FDA approval only for use in ulcerative colitis.

As noted above, it has been difficult to show efficacy for sulfasalazine in preventing relapses of Crohn's disease. Several trials have shown the potential for oral 5-ASA agents to maintain remission in Crohn's disease, but the results have been variable. In one promising trial, 34 percent of patients with Crohn's disease relapsed on Asacol (2.4 g per day) in 1 year compared with 55 percent on placebo. However, these effects were especially pronounced in patients with ileitis, not those with colitis. In another study, 161 patients with inactive Crohn's disease (90 percent of whom had colon involvement) were randomized to receive either Pentasa, 2 g per day, or placebo in a 2 year trial. Only in those patients who began therapy within 3 months of remission was there a significant difference on drug therapy, with ongoing remission rates of 45 percent and 29 percent in the Pentasa and placebo groups, respectively. This efficacy was apparently unrelated to disease location, although not specifically commented on by the authors.

I believe that further clinical experience is needed before we know the true role for the oral 5-ASA agents in Crohn's disease. For now, it seems reasonable to consider long-term maintenance therapy for patients with Crohn's colitis with one of these agents in the same manner as one might use sulfasalazine.

Although 80 to 90 percent of patients intolerant of or allergic to sulfasalazine tolerate either the topical or oral 5-ASA preparations, 10 to 20 percent of patients experience the identical reaction with 5-ASA as noted with sulfasalazine. Side effects reported with the aminosalicylates include anal irritation with the topical preparations, pancreatitis, pericarditis, pneumonitis, nephritis, exacerbation of colitis, and watery diarrhea, seen particularly with olsalazine. Although experience is limited, these agents appear to be safe during pregnancy and nursing.

The mechanism of action of the aminosalicylates and the parent drug sulfasalazine remains uncertain. Most speculation has focused on the role of these agents in inhibiting the lipoxygenase pathway of arachidonic acid metabolism, and thus decreasing the production of chemotactically active leukotrienes and hydroxy fatty acids. Other investigations have pointed to a possible role as oxygen-derived free radical scavengers and as a blocker of certain antibodies toxic to colonic epithelial cells.

Metronidazole and Other Antibiotics

Although not all investigations agree, controlled trials suggest that metronidazole is as effective as sulfasalazine and more effective than placebo in patients with mild to moderate Crohn's colitis and ileocolitis. The drug has not proved effective when only the ileum is involved. Its use as a prophylactic agent for Crohn's disease patients in remission has not been investigated. I turn to metronidazole for the patient with Crohn's colitis who is not responding to or cannot tolerate sulfasalazine or one of the oral aminosalicylates. I give the drug at a dosage of 10 mg per kilogram per day and hope to see a response within 4 weeks. I then usually continue the drug for 4 to 6 months before gradually tapering and stopping it.

As with sulfasalazine, the use of metronidazole is limited by a high incidence of side effects, including nausea, anorexia, metallic taste, furry tongue, and depression. Peripheral neuropathy is a serious problem at higher doses (greater than 1 g per day), but it can occur at lower doses and may persist when the patient is off therapy. Although the potential for carcinogenicity has been raised by in vitro and animal studies, there is no evidence that metronidazole causes malignancy in humans. It should not, however, be used during pregnancy.

The way in which metronidazole works in Crohn's colitis is not clear. By decreasing the anaerobic floral burden, it may be diminishing an antigen stimulus to inflammation or decreasing the production of bacterial toxins injurious to the bowel. However, it is speculated that metronidazole may have anti-inflammatory or immunosuppressive properties independent of its antimicrobial action.

In addition to metronidazole, there has long been advocacy for the use of a wide array of broad-spectrum antibiotics in the management of mild to moderate Crohn's disease regardless of distribution. Ampicillin, tetracycline, and various cephalosporins have been reported anecdotally to be of utility. I have recently had success in treating several patients with Crohn's colitis with oral vancomycin despite negative *Clostridium difficile* toxin titers, and ciprofloxacin has produced dramatic results in a group of my patients with Crohn's ileitis and ileocolitis.

Finally, there is interest in the use of combinations of antituberculous agents. Uncontrolled trials have suggested efficacy for regimens of two and four drugs in refractory active Crohn's disease of small and large bowel, and a placebo-controlled trial showed that a four drug regimen maintained remission in Crohn's patients. I would await the results of further trials, however, before I begin to use antituberculous therapy in any but the most refractory of patients.

Corticosteroids

Both topical and systemic steroids can play an important role in the management of patients with colonic Crohn's disease. As with the topical aminosalicylate preparations, hydrocortisone enemas (Cortenema) should be considered in patients with active Crohn's proctosigmoiditis. I begin them with one enema every night for 2 to 3 weeks and then taper to every other night for 2 to 3 weeks. Some patients continue to have smoldering symptoms and seem to benefit from continued use of the enemas every 2 to 3 nights with few systemic effects. Currently, rapidly metabolized forms of topical steroids, including budesonide and beclomethasone dipropionate, appear promising in studies of patients with distal ulcerative colitis, but their use has not been reported in patients with distal Crohn's colitis.

For patients with more extensive mild to moderate Crohn's colitis who have not fully responded to sulfasalazine, oral aminosalicylates, or metronidazole or cannot tolerate these agents, I add corticosteroids. Although controlled trials give conflicting results with regard to efficacy, most of my patients finish with a combination of steroids and one of the other agents. I begin treatment with prednisone, 40 to 60 mg per day, and hope to see a response to the initial dose within 2 weeks. Once the desired response is obtained, the prednisone dosage is tapered by 5 mg every 7 to 10 days. Since there is no benefit in continuing prednisone as a prophylactic agent once remission is achieved, I try to withdraw patients completely from the prednisone. However, some patients begin to have mild smoldering active disease as the dosage is tapered, and benefit from continued low dosages of the drug, 5 to 10 mg per day or 10 to 20 mg on alternate days. The latter schedule may decrease the frequency of the well-known long-term side effects of steroids, including cataracts, osteoporosis, hypertension, and diabetes.

As with topical preparations, there are now ongoing studies of slow-release forms of oral budesonide. Preliminary results of open trials in patients with Crohn's ileitis and ileocolitis support the efficacy of budesonide, with little or no impact on the pituitary-adrenal access.

Immunomodulators

6-Mercaptopurine (6-MP) and Azathioprine

Resistance to the use of the immunosuppressive drugs azathioprine (Imuran) and its metabolite 6-MP (Purinethol), resulted from the inability of several short-term controlled trials to show efficacy in patients with inflammatory bowel disease (IBD), and from concern over their potential adverse effects. Much of that concern has been allayed by subsequent long-term studies and by an enlarging experience attesting to their relative safety. In a 2-year, double-blind, placebo-controlled cross-over study of patients with Crohn's disease, 6-MP used in conjunction with sulfasalazine and/or prednisone was successful in achieving specific therapeutic goals in two-thirds of patients. Many authors have now published their experiences supporting the use of these agents in patients with Crohn's disease refractory to or dependent on steroids, and the ability to taper steroid dosage and heal fistulas. There is also evidence from controlled observations that these drugs can maintain remission in Crohn's disease.

I turn to 6-MP (the drug is the active metabolite of Imuran and the two can be used interchangeably) in patients with Crohn's colitis refractory to other drugs, those dependent on steroids, those with nonhealing fistulas, and those with early postoperative recurrence. I initiate treatment at 50 mg per day, explaining to patients that the average time for clinical response is about 3 months and that some individuals may not show benefit for 6 to 9 months. I monitor the CBC weekly for the first week of therapy, every other week for the second week, and monthly thereafter. If after 4 weeks there is no therapeutic response (e.g., decrease in symptoms, ability to slowly taper steroids), I raise the dosage but not to exceed 2 mg per kilogram per day. Some authors feel that mild leukopenia must be achieved to get a maximal response, but I lower the dose of drug if the WBC count drops below 4,000 k per microliter.

Once the desired therapeutic response is achieved, the question arises as to how long to continue therapy. This is of concern to all patients, since before beginning therapy they are told of the very small potential risk of malignancy, particularly lymphoma. In most patients, I suggest continuation of the drug for 2 years with an attempt at withdrawal at that point. Those with the most refractory cases of Crohn's who have already had multiple surgeries tend to want to stay on the drug indefinitely. Some can stop it successfully for prolonged periods, while others flare shortly after withdrawal and end up on another protracted course of therapy.

The overall toxicity of 6-MP and azathioprine has been limited, and more than 90 percent of patients treated have not experienced an adverse effect. Mild allergic reactions such as fever and rash are infrequent, as are more serious reactions such as hepatitis and pancreatitis. Bone marrow depression can usually be avoided by careful monitoring, and teratogenicity has not been established, although I discourage women from becoming pregnant while on 6-MP or azathioprine. If conception occurs, the drug is stopped and the pregnancy continued. Thus far, the long-term risk of malignancy in patients with IBD appears to be extremely low.

Methotrexate

Long given to patients with rheumatologic disorders, methotrexate has recently been used with apparent success in patients with IBD. In an open trial of patients with active small bowel and colonic Crohn's disease, 30 of 37 (70 percent) improved or went into remission during a 12 week treatment period, receiving 25 mg per week intramuscularly. Eighty percent of patients previously unresponsive to 6-MP or azathioprine improved on methotrexate.

In a chronic-phase open trial in which 39 patients with Crohn's disease receive 15 mg per week of methotrexate orally with gradual tapering of the dose, 20 (51 percent) remain on methotrexate at a mean follow-up of 69 weeks. Most patients in this group remain dependent on low-dose prednisone. Adverse effects have been limited to a few patients with abnormal liver enzymes, mild leukopenia, and pneumonitis.

In a separate 52-week trial, patients with ileal and colonic Crohn's disease who were steroid dependent were randomized to either methotrexate, 15 mg per week, or placebo. At the end of the trial, there were no differences in the activity index between the two groups. In the course of the study, however, 46 percent of patients in the treatment group had flares compared with 80 percent in the placebo group.

Although more data from controlled trials are awaited, I believe there is a role for methotrexate in the patient with Crohn's colitis who has failed standard treatment, including 6-MP. If there is no evidence of small bowel disease that might compromise absorption, I begin patients on 15 mg per week and hope to see a response within 4 months. I then taper the dosage and maintain it at 5 to 7.5 mg per week for 2 years before attempting to stop it.

Cyclosporine

In a 3 month placebo-controlled trial involving patients with refractory ileal and colonic Crohn's disease, oral cyclosporine was associated with improvement in 59 percent of patients compared with a 32 percent improvement rate on placebo. However, during a 3 month period in which cyclosporine was then gradually withdrawn, only 38 percent of the original responders to cyclosporine remained well. Long-term use of low-dose cyclosporine in patients with Crohn's disease in remission has not been efficacious. Long-term side effects of hirsuitism and paresthesias are common. Hypertension and renal failure are also potential problems for those on chronic cyclosporine therapy. I believe that cyclosporine has a limited role in patients with Crohn's colitis and should be reserved for those with active disease who are refractory to standard therapies and not good candidates for surgery.

OTHER MODALITIES

T-cell apheresis has been reported to achieve remission in 64 of 72 patients with refractory, chronic active Crohn's disease in open trials. The remission lasted 1 year in 24 patients and 5 years in one patient. The investigators report no mortality or immunoincompetence, but sepsis related to central lines was seen. In the one reported controlled trial, T-cell apheresis improved steroid weaning in Crohn's disease but had no effect on the relapse rate.

In an open trial of a small number of patients with active Crohn's disease, infusions of a chimeric monoclonal anti-CD4 antibody appeared to produce remission.

Finally, intravenous immunoglobulin given to a very few patients with active Crohn's disease was associated with improvement in disease parameters and in lowering steroid dosage. Although these modalities can be considered for patients with Crohn's colitis in whom other therapeutic options have been unsuccessful, they should be viewed as experimental and requiring further controlled observations.

ANTIDIARRHEAL, ANTICHOLINERGIC, AND PSYCHOTROPIC AGENTS

Loperamide, diphenoxylate with atropine, and codeine may be of benefit in the setting of mild, chronic diarrhea due to active Crohn's colitis. These agents should not be used in unstable patients with severe degrees of activity because of the risk of precipitating ileus and even toxic megacolon. Occasional patients with Crohn's colitis have symptoms resembling the irritable bowel syndrome, with frequent small stools alternating with constipation associated with a sense of incomplete evacuation. For such patients, hydrophilic mucilloids such as psyllium may be of benefit. Similarly, the crampy pain experienced by such patients may be relieved by anticholinergic drugs such as propantheline, bromide, dicyclomine hydrochloride, and hyoscyamine sulfate given before meals and at bedtime. Although not a substitute for a concerned caregiver, minor tranquilizers such as oxazepam and diazepam, or antidepressants such as amitryptiline and doxepin, may be useful in patients in whom stress appears to be playing a pivotal role in symptom exacerbation. Behavior modification should also be considered in such patients.

NUTRITIONAL THERAPY

It has been difficult to prove that specific diets are effective for patients with Crohn's colitis. I always consider lactose intolerance in such patients and usually perform a lactose breath test to determine whether lactose withdrawal might benefit them. I also ask patients with gas, cramps, and diarrhea to avoid fresh fruit and fresh vegetables, carbonated beverages, and diet gum.

Controlled trials have shown that both total enteral nutrition (TEN) and total parenteral nutrition (TPN) may induce remission in Crohn's disease. Most studies suggest that patients with ileal disease derive greater benefit from this approach than do those with Crohn's colitis. In my experience, most patients have limited tolerance for prolonged TEN, but I use elemental diets to supplement caloric intake in patients with Crohn's colitis. I rarely use TPN in patients with Crohn's colitis, since in my experience the improvements are short-lived and not usually worth the risks of infection with a prolonged central venous line. Such tools are extremely useful, however, in young children with growth failure.

OTHER CONSIDERATIONS

Perineal Disease

For patients with perineal fistulas and abscesses who do not require surgical intervention, or for those who have persistent problems despite surgery, I administer metronidazole, 1 to 2 g per day. For patients who respond, I attempt to slowly lower the dosage, although many require indefinite maintenance therapy at doses of 500 mg to 1 g per day. Ciprofloxacin, 500 mg twice a day, can be used in a similar fashion. Finally, there is evidence from preliminary studies that continuous infusions of cyclosporine (4 mg per kilogram per day) may promptly improve refractory perineal Crohn's disease.*

Fulminant Colitis

A few patients with Crohn's colitis present with severe symptoms and toxicity, with or without megacolon. Such patients are treated in a manner similar to those with severe ulcerative colitis, with intravenous (IV) fluids and electrolyte replacement and bowel rest. I use IV prednisolone as a continuous drip at 60 mg per 24 hours and add broad-spectrum antibiotics (e.g., ampicillin, gentamicin, or metronidazole). For those with dilated colons, I place a nasogastric tube and use the technique of rolling them to a prone position for 15 minutes every 2 hours. For those not improving within 72 hours, surgical intervention is advised. Whether IV cyclosporine, now shown to be of benefit in a controlled trial of patients with severe ulcerative colitis, will be of similar benefit for those with Crohn's colitis is not clear.

A more common acute presentation of the patient with Crohn's colitis is that of an acute appendicitis- or diverticulitis-like picture, with localized peritoneal signs due to a contained microperforation. I avoid corticosteroids in such patients not already on them for fear of masking sepsis, and instead use broad-spectrum antibiotics as primary therapy in such instances.

Colon Cancer

It is becoming increasingly apparent that patients with Crohn's colitis probably have a risk of colon cancer similar to that in their counterparts with ulcerative colitis, given the same extent and duration of disease. Although good prospective trials with large numbers of patients are lacking to support a surveillance program, I have begun to perform colonoscopies with biopsies for dysplasia in patients with Crohn's colitis who have had their disease for over 7 years, and I recommend colectomy for those with high-grade dysplasia. Unlike the situation in patients with ulcerative colitis, colon

*Editor's Note: Although responses to cyclosporine may be dramatic, some form of long-term suppression or immunomodulation is usually needed.

cancer in Crohn's disease may occur in grossly uninvolved areas in up to one-quarter of patients.*

Surgical Options

The indications for surgery in patients with Crohn's colitis include refractoriness to medical therapy, obstruction, perforation, abscess formation, fistulas, and perineal disease. Since many patients have rectal sparing, a segmental resection with anastomosis is often possible, although the recurrence rate is extremely high. For those with disease involving most of the colon, including the rectum, panproctocolectomy is necessary. The ileoanal anastomosis and pouch is not an option for patients with Crohn's colitis because of the very high recurrence rate in the pouch. Almost 75 percent of patients who have a colectomy with ileostomy for Crohn's colitis with no obvious evidence of small bowel Crohn's disease will remain disease free.

---

*Editor's Note: Patients with Crohn's colitis who are first diagnosed after the age of 40 years may have had subliminal illness for years before diagnosis and I therefore start surveillance soon after diagnosis.

SUGGESTED READING

Brynskov J, Freund L, Rasmussen JN, et al. A placebo-controlled double-blind randomized trial of cyclosporine therapy in active chronic Crohn's disease. N Engl J Med 1989; 321:845–850.
Ekbom A, Helmich C, Adams HO. Increased risk of large bowel cancer in Crohn's disease with colonic involvement. Lancet 1990; 336: 357–359.
Kozarek RA, Patterson DJ, Gelfand MD, et al. Long-term use of methotrexate in inflammatory bowel disease. Gastroenterology 1992; 102:A648.
Nyman M, Hansson J, Eriksson S. Long-term immunosuppressive treatment in Crohn's disease. Scand J Gastroenterol 1985; 20: 1197–1203.
Peppercorn MA. Advances in the drug therapy for inflammatory bowel disease. Ann Intern Med 1990; 112:50–60.
Present DH, Korelitz BI, Wisch N, et al. Treatment of Crohn's disease with 6-mercaptopurine. A long-term randomized double blind study. N Engl J Med 1980; 302:981–987.
Roth M, Ueberschoer B, Ewe K, et al. Oral slow release budesonide induced remission in active Crohn's disease with little effect on adrenal function. Gastroenterology 1992; 102:A688.
Singleton J, Gitnick G, Hanauer SB, et al. Response of Crohn's disease to oral Pentasa as a function of disease location and prior therapy. Gastroenterology 1991; 100:A251.
Summers RW, Switz DM, Sessions, JT Jr, et al. National Cooperative Crohn's Disease Study: results of drug treatment. Gastroenterology 1983; 77:847–869.
Ursing B, Alm J, Barany F, et al. A comparative study of metronidazole and sulfasalazine for active Crohn's disease: the cooperative Crohn's disease study in Sweden. Gastroenterology 1982; 83:550–562.

INFLAMMATORY BOWEL DISEASE AND CANCER

ROBERT E. PETRAS, M.D.
RICHARD G. FARMER, M.D., F.A.C.P.

CANCER RISK AND MANAGEMENT OPTIONS IN ULCERATIVE COLITIS

Patients with longstanding ulcerative colitis (UC) are at increased risk for the development of colorectal adenocarcinoma. Those at greatest risk are patients with extensive colitis, defined as contiguous disease from the rectum beyond the splenic flexure, who have had symptoms of colitis for more than 7 to 10 years. Early age at onset of colitis also appears to be associated with an increased cancer risk. Although the principal focus of cancer risk has been on patients with extensive colitis, patients with left-sided colitis also developed colorectal carcinoma at a higher rate but their risk does not become appreciably higher until after symptoms of colitis have been present for more than 20 years.

Estimates of the cancer risk in UC vary considerably. Methodologic problems surround many of the current assessments of cancer risk including use of referral center populations, inclusion of patients already known to have cancer, and projection of cancer risk using relatively small patient numbers. More recent epidemiologic data suggest that patients with UC have six to ten times the risk of developing colorectal adenocarcinoma when compared to the general population. Looking specifically at the subgroup with extensive colitis, the risk is fifteen to nineteenfold.

This increased risk poses a considerable management dilemma for physicians caring for patients not sick enough to require colectomy. Several management options are available. First, physicians can ignore the risk. Many prefer this approach when dealing with an elderly patient or a patient who is not a surgical candidate. A second approach is "prophylactic colectomy" for patients with symptoms of colitis for more than 7 to 10 years. This could be the best approach when dealing with a very young patient because of the expected long duration of cancer risk and the fact that cancer surveillance programs occasionally fail. Furthermore, the results of ileal pouch–anal anastomosis procedures are better in young patients. Although "prophylactic colectomy" theoretically eliminates the cancer problem, several factors have made this approach unacceptable to many patients and physicians. Patients with long-duration extensive colitis are often asymptomatic or only mildly symptomatic. Such patients find it difficult to accept the morbidity and mortality associated with a major surgery or the social implications of a permanent ileostomy should the pelvic pouch fail. Besides, the data suggest that "prophylactic colectomy" would have been unnecessary in most patients because they would not have developed carcinoma.

The third option is colonoscopic surveillance with biopsy. The strategy of this approach is either identification of a marker that signals a subgroup of colitics at greatest risk of carcinoma, or detection of carcinoma in its earliest recognizable and curable phases.

PATHOLOGY OF DYSPLASIA

Dysplasia, the presumed precancerous epithelial change, has been regularly recognized in colons both adjacent to and distant from colitis-associated carcinomas. Circumstantial evidence suggests that dysplasia may not only be a marker for carcinoma, but may itself be the carcinoma in an early preinvasive phase.

Dysplastic epithelium can occur in a grossly flat mucosa, in a mucosa with a villous or plaquelike configuration, or in a nodular growth resembling an adenoma. Dysplasia is recognized by histologic examination of biopsy specimens utilizing well-defined cytologic criteria that include nuclear enlargement with hyperchromasia, increased mitotic figures, and decreased intracellular mucin. Most colitis-associated dysplasias resemble adenomas as seen in the noncolitic patient. The pathologist should use the term *dysplasia* only as a synonym for intraepithelial neoplasia and not in reference to reactive or reparative changes seen with active inflammation. The distinction of repair from dysplasia can be difficult; it takes a degree of experience and sometimes can be impossible. In general, cytologic changes in the presence of active inflammation must be interpreted with caution. The Inflammatory Bowel Disease-Dysplasia Morphology Study Group has proposed a three-tiered classification for biopsy interpretation in inflammatory bowel disease (IBD): positive, negative, and indefinite for dysplasia. Our experience has shown this classification to be useful and reasonably reproducible. Biopsy specimens negative for dysplasia include normal colon and those showing changes of active or quiescent colitis. Positive biopsy specimens are reported as showing either high-grade or low-grade dysplasia, the distinction being based on the degree of cytologic atypia present.

Biopsy specimens are classified as showing changes indefinite for dysplasia when unusual cytologic abnormalities are seen but are of insufficient degree to warrant a diagnosis of true dysplasia. Indefinite changes are usually encountered in a background of active inflammation, in which atypical epithelial changes may represent repair or regeneration rather than dysplasia. The indefinite category also includes odd patterns of epithelial growth that have not yet been observed to give rise to carcinoma (e.g., hyperplastic polyp-like change). This category is a legitimate diagnosis that should alert the treating physician that worrisome cytologic changes are present and may place a patient in a higher risk category, requiring more frequent surveillance.

COLONOSCOPIC SURVEILLANCE

Patients whose biopsy specimens remain negative for dysplasia can safely continue regular surveillance. Most experienced clinicians recommend total colonoscopic examination every 1 to 2 years for patients with extensive colitis who have had symptoms for more than 7 to 10 years. Patients who have colonic epithelial changes indefinite for dysplasia require shorter-term follow-up (6 months to 1 year). Management recommendations for patients with low-grade dysplasia are difficult to make because of the paucity of long-term follow-up information available in this group. Currently, short-term follow-up (3 to 6 months) seems safe for patients with low-grade dysplasia; however, if dysplasia persists or is associated with any suspicious gross lesion or stricture, colectomy should be considered. We have observed the progression of low-grade dysplasia to high-grade dysplasia and cancer in several patients. Therefore, low-grade dysplasia cannot be ignored or allowed to go unobserved if colectomy is not performed. If high-grade dysplasia is encountered, colectomy should be recommended.

Our experience with surveillance biopsy interpretation has shown that true negative results are rarely interpreted as dysplasia, and dysplasia, especially high-grade dysplasia, is rarely missed. However, variations in interpretation do occur; in general, confirmation of a biopsy diagnosis is desirable before colectomy. Any one or more of the following may be considered as adequate confirmation: (1) a finding of dysplasia in repeat biopsy from the same site, (2) a finding of dysplasia in one or more additional sites during the same endoscopic examination, or (3) review and confirmation of the dysplasia interpretation by another pathologist familiar with the classification system.

Surveillance endoscopy with biopsy has a number of limitations. Participation in a surveillance program does not guarantee that a potentially lethal advanced cancer will not develop. Dysplasia is an unusual phenomenon; it is difficult for any one pathologist to acquire experience, and errors in histologic interpretation can occur. Dysplasia can be extremely focal and is therefore subject to considerable sampling error. Most authorities consider dysplasia a neoplastic change and it is extremely unlikely that it ever resolves spontaneously. Thus, a clinician should never be lulled into a false sense of security by negative follow-up biopsies once true dysplasia has been identified. Although dysplasia is invariably found adjacent to carcinomas, dysplasia distant from carcinoma or throughout the large bowel is encountered less frequently. In our experience, a negative rectal biopsy can occur in at least half of patients who have proximal carcinoma or dysplasia; therefore, rectal biopsy alone has no role in a cancer surveillance program in UC.*

Experience from the perspective of a pathologist, as well as the clinician-endoscopist, indicates that surveillance programs are beneficial to patients when compared with no follow-up or with prophylactic colectomy. The incidence of colonic carcinoma is low in patients in whom biopsy specimens have remained negative for dysplasia. In the Cleveland Clinic study of patients undergoing a surveillance program, cancer was not found in any patient in whom surveillance biopsies were negative for dysplasia and who underwent surgery for symptoms. However, the most significant factor in any surveillance program is patient compliance, and despite extensive telephone surveys and patient contact, loss of patients to regular follow-up surveillance colonoscopy continues to be a problem.†

OTHER SURVEILLANCE MARKERS

Many groups have searched for other specific markers for precancer in UC. Mucin histochemistry, lectin binding, carcinoembryonic antigen immunocytochemistry, and analysis for various oncogene products do not reliably differentiate dysplastic from reparative epithelium in UC. Recently, many investigators described significant correlations between DNA abnormalities by flow cytometery and dysplasia/carcinoma in UC. However, only 80 to 90 percent of invasive carcinomas and 50 to 80 percent of the dysplasia lesions demonstrate DNA abnormalities by this technique indicating that DNA analysis is not sensitive enough to be used alone in a cancer surveillance program. As another aspect, many specimens (≥ 6 percent) from patients apparently lacking dysplasia or carcinoma clinically and histologically showed DNA abnormalities, perhaps serving as a predictor of future neoplasia. Technical problems with flow cytometry such as failure to disaggregate nuclear clumps, prolonged exposure of the sample to high temperature, and debris in the sample can explain some of the "false positives". Alternatively, the test may identify a subgroup of patients different from the group identified by histologic dysplasia that show objective chromosomal abnormalities in the absence of recognizable dysplasia. Preliminary evidence suggests, as mentioned above, that abnormal DNA content predicts later development of dysplasia, but until

large prospective studies to determine the usefulness of DNA analysis as a marker of cancer in UC are performed, histologic identification of dysplasia remains the only reliable marker for cancer. DNA analysis can potentially play a role now in cancer surveillance in that patients with normal DNA content and no signs of histologic dysplasia probably can be examined at longer intervals than 1 to 2 years.‡

THE "ADENOMA" IN THE COLITIC PATIENT

A special problem concerns the occurrence of "adenomas" in a patient with colitis. Since both conditions are common, there is probably no theoretical reason why they should not coexist. Since most IBD-associated dysplasias resemble adenomas, the distinction in practice may be impossible. In general, a diagnosis of "adenoma" in a patient with IBD must be viewed with skepticism because the changes probably represent IBD-associated dysplasia, which implies a substantial risk for the development of carcinoma or for coexisting carcinoma. Occasionally an "adenoma" in a colitic patient may be treated by local excision, but only if all the following criteria are met: (1) the patient is in an adenoma age group (>40 years), (2) the dysplasia lesion is pedunculated, (3) the excision is complete, and (4) the mucosa of the stalk lacks dysplasia. We can also accept an "adenoma" in a patient with colitis if the lesion occurs in an area not affected by IBD (e.g., cecal adenoma in a patient with left-sided colitis).

DYSPLASIA AND CARCINOMA IN CROHN'S DISEASE

Increasing clinical and pathologic evidence suggests that patients with Crohn's disease are also at increased risk of intestinal carcinoma. Small bowel carcinomas in our patients with Crohn's disease have occurred, on average, 20 years after the onset of Crohn's disease. Most involve the ileum and have always occurred in areas actively involved with Crohn's disease. The small bowel carcinomas in Crohn's disease are clinically and grossly subtle and often occur in strictured areas that resemble the inflammatory strictures of Crohn's disease. Small intestinal carcinomas in Crohn's disease tend to be poorly differentiated and are associated with poor prognosis. Approximately one-fourth of cases have occurred in bypassed or out-of-circuit segments.

Colonic carcinomas in patients with Crohn's disease have generally developed after about 20 years of disease. The diagnosis has usually been made clinically since a gross intraluminal lesion can often be visualized. The colonic carcinomas have been better differentiated than their small bowel counterparts and the prevalence of

---

*Editor's Note:** The recent paper by Woolrich, Korelitz, and their colleagues at Lenox Hill Hospital in New York shows that dysplasia found on the first colonoscopy sets the stage for invariably (eventually) finding carcinoma over the ensuing years.

†**Editor's Note:** Experience from the Cleveland Clinic, the Lahey Clinic, and Johns Hopkins indicates a significantly better survival rate for those whose cancer was found as a result of some preventive measure (colonoscopy, biopsies, or prophylactic colectomy) than those who presented with colon cancer-related symptoms.

‡**Editor's Note:** As the genetic deletions and alterations associated with neoplasia in IBD are identified, examination of stool (or bowel washing) may provide surveillance markers in the future.

mucinous histologic type is increased. About 20 percent occur in areas of the colon that are not grossly diseased.

Recent reports using current histologic criteria almost invariably note dysplasia in epithelium adjacent to both small bowel and colonic carcinomas in Crohn's disease. Dysplasia distant from carcinomas has also been encountered in specimens exhibiting both colonic carcinoma and Crohn's disease. These features suggest that a dysplasia-carcinoma sequence similar to that proposed for ulcerative colitis also occurs in Crohn's disease.

CANCER SURVEILLANCE IN CROHN'S DISEASE

Opinions vary regarding the usefulness of a cancer surveillance program in patients with longstanding Crohn's disease. In our experience, endoscopic surveillance is of limited value in small-bowel Crohn's disease. The small intestine, in general, is inaccessible by current endoscopic methods. The current histologic marker, dysplasia, is extremely focal. Since only approximately 80 cases of small bowel carcinoma associated with Crohn's disease have been reported, and about one-quarter of these occurred in out-of-circuit segments, the expected cancer or dysplasia yield of a surveillance program would be quite small.

It is possible that endoscopic surveillance could occasionally benefit a patient with colonic Crohn's disease by detecting dysplasia or early carcinoma, but current data lead one to question the efficacy of a regular cancer surveillance program. Colonoscopy may be technically difficult or even dangerous in some patients with Crohn's disease because of strictured areas. The absolute number of colonic carcinomas in Crohn's disease is quite small, so the expected yield of positive cases in a surveillance program would also be small.

Our experience indicates that a patient with recrudescence of colitis-like symptoms and longstanding inactive Crohn's disease should be thoroughly investigated for carcinoma and tests should include colonoscopy. Yearly surveillance of an out-of-circuit rectum seems reasonable considering that approximately 20 percent of the reported cases of cancer in Crohn's disease have occurred in such segments. It may, however,

be better to advise removal of a defunctionalized rectum, especially if reanastomosis is not planned, is not possible, or is contraindicated. The presence of dysplasia, especially high-grade dysplasia, in a biopsy specimen from a patient with Crohn's disease must alert the physician to the possibility of a coexistent invasive malignancy; in this situation, we would recommend colectomy as in UC. Clinicians should also recognize that chronic fistula or anal strictures in Crohn's disease may be complicated by carcinoma.*

SUGGESTED READING

Ekbom A, Helmick C, Zack M, Adami H. Ulcerative colitis and colorectal cancer: A population based study. N Engl J Med 1990; 323:1228–1233.

Mir-Madjlessi SH, Farmer RG, Easley KA, Beck GJ. Colorectal and extracolonic malignancy in ulcerative colitis. Cancer 1986; 58: 1569–1574.

Nugent FW, Haggitt RC, Gilpin PA. Cancer surveillance in ulcerative colitis. Gastroenterology 1991; 100:1241–1248.

Petras RE, Mir-Madjlessi SH, Farmer RG. Crohn's disease and intestinal carcinoma. A report of 11 cases with emphasis on associated epithelial dysplasia. Gastroenterology 1987; 93: 1307–1314.

Petras RE. Non-neoplastic intestinal diseases. In: Sternberg SS, ed. Diagnostic surgical pathology. 2nd ed. New York: Raven Press, 1994:1247.

Riddell RH, Goldman H, Ransohoff DF, et al. Dysplasia and inflammatory bowel disease: Standardized classification with provisional clinical application. Hum Pathol 1983; 14:951–966.

Rosenstock E, Farmer RG, Petras R, et al. Surveillance for colonic carcinoma in ulcerative colitis. Gastroenterology 1985; 89: 1342–1346.

Rubin CE, Haggitt RC, Burmer GC, et al. DNA ancuploidy in colonic biopsies predicts future development of dysplasia in ulcerative colitis. Gastroenterology 1992; 103:1611–1620.

Woolrich AJ, DaSilva MD, Korelitz B. Surveillance in the routine management of ulcerative colitis: The predictive value of low-grade dysplasia. Gastroenterology 1992; 103:431–438.

*_____

*****Editor's Note:** An additional point: four of our patients had colon carcinoma and Crohn's disease diagnosed at the same time. All were over 50. Presumably undiagnosed subtle Crohn's was present for years. Thus surveillance should start as soon as the diagnosis is made in those over 50.

INFLAMMATORY BOWEL DISEASE AND CANCER: DECISION MAKING

JOHN E. LENNARD-JONES, M.D., F.R.C.P., F.R.C.S.

There is no doubt that ulcerative colitis and Crohn's colitis are associated with a risk of colorectal cancer greater than in the general population. Patients with inflammatory bowel disease (IBD) constitute one of the high-risk groups within the wider problem of a universal liability to this form of cancer. The problem is to measure the element of increased liability in IBD and seek to reduce it toward the background level of risk we all face.

For clarity of discussion, ulcerative colitis and Crohn's disease are dealt with separately.

ULCERATIVE COLITIS

Therapeutic Possibilities

For the patient with ulcerative colitis, the big decision is whether at some stage to undergo surgical treatment for removal of the diseased colon. Very often, the correct decision is clear because the inflammation is causing so much trouble that the potential benefits of operation outweigh the possible disadvantages. For cancer prevention, the decision is often difficult because the patient is well.

Colectomy not only cures ulcerative colitis but also removes the carcinoma risk. In past years, patients wished to avoid a permanent abdominal stoma. Nowadays, the proportion of patients with ulcerative colitis who need a permanent stoma is less as reservoir procedures with ileoanal anastamosis are more commonly performed. If the operation were complication free and the patient symptomless afterwards, it would be advised and accepted more commonly than it is. In fact, there is a small postoperative mortality rate, and postoperative complications such as sepsis or obstruction can occur. Furthermore, after a pouch procedure, patients tend to pass several loose stools daily, and there is a liability to recurrent "pouchitis." Every sensible person wishes to avoid the discomfort and the time of restricted activity that major surgery entails. Add to this an element of uncertainty about the postoperative result, and a patient who has few symptoms and little disability understandably requires good evidence to justify advice that surgical treatment is needed. When, if ever, should a clinician advise a patient who is well to accept surgery?

If surgery is neither advised nor accepted, is the risk of carcinoma great enough to warrant regular precautionary measures? Are there grounds for suggesting that the patient should consult a doctor regularly? Should regular investigations be undertaken?

What is the Risk of Developing Carcinoma?

The answer to this question is not easy because it depends on the proportion of the colon inflamed, possibly on the severity of inflammation, on the duration of illness, and on the patient's age.

Extent of Disease

The literature shows that the carcinoma risk is greatest among patients in whom most or all of the colon is, or has been, inflamed. The term "extensive colitis" is widely used but with different definitions. Some series restrict the term to inflammation of the whole colon, up to and including the hepatic flexure; many series take the splenic flexure as the dividing point between "extensive" and "left-sided" colitis; and a few refer to disease proximal to the rectosigmoid as "extensive." This confusion is regrettable, and I propose that in the interests of standardization, the term "extensive colitis" should mean inflammation up to and including the splenic flexure of the colon.

Population studies show that the incidence of colorectal carcinoma among all patients with ulcerative colitis is about eight times that expected. For patients with proctitis, defined as inflammation limited to the rectum, the risk is not greater than average. For those with "left-sided" disease it is about fourfold, and for those with "extensive" disease about 20 times that expected.

Patients with proctitis can therefore be reassured that unless the extent of disease changes, they need not worry about an increased risk of cancer. For those in whom inflammation has never spread above the splenic flexure, the risk is increased but low (e.g., similar to that in healthy people with a relative who developed colorectal cancer at a relatively young age). For those in whom the inflammation has at any time involved the transverse or ascending colon, the increased risk is appreciable.

Severity of Inflammation

The definition of the extent of disease depends on the mode of diagnosis. All series before the early 1970s assessed the extent by barium enema. Originally, a single contrast technique was used that is less sensitive for showing minor mucosal disease than the double air-contrast method introduced during the 1960s. Nowadays, the extent of colitis is generally judged by endoscopy with biopsy. Endoscopic assessment of the extent tends to exceed the corresponding radiologic abnormality. Biopsy evidence of inflammation tends to exceed in extent the visual changes of inflammation. Biopsies may be abnormal throughout much of the colon when the mucosa appears normal.

There is thus a gradient of severity from mucosal ulceration or other structural changes demonstrated by single contrast barium enema to abnormal biopsies but with normal radiologic and endoscopic appearances. Series from which the risks of carcinoma have been calculated mainly relied on radiologic assessment of disease extent. We do not know if the lesser degrees of inflammation shown only by endoscopy or biopsy are associated with an increased risk of carcinoma.

As a practicality, I suggest that the extent of disease be defined from abnormalities of the mucosal line on double contrast barium enema or macroscopic evidence of inflammation seen on endoscopy during or soon after an acute episode.

Duration of Disease

All published series show a very low incidence of carcinoma during the first 10 years of disease. Carcinoma can occur during this period, but the risk is so low that it need not influence clinical decisions.

After the tenth year, patients with extensive colitis have an annual risk of carcinoma of about one in 100 per year. The largest, longest, and most complete follow-up study based on defined populations showed a cumulative increase (CI [confidence interval]) up to 25 years from onset of symptoms of 3.4 percent (CI = 1 to 5.8) at 15 years; 7.2 percent (CI = 3.6 to 10.8) at 20 years; and 11.6 percent (CI = 6.4 to 16.8) at 25 years. Other series have given similar figures at 25 years.

There is controversy over whether the annual risk increases with the passage of time after 10 years. In part, there is confusion because the gradient of life table curves tends to increase with time as the number of patients observed decreases. For the same reason, the confidence intervals widen unacceptably if the number of patients followed is low after 25 years. At present, I regard all estimates over 25 years as approximate and do not base clinical decisions upon them.

Age of Onset

The literature is divided over whether early age of onset leads to a greater cancer risk than onset later in life. Confounding variables include (1) a tendency for colitis to be more often extensive in younger than in older people, (2) the potentially long period of follow-up; and (3) the fact that the relative risk is very high among young people because colorectal cancer is so uncommon in the general population at that age. For practical purposes, the risk of young people with extensive colitis should be regarded as high because they have so many years of life ahead of them. Avoidance of cancer is also particularly important because the development of carcinoma is such a tragedy in a young person.

How Great is the Risk of Dying of Carcinoma?

If cancer can often be cured when it occurs, the pressures for prevention or early diagnosis are reduced. In fact, the likelihood of surgical cure is about the same as that for colorectal carcinoma in the general population. Overall, the crude 5 year survival rate in recent series, including disseminated tumors that are inoperable or treated palliatively, is in the range of 30 to 55 percent. For Dukes A tumors the 5 year survival rate is about 95 percent, for Dukes B 60 to 90 percent, and for Dukes C 20 to 60 percent, depending on the extent of lymph node involvement.

Thus, although the cumulative incidence of carcinoma for a patient with extensive colitis treated medically is about one in eight (12 percent) during the period of 10 to 25 years after onset, the risk of dying is less: 8 percent if 5 year survival is 30 percent and 6 percent if it is 50 percent. Since life tables refer only to patients who survive with an intact colon, mortality from cancer is in practice less because some patients die from an unrelated illness, particularly if colitis begins later in life, e.g., after the age of 50. As discussed earlier, many patients are removed from risk by colectomy.

How Can the Risk of Carcinoma be Minimized?
Prevention by Colectomy Before Development of Precancerous Change or Carcinoma

In my opinion, prophylactic colectomy for symptomless patients without dysplasia is not warranted. However, if patients are endangered by acute disease, socially disabled by chronic disease, or persistently unwell, colectomy is advisable. This is especially the case in young people for whom conservative operations are most appropriate and surgical cure offers many years of good health. The cancer risk is a factor in encouraging operation among such young people. A recent Danish series in which surgical treatment was undertaken for 35 percent of patients with total colitis within 5 years of onset, and an overall colectomy rate of almost 25 percent at 10 years, showed no increased risk of carcinoma in the total series followed for a median of 11.7 (range 0 to 26) years.

Prevention by Colectomy After Detection of Precancerous Changes

At present the only widely used marker of precancerous change is epithelial dysplasia diagnosed on biopsy, or occasionally on cytologic brushings. It is hard to prove that dysplasia if left untreated advances to carcinoma, and if so over what time scale. Recent studies have shown that the finding of low-grade dysplasia by current criteria is followed by the development of high-grade dysplasia or carcinoma in about 50 percent of patients within 5 years. Difficulties in the grading of dysplasia, which involve interobserver variation, suggest that more than one experienced pathologist should independently agree about the presence or absence of low-grade dysplastic changes. Current evidence suggests that a repeated finding of low-grade dysplasia is an indication for colectomy.

High-grade dysplasia or low-grade dysplasia associated with an elevated lesion is subject to less interobserver variation. In general, both have proved to be such a good marker of malignancy that follow-up studies have not been possible for ethical reasons. There is little doubt that either of these findings is an indication of likely present or future malignancy and is an indication for colectomy.

Cure by Colectomy Before Carcinoma has Spread Beyond the Bowel Wall

In general, a carcinoma that presents with symptoms tends to be an advanced tumor. A symptomless carcinoma may be found at a curable stage on endoscopy as an unexpected finding in the colectomy specimen after an operation performed for inflammation, or when an operation is performed for dysplasia. All grades of dysplasia can be a marker of cancer near the site of biopsy or elsewhere in the colon. In most series, high-grade dysplasia or a dysplasia-associated mass lesion are associated with undetected carcinoma in at least 40 percent of cases.

Do Regular Investigations Reduce Cancer Risk?

Screening Colonoscopy

After 8–10 Years of Disease. During the early years of disease, inflammation thought initially to be distal may spread insidiously to involve much of the colon. Such patients tend not to be recognized as in the highest-risk group and thus do not receive the same attention as other patients with extensive colitis. If patients are known to have extensive colitis, a colonoscopy at this stage excludes the presence of adenomas or dysplasia. For these reasons, I recommend a screening colonoscopy for every patient with colitis 8 to 10 years after onset.

After More Than 10 Years of Disease When no Investigation has been Undertaken for Several Years. Several series have shown that colonoscopy performed in these circumstances not only assesses the current extent and severity of inflammation but also may detect dysplasia or a carcinoma. In my own series, three patients were found to have high-grade dysplasia or a dysplastic mass at the first colonoscopy; two of these three patients had an undetected Dukes A carcinoma at operation. Among those who continued in the surveillance program, 38 others with dysplasia at the initial colonoscopy later developed carcinoma, compared with eight of 243 patients without dysplasia initially (p < .01). These findings are similar to those at the Lahey Clinic and show how a screening colonoscopy in patients with a long history of disease can detect a high-risk group.*

---

*Editor's Note: The report from Lenox Hill Hospital in New York by Woulrich, Korelitz, and their colleague also stresses the importance of finding dysplasia on the first examination.

Regular Clinical Supervision

Supervision means regular clinical consultation at yearly or more frequent intervals with a facility for early consultation at other times if new symptoms develop. The object of regular supervision is to ensure optimal use of drug therapy, to encourage patients to accept surgery if their symptoms make this advisable, and to investigate whenever there is a clinical suspicion that inflammation has extended or that a carcinoma may be present. Such supervision probably prevents deaths from acute colitis and may prevent carcinoma by encouraging surgical treatment for severe or chronic inflammation. It has not been shown to benefit the patient by early diagnosis of carcinoma.

Surveillance

Surveillance is based on two premises: (1) that a precancerous phase of colitis is recognizable so that prophylactic colectomy can be undertaken and (2) that regular investigations may detect symptomless carcinoma at a curable stage.

A surveillance program is successful only if it reduces cancer deaths; no program has been shown to achieve this aim, and the efficacy of such programs is controversial. In fact, as already shown, cancer mortality with current methods of management is likely to be low among patients with extensive colitis.

Published series fall into two groups. Series from the United States have shown a high pick-up rate at the first (screening) colonoscopy and thereafter a relatively low detection rate of dysplasia or carcinoma among those who were free of dysplasia at the first examination. Deaths from colorectal carcinoma occurred in all these series, and their value can be questioned for this reason. Studies from Scandinavia have shown a low detection rate of dysplasia and carcinoma, with no deaths, possibly in part because surveillance began at an earlier stage in the disease than in America so that patients showed no evidence of precancer initially. These results from Scandinavia and a series from England raise the issue of cost effectiveness of surveillance, because the few positive findings may not justify the effort and expense involved. My own study from England among 332 patients, all with a disease duration greater than 10 years and all with inflammation proximal to the hepatic flexure seen and followed over 21 years, has given mixed results. Eleven patients were operated on for symptomless carcinoma found at endoscopy, or in the operation specimen after colectomy for dysplasia (Dukes A8, B1, C2); all these patients survive. Twelve patients were also operated on for dysplasia without carcinoma. However, six patients developed a symptomatic carcinoma that led to death in four.†

---

†Editor's Note: There are now three U.S. groups who report prolonged survival for patients whose cancers were found as a result of surveillance, compared with patients who presented with colon cancer-related symptoms. These studies were from the Cleveland Clinic, The Lahey Clinic, and the Johns Hopkins Hospital.

At present, surveillance is not mandatory because its value is not proved. If a patient with extensive colitis wishes to be investigated regularly, and diagnostic facilities and costs allow, such a program probably offers the best way of reducing the cancer risk, although both patient and doctor need to recognize that it is not infallible.

How Should Regular Investigation Be Organized?

Selection of Patients

Those at highest risk are likely to derive the greatest benefit, i.e., patients with extensive inflammation and a total duration of symptoms greater than 10 years.

Mode of Endoscopy

About half the carcinomas in ulcerative colitis, and almost half the biopsies showing dysplasia separate from a tumor, occur in the rectosigmoid. Flexible sigmoidoscopy therefore has a role even as the only mode of examination. Colonoscopy is needed for complete examination of the colon.

Frequency of Endoscopy

In my experience, interval cancers occurred when colonoscopy was arranged every 2 years. Ideally, annual colonoscopy appears advisable, with the interval to the next examination reduced to 6 months if indefinite (probably positive) or low-grade dysplasia in flat mucosa is detected. As an alternative policy, colonoscopy alternating with flexible sigmoidoscopy at yearly intervals would probably be effective.

Number of Biopsies

A recent study suggested that 33 biopsies are needed at colonoscopy to give a 90 percent chance of detecting dysplasia if it is present. This is time consuming. Our practice has been to take an average of nine biopsies at each colonoscopy, and the detection rate of dysplasia has been satisfactory provided that results of successive endoscopies are taken into account. In view of the patchy nature of dysplasia, as many biopsies as practicable should be taken at each examination, probably between 10 and 20.*

Action to be Taken on Finding Dysplasia or Adenoma

Patients need to understand the reason for regular investigation and that, if presumed precancerous changes are found, surgery will be advised. High-grade dysplasia or dysplasia on the surface of a widespread elevated or villous lesion is an indication for operation. An adenoma is, by definition, a polyp with dysplastic epithelium. The problem in colitis is to know whether it is an isolated abnormality, common in middle-aged or elderly healthy people, or a manifestation of dysplasia. A pedunculated polyp or a polyp around which there is no evidence of dysplasia on biopsy, especially if it is found beyond the limit of inflammation and/or in a patient after the fourth decade, can be removed endoscopically and the site observed at follow-up endoscopy at 6 months and annually thereafter. An isolated broad-based polyp situated in the area of colitis in a young person should be regarded with great suspicion, and multiple biopsies should be taken to exclude dysplasia around its base or elsewhere in the colon. The probability is that this lesion is a manifestation of dysplasia in colitis. The finding of more than one such polyp, or the development of further polyps, confirms this impression, and colectomy should be advised.

Low-grade or indefinite (probably positive) dysplasia† is an indication for particularly careful repeat colonoscopy within 6 months at which more biopsies than usual are taken. If low-grade dysplasia is again found, colectomy should be advised, especially if there are any supporting indications. If this advice is not accepted or indefinite dysplasia is found, a policy of annual examination can be resumed.

CROHN'S DISEASE

A population study has shown no excessive cancer mortality in Crohn's disease of the small intestine and an excessive risk in Crohn's disease or ileocolitis similar to that found in left-sided ulcerative colitis: about four times that expected. However, a recent hospital-based study has found a cancer risk in Crohn's colitis equivalent to that in extensive ulcerative colitis. Clinical experience suggests that carcinoma in Crohn's colitis is less common than in ulcerative colitis, perhaps partly because Crohn's colitis tends to be treated by colectomy more often than ulcerative colitis.

Should Cancer Risk Influence Clinical Policy in Small Bowel Disease?

The risk is so low that the only preventive measure needed is to avoid leaving defunctioned inflamed loops of intestine at operation. Small bowel carcinomas complicating Crohn's disease usually involve areas of long-standing disease and tend to be difficult to detect at surgery, or even in an operative specimen; they are generally highly malignant.

---

*Editor's Note: Irreversible strictures in long-standing ulcerative colitis are particularly worrisome and may not permit adequate sampling.

†Editor's Note: In the Western hemisphere, some pathologists are now lumping all indefinites into one category, rather than attempting to distinguish between probably positive and probably negative.

Should Prophylactic Colectomy be Advised?

The same arguments apply as for ulcerative colitis. Dysplasia does occur in Crohn's disease but is a most unusual indication for colectomy.

Do Screening Examinations Have a Role?

When endoscopies are performed, biopsies should be taken and examined for dysplasia. A stricture should be examined with particular care.

Is Regular Supervision Likely to Influence Cancer Mortality?

Cancer can occur in chronic anorectal disease, either as a squamous carcinoma or as an adenocarcinoma of the distal rectum. Digital examination should be performed to search for induration in an anal fistula or an atypical anal ulcer. Sigmoidoscopy with biopsy is useful to seek strictures or dysplasia. When colonoscopic or radiographic investigation of new symptoms is arranged, the possibility of carcinoma should be kept in mind.

Is Regular Surveillance Indicated?

The incidence of carcinoma and of dysplasia is probably less than in extensive ulcerative colitis, and examination can be difficult because of strictures. No controlled evaluation of surveillance is available. At a time when the role of surveillance in ulcerative colitis is uncertain, it seems unwise to adopt a similar program in Crohn's colitis, in which the likelihood of success is less.*

---

*Editor's Note: Crohn's colitis may be subclinical for years, so that carcinoma and Crohn's disease are diagnosed at almost the same time in some patients, especially those over 50 years of age.

Pros and Cons of Options (Table 1)

Active Surgical Policy for Appropriate Patients During the First Few Years of Disease

Pro: If surgical result is good, this leads to cure and eliminates cancer risk.
Con: If surgical result is poor, this leads to persistent or recurrent symptoms. A permanent stoma may be needed.

Colonoscopy for All Patients With Ulcerative Colitis 8–10 Years After Onset

Pro: This may improve medical management of colitis and encourage appropriate patients with severe symptomatic and extensive disease to accept surgery. It provides a good baseline for surveillance if this is decided on.
Con: This increases the workload and may lead to unnecessary alarm among patients, especially those with proctosigmoiditis.

Screening Colonoscopy for Patients With a Long History of Unsupervised Colitis

Pro: This provides good assessment both of inflammation and of possible dysplasia or carcinoma.
Con: Nil.

Regular Clinical Supervision for all Patients With Ulcerative Colitis

Pro: This allows regular assessment of symptoms and disability, checks on growth in young people, detects anemia and treatable complications, permits review of drug therapy, provides encouragement of surgical treatment for patients with severe disability, and maintains contact with patients so that relapses or

Table 1 Pros and Cons of Treatment Options in Crohn's Disease

Options	Pros	Cons	Opinion
Colectomy for disability	Prevents cancer	Postoperative results uncertain	Outcome better than disease
Colectomy for statistical cancer risk (symptomless patient)	Prevents cancer	Postoperative results uncertain	Possible postoperative sequelae unacceptable
Colectomy for dysplasia	Prevents cancer May cure undetected cancer	Postoperative results uncertain	Postoperative sequelae acceptable
Screening colonoscopy and biopsies (occasional investigation)	Detects dysplasia and cancer	Nil	Worthwhile
Clinical supervision (investigation only for symptoms)	Optimizes medical care May encourage surgery Maintains patient contact	Symptomatic cancer tends to be advanced	Worthwhile
Surveillance (regular endoscopy and biopsy)	Colectomy for precancer and/or curable cancer in some patients	Incurable cancers occur Costly	Unproved Optional

new symptoms can be reported and treated or investigated early.

Con: This increases clinical workload and cost. It makes patients dependent on clinicians and may increase anxiety about illness.

Regular Annual Investigation by Endoscopy After 10 Years of Disease in Patients With Extensive Colitis

Pro: This may detect dysplasia and curable carcinoma.

Con: This has uncertain clinical benefit or cost effectiveness. It may reduce but does not eliminate cancer risk; it is labor intensive, and demanding on patients; and it may increase anxiety.

THE FUTURE

The chronic inflammation and rapid epithelial cell turnover associated with ulcerative colitis lead to genetic changes that predispose to carcinoma, and are in many patients manifested as dysplasia. Dysplasia has limitations but is clinically useful; the possible role of the chromosomal change measured as aneuploidy is being investigated. Selected centers should be encouraged to test gene mutations, deletions, and expression as possible future markers of neoplastic potential. New techniques of obtaining DNA for analysis from wide areas of epithelium, e.g., by brushing, washing, or search in the stool, also need investigation.

Editor's Note: The author presents a balanced and reasoned review based on extensive experience. Those of us working exclusively

at tertiary referral centers, and therefore dealing with more patients at high risk, may feel that surveillance or colectomy is essential for those with pancolitis of over 10 years' duration and especially of childhood onset.

SUGGESTED READING

Burmer GC, Rabinovitch PS, Haggitt RC, et al. Neoplastic progression in ulcerative colitis: histology, DNA content, and loss of a p53 allele. Gastroenterology 1992; 103:1602–1610.

Connell WR, Lennard-Jones JE, Williams CB, et al. Factors affecting endoscopic surveillance for cancer in ulcerative colitis. (Submitted for publication)

Ekbom A, Helmick C, Zack M, Hans-Olov A. Increased risk of large-bowel cancer in Crohn's disease with colonic involvement. Lancet 1990; 336:357–359.

Gyde SN, Prior P, Allan RN, et al. Colorectal cancer in ulcerative colitis: a cohort study of primary referrals from three centres. Gut 1988; 29:206–217.

Langholz E, Munkholm P, Davidsen M, Binder V. Colorectal cancer risk and mortality in patients with ulcerative colitis. Gastroenterology 1992; 103:1444–1451.

Lennard-Jones JE. Reply to a selected summary. Gastroenterology 1991; 100:571–572.

Löfberg R, Brostrom O, Karlén P, et al. Colonoscopic surveillance in long-standing total ulcerative colitis: a 15-year follow-up study. Gastroenterology 1990; 99:1021–1031.

Lynch DAF, Lobo AJ, Sobala GM, et al. Failure of colonoscopic surveillance in ulcerative colitis. Gut 1993; 34:1075–1080.

Nugent FW, Haggitt RC, Gilpin PA. Cancer surveillance in ulcerative colitis. Gastroenterology 1991; 100:1241–1248.

Riddell RH, ed. Dysplasia and cancer in ulcerative colitis. New York: Elsevier, 1991.

Rubin CE, Haggitt RC, Burmer GC, et al. DNA aneuploidy in colonic biopsies predicts future development of dysplasia in ulcerative colitis. Gastroenterology 1992; 103:1611–1620.

Taylor BA, Pemberton JH, Carpenter HA, et al. Dysplasia in chronic ulcerative colitis; implications for colonoscopic surveillance. Dis Colon Rectum 1992; 35:950–956.

LOWER INTESTINAL STRICTURES IN INFLAMMATORY BOWEL DISEASE

PANKAJ J. PASRICHA, M.D.
THEODORE M. BAYLESS, M.D.

ETIOLOGY AND GENERAL APPROACH TO DIAGNOSIS

Strictures of the bowel may develop as a complication of many gastroenterologic diseases. The most common cause of ileocolic colorectal strictures are inflammatory bowel disease (IBD), malignancy, diverticular disease, ischemia, and surgical anastomoses. Less common but important causes include medications (particularly nonsteroidal agents and slow-release po-

tassium preparations), radiation injury, and a variety of infectious diseases (lymphogranuloma venereum, tuberculosis, amebiasis, schistosomiasis). Idiopathic IBD is one of the most important causes of intestinal strictures. Several differences are apparent between the strictures of Crohn's disease and those of ulcerative colitis (UC), in keeping with the known pathophysiology of these two diseases (Table 1). As a general rule, strictures in Crohn's disease are far more common than in UC, preferentially involve the small bowel, and are usually benign, and are far more likely to result in intestinal obstruction.

In a broad sense, the term "stricture" applies to almost any narrowing of the bowel that alters the flow of barium or hinders the passage of an endoscope. In the absence of malignancy, the clinical importance of strictures lies in their ability to cause bowel obstruction. Bowel obstruction may be due to extreme narrowing from fibrosis, superimposed inflammation or edema, or impaction of a fibrous bolus (such as celery or corn). The clinical features are determined in large part by the site of the obstruction. Acute small bowel obstruction

Table 1 Strictures Associated With Inflammatory Bowel Disease: Key Features

	Crohn's Disease	Ulcerative Colitis
Overall incidence	30%–50%	10%
Site	Small bowel	Exclusively colon
	Colon (less common)	
Pathology	Active inflammation (transmural)	Muscular hypertrophy
		Pseudopolyps
	Fibrosis	Neoplasia
Associated cancer	Uncommon	10%
Obstruction	Common (30%–40%)	Rare

presents with intestinal pain (colic), abdominal distention, and vomiting. If the obstruction is in the distal ileum, the symptoms may be more gradual in onset. Colonic obstruction is more subtle, with most patients complaining of abdominal cramping and diarrhea. In the case of IBD, these symptoms can often be mistaken for an exacerbation of colitis.

Radiologic studies are extremely important in patients with suspected intestinal strictures and serve not only to identify the site of narrowing but also to provide valuable clues to the nature of the underlying lesion. Plain x-ray films of the abdomen usually provide the initial clue to an obstructing lesion, with the demonstration of air-fluid levels in dilated loops of bowel. However, the radiographic picture may be normal or indeterminate in some cases, particularly if the obstruction is proximally located. Contrast studies remain the mainstay of evaluation of intestinal obstruction. If colonic obstruction is suspected clinically, the first test to be ordered is a barium enema. Barium should not be given orally in this situation because water absorption from the non-obstructed proximal colon may result in the formation of concretions and the conversion of a partial obstruction to a complete one.

If the barium enema does not reveal a colonic obstruction, an attempt can be made to reflux the contrast material into the small bowel and obtain pictures of the distal ileum. In most cases of small bowel strictures, however, oral barium is the preferred contrast agent. Unlike the situation in the colon, barium does not become inspissated in the small bowel because of continuous production of intestinal secretions. However, in cases of suspected perforations, barium should not be used as it may cause an inflammatory response in the peritoneal cavity. Instead, a water-soluble material such as meglumine diatrizoate (Gastrografin) is preferred in this situation. These agents are generally less satisfactory in patients with intestinal obstruction because they do not coat the mucosa well and may become progressively less radiodense as they travel distally as water is drawn into the bowel in response to their marked hypertonicity. A routine small bowel series may fail to define the obstructing lesion in about 25 percent of cases. In such patients, enteroclysis (small bowel enema) is an ex-

tremely valuable tool in the hands of skilled radiologists and may be the procedure of choice in patients with multiple stenotic lesions, who have slow transit and excessive secretions.

Radiologically, an attempt should be made to distinguish extrinsic (e.g., adhesions) from intrinsic causes of obstruction. The former usually result in a smooth extrinsic defect with preservation of normal mucosal patterns. The configuration of an intrinsic stricture may vary with etiology or pathogenesis. The narrowing at a colocolonic anastomosis may be short and symmetric. A similar short stricture can occur at the site of a nonsteroidal anti-inflammatory drug (NSAID)- or potassium-induced ulceration or stricture as well as a lymphoma or a short segment affected with Crohn's disease. Rarely, a NSAID-related stricture takes the form of a web. The usual ileal strictures in Crohn's disease are elongated, at least for 3 or 4 cm, and most are 20 or 30 cm long with thickened mucosa and irregular margins. Primary bowel cancers may produce an apple-core appearance with overhanging edges. Cancer complicating long-standing colitis may result in an asymmetric narrowing; diverticulitis superimposed on Crohn's disease, usually in an elderly patient, may produce a symmetric narrowing.

Colonoscopy is almost invariably attempted in the work-up of strictures of the colon, and in some cases may also be successful in evaluating lesions of the terminal ileum. The pediatric colonoscope or occasionally an upper endoscope is used when the adult colonoscope is unsuccessful in traversing the strictured area. However, care must be exercised to prevent perforation, particularly in the setting of active inflammation. Endoscopy is the only method of obtaining tissue for histologic examination before surgery, and often influences the approach to management by providing information on the presence and severity of underlying inflammation, dysplasia, and malignancy. Fibrotic strictures are often short and bland in appearance, whereas active inflammation is suggested by the presence of ulcers and mucosal edema. Malignant strictures may be associated with an ulcerative or polypoid appearance. When an extremely narrowed stricture prevents direct biopsies, cytologic specimens can often be obtained by means of a brush that is carefully passed distally. Strictures in the small bowel are more problematic, as most remain endoscopically inaccessible. The role of small bowel enteroscopy in the evaluation of ileal disease remains to be fully established, but it is conceivable that in the near future, improvements in instrument design will provide new and more accurate means to evaluate this difficult group of patients. There is a separate chapter on small bowel enteroscopy. Endoscopic treatment of stricturing lesions is discussed later in this chapter.

GENERAL APPROACH TO MANAGEMENT

When confronting a stricture, the physician has to deal with several issues, the most important of which are the possibility of a neoplasm, the presence or absence of a reversible or inflammatory component, and the need for treatment. The relative importance of these questions depends in part on the nature of the underlying disease, but most often the approach to management has to be tailored to each individual case.

Ulcerative Colitis

Colonic Strictures

Ulcerative colitis can produce colonic strictures in up to 13 percent of patients but rarely results in significant obstruction (less than 1 percent of all cases of colitis). Colonic strictures in UC tend to be short (less than 3 cm) and most frequently involve the rectum and sigmoid. Because strictures secondary to UC rarely cause obstruction, the most important issue in these cases is the exclusion of cancer. Although 80 to 90 percent of radiologic strictures prove benign, any stricture in patients with ulcerative colitis should be viewed with great suspicion. Gumaste and colleagues described 70 strictures in 49 (5 percent) of 1156 UC patients; 17 were malignant. The principal features distinguishing malignant from benign strictures were

1. An appearance late in the course of UC. There was a 61 percent probability of malignancy in strictures developing after 20 years compared with 6 percent in those with a shorter duration.
2. A location proximal to the splenic flexure, which led to a 80 percent probability of malignancy compared with 4 percent in the sigmoid and 10 percent in the rectum.
3. A symptomatic large bowel obstruction, which was associated with a 100 percent probability of malignancy compared with only 14 percent in patients without obstruction or constipation.

As one might have expected, the cancers associated with strictures were more advanced: 76 percent stage D compared with only 18 percent stage D in cancers in patients without stricture.

The duration of colitis is a major risk factor for cancer, but in practice it may be difficult to assess this precisely. The illness may be present for months and sometimes years before the symptoms become obvious enough to bring the patient to effective medical attention. The extensive UC associated with primary sclerosing cholangitis may also be quite subtle clinically, and dysplasia or cancer will not be discovered if one relies on the usual colonoscopic surveillance program starting 8 years after the diagnosis of IBD.

With the above caveats in mind, a useful approach to these cases can be determined given some idea of the duration of disease. In patients with UC of relatively short duration (less than 5 years), most strictures are due to associated muscular spasm with moderate or severely active colitis. If the colitis has lasted for more than 5 years and the narrowing does not decrease

with glucagon nor improve with several months of treatment of the colitis and is present on repeat examinations, the concern for the possibility of neoplasia should increase. Sometimes, the decrease in inflammation enables the pathologist to more clearly separate the atypia due to intense inflammation and regeneration from true dysplasia. Fixed strictures in UC must be taken very seriously. If dysplasia or cancer is found or if adequate biopsies cannot be performed, colectomy is usually indicated. The absence of dysplasia in a few biopsies may be misleading. It is advisable to take multiple biopsies on either side of the narrowing as well as within the stricture. Cytologic brushings may also help. It is also helpful, if possible, to obtain multiple biopsies (e.g. three) from each of at least eight other areas of the entire colon. The most conservative and probably safest approach is to resect a persistent stricture in the colon of a patient with long-standing UC. The future availability of genetic or biochemical markers would help identify aneuploidy or dysplastic areas and, perhaps, patients at greatest risk.

Distal Colorectal Strictures

Patients with ulcerative proctosigmoiditis are not thought to be at increased risk of carcinoma. Therefore, a malignant stricture in the left colon clearly above the area of chronic proctosigmoiditis in a patient over 60 years of age may be an "incidental" carcinoma, perhaps independent of the limited IBD. In the usual kind of stricture, the decisions usually revolve around whether or not to perform a total colectomy and ileostomy. The presence of dysplasia anywhere in the large intestine usually leads to a colectomy. Some patients, especially those with already widespread carcinoma, may be best served by a palliative anterior resection of the left colon.

Crohn's Disease

Small Bowel Strictures

The differential diagnosis of Crohn's disease obstructing the terminal ileum is important to keep in mind, because we are often dependent on the radiographic appearance in disease of short duration. Other disorders that can lead to narrowing of the terminal ileum and perhaps the cecum include periappendiceal abscess, chronic appendicitis, foreign body perforation, NSAID-induced ulceration, yersinosis, aspergillosis, amebiasis, tuberculosis, histoplasmosis, carcinoma, and lymphoma. In older patients and in those on oral contraceptives, ischemia can also cause bowel narrowing.

It is useful to try to divide patients with ileal disease into three groups: (1) those with primary inflammatory disease, (2) those who have stricturing and obstruction after 8 to 10 years, and (3) those who have aggressive fistulizing disease, often requiring surgery in the first 3 or 4 years of disease.

Strictures of 5 cm or more in length that cause symptoms and signs of partial obstruction in the first 3 years of Crohn's disease or in the first few years after ileocolonic resection may be due in part to inflammatory reactions. A computed tomographic (CT) scan can often detect a phlegmon or abscess formation. Conventional radiography is also usually needed for planning management. When there is a very narrowed segment of ileum, decision making includes concerns over how much of the luminal narrowing is due to muscle hypertrophy, fibrosis, and fixed obstruction. It is sometimes assumed that fibrotic stricturing will not cause obstruction until about 7 years after the onset or postoperative recurrence of Crohn's disease. Unfortunately, this is not always true. Dilatation of the bowel proximal to a stricture suggests a prolonged duration of that narrowing even if the patient is not completely obstructed.

Treatment of the inflammatory component of a Crohn's stricture may include bowel rest with total parenteral nutrition or an elemental diet. Medical therapy may include adrenocortical steroids and antibiotics, such as metronidazole or tetracycline. Even coexistent fistulas into the adjacent mesentery or into nearby loops of ileum or colon can become quiescent as the underlying inflammation in the ileum is lessened.

An alternative approach to a terminal ileal stricture early in the course of Crohn's disease, especially if there is diagnostic uncertainty, is surgical resection. It has been argued by some that even early in Crohn's disease, this usually assures the patient a rapid recovery and spares the potential problems of steroid side effects and the subsequent prolonged need for medications. An added argument in prepubescent adolescents is the desire to eliminate a focus of inflammation that, along with inadequate nutrition, could further delay their growth. Surgical resection is discussed in a separate chapter. An approximately 50 percent chance of recurrence of ileitis has usually been cited as the reason for not recommending "early" ileal resection for more patients with very active "ileitis." Some data suggest that the recurrence rate is higher in younger patients, especially if the resection is done early in the course of the disease and for a long segment.

Almost 50 percent of patients in the "stricturing" or "nonperforating" group who have been followed in the long term appear to need a second surgery for recurrent obstruction in the neoterminal ileum. There has often been an 8 to 9 year time lag between the first surgery for obstruction and the second. Care must be taken not to push high dose anti-inflammatory or immunomodulator therapy in the face of recurrent partial obstruction or complete obstruction. Secondary fistula and sometimes perforation and abscess formation can occur at the site of fixed obstruction. Since a purulent complication may require drainage and/or a temporary ileostomy, it seems better to advise elective resection of the narrowed ileum as well as the fistulas that often arise from a very short segment. While some patients endure multiple episodes of partial or even complete obstruction, a complication necessitating emergency surgery and ileostomy may occur. Physicians and patients should recognize when underlying fixed obstruction is the process that requires correction. This is not the time to try new or hopefully more effective anti-inflammatory agents.

Adenocarcinoma occurs more often than expected within strictures in the distal ileum. The duration of disease is the key risk factor. Strictures either bypassed or still in continuity with the fecal stream are at increased risk. The average patient has had Crohn's disease for at least 20 years. Although dysplasia has been found within strictures associated with cancer, a practical surveillance program does not currently seem feasible. In the future, genetic markers within intestinal lavage or in feces may prove helpful. Unfortunately, most of the cancers are found incidentally at the time of stricture resection and are usually in an incurable stage. 5 year survival is unusual. Occasionally, lymphoma of the ileum complicating Crohn's disease is encountered.

In terms of prophylaxis after ileocolonic resection, there is no evidence that sulfasalazine, locally released newer 5-aminosalicylic acid (5-ASA) agents, or prednisone will prevent repeat stricturing. Although a trial of 6-mercaptopurine (6-MP) for prevention of postoperative recurrences is under way, it has not been our experience that azathioprine prevents recurrent obstruction in patients who appear to be predisposed to this complication.

Ideally, anticytokine agents effective in lessening muscle hypertrophy and fibrosis will become available in the future. These might be combined with current anti-inflammatory agents, perhaps locally released 5-aminosalicylates or rapidly metabolized steroids such as budesonide or metronidazole. The latter agent may be helpful if, as we suspect, colonic bacteria play a role in localization of recurrences in the neoterminal ileum.

Since surveillance for dysplasia in patients with ileal strictures is not yet feasible, resection of long-standing strictures whenever possible and avoidance of leaving bypassed segments of bowel out of the fecal stream seem to be reasonable preventive measures. Laparoscopy-assisted ileocolonic resections appear to be feasible and may solve some diagnostic dilemmas. This is discussed in the chapter on laparoscopic surgery.

Colonic Strictures

When Crohn's disease affects the colon, it is less likely to produce strictures and bowel obstruction than when it involves the small bowel. Thus, only about 20 percent of patients with Crohn's colitis develop intestinal obstruction as opposed to 40 to 50 percent of those with small bowel Crohn's. Colonic strictures in Crohn's disease have somewhat different implications from those in UC. Clinically significant obstruction is more likely in Crohn's than in UC. By contrast, the risk of developing dysplasia or adenocarcinoma in Crohn's colitis is increased compared with the control population, but probably to a lesser extent than in UC. The role of dysplasia and cancer surveillance for colonic lesions in Crohn's is controversial, and no firm guidelines are available. The onset of Crohn's may be very subtle, and therefore any surveillance program should begin at the time of diagnosis in patients over 50 years of age. Since about 25 percent of cancers occur in grossly uninvolved areas, the entire colon and accessible ileum should be sampled.

The general principles outlined above for ileal strictures apply to the management of colonic strictures in Crohn's disease. These lesions are somewhat less problematic, however, because of greater endoscopic accessibility for both diagnostic and therapeutic purposes. Balloon dilatation of colonic strictures is still in its adolescence (see below) but represents an attractive option in patients who have symptomatic colonic strictures without dysplasia.

Anorectal Strictures

Although many of the carcinomas that develop in patients with long-standing Crohn's disease are in the rectum, benign rectal strictures just inside the anal canal are not uncommon in patients with persistent rectal or perianal Crohn's disease. Most low rectal strictures are benign and secondary to laterally aggressive Crohn's disease, but this does not assure the benign nature of the stricture, especially if the patient has had Crohn's disease for over 20 years. Perhaps, as more experience accumulates, endoscopic ultrasonography may prove helpful. Squamous cell carcinoma or adenocarcinoma can occur in longstanding fistulas, sometimes without coexisting colonic or rectal dysplasia. Firm anorectal strictures are sometimes best biopsied by surgeons with the patient under anesthesia.

Conventional dilators have long been used for anorectal strictures complicating Crohn's disease, which are usually short and membranous and can often be dilated with the finger or a rigid dilator. Most can be managed by one or two dilatations. Some surgeons prescribe daily dilatation by the patient after local incisions in the stricture. We have usually continued metronidazole and/or azathioprine administration in such patients if we are convinced of the benign nature of the stricture. Rectal strictures in patients with Crohn's disease may be accompanied by aggressive and progressive perianal disease. This can result in poor healing of perineal wounds after proctocolectomy. In a British study by Linares and colleagues of 44 patients with anorectal strictures complicating Crohn's disease, 98 percent had proctitis and 93 percent had severe perianal disease with fissures, fistulas, and ulcers. Thus, control of inflammation is a necessary measure along with attempts to treat the stricture itself. If the perianal and perineal complications continue to advance despite local surgical drainage procedures, antibiotics, and anti-inflammatory therapy, perhaps including azathioprine, 6-MP, and even methotrexate or cyclosporine, many surgeons will recommend diversion of the fecal stream. This may be by

means of a colectomy and ileostomy or a colostomy with retention of the rectum. However, if the rectum is markedly diseased and contracted, its removal and a permanent colostomy are often reasonable.

In practice, if there is extensive ileal disease with varying degrees of activity, we have usually advised removal of the ileal or ileocolonic disease at the time of fecal diversion. This is based on the assumption that perianal disease may at times be the earliest manifestation of ileal Crohn's disease. The purpose of a "temporary" fecal stream diversion is presumably eventual reanastomosis of ileocolonic or colocolonic continuity. The absence of intensive rectal involvement may prove to be a key deciding factor in future successful reconnection. As a word of caution, the bypassed ileum and colon appear to be liable to perforation at the time of colonoscopy, either through ulcerated and thinned areas or through old fistulous tracts.

Anastomotic Colocolonic or Ileocolonic Strictures

Short, symmetric strictures at the site of anastomosis after a segmental colonic resection are usually benign. Again, one must remember that reliance on only a few colonic biopsies may miss dysplasia or carcinoma. When further scarring and narrowing prevents both dilatation and thorough surveillance of the entire remaining colon in a patient with 15 or more years of Crohn's disease, one is looking for any excuse to remove the strictured area.

ENDOSCOPIC BALLOON DILATATION OF STRICTURES

It is only natural that the rapidly growing therapeutic armamentarium available to endoscopists has aroused interest in nonsurgical alternatives to treat IBD-related complications such as strictures. Endoscopic dilatation of many colonic and anastomotic strictures is now technically feasible. This procedure is particularly relevant to Crohn's disease rather than UC for several reasons. Although they are usually asymptomatic, the risk of neoplasia in strictures associated with UC provides a strong impetus for surgical resection, particularly since colectomy also results in a cure for the disease. By contrast, Crohn's strictures are often symptomatic, and resection is associated with a high rate of recurrence at the anastomotic site, requiring additional surgery.

The availability of through-the-scope (TTS) balloon dilators has been a major advance in the treatment of gastrointestinal (GI) strictures. These dilators have several advantages compared with the traditional Savary or Eder-Puestow systems. They do not require fluoroscopy or a guidewire, are flexible, and avoid the potential of shear injury resulting from the generation of longitudinal forces.

The technique of balloon dilatation is fairly straightforward and similar to that used in other areas of the gut.

It is based largely on empirical principles, and there are few data to favor any particular approach. An 18 mm balloon is usually employed at the onset, although in some cases diameters up to 25 mm have been used (the latter require a 4.2 mm channel, which is not available in the standard adult colonoscope). Balloons are available in various lengths (3 to 8 cm); the longer balloons are technically easier to maintain within the stricture. An 18 mm TTS balloon that is often used for esophageal dilatation often suffices. After correct placement of the balloon across the stricture, it is inflated by air or water (the latter is preferred, because it is not compressible) to the maximal specified pressure (35 psi for an 18 mm balloon) and held in place for usually 1 to 3 minutes. The procedure may be repeated up to as many as four times per session. Occasionally, in difficult cases, a guidewire has to be passed initially through the stricture and the balloon catheter introduced over it.

The largest series to date in this evolving field have been reported from Europe and are summarized in Table 2. Favorable factors that predicted long-term success in these studies were a long interval between the resection and development of symptomatic stenosis (presumably representing less aggressive disease) and the absence of active disease at the stricture. Local disease activity almost invariably resulted in poor long-term outcome.

A word of caution is due about transendoscopic balloon dilatation of colonic strictures at any locale. If the stricture is at the site of a previous fistula, there is a risk of perforation and reopening of the fistulous tract. Abdominal CT scans, barium enemas, and/or upper GI–small bowel series are sometimes performed, but are not essential, before dilatation to assess disease elsewhere and to avoid dilating the site of an unexpected small bowel fistula.

Although balloon dilatation has most commonly been applied to anastomotic strictures, it is increasingly being used at other sites of involvement in Crohn's disease, including duodenal, colonic, and anorectal strictures.

Other Endoscopic Techniques

Some authors have attempted to treat difficult strictures with more aggressive measures, including the use of electrocautery incision (using a needle-knife or standard papillotome) and neodymium: yttrium-aluminum-garnet (Nd:YAG) laser. Two or three short radial incisions are made and the stricture may then be dilated by a balloon. However, although these procedures are intriguing, there is not enough information on their safety and efficacy for them to be recommended for general use.

RECOMMENDATIONS

Lower intestinal strictures in a patient with presumed IBD pose a series of questions for the physician and surgeon. Is the patient symptomatic from the strictures? What is the nature of the underlying bowel disease? What is the cause of the stricture, whether it be active disease, scarring, or neoplasm? Is exploratory laparotomy and resection necessary for diagnosis? What is the best management strategy? Resection? Balloon dilatation? If treatment is safe and successful, how long will the benefit last? What is the ideal management for the underlying disease? In the future, can this type of stricture be prevented? Strategies vary for strictures in the colon, rectum, and ileum. Duodenal, jejunal, and ileal strictures are discussed in the chapter on surgery for Crohn's disease. Distal ileal strictures early in the course of the illness may not need to be resected, in contrast to the usual ileal stricture 8 to 10 years after onset of the disease or after a previous resection. Anastomotic stricturing may require different approaches depending on the time since surgery and the length of the stricture. Transendoscopic balloon dilatation can be helpful for long-duration, short-length anastomotic strictures that are not in an area of active disease.

Table 2 Results of Endoscopic Balloon Dilatation of Bowel Strictures

	Brysem et al	Blomberg et al	Total
Total no. of patients	18	27	45
Anastomotic	14	27	
Terminal ileum	4		
Total procedures	26	139	165
Technical success	16	27	43 (96%)
Short-term improvement	14	27	41 (91%)
Long-term (>1 yr) improvement	8	18	26 (58%)
Median follow-up	25 mo	19 mo	
Complications	0	Perforation, 1 Hemorrhage, 2	3 (7%)

SUGGESTED READING

Bedogni G, Ricci E, Pedrarolli C, et al. Endoscopic dilation of anastomotic colonic stenosis by different techniques: an alternative to surgery. Gastrointest Endosc 1987; 33:21–26.
Blomberg B. Endoscopic treatment modalities in inflammatory bowel disease. Endoscopy 1992; 24:578–581.
Blomberg B, Rolny P, Jarnerot G. Endoscopic treatment of anastomotic strictures in Crohn's disease. Endoscopy 1991; 23:195–198.
Breysem Y, Janssens JF, Coremans G, et al. Endoscopic balloon dilation of colonic and ileo-colonic Crohn's strictures: long-term results. Gastrointest Endosc 1992; 38:142–147.
Dinneen MD, Motson RW. Treatment of colonic anastomotic strictures with "through the scope" balloon dilators. J R Soc Med 1991; 84:264–266.
Fregonese D, DiFalco G, DiToma F. Balloon dilatation of anastomotic intestinal stenoses: long-term results. Endoscopy 1990; 22:249–253.
Graham M. Stricture formation: pathophysiologic and therapeutic concepts. In: MacDermott RP, Stenson WF, eds. Inflammatory bowel disease. New York: Elsevier Press, 1992:323–336.
Gumaste V, Sachar DB, Greenstein AJ. Benign and malignant colorectal strictures in ulcerative colitis. Gut 1992; 33:938–941.
Kozarek RA. Hydrostatic balloon dilation of gastrointestinal stenoses: a national survey. Gastrointest Endosc 1986; 32:15–19.

Lashner RA, Turner BC, Bostwick D, et al. Dysplasia and cancer complicating strictures in ulcerative colitis. Dig Dis Sci 1990; 35:349–352.

Linares L, Moreira LF, Andrews H, et al. Natural history and treatment of anorectal strictures complicating Crohn's disease. Br J Surg 1988; 75:653–655.

Neufeld DM, Shemesh EI, Kodner IJ, Shatz BA. Endoscopic management of anastomotic colon strictures with electrocautery and balloon dilation. Gastrointest Endosc 1987; 33:24–26.

Williams AJ, Palmer KR. Endoscopic balloon dilatation as a therapeutic option in the management of intestinal strictures resulting from Crohn's disease. Br J Surg 1991; 78:453–454.

ACUTE COLONIC PSEUDO-OBSTRUCTION (OGILVIE'S SYNDROME)

DAVID T. WALDEN, M.D.
NORMAN E. MARCON, M.D., F.R.C.P.C

Acute colonic pseudo-obstruction (ACPO) is a dangerous complication of serious medical and surgical diseases that occurs in hospitalized patients. Luminal dilatation compromises arterial circulation and thus may lead to ischemic injury, mural necrosis, and perforation. The diagnosis of ACPO is suggested by x-ray films obtained to investigate progressive abdominal distention and mild pain along with a reduction in stool volume. Radiographically, a dilated, gas-filled cecum and proximal colon are seen. Risk factors and conditions associated with the development of ACPO are listed in Table 1.*

THERAPEUTIC GOALS

The goal of therapy for ACPO is prevention of colonic perforation, with its mortality rate of 43 to 75 percent, while exacerbating factors are removed and the precipitating disorder is aggressively managed. Early recognition requires a high index of suspicion in susceptible patients. Risk factors for increased mortality from ACPO include advanced age, a cecal diameter greater than 14 cm, distention lasting more than 7 days, and the need for surgical therapy. Assessment of cecal diameter and exclusion of mechanical obstruction are necessary in order to select the most appropriate initial management.

Exclusion of mechanical obstruction or volvulus is made either radiologically or at colonoscopy. A water-soluble contrast enema (Gastrografin) should be administered, and the examination terminated once the dilated segment is reached. The high osmotic character of this agent helps promote evacuation of the distal bowel, with a subsequent decrease in distention. Barium should be avoided because it interferes with visualization if colonoscopy becomes necessary.

MANAGEMENT SELECTION

Cecal diameter is normally 3.5 to 8.5 cm. The perforation risk is low when the diameter is less than 12 cm, but has occurred in 23 percent of patients with diameters greater than 14 cm. Cecal diameters of up to 25 cm have been reported without subsequent perforation in some cases of ACPO. Because of the imperfect correlation between cecal diameter and perforation risk, thresholds ranging from 9 to 14 cm have been arbitrarily chosen above which early decompression is advocated. In contrast, a series of 24 cancer patients with ACPO has been reported in which conservative management alone resolved dilatation in 96 percent of cases without the need for decompression.

As there is no consensus regarding management

Table 1 Conditions Associated With Acute Colonic Pseudo-Obstruction

Medical	Surgical
Sepsis	Coronary bypass
Pneumonia	Craniotomy
Meningitis	Lumbar laminectomy
Myocardial infarction	Spinal surgery
Congestive heart failure	Fracture reduction
Acute pancreatitis	Hip replacement
Acute cholecystitis	Nephrectomy
Acute appendicitis	Cystectomy
Renal failure	Herniorrhaphy
Liver failure	Cesarean section
Metastatic carcinoma	Therapeutic abortion
Systemic lupus erythematosus	Hysterectomy
Drugs	Metabolic/toxic
Narcotic analgesics	Hypokalemia
Anticholinergics	Hyponatremia
Tricyclic antidepressants	Hypocalcemia
Calcium channel blockers	Hypomagnesemia
Clonidine	Hypophosphatemia
	Hypothyroidism
Neurologic	Diabetes
Stroke	Alcoholism
Organic brain syndrome	Lead poisoning
Parkinson's disease	
Guillain-Barré syndrome	Miscellaneous
Multiple sclerosis	Idiopathic
Myotonic dystrophy	Trauma
	Burns
	Mechanical ventilation

*****Editor's Note:** Lest we forget, Ogilvie's patients had metastatic carcinoma thought to be causing neurogenic colonic distention.

selection, we have adopted the following approach based on clinical evaluation and radiologic criteria. Stable patients presenting with cecal diameters of 9 to 12 cm are managed conservatively (see below) and are followed with plain abdominal films every 12 hours. Patients with initial cecal diameters of 12 to 18 cm may also be given a brief trial of conservative management provided that they are clinically stable, but should undergo colonoscopic decompression if a response is not evident within 12 to 24 hours. Prompt colonoscopic decompression is indicated for patients in whom there is massive distention (cecal diameter greater than 18 cm), progressive dilatation despite conservative measures, or deterioration in clinical status as manifested by increased distention or pain. Peritoneal signs or radiographic evidence of perforation are indications for urgent laparotomy.

MEDICAL MANAGEMENT

Initial supportive measures are appropriate in all cases of nonperforated ACPO and are summarized in Table 2. A nasogastric tube is placed to low intermittent wall suction and patients are given nothing by mouth. Volume status is optimized and electrolyte disturbances are addressed. Of particular importance are identification and correction of potassium, calcium, phosphorus, and magnesium deficiencies. Drugs known to interfere with bowel motility, including narcotic analgesics, anticholinergics, phenothiazines, tricyclic antidepressants, calcium channel blockers, and clonidine, are discontinued. Oral laxatives have no role in the management of ACPO, but gentle tap water enemas are helpful if formed stool is present in the rectum or left colon. Unless there is evidence of sigmoid distention, a rectal tube is not required. Decompression may be aided by rolling the patient from side to side and into the prone position. There have been isolated reports of successful resolution of ACPO after pharmacologic therapy with erythromycin (a motilin agonist), 250 mg intravenously (IV) every 8 hours in one patient and cisapride, 10 mg IV every 4 hours in another. Metoclopramide has not been useful.

Conservative management alone is effective in resolving dilatation in 32 to 96 percent of cases of ACPO

Table 2 Initial Management of Acute Colonic Pseudo-Obstruction

EXCLUDE MECHANICAL OBSTRUCTION	Discontinue offending drugs, especially narcotic analgesics
PLAIN ABDOMINAL FILMS EVERY 12–24 HR	Tap water enema +/− without rectal tube
NPO	Frequent changes in patient position
Nasogastric suction	?Erythromycin
Optimize volume status	?Cisapride
Correct metabolic disturbances: Potassium, calcium, phosphorus, magnesium	

but is associated with a recurrence rate of about 30 percent. Patients should be examined frequently and followed with plain films of the abdomen every 12 to 24 hours until decompression is documented. Colonoscopic decompression is indicated if the cecal diameter remains above 12 cm for more than 24 hours, if progressive dilation occurs, or if there is worsening abdominal distention or pain.

COLONOSCOPIC DECOMPRESSION

Colonoscopic decompression (CD) of ACPO was first described in 1977. Placement of a transanal decompression tube at the time of the initial procedure allows ongoing decompression, minimizes the risk of recurrence, and should be performed in all cases in which CD is attempted. Percutaneous endoscopic cecostomy has been described, but experience with this technique will be limited given the success of CD with tube placement. It should be emphasized that decompression techniques do not provide specific therapy for ACPO but instead reduce the risk of complications while the underlying precipitating factors are addressed. Decompression techniques are not appropriate when there is peritonitis or suspected perforation.

Technique

CD is performed in the unprepared bowel, but tap water enemas may be given shortly before the procedure to eliminate formed stool from the rectum and left colon. Oral bowel preparation is contraindicated. Fluoroscopy is highly recommended to facilitate decompression tube placement, but CD may be successfully performed without fluoroscopy in patients who cannot be transported.

If available, a large-channel therapeutic colonoscope allows more effective irrigation and suctioning. The colonoscope is advanced using minimal air insufflation and copious irrigation. Insertion to the cecum usually proceeds in a timely manner but can be tedious. The dilated proximal colon may be reached in most cases; insertion to at least the hepatic flexure is usually necessary to achieve effective decompression.

The mucosa of the proximal colon and cecum should be evaluated for signs of ischemic injury such as duskiness or ulceration. If ischemia is encountered, decompression should be carried out without further advancement and prompt surgical consultation obtained. Mucosal ischemia seen at colonoscopy is an ominous finding. Clearly, some patients with ischemia do not require surgery, but the characteristics that define these individuals have not been delineated. Most patients with extensive ulceration are best treated surgically, as they are poorly tolerant of perforation and its sequelae.

Simple decompression may be achieved by slowly withdrawing the colonoscope while applying suction until luminal collapse is observed. This traditional technique alone will decompress the dilated segment in about 85 percent of cases, but a recurrence rate of about 50 percent limits its usefulness.

Transanal Tube Placement

To prevent recurrences, transanal decompression tube placement should be performed whenever CD is carried out. Although it adds a few minutes to the procedure time, this modification is technically simple. With the colonoscope positioned in the right colon or cecum, a 480 cm (0.035 inch) endobiliary wire sheathed inside a 6 Fr biliary stent introducer catheter for added stiffness is advanced into the lumen. With fluoroscopy to confirm position of the wire tip, the colonoscope is removed over the sheathed guidewire while suctioning is employed to effect initial decompression. The choice of decompression tube may include a commercially available device specifically designed for this purpose, or an enteroclysis tube or nasogastric tube at least 140 cm in length with additional holes cut near the tip. The tube is lubricated and inserted over the wire with fluoroscopic guidance. Should looping occur, axial rotation of the tube about the guidewire may facilitate passage. If fluoroscopy is not available, tube decompression may be achieved by direct insertion of a 250 cm, 10 Fr nasobiliary catheter modified with additional holes through the biopsy channel of the colonoscope into the cecum or right colon without the need for a guidewire. In this case, appropriate tube position may be confirmed with a portable abdominal film.

After the procedure, the guidewire is removed and the tube secured to the inner thigh with tape. The tube is connected to low intermittent suction and irrigated with 100 ml of water every 2 hours or whenever there is a suspicion of clogging. Cecal diameter and tube position should be verified by daily plain films of the abdomen until dilation has resolved, which usually occurs in 3 to 6 days. The tube may be safely left in place for longer periods if necessary and often passes spontaneously once colonic motility resumes. If dilation persists or recurs, migration or clogging of the tube should be considered and repeat CD performed as necessary.

The reported complication rate of CD is approximately 3 percent, with perforation occurring in about 1 percent of cases. There have been no complications in our series of 30 patients undergoing CD. The overall mortality rate of CD is 1 percent, which compares favorably with about 25% in nonperforated ACPO patients undergoing surgical decompression.

SURGICAL THERAPY

Because CD is effective, is widely available, and may be repeated as necessary, surgical decompression is rarely required. In cases in which decompression is indicated but colonoscopy is unavailable or has been unsuccessful, tube cecostomy may be performed, taking into account the same indications as outlined earlier for CD. The procedure may be carried out under local anesthesia and provides effective decompression through a large-caliber tube, but carries a mortality rate of 12 to 30 percent. When no longer necessary, the tube may be removed with the expectation of spontaneous stoma closure. The recent development of laparoscopic cecostomy awaits further evaluation.

Laparotomy is required when there is clinical or radiographic evidence of perforation, and in most patients in whom ischemic changes are identified at colonoscopy. The extent of ischemic injury and the presence or absence of fecal soilage determine the choice of procedure. In some patients, resection of a limited area of ischemic cecum with exteriorization may suffice, whereas complete cecal resection by right hemicolectomy is required in individuals with more extensive injury. The mortality rate of laparotomy is approximately 40 percent, largely attributable to severe concurrent illness in many patients.

OTHER TECHNIQUES

Percutaneous computed tomography–guided needle decompression of the cecum by the retroperitoneal approach has been described as an adjunct to therapy for ACPO, but it is unlikely that this technique will ever become widely used given the ease and availability of CD. Epidural anesthesia had a beneficial effect in about 50 percent of patients with refractory ACPO in a small series, but this requires further evaluation before it can be recommended.

SUGGESTED READING

Bachulis BL, Smith PE. Pseudoobstruction of the colon. Am J Surg 1978; 136:66–72.

Dorudi S, Berry AR, Kettlewell MGW. Acute colonic pseudo-obstruction. Br J Surg 1992; 79:99–103.

Fausel CS, Goff JS. Nonoperative management of acute idiopathic colonic pseudo-obstruction (Ogilvie's syndrome). West J Med 1985; 143:50–54.

Gosche JR, Sharpe JN, Larson GM. Colonoscopic decompression for pseudo-obstruction of the colon. Am Surg 1989; 55:111–115.

Harig JM, Fumo DE, Loo FD, et al. Treatment of acute nontoxic megacolon during colonoscopy: tube placement versus simple decompression. Gastrointest Endosc 1988; 34:23–27.

Sloyer AF, Panella VS, Demas BE, et al. Ogilvie's syndrome. Successful management without colonoscopy. Dig Dis Sci 1988; 33:1391–1396.

Vanek VW, Al-Salti M. Acute pseudo-obstruction of the colon (Ogilvie's syndrome). Dis Colon Rectum 1986; 29:203–210.

COLLAGENOUS AND LYMPHOCYTIC (MICROSCOPIC) COLITIS

WILLIAM J. TREMAINE, M.D.

DIAGNOSIS AND CLINICAL FEATURES

Collagenous colitis and lymphocytic (microscopic) colitis are syndromes characterized by chronic watery diarrhea and specific histologically seen abnormalities of the colonic mucosa. In both, there are increased numbers of lymphocytes in the colonic surface epithelium and crypt epithelium, and a mixed but predominantly mononuclear infiltrate in the lamina propria. Also, in patients with collagenous colitis, there is a collagen band beneath the surface epithelium. Because of the identical symptoms and the similar histologic features in collagenous colitis and lymphocytic colitis, there is controversy over whether these syndromes are different manifestations of the same disease process or different diseases. The pathogenesis of these disorders is unknown, but the association of collagenous colitis with celiac sprue, inflammatory arthritis, autoimmune thyroid disease, diabetes, chronic hepatitis, and type A atrophic gastritis suggests an immune disorder triggered by foods, infection, medication, or environmental toxin. In some studies, serologic markers of autoimmune disease are more common in collagenous colitis than in lymphocytic colitis. However, immunoglobulin and complement deposits have not been found in tissue to confirm that these are primarily autoimmune disorders.

Collagenous colitis and microscopic colitis may be considered as idiopathic inflammatory bowel diseases, but there is no evidence that either predisposes to the development of ulcerative colitis or Crohn's disease. Collagenous colitis occurs more commonly in women. In contrast, women and men develop lymphocytic colitis with equal frequency. Middle-aged adults are most commonly affected, although there are reports of microscopic colitis in children as young as 1.5 years, and either condition may develop in older adults, even those in their 80s. A familial occurrence with one first-degree relative affected has been reported in two families. Symptoms include watery diarrhea with three to seven stools a day on average, although some patients may have profuse diarrhea with 1 to 2 L per day of stool and cramping abdominal pain of mild to moderate severity. Hematology and blood chemistry study results are usually normal or mildly and nonspecifically abnormal. Recent studies show an increased frequency of positive anti-nuclear cytoplasmic antibodies (ANCAs) in patients with collagenous colitis compared with normals or patients with infectious colitis, but the frequency is not as high as in patients with ulcerative colitis or Crohn's disease. Currently, ANCA positivity is not helpful in the diagnosis but may be a clue to the pathogenesis. On colonoscopic or flexible sigmoidoscopic examination, the colonic mucosa appears normal in about 50 percent of cases; in the remainder there are mild abnormalities with patchy erythema, edema, or granularity. Histologically apparent abnormalities may be patchy and in some patients are noted just in the right side of the colon. Rectal biopsies alone can miss the diagnosis of collagenous colitis in up to 20 percent of cases.

TREATMENT STRATEGIES

Medical therapy for collagenous and lymphocytic colitis is empiric; no controlled treatment trials have been performed for either. Although symptoms may resolve spontaneously, they usually persist for several years and necessitate intervention. Enthusiasm for medical treatment should be tempered by the risks of side effects from long-term treatment with some medications, particularly corticosteroids. The histologic abnormalities essential to the diagnosis of these conditions may resolve completely. Usually, when the histologic picture has normalized, the symptoms have also resolved. The symptoms of collagenous and lymphocytic colitis are often indistinguishable from those of irritable bowel syndrome (IBS). As a consequence, some patients with collagenous or lymphocytic colitis may have persistent bowel symptoms despite normalization of histologic appearance because of pre-existing IBS. Therefore, a decision to discontinue specific therapy should be based on both histologic and symptomatic resolution. The histologic abnormalities may be patchy, and biopsies should be taken from several sites at follow-up examinations to minimize the risk of a sampling error.

Symptomatic Therapy

If the symptoms are mild, nonspecific treatment is worth a try. However, patients who respond to symptomatic therapy usually do not obtain complete relief. Patients may improve with bulk agents such as psyllium, hemicellulose, or cellulose, 1 or 2 tsp twice a day. Antimotility agents such as diphenoxylate hydrochloride and atropine (Lomotil), loperamide hydrochloride (Imodium), or deodorized tincture of opium may be used alone or in combination with bulk agents. Some patients improve with cholestyramine, 2 to 4 g three times a day. The antidiarrheal effect of cholestyramine has been attributed to its ability to bind bile acids, but a recent report raised the possibility that in collagenous colitis cholestyramine controls diarrhea by binding a yet-to-be-identified bacterial cytotoxin. Pepto-Bismol has been effective in some patients.

Other medications that can also cause diarrhea should be discontinued if possible. In particular, nonsteroidal anti-inflammatory drugs may induce diarrhea and endoscopic and histologic abnormalities in the colon. Other agents such as antibiotics, diuretics, antihypertensives, and cardiac medications may worsen the diarrhea because of underlying collagenous or lymphocytic colitis. The possibility of coexisting lactose intolerance or of a high dietary intake of fructose or caffeine should be considered.

Anti-Inflammatory Therapy
Sulfasalazine and Other 5-Aminosalicylates

Most of the anti-inflammatory agents used to treat ulcerative colitis and Crohn's disease have also been employed for collagenous and microscopic colitis. Sulfasalazine, 2 to 4 g per day in divided doses, appears to be effective in a number of uncontrolled studies. The dosage can be gradually increased from one 500 mg tablet the first day by adding an additional tablet daily up to the final dose. Folic acid, 1 mg daily, may be given along with sulfasalazine to avoid deficiency due to competitive inhibition of absorption of folate. Blood counts may be checked after 1 week of treatment to identify the rare patient who develops anemia or leukopenia; counts can then be monitored at 6 month intervals. Patients who respond usually improve within 2 to 3 weeks. If symptomatic remission is achieved, the dose may be tapered after 3 months by one tablet every 2 weeks to the lowest effective dose, or as low as 1 g twice a day. About 50 percent of patients treated with sulfasalazine improve on treatment.

Side effects with sulfasalazine are common. Dose-related symptoms occur in about 20 percent of patients and include anorexia, nausea, headache, and dyspepsia. Other less common adverse reactions are fever, rash, hepatitis, pancreatitis, alveolitis, and cytopenia. Reversible male infertility may also occur. For patients with a history of sulfa allergy and those who have had adverse reactions to sulfasalazine, other 5-aminosalicylic acid (5-ASA) compounds may be used. Three oral preparations, olsalazine (Dipentum) and mesalamine (Asacol and Pentasa), are available for prescription use in the United States to treat ulcerative colitis. Each has been used in patients with collagenous and lymphocytic colitis with apparent benefit, although no controlled trials have been made and none is approved by the Food and Drug Administration for these indications. The usual dose of Dipentum is 500 mg twice a day, for Asacol 800 mg three times a day, and for Pentasa 500–1,000 mg b.i.d. to q.i.d.; the dosage of each can be increased to 3 to 4.8 g per day if necessary to control symptoms. Patients who respond usually improve within 2 to 3 weeks. Once symptomatic control is achieved, the dose may be gradually tapered. Side effects occur with the oral 5-ASA drugs in less than 10 percent of patients. Since collagenous colitis and lymphocytic colitis often involve the proximal colon, 5-ASA enemas and suppositories are unlikely to be effective.

Corticosteroids

Oral corticosteroids may be used alone or in combination with sulfasalazine or the 5-ASAs. Prednisone in a single morning dose of 20 to 30 mg controls symptoms in most patients. Those who respond usually improve within 1 week. After 4 weeks of symptomatic remission, the dose may be tapered by 5 mg each 2 weeks to the lowest effective dose. For patients with recurrent symptoms, the dose may be increased again by 5 to 10 mg to control symptoms, and then maintained at that level. After about 3 months of treatment, the colon biopsies should be repeated. If resolution is seen histologically, the dose of prednisone can be tapered again. For patients also on sulfasalazine or oral 5-ASA, the prednisone can usually be tapered and discontinued without an immediate recurrence of symptoms, although exacerbations requiring repeat courses of steroids may occur. Alternate-day steroids can be considered, particularly for patients who are unable to taper and discontinue therapy because of recurrent symptoms. For the rare patient who requires hospitalization for intravenous (IV) fluids because of severe diarrhea with dehydration, IV steroids such as methylprednisolone, 30 mg twice a day, are indicated. Corticosteroid enemas would probably not be effective in view of the typical generalized colonic involvement. Because of the great potential for side effects with prolonged corticosteroid use, particularly in the older age group that usually develops collagenous or lymphocytic colitis, alternative therapies such as 5-ASA should be started once a symptomatic response is achieved and continued as prednisone is tapered and discontinued. Therapy should continue until follow-up biopsies confirm histologic resolution.

Other Specific Treatments

Antisecretory therapy has been attempted with the somatostatin analog Sandostatin, and also with clonidine and indomethacin, all without success. Perhaps this reflects a multifactorial cause of the diarrhea in these conditions. Chlorpheniramine, 32 mg per day, has been effective in the treatment of microscopic colitis in a patient with increased mast cells in the ileal and colonic mucosa. Metronidazole, 250 mg three or four times a day, appeared to be effective in some patients, although the appropriate duration of therapy is unclear. The antimalarial agent quinacrine improved the symptoms in some patients, but the potential side effects, such as fatal aplastic anemia, make it an unlikely choice for treatment. Mepacrine has also been said to be useful.

The immunomodulatory agents 6-mercaptopurine, azathioprine, and cyclosporine are used to treat other inflammatory bowel diseases. So far, there are no reports of the use of these drugs for collagenous or lymphocytic colitis. Rarely, patients may have severe symptoms with these conditions despite medical therapy. Nevertheless, there appears to be no role for colectomy, diverting ileostomy, or other surgical intervention.

TREATMENT OF ASSOCIATED DISORDERS

As noted, a number of other medical conditions have occurred in association with collagenous and lymphocytic colitis. For some of these, diarrhea is a common feature, and treatment may ameliorate the symptoms of collagenous or lymphocytic colitis. Celiac sprue and nonspecific small intestinal villous atrophy have been reported in association with collagenous colitis. Patients with collagenous or lymphocytic colitis who have steatorrhea or other evidence of malabsorption should undergo small intestinal biopsies to search for these conditions. Even when there is no other evidence of malabsorption, a small bowel biopsy should be considered in a patient with collagenous colitis who fails to respond to the usual therapies. If villous atrophy is found, small bowel bacterial overgrowth and giardiasis should be excluded. Thereafter, a gluten-free diet is indicated, in addition to standard therapy for collagenous colitis. Conversely, a patient with celiac sprue who fails to respond to diet restrictions should be evaluated for coexistent collagenous or lymphocytic colitis. Protein-losing enteropathy has been found in a patient with collagenous colitis, apparently due to marked protein loss from the abnormal colonic mucosa. In such a patient, the fecal alpha$_1$-antitrypsin level as well as the colonic histologic picture could be followed to assess the response to treatment. Both hyperthyroidism and hypothyroidism have been reported in patients with collagenous and lymphocytic colitis, and either condition may complicate therapy. Patients who also have diabetes mellitus are at risk for bacterial overgrowth, celiac sprue, pancreatic insufficiency, or diabetic diarrhea.

Although there is no proof that they are predisposed to develop other bowel diseases, a few patients with collagenous or lymphocytic colitis have been reported with coexistent inflammatory bowel disease or colorectal cancer. With this in mind, a complete evaluation of the colon should be performed at the time of diagnosis of collagenous or microscopic colitis, either with colonoscopy or flexible sigmoidoscopy plus barium enema, to rule out other pathology. Once the diagnosis is made, follow-up evaluations of the entire colon depend on the patient's response to treatment and the clinical course. At present, there are no data to suggest that patients with collagenous colitis or lymphocytic colitis are at increased risk for malignancy of the colon, and intensive periodic surveillance for dysplasia or malignancy does not appear justified.

SUGGESTED READING

Baum CA, Bhatia P, Miner PB. Increased colonic mucosal mast cells associated with severe watery diarrhea and microscopic colitis. Dig Dis Sci 1989; 34:1462–1465.

Carpenter HA, Tremaine WJ, Batts KP, Czaja AJ. Sequential histologic evaluations in collagenous colitis. Correlations with disease behavior and sampling strategy. Dig Dis Sci 1992; 37: 1903–1909.

DuBois RN, Lazenby AJ, Yardley JH, et al. Lymphocytic enterocolitis in patients with "refractory sprue." JAMA 1989; 262:935–937.

Giardiello FM, Lazenby AJ, Bayless TM, et al. Lymphocytic (microscopic) colitis. Clinicopathologic study of 18 patients and comparison to collagenous colitis. Dig Dis Sci 1989; 34:1730–1738.

Stark ME, Batts KP, Alexander GL. Protein-losing enteropathy with collagenous colitis. Am J Gastroenterol 1992; 87:780–783.

van Tilburg AJP, Lam HGT, Seldenrijk CA, et al. Familial occurrence of collagenous colitis. A report of two families. J Clin Gastroenterol 1990; 12:279–285.

Wang KW, Perrault J, Carpenter HA, et al. Collagenous colitis: a clinicopathologic correlation. Mayo Clin Proc 1987; 62:665–671.

SOLITARY RECTAL ULCER SYNDROME

MALCOLM G. ROBINSON, M.D.
HATTON SUMNER, M.D.

DEFINITION, DIAGNOSIS, AND SYMPTOMS

Although the initial description of solitary rectal ulcer syndrome (SRUS) included the presence of rectal ulceration ascribed to mucosal damage from inspissated stool, it is now known that the syndrome can occur in the absence of ulceration in up to one-third of patients or may involve multiple ulcers in a similar number. If ulcers are present, they tend to occur 7 to 10 cm above the anal verge, with white, gray, or yellow bases and surrounding hyperemic mucosa. Patients without ulcers may have mucosal nodularity or actual polypoid lesions. Diagnosis is dependent on endoscopic or surgical biopsy in this somewhat variable clinical setting.

The biopsy appearance is usually characteristic, especially in the early or preulcer phase of the disease. The features include hypertrophy of the muscularis mucosae, fibromuscular obliteration of the lamina propria, and hyperplasia of the crypt epithelium. Ulcers or more superficial surface erosions are superimposed on these early diagnostic features in most, although by no means all, patients.

Rectal bleeding is present in over 90 percent of patients with SRUS, together with very frequent dyschezia, anorectal pain, mucorrhea, diarrhea, or constipation. Many patients admit to self-digitation in an attempt to facilitate defecation. Mucosal prolapse is common and should be diligently sought, including examination of patients squatting and straining.

The pathophysiology of SRUS in many patients appears to be related to repeated mucosal trauma from prolapse due to straining during defecation. This can sometimes be demonstrated by defecography.

NATURAL HISTORY AND DIFFERENTIAL DIAGNOSIS

Rectal ulceration varies over time, but complete healing occurs in less than 10 percent of patients. Symptoms do not correlate with the presence or absence of ulceration. SRUS must be differentiated from a variety of diseases both inflammatory and neoplastic. A major feature distinguishing SRUS from Crohn's disease or ulcerative proctitis is that the latter entities, in addition to possessing clinical and pathologic features of their own, do not typically show the fibromuscular obliteration of the lamina propria so characteristic of SRUS. In some patients, epithelial hyperplasia is a prominent histopathologic feature of the biopsy, causing consideration of a neoplastic process. The hyperplastic epithelium can assume a somewhat villous configuration and be mistaken for a villoglandular polyp, especially if the lesion appeared polypoid endoscopically. A few patients show epithelial glands displaced deeply into a fibrotic submucosa (colitis cystica profunda), which can mimic an invasive carcinoma. The inflammatory cloacogenic polyp presenting at the anorectal transition zone is another variant of this syndrome.

TREATMENT

Various medical therapies have been advocated for this syndrome, but there is no evidence to support use of diet, avoidance of "straining," topical steroids, or 5-aminosalicylic acid.

Local surgical excision of ulceration and cauterization techniques have been advocated, but results have been variable and long-term follow-up data are minimal. Diverting colostomy has been undertaken for severely symptomatic patients and produced satisfactory alleviation of symptoms. In the presence of documented mucosal prolapse, surgical prolapse repair seems at least theoretically justified. However, the existence of over 100 different surgical procedures for rectal prolapse suggests that no procedure is ideal for all patients. At least one report from St. Mark's Hospital describes favorable results from combined anteroposterior rectopexy in the particularly difficult group of symptomatic patients who have SRUS without overt rectal prolapse.

SUGGESTED READING

Andrews NJ, Jones DJ. ABC of colorectal diseases. Rectal prolapse and associated conditions. Br Med J 1992; 305:243–246.

Bogomoletz WV. Solitary rectal ulcer syndrome. Mucosal prolapse syndrome. Pathol Annu 1992; 27:75–86.

Ford MJ, Anderson JR, Gilmour HM, et al. Clinical spectrum of "solitary ulcer" of the rectum. Gastroenterology 1983; 84:1533–1540.

Levine DS. "Solitary" rectal ulcer syndrome. Are "solitary" rectal ulcer syndrome and "localized" colitis cystica profunda analogous syndromes caused by rectal prolapse? Gastroenterology 1987; 92:243–253.

Nicholls RJ, Simson JNL. Anteroposterior rectopexy in the treatment of solitary rectal ulcer syndrome without overt rectal prolapse. Br J Surg 1986; 73:222–224.

FECAL INCONTINENCE

ARNOLD WALD, M.D.

Fecal incontinence is an embarrassing and often socially incapacitating problem that occurs in all age groups. Incontinence may occur in otherwise healthy individuals with acute severe diarrhea, but most patients with chronic fecal soiling exhibit abnormalities of one or more of the following: mental status, stool consistency, defecation, rectal sensation, rectal storage capacity, function of the anal sphincters or anorectal reflexes, and pelvic floor muscles.

A careful medical history and physical examination should suggest the cause of fecal incontinence as well as the possible pathophysiology in most patients. In many cases, additional information of value may be obtained from diagnostic evaluation using anorectal manometry, dynamic radiographic studies of the anorectum, and neurophysiologic testing of the pelvic floor and anal sphincters.* Manometry accurately measures anorectal sensory and motor function, including rectal sensation and compliance, resting anal sphincter tone, and squeeze pressures. Proctography employs cinefluoroscopic techniques to evaluate anorectal structure and function during rectal retention and defecation, whereas electromyographic (EMG) studies can assess the innervation of the external anal sphincter and puborectal muscles after traumatic injury, and identify reinnervation of these muscles in patients with suspected pelvic neuropathy. In addition, measurements of pudendal nerve conduction help to identify the presence of peripheral neuropathy. Such information helps in planning treatment for many patients with fecal incontinence and in clarifying the pathogenesis of fecal soiling associated with a variety of disorders (Table 1). Interpretation of these techniques is best when experienced individuals are available to perform and analyze the studies.

---

*__Editor's Note:__ Endoscopic ultrasonography may prove helpful in the future, especially when considering surgical repairs. (Sultan AH, et al. Anal endosonography in fecal incontinence: the new gold standard in diagnosing sphincter defects. Gastroenterology 1993; 104:589.)

Table 1 Rectosphincteric Abnormalities Associated With Fecal Incontinence

Groups	Reservoir	Sensory	Sphincter
Adults			
Sphincter trauma	N	N	A
Pelvic neuropathy	N	N	A
Diabetes mellitus	N	A	A
Neurogenic	N	A	A
Inflammatory bowel disease	A	N	N
Ileoanal anastomosis	A	N	N
Children			
Encopresis	N	A	N
Spina bifida	N	A	A
Imperforate anus	A	N	A

N = often or always normal; A = often or always abnormal.

TREATMENT STRATEGIES IN ADULTS

The management of fecal incontinence involves strategies designed to correct abnormal continence mechanisms and to ameliorate diarrhea, if present. These approaches include measures to alter colonic function, enhance puborectal and anal sphincter function, improve rectal sensation, and correct anorectal anatomic derangements. Optimal management requires careful assessment of possible causes of fecal incontinence in each patient.

Anal Sphincter Dysfunction

Patients with rectosphincteric abnormalities include those who have sustained sphincteric trauma through injury or surgery and many patients with pelvic floor neuropathy; the latter often exhibit weakness of the puborectal muscle as well.* Generally, these patients have normal rectal sensation and storage capacity and may present with or without diarrhea.

Biofeedback

Biofeedback based on the classic techniques of Engel and associates is a simple and effective treatment for patients in this category. The method utilizes the manometer used for diagnostic studies; the recording apparatus provides information (biofeedback) about anorectal responses so that the patient can tell whether anal sphincter responses are being performed appropriately. Thus, biofeedback is a trial-and-error learning

---

*Editor's Note: There are some recent endosonographic studies of incontinence following childbirth- or episiotomy-associated sphincter/pelvic floor injuries. Hopefully, additional therapeutic concepts can be applied for these often quite symptomatic women. (Sultan et al. Anal sphincter damage occurs in 80% of forceps but only 24% of vacuum deliveries: a major determinant for the development of fecal incontinence. Gastroenterology 1993; 104:588.)

process using a visual display to monitor anal sphincter responses.

Before biofeedback is performed, the importance of the external sphincter to fecal continence is explained and patients are shown how their sphincteric responses differ from normal. Biofeedback conditioning is then carried out in three phases (Fig. 1).

Phase 1. Patients are asked to contract the external anal sphincter while they watch the recording of the sphincteric responses. A normal response is illustrated and patients are praised when they produce an appropriate contraction. The ability to make an appropriate contraction is achieved through trial and error; the first phase ends when the subject produces that response repeatedly on request.

Phase 2. The appropriate contraction response is then synchronized with rectal distention (which also elicits internal sphincter relaxation). Responses are monitored by having patients watch the recording to ensure appropriate synchronization with internal sphincter relaxation.

Phase 3. Patients are weaned from the instrument by blocking their view of the recordings. During this phase, patients are informed by the instructor when sphincteric responses are appropriate. When this occurs repeatedly, the training session ends; sessions last approximately 30 to 60 minutes.

Subsequently, patients are instructed to practice sphincter contraction exercises three to four times daily and to contract the sphincter whenever they sense rectal distention or urgency. Routine reinforcement sessions are infrequently needed for adults and are reserved for those whose initial response is suboptimal or in whom relapses occur.

Prerequisites for successful biofeedback include appropriate motivation, ability to comprehend and follow directions, a threshold of sensing rectal distention in the normal range, and ability to contract the external anal sphincter or gluteal muscles. Success has been achieved in more than 70 percent of patients who meet these requirements.

Surgery

In general, surgery for incontinence should be considered only after conservative measures have failed. Exceptions are gross rectal prolapse, since surgical resuspension restores continence in approximately half of these patients, and acute damage to the external anal sphincter, which is best managed by direct primary repair. There is a separate chapter on surgical aspects of incontinence.

The large number of surgical procedures advocated for fecal incontinence suggests that no single technique is best for all cases. Most sphincter repairs are performed at a time remote from an identifiable injury or in the absence of an identifiable cause. After surgery, approximately 80 percent of patients regain continence of solid stool, but note somewhat poorer results with liquid stool. Because poor surgical results are associated

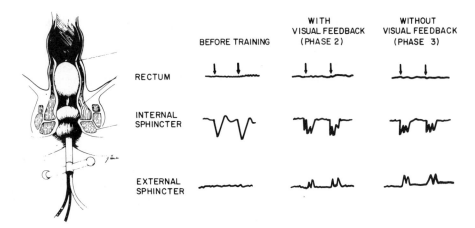

Figure 1 Three phases of biofeedback training for patients with anal sphincter dysfunction.

with neuropathy of the pelvic floor, preoperative EMG and nerve conduction studies may help identify those patients who might do poorly with sphincter repair only.

Postanal repair had been advocated in the United Kingdom to treat patients with a poorly functioning but anatomically intact sphincter. The levator ani, puborectal, and external sphincter muscles are plicated posteriorly to restore the anorectal angle and tighten the anal canal. Early studies reported that continence was satisfactory in 80 percent of patients, but subsequent studies with a longer follow-up indicated less satisfactory results. Anterior repair has been the preferred approach in the United States; satisfactory outcomes have been reported in 62 percent of patients with idiopathic fecal incontinence and 71 percent of those with a traumatic etiology. The chapter on surgical aspects provides more information.

Incontinence with Diarrhea

In some patients, fecal incontinence develops only with the occurrence of diarrhea. Liquid stool may be more difficult to perceive and, particularly when associated with urgency, more difficult to retain. Thus, diarrhea may uncover underlying abnormalities of anorectal continence mechanisms that result in fecal soiling. Rarely, massive diarrhea may overwhelm normal continence mechanisms.

Despite the presence of anorectal dysfunction, fecal incontinence can often be controlled by successfully treating the diarrhea. If a specific cause of diarrhea cannot be identified, nonspecific approaches to alter stool consistency or colonic motility often prove helpful. Therapeutic approaches include bulk laxatives, anticholinergics, antidiarrheal agents, and bile acid–binding resins.

In disorders such as diarrhea-predominant irritable bowel syndrome (IBS) and idiopathic low-volume diarrhea, bulk laxatives may help regulate bowel habits and decrease stool water content. Drinking smaller amounts of water than is usually recommended when consuming bulk laxatives may be helpful in this regard. Although anticholinergic drugs may decrease colonic motility and abdominal cramping, side effects are not uncommon. I prefer agents such as loperamide, which is prescribed in doses of 2 to 4 mg and adjusted according to the clinical response rather than administered after each episode of diarrhea. The maximum dose of 4 mg four times a day is rarely necessary, and a single morning or nighttime dose is often sufficient. I prefer diphenoxylate as a second-line agent and avoid codeine for long-term control because of its potentially addictive properties. There is some evidence that loperamide, but not diphenoxylate, improves anorectal continence mechanisms as well.

It has been suggested that bile acid–binding agents such as cholestyramine and colestipol hydrochloride may be helpful in ameliorating diarrhea and fecal incontinence in patients with radiation enteritis, IBS, choleretic enteropathy, and idiopathic diarrhea with previous cholecystectomy. Appropriate doses are 4 g cholestyramine resin or 5 g colestipol hydrochloride in the morning, or at night if the patient has undergone cholecystectomy.

Diabetes-Associated Fecal Incontinence

Fecal incontinence occurs in up to 20 percent of diabetic patients, most of whom have diarrhea as well as peripheral and autonomic neuropathy. Most of these patients have rectosphincteric abnormalities, and more than 50 percent have impairment of conscious rectal sensation.

I begin biofeedback in diabetic patients by employing rectal sensory conditioning in those who have abnormal conscious rectal sensation. I attempt to decrease the threshold of conscious rectal sensation in the following manner. Once the smallest volume of rectal distention sensed by the patient is determined, progressively smaller distention volumes are administered in decrements of 1 to 5 ml of air. When a given distention volume is sensed repeatedly, the volume is decreased and the process repeated until no further improvement can be achieved.

After sensory discrimination training, the biofeedback program proceeds in a manner identical to that for patients with normal rectal sensation. Loperamide may be helpful in those who do not respond to biofeedback. Good to excellent results have been obtained in more than 70 percent of a relatively small number of diabetic patients.

Neurogenic Injury

Fecal incontinence may occur with injury to the sacral or suprasacral spinal cord. Rectal sensation is frequently lost and external sphincter denervation is common. Sensory and motor function should be assessed by manometry in patients who appear to retain some muscle and sensory function.

Treatment of suprasacral lesions consists of attempting bowel retraining using planned regular defecation. If patients have recognizable warning symptoms of impending defecation such as dizziness or piloerection, they may be able to anticipate defecation and transfer to a toilet. In others, digital rectal stimulation or a glycerin suppository may stimulate evacuation. If such measures are ineffective, a stimulant laxative suppository such as bisacodyl may be required. If all these measures prove unsatisfactory, a low-bulk diet combined with a stool softener and small amounts of loperamide to produce constipation may decrease unwanted soiling. A weekly enema, followed if necessary by a bisacodyl suppository (Dulcolax, 10 mg) to promote colonic evacuation, should be administered to prevent fecal impaction.

Patients with sacral lesions often have fecal retention because of poor contractility of the distal colon and rectum. I prefer a low-bulk diet with stool softeners (see above) to minimize stool build-up. Bisacodyl suppositories are administered every 2 to 3 days to promote rectal emptying. This can be supplemented by digital evacuation daily to minimize fecal build-up. If continence cannot be established, a diverting colostomy can be created.

Impaired Reservoir Capacity

Patients with impaired reservoir capacity include those with idiopathic inflammatory bowel disease involving the rectum, radiation proctitis, chronic rectal ischemia, colectomy with ileoanal anastomosis, and sphincter-saving procedures for rectal lesions. Therapeutic approaches depend on the underlying disease processes. Rectal urgency and incontinence due to idiopathic proctitis often respond to steroid or 5-aminosalicylate retention enemas.* These may be supplemented with loperamide or diphenoxylate to control

diarrhea and cramping. Patients with soiling associated with ileoanal anastomosis often lack localizing rectal sensation. Therapeutic approaches include reducing fecal volume through fiber restriction, use of loperamide or diphenoxylate to prolong transit and promote fluid and electrolyte intestinal absorption, and attempted defecation after meals. With time, rectal or ileal capacity may improve to restore continence in some patients.

"Overflow" Incontinence

"Overflow" soiling associated with fecal impaction is not infrequent in elderly patients who are physically immobilized. Liquid stools that seep around the obstructing fecal bolus may be misdiagnosed as diarrhea. A rectal examination to rule out impaction is mandatory before treating diarrhea or incontinence in an elderly or debilitated patient.

Treatment consists of phosphate enemas (Fleet), given once or twice daily until there is no fecal return. If the impaction is hard, a mineral oil enema (Fleet) to soften the stool should be administered. Digital removal, an unpleasant task, is rarely necessary. Failure to evacuate the colon adequately is the most frequent reason for treatment failure.

Once evacuation is complete, preventive measures should be taken. Once a week, a phosphate enema or a bisacodyl suppository will ensure periodic colonic evacuation and prevent recurrence of soiling.

TREATMENT STRATEGIES IN CHILDREN†

Encopresis

Most children with encopresis have constipation and overflow soiling, often associated with megarectum or megacolon. The correct diagnosis is made by rectal examination or abdominal x-ray films. As with adults, initial management consists of thorough colonic evacuation with enemas. I administer twice daily enemas (4 ½ ounce disposable phosphate or 1 quart of warm tap water administered by bag drip) for 2 to 3 days; occasionally, children must be hospitalized to accomplish this critical task.

After colonic evacuation, 1 or 2 tbsp of lactulose (Chronulac) are given twice daily to produce one or two soft, formed stools per day. Sorbitol in equivalent doses is an excellent low-cost substitute. This is combined with a bowel training program in which the child is instructed to sit on the toilet 20 minutes after a selected meal (preferably breakfast) to take advantage of the gastrocolic reflex. A footstool should be used so that the child's legs are firmly supported. A calendar is kept to record the patterns of defecation and soiling. Punishment is forbidden at any time. The lactulose or sorbitol is

---

*Editor's Note: Patients with proctitis may be unable to retain an entire 5-aminosalicylate 100 ml enema when first instituted. Use of 500 mg suppositories or half of an enema for a few days may lessen inflammation and increase retentive capacity.

---

†Editor's Note: Although this section is also in the chapter on childhood constipation, I thought that two somewhat different approaches could be interesting.

tapered and eventually discontinued after continence has been maintained for about 6 months. However, recurrences are not uncommon and treatment must be reinstituted. Thus, careful follow-up for recurrent problems is required for such children.

Office counseling is generally sufficient if individual or family problems are uncovered, but more formal psychotherapy may be necessary in some cases. Fecal incontinence in children without constipation or fecal impaction suggests severe underlying psychopathology and responds poorly to treatment.

Spina Bifida

Fecal incontinence is often associated with constipation in children with spina bifida. Sphincter denervation and decreased anal tone occur in most children, and rectal sensation is often impaired. With good bowel programs, fecal impaction can be avoided and satisfactory continence is often achieved.

Toilet training should be started at age 2 or 3 years by placing the child on a commode 20 to 30 minutes after a meal. Rectal evacuation can be aided by manually increasing abdominal pressure or by the Valsalva maneuver. Insertion of a glycerin suppository shortly after the child eats may promote defecation. If such measures are unsuccessful, a 2 ¼ ounce disposable phosphate enema is administered 30 minutes after meals to evacuate the distal colon.

In some patients, toilet training is unsuccessful or diarrhea is a problem. A constipating diet low in fiber and lactose (in lactose-intolerant children), supplemented by small doses of loperamide or diphenoxylate to reduce stool frequency, may be helpful. Phosphate or warm tap water enemas once or twice a week will prevent fecal impaction. Laxatives and cathartics should be avoided unless enemas cannot be retained or are ineffective.

Some children with spina bifida have been successfully treated with biofeedback techniques in which gluteal muscle contraction substitutes for the external sphincter. Although few children are eligible, a successful outcome can be gratifying in terms of independence and control over a bodily function. Potential candidates should be strongly motivated and able to learn, be capable of standing or ambulating without full leg braces, and have normal rectal sensation by objective testing. Approximately four to six reinforcement sessions at 2 week intervals are required, unlike biofeedback training in adult patients.

Imperforate Anus

Fecal incontinence may be variously associated with a decrease in rectal compliance, anal sphincter weakness or dysfunction due to poor surgical placement, or stricture with fecal impaction and overflow incontinence. A full diagnostic evaluation is necessary, since treatment approaches differ according to the abnormalities present. Biofeedback may be effective for external sphincter dysfunction alone; anal dilation, bowel cleansing, and bowel training as previously detailed are effective if constipation and impaction are present. Decreased rectal compliance or capacity is difficult to correct surgically. Measures to reduce stool volume, combined with constipating drugs and weekly or twice weekly enemas, may be employed in such patients.

SUGGESTED READING

Caruana BJ, Wald A, Hinds JP, et al. Anorectal sensory and motor function in neurogenic fecal incontinence. Gastroenterology 1991; 100:456–470.

Engel BT, Nikoomanesh P, Schuster MM. Operant conditioning of rectosphincteric responses in the treatment of fecal incontinence. N Engl J Med 1974; 190:645–649.

Madoff RD, Williams JG, Caushaj PF. Fecal incontinence. N Engl J Med 1992; 326:1002–1007.

Miller R, Orrom WJ, Corness H, et al. Anterior sphincter plication and levatorplasty in the treatment of faecal incontinence. Br J Surg 1989; 76:1058–1060.

Read M, Read NW, Barber DC, et al. Effects of loperamide on anal sphincter function in patients complaining of chronic diarrhea and fecal incontinence and urgency. Dig Dis Sci 1982; 27:807–814.

Wald A, Tunuguntla AK. Anorectal sensorimotor dysfunction in fecal incontinence and diabetes mellitus: modification with biofeedback therapy. N Engl J Med 1984; 310:1282–1287.

ANORECTAL DISORDERS

LEE E. SMITH, M.D.

INTERNAL AND EXTERNAL HEMORRHOIDS

Please see the subsequent chapter on hemorrhoids.

ANAL FISSURE

Ordinarily, the patient with a fissure has pain, which is noted during a bowel movement or just after a bowel movement. The pain is self-limited and wanes until the next bowel movement when the pain may recur. The patient may note that there is a small amount of blood, usually bright red, but this is not always present. The patient may also note that there is a small lump on the margin of the anus which they often confuse with a "hemorrhoid." They specifically blame this skin tag, the sentinel tag, for the pain. Actually, the fissure site is just inside the anal margin from the tag.

Examination of these patients is your chance to make a friend. The patient is extremely anxious that you are going to hurt him or her with a digital or endoscopic examination. If the proper symptoms are present, the examination can stop as soon as the fissure is identified. Of course, anoscopy and sigmoidoscopy may be performed later when there is no pain. By simply separating the buttocks, one may see the sentinel tag if it is present, and the fissure will be obvious with a little retraction at the margins of the anus to separate the skin in the midline. The classical place for a fissure is in the midline, usually posterior. A few occur in the anterior midline, especially in females. The classic triad includes the finding of the sentinel skin tag, the fissure and a hypertrophied anal papilla inside at the level of the fissure. The fissure ordinarily occurs over the distal margin of the internal sphincter. This is not variable. If the fissure is found more proximal near the dentate line or on the perianal skin or in a lateral position, then think of other pathologies that might be represented by an ulcer.

The course of an acute fissure is one of healing, and there is a chance that it may stay healed. Frequently, hard bowel movements will crack open the fissure again. Pain results in some spasm, and the spasm results in some pain. The finding of a *tense internal anal sphincter* is part of the basic pathophysiology. This tense sphincter permits laceration of the anoderm in the anterior or posterior midline. Diarrhea enhances sphincter tone as the patient tries to cope with the loose stool. Often the patient has repeated episodes of acute fissuring with healing, and eventually the margins of the ulcer become scarred and white, showing its chronicity. Likewise, the skin tag and the papilla begin to form. The white chronic appearance is different from the initial acute red fissure that is noted.

I initially treat the patient with warm sitz baths and a bulk-type stool softener. It is important to keep the patient from having a hard stool or having diarrhea. A bulk stool softener offers the patient the best chance of healing. The patient has one month to heal the fissure, or he may opt for a partial internal sphincterotomy. If healing ensues but recurs, the patient may want to have an operation anyway.

When medical management has failed, a partial lateral internal sphincterotomy may be performed in either an open or closed fashion under local anesthesia in the office. It is a very straightforward operation for someone who knows the anatomy well.

ANORECTAL ABSCESS

Correct diagnosis is key to directing the patient to the proper management. The patient with an abscess complains of pain, but it is usually somewhat slower in onset, is not necessarily associated with a bowel movement, and is not necessarily associated with discharge but is progressively more agonizing and painful. The pain may be throbbing, and it often keeps the patient from sleeping. Physical examination usually reveals a red, hot, swollen, tender site where the patient directs your attention. An exception is the deep posterior anal space abscess. The patient points to the posterior aspect of the anus where one might expect to find a fissure, but nothing is evident. However, the throbbing pain is exaggerated when a digital examination is tried, and a tender, bulging site is found in the posterior midline, high in the anal canal.

Incision and drainage is appropriate whenever an abscess is identified. Most abscesses can be treated in the office. Only about 10 percent are so large or deep that the formal operating room is necessitated. Antibiotics and sitz baths are not appropriate to buy time or to "allow the abscess to become fluctuant." When an abscess is suspected, it should be drained within the day.

The drainage of an abscess is straight forward. The most fluctuant or central site on the abscess is chosen. A quick-acting local anesthetic solution such as 1 percent lidocaine or 1 percent chloroprocaine with epinephrine may be employed. A fine 30 gauge needle may be used to inject the solution at the designated site. An area about the size of a quarter should be infiltrated. The epinephrine will blanche the tissue so that the surgeon can see where the anesthetic lies. In the face of an infection, an unusually large amount of anesthetic is required, because in the acid pH found in the area of an infection, the basic anesthetic solution is readily neutralized. Having numbed the site, a cruciate incision is made and is carried down into the abscess cavity. The purulence will rush out when the cavity is entered. The cruciate incisions are made 2 cm long. This "X" shape creates four corners which can be trimmed off to be certain that the wound does not tend to close and coapt, possibly allowing recollection of pus. Occasionally, I place a small gauze wick into the abscess cavity. Should there be bleeding, it might be packed tightly. I have never taken a patient to the formal operating room for additional drainage if it has been localized to one quadrant of the anus. If the infection seems to extend across midline, suggesting a horseshoe abscess, then it is appropriate to get better anesthesia for multiple incisions and drainages.

FISTULA IN ANO

A fistula is the result of an abscess that has been drained either by surgical means or spontaneously. The origin of the abscess is generally a closed infection of the crypts and glands at the level of the dentate line. Infection of these anal glands results in a pocket of pus which may empty back into the anal canal or which may track between the sphincter muscles creating a path which becomes the fistula. The fistula is like a tunnel which extends from a point within the anal canal, usually at the dentate line, to a point on the skin. The difficult and most important distinction is how much muscle is involved between the two openings. The chance that an abscess will heal spontaneously after it is drained is about 50 percent. Fistulas may heal at the skin level and reabscess subsequently.

The treatment for a fistula is surgical. The critical determination is how much muscle can be cut without creating gross incontinence. Generally speaking, fistulas that lie below the dentate line may be incised, even if it includes both internal and external sphincters. Muscle above the dentate line should be spared during the procedure. The most common type fistula is called intersphincteric in which the track runs from the internal opening between the internal and external sphincter to the skin. The internal sphincter can be laid open readily with minimal dysfunction. A transphincteric fistula traverses both the internal and external sphincter muscles. If it lies below the dentate line, it can be incised. High lying tracks which run to a point above the dentate line often have side tracks from the posterior midline in the horseshoe fashion and usually require staged operations.

At the first operation all of the track except for the sphincter muscle are layed open. Sometimes a seton is looped through the track and left in place. The wound heals down around the seton leaving a fine track. At a second operation, the muscle can be incised. Most simple fistulas below the level of the dentate line can be performed with sedation and local anesthesia. The more complex fistulas require general anesthesia and often require evaluation under anesthesia for staging and completion of the fistulotomy.

RECTAL PROLAPSE

In this predominantly female disorder, the rectum everts out through the anus and may be visualized by the examining physician. The patient may need to strain while sitting on a toilet to make it intussuscept out. It is important to differentiate a true rectal prolapse from a mucosal or hemorrhoidal prolapse. In true prolapse the folds of mucosa appear as concentric rings. Constant manual pressure almost always reduces it. In the mucosal or hemorrhoidal prolapse the individual hemorrhoidal columns evert out as separate mounds of tissue creating visible clefts between the bundles of tissue. The occult rectal prolapse is not easy to detect because the patient complains of straining with bowel movements and a sense of incomplete evacuation; yet it can only be suspected by digital examination and sigmoidoscopy. Cine radiography usually shows the intussusception. Before repair is considered, the symptoms should be significantly incapacitating. Solitary rectal ulcer may be noted in some patients who have prolapse. True rectal prolapse is an intussusception of the full thickness rectal wall. As the intussusception progresses, traction on the adjacent nerve results in a neuropathy, which in turn, leads to an incompetent sphincter. A digital examination will help define how competently the sphincter squeezes and how much tone is present. Because of the possible loss of continence, the prolapse should be repaired electively after it is discovered. The issue of a solitary rectal ulcer and prolapse is discussed in a separate chapter.

There is no good medical management. Patients who are reasonable risks for a general anesthesia should have a repair by abdominal approach. I prefer to perform a rectopexy and an anterior resection which both fixes the rectum and takes out the redundancy which permits the intussusception to occur. The recurrence rate is minimal. Most recently, laparoscopy offers a minimally invasive approach to the abdomen for these repairs.

Some surgeons use a mesh to fixate the rectum to the sacrum posteriorly. I have found that obstruction may result, and constipation is often worsened.

In elderly and poorer risk patients, a perineal procedure may be a good alternative. Perineal rectosigmoidectomy may be performed with good relief of symptoms. In this procedure, the prolapse is extracted as far as it can be pulled, and carefully excised. Then the cut edges are reapproximated and inverted back through the anus into the pelvis.

In bedridden patients, who are nursing problems, an anal loop may be placed to encircle the anus and narrow the anal opening. Local anesthesias may be employed. This holds the rectum up above the levator sling. Failure occurs if they erode and become infected; however, after healing, the anal loop may be reapplied.

PRURITUS ANI

Pruritus ani is an unpleasant perianal sensation characterized by itching. This occurs more often in men, and is usually idiopathic. Poor anal hygiene seems to be a major contributing factor, although neurogenic, psychogenic and local allergic reactions play a role. On physical examination the skin may be normal, red and excoriated, or white and lichenified. Seek first a primary etiology, such as infection with fungi, yeast, or bacteria, local superficial neoplasm or primary disease for which the itching is simply a peripheral manifestation.

Treatment is usually symptomatic. Assure the patient that there is no significant underlying pathology, especially cancer, if this has been verified, and instruct him to carefully clean and dry the perineum at least two times or more without scratching or rubbing which may excoriate the skin even more. Use of a hair dryer or patting to dry is preferable to rubbing with a towel or dry toilet tissue. A water soluble 1 percent hydrocortisone cream often alleviates the acute flare up. Avoid fluorinated or over 1 percent hydrocortisone topicals, because it may atrophy the skin with chronic use. Some foods, especially coffee, tea, dairy products, beer, chocolate, cola, citrus fruit and alcohol have been named as contributing "dietary allergens." An elimination diet to see whether there is improvement as possible offending substances are deleted from the diet, may help the patient to find a food which might better be permanently discontinued. In extreme cases, antihistamines may be of value. Diphenhydramine hydrochloride (Benadryl) 25 mg four times per day may suffice. There is no place for surgical treatment in these patients who simply itch.*

ANAL CROHN'S DISEASE

Crohn's disease may present as isolated anal disease but more frequently it is associated with other sites of involvement. About 25% of patients with ileal Crohn's disease also have anal manifestations. By contrast, 75 percent of patients with Crohn's colitis also have anal Crohn's disease. If the rectum is involved, the anus is almost always involved as well. The patient mainly complains of pain, discharge, and soiling. Examination reveals local skin tags, fissures, abscesses, and/or fistulas. In time these conditions may lead to incontinence. In general, treatment is directed at the complications of the disease as conservative management fails. A collection of pus should be drained. These patients do not heal well and sometimes antibiotics promote more rapid resolution of the local inflammation. Patients usually have diarrhea and there is need to slow bowel motility. Loperamide (Imodium) or diphenoxylate hydrochloride (Lomotil) may be employed to slow the bowel. Sulfasalazine, 5-amino-salicylic acid, steroids, or immunosuppressive agents may be added when the disease flares. Restricting the diet or using total parenteral nutrition may reduce the fecal output and enhance healing. Oral metronidazole has been touted as a fistula-healing medication, but the value is far less than initial reports suggested.

For patients who have painful fissures that do not

abate under good medical management, examination under anesthesia is used to identify fissures that may respond to sphincterotomy and abscesses that may be drained. In patients who have complex fistulas traversing the sphincter muscles, the muscles should be preserved and setons (drains) may be placed through the fistula tracts. The seton is a fixed, passive drain which offers the possibility of reduction in abscess pain.

Rectovaginal fistulas may be left untreated if they are causing minimal symptoms. On the other hand, symptomatic fistulas may be improved by advancement of a flap of mucosa to cover the defect. The success rate for Crohn's patients is lower than in patients who are otherwise normal. Unroofing of fistulas may result in poor healing when the disease is active. Division of muscle should be avoided in these poor healing patients.

Ultimately, incontinence is likely when there is extensive disease affecting the sphincter. Disease that is unresponsive to medication or local surgery may require proctectomy or proctocolectomy to deal with the severe unrelenting symptoms. Unlike ulcerative colitis, if the colon, rectum, or portions of the colon appear to be normal, they may be spared.†

AIDS AND ANORECTAL DISEASE

Fifty percent of patients who subsequently are diagnosed as having Acquired Immunodeficiency Syndrome (AIDS) present with anorectal pathology; sometimes this is the first symptom. This manifestation is usually an infection, such as an abscess, a fistula, a proctitis, or a fissure. Other opportunistic infections may attack the anal area as well as the rest of the gastrointestinal tract as the immune mechanism fails. Malignancies of the anorectum are being reported with increasing frequency. Thus ulcers or indurated sites merit biopsy. The use of surgery for these patients should be carefully weighed because healing is often poor. If the immune mechanism is adequate, minor surgical procedures might be entertained to treat fissures that are severely painful. Incision and drainage is indicated for discrete abscesses. If AIDS is the diagnosis, consider and test for other sexually transmitted diseases. Various spirochetes, bacteria, viruses, and parasites find their way to the anorectum. For fistulas and abscesses, setons may be placed through the tracks and tied, to be left in place permanently. These permanent drains may avert the recollection of pus and the attending pain. I use the soft rubber vessel loops as setons.

SEXUALLY TRANSMITTED DISEASES

Sexually transmitted diseases (STD) seem to be exceeded only by the common cold and influenza in

---

*Editor's Note: Breaking the cycle of excessive use of topical anesthetic creams, which can be sensitizing agents, may be helpful.

†Editor's Note: Endoscopic ultrasound may provide useful preoperative and intraoperative information. Also defunctionalization via colostomy has apparently been helpful in some patients.

Table 1 Diagnostic Tests for Enteric STDs

Pathogen	Test
Spirochete	
Treponema pallidum	Dark field microscopy, FTA, VDRL serology
Bacteria	
Neisseria gonorrhoea	Gram stain, culture
Chlamydia trachomatous	Monoclonal antibody, culture
Shigella sp.	Stool culture
Campylobacter fetus	Stool culture
Salmonella typhimurium	Stool culture, blood culture
Mycobacterium avium	Mucosal biopsy and culture, acid fast stain of stool
Virus	
Condyloma acuminata	Clinical identification, biopsy
Herpes simplex	Biopsy, culture, monoclonal ab.
Cytomegalovirus	Biopsy, culture
Human immunodeficiency	ELISA, Western blot
Yeast	
Candida	Culture
Cryptosporidiosis	Biopsy, acid fast stain of stool
Isospora	Biopsy, acid fast stain of stool
Protozoa	
Entamoeba histolytica	Stool examination
Giardia lamblia	Stool examination

FTA = fluorescent treponemal antibody absorption test; VDRL = Venereal Disease Research Laboratory; ELISA = enzyme-linked immunosorbent assay.

Table 2 Suggested Treatment of Sexually Transmitted Disease

Neisseria gonorrhea proctitis	Ceftriaxone 250 mg IM once, plus doxycycline 100 mg po b.i.d. for 7 days
Chlamydia trachomatis	Doxycycline 100 mg b.i.d. for 7 days, or tetracycline 500 mg q.i.d. for 7 days
Campylobacter	Erythromycin 500 mg q.i.d. for 7 days, or ciprofloxacin 500 mg q 12h for 7 days
Shigella	Trimethoprim-sulfamethoxazole double strength po b.i.d. for 5 days
Hemophilus ducreyi	Erythromycin base 500 mg po q.i.d. for 7 days, or ceftriaxone 250 mg IM once
Danovania granulomatis	Tetracycline 500 mg q.i.d. for 10 days
Syphilis	Penicillin G 2.4 million units IM, or tetracycline 500 mg q.i.d. for 30 days
Herpes proctitis	Acyclovir 400 mg 5 times per day for 5 days
Hepatitis	Symptomatic
Entamoeba histolytia	Metronidazole 750 mg t.i.d. for 10 days plus diloxanide furoate 500 mg t.i.d. for 10 days
Giardia lamblia	Metronidazole 250 mg po t.i.d for 7 days

frequency! Homosexuality and promiscuity have created this apparent high incidence. The most common STDs in homosexuals are gonorrhea, syphilis, and condyloma acuminata. Proctitis is often caused by specific organisms, especially *Neisseria gonorrhoeae, Chlamydia trachomatis, Treponema pallidum,* and herpes virus type 2 (herpes simplex). When proctitis, usually associated with anal pain and discharge, is diagnosed, testing for STDs is necessary. As part of the anoscopy and sigmoidoscopy, culture, smears, and biopsies should be taken appropriately. Serologic tests for syphilis should be included as well as an enzyme-linked immunosorbent assay (ELISA) to detect antibodies of the human immunodeficiency virus (HIV). Table 1 lists enteric STDs and the tests for them. Once the diagnosis is made, most STDs can be treated as in Table 2.

Special mention will be made of condyloma acuminata. The papilloma virus is the causative agent with an incubation period of 1 to 6 months. The cauliflower-like masses are found on the genitals or perianal area. An anoscope must be used to look for these lesions on the dentate line. Currently, the only treatment methods that have been effective require destruction of the lesions individually. I prefer to use bichloroacetic acid in the office for a few scattered genital warts or electrocautery under local anesthesia. For extensive condyloma, anesthesia for electrocautery or laser destruction is necessary. The difficulty is assuring cure. Recurrence is frequent and the patient is followed at 1 or 2-month intervals with treatment whenever new warts are found.

Discharge from follow-up comes after no new lesions have been found for 6 months.

INCONTINENCE

Continence is the ability to defer defecation to an appropriate time; the inability to do this is incontinence, a disorder that frequently leads to a nursing home. Prevalence of incontinence is not known, but multiple etiologies, including vaginal delivery, vaginal hysterectomy, and diarrheal disorders contribute to incontinence (Table 3); therefore, it is easy to understand a high incidence. The chapter *Fecal Incontinence* provides additional information.

Diagnosis is predicated upon careful history and physical followed by specific diagnostic tests. The pertinent history includes questions about onset, possible etiologic factors, and stool characteristics. Is the patient able to control gas, liquid and solid? Does the patient require a pad? Is the patient continent at night? Are there contributing diseases or neurologic disorders? Has the patient had trauma, surgery, pregnancy or gynecological problems and treatments?

At physical examination a patulous anus may be seen, and sphincter tone and strength of voluntary squeeze may be tested by digital examination. An

Table 3 Causes of Incontinence

Primary
Nervous system
  Upper motor neuron lesions
    Dementia
    Cerebrovascular disease
    Hydrocephalus
    Multiple sclerosis
    Tumors
    Infections
  Spinal cord lesions
    Trauma
    Cord compression
    Multiple sclerosis
    Ischemia
  Lower motor neuron lesions
    Conus medullaris tumor
    Multiple sclerosis
    Meningomyelocele
    Tabes dorsalis
  Cauda equina lesions
    Lumbosacral trauma
    Lumbosacral disc prolapse
    Lumbar canal stenosis and spondylosis
    Ankylosing spondylitis
  Peripheral nerve lesions
    Pudendal neuropathy
    Pelvic neoplasms
    Diabetic neuropathy
    Autonomic neuropathy

Acquired
  Rectal prolapse
  Anorectal infection
  Aging

Traumatic
  Obstetric
  Operative
    Anal dilatation
    Fistula
    Sphincterotomy
    Anal anastomoses
    Hemorrhoidectomy
    External penetrating trauma

Congenital
  Hirschsprung's disease

Meningomyelocele

Secondary
  Diarrhea
  Disease involving sphincter
  Inflammatory bowel disease
  Fecal impaction
  Laxative abuse
  Diabetes
  Metabolic
  Psychiatric
  Rectal neoplasm

impaction may be noted. A local neurological examination can test pain perception by pinprick, and touch and the anal cutaneous reflex by a cotton tipped applicator. Ordinarily, evaluation of the anus, rectum, and colon by endoscopy and barium enema may define a primary contributing pathology. A simple office test for continence is performed by inserting a 200 ml tap water enema and having the patient walk about to see whether they can hold it within the rectum for a few minutes. A person who has severe incontinence cannot hold this enema.

If incontinence is present, the dysfunction may be better defined by physiologic testing, as discussed in other chapters. Manometry will determine basal pressure, squeeze pressure and the presence of the rectoanal inhibitory reflex. Defecography shows whether the anorectal angle is maintained. Electromyography may point out injury potentials associated with muscle or nerve injury. Rectal compliance testing verifies adequacy of reservoir and volume tolerance. Finally, anal ultrasound detects breaks in the sphincter muscles.

Medical management is based on the treatment of specific diseases that are identified, such as diabetes or inflammatory proctitis. General methods to control incontinence include bulking agents and foods containing pectin to give the stool solidity, because watery stool is difficult to hold. Lactose deprivation will help those who are found to be lactose intolerant. Increased bowel motility may be controlled by use of anticholinergics and opiates.

Biofeedback is a painless and inexpensive conditioning technique to help well-motivated patients enhance their sphincter mechanism. The patient may be aided to sense stool within the rectum better and then react by closing the sphincter to control the stool in a timely fashion. This technique is described in detail in the chapter on incontinence.

Some surgical procedures may be of help in specific abnormalities. Eighty to ninety percent of patients who have an obstetrical injury can be treated successfully by simply repairing the sphincter muscle. For patients who have a neuropathy of the pelvic floor, the postanal repair reconstructs the anorectal angle. This method has not been reported to be uniformly successful throughout the world. In recent years, muscle transpositions of the gracilis muscle or the gluteus muscle have been used to create neosphincters; muscle stimulators have been employed to enhance activity in the transposed muscles. An unproven, but rational, artificial sphincter has been tried in a limited number of patients with some success. The long-term follow-up will determine whether this is a viable option.

Finally, if diet, medication and surgery have failed, a colostomy may be a solution. The control that the patient seeks is offered by the appliance that is always present to collect the fecal matter. Hence, they can confidently leave the home without plotting where the bathrooms are.

SUGGESTED READING*

Gordon PH, Nivatvongs S, eds. Principles and Practice of Surgery for the Colon, Rectum, and Anus. St. Louis: Quality Medical Publishing, 1992.
Smith L, ed. Practical Guide to Anorectal Testing. New York: Igaku-Shoin, 1990.

*Editor's Note: Please see other relevant chapters for additional references.

HEMORRHOIDS

RAMA P. VENU, M.D.
JOHN A. LoGIUDICE, M.D.
STEPHEN F. DEUTSCH, M.D.
GAYLE M. ROSENTHAL, M.D.

Hemorrhoids are dilated veins located at the lower rectum and anal canal. Although not a serious illness, hemorrhoids constitute the most common abnormality affecting the anorectal region. Approximately 10 million people in the United States are affected by hemorrhoids at any time with a prevalence rate of 4.4 percent. It is estimated that about 50 percent of the population above 50 years of age suffer from hemorrhoids, costing more than 100 million dollars annually for over-the-counter hemorrhoidal medications.

ANATOMICAL CONSIDERATIONS

The anorectal area is a highly vascular region enriched by hemorrhoidal vessels. Internal hemorrhoids arise from the superior hemorrhoidal plexus situated above the dentate line. The dentate line is an important landmark in the anorectal region for a variety of reasons. (1) It separates the mucosal surface from the cutaneous surface. (2) Autonomic nerves innervate the mucosa while the cutaneous surface below the dentate line is chiefly innervated by somatic nerves and, therefore, is very sensitive to painful stimuli. This is an important practical point to be kept in mind when nonoperative therapies are undertaken. Application of coagulation current, laser, or infrared beam in this region can cause severe pain and discomfort to the patient. (3) External hemorrhoids arise from the inferior hemorrhoidal plexus located below the dentate line.

Internal hemorrhoids are usually located at three primary sites: (1) left lateral, (2) right anterior, and (3) right posterior; at the 2 o'clock, 5 o'clock, and 9 o'clock positions of the anal ring.

PATHOGENESIS

The mechanism leading to hemorrhoid formation is not well understood. Since hemorrhoidal bleeding is characteristically bright red, hemorrhoids are considered to be a form of arteriovenous malformation. A defective anchoring mechanism resulting from submucosal connective tissue abnormalities is another postulated mechanism for hemorrhoids. Yet another view focuses on abnormality in the internal anal sphincter mechanism. Spasm involving the internal sphincter can raise rectal pressure which in turn pushes the hemorrhoidal plexus downwards. As a proof of this theory the association between hemorrhoids and situations of high rectal pressure are often quoted. Thus, hemorrhoids are frequently seen in subjects with pregnancy, pelvic tumors, and constipation.

CLASSIFICATION

Hemorrhoids are classified as external or internal based on their anatomical location. Thus, internal hemorrhoids are located above the dentate line while external hemorrhoids are located below this line. Most hemorrhoids remain asymptomatic. A clinical classification is adopted for internal hemorrhoids on the basis of their protrusion into the lumen, prolapse through the anal canal, and reducibility.

First degree internal hemorrhoids merely protrude into the lumen. Second degree internal hemorrhoids prolapse through the anus during straining of defecation, but reduce spontaneously. A third degree hemorrhoid prolapses through the anal canal and requires manual reduction. Fourth degree hemorrhoids prolapse through the anal canal and are irreducible. This classification is useful in the proper selection of patients for appropriate therapy and to assess the efficacy of various therapeutic modalities in clinical trials.

CLINICAL MANIFESTATIONS

Internal Hemorrhoids

Bleeding per rectum is the most common and alarming symptom associated with internal hemorrhoids. Bleeding often manifests as red spots on the toilet tissue. Dripping of blood after bowel movement may also occur. Massive rectal bleeding requiring blood transfusion or chronic low grade bleeding with iron-deficiency anemia are seldom encountered among patients with internal hemorrhoids. Pruritus ani, fecal soiling, mucous drainage, and protrusion of hemorrhoids are not uncommon symptoms associated with internal hemorrhoids. Although mild anorectal discomfort may be present with all degrees of internal hemorrhoids, strangulated hemorrhoids cause significant pain in the anorectal area. If untreated, this can lead to gangrene formation, ulceration, and infection.

External Hemorrhoids

Similar to internal hemorrhoids, external hemorrhoids often produce swelling and mild discomfort in the anal area. However, thrombosis of the external hemorrhoid can cause severe pain. The skin overlying the hemorrhoidal cushion often becomes reddened and swollen. If untreated, ulceration, infection, and abscess formation can occur. Organization of the thrombus can result in external skin tags. Such cutaneous tags are also seen in association with inflammatory bowel disease or in patients following hemorrhoidectomy.

DIAGNOSIS

Inspection

The first step in the diagnosis of anorectal abnormality is proper inspection of the perineal area. The patient should be examined in a comfortable knee-chest position. The anus and the perianal area should be examined visually after spreading the buttocks area. Inspection can be extremely helpful in differentiating hemorrhoids from other not so rare conditions such as condyloma acuminata, perianal fistulae, thrombosed external hemorrhoids, and perirectal abscesses.

Digital Examination

A proper digital examination should follow the inspection. During digital examination, hemorrhoids, polyps, and malignancy can be identified. Distinguishing a thrombosed hemorrhoid from a perianal fistula or abscess can be difficult.

Anoscopy

Anoscopic examination is the most useful procedure for the diagnosis and classification of hemorrhoids. The anoscope with the obturator in place is gently introduced into the anal canal. The obturator is then removed. The anal canal is then inspected under adequate illumination. The hemorrhoidal cushion can be seen bulging through the anoscope. All quadrants of the anal canal should be examined by reintroducing the scope.

Flexible Sigmoidoscopy

Any patient presenting with rectal bleeding or other anorectal symptoms should be carefully evaluated to rule out adenoma, adenocarcinoma or other neoplastic disorders involving the anorectal area. Therefore, every patient with suspected hemorrhoids should eventually have flexible sigmoidoscopic examination, perhaps followed by colonoscopy or barium enema. It should always be kept in mind that all that bleed are not hemorrhoids.

MANAGEMENT

General Guidelines

Irrespective of the stage of internal hemorrhoids, all patients presenting with hemorrhoidal symptoms should follow certain general guidelines consisting of (1) diet, (2) anorectal hygiene, and (3) local therapy.

Diet

A diet rich in fiber seems to be beneficial for most patients with hemorrhoids. High-fiber diets can be useful in regulating bowel movements, thus avoiding straining during defecation. Quite often hydrophilic bulk agents such as psyllium or mucinoids may be necessary in addition to a standard high-fiber diet. Elimination of certain foods such as spices, citrus fruits, alcohol, caffeine, chocolate, and tomatoes may be beneficial.

Perianal Hygiene

Adequate anal hygiene can be extremely helpful for symptomatic relief. Perianal irritation and pruritus ani are often associated with residual stool soiling. After each bowel movement, moistened white toilet paper should be used for proper swabbing of the anal region. Vigorous wiping should be avoided. Cleansing pads or Tucks and perianal cleansing lotions, such as Baleonol, will provide a soothing effect. Sitz baths once or twice a day, preferably after a bowel movement, are especially useful to cleanse the perianal area and to facilitate relaxation of the internal sphincter.

Pharmacotherapy

Topical Agents

Several pharmacological agents are available for topical use in patients with hemorrhoids. Two major components of these agents are hydrocortisone acetate and local anesthetic agents from one of the "caine" families. These agents are dispensed as ointment, cream, or foam. Such topical agents may be applied digitally using a fingercot "glove" or applicator. Although well-controlled studies are lacking, many patients claim some symptomatic improvement with these pharmacological agents. In an occasional patient, severe allergic reaction may occur from the "caine" topical anesthetics.

Suppositories

Besides the topical agents, a variety of suppositories are also available. The chief ingredients in these suppositories are similar to the topical agents. The suppositories melt in the rectum and gravitate to the anal canal. A suppository is best utilized at bedtime. Efficacy of anal suppositories is not well studied.

Local Injection

Submucosal injection of a variety of sclerosants such as 5 percent phenol, sodium morrhuate, or hypertonic saline adjacent to the hemorrhoidal vein is one of the earliest therapies utilized for internal hemorrhoids. Some reports indicate significant success with injection therapy especially in patients with first and second degree internal hemorrhoids. However, pain at the site of injection, infection, and abscess formation may complicate injection therapy.

Nonsurgical Treatment

Cryotherapy

Cryotherapy of hemorrhoids is accomplished by specially designed cryoprobes activated by liquid nitrogen, carbon dioxide, or nitrous oxide. Rapid freezing followed by rapid thawing leads to tissue destruction from necrosis. However, the extent of tissue necrosis is often uncontrolled, causing delayed healing and prolonged drainage or pain.

Rubberband Ligation

Rubberband ligation is the most common outpatient therapy employed in patients with symptomatic internal hemorrhoids. In this technique, the hemorrhoidal tissue is grasped, gently pulled, and a rubberband is slid over the tissue which eventually leads to necrosis and destruction of the hemorrhoidal cushion. No anesthetic agent is required, and the procedure can be performed through an anoscope. Complications such as bleeding, fever, pain, infection, and drainage are rare.

Photocoagulation

Thermal injury through photocoagulation is utilized in some of the newer, nonoperative therapies such as infrared coagulation (IRC) and lasers.

Infrared Coagulation. A rigid light guide with a curved tip is used for IRC. A special polymer that is transparent to infrared placed at the tip of the probe allows tissue contact. A low voltage, tungsten halogen lamp (15 volt) is the source of the infrared beam. The optimal amount of energy to be delivered to the tissue can be preset using a timer. The probe is fitted onto a handle with a switch which is easy to operate. The tip can be rotated and the contact tip is replaceable.

Coagulation of the hemorrhoidal cushion causes fixation of the tissue to the submucosa with scarring and retraction. Most patients experience a sensation of heat, but severe pain is unusual. Bleeding, pain, thrombosis, and anal fissure are some of the rare complications of IRC.

Bipolar Coagulation. The equipment for Bipolar coagulation (bicap) consists of a rigid rod with the active electrode at its tip. No grounding of the patient is required in this technique. The electrical energy delivered is controlled by a foot pedal. Coagulation is generated at the base of the hemorrhoidal tissue in 1 or 2 second pulses. Similar to IRC, bipolar coagulation may be occasionally associated with pain, infection, bleeding, or thrombosis.

Direct Current Coagulation. Coagulation with direct current coagulation (DC), on the other hand, requires a grounding plate. After the electrode is applied at the base of the hemorrhoid, low-voltage current is gradually increased to 16 mA. Although DC is as effective as bicap, it takes more time and may be occasionally painful.

Surgical Therapy

Hemorrhoidectomy is the most definitive form of surgical therapy for internal hemorrhoids. It is especially indicated in most patients with third degree hemorrhoids, all patients with fourth degree hemorrhoids, strangulated hemorrhoids, and when other nonsurgical therapies are unsuccessful. However, fecal incontinence may be a rare complication from surgical therapy. This may be a problem especially with loose or watery stools.

Ablation of the internal anal sphincter is another surgical technique sometimes employed in the treatment of internal hemorrhoids. It is especially useful in patients who have a high resting anal sphincter pressure associated with internal hemorrhoids.

Thrombosis of an external hemorrhoid often requires surgical intervention. If severe pain persists more than 24 to 48 hours in patients with thrombosed external hemorrhoids, surgical evacuation is also advocated by some experts to prevent recurrent thrombus formation. The chapter on perianal surgery provides more details.

SUGGESTED READING

Ambrose NS, Morris D, Alexander-Williams J, et al. A randomized trial of photocoagulation or injection sclerotherapy for the treatment of first- and second-degree hemorrhoids. Dis Colon Rectum 1985; 28:238.

Buls JG, Goldberg SM. Modern management of hemorrhoids. Surg Clin North Am 1978; 58:469.

Dennison AR, Whiston RJ, Rooney S, Morris DL. The management of hemorrhoids. Am J Gastroenterol 1989; 84:475–481.

Leicester RJ, Nichols RJ, Mann CV. Infrared coagulation: A new treatment for hemorrhoids. Dis Colon Rectum 1981; 24:602–605.

Lieberman DA. Common anorectal disorders. Ann Internal Med 1984; 101:837–846.

Russell Y, Migi KB, Pacher J, Loren L. Randomized, prospective trial of direct current versus bipolar electrocoagulation for bleeding internal hemorrhoids. Gastrointest Endosc 1993; 39:766–769.

ILEOSTOMY AND OSTOMY MANAGEMENT*

ROBIN S. McLEOD, M.D., F.R.C.S.C., F.A.C.S.
ZANE COHEN, M.D., F.R.C.S.C., F.A.C.S.

From estimates of United Ostomy Association membership, there are over 15,000 ostomates in the United States. The most common indicators for an ileostomy are ulcerative colitis and Crohn's disease; the most common indication for a colostomy is carcinoma of the rectum. Although the quality of life of most ostomates is normal or only minimally affected by the stoma, most patients are anxious preoperatively about both the surgery and the stoma. There may be concerns about management of the appliance, diet, work, and activity restrictions as well as psychological concerns about sexuality and body image. Thus, the management of patients with a stoma must begin before the operation. At our institution, the surgical procedure is discussed, printed materials and names of individuals who have a stoma are given to the patient, and, if possible, all patients are seen by an enterostomal therapist before hospitalization.

The other aspect of ostomy management that must be considered preoperatively is stomal siting. Our studies have shown that the most common reason for ostomates having a poor quality of life is poor stoma function. In most instances, this problem can be avoided by proper marking of the stoma preoperatively, even in patients requiring emergency surgery. This is best done by the enterostomal therapist, who views the patient both sitting and lying to observe the abdominal contour and landmarks. Consideration should also be given to the patient's activities and clothing preferences when selecting the site.

ILEOSTOMY

Postoperative Management

The stoma is typically edematous immediately postoperatively, but this resolves within a few days to a few weeks. The normal color of the mucosa ranges from pink to deep red. If there is concern about the viability of the stoma, it is important to determine whether the ischemia is limited to the extrafascial bowel or whether the intra-abdominal bowel is affected. If it is the former, intervention is unnecessary, whereas if it is the latter, surgery is required. The viability of the stoma may be assessed by pricking the mucosa lightly with a small-gauge needle to check whether there is arterial bleeding.

To determine the line of demarcation, a light may be shone into the stoma while a test tube is gently inserted into the proximal limb of the stoma. Alternatively, the ileostomy may be gently endoscoped. If only the stoma is affected, there may be sloughing of the mucosa only, and this will lead to no permanent complication. If there is full-thickness necrosis, the stoma may stricture and a stoma revision may be required at a later date.

Intestinal peristalsis usually recommences 2 to 5 days after the surgery. Not infrequently, there is an early output of intestinal content from the ileostomy while there is still an ileus in the upper intestinal tract. However, oral ingestion should not be started until there are signs, e.g., the passage of air and resumption of bowel sounds, that the ileus has resolved. Occasionally, there may be edema at the fascial level leading to a partial obstruction. Insertion of a large Foley catheter may help relieve the obstruction while the edema resolves. The normal output from an ileostomy should range between 500 and 1,000 ml. Patients need to be aware of their ileostomy output. Low outputs may indicate an obstruction; higher outputs may result in dehydration.

While in the hospital, the patient should be taught how to care for the ileostomy in order to be proficient and confident in managing the appliance before discharge. It may also be beneficial to have a visiting nurse provide assistance following discharge.

Approximately 50 percent of patients experience some dietary restrictions postoperatively, but these are severe in only about 10 percent. Initially, patients should be advised to take a low-residue diet, but within a few weeks they can begin to introduce other foods into their diet. Foods that commonly affect patients are nuts, popcorn, corn, Oriental vegetables, cabbage, and mushrooms.

Skin care is an important component of management of ileostomates. Dermatitis caused by the leakage of stool onto the peristomal skin is the most common skin problem associated with an intestinal stoma. Ileostomy effluent is very irritating to the skin because it contains pancreatic proteolytic enzymes, bile acids, and a high concentration of alkali. Leakage may cause erythema, ulceration, and, with prolonged exposure, pseudoepitheliomatous hyperplasia of the skin. This is characterized by reddish-brown nodules that may become confluent at the mucocutaneous border and may prevent adequate maintenance of the appliance because of pain and mucous sequestration. A properly fitting appliance usually allows this condition to resolve. Occasionally, a convex face plate and belt may be needed to maintain a seal around the stoma, and rarely the stoma must be resited.

Folliculitis under the face plate may occur after the hair around the stoma has been shaved with a razor blade, or if the hair follicles are injured when the face plate of the appliance is repeatedly pulled off. The condition usually resolves with local treatment and clipping of the hair with an electric razor or scissors. Contact dermatitis may occur from an allergic reaction to the appliance or tape; this should be suspected if the

---

***Editor's Note:** This chapter presents practical information that will prove useful, especially to the nonsurgeons among us.

irritation follows the pattern of the appliance or tape. A different skin barrier may afford equal protection and eliminate the allergic reaction. Skin testing for sensitivity to appliance materials may reduce this problem in patients who have had an allergic reaction. The other common skin lesion is *Monilia* infection, which can be recognized by its characteristic appearance of well-circumscribed erythema with satellite papules and pustules. It usually responds to dusting the skin with nystatin powder before fitting the appliance.

Postoperatively, most ileostomates achieve a satisfactory quality of life and the overwhelming majority feel that they lead normal lives or experience only minor restrictions because of the stoma. Their improved physical well-being is probably the major reason for their high degree of satisfaction. In fact, it is not uncommon for patients to comment that they wished they had had surgery much earlier in their disease course. Despite these feelings, a few patients complain of problems with noise and odor. It may be difficult to eliminate these difficulties completely, but avoidance of gas-producing foods and the use of charcoal and chlorophyll tablets may be beneficial. High-volume ileostomy output is uncommon unless the patient has had a concomitant small bowel resection. However, ileostomates are prone to dehydration in hot weather or during a flu-like illness and should be cautioned to increase their intake of fluid and salt at those times. Other causes of high output are recurrent Crohn's disease and partial small bowel obstruction.

From a psychological standpoint, most patients adapt well to the ileostomy. However, a few have a poor body image and may experience negative feelings from family, friends, and employers. These patients may benefit from counseling or referral to a local ostomy chapter.

Late Complications

Many patients may experience problems related to the ileostomy, but complications tend to be temporary or minor and are often eliminated by a change in appliance. However, 15 to 25 percent of patients require revisional surgery to the ileostomy. Such surgery is required more frequently in patients with Crohn's disease owing to recurrence of disease. Otherwise, the most common indications for surgery are retraction or prolapse of the stoma, stenosis, and fistula formation. Some patients may require resiting of the stoma because of problems related to leakage, a complication that should be avoided by proper placement initially. Unlike the situation with colostomies, parastomal hernia formation is infrequent.

Cases of retraction and prolapse of the stoma can be divided into those that are fixed and those that are intermittent. If the stoma is constantly retracted, it is usually because there was tension and insufficient length of bowel to evert the stoma when it was constructed. A convex appliance may be sufficient to obviate the commonly associated problem of leakage; if not, surgical revision may be necessary. A local skin level revision is

often successful, but sometimes a laparotomy is required to mobilize the small bowel adequately. Retraction of the bowel at a later date often signifies recurrent Crohn's disease. Removal of the appliance and close inspection of the stoma may reveal aphthous ulcers and other features typical of Crohn's disease; if so, treatment should be directed toward the Crohn's disease. The other situation is that of the stoma intermittently retracting and prolapsing. Again, difficulty in maintaining an appliance and leakage are the most common complaints. This is usually associated with a large stomal aperture and failure of the two serosal surfaces of the bowel to fuse, allowing the bowel to intermittently retract and prolapse. A local skin level procedure, with tightening of the fascial defect and amputation of the excess bowel, may be performed. Often, however, this is unsuccessful and resiting of the ileostomy is required. Retraction and prolapse may also be associated with a parastomal hernia, which is likewise best treated by resiting the stoma.

Peristomal fistulas are uncommon and almost always a manifestation of recurrent Crohn's disease. Occasionally a fistula may occur in the absence of Crohn's disease as a result of a suture pulling out at the time of maturing the stoma. A fistula may pose a difficult problem because it typically lies at the skin level, so there is constant leakage of stool with undermining of the appliance. Medical therapy is rarely of benefit, and a laparotomy with resection of the involved bowel and resiting of the stoma is usually necessary. If there is an associated abscess, it should be drained and treated with antibiotics, if possible, before surgery.

Peristomal ulceration most commonly occurs in patients with Crohn's disease and often suggests activation of disease. Occasionally, it may be due to continued skin irritation. Treatment may be difficult, especially if there is active disease. The enterostomal therapist plays an important role in the management of these patients. The ulcer should be treated with a debriding agent and packed with gauze, and an appliance applied. The dressing and appliance should be changed daily. Often, different agents and dressings may need to be tried, as these can be quite resistant to treatment. If there is a septic component, antibiotics may be beneficial. In resistant cases, stomal resiting is necessary, with or without concomitant resection of the bowel.

Stomal blockage, which occurs not infrequently, is usually caused by ingestion of high-fiber foods such as nuts, popcorn, string vegetables, raw vegetables, corned beef, cabbage, oranges, or fruit peels. The patient experiences cramping abdominal pain, nausea and vomiting, and cessation of ileostomy output. Treatment involves rehydration with intravenous fluids and nasogastric decompression. The obstruction can occasionally be relieved by irrigating the stoma with a large-bore Foley catheter placed into the stoma. Food bolus obstructions almost always resolve spontaneously within 24 hours; if not, one should suspect a blockage from another cause (e.g., adhesions) and treat the patient accordingly.

KOCK POUCH

The Kock pouch or continent ileostomy consists of a reservoir and nipple valve constructed from the distal small bowel and brought out to the surface as a flush stoma. The advantage of this procedure is that the ileostomy is continent, so the need for an appliance is eliminated. Although this was a significant advance, the procedure is now performed relatively infrequently because the surgical complication rate is high and patients are still left with a stoma. Thus, for patients wishing to avoid an ileostomy, the ileoanal pouch procedure is usually preferred.

The immediate postoperative care of these patients is similar to that of anyone undergoing a major abdominal procedure. In addition, the catheter that is left in situ at surgery must be irrigated frequently, and the stoma must be checked for signs of ischemia. Most surgeons leave the catheter in place for several weeks to decompress the pouch and in hopes of allowing better fixation of the pouch and nipple valve. After this, the patient must be taught how to intubate the pouch; thereafter, the pouch may be intubated as necessary, usually three or four times a day. Between times, a gauze patch or Band-Aid may be used to cover the stoma. Rarely, patients have trouble with excessive mucous discharge from the efferent limb. Little can be done for this except to ensure that the bowel is flush with the skin and to change the bandage more frequently. If patients have trouble emptying the pouch because the stool is thick, they should be told to increase their fluid intake and drink prune juice. The pouch may also be irrigated. Dietary restrictions, if any, are usually similar to those experienced by patients with conventional ileostomies.

Complications tend to be related to the nipple valve, which is formed by intussuscepting a 10 to 12 cm segment of nipple valve. Dessusception of the valve, known as valve slippage, has been the Achilles heel of the operation, and despite modifications still occurs in 10 to 15 percent of patients. Usually, patients complain of difficulty in intubating the pouch and incontinence. The history is usually adequate to suggest the diagnosis, but it can be confirmed with a pouchogram. If the valve has slipped, surgical revision to reconstruct it is necessary. "Valve prolapse" is the term used for the situation in which the valve is intact but prolapses through the stomal aperture. This is the result of an excessively large fascial opening, and it can be corrected by a skin level revision in which the fascial defect is tightened.

One of the unique complications of both the Kock pouch and the ileoanal pouch procedures is pouchitis, which is a nonspecific inflammation of the pouch mucosa. The risk is variable, depending on the series, and ranges from 10 to 35 percent. Typically, there is an acute onset of symptoms, which include increased ileostomy effluent, fever, abdominal tenderness, nausea and vomiting, and malaise. Endoscopically, the mucosa is fiery red and edematous with areas of ulceration and punctate hemorrhages. Although the cause of pouchitis is unknown, there is evidence that the condition is due to bacterial overgrowth; patients respond well to a short course of a broad-spectrum antibiotic. Pouchitis rarely has a more chronic course; if so, Crohn's disease should be suspected. Other inflammatory agents have been used in these situations, but often with little benefit. In recalcitrant cases, excision of the pouch may be necessary.

ILEOANAL POUCH PROCEDURE

The ileoanal pouch or pelvic pouch procedure has been a major advance for patients with ulcerative colitis requiring surgery. The major advantage of this operation is that patients do not have a permanent stoma and they evacuate by the normal route; neither catheters nor appliances are necessary.

After surgery (or closure of the ileostomy), stool frequency tends to be erratic for about 3 months, during which time patients may evacuate 10 to 15 times per 24 hours. Bulk agents with psyllium and antidiarrheal agents such as loperamide may help decrease the number of bowel movements. Problems with perianal skin irritation because of excessive diarrhea are common. Careful hygiene and use of creams and barrier agents such as petroleum jelly and zinc oxide are usually adequate. After 3 months, the pattern of bowel evacuation stabilizes and usually does not interfere with the patient's daily activities. By 12 months, bowel function has usually stabilized at, on average, five or six bowel movements a day. Approximately one-third of patients require long-term antidiarrheal and bulk agents.

As with the other procedures, most patients do not have dietary restrictions. Initially, they should avoid high-residue foods, but these can be gradually introduced after a few weeks. If patients have had no problems with any foods while having an ileostomy, it is unlikely that they will experience difficulties with the pelvic reservoir. However, food ingestion may increase stool frequency, and some patients modify their intake accordingly. In addition, some (usually gas-producing) foods may increase stool frequency. On the other hand, bananas, mashed potatoes, boiled rice, tapioca, peanut butter, applesauce, and cheese tend to decrease stool frequency.

Complications after this procedure occur frequently. The list includes those seen with other major abdominal procedures: small bowel obstruction, intra-abdominal sepsis, and cardiac, respiratory, urinary, and thrombotic difficulties. There are also complications specific to this operation, the most significant being a leak from the ileoanal anastomosis. This may manifest as a pelvic, intra-abdominal, or perianal abscess or as a fistula to the perianal skin, abdomen, or vagina. Although it usually manifests soon after surgery, a small leak may not be detected initially, either clinically or radiologically. One should suspect a leak in patients who have poor functional results. Treatment varies, depending on the size of the anastomotic dehiscence and the symptoms.

One late complication is ileoanal anastomotic stricture. Treatment, consisting of anal dilatation, is usually necessary only in patients who have difficulty evacuating. Perianal complications such as abscesses and fistulas may occur, but if they do, one Crohn's disease must always be suspected. Generally, abscesses can be drained and superficial fistulas laid open. However, one should always be cautious about dividing even part of the anal sphincter in these patients. The other late complication of significance is pouchitis, which is manifest in a way similar to that seen in patients with Kock pouches. Again, broad-spectrum antibiotics are usually effective treatment.

COLOSTOMY

The early management of a colostomy is similar to that for an ileostomy. Preoperative stoma siting and counseling are as important for this group of patients as for those undergoing ileostomy surgery. However, the concerns of these patients often differ from those of ileostomates, since they are often elderly and the diagnosis is usually cancer.

As with most abdominal surgery, there tends to be an ileus that resolves several days after surgery. However, whereas one should wait until the ileostomy has passed gas and effluent before oral intake is initiated, the colostomy must often be stimulated by the ingestion of food before it begins to function. Vascular insufficiency tends to occur with greater frequency in colostomies because of abdominal wall thickness, tension placed on the mesentery, and poorer vascular supply of the colon. Steps to assess the vascular supply are similar to those described for ileostomies. Superficial necrosis of a portion of the stoma may be managed with observation in the realization that a stricture may occur and need to be revised later. Separation of the stoma at the mucocutaneous junction may arise, especially if there is tension or vascular compromise. In virtually all situations, these should be treated nonoperatively, and healing will occur with time. A stricture may result, but the stoma can be revised at a later date if it is symptomatic.

The colostomy effluent is usually solid and nonirritating, so the colostomy can be made flush with the skin unless there has been a significant bowel resection previously or there is underlying disease in the colon or small bowel. Function through a descending colostomy is similar to normal bowel function. Some patients may suffer from constipation or even fecal impaction, particularly if there is a preoperative history of constipation or irritable bowel syndrome. Bulk agents may help regulate the stoma. Fecal impaction may require treatment with a retention enema of cottonseed oil and water.

For patients wishing to eliminate the use of an appliance, there are two possible alternatives: a continent colostomy ring (such as the Erlangen magnetic colostomy device) or colostomy irrigation. Although the concept of a continence device has appeal, it has in fact had limited success. Some patients may wish to try colostomy irrigations, but these are possible only in patients with end-sigmoid colostomies. They must also be well motivated. The advantage of irrigation is that there is no soiling of stool throughout the day, so a cap can be worn. However, the irrigation procedure often takes 1 or 2 hours to complete and must be done regularly at the same time each day.

An enterostomal therapist should be consulted to instruct the patient. Usually, 1,000 ml of lukewarm water is inserted through a soft-tipped cone gently inserted into the colostomy. Caution is required to ensure that the colostomy is not injured during insertion.

Late Complications

The late complications associated with a colostomy are similar to those with an ileostomy, but they differ in frequency. Food blockages and skin irritation are uncommon in patients with colostomies, whereas parastomal hernia formation often occurs, particularly if the colostomy is of long standing. Stricture also occurs more frequently, probably because of the more tenuous blood supply. Prolapse of the stoma is commonly seen with loop colostomies, especially transverse loop colostomies, but otherwise occurs infrequently.

Stomas placed outside the rectus sheath, or those in which the fascial aperture is large, are predisposed to the formation of paracolostomy hernias. Often the colon proximal to the stoma bulges into the subcutaneous tissue and may become obstructed. The indications for surgical repair are symptoms related to entrapment of the intestine, difficulty in irrigating the stoma, parastomal pain, and problems in maintaining the appliance. The treatment of choice is to move the stoma to another site on the abdomen. This may be difficult when there are multiple previous incisions or repairs. In these situations, the stoma can be safely brought out through a synthetic mesh.

SUGGESTED READING

MacKeigan JM, Cataldo PA, eds. Intestinal stomas. Principles, techniques and management. Quality Medical Publishing, St. Louis: 1993.

McLeod RS, Lavery IC, Leatherman JR, et al. Factors affecting quality of life with a conventional ileostomy. World J Surg 1986; 10:474–480.

Morowitz DA, Kirsner JB. Ileostomy in ulcerative colitis. A questionnaire study of 1,803 patients. Am J Surg 1981; 141:370–375.

Nicholls RJ, Bartolo DCC, Mortensen NJ, eds. Restorative proctocolectomy. London: Blackwell Scientific, 1993.

Pemberton JH. Management of conventional ileostomies. World J Surg 1988; 12:203–214.

ILEOSTOMY ALTERNATIVES

JAMES V. SITZMANN, M.D.

The Brooke ileostomy is the standard terminus after total abdominal colectomy and proctectomy for inflammatory or malignant disease. It is relatively simple and straightforward to construct and quite safe. The drawbacks of end-ileostomy are (1) the social stigma; (2) in the absence of a colon, the limited ability to absorb water; and (3) because of its fixed attachment to the anterior abdominal wall, a propensity for bowel obstruction, which can be either spontaneous or diet induced by high-fiber intake. The problem of dehydration can become acute, depending on the patient's dietary habits or the climatic changes. The social issues, while less of a concern medically, tend to be the chief concern of the patient.

A Brooke ileostomy is incontinent of gas and stool. The appliance, although far safer than in the past, does not always fit well and can leak and cause marked peristomal skin irritation or breakdown. Lastly, the noises and odors of evacuation cannot be well controlled with a stoma and can lead to episodes of acute social compromise. It is with this background that continent alternatives to ileostomies have been developed. While rarely addressing the issues of propensity to dehydration or bowel obstruction, they solve the problem of uncontrolled random evacuation of stool, gas, and liquid.

Strictly speaking, there are four alternatives to ileostomy: (1) an ileoanal pull-through procedure after a total abdominal colectomy and a mucosal proctectomy, (2) the continent ileostomy (Kock pouch), (3) the continent ostomy device, and (4) finally, but not technically a true alternative because it spares the rectum, the ileorectostomy. The indications for these operations are generally confined to patients with documented ulcerative colitis, familial adenomatosis polyposis, or colonic polyposis. Patients with Crohn's disease, indeterminate colitis, or rectal cancer are generally not candidates for the ileoanal pull-through procedure.

Patients with Crohn's disease have a high risk of recurrent small bowel disease in the newly constructed pouch, be it an ileoanal pull-through or a continent Kock pouch. In patients with rectal cancer, mucosal stripping is technically not possible if adequate margins are to be achieved around the cancer. Finally, if the patient should need adjuvant radiation therapy with an ileal pouch in the field, functional results might be compromised.

THE TEAM APPROACH

Role of the Ostomy Nurse

Any patient with severe ulcerative colitis or familial polyposis being considered for surgery should have a consultation with a dedicated ostomy nurse. Such a nurse is either a clinical practitioner or a clinical nurse specialist who brings special skills to the care, education, and emotional support of patients and their families considering ostomies. All patients with ulcerative colitis or polyposis who are considering surgery need to understand clearly that they may very well have no choice and may end up with a permanent Brooke ileostomy.

A discussion of an ostomy, either temporary or permanent, and ostomy alternatives is best done with a nurse who has audiovisual materials, simulated ostomies that can be placed on the skin, and an array of ostomy appliances and ostomy aids for the patient to examine and with which to become familiar. The ostomy nurse will also facilitate the introduction of the patient to the various ostomy societies, e.g., the Ostomates Club, the Ostomy Society, or the Crohn's and Colitis Foundation (CCFA) local branch, as well as to other patients the surgeon has operated on or to patients of other surgeons. Patients find it invaluable to speak with other patients about their ostomy experiences. This tends to reduce the level of anxiety and fear associated with this dramatic change in body image. They can also be introduced to patients with other specific continent-saving procedures, and learn, firsthand, from their experiences. The surgeon has nothing to fear from this ad hoc, uncensored patient appraisal of these various options. It is typical for surgeons to over- or underestimate various aspects of the continence alternatives. Patients are able to make a far more intelligent choice if they can review their options not only with the surgeon and the nurse, but also with other patients.

Finally, the ostomy nurse can assist the patient in the peri- and postoperative periods, especially with the local skin care around the stoma or the perianal region after pull-through procedures, and provide another voice of general support. The services of the nurse are essential for properly marking the ostomy site and testing various appliances with the patient for either temporary or continent ostomies, as the supine, anesthetized abdomen rarely configures to the upright or sitting position.

Role of the Gastroenterologist

It is important that an identified gastroenterologist work with the surgical team at the institution performing the procedures. Gastroenterology expertise should include experience in treating patients with continent ileostomies, ileal pull-throughs, or Kock pouches. The gastroenterology team should also be well versed in the treatment and management of irritable bowel syndrome (IBS), "pouchitis," Crohn's disease, and malabsorptive states and the differentiation of these diseases.

A gastroenterologist with specific interest in polyposis is advisable for polyposis patients, as is an appropriate polyposis tumor registry. Polyposis patients and their families require special care, genetic counseling, and lifelong upper and lower gastrointestinal surveillance. Thus, while the gastroenterologist's role is less prominent during the actual performance of the operation and the postoperative care, he or she is very important in the discussion of operative alternatives and the choice of procedure, as well as the long-term follow-up. It is not uncommon for patients to have dramatic misconceptions and expectations about these procedures. A gastroenterologist with wide experience and familiarity with the surgical techniques, as well as the surgical staff, is an invaluable aid in correcting any misperception before operative therapies are begun.

Role of the Surgeon

Surgeons should be willing to place themselves in the context of a caregiver who is a member of a team consisting of the ostomy nurse specialist, gastroenterologist, and family practitioner, if present. Surgeons should explain the ostomy alternatives in a realistic, unbiased, and unhurried manner. Attempts to "sell" various alternatives as in the patient's best interest typically lead to inappropriate expectations. Finally, surgeons should never rush or pressure a patient into making a decision. The underlying disease state is the potentially lethal process threatening the patient's life. Surgeons should make clear to the patient that they are primarily treating the disease process with a proctocolectomy. The subsequent issues of continence-sparing procedures, and the choice of procedure, can almost always be decided at the patient's leisure. Thus, while it is medically advisable to minimize the number of procedures necessary to treat any disease state, it is important for the patient to know that temporizing intermediate procedures can be performed to control the disease while retaining the patient's choice and options. This is especially important for patients who feel terribly victimized by their disease. The sense of loss of control of their lives and bodies is severe, especially in younger patients under 30 years of age. It is a severe blow to their confidence and their body image, reflecting on their total personality. It is in the patients' best interest for surgeons not to reinforce the sense of victimization by removing or minimizing patients' choices.

ILEOANAL POUCH AND ANASTOMOSIS

Ileoanal pouch and anastomosis is the preferred operative approach for ulcerative colitis and polyposis coli in most major institutions. The basic operation consists of total abdominal colectomy with mucosal proctectomy. The level at which the proctectomy ends is debatable, but most surgeons favor mucosectomy to at least the dentate line; in my institution, mucosectomy to the squamous perianal epithelium is favored. This is combined with the construction of a J, S, or W pouch (the most common being the J pouch), with an ileoanal anastomosis. Coupled with this is a temporary ileostomy. The advantages of the operation are that it preserves sphincter function and anal continence, and there is no permanent ileostomy. It preserves the reservoir function of the colon as well as rectal and anal functions. It does not replace the water-absorptive capability of the colon completely, however, and this is a major source of the postoperative problem of watery, somewhat soft stools.

Editor's Note: Two key decisions are (1) whether to leave 1.5 cm of mucosa when doing a stapled anastomosis and (2) whether to perform a defunctioning ileostomy. Proponents of leaving 1.5 cm of mucosa claim complete continence, with a minority of patients staining or soiling. Those favoring complete mucosectomy and hand-sewn anastomosis (the author of this chapter) cite continence in all patients, also without the potential risk of leaving 1.5 cm of ulcerative colitis and potential dysplasia or cancer behind. Each view has its boosters.

Proponents of a defunctioning ileostomy believe that this lessens the likelihood of leakage, infections, or hemorrhage, which may compromise the capacity and distensibility of the pouch. They choose to "protect" everyone. Recently, several groups have advocated a one-step procedure without a defunctioning ileostomy; they claim that this is usually possible, even with fulminant colitis, and safe.

Indications

Indications for the ileoanal pull-through procedure are ulcerative colitis, familial polyposis, or multiple synchronous colon cancers. Specific operative indications for patients with ulcerative colitis include intractability, high-grade dysplasia, and cancer on colon biopsy.* Contraindications to the operation include morbid obesity (more than 80 to 100 pounds above the ideal body weight), rectal cancer, Crohn's disease, previous incontinence, and sphincter injury. Relative contraindications include a history of systemic disease such as sclerosing cholangitis, which may require liver transplant, or in the case of polyposis patients, duodenal polyps, which may require pancreaticoduodenectomy. The operation typically is performed in young adults up to middle age. Patients older than 55 are generally not candidates because their anal sphincter tends to be less competent and they tolerate the rigors of multiple operations less well.

Operative Preparation

In the elective situation, the patient can have a clear liquid diet for 48 hours, coupled with an oral antibiotic and a cathartic. Antibiotics typically consist of neomycin, 250 mg four times a day, and erythromycin-base, 250 mg four times a day. Intravenous (IV) second- or third-generation cephalosporin is given on call to the operating room.

---

*Editor's Note: I try to counsel patients who had symptomatic IBS before the onset of ulcerative colitis to avoid an ileoanal pouch because the ileum is as spastic as the colon was.

Procedure

In the urgent situation, such as fulminant colitis, patients are typically offered total abdominal colectomy with a Hartmann pouch and an end-ileostomy. In the elective situation, they are offered colectomy and proximal proctectomy. The proximal rectum is mobilized, staying close to the rectal wall. Specifically, bifurcation of the aorta and iliac vessels is avoided to minimize the risk of sympathetic nerve injury and subsequent ejaculatory dysfunction in males. The rectum is dissected to the level of the coccyx posteriorly and laterally, and anteriorly to the prostate in males, or one-third of the distance from the apex of the vagina in females. It is then divided with a TA-55 stapler.

The ileal J pouch is constructed by retroflexing 18 cm of terminal ileum back on itself, creating an enterotomy at the apex, placing a GIA stapler into each limb of the bowel, approximating the device, and firing it. The staple line is reinforced with a layer of seromuscular 3-0 interrupted silk sutures. The surgeon then moves to the rectum to begin mucosal stripping. I typically do not begin stripping at the dentate line but rather at the perianal skin, and lift up the anocuticular verge with electrocautery over the hemorrhoidal plexus and up to the dentate line. At this point, I grasp the stapled end of the rectum from within, evert it all onto the perineum, and finish the stripping. Pelvic drains are placed, the J pouch is pulled down to the anus,* and the perianal skin is sutured in full-thickness fashion to the small bowel wall. A proximal diverting loop ileostomy is constructed in the right lower quadrant.

The patient is allowed to recover for 2 to 3 months. Before ileostomy take-down, a barium study is done via the anus to confirm the integrity of the pouch, and the closed loop ileostomy is removed through a small elliptical incision around the stoma 2 to 3 months after the original procedure.

Postoperatively, patients are begun on a diet, and usually loperamide (Imodium), 2 or 4 mg three or four times daily with meals and at bedtime, and psyllium fiber (1 or 2 tsp) are added. The dietary instructions are quite specific. Patients are kept on a low-fiber, lactose-free, low-fat, caffeine- and chocolate-free diet. Loperamide and psyllium can frequently be tapered over 6 to 12 months. Early in the postoperative period, especially in the first month or two, patients pass large quantities of stool. As the small bowel adapts to its new role as a neorectum, increases its water-absorptive capability, and increases the size of the reservoir, stool frequency decreases, often by 50 percent over the first 6 to 12 months. Mean stool output 1 year after surgery is approximately 4.5 stools per day (in my 105 patients).

Some individuals have a higher output, depending on diet and the presence or absence of IBS.†

Complications

The main complications reported in the literature are pelvic sepsis from a pouch leak and intestinal obstruction. Perianastomotic sepsis is minimized with diverting ileostomies. Intestinal obstruction is also minimized by meticulous closure of all potential hernia spaces. Long-term complications include anal stricture and "pouchitis." Pouchitis is a poorly defined entity that may consist of several overlapping disease states, such as IBS or even Crohn's. Most pouchitis, however, is believed to be a reaction of the small bowel mucosa to anaerobic bacterial overgrowth. Pouchitis is defined clinically as an increase in stool frequency, a decrease in stool consistency (i.e., more watery stools), pelvic pain, tenesmus, and occasionally fever. Patients are treated with a broad-spectrum antimicrobial agent that eradicates or minimizes anaerobic bacteria flora, e.g., metronidazole (250 mg three times daily), ciprofloxacin (500 mg twice daily), or tetracycline (250 mg three or four times daily).

Long-Term Follow-Up

The long-term follow-up should include a routine ileopouchoscopy. This can be done with mild IV sedation and a flexible adult sigmoidoscope. I routinely survey patients at 3 to 6 month intervals for the first 18 months, and if there is any suspicion of pouchitis or change in bowel habits, surveillance can be increased in frequency. This allows good assessment of baseline pouch function, and long-term surveillance will ensure no recurrence of inflammatory or polypoid changes in the pouch. There have been reports of colonization of the ileoepithelium, and a few scattered reports of cancer development in the ileomucosa of the pouch.‡

My current recommendation is to continue long-term ileopouchoscopy.

Outcome

Overall satisfaction with this procedure is extraordinarily high among most patients. The rare to occasional nocturnal leakage that occurs in 20 to 30 percent of patients in our care is well tolerated by those patients who are happy to be rid of their underlying disease, off their steroids, and free of the risk and anxiety of cancer.§

---

*Editor's Note: It is the "pulling down" of the ileal pouch that is reportedly difficult in hefty, "linebacker-type" men with a small pelvis. Any vascular compromise endangers subsequent satisfactory results from the pouch.

---

†Editor's Note: Patients who have eight or nine stools per 24 hours often soil or stain at night, necessitating the use of a pad.

‡ Editor's Note: Dysplasia and cancer from the Brooke ileostomy, although rare, do occur. Presumably the presence of dysplasia or cancer in the removed colon may increase the risk.

§Editor's Note: Patients with familial polyposis, who were entirely asymptomatic before colectomy, may not be as "grateful" as patients with intractable ulcerative colitis.

Bowel function typically ranges from two to eight bowel motions per day in 90 percent of patients.

CONTINENT ILEOSTOMY (KOCK POUCH)

The continent ileostomy, called a Kock pouch after its inventor, consists of an ileal pouch connected to a special valve of terminal ileum that prevents the pouch from emptying unless intubated. The rationale of the procedure is that in patients who have had total abdominal colectomy and proctectomy, it will prevent the ileum from evacuating its contents without the direct action of self-intubation. A tube must be placed through the stoma, the valve of the pouch, and then into the pouch itself, several times a day to empty the contents. The catheter is then removed, rinsed, and placed into a purse or pocket to be carried with the patient. A small dressing or Band-Aid is placed over the stoma itself (about the size of a nickel) to prevent mucus. In theory, no gas or stool leaks between intubations and no external ileostomy appliance need be worn.

Indications and Contraindications

The operation is best suited to young or middle-aged adults who have had a total proctocolectomy for ulcerative colitis or polyposis coli. Typically, these patients have not been candidates for ileo pull-through procedures because of either cancer in the rectum or severe perineal disease that has prevented or compromised mucosectomy. Unfortunately, the morbidly obese are poor candidates for this operation, as well as for the ileoanal pull-through procedure. Patients over 70 and those patients with psychiatric disability who do not understand the need to catheterize themselves periodically are also poor candidates.

Procedure

The operation is generally performed as a one-stage procedure, although some surgeons prefer, in patients with ulcerative colitis, to do it in two stages—removing the colon and rectum first, weaning the patient off steroids, and then creating the pouch. Similarly, for patients with cancer of the rectum or colon with familial polyposis, the colectomy/proctectomy is performed, any adjuvant radiation or chemotherapy is delivered, and then the pouch is created.

There is some benefit to a delay in performing a two-stage rather than one-stage procedure. Many patients, after having a Brooke ileostomy for 6 months or longer, elect to keep this method of bowel evacuation rather than undergo another complex procedure, which is a variant on an incontinent ileostomy. This allows patients to become more confident in their choice and minimizes the risk of a complex procedure that is not right for a given patient.

The technical performance of the procedure has been moderately standardized, with several variations in the creation of the nipple valve. The pouch is fashioned with 45 cm of terminal ileum, using either a stapler and seromuscular reinforcements or a continuous 2-0 chromic catgut layer in two layers. The terminal ileum is then intussuscepted into itself for 5 cm and anchored into place with the GIA stapler without the blade, as well as with 4-0 Dacron sutures at the exit of the efferent limb from the pouch, to anchor the valve in place. Many surgeons also score the serosa with electric cautery to further induce scarring of the bowel to itself. Lastly, in a new technique, some surgeons wrap the valve with a loop of bowel as a form of Nissen valve around the exit valve: a type of physiologic sling to further improve the valve's continence function. The efferent ileal limb leading to the cutaneous stoma is as short as possible, and the stoma is placed just above the hairline in the right lower quadrant. The pouch is tacked to the anterior abdominal wall beneath the stoma and situated in the right pelvic gutter, so that when full, it is held in place by the pelvis laterally, posteriorly, and inferiorly. This is important, as if the pouch is full of stool and not properly anchored or supported, it will pull away from the anterior abdominal wall, and nipple valve incompetence will ensue. The cutaneous stoma is made flush with the skin, and the rest of the pouch is tacked to the space lateral to the pouch. It is important to close all the space around the ileal mesentery, so that there is no potential for pouch volvulus or peripouch herniation. Postoperatively, the pouch is intubated for 1 month to ensure that the pouch and valve remain in the appropriate position while the normal scar tissue fixes the pouch in proper position.

The patient should begin intubations every 2 hours during the day, and the catheter should be left in place overnight for approximately 1 month. During the second month the patient can begin intubations four times a day and leave it closed at night. In general, patients need no medication. Dietary control is again important, and dietary fiber should be tightly controlled. Indigestible foods such as cabbage, beans, corn on the cob, and nuts can plug the catheter during intubations and may even form a sediment at the bottom of the pouch. Typically, the patient should be instructed about a low-fiber diet.

The results of the procedure are well accepted by patients, who have been carefully informed of the outcome and accept that they will have an ostomy, need to intubate themselves, and be in close contact with and perhaps handle their own stool. Patients who wish to deny that they have a stoma, find handling stool offensive, or will not empty their pouch regularly are not good candidates for this procedure. Such an attitude can result in nipple valve malfunction, pouchitis, and diarrhea.

Complications

The main complication of the Kock pouch is valve dysfunction, which results from the breakdown of the intussusception of the nipple valve. When this occurs, the patient experiences leakage of pouch contents and has difficulty in intubating the pouch. Reoperation is required to reconstruct the valve. Approximately 20 percent of patients require nipple valve reconstruction. Reoperation does not guarantee that the valve will function, and a second reoperation is required in 15 to 20 percent of these patients. Pouchitis can usually be managed with antibiotics.

ILEOSTOMY OCCLUDING DEVICE

The artificial ileostomy occluder is a simple mechanical device that causes bowel obstruction at the ileostomy. The bowel proximal to this then dilates and forms a somewhat tortuous reservoir. The device is a 28 Fr catheter with a soft inflatable balloon on the end that is inserted into the bowel; an anterior abdominal wall disc is placed to hold the catheter and balloon in place so that it is not extruded by peristalsis. The device can be used in elderly and obese patients who are not candidates for the ileoanal pull-through procedure or continent ileostomies. It is generally used with a pouch, which is constructed in the same fashion as a Kock pouch except that a nipple valve is not made. The exit limb from the pouch is simply brought to the abdominal wall. The device is positioned into the bowel just below the fascia and connected to straight drainage for 1 month to allow the pouch to heal. Intermittent occlusions with the device are begun thereafter, much as the graded, periodic intubations are done with the Kock pouch. Only short periods of occlusion can be tolerated at first, because the device is causing bowel obstruction, and patients experience cramps and abdominal pain of varying severity.

Outcome

The main advantage is simplicity. The device can be removed and inserted at will. The disadvantages are that the patient needs to wear an unsightly appliance and there is a moderate amount of weeping mucus from the terminal ileum, so that absorbent pads must be worn between the appliance and the skin.

ILEORECTOSTOMY

Ileorectostomy is generally mentioned by surgeons who perform continent-sparing procedures only to be condemned. It does have a place, however, in the armamentarium of the colorectal surgeon, despite its limited use.* The operation leaves rectal mucosa in place, which is susceptible to the underlying disease that was the indication for the colectomy and proximal proctectomy. Thus, ileorectal anastomosis is not a definitive treatment for ulcerative colitis or familial colonic polyposis. However, for patients with multiple synchronous colon cancers or multiple colonic polyposis (as opposed to the familial variety), it is a procedure to

be used in those who cannot have the ileoanal pull-through or continent ileostomy. These patients are generally morbidly obese or lack the social, emotional, or intellectual skills to adapt to continent ileostomies or ileoanal pull-through procedures.

Procedure

The operation is carried out in the standard fashion with colectomy and proximal proctectomy. After excision of the proximal rectum, the ileum can be anastomosed end to end or end to side to the rectum, using either the EEA stapler or a hand-sewn anastomosis with a 3-0 running Vicryl suture on the inner layer and 4-0 interrupted silk for the outer layer. Some surgeons create an ileal J pouch and anastomose this to the rectal stump.

Outcome

After this procedure, most patients have upward of four stools per day and some as many as 12 per day. Most are continent, but the loss of colonic reservoir capacity and the water-absorptive capacity of the colon is the limiting factor of this procedure. Patients often require treatment with loperamide and bulk-forming, water-absorbing psyllium fiber. Thus, ileorectostomy is not a good operation for patients over the age of 70 who may have crippling incontinence and diarrhea.

Long-Term Follow-Up

Patients require close long-term surveillance because they have a residual rectum at risk of disease, and need to have 6 monthly to yearly proctoscopy follow-up for life. A 20 percent incidence of colon cancer has been reported in some series with extensive follow-up.

SUGGESTED READING

Becker JM, Raymond JL. Ileal pouch anal anastomosis, a single surgeon's experience with 100 cases. Ann Surg 1986; 204:375–383.

Braun J, Treutner KH, Harder M, et al. Anal sphincter function after intersphincteric resection and stapled ileal-pouch anal anastomosis. Dis Colon Rectum 1991; 34:8–16.

Dozois RR, ed. Alternatives to conventional ileostomy. Chicago: Year Book, 1985.

Dozois RR, Kelly KA, Welling DR, et al. Ileal pouch anal anastomosis: comparison of results in familial adenomatous polyposis and chronic ulcerative colitis. Ann Surg 1989; 210:268–273.

Lohmuller JL, Pemberton JH, Dozois RR, et al. Pouchitis and extraintestinal manifestations of inflammatory bowel disease after ileal pouch anal anastomosis. Ann Surg 1990; 211:622–627.

Madden MV, Farthing MJG, Nicholls RJ. Inflammation in ileal reservoirs: "pouchitis." Gut 1990; 31:247–249.

Sugarman HJ, Newsome HH, Decosta G, et al. Stapled ileoanal anastomosis for ulcerative colitis and familial polyposis without a temporary diverting ileostomy. Ann Surg 1991; 213:606–617.

---

*Editor's Note: Some groups, notably the Cleveland Clinic, still advocate this procedure as an ileostomy alternative.

COLORECTAL CANCER SCREENING

NEIL D. HERBSMAN, M.D.
SIDNEY J. WINAWER, M.D.

Colorectal cancer is one of the leading causes of cancer-related morbidity and mortality, resulting in approximately 160,000 new cases and 60,000 deaths per year in the United States. Early detection can reduce mortality rates and provide a better quality of life. Survival is significantly improved in patients who undergo surgical resection at an early stage. The advent of colonoscopy in the 1970s provided an accurate means of making the diagnosis of early colon cancer, and the development of fecal occult blood testing has made possible the identification of individuals likely to have colorectal cancer. Cancers of the rectum and colon are believed to arise over the course of many years from adenomatous polyps. The ability to detect and remove these polyps endoscopically further supports the rationale for using screening tests to detect early colorectal cancer and adenomatous polyps. With the judicious use of screening tests, improved detection of adenomatous polyps and early colorectal cancer should be possible.

SCREENING AND DIAGNOSTIC TESTS

Screening Concepts

Testing for the early detection of cancer in asymptomatic people can be accomplished by one of two methods: case finding or screening. Case finding involves the use of tests for cancer carried out as part of a comprehensive medical examination. The physician can use other information about the patient's risks and health as well as other tests to complement screening tests. Screening is performed in large outreach programs where the general public can undergo tests to identify those likely to have colon cancer.

To be effective, screening tests for the early detection of cancer in average-risk people have a high sensitivity and specificity, detect disease early enough to influence morbidity and mortality, and be relatively safe, convenient, and inexpensive. Guidelines for the use of screening tests are intended for average-risk people. Persons with signs or symptoms of cancer require a careful diagnostic work-up. In addition, groups at high risk for the development of colorectal cancer require screening guidelines that are different from those in people with average risk.

History

A thorough personal and family history can provide valuable information to identify those at increased risk for developing colorectal cancer. These groups are discussed in a later section of this chapter.

Rectal Examination

A digital rectal examination should be included in the general physical examination of people over 40 years of age. Because of the proximal anatomic migration of colorectal cancer in recent years, however, less than 10 percent of neoplasms are detectable by digital rectal examination. The low sensitivity of this examination is somewhat offset by its safety and low cost. Obviously, examination of the prostate should be performed in men at the same time.

Fecal Occult Blood Testing

The most commonly used test for occult blood in the stool employs guaiac-impregnated paper that undergoes oxidation to a blue compound by the peroxidase-like activity of hemoglobin. Compounds that have peroxidase activity other than hemoglobin, primarily found in uncooked vegetables and fruit, can cause false-positive results. Consumption of red meat can also produce false-positive results from guaiac cards, especially if the slides are rehydrated. Vitamin C inhibits the guaiac reaction and causes false-negative results. Iron and laxatives can have an unpredictable effect on the guaiac test. To obtain optimal sensitivity and specificity, certain dietary guidelines should be followed in the 48 hours before collection of the stool samples.

Fecal occult blood testing also has other limitations. A negative test for occult blood does not rule out colorectal cancer or a polyp, since these may bleed only intermittently.* Storage of the slides for more than 4 to 6 days may cause a weakly positive test to become negative. Despite these limitations, controlled trials of stool blood testing in screening for colorectal cancer have shown that a significantly larger percentage of colorectal cancers are Dukes A or B in patients who screened than in control groups. Some of these studies have also shown a significant survival advantage and reduction in mortality rates from colorectal cancer in the screened groups. Sensitivity of nonhydrated slides for colorectal cancer has been estimated to be 70 to 80 percent. Rehydration of the slides increases sensitivity but at the expense of a loss of specificity, so this technique has not been recommended in the past. This could change with the recent report of a mortality reduction in colorectal cancer with use of rehydrated slides.†

---

*Editor's Note: It is said that only half of the colon cancers will be detected if only one guaiac test is made. Polyps less than 2 cm in size rarely give a positive stool test; even 2 cm polyps give positive results only 30 percent of the time.

†Editor's Note: Hemoccult Sensa cards are more sensitive than Hemoccult cards. Patients using the former should be instructed to avoid red meat.

To obtain maximal effectiveness of the stool blood test, patients should receive cards for preparation of specimens at home. Ideally, patients should be given three double cards, and over a 3 day period six samples from three stools should be obtained. Each card contains two windows, and a small amount of stool should be smeared on each window with an applicator. Diagnostic investigation is warranted if even a single test is positive. If the patient's medical situation permits, this should be done with colonoscopy.

Stool blood tests other than the standard guaiac have been introduced, including immunochemical tests specific for human hemoglobin and quantitative tests based on the fluorescence of heme-derived porphyrins (Hemoquant). These tests are not affected by iron, vitamin C, or diet. The Hemoquant test is limited by its cost and a loss of specificity with its increased sensitivity, which makes it unsuitable for screening. The immunochemical tests hold out more promise for maintaining high specificity with increased sensitivity, but require more evaluation.

Sigmoidoscopy

Sigmoidoscopy offers the ability to detect a large proportion of colorectal cancers. A 25 cm rigid sigmoidoscope can be inserted to approximately 20 cm, significantly increasing the number of colorectal cancers detected compared with digital rectal examination. However, the discomfort of the procedure and the limited depth of insertion detract from its suitability as a screening test. The rigid sigmoidoscope has been almost completely replaced by flexible sigmoidoscopes ranging in length from 35 to 60 cm. The yield of flexible sigmoidoscopy is two to three times greater than that of rigid sigmoidoscopy. In theory, a 60 cm flexible sigmoidoscope could detect 50 to 60 percent of colorectal cancers. The actual percentage detected is probably slightly lower since the average depth of insertion is between 40 and 50 cm, and there has been a recent trend toward proximal migration of colorectal cancer. Two recent case control studies found a 60 percent reduction in the risk of fatal distal colorectal cancer in patients who had undergone sigmoidoscopic screening.

The incidence of perforation during sigmoidoscopy has been reported at one in 10,000, making this a relatively safe procedure. Preparation is simple: usually one tap water or Fleet enema 2 hours before the procedure is sufficient.

Colonoscopy

In the asymptomatic person at average risk for development of colorectal cancer, there is no role for the routine use of colonoscopy as a screening test. However, colonoscopy is indicated as a screening test in high-risk groups. Furthermore, colonoscopy should be the primary method for diagnostic investigation after a positive fecal occult blood stool test, because it is more sensitive than

barium enema and because of its potential for polypectomy and biopsy. Patients with the finding of colorectal cancer or adenomatous polyps on sigmoidoscopy should undergo colonoscopy to evaluate the entire colon for any synchronous (additional) lesions.

Biomarkers

Carcinoembryonic antigen (CEA) levels have been used to monitor patients with colorectal cancer postoperatively. The low sensitivity and specificity of this test make it a very poor method for identifying patients with colorectal cancer initially, especially early cancer or polyps. CEA should not be used to screen asymptomatic patients for colorectal cancer.

SCREENING GUIDELINES

Guidelines for colorectal cancer screening must take into account the level of risk in the groups being screened. People at increased risk should be screened differently from the asymptomatic average-risk people. Everyone should be encouraged to enter the health care system. Patients can then be categorized as either average risk or high risk and the appropriate screening recommendations made.

Average-Risk Patients

People who are at average risk for colorectal cancer and asymptomatic should undergo fecal occult blood testing of the stool annually, starting at the age of 50. Flexible sigmoidoscopy should be performed every 3 to 5 years, also beginning at age 50. A positive stool blood test or the finding of an adenomatous polyp on sigmoidoscopy necessitates colonoscopy to evaluate the entire colon.

High-Risk Patients

History of Polyps

Adenomatous polyps are believed to be the precursor lesions for colorectal cancer. Patients with a history of adenomatous polyps are at increased risk for development of new adenomas. After polypectomy, the physician should have a high degree of confidence that the colon is free of adenomas before recommending long-term follow-up. In certain circumstances, repeat examinations may be indicated, including (1) incomplete removal of a large or sessile polyp, (2) the presence of numerous polyps, and (3) an unsatisfactory first examination of the colon. After removal of a malignant polyp, repeat examination may be needed after 3 to 6 months and 1 year before starting a long-term program, depending on the nature of the pathologic condition. Once the physician is satisfied that the colon is clear, long-term surveillance can be initiated consisting of colonoscopy every 3 years. The interval can be lengthened after one or two normal examinations.*

History of Colorectal Cancer

Patients with a history of colorectal cancer are not only at increased risk for development of an anastomotic recurrence of the original cancer but also at risk for developing a second primary tumor from an adenomatous polyp. Colonoscopy should be performed 6 to 12 months after surgery and then yearly for 1 or 2 years. After this, if there is no evidence of recurrent colorectal cancer or adenomas, long-term surveillance can be carried out in a manner similar to that for patients with adenomatous polyps (colonoscopy every 3 years).

Inflammatory Bowel Disease

Inflammatory bowel disease (IBD) is discussed in greater detail in the chapter on neoplasia in IBD. Approximately 8 years after the diagnosis of ulcerative colitis, the risk of developing colorectal carcinoma begins to increase in patients with universal colitis involving the entire bowel. At that time, colonoscopy is indicated every 1 to 2 years. Multiple biopsies should be taken every 10 to 12 cm from normal-appearing mucosa and examined for dysplasia. Dysplastic-appearing lesions should also be biopsied. In contrast to most other patients at increased risk for colorectal cancer, patients with ulcerative colitis can develop carcinoma in flat mucosa. Patients with only distal colitis should have colonoscopy every 1 to 2 years, starting 15 years after the initial diagnosis. Colonoscopy should not usually be performed in patients with active IBD, since it may be difficult to evaluate biopsies for dysplasia during this period. An increased risk of colon cancer has also been noted in patients with Crohn's disease, although this risk is less than in ulcerative colitis.†

HNPCC

Approximately 5 percent of colorectal cancers can be attributed to the hereditary nonpolyposis colorectal cancer syndromes (HNPCC). These syndromes are inherited in an autosomal dominant pattern. Patients who have three or more first-degree relatives with colorectal cancer, at least one being first degree (siblings, parents, or children), one under age 50, and with two generations affected, should be considered to have HNPCC. In these kindreds, colorectal cancer usually occurs at a younger age than sporadic colorectal cancer

and more often on the right side of the colon. Family members of a kindred with HNPCC should have colonoscopy every 2 years from the ages of 21 to 35 and annually thereafter.

Family History of Colorectal Cancer or Adenomatous Polyps

There is good evidence that inheritance plays a role in the development of most sporadic colorectal cancers. Colon cancer has been demonstrated to occur approximately three times more often than expected in first-degree relatives of patients with colorectal cancer. First-degree relatives of patients with colonic adenomas are also at increased risk for cancer of the colon. Patients with one or two first-degree relatives with colorectal cancer should undergo colonoscopy every 3 to 5 years beginning at age 35 to 40 or at an age 5 years earlier than the age of the youngest relative with colon cancer, whichever comes first. In the past, standard screening with stool blood testing and sigmoidoscopy was the recommended approach when only one first-degree relative had colorectal cancer. However, the high lifetime risk of 18 percent has resulted in a change in these guidelines.

Familial Adenomatous Polyposis

Familial adenomatous polyposis is an inherited syndrome in which patients have hundreds to thousands of polyps in the colon and rectum. This disease is inherited in an autosomal dominant pattern with high penetrance. Gardner's syndrome has gastrointestinal (GI) manifestations identical to those of familial adenomatous polyposis, with the addition of various extracolonic findings such as osteomas of the skull, epidermal cysts, and desmoid tumors. Both of these diseases have a high incidence of associated colorectal cancer. Recently, the gene for these disorders has been identified on chromosome 5 and termed the APC gene. Since this is an inherited germ line alteration, it can be identified in peripheral blood cells. Members of affected families with the gene should be screened with sigmoidoscopy every year beginning at puberty. Colectomy is advised once adenomatous polyps have been observed.

Nonadenomatous Polyposis Syndromes

Peutz-Jeghers syndrome is an autosomal dominant disorder in which there are characteristic mucocutaneous pigmentation and GI hamartomatous polyps, which can occur in the stomach, small intestine, or colon. There is evidence that these polyps have a small but definite association with GI malignancy. Familial juvenile polyposis is an additional syndrome characterized by non-neoplastic hamartomatous polyps that is inherited in an autosomal dominant pattern in approximately 25 percent of cases. Juvenile polyposis is also associated with a small but definite increased risk of GI malignan-

---

*Editor's Note: The 1993 *New England Journal of Medicine* article cited in the Suggested Reading provides support for these statements.

†Editor's Note: Patients with proctosigmoiditis are not thought to be at increased risk of colon cancer in the noninvolved colon. After one colonoscopy at 8 to 10 years to ascertain histologic proof of distal localization, flexible sigmoidoscopy every 3 to 5 years should be sufficient.

cies. The risk of colorectal cancer in both of these syndromes is not as great as in familial adenomatous polyposis, so prophylactic colectomy is not recommended. In patients at risk for these syndromes, screening should be started in the second decade of life, with yearly fecal occult blood testing and flexible sigmoidoscopy every 3 years. Periodic screening of the upper intestinal tract with endoscopy and small bowel x-ray examination should also be performed every 3 to 5 years.

RECOMMENDATIONS

For the purpose of colorectal cancer screening, patients should be identified as at either average risk or high risk for developing colorectal cancer. Once this distinction has been made, the physician can make recommendations regarding specific screening tests and their frequency. Average-risk patients should be screened with flexible sigmoidoscopy and fecal occult blood tests. High-risk patients should be screened initially with colonoscopy, with subsequent examinations from yearly to every 3 to 5 years, depending on the risk factors. The expectation is that with more widespread judicious application of screening, a resultant decline in morbidity and mortality from colorectal cancer will be seen. Recent research has begun to unravel the genetic mechanisms responsible for those at high risk for developing colorectal cancer. In the future, genetic screening tests using these developments may help to identify a greater percentage of high-risk individuals. Periodic colonoscopy could then be targeted to this small subset of the general population to find and remove adenomatous polyps. More complete prevention of colorectal cancer could result from this approach.

SUGGESTED READING

Burt RW, Bishop DT, Lynch HT, et al. Risk and surveillance of individuals with heritable factors for colorectal cancer. Bull World Health Organ 1990; 68:655–665.

Eddy DM. Screening for colorectal cancer. Ann Intern Med 1990; 113:373–384.

Mandel JS, Bond JH, Church TR, et al. Reducing mortality from colorectal cancer by screening for fecal occult blood. N Engl J Med 1993; 328:1365–1371.

Selby JV, Friedman GD, Quesenberry CP Jr, Weiss NS. A case-control study of screening sigmoidoscopy and mortality from colorectal cancer. N Engl J Med 1992; 326:653–657.

Winawer SJ, Flehinger BJ, Schottenfeld D, et al. Screening for colorectal cancer with fecal occult blood testing and sigmoidoscopy. J Natl Cancer Inst 1993; 85:1311–1318.

Winawer SJ, Schottenfeld D, Flehinger BJ. Colorectal cancer screening. J Natl Cancer Inst 1991; 83:243–253.

Winawer SJ, Zauber AG, O'Brien MJ, et al. Randomized comparison of surveillance intervals after colonoscopic removal of newly diagnosed adenomatous polyps. N Engl J Med 1993; 328:901–906.

COLORECTAL POLYPS AND POLYPOSIS SYNDROMES

FRANCIS M. GIARDIELLO, M.D.

A polyp is defined as any tissue protrusion above the normal, flat, colorectal mucosal surface. Polyps are clinically important for two reasons. First, they can cause symptoms including bleeding and occasionally intussusception. Second, some polyps are premalignant lesions that can degenerate over time to adenocarcinoma, while others may already harbor adenocarcinoma.

It is essential to determine the histopathology of the polyp for proper patient management. The number of polyps and any patient and family history of polyps or colorectal cancer should also be ascertained. With these data, decisions concerning work-up, treatment, and follow-up can be made. Table 1 classifies polyps according to histopathology.

Table 1 Histologic Classification and Inheritance of Polyps and Polyposis Syndromes

Adenomatous polyps (tubular, tubulovillous, villous)
Adenomatous polyposis syndromes
  Familial adenomatous polyposis coli*
    (familial polyposis/Gardner's syndrome)
  Turcot's syndrome*
Hamartomatous polyps
  Peutz-Jeghers syndrome*
  Solitary juvenile polyp/familial juvenile polyposis*
  Ruvalcaba-Myhre-Smith syndrome*
  Cronkhite-Canada syndrome
  Cowden's disease*
  Intestinal ganglioneuromatosis*
  Devon family syndrome*
Hyperplastic polyps/hyperplastic polyposis
Nodular lymphoid hyperplasia
Lymphomatous/leukematous polyposis
Inflammatory polyps
Miscellaneous

*Inherited conditions.

ADENOMATOUS POLYPS

Clinical Aspects

Most authorities believe in the adenoma-carcinoma sequence in which perhaps 10 to 30 percent of premalignant adenomas progress to carcinoma. Adenomas can be histologically divided into tubular, tubulovillous, or villous, each with increasing malignant potential and increasing risk of harboring carcinoma. Also, the larger the adenoma, the greater the chance of concomitant cancer (<1 cm ≥ 1 percent risk; 1 to 2 cm = 10 percent risk; >2 cm = >40 percent risk). Sixty percent of adenomas are found in the left colon (the splenic flexure to the anus). Synchronous adenomas are encountered 20 to 50 percent of the time. Endoscopically, polyps can appear sessile or pediculated.

Management

Since adenomas can progress to adenocarcinoma and may already harbor cancer, they should be removed. This rule also applies to diminutive lesions (adenomas under 6 mm in size). Whenever one colorectal adenomatous polyp is discovered, total colonoscopy is mandatory to exclude synchronous lesions.

Management of colorectal adenomas depends on the number of polyps found. Patients with more than 10 to 20 adenomas but fewer than 100, with no family history of familial adenomatous polyposis (FAP), should be considered for subtotal colectomy with ileorectal anastomosis, and the condition viewed with suspicion as a variant of FAP (see later). When clinically available, these individuals should be genotypically tested for the mutated adenomatous polyposis coli (APC) gene. Patients with more than 100 adenomas have FAP (see later).

For patients with fewer than ten adenomas, these polyps can be safely removed by colonoscopy and polypectomy. The technique of polypectomy is discussed in another chapter. Laser ablation with the neodymium: yttrium-aluminum-garnet laser is an alternative and has been used to remove the multiple adenomas that can occur in the retained rectal segment of patients with FAP. Laser therapy is an option in patients deemed nonsurgical candidates who have adenomas that cannot be removed by colonoscopic polypectomy. The disadvantages of laser ablation include the risk of colonic perforation and the fact that no specimen is retrieved for pathologic examination, raising the concern that all neoplastic tissue may not have been destroyed.

When a large sessile polyp cannot be removed endoscopically, surgical resection is indicated. Laparotomy with segmental resection is usually performed, although an innovation with laparoscopic colectomy has been performed in some centers. Alternatively, some rectal adenomas can be removed by transanal excision, avoiding laparotomy.

Upon pathologic review, polypectomy specimens may contain invasive carcinoma. If the following criteria are fulfilled, subsequent colectomy can be avoided: (1) the polyp is not sessile, (2) cancer was not at the margin of the polypectomy burn, (3) cancer did not invade the lymphatics or blood vessels, (4) the cancer was well or moderately well differentiated, and (5) repeat colonoscopy 3 months later reveals no further tumor. Colectomy is advocated if any of the above criteria are violated. When colectomy is required, a formal cancer operation with lymph node dissection is advocated.

Follow-Up

Colonoscopic examination is recommended 6 months to 1 year after initial polypectomy. This frequency is repeated until the colon is polyp free. Subsequent surveillance with annual stool occult blood testing and colonoscopy every 3 years, and sooner if stool is positive for blood, is advocated. Patients operated on for invasive cancer should be followed every 3 months for the first 3 years with physical examination, complete blood count, serum alkaline phosphatase levels, and pre- and postsurgical carcinoembryonic antigen (CEA) levels. Repeat colonoscopy should be done 6 months to 1 year after surgery with biopsies of the anastomotic site. Once the colon has been free of neoplasm for 3 years, surveillance as for adenoma is sufficient.

ADENOMATOUS POLYPOSIS SYNDROMES

Familial Adenomatous Polyposis (Familial Polyposis/Gardner's Syndrome)

Clinical Aspects

FAP is an autosomal dominant syndrome with high penetrance caused by mutation of the APC gene on the long arm of chromosome 5. Patients develop hundreds to thousands of adenomas diffusely throughout the colorectum, usually in teenage years. Colorectal cancer is inevitable by the fifth decade of life if colectomy is not performed.

Extracolonic Lesions

FAP patients can develop both benign and malignant extracolonic lesions. Previously, FAP without extracolonic manifestations was called familial polyposis, and FAP with extracolonic manifestations was termed Gardner's syndrome. Benign lesions include osteomas of the jaw and long bones, skin lipomas, skin cysts, desmoid tumors of the abdomen and extremities, pigmented ocular fundus lesions, clinically occult osteosclerotic jaw lesions, gastric fundic gland retention polyps, gastric adenomas, and duodenal adenomas. FAP patients are at increased risk for malignancies of the duodenum, ampulla of Vater, thyroid, pancreas, and liver (exclusively, hepatoblastoma a rapidly progressive hepatic tumor occurring before age 5). In fact, cancer of the duodenum is the second most common cause of death in this population after colorectal cancer.

Diagnosis

In the setting of a family history of FAP, the diagnosis of FAP is confirmed by finding more than 100 *adenomatous* polyps on endoscopic examination of the colon (sigmoidoscopy is usually sufficient, since FAP affects the colon diffusely). Importantly, approximately one-third of newly diagnosed patients are new mutations with no family history of adenomatous polyposis. In an at-risk patient, the finding of more than three pigmented ocular fundus lesions on indirect ophthalmoscopic examination has a 100 percent positive predictive value for the diagnosis of FAP. Recently, genotyping by DNA linkage analysis to diagnose presymptomatic patients has become available, and direct DNA genotypic analysis will be clinically obtainable shortly.

Screening

At-risk individuals (first-degree relatives of affected patients) should undergo screening with yearly sigmoidoscopy starting at age 12 years. This frequency is reduced to every 2 years after age 25 and every 3 years after age 35. After age 50, patients are advised to follow the American Cancer Society guidelines for screening average-risk patients (flexible sigmoidoscopy at age 50, if negative at age 51, and then every 3 to 5 years; three stool Hemoccult tests every year starting at age 50).

When clinically available, direct genotypic testing should be conducted in all at-risk individuals. If they do not have the mutated APC gene, the need for screening by flexible sigmoidoscopy can be reduced to three time points: ages 18, 25, and 35 years. Although DNA testing should have a virtually 100 percent positive and negative predictive value if the exact pedigree mutation is known, I still recommend several sigmoidoscopies as noted above to ensure that patients with false-negative results are diagnosed.

Hepatoblastoma occurs in about one in 300 at-risk persons under the age of 5 years. By means of defining which offspring actually have FAP by genetic testing, the risk is increased to about one in 150 individuals. Because of the magnitude of hepatoblastoma risk and its potential curability by early surgery, it may be prudent to perform screening with serum alpha-fetoprotein levels and possibly computed tomography of the abdomen in infants and young children of parents affected with FAP.

Treatment

Colectomy is the only effective therapy that eliminates the inevitable risk of colorectal cancer in FAP patients. Before surgery, upper endoscopy should be performed to assess the upper gastrointestinal (GI) tract for adenomas (large adenomas of the duodenum may be removed during laparotomy for colectomy). In patients older than 25 to 30 years with large polyps (greater than 1 cm) or villous adenomas, colonoscopy is useful to evaluate for concomitant colorectal cancer that might alter the choice of surgical procedure.

Surgery should be performed at the time of diagnosis of FAP to minimize any risk of colorectal cancer. However, if the patient is in the second decade of life and the polyps are small (less than 5 mm) and infrequent, surgery may be delayed to accommodate work and school schedules.

Surgical options include subtotal colectomy with ileorectal anastomosis, total colectomy with Brooke ileostomy (or continent ileostomy), and colectomy with mucosal proctectomy and ileoanal pull-through (with pouch formation).

Since colorectal cancer can occur in the rectal segment even under close endoscopic observation, I favor ileoanal pull-through or total colectomy with ileostomy; these procedures remove all at-risk mucosa. Also, I question the wisdom of ileoanal anastomosis operations performed in one step in which a strip of potentially neoplastic rectal mucosa is left 1 cm above the dentate line. In my experience, most young adult patients choose the ileoanal pull-through operation for cosmetic reasons, and if this is performed by a seasoned surgeon, most have excellent results. On the other hand, on the basis of their experience, clinicians at St. Mark's Hospital, London continue to recommend ileorectal anastomosis.*

Postoperative Follow-Up

Patients with subtotal colectomy require routine endoscopic surveillance of the remaining rectum about every 6 months for recurrent adenomas or carcinoma. Some authorities ablate recurrent adenomas with electrocautery or laser therapy. When adenomas are uncontrollable or carcinoma is found, the rectum should be removed. Ongoing trials are investigating the usefulness of medical therapy with oral sulindac to prevent or eliminate polyps in the retained rectum. Preliminary results have been encouraging, but sulindac's role in treatment is not yet clear.

Since the long-term risk of neoplastic transformation in the ileoanal pouch of patients with ileoanal pull-throughs is not known, endoscopic biopsy surveillance at 3 to 5 year intervals should be considered.

Duodenal and periampullary carcinoma is estimated to occur over a lifetime in one of 21 FAP patients. Therefore, although the cost benefit has not been established, most authorities recommend upper endoscopic surveillance (with biopsy and brushing) of the stomach, duodenum, and periampullary region with front and/or side viewing endoscopes every 4 years. In patients with upper tract adenomas, surveillance at yearly intervals is recommended. Gastrectomy is not indicated in patients with fundic gland retention polyps of the stomach; these are considered benign lesions. Moreover, gastric adenocarcinoma in FAP patients is

---

*Editor's Note: Although ileoanal pouch anastomoses are usually successful with a very low rate of pouchitis, patients are still not thrilled to trade one bowel movement per day for an average of five per day. I imagine one-stage surgery will be more common in the future.

not increased over the general population, and adenomas of the stomach alone are not an indication for gastrectomy.

FAP patients are also at risk for neoplasms of the thyroid (usually in the third decade of life) and pancreatic cancer (the lifetime risk is about one in 47 and one in 59 persons, respectively). Screening for pancreatic cancer may not be worthwhile with currently available methods, but careful physical examination of the thyroid is warranted along with consideration of ultrasonography.

Turcot's Syndrome

Clinical Aspects

Turcot's syndrome can be considered simply as FAP with extracolonic manifestations in which the extracolonic lesion is a brain tumor. Of note, some patients may not fully express the polyposis phenotype and have as few as ten colorectal adenomatous polyps. Brain neoplasms noted in Turcot's syndrome include primarily medulloblastomas but also glioblastomas and astrocytomas. These tumors usually present in the second decade of life. Although brain neoplasms generally involve only one individual in an FAP pedigree, several families have had multiple offspring affected.

Management

Management of Turcot's syndrome is identical to that of FAP with the addition of careful neurologic examinations as part of routine surveillance.

HAMARTOMATOUS POLYPOSIS SYNDROMES

Hamartomatous polyps and polyposis syndromes are less common than the adenomatous lesions. Previously, these hamartomatous conditions were thought to harbor little if any malignant potential, but recent evidence supports neoplastic sequelae in some of these syndromes.

Peutz-Jeghers Syndrome

Clinical Aspects

Peutz-Jeghers syndrome is an autosomal dominant condition in which Peutz-Jeghers polyps occur primarily in the small intestine, but they may also be in the colon and stomach. The polyps usually number between one and 20 per intestinal segment and have a unique histopathology, with polyp epithelium supported by an arborizing framework of smooth muscle. The characteristic physical finding is macular melanin pigmentation on the lips and buccal mucosa but also on the digits of the hands, feet, and eyelids.

The primary complication of this disorder in childhood is small intestine intussusception; intestinal bleeding can also occur. Adults are at a strikingly increased risk, at relatively young age, for both GI and non-GI cancers (breast, ovary, endometrium, pancreas). Subsets of patients have both intestinal adenomas and hamartomas. Unusual tumors found are Sertoli cell tumor of the ovary and adenoma malignum of the cervix in women, and testicular cancer in prepubescent boys.

Management

At-risk individuals (first-degree relatives of affected individuals) should be screened at least once early in the second decade of life for Peutz-Jeghers syndrome with upper GI endoscopy and small bowel follow-through radiography.

When diagnosed, affected patients should have at least an initial upper and lower GI endoscopy biopsying all polyps to search for concomitant adenomas (the probable major source of GI neoplasms). All adenomas should be removed. Some authors recommend repeating these endoscopic and small bowel x-ray studies every 2 years. These authorities suggest endoscopic polypectomy of Peutz-Jeghers polyps that are hemorrhagic or over 1 cm in size. Surgery has been recommended for symptomatic small intestinal polyps or those over 1.5 cm. During laparotomy, an attempt to clear the small intestine of polyps should be made by concomitant endoscopic polypectomy or, in the case of larger polyps, enterotomy.

Additional screening in affected patients should include annual history and physical examinations with routine laboratory tests; mammography with a baseline examination at age 25, and then yearly at age 40; and annual gynecologic examination with pelvic ultrasonography starting in adolescence. Patients should be encouraged to perform self-examinations of the breast and testicles.

Solitary Juvenile Polyps/Familial Juvenile Polyposis

Clinical Aspects

Juvenile polyps are hamartomatous lesions with a histopathologic appearance characterized by edematous mucosa and dilated, mucus-filled cysts.

Most patients with solitary juvenile polyps present on average at 4 years of age with rectal bleeding or anal prolapse of a polyp. Patients with solitary juvenile polyps, the vast majority of individuals affected by this lesion, have a nonfamilial condition, and removal of the polyp is sufficient treatment.

On the other hand, patients with more than two rectosigmoid juvenile polyps or with a family history of juvenile polyps should be suspected of having familial juvenile polyposis. These patients present on average at 9 years of age (although they can be preschoolers) with anemia, rectal bleeding, failure to thrive, and abdominal pain. In this syndrome, polyps, numbering from a dozen to hundreds, occur primarily in the colon but also in the small intestine and stomach. This may be an autosomal dominant condition.

Of concern in familial juvenile polyposis patients is the high incidence of colorectal neoplasia (dysplasia and adenocarcinoma) found in up to 20 percent of patients at relatively young ages (average 37 years, but dysplasia has been found in the colectomy specimens of several patients under 5 years of age). Colorectal neoplasia can be found in the juvenile polyps as well as the flat mucosa. Gastric, duodenal, and pancreatic cancers have also been reported.

Management

Rarely, patients with solitary juvenile polyps develop colorectal neoplasia. Therefore, these lesions should usually be removed, even if asymptomatic. In patients with a solitary juvenile polyp and no family history of juvenile polyps, this is sufficient treatment.

In contrast, I recommend that, when possible, juvenile polyp patients with multiple such polyps (three or more rectosigmoid polyps) or a family history of juvenile polyps should have complete upper and lower GI endoscopy and small bowel radiography examinations to determine whether familial juvenile polyposis is present. In affected individuals, periodic surveillance by colonoscopy with multiple random biopsies of both polyps and flat mucosa (as done in ulcerative colitis surveillance) every 1 to 3 years is recommended. The upper tract probably should also be surveyed. Removal of dysplastic juvenile polyps can be accomplished by endoscopic polypectomy in those with a small number of polyps. At times, colonoscopy surveillance may be difficult, especially in patients with numerous lesions. Colectomy is a consideration in these individuals because neoplasia may not be sampled by biopsies and polypectomies. Currently, there appear to be insufficient data to justify prophylactic colectomy solely for the risk of colorectal carcinoma, as is done in FAP. However, when there are any other indications such as persistent rectal bleeding or refractory protein loss, subtotal colectomy with ileorectal anastomosis is appropriate.

Screening

An initial screening of first-degree relatives at 12 years of age with colonoscopy is prudent because of the difficulty in recognizing asymptomatic affected individuals. Some authorities recommend subsequent screening with flexible sigmoidoscopy and Hemoccult testing every 3 to 5 years.

Ruvalcaba-Myhre-Smith Syndrome

Ruvalcaba-Myhre-Smith syndrome is very rare and may be a variant of juvenile polyposis. Affected individuals have unusual craniofacial appearance, developmental delay, macrocephaly, and pigmented macules on the shaft and glans of the penis. Intussusception is a complication.

Cronkhite-Canada Syndrome

Clinical Aspects

Cronkhite-Canada Syndrome is a nonfamilial disorder characterized by multiple juvenile polyps noted throughout the GI tract (except the esophagus). In contrast to juvenile polyposis, the mucosa between polyps is also abnormal with edema, congestion, and inflammation of the lamina propria and focal glandular ectasia. Clinical features include cutaneous hyperpigmentation, hair loss, and nail dystrophy (thinning, splitting, and onycholysis). Presenting symptoms are diarrhea from protein loss, variable degrees of fat and disaccharide malabsorption, weight loss, and peripheral edema. The juvenile polyps have been reported to undergo adenomatous and carcinomatous degeneration.

Management

Among the 60 reported cases, there are no controlled medical trials in this disorder. A variety of treatments, including corticosteroids, antibiotics, surgery, and hyperalimentation have been tried with varying success, and some patients appear to improve spontaneously. The current recommendations are for supportive therapy with enteral or parental hyperalimentation. Corticosteroid treatment is suggested if the patient deteriorates. Antibiotics have questionable value. Surgery of the GI tract is used to treat bleeding, malignancy, and intussusception. Screening with colonoscopy for colorectal dysplasia and carcinoma should be performed periodically.

Cowden's Disease

Clinical Aspects

Cowden's disease is rare with fewer than 100 cases reported. This syndrome is autosomal dominant and characterized by multiple facial trichilemmomas occurring around the mouth, nose, and eyes but also on the distal extremities, including the palms and soles. About 35 percent of patients have GI hamartomatous polyps that can occur throughout the intestinal tract, including the esophagus. The histopathologic appearance of these lesions varies widely and may reveal lipomas, juvenile polyps, inflammatory polyps, ganglioneuroma, and lymphoid hyperplasia. Extraintestinal lesions include nodular hyperplasia or follicular adenomas of the thyroid in two-thirds of affected individuals, thyroid cancer in 10 percent, fibrocystic disease and fibroadenomas of the breast in 75 percent of women, and breast cancer in almost 50 percent. A variety of other benign soft tissue tumors and congenital abnormalities have been observed.

Management

Recognition of this syndrome provides the clinician the opportunity to screen for thyroid and breast cancer.

If GI symptoms are absent, investigation of the GI tract is not necessary.

Intestinal Ganglioneuromatosis

Polypoid lesions from overgrowth of nerve tissue in the mucosa, submucosa, or muscle layers of the GI tract can occur in von Recklinghausen's neurofibromatosis, in multiple endocrine neoplasia type II, and as an idiopathic abnormality.

Devon Family Syndrome

A single female family member in three successive generations of a pedigree developed multiple inflammatory polyps of the ileum that precipitated intussusception in each affected individual. The polyps were proliferations of histiocytes.

HYPERPLASTIC POLYPS/HYPERPLASTIC POLYPOSIS

Clinical Aspects

Hyperplastic polyps are considered non-neoplastic lesions and account for approximately 20 percent of all colorectal diminutive polyps (polyps less than 6 mm in size). Often, they are single lesions in the rectosigmoid region. In 10 percent of cases, polyps are multiple; in a few patients, hundreds of hyperplastic polyps have been noted simulating FAP.

Management

Although the question is debatable, most authorities agree that the presence of a hyperplastic polyp on flexible sigmoidoscopy is not a marker of more proximal adenomatous lesions, and therefore not an indication for further evaluation by colonoscopy. In patients with multiple lesions, biopsy and histologic review are necessary to distinguish hyperplastic polyposis from FAP. Hyperplastic lesions can be treated conservatively with removal of symptomatic lesions.

NODULAR LYMPHOID HYPERPLASIA

Clinical Aspects

Nodular lymphoid hyperplasia is a rare disorder usually found in the terminal ileum of patients with FAP, common variable immunodeficiency, and (rarely) intestinal lymphoma and often in healthy children. The polyps are usually 1 to 3 mm in size.

Management

This condition requires no specific treatment per se. Confusion with adenomatous polyps is common in FAP patients with ileorectal anastomosis. The confusion can be eliminated if these lesions are biopsied for histo-

pathologic review. The association with other disorders should be considered.

LYMPHOMATOUS/LEUKEMATOUS POLYPOSIS

Multiple nodular lesions with diffuse involvement of the GI tract can be seen in extranodal lymphoma, Mediterranean-type lymphoma, and chronic leukemia. Polyp size ranges between 3 and 7 mm and the condition can be confused with FAP.

INFLAMMATORY POLYPS

In idiopathic inflammatory bowel disease (ulcerative colitis, Crohn's disease) as well as infectious colitides, islands of regenerated mucosa may appear polypoid. Also, colitis cystica profunda may be noted in inflammatory colitis. These are sessile polyps that consist of dilated and epithelium-lined mucous cysts within the muscularis mucosae. These inflammatory "pseudopolyps" are non-neoplastic and do not require specific treatment.

MISCELLANEOUS

Pneumatosis cystoides intestinalis presents as multiple air-filled cysts within the submucosa of the colorectum or small intestine. Characteristically, when biopsied, these cysts often deflate. The cysts may be associated with chronic obstructive pulmonary disease and scleroderma, and can be treated with nasal canula oxygen. Pneumatosis cystoides intestinalis can also be seen with fulminant intestinal ischemia.

Lipomas are yellow-appearing submucosal lesions usually found in the cecum. Biopsy may reveal normal overlying mucosa. The endoscopist should not try to treat these benign lesions.

SUGGESTED READING

Boland CR, Itzkowitz SH, Kim YS. Colonic polyps and the gastrointestinal polyposis syndromes. In: Sleisenger MH, Fordtran JS, eds. Gastrointestinal disease; pathophysiology, diagnosis, and management. 4th ed. Philadelphia: WB Saunders, 1989:1500–1507.

Burt RW. Polyposis syndromes. In: Yamada T, ed. Textbook of gastroenterology. Philadelphia: JB Lippincott, 1991:1674–1695.

Giardiello FM, Hamilton SR, Kern SE, et al. Colorectal neoplasia in patients with juvenile polyposis or juvenile polyps. Arch Child Dis 1991; 66:971–975.

Giardiello FM, Offerhaus GJA, Krush AJ, et al. The risk of hepatoblastoma in familial adenomatous polyposis. J Pediatr 1991; 119:766–768.

Giardiello FM, Welsh SB, Offerhaus GJA, et al. Increased risk of cancer in Peutz-Jeghers syndrome. N Engl J Med 1987; 316: 1511–1514.

Luk GD. Colonic polyps: benign and premalignant neoplasm of the colon. In: Yamada T, ed. Textbook of gastroenterology. Philadelphia: JB Lippincott, 1991:1645–1674.

Offerhaus GJA, Giardiello FM, Krush AJ, et al. The risk of upper gastrointestinal cancer in familial adenomatous polyposis. Gastroenterology 1992; 102:1980–1982.

COLORECTAL CANCER

JAMES M. STONE, M.D.
JOHN E. NIEDERHUBER, M.D.

EPIDEMIOLOGY AND PATHOLOGY

Colorectal cancer is the second most common visceral malignancy in the United States; approximately 160,000 new cases will occur this year. There is strong evidence that both environmental and genetic factors are involved in the genesis of colorectal cancer. Epidemiologic studies demonstrate a wide variation in the incidence of colorectal cancer in different populations, however, migration studies show that the incidence rates of immigrant populations readily equalize with the host population. Diet is believed to be the dominant environmental factor, and populations that ingest diets high in fat and low in fiber have the highest rates, while western vegetarians and those in developing nations have the lowest rates.

The genetic predisposition to colorectal cancer is most clearly demonstrated in the familial adenomatous polyposis (FAP) syndrome. In this autosomal dominant, heritable syndrome, essentially 100 percent of affected individuals develop colorectal cancer. The genetic locus linked to FAP has been mapped to a specific chromosome (5q). Colorectal cancer may also be inherited in an autosomal dominant fashion in the hereditary nonpolyposis colon cancer syndrome (HNPCC). This syndrome is characterized by early age of cancer onset, predominance of right-sided lesions, and frequent synchronous and metachronous cancers in the absence of multiple polyps. Approximately 5 percent of patients with colorectal cancer have the HNPCC syndrome while an even larger proportion will have a positive family history for colorectal cancer. Persons with a single first-degree relative with colorectal cancer have a three-fold increase in risk of colorectal cancer compared with the general population; two first-degree relatives confers a nine-fold increase in risk. There is a separate chapter on colonic polyposis.

Vogelstein and others have outlined a sequence of genetic abnormalities leading to malignant neoplasia of the colon. Some genetic abnormalities are inherited while others reflect spontaneous somatic mutations or the carcinogenic effect of environmental factors. Eventually, the accumulated activation of oncogenes and inactivation of tumor suppresser genes leads to step-wise transformation of colonic epithelium. The identification of genetic alterations in colon cancer holds great promise in the prevention and early diagnosis of colorectal cancer.

Epidemiological and pathologic data have long supported the concept that the great majority of colorectal cancers arise from benign polyps. The validity of the polyp to cancer sequence has been supported by recent molecular genetic studies: adenomas usually have one mutation or deletion, in situ carcinomas may have two, invasive cancers may have three or four. Colorectal polyps therefore are an important marker for genetic abnormality and cancer risk.

Ninety-five percent of colorectal cancers are adenocarcinomas. On rare occasions lymphomas, malignant carcinoid, melanoma, leiomyosarcomas, or squamous cancers may also arise from the large bowel. The large bowel is rarely the site of metastatic disease, however, melanoma, lymphoma, and carcinomas of the breast, ovary, lung, and stomach occasionally involve the colon. Usually such metastases occur late in the course of disease. Prostate cancer in rare cases invades the rectum by direct extension.

Colorectal cancers are termed invasive when they grow through the muscularis mucosa into the submucosa. Prior to this point, hematogenous or lymphatic metastases are very uncommon. The growing tumor mass may extend circumferentially around the lumen to give the typical "apple-core" appearance seen on barium enema. Intramural spread of the tumor, parallel to the long axis of the bowel, generally does not occur. Recognition of this pattern of tumor growth has enabled surgeons to perform sphincter-sparing, low anterior resection for tumors in the mid to lower rectum.

The pattern of spread of colorectal tumors depends on the anatomy of the involved bowel segment, as well as its lymphatic and vascular supply. The rectum is generally divided into upper, middle, and lower thirds. The tight anatomic confines of the bony pelvis, the diffuse nature of the lymphatic drainage, and the dual blood supply of this area make the pattern of spread from the extraperitoneal rectum different from the intraperitoneal rectum or the colon. Cancers in the lower third of the rectum may spread either via the superior hemorrhoidal veins to the portal system and the liver, or via the middle hemorrhoidal veins to the systemic circulation and the lung. Pulmonary metastases, without intervening liver metastases, are unusual in patients with primary tumors proximal to the lower rectum. Tumor cells of the extraperitoneal rectum may also enter the prevertebral venous plexus and result in thoracic or lumbar spinal metastasis. Tumor cells of the extraperitoneal rectum commonly invade the vagina by direct extension, and on occasion may also directly invade the seminal vesicles, prostate, uterus, urinary bladder, pelvic floor, or sphincter mechanism.

The natural history of tumors arising in the colon and upper rectum are similar. Lymph node metastases generally parallel the arterial supply of the colon, and hematogenous metastases almost always present first in the liver. Tumors that erode through the serosal surface may spread to adjacent or distant peritoneal surfaces. Ovarian metastases occur in approximately 5 percent of women with colon cancer.

Dukes' correlated the degree of tumor invasion at the time of resection with survival and proposed the following classification in 1929: tumor confined to the

Table 1 Classification of Colorectal Cancer

Dukes'		Astler-Coller		5-Year Survival
A	Limited to bowel wall	**A**	Limited to mucosa	90%–95%
B	Through bowel wall	**B1**	Into muscularis propria	60%
		B2	Through serosa	50%
C	Regional node metastasis	**C1**	Into musc. propria, lymph node metastasis	40%
		C2	Through serosa, lymph node metastasis	25%

Table 2 TNM and Endorectal Ultrasound Classification of Colorectal Cancer

TNM Classification	Description	ERUS Classification
Tis	Carcinoma in situ	uT0
T1	Tumor invades submucosa	uT1
T2	Tumor invades muscularis propria	uT2
T3	Tumor invades subserosa or nonperitonealized pericolic or perirectal tissue	uT3
T4	Tumor perforates visceral peritoneum or directly invades other structure	uT4
N0	No regional node metastases	uN0
N1	1-3 pericolic or perirectal nodes involved	uN1
N2	>4 pericolic or perirectal nodes involved	uN1
N3	Node metastasis along major vascular trunk	—
M0	No distant metastasis	—
M1	Distant metastasis	—

Stage 0: Tis, N0, M0; Stage I: T1-2, N0, M0; Stage II: T3–4, N0, M0; Stage III: T1–4, N1–3; M0; Stage IV: T1–4; N1–3; M1.
ERUS = endoluminal rectal ultrasound

bowel wall (stage A); tumor through the bowel wall, no lymph node metastases, (stage B); lymph node metastases (stage C). Although Dukes' classification was originally derived from patients with rectal cancer, it has been useful in staging patients with colon cancer as well. Numerous modifications of Dukes' classification have been proposed with the intent of increasing its prognostic value. The most popular of these is the Astler-Coller system (Table 1). To provide a uniform and orderly classification for cancer of the colon and rectum, the American Joint Committee on Cancer Staging has proposed a TNM classification (Table 2). Accurate classification is essential for determining prognosis, entering patients into therapeutic trials, and determining the outcome of therapy.*

PREVENTION AND SCREENING

Primary prevention of colorectal cancer through interventions that reduce or eliminate the genetic changes responsible for malignant transformation is not yet available, but is the goal of much of today's research. Secondary prevention of colon cancer, however, is possible through the elimination of colon polyps. Colonoscopy is the most reliable method for detecting colorectal polyps and it offers the opportunity to remove polyps and subject them to histologic review. However, colonoscopy is impractical as a screening test because it is expensive, time-consuming, and likely to cause complications.

Current screening techniques are primarily designed to detect colorectal cancer while it is in a curable stage, however, an attempt should also be made to eliminate colon polyps when they are found. Recently published data from the University of Minnesota shows that screening a normal risk population for colon cancer with the fecal occult blood test diminishes the likelihood of dying of colorectal cancer by 33 percent. In 1992 the American Cancer Society revised its recommendations for screening for colon and rectum cancer. Asymptomatic individuals should undergo digital rectal examination starting at age 40 and beginning at age 50, should have yearly fecal occult blood tests and sigmoidoscopy (preferably flexible) repeated at 3- to 5-year intervals. Individuals with one or more first-degree relatives who have colon or rectum cancer before the age of 55, should

*__Editor's Note:__ Although there are similar tables in other chapters, the variations used here seemed worthy of some duplication.

undergo colonoscopy or barium enema examination at 5-year intervals, starting at 35 to 40 years of age. If occult blood is found or if an adenomatous polyp is present at flexible sigmoidoscopy, colonoscopy or air contrast barium enema (ACBE) should be performed. If a cancer of the distal colon or rectum is found on flexible sigmoidoscopy, colonoscopy or ACBE should be performed in the perioperative period.

As suggested in the American Cancer Society recommendations, patients with higher than normal risk of developing colon cancer (Table 3) should be screened more aggressively, preferably with interval colonoscopy (Tables 4 and 5). Screening is discussed in more detail in the chapter *Colorectal Cancer Screening.*

Table 3 Patients at Increased Risk for Colorectal Cancer

Personal history of:
   Colorectal cancer
   Adenoma
   Ureterosigmoidostomy
   Radiation therapy involving large bowel
   Ulcerative colitis

Family history of:
   Colorectal cancer
   Polyposis syndrome
   Hereditary nonpolyposis colon cancer syndrome

DIAGNOSIS AND EVALUATION

The signs and symptoms of colorectal cancer are determined by the location, size, and invasiveness of the primary tumor. Rectal cancers usually present with bright red rectal bleeding. In later stages, they may cause tenesmus, fecal urgency, a sense of incomplete evacuation, and the need to have frequent small bowel movements. Large tumors may cause symptoms of colonic obstruction. Invasion of adjacent structures may result in fecal incontinence, rectovaginal or rectovesical fistula, or sacral pain.

Tumors in the distal colon tend to cause obstructive symptoms because the lumen is relatively narrow and the stool is more solid. Conversely, tumors of the proximal colon are slower to cause obstruction because of the larger size of the lumen and the more liquid nature of the stool. These tumors are more likely to manifest with the symptoms of anemia or an abdominal mass. An exception is tumors arising at the ileocecal valve, which tend to cause obstruction of the narrow terminal ileum. These patients present with symptoms of distal small bowel obstruction or right lower quadrant pain, and may come to operation with a diagnosis of adhesive band obstruction, inflammatory bowel disease, or acute appendicitis.

When colorectal cancer is suspected because of clinical signs or symptoms the preferred diagnostic test is total colonoscopy. If colonoscopy cannot be performed

Table 4 American Cancer Society Recommendations for Early Detection of Colorectal Cancer — Normal Risk

Test or Procedure	Gender	Age	Frequency
Sigmoidoscopy, preferably flexible	M & F	50 yr and over	Every 3-5 yr
Fecal occult blood testing	M & F	50 yr and over	Every yr
Digital rectal examination	M & F	40 yr and over	Every yr

Table 5 American Cancer Society Recommendations for Early Detection of Colorectal Cancer — Increased Risk

Risk factor	Test	Age	Frequency
1st-degree relative with colorectal cancer onset <55 yr old	Colonoscopy or ACBE	35-40 yr	5-yr intervals
Family hx of familial adenomatous polyposis	Proctoscopy	13 yr	Yearly to 45 yr old
Familial adenomatous polyposis trait	Colonoscopy and biopsies	Discovery to time of colectomy	Yearly
Ulcerative pancolitis	Colonoscopy and biopsies	10 yr after onset of disease	Yearly
Ureterosigmoidostomy	Flexible sigmoidoscopy	5 yr after ureterosigmoidostomy	Yearly
Radiation proctosigmoiditis	Flexible sigmoidoscopy	10 yr after radation	Yearly
Hereditary nonpolyposis cancer syndrome	Colonoscopy or ACBE	5 yr before the onset of earliest cancer	Yearly

ACBE = air contrast barium enema
Adapted from Levin B, Murphy GP. Revision in American Cancer Society recommendations for the early detection of colorectal cancer. CA Cancer J Clin 1992; 42:296-299; with permission.

or is incomplete, sigmoidoscopy followed by ACBE is the required evaluation. Sigmoidoscopy is important to prevent the inadvertent infusion of barium above a distal obstructing lesion and because most of the lesions missed on ACBE are in the rectum or sigmoid colon. The area of rectum posterior and immediately proximal to the sphincter mechanism falls back into the sacral hollow and is not seen well during routine colonoscopy. This area should be palpated by digital examination before inserting the colonoscope. The ACBE is preferred over a full-column barium study because it is more sensitive. Complete colonoscopy should be the goal even if an obvious cancer is identified because the incidence of synchronous cancers is 2 to 4 percent and the incidence of concomitant adenomatous polyps is nearly 50 percent. If colonoscopy cannot be completed preoperatively because of an obstructing lesion, it should be completed after the patient recovers from excision of the obstructing lesion.

After the diagnosis of colon or rectum cancer is established, certain laboratory and radiologic studies may be of use in planning therapy. Measurement of the hematocrit determines the presence of anemia and the ability of the patient to donate autologous blood. The blood carcinoembryonic antigen (CEA) level is determined preoperatively. If the preoperative CEA level is greatly elevated, liver metastasis should be strongly suspected. A rising CEA level in the postoperative period may be an early indication of cancer recurrence. A chest radiograph will reveal lung metastasis. Although the cost effectiveness of routine preoperative computed tomography (CT) remains unproved, several factors support the use of CT as part of the preoperative evaluation. If resectable liver metastases are found, the surgeon should be prepared to resect them at the same time that the primary tumor is resected. Patients with multiple metastases may be candidates for hepatic artery infusion therapy. Preoperative CT scans demonstrating multiple liver metastases prepare the patient and the surgeon for placement of an infusion device at the time of the initial operation. The CT scan may also provide information about invasion of the primary tumor into adjacent structures which is important for planning the operative approach. The scan serves as a baseline for patients with high-risk lesions who will be followed for recurrence by serial CT scans.

Although CT scans are more sensitive than palpation for identifying liver metastases deep within the liver, the most sensitive method of identifying liver metastases is intraoperative hepatic ultrasound combined with palpation to identify small surface lesions. Intraoperative ultrasound is not performed on all patients operated on for colon and rectum cancer because of the time, cost, and need to surgically expose the liver. Intraoperative ultrasound is very useful in patients with planned hepatic resection to identify previously unsuspected lesions, and to more precisely understand the relationship between the tumor(s) and major intrahepatic structures, to better delineate CT findings that are suspicious but inconclu-

sive, and in patients with suspected liver metastases but normal CT scans (CEA greater than 100 ng per deciliter, or prior to resection of a pulmonary metastasis from colon cancer). There is a separate chapter on resection of liver metasteses.

THERAPY

The most effective therapy for primary colon and rectum cancer remains surgical resection. The goals of surgical resection are removal of the primary tumor with an adequate margin of normal proximal and distal colon along with the lymphatics draining the involved bowel. Recently, postoperative adjuvant therapy has been shown to diminish the likelihood of tumor recurrence and to increase survival in patients with certain stages of colon or rectum cancer. Although colon and rectum tumors are histologically indistinguishable, differences in regional anatomy, venous and lymphatic drainage, accessibility, and response to treatment cause them to be managed in very different ways.

Colon Cancer

The blood supply and concomitant lymphatic drainage are the major determinants of the extent of resection performed for colon cancer. Traditional radical lymphadenectomy involves ligation of the appropriate colic vessel(s) as close as possible to their origin off of the superior mesenteric artery for the right and transverse colon, or the aorta for the left colon. A further consideration is the ability to bring two healthy bowel ends, with good arterial blood supply, together without tension. Tumors arising in the left colon may require resection back to the transverse colon solely for this purpose. The adequacy of proximal and distal colon margins is rarely a consideration because proper lymphatic resection necessitates a generous resection of normal proximal and distal colon. Although there is no prospectively-derived, controlled evidence that radical lymphadenectomy enhances the cure rate in patients with colon cancer, there is good reason to continue the practice. Radical lymphadenectomy is likely to be helpful because (1) the best chance to cure a colon cancer is at the time of the first operation; (2) many patients with excised lymph node metastases will be cured; (3) lymph node metastases are only reliably diagnosed by histologic examination; (4) the presence or absence of lymph node metastases has important prognostic implications and guides effective, but toxic, adjuvant therapy, and traditional radical lymphadenectomy adds little to morbidity.

The anastomosis may be effected by either a sutured or stapled technique. Although it is not difficult to find vigorous proponents of one technique over the other, in the intraperitoneal colon, either technique properly performed will give equivalent results. We prefer to perform intraperitoneal anastomosis by an end-to-end sutured technique. A sutured anastomosis can be performed almost as quickly as a stapled anastomosis and eliminates the cost of the three to four stapler firings used in a typical anastomosis. The anastomosis may be performed via an end-to-end, end-to-side, side-to-end, or stapled "functional" end-to-end technique. The colonoscopist should understand the various techniques, so that they may be recognized at the time of follow-up endoscopy.

Obstruction or perforation of the primary tumor may create special situations which necessitate changes in the operative approach. Ten to 20 percent of colon and rectum cancers present with signs of obstruction. Management is determined by the degree of luminal obstruction, the location of the lesion, and the overall condition of the patient. Most patients with partial obstruction can undergo elective resection, and obstructing cancers in the right colon can usually be managed with a standard right hemicolectomy. The treatment of obstruction distal to the splenic flexure has been associated with higher complication rates so a greater variety of management strategies have been developed. The traditional three-stage approach, proximal colostomy, resection, and anastomosis in three separate operations, is now rarely performed. When there is complete distal colonic obstruction and the patient's condition precludes resection, a loop colostomy should be performed. Unless there is evidence of perforation, the colostomy can be performed through a limited incision under local or general anesthesia. Approximately 1 week later, resection of the tumor—carried back to the colostomy—and primary anastomosis is possible.

If the patient with a distal obstruction can tolerate a laparotomy and the amount of intestinal distention does not preclude a standard lymphadenectomy, resection with anastomosis and a proximal loop colostomy may be performed. The colostomy is closed after healing of the anastomosis has been confirmed by contrast enema. Since the ileocecal valve usually protects the ileum from the effects of distention, one modern approach has been to carry the resection back to the terminal ileum and perform a primary ileorectal or ileosigmoid anastomosis. Although anastomotic leaks are rare with this approach, an extensive operation is required and functional results are often poor. Recently, some surgeons have advocated resection followed by on-table bowel prep and primary anastomosis. This approach has been successful but should only be attempted when two healthy, well-vascularized bowel ends can be brought together without tension.

Perforation occurs most commonly in the cecum, the most easily distended part of the colon, or at the site of the tumor itself. Perforation is a surgical emergency and is managed by prompt resuscitation and resection of the perforated area. Performing proximal colostomy and drainage of the area of perforation does not reliably control sepsis and should only be used in the most desperate situations. If at all possible the area of perforation should be resected. If the peritoneal soilage is localized away from the anastomosis, the bowel may be reconnected in a standard fashion. An unprotected anastomosis should not be performed in a region of established peritonitis.

Laparoscopic colectomy is increasingly popular; however, claims that the extent of lymphadenectomy, morbidity, and ultimate survival are equivalent to conventional techniques remain unsubstantiated. Currently, most "laparoscopic" colectomies are actually performed through a combination of conventional and laparoscopic techniques (laparoscopic-assisted colectomy). A limited incision is necessary to remove the specimen, and to re-establish bowel continuity because intracorporeal anastomotic techniques are cumbersome and unreliable. It is likely that improvements in instrumentation and technique will increase the application of minimal access surgery in colon cancer in the future.

Adjuvant Therapy

An indication that many patients have undetected spread beyond the margins of resection is that 40 to 50 percent of patients who undergo an attempted curative resection eventually die of disseminated disease. The need to eliminate these microscopic metastatic deposits before they can grow into overt metastases has led to an extensive search for effective adjuvant therapy. The success of combined 5-fluorouracil (5-FU) and levamisole in trials from the Mayo Clinic and the North Central Cancer Treatment Group (NCCTG), led to a large multicenter trial of 5-FU and levamisole in stage II and stage III colon cancer in 1985. Over 2 years, 1,296 patients were randomized into groups receiving levamisole alone, levamisole and 5-FU, or no treatment beyond surgery. With a median 3 year follow-up, there was a significant reduction in disease recurrence and a significant improvement in overall survival in the stage III patients who received 5-FU and levamisole. There was no benefit demonstrated in the stage II patients. These results generated a clinical alert from the NIH which recommended the 5-FU-levamisole regimen for "nearly every" patient with colon cancer and lymph node metastases. Although the local recurrence rate for high risk colon tumors (T3 tumors, especially in the retroperitoneal colon) is almost 40 percent, there has been little role for radiotherapy in colon cancer. This is because colon tumors, which are relatively radioresistant, are surrounded by radiosensitive organs such as the small bowel, kidney and liver which limit radiation dose. Adjuvant therapy of colon cancer is discussed in greater detail in the next chapter.

Rectal Cancer

While the surgical treatment of colon cancer has changed little in the past 50 years, the treatment of extraperitoneal cancer of the rectum has been changing rapidly over the past 10 years. As with colon cancer, the time-honored approach to rectal cancer is radical excision which involves removal of the tumor-bearing rectum along with its lymphatic drainage, and an acceptable distal margin. Since the appearance of circular staplers in the early 1980s, the generally accepted paradigm has been: cancer of the upper and middle rectum—perform sphincter sparing (low anterior) resection; cancer of the lower third of the rectum—perform abdominal-perineal resection (APR) with permanent colostomy. Radical excision was felt to be necessary because there was no way of knowing preoperatively which tumors were confined to the bowel wall (curable with a local excision), and which had metastasized to regional nodes (require radical lymphatic excision for cure). On the other side of the equation, cancer recurred in the operative field in 20 to 40 percent of patients with advanced primary cancers. This suggested that standard radical surgical techniques were insufficient to provide local control in some circumstances.

The advent of effective adjuvant therapy, and the ability to more accurately stage tumors preoperatively, has further modified thinking about the treatment for rectum cancer. The current trend is best categorized as an attempt to match the invasiveness of the therapy to the risk from the tumor. Low-risk cancers are treated with minimal operations such as transanal local resection, while tumors at the highest risk for local or distant failure are treated with radical excision, radiation, and chemotherapy. The challenge posed by this treatment model is that there must be a way to differentiate high-risk from low-risk cancers preoperatively.

Pathology studies, performed on radical excision specimens, have shown a strong correlation between the depth of primary tumor invasion and lymph node metastases (Table 6). Today, depth of invasion of the primary tumor is determined with greater than 90 percent accuracy by ERUS. This technique utilizes a 7 MHz probe which is inserted into the rectum, above the tumor, through a modified proctoscope. A five layer image of the rectal wall is obtained and the probe is pulled down over the tumor (Fig. 1). The depth of tumor invasion is determined by the disruption of the normal tissue interfaces within the rectal wall. Lymph nodes in the perirectal area may also be imaged in this way, however, the accuracy of determining lymph node metastasis with ERUS is only about 66 percent. An ERUS staging system has been devised that parallels the TNM system (Table 2). One of the major advantages of preoperative staging with ERUS is the ability to select good-risk candidates for local excision. Full-thickness excision of the extraperitoneal rectal wall may be performed with minimal morbidity via the transanal route. In this technique, a retractor is placed in the anus, the rectal wall is pulled down with stay sutures, and a full thickness disk of the rectal wall encompassing the tumor is removed (Fig. 2). The defect is repaired by suturing. The operation generally requires a general or regional anesthetic and a full bowel prep. Many of the problems with conventional radical surgery such as impotence, small bowel obstruction, incontinence, need for transfusion or colostomy are avoided. Other perineal ap-

Table 6 Rectal Cancer: Depth of Primary Tumor Invasion and Incidence of Lymph Node Metastases

Depth of invasion:	T0	T1	T2	T3
Lymph node metastases:	≥ 0	5%	20%	35%–55%

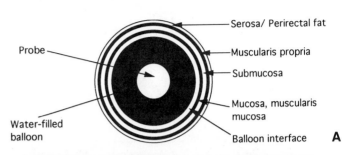

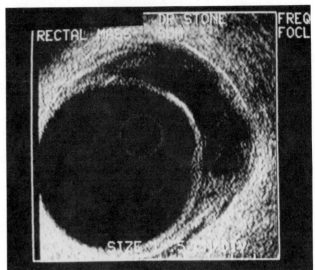

Figure 1 *A,* Five layer model of the rectal wall. Obliteration of normal interface echoes indicates depth of invasion into the rectal wall. *B,* Lesion—note break in second bright line, thickening of outer dark line, and maintenance of outer bright line, interface between muscularis propria, and perirectal tissue.

proaches such as the transsacral or transsphincteric approach give somewhat wider exposure but at the price of higher complication rates. In general, local excision is preferred over nonresectional therapies such as electrofulgeration, laser photoablation, or endocavitary radiation because excision allows complete pathologic examination of the tissue.

Tumors which are accessible through one of the perineal approaches should be treated by local excision if they are well or moderately well differentiated, and do not invade beyond the submucosa (uT1). Tumors that invade into, but not through the muscularis propria (uT2), have a local recurrence rate of approximately 20 percent when treated by local excision. These patients typically are treated with radical resection, however, preliminary work suggests that adjuvant therapy improves the success rate of local excision to approximately

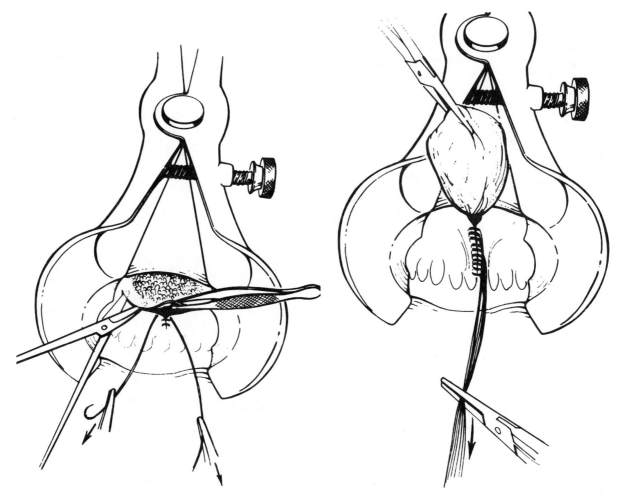

Figure 2 Technique of transanal excision. An anoscope is placed and stay sutures adjacent to the tumor are used to pull the rectal wall distally. An incision is made at the distal end of the tumor. The incision is closed as dissection proceeds into the more proximal rectum. The sutures are left long and are used to place further traction on the rectal wall.

90 percent in patients with T2 tumors. Consideration should be given to local excision in patients with uT2 tumors who are poor operative risks. Tumors that invade into the perirectal fat (T3) must be treated by radical excision because the failure rate of local excision is greater than 50 percent.

Radical excision of low rectal tumors traditionally has included excision of the anus, rectum, and distal sigmoid colon along with its mesentery and creation of a permanent end-colostomy (abdominal-perineal resection). The introduction of circular stapling devices, along with the understanding that distal spread along the bowel wall is rare, has greatly diminished the number of APRs performed. Indications for APR now are inability to obtain a 2 cm unstretched distal margin, poorly differentiated tumors of the lower rectum, pre-existing fecal incontinence, or invasion of the sphincters or adjacent organs. If APR is not necessary, an anastomosis from the proximal colon to the rectum is performed. When the anastomosis is below the peritoneal reflection it is termed a low anterior resection. Anastomosis to the extraperitoneal rectum is best performed with a circular

stapling device. If the anastomosis is not technically perfect or the health of the bowel is questioned, a temporary colostomy or ileostomy may be created. The stoma is closed 6 weeks later after healing has been confirmed by a contrast enema.

Adjuvant Therapy

Although several studies have shown adjuvant radiation therapy to be effective in decreasing the incidence of local failure, it has not been possible to demonstrate that there is a survival benefit from adjuvant radiation alone. An improvement in local control, however, is a worthwhile goal because local recurrence of rectal cancer is a very morbid process (sacral pain, fistulae, obstruction) for which there is no effective therapy.

Combined adjuvant radiation and chemotherapy has been shown to provide a survival benefit in recent studies (Table 7). The Gastrointestinal Tumor Study Group (GITSG) data showed a survival benefit to patients treated with adjuvant combined chemotherapy

Table 7 Adjuvant Radiation and Chemotherapy Studies for Rectal Cancer

Study	Included	Treatment (N)	5-Year Survival
GITSG	B2 or C <12 cm	Observation (58) ChemoRx (48) Radiation (50) Chemo-Rad (46)	45% 54% 52% 67%*
NCCTG	T3 or T4 and N1 or N2	Radiation (100) Chemo-Rad (104)	48% 58%
NSABP R-01	B2 or C	Observation (184) Radiation (184) ChemoRx (187)	43% 41% 53% ($p = 0.05$, men only)

*$p < 0.05$.

and radiation over those treated with adjuvant chemotherapy or radiotherapy alone. A multi-center study performed by the NCCTG compared radiation and chemotherapy with radiation alone and again found a survival benefit to the combined regimen. The NSABP R-01 study is significant because it supported the efficacy of chemotherapy by showing a survival benefit over radiation therapy alone (albeit only in men and at the $p = 0.05$ level). Based on these studies, the National Cancer Institute (NCI) issued a clinical announcement in March 1991 recommending combined 5-FU and postoperative radiation therapy for extraperitoneal rectal tumors that penetrated through the full thickness of the rectal wall or had regional lymph node metastases. Semustine (MeCCNU) was used in addition to 5-FU in all three studies, but was omitted from the NCI recommendations because of the risk of leukemia and renal failure, and the finding in subsequent studies (GITSG 7180, NSABP R-02) that it added no benefit to 5-FU. Adjuvant therapy of rectal cancer is also discussed in the next chapter.

FUTURE CONSIDERATIONS

At present almost one-half of patients treated for colon and rectum cancer will eventually die of their disease. Epidemiologic studies suggest that in the United States, modest dietary changes including a one-third reduction in dietary fat, would result in a substantial decrease in the incidence of colon and rectum cancer. Improvement in secondary prevention may come from detection of genetic markers in stool. Although the maturation of minimal access techniques will probably diminish the length of hospitalization and allow people to return to work sooner, it is unlikely that changes in surgical technique will have a major impact on survival.

Improvements in preoperative staging through the use of intrarectal magnetic resonance imaging, ultrasound, and laparoscopy will allow the extent of surgery to be better matched to the risks presented by the tumor, and thereby improve outcome. The development of new multi-agent chemotherapy regimens, optimization of dosage, and delivery regimens for 5-FU, as well as improved modulation of 5-FU with other agents such as leucovorin, will also likely lead to improvement in outcome. Radiolabeled monoclonal antibodies have been developed that can be used in the detection of metastatic lesions from colon and rectum cancer. The new approach of immunotargeted therapy links the same antibodies to cytotoxic agents with the intent of killing metastatic deposits. Attempts to modulate the host immune system via nonspecific immune stimulants or transfer of sensitized lymphocytes may also prove useful. In the future, elucidation of the genetic and protein abnormalities involved in colon carcinogenesis will present new intracellular targets for therapy.

SUGGESTED READING

Fearon ER, Vogelstein JB. A genetic model for colorectal tumorogenesis. Cell 1990; 61:759–767.

Krook JE, Moertel CG, Gunderson LL, et al. Effective surgical adjuvant therapy for high risk rectal carcinoma. N Engl J Med 1991; 326:709–715.

Levin B, Murphy GP. Revision in American Cancer Society Recommendations for the early detection of colorectal cancer. CA Cancer J Clin 1992; 42:296–299.

Mandel JS, Bond JH, Church TR, et al. Reducing mortality from colorectal cancer by screening for fecal occult blood. N Engl J Med 1993; 328:1365–1371.

Moertel CG, Fleming TR, MacDonald JS, et al. Levamisole and flourouracil for adjuvant therapy of resected colon cancer. N Engl J Med 1990; 322:352–358.

COLORECTAL CANCER: ADJUVANT THERAPY

PAUL C. SCHROY III, M.D.
PAUL J. HESKETH, M.D.

Colorectal cancer is a major worldwide health problem, especially in westernized countries. In the United States, it is the second leading cause of cancer-related death and will account for nearly 60,000 deaths in 1993. Although 5 year survival rates have improved significantly over the past four decades, patients with locally advanced disease amenable to "curative" surgical resection remain a formidable challenge. The substantial rate of postoperative tumor recurrence and death in such patients argues strongly for additional therapeutic modalities (adjuvant therapy) combined with surgery as a means of attaining better disease control. In this chapter, we assess the current status of adjuvant therapy in colorectal cancer, beginning with a brief review of completed randomized controlled trials reported in the English language. Promising new approaches currently being evaluated or planned are also described. Finally, we offer recommendations for adjuvant treatment based on our interpretation of existing data.*

RATIONALE

The development of effective adjuvant regimens for colorectal cancer is contingent on a clear understanding of the natural history of the disease, precise surgical and pathologic staging, and reliable prognostic indices. Various classification systems have been developed to aid the selection of patients most likely to benefit from adjuvant therapy. Since Dukes' original staging system for rectal cancers in 1922, numerous modifications have been made in an attempt to incorporate additional prognostic information. The most useful systems are based on pathologic features that have independent prognostic significance, including depth of penetration through the bowel wall and lymph node involvement (see other chapters on colon cancer). Patients with tumors confined to the mucosa or submucosa constitute a good prognostic subgroup with expected 5 year survival rates after surgical resection in excess of 90 percent. Such patients are unlikely to benefit from adjuvant intervention unless it is extremely effective and carries minimal toxicity. On the other hand, patients with penetration through the bowel wall and/or lymph node involvement

constitute a more appropriate subgroup to treat, given their relatively high risk of relapse and death after curative resection. Up to 50 percent of such patients ultimately die of their disease after surgery alone. Effective adjuvant therapy for this subgroup, which makes up the majority of newly diagnosed cases, would have a substantial impact on overall colorectal cancer mortality.

HISTORICAL PERSPECTIVES

More than 10,000 patients have been entered into randomized surgical adjuvant studies over the past 30 years. Until recently, most such studies failed to demonstrate a significant impact on either disease-free survival or overall survival rates. Over the past few years, however, prospective multi-institutional randomized trials have provided credible evidence supporting the role of adjuvant therapy, especially for rectal cancer. In reviewing the current status of adjuvant therapy, it is important to keep in mind that cancers arising in the rectum exhibit a different natural history and response to therapy from those of colon cancers arising more proximally. For this reason, the two diseases are discussed separately whenever possible.

Colon Cancer

Chemotherapy

The availability of several new cytotoxic agents in the early 1950s was one of the primary motivating forces behind the concept of surgical adjuvant therapy in colorectal cancer. The initial studies often employed *single-agent* chemotherapy and studied rather heterogeneous patient populations without appropriate (untreated) control groups. At least 13 randomized controlled trials have been reported since 1956 comparing adjuvant single-agent chemotherapy with surgery alone in patients with Dukes B2 and C lesions. None of the agents studied, including nitrogen mustard, thiotepa, razoxane, and the fluorinated pyrimidines (fluorouracil or floxuridine), demonstrated a significant impact on survival compared with surgery alone. Three cooperative group studies, however, demonstrated a nonsignificant survival benefit varying between 5 and 10 percent with fluorouracil, the most active agent in advanced colorectal cancer. A recently reported meta-analysis of all controlled randomized trials also confirms a small but consistent benefit from treatment with fluorinated pyrimidines. If the comparison is limited to trials in which fluorinated pyrimidines were administered for at least 1 year, the treatment benefit becomes significant, with a 17 percent reduction in the chance of dying in the chemotherapy-treated group compared with the control group.

The recognition that the therapeutic benefits of single-agent chemotherapy were modest at best, along with data suggesting the superiority of combination

*Editor's Note: Please forgive some duplication with other chapters on colorectal cancer, but I felt that the authors of each of the chapters should be able to explain their rationale for decision making for an illness that is the leading cause of death among gastrointestinal diseases.

chemotherapy in the adjuvant or advanced disease setting in several other malignant diseases, provided a strong rationale for studying the role of adjuvant *combination* chemotherapy in colorectal cancer. The combination of fluorouracil and semustine, or methyl chloroethyl-cyclohexyl-nitrosourea (methyl-CCNU), evoked the greatest interest during the 1970s and early 1980s. This interest was predicated on strong preclinical data and early clinical trials demonstrating a superior response rate with a fluorouracil-semustine combination compared with fluorouracil alone in patients with advanced disease. At least six prospective randomized trials have been reported comparing the combination of fluorouracil-semustine, either alone or combined with another chemotherapeutic agent (e.g., vincristine) or the nonspecific immunostimulant bacille Calmette-Guérin (BCG), with surgery. Long-term follow-up data have appeared on four of these studies (Table 1). The only trial to show a significant overall benefit for chemotherapy was conducted by the National Surgical Adjuvant Breast Project (NSABP) between November 1977 and February 1983. In this study, 1,166 patients with colon cancer were randomized after curative surgical resection to observation, fluorouracil-semustine combined with vincristine (Oncovin) administered for 80 weeks, or BCG administered by scarification over a similar period. Chemotherapy-treated patients experienced significantly improved disease-free survival (P = .02) and overall survival (67 percent versus 59 percent; P = .05) compared with control patients. Of note, patients receiving BCG also experienced an improved overall but not disease-free survival, possibly reflective of a protective effect from death due to cardiovascular disease rather than an effect on the recurrence rate of cancer. The discrepancy between the results of this study and those of the other trials that failed to demonstrate significant sur-

vival benefit is best explained by differences in sample size. In light of these inconclusive data and the enhanced toxicity, particularly the potential leukemogenicity associated with semustine, interest in combination chemotherapy with fluorouracil-semustine in the adjuvant setting rapidly declined. A National Cancer Institute (NCI) survey found that the relative risk of leukemia or preleukemia was 12.4 times greater for patients with gastrointestinal neoplasms treated with semustine.

To date, the combination of fluorouracil and levamisole has demonstrated the most significant activity of any adjuvant chemotherapeutic regimen for colorectal cancer (Table 2). Levamisole is an anthelmintic agent with putative immunostimulatory effects. Interest in levamisole for treatment of colorectal cancer stemmed from the results of a small trial reported by Verhaegen and colleagues in 1982 in which levamisole-treated patients survived significantly longer than untreated patients after curative resection. On the basis of these data, three randomized trials have been carried out to assess the therapeutic efficacy of adjuvant levamisole-fluorouracil. The North Central Cancer Treatment Group (NCCTG) trial compared levamisole alone for 1 year, or levamisole plus fluorouracil for 1 year, after curative surgical resection with surgery alone in 401 randomized patients with Dukes B and C cancers. At a median follow-up of nearly 8 years, disease-free survival was significantly prolonged in both treatment arms compared with controls. A trend toward improved overall survival was also observed, but this achieved statistical significance only for patients with Dukes C lesions (positive nodes) treated with the combination. Toxicity levels were acceptable. A smaller adjuvant trial reported by Windle and colleagues also demonstrated a significant survival advantage for a different levamisole-fluorouracil regimen

Table 1 Randomized, Controlled Trials With Adjuvant Semustine-Fluorouracil in Colorectal Cancer

Group	Regimen	Evaluable Patients	Five-Year Survival (%)	Difference
VASOG-27A	MF	645	53	NS
	S		50	
GITSG 6175	MF	572	61*	NS
	BCG-MER		59	
	MF/BCG-MER		58	
	S		62	
NSABP C-01	MOF	1,116	67	P = .05
	BCG		67	P = .03
	S		59	
SWOG 7510	MF	560	56*	NS
	MF/BCG		61	
	S		59	

VASOG = Veterans Administration Surgical Oncology Group; GITSG = Gastrointestinal Tumor Study Group; NSABP = National Surgical Adjuvant Breast Project; SWOG = Southwest Oncology Group; MF = semustine-fluorouracil; S = surgery only; MOF = semustine-fluorouracil-vincristine; BCG = bacille Calmette-Guérin; BCG-MER = methanol extraction residue of bacille Calmette-Guérin; NS = not significant.
*Approximate values from survival curves.
From Hesketh PJ, Bulger KN. Role of adjuvant therapy in colorectal cancer. Adv Intern Med 1991; 36:219–247; with permission.

Table 2 Adjuvant Levamisole-Fluorouracil in Colorectal Cancer

Group	Regimen	Patients	Findings
Windle et al	Fluorouracil	45	Death from tumor recurrence at minimal follow-up
	Fluorouracil-levamisole	47	of 5 yr: fluorouracil, 44%; fluorouracil-
	Control	49	levamisole, 32%; controls, 52%
NCCTG	Levamisole	130	Prolonged DFS with levamisole and fluorouracil-
	Fluorouracil-levamisole	136	levamisole; significantly better survival with
	Control	135	fluorouracil-levamisole in stage C
Intergroup	Levamisole	1,296	Interim analysis 9/1/89: survival benefit in stage C
	Fluorouracil-levamisole		comparable with NCCTG trial
	Control		

Intergroup = Eastern Cooperative Oncology Group (ECOG), Southwest Oncology Group (SWOG), and North Central Cancer Treatment Group (NCCTG); DFS = disease-free survival.

From Hesketh PJ, Bulger KN. Role of adjuvant therapy in colorectal cancer. Adv Intern Med 1991; 36:219–247; with permission.

compared with the control and fluorouracil-alone arms.

On the basis of these encouraging results, a national intergroup study was undertaken in 1984 involving the Southwest Oncology Group (SWOG), the Eastern Cooperative Oncology Group (ECOG), and the NCCTG. The study design was similar to that of the preliminary NCCTG trial, with two notable exceptions. First, patients with Dukes B2 and C tumors were prospectively analyzed separately. Second, only patients with colon cancer were studied; those with rectal cancers were excluded. A total of 1,296 patients were entered. Preliminary results, released in the fall of 1989, confirmed the efficacy of combined treatment with levamisole and fluorouracil in patients with Dukes C disease, with a 41 percent reduction in tumor recurrence rate and death. Unlike the earlier NCCTG trial, levamisole alone provided no benefit. The data regarding Dukes B2 patients were inconclusive. On the basis of these interim results, the NCI obtained permission from the Food and Drug Administration to confer group C status on levamisole, thereby allowing it to be distributed to individual practitioners on request for use in combination with fluorouracil in patients with Dukes C colon cancer. It was also decided that a postsurgical observation-only arm was no longer justifiable in NCI-sponsored adjuvant studies for patients with Dukes C disease. Levamisole subsequently became commercially available.

Radiotherapy

The role of adjuvant irradiation for cancers arising above the peritoneal reflection remains poorly defined. In contrast to rectal cancers, no randomized controlled trials have been carried out to date. A local control advantage was seen with postoperative irradiation in selected subsets of patients treated at the Massachusetts General Hospital in comparison with historical controls. Confirmation of these data awaits future randomized controlled trials.

Rectal Cancer

Chemotherapy

The impact of *single-agent* adjuvant chemotherapy in patients with rectal cancer is difficult to ascertain. Many of the abovementioned studies for colon cancer included relatively few patients with rectal cancers, variably defined the anatomic extent of the rectum, and often did not analyze their results with respect to the primary site. Available data, however, suggest that adjuvant chemotherapy with fluorouracil provides a small survival advantage in rectal cancer patients.

Cooperative trials have been undertaken to assess the independent role of adjuvant *combination* chemotherapy for rectal cancer. Two such trials have suggested a benefit. The GITSG observed a trend toward improved survival at 5 years in patients treated with fluorouracil-semustine for 18 months, albeit less than that seen with combined therapy (radiation plus fluorouracil-semustine), as discussed below. The NSABP observed significant improvement in disease-free survival with semustine-fluorouracil-vincristine (MOF). Curiously, improvement in overall survival was noted only in men, particularly those under age 65.

In terms of currently available data, it remains unclear whether adjuvant chemotherapy alone confers greater benefit in rectal or in colon cancer. Perhaps the greatest utility for chemotherapy in rectal cancer is achieved when it is combined with radiotherapy.

Radiotherapy

Cancers of the rectum have been associated with much higher local recurrence rates than tumors arising above the pelvic peritoneal reflection. Local failure rates of 25 and 50 percent can be expected with Dukes B and C rectal tumors, respectively, when surgery alone is employed. Such recurrences are often associated with significant morbidity, such as severe pain and bowel or bladder dysfunction. Not surprisingly, there has been considerable interest in the role of radiotherapy com-

Table 3 Combined Radiotherapy-Chemotherapy Trials in Rectal Cancer

Group	Patients	Treatment	Local Relapse (%)	Five-Year Survival (%)	Severe Toxicity (%)
GITSG	204	Surgery alone	21	46*	–
		Radiotherapy	20	52	20
		MF	27	56	31
		RT/fluorouracil, then MF	11	59	61
NCCTG	200	Radiotherapy	25	47*	6
		MF, then RT/fluorouracil, then MF	13.5	57	7

GISTG = Gastrointestinal Tumor Study Group; NCCTG = North Central Cancer Treatment Group; RT = radiotherapy; MF = semustine-fluorouracil.
*Estimated from survival curves.
From Hesketh PJ, Bulger KN. Role of adjuvant therapy in colorectal cancer. Adv Intern Med 1991; 36:219–247; with permission.

bined with surgery to improve local control. Adjuvant irradiation has been employed both preoperatively and postoperatively, alone or in combination with chemotherapy.

Preoperative adjuvant (neoadjuvant) radiotherapy has been studied in nine randomized controlled trials. Six studies using low-dose levels (<3,200 cGy) with small fraction size observed little or no treatment benefit. However, three trials employing either larger total radiation doses (>3,400 cGy) or larger fraction size reported more promising results. The European Organization for Research on Treatment of Cancer (EORTC) trial demonstrated both a reduction in 5 year local recurrences and improved 5 year survival in patients receiving adjuvant radiotherapy. The Stockholm Rectal Cancer Study Group, using a relatively low total radiation dose (2,500 cGy) but a large fraction size (500 cGy), also noted a reduction in local recurrences. Unlike the EORTC trial, no survival benefit was noted; in fact, a significant increase in mortality was observed in the radiation arm in patients over 75 years of age. Lastly, a small series from Yale demonstrated increased survival in patients given 4,600 cGy preoperatively.

Three major randomized trials have examined the role of postoperative adjuvant radiation. Nonsignificant trends toward better local control were noted in all three studies, and one study also showed a trend toward improved survival. Severe radiation toxicity was seen in 0, 10, and 20 percent of patients, respectively.

Combined Radiotherapy and Chemotherapy

As it became increasingly apparent that local radiotherapy alone was unlikely to improve survival, trials were undertaken to assess combination systemic chemotherapy and radiation therapy. Besides addressing the issue of systemic relapse, the use of certain chemotherapeutic agents with radiosensitizing properties (e.g., fluorouracil) had the potential to improve local control when combined with radiation. To date, two major trials combining chemotherapy and postoperative radiotherapy have been performed (Table 3). The GITSG trial randomized patients to four treatment arms: surgery alone, radiotherapy alone (4,400 to 4,800 cGy), chemotherapy alone with semustine-fluorouracil for 18 months, or the same chemotherapy-radiotherapy combined. Combined therapy demonstrated the greatest activity, with highly significant improvements in local recurrence rates, disease-free survival, and overall survival compared with surgery alone, but at the expense of enhanced treatment-related toxicity. Severe or life-threatening acute toxicities were noted in 61 percent of patients in the combined modality arm compared with 20 and 31 percent in the radiation and chemotherapy arms, respectively. There were also two late treatment-related deaths from radiation enteritis in the combined-modality arm compared with one from acute nonlymphocytic leukemia in the chemotherapy-alone arm. Concern about the potential leukemogenicity of semustine led the GITSG to perform a subsequent trial that demonstrated no additional therapeutic benefit when semustine was added to fluorouracil compared with fluorouracil alone. The NCCTG trial also reported significant improvements in local recurrence rates, disease-free survival, and overall survival with combined therapy. Severe, delayed treatment-related complications, most notably small bowel obstruction, occurred in 6 percent of patients receiving radiation and 6.7 percent of patients receiving combination therapy. On balance, these results strongly suggest that a combined-modality approach with chemotherapy and radiotherapy represents a major therapeutic advance in the adjuvant treatment of rectal cancer.

Regional Adjuvant Therapy

Portal Vein Infusion

Up to 50 percent of patients who relapse after curative resection develop metastatic disease in the liver. Hepatic infusion of cytotoxic agents via the portal vein has been advocated as a rational means of addressing this problem. Studies to date have explored the role of perioperative infusion, based on the observation by Fischer and Turnbull that malignant cells were present in the portal circulation of one-third of patients undergoing large bowel resections for colorectal cancer. A trial by Taylor and colleagues was the first to report a positive impact on both liver recurrence rates and survival. Subsequent to this report, at least seven multicenter trials of adjuvant intraportal chemotherapy have been undertaken. Three of these trials included heparin- or urokinase-only arms in light of data suggesting that anticoagulation may have an impact on the development of metastatic disease. Preliminary results from four studies all demonstrate a benefit from treatment with liver perfusion.

Intraperitoneal Chemotherapy

The administration of adjuvant chemotherapy via the intraperitoneal route has also been studied. Available data suggest that intraperitoneal chemotherapy may have an impact on local recurrence rates but not on survival. These data argue against its use as a single modality but suggest a possible role in combination with systemic therapies.

FUTURE DIRECTIONS

Many ongoing and completed, but as yet unreported, trials have been designed to address unresolved questions about adjuvant therapy for colorectal cancer. Attempts to enhance the activity of fluorouracil, the most active single agent in this disease, through pharmacologic modulation with reduced folates (e.g., leucovorin) has been an area of intense interest. Phase III trials in advanced colorectal cancer have shown significantly superior response rates for fluorouracil-leucovorin combinations compared with fluorouracil alone. In view of these data, several studies have been undertaken to examine the role of fluorouracil-leucovorin in the adjuvant setting (see below).

Another promising area that warrants further study is the fluorouracil-levamisole combination. Important questions need to be answered regarding optimal dosage, schedule, routes of administration, and the role of additional agents (e.g., leucovorin) or modalities. Preliminary results from a large NSABP trial comparing fluorouracil-leucovorin with fluorouracil-levamisole should be available soon. Conclusive data regarding the efficacy of fluorouracil-levamisole in patients with Dukes B2 lesions is also needed.

In rectal cancer, further definition of the relative roles of radiotherapy alone, chemotherapy alone, and combined therapy remains an area of ongoing investigation. Again, issues such as optimal dosage and schedule need to be defined. The role of "sandwich" radiotherapy (pre- and postoperative) is also being examined.

In addition to better-defined guidelines for the use of conventional therapies, there is an obvious need for innovative and potentially more effective strategies. Immunotherapeutic approaches employing tumor vaccines or immunomodulatory agents such as interferon and interleukin have engendered considerable interest. Other novel approaches including the use of genetically engineered fusion toxins, differentiation agents, and various biologic response modifiers are also under consideration.

RECOMMENDATIONS

Despite nearly three decades of consistently disappointing data regarding the role of adjuvant therapy in resectable colorectal cancer, recently emerging results offer some basis for cautious optimism. For patients with tumors arising proximal to the peritoneal reflection, adjuvant fluorouracil-containing regimens appear to confer a modest treatment benefit after curative surgical resection. The two most promising chemotherapy regimens at present appear to be fluorouracil-levamisole and fluorouracil-leucovorin. The optimal schedule and dosage of these agents remains to be determined. Portal vein chemotherapy infusion studies have yielded promising but inconclusive results to date. As data from completed or ongoing large group studies become available, the role of this modality will be better clarified.

In rectal cancer, available data suggest that adjuvant radiotherapy alone has a modest but consistent ability to reduce local recurrence without demonstrating any survival advantage. The optimal dosage and sequencing of radiotherapy remains poorly defined. Two completed cooperative group studies strongly suggest that the ideal use of radiotherapy is in combination with chemotherapy. The independent role of chemotherapy in rectal cancer remains unclear. There is evidence suggesting that adjuvant chemotherapy alone may be more effective with rectal cancer than with primary tumors arising proximal to the peritoneal reflection.

Despite the large number of unresolved questions that remain, we believe that interim treatment recommendations can be made:

1. Patients with Dukes' B2 and C rectal and colonic adenocarcinomas should be entered into an appropriate adjuvant clinical trial when feasible.
2. Outside the setting of a protocol, there is a sound rationale to treat Dukes' B2 and C rectal cancer with combination chemotherapy and postoperative radiotherapy. The chemotherapy might consist of fluorouracil either alone or combined with levamisole. To lessen the potential of radiation-induced toxicity, techniques such as meshing the small bowel out of the pelvis, bladder distention, or the use of multiple radiation portals may be employed.
3. In more proximal colonic tumors (above the pelvic-peritoneal reflection), adjuvant chemotherapy with fluorouracil-levamisole or fluorouracil-leucovorin should be administered to patients with Dukes' C tumors. The inconclusive results to date of adjuvant chemotherapy for patients with Dukes' B disease, combined with recently described improvements in survival for this disease stage, suggest that adjuvant therapy

should be withheld in this group outside the setting of a clinical study.

ADDENDUM

The NSABP recently reported their results of a randomized trial designed to assess the efficacy of adjuvant therapy with fluorouracil-leucovorin in patients with Dukes' B and C colorectal cancer. The fluorouracil-leucovorin combination was significantly superior to MOF in prolonging the disease-free survival and overall survival in both groups of patients. The differences in disease-free survival and overall survival were of similar magnitude to those previously reported with fluorouracil-levamisole. Hence, pending the results of an ongoing NSABP trial comparing the two regimens, these recent data support the use of fluorouracil-leucovorin as adjuvant therapy for patients with Dukes' C, and possibly Dukes' B, tumors. (See Wolmark et al. 1993 reference in the Suggested Reading section.)

SUGGESTED READING

Douglas HO, Moertel CG, Mayer RJ, et al. Survival after postoperative combination treatment of rectal cancer. N Engl J Med 1986; 315:1294–1295.

Gastrointestinal Tumor Study Group. Adjuvant therapy of colon cancer. Results of a prospectively randomized trial. N Engl J Med 1984; 310:737–743.
Hesketh PJ, Bulger KN. Role of adjuvant therapy in colorectal cancer. Adv Intern Med 1991; 36:219–247.
Krook JE, Moertel CG, Gunderson LL. Effective surgical adjuvant therapy for high-risk rectal carcinoma. N Engl J Med 1991; 324:709–715.
Moertel CG, Fleming JR, MacDonald JS, et al. Levamisole and 5-fluorouracil for adjuvant therapy of resected colon carcinoma. N Engl J Med 1990; 322:352–358.
Taylor I, Machin D, Mullee M, et al. A randomized controlled trial of adjuvant portal vein cytotoxic perfusion in colorectal cancer. Br J Surg 1985; 72:359–363.
Wolmark N, Fisher B, Rockette H, et al. Postoperative adjuvant chemotherapy or BCG for colon cancer. Results from NSABP protocol C-01. J Natl Cancer Inst 1988; 80:30–36.
Wolmark N, Rockette H, Fisher B, et al. The benefit of leucovorin-modulated fluorouracil as postoperative adjuvant therapy for primary colon cancer; results from National Surgical Breast and Bowel Project protocol C-03. J Clin Oncol 1993; 11:1879–1887.

SEVERE LOWER GASTROINTESTINAL BLEEDING

THOMAS J. SAVIDES, M.D.
DENNIS M. JENSEN, M.D.

Lower gastrointestinal (GI) bleeding in adults is usually mild and self-limited and can be evaluated on an outpatient basis. Such bleeding is usually due to internal hemorrhoids, colonic polyps, colon cancer, or inflammatory bowel disease. At times, however, hematochezia can be severe and ongoing, requiring hospitalization, resuscitation, and therapeutic intervention. This chapter focuses on our approach to the colonoscopic diagnosis and treatment of these patients with severe lower GI bleeding.

The clinical and laboratory research reported in this chapter was supported in part by a NIH CORE grant to CURE (NIH NIDDK 41301–Human Subjects Core), and Veterans Administration Research Funds (Merit Review–Dr. Jensen).

DEFINITIONS

Hematochezia is passage per rectum of bright red blood, clots, or burgundy stools. It can originate from bleeding lesions in the upper gastrointestinal (UGI) tract, small intestine, or colon. We previously evaluated 80 consecutive patients with hematochezia who were admitted to our intensive care unit. Severe GI bleeding was associated with shock or hypotension, required intensive care unit (ICU) management for resuscitation, and needed red blood cell (RBC) transfusions. Our definition of ongoing hematochezia was continued blood per rectum for at least 4 hours while under ICU observation. These patients were elderly, with a mean age of 77 years, and two-thirds were male; 90 percent had other medical or surgical problems. They were evaluated with panendoscopy and urgent colonoscopy after purge. The diagnosis of a bleeding site was based on (1) active bleeding from the lesion; (2) stigmata of recent hemorrhage, such as a visible vessel or adherent clot resistant to washing with an endoscopic catheter; or (3) blood in the area and a clean lesion without other lesions in the bowel segment to explain the bleeding. The causes of bleeding are shown in Table 1. The most common bleeding lesions were colonic angiomas and diverticula.

Table 1 Etiology of Severe Hematochezia in 80 Patients

Lesion Site	Percentage of Patients
Colonic	74
Angiomas	30
Diverticulosis	16
Polyps or cancer	11
Colitis	9
Rectal lesions	4
Bleeding polyp stalk	3
Endometriosis	1
Upper gastrointestinal	11
Small bowel*	9
No site found	6

*Diagnosis of small bowel source made when upper endoscopy and colonoscopy results were negative, but fresh blood or clots seen coming through the ileocecal valve.

INITIAL MANAGEMENT AND DIAGNOSTIC APPROACH

Patients with severe hematochezia are admitted to an ICU and resuscitated as necessary with fluids and correction of coagulopathy or thrombocytopenia. Anoscopy with a slotted anoscope is performed to evaluate obvious rectal lesions. A nasogastric (NG) tube is placed to determine whether there is fresh blood, clots, or "coffee grounds" to implicate an UGI source. A NG lavage negative for blood does not exclude an UGI source; 11% of our patients in whom NG lavage revealed no blood still had an UGI source for the bleeding. However, no hematochezia patient with bile in the NG aspirate (and no blood, clots, or coffee grounds) had an UGI source. Therefore, bile and absence of blood are required to rule out an UGI source for ongoing hematochezia.

Patients with massive bleeding and shock who cannot be stabilized with ICU resuscitation should undergo urgent surgical exploration. However, nearly all patients become hemodynamically stable with fluid or transfusion resuscitation in the ICU and undergo urgent endoscopic evaluation. Figure 1 shows our algorithm for management of patients who are medically stable.

Colonoscopy and Upper Endoscopy

We perform urgent colonoscopy after a sulfate purge in hemodynamically stable patients with severe hematochezia who have a negative NG lavage and anoscopy. While in the ICU, the patient either drinks or receives 4 to 6 L of polyethelene-sulfate purge via a NG tube over 3 to 5 hours until the rectal effluent is clear of stool, blood, and clots. Metoclopramide, 10 mg intravenously given before the purge and repeated every 3 to 4 hours, may facilitate gastric emptying and reduce nausea. During the purge, the patient receives cardiac monitoring and is transfused packed RBCs, fresh-frozen plasma, and platelets as needed.

Colonoscopy is usually performed at the bedside in the ICU. Diagnosis of a colonic bleeding site is made only if active bleeding, a nonbleeding visible vessel, or a

ER/ICU
Resuscitation/stabilization
History and physical examination
Laboratory studies
Anoscopy
Gastroenterology and surgical consultations
↓
Nasogastric aspirate→Blood or no bile→Upper endoscopy
↓
Negative
↓
Sulfate purge and colonoscopy→If site, treat
↓
Negative
↓
Upper endoscopy→If lesion, treat
↓
Negative
↓
Push enteroscopy with colonoscope→If lesion, treat
↓
Technetium-labeled red cell scan→If positive, repeat endoscopy or angiography

Figure 1 Diagnostic and therapeutic approach to severe lower gastrointestinal bleeding.

clot on a lesion resistant to washing is found. If colonoscopy does not reveal a bleeding source, an upper endoscopy is immediately performed. When fresh blood or clots are seen coming from the ileocecal valve and no lesion is found on colonoscopy or upper endoscopy, the small bowel is presumed to be the bleeding site.

Push Enteroscopy

Less than 10 percent of the time the bleeding site remains obscure after urgent upper endoscopy and colonoscopy in patients with ongoing hematochezia. If the patient has stopped bleeding and is hemodynamically stable, we re-examine the UGI tract using a 180 cm long video colonoscope to evaluate the distal duodenoum and proximal jejunum 80 to 100 cm beyond the ligament of Treitz. This "push enteroscopy" technique allows determination of lesions in 19 to 52 percent of patients with obscure bleeding sites. We do not use the currently available 280 cm or longer sonde enteroscopes in patients with acute bleeding because of the prolonged time needed for these examinations, the requirements for overtubes, and the need for fluoroscopy. Although hemostasis or biopsies cannot be performed through the sonde instrument, it is possible through longer push instruments. These techniques can be useful in determining the cause of chronic GI bleeding of obscure origin, particularly in ambulatory patients. There is a separate chapter on enteroscopy.

Technetium-99m Red Blood Cell Scanning

In patients who have intermittent lower GI bleeding in the hospital and negative endoscopic evaluations, we obtain a technetium-labeled RBC scan during the next acute bleeding episode. This test can be useful for

Table 2 Diagnostic Yield of Emergency Colonoscopy versus Angiography in Patients With Ongoing Hematochezia

	Colonoscopy (%)	Angiography (%)
Angioma	80	20
Diverticula	75	25
Bleeding tumor or polyp	100	0
Small bowel lesions	100	0
Blind rectal lesions	100	12
Total	82	12

Table 3 Palliative Results in 66 Patients with Colonoscopic Hemostasis of Colonic Angiomats

	Before Treatment	After Treatment
Mean period of comparison (yr)	2	2
Mean hematocrit (%)	26.8	37.3
Mean lower GI bleeding episodes per yr	1.3	0.6
Units of red blood cells transfused per yr	4.3	1.3

determination of the bleeding site if the bleeding rate is more than 0.1 ml per minute. It also has a good chance of detecting an intermittently bleeding lesion, because the long intravascular half-life of the labeled RBCs allows repeated scanning to be performed over at least 24 hours without further injection of isotope. Technetium-99m RBC scanning has demonstrated active bleeding sites in 44 to 72 percent of patients with ongoing lower GI bleeding, with a sensitivity of 93 to 100 percent and a specificity of 85 to 95 percent. However, labeled RBC scans are less accurate for evaluating patients with occult or less severe lower GI bleeding, for whom a definite source of bleeding is often difficult to determine. In one study of the outcome in 19 patients with lower GI bleeding, it was concluded that there was incorrect localization of bleeding sites in 25 percent of patients, and that performance of a surgical procedure that relied exclusively on localization by red cell scintigraphy resulted in the wrong operation in at least 42 percent of cases.

Angiography

We rarely use selective visceral angiography as the initial test for diagnosing the site of severe lower GI bleeding. This is able to determine a source of bleeding only if there is an active arterial bleeding rate greater than 0.5 ml per minute. The diagnostic yield depends on patient selection, the timing of the procedure, and the skill of the angiographers, with positive tests ranging from 12 to 69 percent. The sensitivity for detecting a bleeding site was 36 percent with angiography compared with 100% for technetium-labeled scanning in one comparative study. When we compared emergency angiography with urgent colonoscopy for severe colonic or small bowel bleeding, angiography identified the lesion only 12 percent of the time compared with 82 percent with colonoscopy (Table 2). Complications of angiography can include hematomas, arterial embolization, bowel ischemia or infarction, and renal failure.

TREATMENT OF SEVERE HEMATOCHEZIA

Bleeding stops spontaneously in 70 to 90 percent of ambulatory patients with acute lower GI bleeding. This allows elective diagnosis and treatment in most cases. For the 10 to 30 percent with ongoing or recurrent

hematochezia, urgent diagnosis and treatment are required to control the bleeding. In our large series of patients with ongoing hematochezia, 64 percent required some intervention including endoscopy (39 percent), angiography (1 percent), or surgery (24 percent) for control of continued bleeding or rebleeding.

Colonic Angiomas

Colonic angiomas can be coagulated endoscopically with bipolar electrocoagulation, monopolar electrocoagulation, heater probe, yttrium-aluminum-garnet (YAG) laser, or argon laser. In previous studies we have shown that endoscopic coagulation can definitively control colonic angioma bleeding in 80 percent of patients. These patients often have rebleeding, and 20 percent require more than one colonoscopic treatment. However, with follow-up of over 1 year, these patients showed a significant decrease in frequency of bleeding episodes and the number of units of packed RBCs transfused per year, and an increase in mean hematocrit values (Table 3).

There have been no comparative studies in humans of the different colonoscopic modes of coagulation, nor of colonoscopic hemostasis compared with surgery. We evaluated colonic injury in a canine right colon model to simulate treatment of angiomas with various thermal modalities. These studies revealed that more frequent transmural injury and a higher rate of perforation occurred with monopolar hot biopsy forceps (HBF), monopolar probe electrocoagulation, and YAG laser than with bipolar electrocoagulation, heater probe, or argon laser. There have been reports of high complication rates from use of YAG laser and monopolar HBF in the right colon, although some experienced endoscopists have reported safer results. In view of the laboratory data and clinical reports, we advise against using YAG laser or monopolar electrocautery to treat colonic angiomas, especially in the right colon.

There have been reports of successful use of monopolar HBF to treat colon angiomas, but there have been no long-term follow-up studies of their efficacy or safety. Experimental studies in the canine right colon have shown that monopolar HBF caused greater rates of transmural injury than heater probe or bipolar electrocoagulation. A large survey of endoscopists who used monopolar HBF reported that 16 percent of patients had major complications, including significant bleeding, perforation, postcoagulation syndrome, and death.

Table 4 Comparison of Treatment Techniques for Colonic Angiomas and Peptic Ulcers Using a Bipolar Probe and a 50-watt Generator

	Colonic Angiomas	Peptic Ulcers
Pressure	Light	Firm
Power	2–3	3–4
Pulse	2–3 1 sec pulses	Continuous for 10 sec

Our current technique for treating actively bleeding colonic angiomas is to irrigate the area and then tamponade and coagulate the bleeding point. We use gentle pressure rather than the firm pressure used in treating peptic ulcers. When there is no active bleeding, we coagulate the central feeding vessels first, then coagulate the remainder of the angioma. These techniques are different from those used for treating peptic ulcers, as shown in Table 4.

The main risks of colonoscopic coagulation of angiomas are perforation, postcoagulation syndrome, and delayed bleeding. In a review of 98 patients treated for colonic angioma with an average of two treatment sessions per patient, none had perforations. Postcoagulation syndrome, as defined by abdominal pain, focal rebound tenderness, fever, and leukocytosis without evidence of perforation, occurred in 2 percent of patients. Delayed bleeding was noted in 4 percent of patients, mostly those with coagulopathies.

Diverticula

Colonic diverticular bleeding is usually self-limited but may be severe. When barium enema alone was used alone for diagnosis of diverticular hemorrhage in 50 patients with hematochezia requiring transfusions, 58 percent stopped bleeding during hospitalization and had no further short-term bleeding, 20 percent had recurrent bleeding in the hospital, and 22 percent had ongoing bleeding requiring surgery. Overall, 70 percent of patients stopped bleeding with conservative management, and of those 22 percent experienced subsequent bleeding events. The authors concluded that elective surgery should be considered only in patients who had had a second massive hemorrhage.

Mesenteric angiography has been used for diagnosis and treatment of diverticular hemorrhage. Selective arterial infusion of vasopressin can provide immediate hemostasis in massive colonic hemorrhage. However, in one study, more than 50 percent of these patients then underwent surgery for either elective resection or rebleeding. Transcatheter embolization has also been reported to stop diverticular bleeding in a few cases.

Colonoscopic treatment of bleeding diverticula was first reported in 1986, with heater probe in four patients to achieve definitive hemostasis. We recently described three patients with recurrent in-hospital lower GI bleeding from visible vessels at the necks of colonic diverticula. Because of the rebleeding, the concern over further rebleeding, and the risks involved in surgery in these elderly patients, we coagulated the visible vessels with bipolar electrocoagulation. There were no complications with treatment and none of the patients have had rebleeding with follow-up from 4 to 16 months. There have also been reports of treatment of bleeding diverticula with epinephrine injection directly into the base of the diverticulum. These colonoscopic techniques are still experimental and need to be compared with surgical resection with long-term follow-up. However, they offer a promising new nonsurgical approach to management of elderly patients with diverticular bleeding in whom surgery presents a high risk.

Polyps or Cancer

Focal ulcerations on large polyps or colonic cancers were the third most common diagnosis in our series of patients with severe hematochezia. Diagnosis and hemostasis via urgent colonoscopy are feasible with various accessories such as snares, electrocoagulation, or epinephrine injection. Patients with bleeding polyps can be definitively treated, and those with ulcerated colonic cancer can be stabilized and staged before elective surgical resection.

Ischemic Bowel Disease

Rarely, we encounter elderly patients with a history of atherosclerotic disease who present with hematochezia and on urgent colonoscopy are found to have sparing of the rectum, with sharp demarcation of abnormal mucosa, swelling, and friability. This is consistent with ischemic bowel disease. These patients are managed with supportive medical therapy only, since less than 2 percent of them will proceed to colonic gangrene.

COMMENTS

With currently available video colonoscopes and accessories, and the routine use of colonic purging during medical stabilization, a well-trained colonoscopist can perform a successful diagnostic colonoscopy in most patients with severe hematochezia. If no colonic bleeding site is found, upper endoscopy, push enteroscopy, RBC scanning, and angiography are important additional diagnostic tests to consider for selected patients. Therapeutic colonoscopy can achieve hemostasis of bleeding angiomas, polyps, and cancers and holds promise for treatment of some cases of diverticular bleeding.

SUGGESTED READING*

Farrands PA, Taylor I. Management of acute lower gastrointestinal haemorrhage in a surgical unit over a 4-year period. J R Soc Med 1987; 80:79.

---

*Editor's Note: The authors have a version of this chapter with detailed references. Readers who wish to receive a copy may contact the authors directly.

Jensen DM, Machicado GA. Diagnosis and treatment of severe hematochezia. Gastroenterology 1988; 95:1569–1574.

Jensen DM, Machicado GA. Techniques of hemostasis for lower GI bleeding. In: Jensen DM, Brunetaud JM, eds. Medical laser endoscopy. Dordrecht: Kluwer Academic Publishers, 1990:99–107.

Markisz JA, Front D, Royal HD, et al. An evaluation of 99m Tc-labelled red blood cell scintigraphy for the detection and localization of gastrointestinal bleeding sites. Gastroenterology 1982; 83:394–398.

McGuire HH, Haynes BW. Massive hemorrhage from diverticulosis of the colon: guidelines for therapy based on bleeding patterns observed in fifty cases. Ann Surg 1972; 175:847–853.

Nicholson ML, Neoptolemos JP, Sharp JF, et al. Localization of lower gastrointestinal bleeding using in vivo technetium-99m-labelled red blood cell scintigraphy. Br J Surg 1989; 78:358–361.

Schrock TR. Colonoscopic diagnosis and treatment of lower gastrointestinal bleeding. Surg Clin North Am 1989; 69:1309–1325.

Wadas DD, Sanowski RA. Complications of the hot biopsy forceps technique. Gastrointest Endosc 1988; 34:32–37.

DIVERTICULAR DISEASE OF THE COLON

RANDOLPH M. STEINHAGEN, M.D.
ARTHUR H. AUFSES, Jr., M.D.

Diverticular disease of the colon has emerged as a significant clinical and pathologic entity only during the twentieth century. In the United States, diverticulosis is now the most common condition affecting the large intestine. The incidence of diverticula increases with age. It has been estimated that by age 80, 50 percent of the U.S. population is affected. Most are asymptomatic, but inflammatory or bleeding complications occur in 15 to 20 percent of those at risk, and approximately 30 percent of these affected individuals require surgical intervention. Diverticular disease is seen almost exclusively in populations that consume the low-fiber diet typical of Western societies. Diverticulosis usually involves the sigmoid colon, and this is frequently the only segment involved. The rectum is almost never affected.

DIVERTICULOSIS

Diverticula become symptomatic when complications, such as infection or hemorrhage, supervene. The symptoms frequently attributed to uncomplicated diverticular disease are similar to those of the irritable bowel syndrome. Although increasing the fiber content of the diet does seem to reduce complaints, a corresponding decrease in the rate of complications or the recurrence rate of acute attacks has not been conclusively established.

Barium enema examination and colonoscopy are the mainstays of the diagnostic evaluation, but in the presence of diverticula there may be considerable diagnostic error. Colonoscopy is more accurate, but because of fixation, spasm, or narrowing it may be technically impossible to complete the examination. Occasionally, it is impossible to determine whether the etiology of a stricture is benign or malignant, and this may constitute the indication for surgery.

The treatment of uncomplicated diverticular disease is medical. High-fiber diets are effective in reducing symptoms. Anticholinergic agents and antispasmodics are also frequently used, but without solid evidence for their effectiveness we generally avoid them. Surgical resection for pain relief, in the absence of documented inflammatory complications, is associated with a high rate of recurrent symptoms. In general, surgery should be reserved for patients who develop recurrent attacks of acute diverticulitis and for those who develop complications. The subset of patients at increased risk of developing complications (those under age 40 and those who are immunocompromised) should be treated aggressively and undergo early surgery to provide the best chance of a favorable outcome.

ACUTE DIVERTICULITIS

Approximately 10 to 25 percent of people with diverticula develop diverticulitis at some time during their lifetime; however, less than 20 percent of these afflicted individuals require hospitalization. While perforation may occur, resulting in peritonitis, abscess formation, or fistula, the inflammatory process frequently resolves or is contained by fibrosis and becomes chronic. Recurrent acute attacks are common. With each attack the pericolonic fibrosis increases until the wall becomes encased by a fibrous tissue reaction, sometimes leading to obstruction.

The incidence of complications associated with both initial and subsequent attacks of acute diverticulitis, and the likelihood of recurrent attacks, are critical factors in determining how patients with acute diverticulitis should be treated and when surgery should be recommended. Approximately 20 percent of patients develop complications associated with the first attack of diverticulitis, and this rises to 60 percent with recurrent attacks. The incidence of recurrent attacks has been estimated at approximately 30 percent, most within 5 years. In patients under 40 years of age, the incidence of recurrence approaches 50 percent. Each attack of diverticulitis predisposes to an increased risk of future attacks, and the risk of complications rises with each episode.

The clinical spectrum of acute diverticulitis is wide. In mild cases, spontaneous resolution is common and the patient may remain out of hospital. Treatment generally consists of dietary restriction, limiting intake to fluids and oral antibiotics. At the other end of the spectrum, the patient may be acutely ill with signs of systemic sepsis, peritonitis, and hypovolemia. A trial of medical management is always indicated unless free perforation with diffuse peritonitis is present. Bowel rest, intravenous (IV) fluids, and antibiotics form the mainstay of initial therapy. Broad-spectrum antibiotics covering gram-negative bacilli as well as anaerobes are chosen. Most patients recover from the acute attack. Failure to respond within 48 hours often indicates a complication such as perforation or abscess. Once much of the tenderness and guarding has resolved, a distinct mass may become apparent.

Barium enema studies are not indicated in the early stages of acute diverticulitis when the diagnosis is unequivocal. We have found that computed tomographic (CT) scans of the abdomen and pelvis at the time of initial evaluation are extremely useful. The scans should be done with oral and IV contrast material, and rectal contrast can be administered if only very low instillation pressures are used. Since the inflammatory process is in the bowel wall and pericolonic tissues, CT is highly accurate in confirming the diagnosis; if an abscess is identified, percutaneous drainage may be considered.

It is our policy to recommend surgery, after resolution of uncomplicated acute diverticulitis, for patients with a history of attacks or after the initial episode in patients under age 40.* In the absence of contraindications, patients who develop complications should be treated surgically even if they seem to recover completely. The interval between resolution of an acute attack and planned resection should be sufficient to allow the inflammatory reaction in the pericolic tissues to subside. In general, a minimum of 6 weeks is required, but 3 to 6 months is not an inordinately long interval. Associated medical conditions and the overall status of the patient must also be considered.

At surgery the sigmoid colon should be resected. While it is not necessary to remove all diverticula-containing segments of the colon, the entire segment of thickened, shortened bowel should be removed. This may necessitate resecting all or part of the descending colon and mobilizing the splenic flexure in order to construct an anastomosis. As long as there is no doubt about the diagnosis, wide mesenteric dissection should be avoided, thereby preventing inadvertent injury to retroperitoneal structures. The distal margin of resection should be in the rectum. After surgery, it is rare for diverticular disease to progress into the proximal bowel and cause recurrent symptoms. Recurrent diverticulitis after surgery is most frequently associated with inadequate distal resection.

---

*Editor's Note: The recommendation for surgery after the first uncomplicated attack for persons under 40 is interesting. This differs from the commonly given advice of surgery after the second attack that results in hospitalization.

GENERALIZED PERITONITIS

Diffuse peritonitis as a consequence of diverticulitis occurs as the result of either perforation of an inflamed diverticulum, or intraperitoneal rupture of a previously contained abscess. When a diverticulum ruptures freely, fecal peritonitis, often with pneumoperitoneum, results. Rupture of a diverticular abscess produces local or diffuse purulent peritonitis.

The three-stage procedure, which consists of initial diverting colostomy and drainage, followed by delayed resection and subsequent colostomy closure, had been the accepted standard for the treatment of perforated diverticulitis since the 1940s. This has now changed. When possible, the perforated segment should be resected at the time of the initial procedure and the ends used to construct an end-colostomy and mucus fistula (or Hartmann closure). In our view, resection with anastomosis has no role in the emergency treatment of a patient with diffuse peritonitis.

Occasionally, the surgeon is forced to operate on a patient who is too ill and too unstable to undergo anything but the most minimal and expeditious surgical procedure. Alternatively, mobilization of the perforated segment may be extraordinarily difficult or dangerous, especially for a surgeon with relatively little experience in colonic resection. In these circumstances, it is prudent to remember that colostomy and drainage almost always deals effectively with the immediate septic emergency.

Special attention must be given to the subset of patients who are immunosuppressed because of other diseases or as the result of medications used to treat other conditions. Steroids, chemotherapy, and immunosuppression after transplant surgery place the patient at increased risk for diverticular perforation. Should perforation occur, many of the usual signs of sepsis and peritonitis may be absent. These patients must be approached with a high index of suspicion and must undergo early surgery if they are to survive. It is crucial that immunosuppression be stopped or reduced to physiologic levels as quickly as possible in order to produce the best chance for a favorable outcome.

PERFORATION WITH ABSCESS

Frequently, inflammation is present for a period before actual perforation sufficient to allow the body time to "wall off" and contain the inflammatory process. Under these circumstances, a localized abscess results and generalized peritonitis is thus prevented. At times the abscess contains frank pus, but often it is only a phlegmonous mass consisting of inflamed colon and the inflamed, edematous structures surrounding it.

Initial management should be directed at correcting fluid and electrolyte abnormalities, rehydration, and instituting therapy with broad-spectrum IV antibiotics that cover gram-negative and anaerobic organisms. Plain x-ray films of the abdomen are usually of little diagnostic help but should be taken to evaluate the degree of obstruction present and to look for air outside the intestinal lumen. Occasionally, streaks of gas can be seen tracking in the bowel wall or between the loops. Air within the abscess cavity can sometimes be appreciated. Contrast radiography of the colon should be avoided during the acute phase of the illness, especially when there is a palpable mass and a strong suspicion of an abscess. CT has proved an extremely useful diagnostic and therapeutic modality. When a fluid-filled abscess cavity is visualized, percutaneous drainage should be considered. If technically feasible, this technique may help control systemic sepsis and allow what would otherwise have to be a multiple-stage emergency procedure to be carried out semielectively in a single stage. We have reserved its use for patients who are not improving on medical management alone and in whom CT demonstrates a fluid collection accessible to drainage by the interventional radiologist.

Most patients improve on the regimen of bowel rest, IV fluids, and antibiotics. The signs of systemic sepsis abate, the local tenderness lessens, and the mass shrinks or disappears completely. Failure to improve within 48 to 72 hours mandates emergent surgical intervention. After improvement, antibiotics should be continued for at least 7 days. In most cases, surgery should be recommended during the same hospitalization. The bowel can be prepared, the abscess resected together with the colon, and a primary anastomosis constructed.

If surgery is required during the acute illness without adequate preparation, or if the inflammatory process is found to be too widespread to permit safe anastomosis, we prefer resection with end-colostomy and Hartmann closure of the rectum. Occasionally, diverting colostomy and drainage of the abscess alone is mandated by the patient's condition or the severe inflammatory process, which would make resection unsafe. Fortunately, this is rarely necessary.

FISTULA

Approximately half of the fistulas from diverticulitis are into the bladder, and a colovesical fistula is present in 10 to 15 percent of patients who require surgical treatment for diverticulitis. Other fistulas seen in diverticulitis are colovaginal, coloenteric, and colocutaneous. Less commonly, colo-ureteral and colouterine fistulas have been observed.

Colovesical fistulas are much more common in men than in women, presumably because of the protection afforded by the intervening uterus. Although the patient may present with symptoms referable to the primary diverticular disease, urinary complaints may be the only manifestation of the diverticulitis. Pneumaturia, fecaluria, cystitis, urgency, and dysuria are common. Sepsis from an upper urinary tract infection, especially if there is obstruction to the distal urinary outflow (i.e., prostatic hypertrophy), may occur, but ascending pyelonephritis is rare. Recurrent urinary tract infections, especially with multiple organisms, in an elderly male should arouse the

clinician's suspicions. We have found CT extremely useful in diagnosing colovesical fistula. Thickening of both the colonic and bladder walls with adherence of these two structures is commonly seen. The presence of air or rectally administered contrast material within the bladder is diagnostic.

Although it has been suggested that patients with colovesical fistula can be treated safely for long periods without operation, we believe that unless there are strong medical contraindications, these patients should undergo elective surgical correction. The bowel can be prepared for resection and reanastomosis, and the patients are rarely acutely ill. It is unusual to find acute inflammation or an abscess, and the procedure can almost always be done in a single stage. The actual defect in the bladder may not be easily identifiable, but it is not imperative to do so; if seen, it should be oversewn with absorbable sutures. Excision of the thickened fibrous portion of the bladder wall is not necessary and may be detrimental. A urinary catheter should be left in the bladder for 7 to 10 days postoperatively. If adequate sigmoidectomy is performed, an excellent result may be anticipated.

Colovaginal fistula occurs almost exclusively in women who have undergone previous hysterectomy. Surgical treatment is identical to that described for colovesical fistula. Colocutaneous fistulas, while occasionally spontaneous, most often occur in the setting of previous colonic resection or drainage. These patients are much more likely to present with septic complications and malnutrition. The prognosis frequently depends on the degree of malnutrition present, which is often a function of the volume of fistula output. Preoperative total parenteral nutrition is advised in the setting of high output (more than 200 ml per day) fistulas, and surgical resection, often in stages, is usually necessary. Recurrent fistula formation of any sort after apparently adequate surgical resection should raise suspicion that the cause of the fistula is Crohn's disease, rather than diverticulitis.*

OBSTRUCTION

Complete colonic obstruction is relatively uncommon as a result of diverticulitis. Making the distinction from carcinoma may be a significant problem. Obstruction virtually always occurs in the sigmoid or distal

---

*Editor's Note: A word of caution: we have encountered at least eight individuals in their sixth to eighth decades presenting with symptoms of complicated diverticulitis who also have well-documented but subtle, often previously subclinical, Crohn's disease of the sigmoid and descending colon. If a diverting colostomy has been performed, the issue of diversion colitis versus subtle inflammatory bowel disease in the retained rectal pouch sometimes arises. At times, the pathologist can help resolve the dilemma by reviewing the resected specimen or by reviewing rectal biopsies. Very rapid improvement with short-chain fatty acid enemas would tend to favor diversion colitis (but some ulcerative colitis patients gradually improve with weeks of short-chain fatty acid enemas).

descending colon and is due to repeated attacks of acute, or subacute, diverticulitis, which leads to progressive scarring, fibrosis, thickening of the colonic wall, and narrowing of the lumen.

The onset of obstruction may be rapid, in association with an attack of acute diverticulitis. Here, there is usually a significant component of mucosal edema contributing to blockage of the lumen, and as the acute inflammation resolves on treatment with antibiotics and bowel rest, the obstruction usually resolves as well. At this point the patient should be considered for elective resection based on the criteria already outlined. If significant symptoms persist or there is a narrowed segment that cannot be completely evaluated, resection is indicated. If the obstruction is no longer complete and bowel preparation can be accomplished, this can be done as a single-stage procedure.

Persistent complete obstruction mandates emergent surgical intervention. In this situation, we favor a preliminary transverse colostomy, with limited simultaneous exploration. After decompression and bowel preparation, sigmoid resection is performed within 10 to 14 days. If the colostomy has been constructed on the left side of the transverse colon, consideration may be given to extending the resection to include the stoma as well as the obstructed segment. This avoids a third procedure for colostomy closure. This technique is especially suited to those situations when it has not been possible to completely clean or evaluate the segment between the colostomy and the obstruction, since it will also be resected.

HEMORRHAGE

Diverticular hemorrhage is usually self-limited. It almost always occurs without inflammation, and patients frequently report being asymptomatic until they pass a large amount of bright red or maroon-colored blood. They may have one or two more such movements and then no more, or the bleeding may continue for several days. Initial management consists of resuscitation. Large-bore IV lines and a urinary catheter are inserted. Central venous or pulmonary artery (Swan-Ganz) catheters are placed if mandated by the overall condition of the patient. Serial hematocrit levels should be checked every 2 to 4 hours. Patients with massive, active bleeding require observation in an intensive care unit.

Rigid proctosigmoidoscopy should be performed early to exclude bleeding sources in the rectum and distal sigmoid colon. The extraperitoneal rectum is almost impossible to evaluate intraoperatively and is the area to be left in situ should "blind" resection be necessary; it is therefore vital to be certain preoperatively that this is not the bleeding site.

Rarely is a patient with massive lower intestinal hemorrhage too unstable to undergo further diagnostic evaluation. Most, in fact, stop bleeding, at least intermittently. If bleeding does stop, total colonoscopy should be undertaken expeditiously. Emergency surgery, with-

out additional diagnostic evaluation, should be avoided if at all possible. If bleeding continues, we prefer to proceed with technetium scanning. The tagged cells remain circulating for up to 24 to 36 hours, and thus repeated scanning can detect intermittent bleeding. Because of intestinal peristalsis, exact anatomic localization of the bleeding site is much less precise when only the delayed scans are positive.

If the bleeding scan is negative, angiography is not likely to be helpful and therefore is not performed. In this situation, colonoscopy, especially after a gentle but rapid preparation, is of greatest usefulness. When the bleeding scan is positive, angiography may provide additional diagnostic information or more precise localization. It may also be used therapeutically by means of vasopressin infusion or embolization into the artery supplying the bleeding site. This is not entirely without risk and in our experience has rarely been successful.

If, and when, bleeding ceases, colonoscopy should be performed after the colon has been cleaned. Vascular ectasia can be cauterized and polyps can be removed. There is no reliable endoscopic treatment for bleeding presumed to be of diverticular origin. Recurrent bleeding is managed in similar fashion. If, however, the segment of origin has been identified, strong consideration should be given to segmental resection when bleeding recurs.

If bleeding does not stop, surgery is necessary. If the bleeding site has been localized with confidence preoperatively, we favor segmental resection or hemicolectomy, usually with primary anastomosis if the patient is stable. If localization has been unsuccessful, emergent subtotal colectomy is the procedure of choice. "Blind" hemicolectomy can be expected to fail in approximately 30 percent of cases. Usually, primary ileorectal anastomosis can be accomplished safely, but in the unstable patient there remains a place for subtotal colectomy with end-ileostomy and Hartmann closure of the rectal segment.

DIVERTICULITIS OF THE CECUM AND ASCENDING COLON

On the right side of the colon, true diverticula, which contain all layers of bowel wall, have been noted. These are often solitary, in the region of the cecum, and may be congenital in origin. When these diverticula become inflamed, the clinical presentation is virtually indistinguishable from acute appendicitis. In more than 75 percent of patients who are found to have cecal diverticulitis at surgery, the preoperative diagnosis was acute appendicitis, and in fewer than 10 percent is the correct diagnosis made preoperatively. CT may be helpful in this regard. Approximately 50 percent of cases contain a fecalith. Intraoperative recognition of the nature of the problem is also difficult. The appendix can usually be identified as being normal. In most instances, there is a firm indurated mass involving the cecum or ascending colon, and surgeons may have great difficulty determining that they are not dealing with a perforated carcinoma. Cecal diverticulitis is correctly identified intraoperatively in less than 60 percent of cases.

The treatment for right-sided diverticulitis is controversial. In those rare instances in which the diagnosis can be made with certainty before surgery, conservative management with IV antibiotics, similar to the treatment for acute left-sided diverticulitis, has been recommended. The vast majority require laparotomy because of diagnostic uncertainty. When the nature of the condition is recognized, diverticulectomy and closure of the defect in the cecum has been recommended. In our experience, the inflammatory process is rarely so well localized as to make this feasible. In practice, right hemicolectomy is usually the procedure of choice. Primary anastomosis between noninflamed ileum and transverse colon is almost always possible.

SUGGESTED READING

Almy TP, Howell DA. Diverticular disease of the colon. N Engl J Med 1980; 302:324–331.

Eng K, Ranson JCH, Localio SA. Resection of the perforated segment. A significant advance in treatment of diverticulitis with free perforation or abscess. Am J Surg 1977; 133:67–72.

Hackford AW, Veidenheimer MC. Diverticular disease of the colon. Current concepts and management. Surg Clin North Am 1985; 65:347–363.

Hulnick DH, Megibow AJ, Balthazar EJ, et al. Computed tomography in the evaluation of diverticulitis. Radiology 1984; 152:491–495.

Killingback M. Management of perforative diverticulitis. Surg Clin North Am 1983; 63:97–115.

Mueller PR, Saini S, Wittenburg J, et al. Sigmoid diverticular abscesses: percutaneous drainage as an adjunct to surgical resection in 24 cases. Radiology 1987; 164:321–325.

Nagorney DM, Adson MA, Pemberton JH. Sigmoid diverticulitis with perforation and generalized peritonitis. Dis Colon Rectum 1985; 28:71–75.

Steinhagen RM, Aufses AH Jr. Diverticular disease. In: Moody FG, ed. Surgical treatment of digestive disease. 2nd ed. Chicago: Year Book, 1990:740–753.

Treat MR, Forde KA. Colonoscopy, technetium scanning, and angiography in acute rectal bleeding—an algorithm for their combined use. Surg Gastroenterol 1983; 2:135–138.

THE LIVER

THERAPEUTIC IMPLICATIONS OF THE EVALUATION OF LIVER ENZYMES

NORMAN M. GITLIN, M.D., F.R.C.P. (Lond), F.R.C.P.E. (Edin)

Since the advent of screening biochemical panel tests, the number of patients detected with an elevation of serum alkaline phosphatase (ALP) or aminotransferase levels has risen sharply. Many of these patients are asymptomatic, and detection of these raised levels generates diagnostic and investigative dilemmas, especially if they are the sole biochemical abnormality.

ALP has been noted to be elevated in 4 to 45 percent of patients in a number of screening studies. Elevation of the ALP may be the initial or only sign of occult disease involving mainly the hepatobiliary and skeletal systems. There is a tendency to disregard and neglect slight elevations of ALP (less than twofold), but all ALP abnormalities should be investigated to identify the small group of patients harboring a treatable, curable form of liver disease. The extent of the investigations should be determined by a number of factors, such as age, overall health, medication regimen, the severity and duration of the elevation, and the availability of appropriate investigations and therapy. In an era of fiscal restraint, one should endeavor to avoid widespread investigations and focus only on relevant studies that offer the highest probability of meaningful results.

ALKALINE PHOSPHATASES

Knowledge of the diverse origins of ALP in the human body helps prevent an erroneous conclusion in a patient with elevated ALP. The ALPs are isoenzymes found in many human tissues, including liver, bones, intestine, kidney, placenta, and white blood cells. In health, serum ALP is derived mostly from liver, bone, and (to a much lesser extent) intestine. During the second and third trimesters of a normal pregnancy, placental ALP enters the serum and can often cause an elevation of the ALP. This persists until 2 weeks after childbirth.

The function of ALP is unknown. Results are expressed in international units (IU) per liter. Levels vary during life; females generally have slightly lower levels than males. The biologic half-life of circulating skeletal ALP is between 1 and 2 days. The mechanism whereby ALP is elevated in association with hepatic diseases has been debated for years. The dilemma as to whether the increase reflects induction of liver ALP or a failure of the normal excretion because of mechanical obstruction has been resolved in favor of the former pathogenesis. Studies using radioactive-labeled leucine (^{3}H-leucine) incorporated into ALP demonstrated that biliary tract obstruction elevates ALP in the serum by enhancing its synthesis through enzyme induction. ALP is released from the bile duct cell membranes by the detergent effect of the retained bile acids. Once ALP synthesis is induced, it takes weeks for the enzyme to revert to normal. This accounts for the observation in reversible space-occupying hepatic masses (pyogenic abscess or amebic abscess) that ALP rises relatively late in the disease and takes weeks to revert to normal after the pathologic condition has resolved.

Causes of Elevated ALP

The most common causes of elevated ALP are diseases of the liver and biliary system and bone disorders. Other conditions that require consideration are adverse response to medications, cholestasis of sepsis, normal physiologic states (puberty, pregnancy, or multiple fractures), and (rarely) genetic entities such as benign recurrent cholestasis (Table 1).

The hepatic disorders associated with raised ALP include chronic hepatitis (due to hepatitis B or C virus) and alcoholic liver disease ranging from fatty liver to alcoholic hepatitis and cirrhosis. All of these can manifest solely as raised ALP, and there is usually also an associated elevation of aminotransferase levels. Hepatic malignancies (primary or secondary) are invariably associated with elevated ALP levels. Obesity, with associated hepatic steatosis, has become recognized as a common cause of elevated ALP. The list of medications that can cause a reversible elevation of ALP is formi-

Table 1 Common Causes of Elevated
Alkaline Phosphatase

Source	Cause
Hepatic	Infections (viral abscess)
	Alcoholic fatty liver or hepatitis
	Cirrhosis
	Malignant tumors (primary, secondary)
	Immune disorders (primary biliary cirrhosis, primary sclerosing cholangitis)
	Steatosis
	Drug induced
	Metabolic (uncontrolled diabetes)
	Infiltrates (granuloma, amyloid)
	Vascular (cardiac failure)
	Cysts (polycystic disease, Caroli's syndrome, hydatid)
	Hyperalimentation
	Rejection post-transplantation
Biliary	Cholangitis
	Duct obstruction (calculus, neoplasm, stricture)
Bone	Paget's disease
	Osteomalacia, rickets
	Metastatic neoplasia to bone
	Hyperparathyroidism
	Osteogenic sarcoma
Septicemia	Cholestasis of sepsis
Physiologic	Puberty
	Pregnancy
	Healing fractures
Genetic	Benign recurrent cholestasis
	Familial elevated ALP
Pseudoelevation	Regan's isoenzyme

Table 2 Medications That Can Cause Elevation of
Alkaline Phosphatase ·

Anabolic steroids (methyltestosterone, norethandrolone)
Antithyroid agents (methimazole)
Chlorpromazine hydrochloride
Clofibrate
Erythromycin estolate
Immunosuppressive agents (cyclosporine, azathioprine)
Oral contraceptives (containing estrogens)
Oral hypoglycemics (especially chlorpropamide)

Table 3 Hepatic Complications of Inflammatory
Bowel Disease

Fatty liver
Pericholangitis
Liver abscess
Drug hepatitis
Sclerosing cholangitis
Cholangiocarcinoma
Immunopathic chronic active hepatitis
Amyloidosis
Viral hepatitis
Cholelithiasis

dable and growing (Table 2). A drug-related etiology should always be considered in any patient on medication and manifesting an abnormality of hepatic biochemistry. Immune diseases (primary biliary cirrhosis or sclerosing cholangitis) are often asymptomatic, and their initial detection is because of an asymptomatic elevated ALP level. Metabolic diseases, especially uncontrolled diabetes, with glycogen and fat in the liver are associated with elevated ALP. Hyperalimentation, rejection after transplantation, vascular disease (Budd-Chiari), and extensive hepatic cystic disease can reflect elevated ALP levels.

Biliary disease, cholangitis, obstruction (due to calculi, stricture, neoplasia, or secondary biliary cirrhosis) can often manifest solely as elevated ALP in the initial stages. A commonly misdiagnosed cause of elevated ALP is Paget's disease (osteitis deformans). This should be considered in all middle-aged patients noted to have incidental elevated ALP.

The association between bacterial infection (overt or latent) and abnormalities of ALP is well documented but often unrecognized. It occurs especially in association with gram-negative infections and it may be associated with a cholestatic biochemical picture. The pathogenesis of the cholestasis in this setting is suspected to relate to circulating endotoxins from the bacteria. Legionnaires' disease has also been noted in connection with ALP elevation. Asymptomatic inflammatory bowel disease (IBD) (either ulcerative colitis or granulomatous colitis) can be associated with a diverse spectrum of hepatobiliary disorders (Table 3). It is important not to overlook normal physiologic states: puberty, pregnancy, and post-trauma status are all associated with ALP elevation. Rarer familial and genetic conditions can manifest with ALP elevations (e.g., idiopathic familial elevation of ALP and benign recurrent cholestasis) and seldom offer a significant diagnostic challenge except at initial presentation. Pseudoelevation of ALP due to an isoenzyme indistinguishable from placental ALP was recognized in patients with lung cancer. It bears the name of the first patient in whom it was detected: Regan's isoenzyme.

Investigation and Management of Asymptomatic Patients With Isolated Elevated Hepatic ALP

The hepatobiliary enzymes gamma-glutamyltranspeptidase (GGTP) and/or 5'-nucleotidase (5-NT) are extremely useful to confirm or exclude an hepatic origin of elevated ALP. Elevated 5-NT is specific for hepatobiliary disease. GGTP is helpful in deciding the origin of ALP, as it closely parallels hepatic ALP. Both GGTP and 5-NT can be used to help distinguish the increased ALP of bone or placental origin from that of liver origin. GGTP is a sensitive indicator of liver disease but is not specific, and it can be raised in a number of conditions, including minor hepatic dysfunction, renal disease and cardiac disease and in postsurgical patients. It is often elevated in nonspecific viral illnesses (not associated

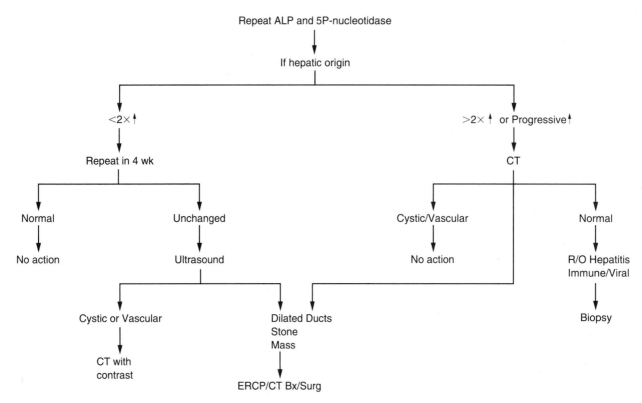

Figure 1 An approach to isolated elevated alkaline phosphatase in an asymptomatic patient. ERCP = endoscopic retrograde cholangiopancreatography; ALP = alkaline phosphatase.

with hepatitis) and is elevated in association with a number of drugs.

Separation of ALP isoenzymes by electrophoresis can help differentiate hepatobiliary from osseous ALP. Isoenzyme 1 arises from the liver, isoenzyme 2 from bone. However, isoenzyme identification is seldom used, and in most instances a concurrent elevation of GGTD or 5-NT is used to establish the origin of elevated ALP. Techniques used to differentiate ALP by utilizing selective inactivation of ALP via heat or urea denaturation are no longer used. Leucine aminopeptidase is also rarely used to assist in the evaluation of hepatobiliary disease.

Once a hepatic origin for increased ALP has been established and confirmed, management initially depends on the height of the elevation. A less than twofold elevation in an asymptomatic patient without other abnormal biochemical markers is best assessed by repeating the ALP test after 2 to 4 weeks. If the level is unchanged, serious hepatic disease is most unlikely and an ultrasound image of the hepatobiliary system is recommended. Possible entities that may account for elevated ALP include multiple congenital cysts, hemangiomas, acquired noninfectious granulomas, and medication-induced causes. Computed tomography (CT) of the abdomen with contrast material usually distinguishes hepatic cysts from hemangiomas or solid tumor masses. No further action is indicated in most patients, but a CT-guided needle biopsy is appropriate if

a solid, nonvascular mass is diagnosed. Evidence on ultrasonography of dilated extrahepatic or intrahepatic bile ducts, a dilated gallbladder, or a biliary calculus requires endoscopic retrograde cholangiopancreatography (ERCP) with possible subsequent surgical exploration of a tumor, stricture, or impacted stone not amenable to ERCP management.

An entirely different approach is advocated if the initial ALP elevation is greater than twofold above the normal laboratory value or if serial estimates show progressive elevation. In both circumstances, a progressive hepatic disease must be confirmed or excluded to permit timely appropriate therapy to commence. A CT scan with contrast of the hepatobiliary system is more informative than an ultrasound evaluation in this situation. On rare occasions, the CT scan can appear normal despite an underlying diffuse hepatocellular carcinoma or diffuse metastatic neoplasm in the liver. If either possibilities are favored, a radioactive isotope scan of the liver parenchyma is also recommended.

Once a solid space-occupying nonvascular mass is identified, a CT-guided needle biopsy/aspiration should be performed. If the mass (or masses) appears cystic or vascular on CT, biopsy is contraindicated, and an arteriogram or tagged red cell scan is helpful. A needle aspiration in the presence of a hydatid cyst, Caroli's syndrome, hemangioma, or a very vascular neoplasm can result in a major complication associated with hemorrhage, anaphylactic shock, or disseminated sepsis. Patients with elevated ALP greater than twice normal yet whose CT scan is normal should be evaluated for a diffuse parenchymatous disease such as primary biliary cirrhosis or primary sclerosing cholangitis. Determination of the titer of antimitochondrial antibody (AMA), smooth muscle antibody (SMA), and antinuclear antibody (ANA) is often diagnostic. ERCP is also indicated in such patients, and a subsequent liver biopsy will complete the evaluation. If the immunologic markers are negative for a diagnosis of primary biliary cirrhosis or an autoimmune disorder, a liver biopsy will help diagnose metabolic conditions with hepatic infiltration, e.g., glycogen/fat in an uncontrolled diabetic, fat/steatosis in steatohepatitis, drug hepatotoxicity, alcoholic fatty liver, or hepatic infiltrates (due to granulomas or amyloid).

A liver biopsy can be extremely helpful and informative in establishing not only the diagnosis, but also the severity of the disease process and the extent of involvement. It is not indicated in all instances; in fatty liver infiltration, ultrasonography is often almost diagnostic with its increased echogenicity. An algorithmic approach to the above decision making is summarized in Figure 1.

AMINOTRANSFERASES

The aminotransferases, formerly known as transaminases, are very sensitive markers of hepatocyte damage. Aspartate aminotransferase (AST), previously SGOT, is a mitochondrial enzyme present in large quantities in the heart, liver, skeletal muscles, and kidney. Alanine aminotransferase (ALT), previously SGPT, is a cytosol enzyme present in the liver, heart, and skeletal muscles. The absolute quantity of ALT in hepatocytes is less than that of AST, but a larger proportion of body ALT is found in the liver than in any other body organ, making it more specific for hepatocyte damage than AST. ALT is present only in hepatocyte cytosol.

AST is found more in hepatocyte mitochondria than in cytosol. Knowledge of these distributions has been used for the diagnostic and prognostic interpretations of a number of diseases involving the liver.

Conditions Associated With AST Elevation Higher Than ALT

Alcohol is predominantly a mitochondrial toxin. In alcoholic hepatitis the AST level is usually higher than the ALT level. Neither is strikingly elevated and they are seldom raised higher than five times the normal range. The ALT elevation is often minimal. An AST-to-ALT ratio greater than 2:0 is most suggestive of alcoholic hepatitis if the absolute elevations are less than fivefold. Such a ratio is rarely encountered in viral hepatitis, drug hepatitis, or steatohepatitis or as a consequence of toxins (e.g., *Amanita* poisoning).

In fulminant hepatic failure due to viral hepatitis, an AST-to-ALT ratio greater than 2:0 can occur. However,

the absolute aminotransferase levels are usually significantly elevated into the range of thousands. This is not seen in uncomplicated viral hepatitis, in which characteristically the exact reverse is noted: ALT much higher than AST. Fulminant hepatic failure associated with Wilson's disease can also manifest an AST-to-ALT ratio greater than 4:0; this can be of diagnostic assistance in recognizing new-onset cases of Wilson's disease. There is a separate chapter on Wilson's disease.

Conditions Associated With ALT Elevation Greater Than AST

Chronic mild to moderate aminotransferase elevation two- to eightfold above normal in asymptomatic patients is a common experience. This is especially evident as a consequence of screening biochemical panel tests for routine physical and insurance examinations and as part of blood donor screening. It is often a dilemma for the physician to decide on the course of further evaluations. Published reports addressing this issue have noted that the common identifiable causes for elevated aminotransferases include chronic viral hepatitis (due mostly to hepatitis C virus but occasionally to hepatitis B), steatohepatitis (associated with obesity), alcoholic fatty liver or alcoholic hepatitis, drug hepatoxicity and, less commonly, metabolic disorders (hemochromatosis, Wilson's disease) or sclerosing cholangitis. Uncontrolled diabetes is fairly often associated with raised aminotransferase and ALP levels.

Differentiation of alcoholic hepatitis from steatohepatitis can be very difficult even at the histologic level. Useful pointers in separating these two conditions are that in steatohepatitis the serum albumin is rarely less than 3.5 g per deciliter, the prothrombin time is rarely greater than 2.0 seconds above the control, the AST-to-ALT ratio is often less than 2.0, and the histologic picture shows less polymorphs and hyaline than is encountered in alcoholic hepatitis.

Extremely high levels of AST and/or ALT in excess of eight times normal are often easier to evaluate than are milder elevations. The underlying pathology that accounts for the marked aminotransferase elevation is usually obvious and acute. Milder elevations are often due to chronic, insidious disorders. Acute viral hepatitis, drug hepatitis, or toxic hepatitis (due to toxins, chemicals, or mushrooms) can cause a severe rise in aminotransferase levels. There is often an accompanying history of exposure, and the acute nature of the disease, the symptoms, and the physical findings are all very compatible and suggestive of an acute hepatic insult. Ischemic hepatitis, a sequel to recent severe hypotension (whether documented or suspected from the history), usually produces a meteoric rise in aminotransferases (up to 20,000 IU) as well as lactic dehydrogenase (LDH). The ALP, bilirubin, and albumin levels alter slightly. Jaundice and a mild coagulopathy can occur. Once the hypotension is corrected (by improving the cardiac status or by correction of the hypovolemia), there is an equally rapid resolution of the enzymes within 5 to 7 days.

It is important to realize that drug interactions or drug-alcohol interactions can result in unanticipated severe, acute liver injury. The combination of alcohol and acetaminophen or isoniazid and acetaminophen can result in severe acute acetaminophen hepatotoxicity as a result of their common drug metabolism by the cytochrome P-450 11E enzyme subset. High aminotransferase levels (above 1,000 IU) and early coagulopathy point to a diagnosis of acetaminophen hepatotoxicity rather than alcoholic hepatitis.

Investigation and Management of Mild to Moderate AST Elevation in Asymptomatic Patients

The initial step is to repeat the aminotransferase tests combined with a full liver chemistry profile, complete blood count, platelet count, and prothrombin time. At the same time, serologic studies using the latest techniques for acute and chronic infection with HCV or HBV are indicated. The evaluation should also include tests for autoimmune markers, including ANA, SMA, serum ferritin, serum iron, iron-binding assays, and percentage saturation. Serum ceruloplasmin and alpha^1-antitrypsin assays should be measured. This initial approach covers the most common causes of mild or moderately elevated aminotransferases.

If the biochemical testing shows evidence of chronic liver disease (low albumin, high globulin, raised prothrombin time, low platelet count), a CT scan is indicated, followed by a liver biopsy if not contraindicated by coagulopathy. If the biochemical tests point to cholestasis, ultrasonography is appropriate, followed by ERCP if there is ductal dilation. A liver biopsy is recommended if the biliary ducts are of normal size. If sclerosing cholangitis is suspected (because of associated IBD, pruritus, or cholestasis) ERCP is strongly recommended. If an infiltrative process of the liver is suspected (amyloid, fat, metastatic cancer), a liver biopsy aided by a CT-guided technique will be rewarding.

If the only abnormality on the screening tests is a mild elevation of AST and/or ALT, and if the patient is symptomatic and tests negative for all other above-mentioned markers, one should retest in 4 months after possible causative factors are adjusted (obesity is corrected, alcohol abstinence is enforced, or medications are discontinued). If the aminotransferases remain elevated for more than 6 months, a CT scan and liver biopsy are recommended. (Table 4 summarizes the above approach.)

Clearly, once the underlying pathology has been documented, the therapeutic approach should be specific to the disorder (venesections for hemochromatosis, penicillamine for Wilson's, consideration of interferon therapy for chronic hepatitis B or C, ursodeoxycholic acid for sclerosing cholangitis, methotrexate and/or ursodeoxycholic acid for primary biliary cirrhosis, steroids for immunopathic chronic active hepatitis, antimicrobial agents for sepsis, and surgery for calculi, strictures, abscesses, and neoplasia). These therapies have

Table 4 Investigation and Management of Mild to Moderate* AST Elevation in Asymptomatic Patients

Repeat AST, ALT with complete liver chemistry panel; perform complete blood count, platelet count, and prothrombin time

Perform serologic tests for HBV, HCV

Perform autoimmune tests for antinuclear antibodies, smooth muscle antibodies, as well as ferritin, serum iron, iron binding, saturation, ceruloplasmin, and α_1-antitrypsin assays

If chronic liver disease is suspected (low albumin, high globulin, prolonged prothrombin time, low platelets), perform CT and if possible liver biopsy

If cholestasis is detected, arrange ultrasonography, ERCP

If sclerosing cholangitis is suspected, arrange ERCP

If infiltration is suspected (neoplasia, fat, amyloid), arrange CT followed by guided liver biopsy

If only abnormality is mildly elevated AST/ALT, retest in 4–6 months after adjustments (weight loss, alcohol abstinence, medication withdrawal); if still elevated at that stage, consider liver biopsy

*Two- to eightfold.
HBV = hepatitis B virus; HCV = hepatitis C virus; ERCP = endoscopic retrograde cholangiopancreatography.

been covered in depth in other chapters. It is wise to remember that tests are best used as a guide in the art and science of medicine; they should not be interpreted as infallible and they should not become our masters and rule us.

SUGGESTED READING

Berman DH, Leventhal RI, Gavaler JS, et al. Clinical differentiation of fulminant wilsonian hepatitis from other causes of hepatic failure. Gastroenterology 1991; 100:1129.

Cohen J, Kaplan M. The SGOT/SGPT ratio: an indicator of alcoholic liver disease. Dig Dis Sci 1979; 24:835.

Diehl AM, Goodman Z, Ishak KG. Alcohol-like liver disease in nonalcoholics: a clinical and histologic comparison with alcohol-induced liver injury. Gastroenterology 1988; 95:1056.

Fang MH, Ginsberg AL, Dobbins WO. Marked elevation in serum alkaline phosphatase activity as a manifestation of systemic infection. Gastroenterology 1980; 78:592.

Gitlin N. The serum glutamic oxaloacetic transaminase/serum glutamic pyruvic transaminase ratio as a prognostic index in severe acute viral hepatitis. Am J Gastroenterol 1982; 77:2.

Hay JE, Czaja AJ, Rakela J, et al. The nature of unexplained chronic aminotransferase elevations of a mild to moderate degree in asymptomatic patients. Hepatology 1989; 9:193.

Kaplan MM. Induction of rat liver alkaline phosphatase by bile duct ligation. Yale J Biol Med 1979; 52:69.

Lai CL, Ng RP, Lok ASF. The diagnostic value of the ratio of serum gamma-glutamyl transpeptidase to alkaline phosphatase in alcoholic liver disease. Scand J Gastroenterol 1982; 17:41.

Nalpas B, Vassault A, Charpin S, et al. Serum mitochondrial aspartate aminotransferase as a marker of chronic alcoholism: diagnostic value and interpretation in a liver unit. Hepatology 1986; 6:608.

ACUTE HEPATITIS: MANAGEMENT AND PREVENTION

DOMINIQUE Q. PHAM, M.D.
LEONARD B. SEEFF, M.D.

Advances in the treatment of acute viral hepatitis have not kept pace with the serologic and epidemiologic progress achieved over the past 2 decades. The only new efforts regarding treatment are several recent but limited studies involving interferon administration to patients with acute hepatitis B and C. The results of these studies at present are too preliminary to form an opinion with regard to efficacy. The mainstay of hepatitis management, therefore, continues to be supportive care, avoidance of liver-damaging events, and observation for progression to fulminant or subfulminant hepatitis. Indeed, the primary gains in treatment have been the omission of certain approaches that were common previously—mandatory hospitalizations, mandatory bedrest, special diets, and treatment with corticosteroids in certain circumstances. Prevention of the disease, however, has made significant progress, and if fully implemented, could potentially eliminate or at least dramatically reduce the prevalence of some hepatitis types.

EVALUATION

There is no feature that is pathognomonic of acute viral hepatitis. In most instances, a presumptive diagnosis can be made from the accumulation of historical facts, physical findings, biochemical alterations, and serologic markers. In gathering the patient's history, it is important to focus on circumstances that favor exposure to viral hepatitis and on the use of all medications (prescription and over-the-counter). It must be remembered that the illness can be mimicked by drug hepatotoxicity, congestive heart failure, sudden hypotension, and acute choledocholithiasis. A similar though generally distinguishable presentation can result from infections by other agents such as cytomegalovirus, Epstein-Barr virus, autoimmune hepatitis, and metabolic disorders (Wilson's disease, alpha$_1$-antitrypsin deficiency). Physical examination should include evaluation of mental status and a search for features that might suggest the presence of chronic liver disease (spider angiomata, collateral venous pattern, gynecomastia, ascites, peripheral edema), since acute reactivation or superinfection of chronic liver disease may simulate a bout of acute hepatitis.

Minimal biochemical and serologic testing should include the serum aminotransferases, bilirubin, alkaline phosphatase, serum proteins, prothrombin time (PT), IgM anti-HAV, HBsAg, IgM anti-HBc, and anti-HCV. Additional serologic markers can be sought as necessary. Among the biochemical tests, the PT and the serum bilirubin are the most important prognostic indicators. Prolongation of the PT by more than 3 seconds and a serum bilirubin level that is greater than 20 mg per deciliter suggest the potential for the development of severe, progressive disease. Serum bilirubin values at this level should also trigger consideration of hemolysis, such as may occur in patients with underlying G6-PD deficiency or sickle cell anemia. Biochemical screening is warranted twice a week when enzyme values are rising, weekly after they have plateaued, and at 1- to 2-week intervals during the subsiding phase. Ideally, completion of evaluation requires identification of loss of HBsAg, to exclude advance to the carrier state, and return of enzymes to normal, to exclude progression to chronic hepatitis.

A routine liver biopsy is unnecessary. It can be considered when there is reason to suspect that the diagnosis might be an exacerbation of pre-existing chronic liver disease or when the disease runs an atypical, protracted course (persisting symptoms or severe biochemical abnormalities for more than 6 weeks). The finding of bridging or submassive necrosis might lead to the consideration to contact a liver transplant center.

THERAPY

Treatment Environment

Provided there is adequate family and medical support, most patients with uncomplicated acute viral hepatitis can be treated at home. Hospitalizations for isolation purposes is not warranted because the most infectious period for hepatitis A and B precedes the development of clinically apparent disease. Adequate care implies that there is a household member willing to observe the patient daily for any signs of unusual physical or mental change, to supply the necessary nursing and subsistence support, and to ensure patient compliance with medical follow-up. Hospitalization will, however, need to be considered if the patient has protracted vomiting with the threat of dehydration, disturbing mental status changes, or worsening biochemical tests. The latter include rising serum bilirubin values, particularly if accompanied by rapidly declining serum enzyme activity, an increasing PT, and falling albumin levels. Elderly patients and those with significant medical problems may need to be hospitalized.

Bedrest

There is now general agreement that complete bedrest is not essential. This decision derives from studies which showed no differences in clinical outcomes when convalescing patients were subjected to strenuous activity or assigned to bedrest. However, these studies involved young and otherwise healthy men, mostly military personnel, and it is uncertain whether these results apply to older and more frail populations. The following program seems to be a reasonable approach. Bedrest with bathroom privileges should be advised when the bilirubin level is rising, if the PT is prolonged by more than 3 seconds, if the patient is severely symptomatic, or if the patient is more than 40 years of age. Gradual return to normal activity is permitted when symptoms and biochemical tests begin to improve. Patients can return to work when their biochemical tests show consistent improvement (consistent reduction of the serum enzymes preferably to less than 100 IU per liter) and they have no symptoms or jaundice.

Diet

Under normal circumstances, no specific diet restriction seems necessary. A nutritious diet should be encouraged which need not include vitamin supplementation unless there is evidence of a specific deficiency. The challenge is to induce patient to eat when anorexia and nausea are present. Because anorexia and nausea typically are least severe in the morning, it is useful to offer the major proportion of calories at this time and to provide the remainder in frequent small meals during the rest of the day. This might be accomplished with the aid of high calorie liquid formulas. Some believe a high protein diet is beneficial but there is no obvious long-term benefit. Fatty foods need not be restricted unless they produce nausea. Severe, continued vomiting will obviously necessitate fluid and electrolyte replacement.

Drugs

As a general rule, all drugs, particularly narcotics, analgesics, and tranquilizers, should be avoided during the course of acute hepatitis. Protracted nausea and vomiting may require judicious use of small doses of metoclopramide. If sedation is necessary, oxazepam is preferred because its metabolism is not impaired by acute liver damage. Rarely, pruritis may be sufficiently severe to warrant the use of medication, such as hydroxyzine or cholestyramine. The use of vitamin K is of no benefit in acute hepatitis although it may improve abnormal PTs in patients with cholestatic liver disease. Data regarding the effects of alcohol in patients with acute hepatitis are conflicting, but the prudent approach is to proscribe its use during the acute and convalescent phase so as to reduce confusion about the meaning of subsequent enzyme abnormalities. Oral contraceptives can be continued without deleterious effect. Early studies suggested that the use of corticosteroids could hasten recovery from acute viral hepatitis accompanied by rapid reduction in serum bilirubin. Later studies comparing corticosteroids with placebos failed to substantiate a beneficial effect. Furthermore, it has been suggested that corticosteroid treatment may predispose to a higher rate of relapse and interfere with the normal immune response, particularly in persons with acute hepatitis B, and hence may promote the development of chronic hepatitis. Accordingly, the use of corticosteroids for uncomplicated viral hepatitis is neither justified nor helpful.

Elective Surgery

Unequivocal objective evidence of the dangers of surgery is scanty. In one commonly-cited study, of the 42 patients with acute viral hepatitis who were subjected to surgery, five died within 3 weeks of surgery and nonfatal major complications developed in five other patients. Elective surgery should be avoided during acute viral hepatitis.

New Forms of Treatment

A variety of specific treatment modalities have been tested in the treatment of acute viral hepatitis. Their effects are aimed directly at inhibition of viral synthesis or at alteration of the immune response. Efforts have been made to treat patients with acute viral hepatitis with ribavirin, isoprinosine, (+)-cyanidanol-3, levamisole, and anti-HBs hyperimmune globulin, with little success. Recently, based on the evidence of the partial benefit of interferon treatment in patients with chronic hepatitis B and C, efforts have begun to evaluate its efficacy for treatment of the acute illness. In one randomized, placebo-controlled trial of interferon alpha in acute hepatitis B, interferon was well tolerated. Treatment in this study appeared to shorten the period of clinical disease and induce higher titers of anti-HBs antibodies. However, there were no differences in the overall clinical and biochemical outcomes among the control and treated groups. Some preliminary studies have supported the use of interferon during acute hepatitis C infection to prevent progression to the chronic stage. These studies involved a limited number of patients, used different types and doses of interferon, and had varying durations of follow-up. Thus, it is difficult to draw any firm conclusion regarding the efficacy of interferon in preventing the progression of HCV infection to chronicity. At the present time, interferon is not recommended for treatment of acute hepatitis B or C until more data become available.

GENERAL PREVENTION OF VIRAL HEPATITIS

The institution of appropriate preventive public health measures depends on a thorough knowledge of the modes of transmission of hepatitis. Hepatitis A is primarily transmitted by person-to-person contact, generally through fecal contamination and oral ingestion; hence those at risk are susceptible to household or institutional contacts. The virus reaches its highest concentration in the feces from the latter half of the incubation period to approximately the time of peak illness, generally within 1 week of onset of disease.

Because of this pattern of viral excretion, many of the contacts are likely to have been exposed by the time the index case is brought to medical attention. Nevertheless, to curtail further spread, the modes of disease transmission should be discussed with the patient, and strict standards of personal hygiene should be imposed. This includes regular hand washing, particularly after using the toilet (separate facilities are not required); a warning against intimate contact; and a prohibition of the sharing of food and drink. Food can be eaten using paper plates or disposable utensils although household implements are perfectly safe if washed in a dishwasher. When hospitalization is required, there is no need to impose reverse isolation procedures or enforce the use of separate bathroom facilities. Universal precautions as recommended by the Occupational Safety and Health Administration (OSHA) should be applied. Transmission of hepatitis A virus by the percutaneous route has been reported but is uncommon.

The hepatitis B virus is present in blood and in all body fluids, with the exception of the stool; presumably the same holds true for the viruses of hepatitis C and the delta agent. Thus, blood and body secretions are the source of transmission and high-risk individuals are those who are likely to come into contact with blood and its products or who have intimate contact with the index case. However, sexual transmission of hepatitis C, unlike hepatitis B, seems to be minimal. Nonpercutaneous transmission other than sexual contact also occurs but the precise mechanism often cannot be established. Consequently, preventive measures that can be adopted include the application of universal precautions, i.e., the consistent use of gloves, gown, and face mask when contamination is anticipated; the requirement that needles be properly disposed of; and that instruments in contact with blood and secretions be adequately cleaned (with soap and water), disinfected (sodium hypochlorite, formalin, glutaraldehyde), and sterilized (autoclaving, ethylene oxide). Other efforts include reduction of the number of blood transfusions; development and maintenance of hospital surveillance to identify HBsAg carriers; and the recommendation that sexual abstinence be followed during the acute disease and that sexual contact be limited by the carrier. As will be discussed, many of these problems could be avoided if immune prophylaxis is provided for all susceptible high-risk individuals.

IMMUNOPROPHYLAXIS

Hepatitis A

Pre-Exposure Prophylaxis

Immune globulin (IG) is recommended for all susceptible travelers to developing countries, especially those who live in or visit rural areas, or frequently eat or drink in settings of poor sanitation. A single dose of IG of 0.02 ml per kilogram of body weight is recommended if travel is for less than 3 months. For prolonged travel

Table 1 Recommendations for Hepatitis A Prophylaxis*

	IG Doses	Groups Exposed
Pre-exposure	0.02 ml/kg bw† × 1	Travelers <3 months
	0.06 ml/kg bw q5 months	Travelers >3 months
Postexposure	0.02 ml/kg bw within 2 weeks	Household, sexual, day care center contacts; outbreaks in institutions

*ACIP, CDC, 1990.
†Body weight.

or residence in developing countries, 0.06 ml per kilogram should be given every 5 months (Table 1).

Inactivated hepatitis A vaccine in clinical trials has been shown to be well tolerated and immunogenic. It may supersede the use of immunoglobulin for pre-exposure prophylaxis against hepatitis A. In the United States, recommendations for the use of inactivated hepatitis A vaccine will be developed in the near future.

Postexposure Prophylaxis

For postexposure IG prophylaxis, a single intramuscular dose of 0.02 ml per kilogram is recommended within 2 weeks of exposure for all household and sexual contacts, for contacts in day care centers, and for residents in institutions for custodial care (see Table 1). Serologic confirmation of the index case is recommended before contacts are treated. Serologic screening of contacts for anti-HAV is not recommended because of the cost of screening and the delay in prophylaxis administration.

Hepatitis B

Pre-Exposure Prophylaxis

Two types of hepatitis B vaccines currently licensed in the United States are (1) Plasma-derived vaccine (Heptavax-B) which is no longer being produced and the use of which is now limited to hemodialysis patients, other immunocompromised hosts, and persons with known allergy to yeast; and (2) recombinant vaccine (Recombivax HB and Engerix-B). Primary vaccination consists of three intramuscular doses of vaccine at 0, 1, and 6 months. Adults and older children should be given a full 1.0 ml dose, while children less than 11 years of age should be given half (0.5 ml) this dose. Hepatitis B vaccine should be given only in the deltoid muscle for adults and children or in the anterolateral thigh muscle for infants and neonates. For hemodialysis patients and those who are immunocompromised, higher vaccine doses or an increased number of doses are required (see Table 2 for recommended doses and schedules of currently available vaccines).

Previously, groups recommended for pre-exposure vaccination included persons with occupational risk,

Table 2 Recommended Doses of Currently Licensed Hepatitis B Vaccines*

	Dose mg/ml†		
Groups	Heptavax-B‡	Recombivax HB	Engerix-B§
Infants of HBV-carrier mothers	10 (0.5)	5 (0.5)	10 (0.5)
Other infants and children <11 yr	10 (0.5)	2.5 (0.25)	10 (0.5)
Children and adolescents 11–19 yr	20 (1.0)	5 (0.5)	20 (1.0)
Adults >19 yr	20 (1.0)	10 (1.0)	20 (1.0)
Dialysis and immuno-compromised patients	40 (2.0)	40 (1.0)	40 (2.0)

*ACIP, CDC, 1990.

†Usual schedule: three doses at 0, 1, 6 months

‡Heptavax-B: Available only for hemodialysis, immunocompromised patients, and persons with known allergy to yeast.

§Alternative schedule for Engerix-B: 0, 1, 2, 12 months or 0, 1, 2, 6 months for dialysis and immunocompromised patients.

Table 3 Recommendations for Hepatitis B Postexposure Prophylaxis*

Exposure	HBIG	Vaccine	Timing
Perinatal	0.5 ml IM × 1	0.5 ml IM followed by usual schedule	Within 12 hr of birth
Sexual	0.06 ml/kg bw IM × 1	1.0 ml IM followed by usual schedule	Within 14 days of last sexual contact
Infants <12 months (household contact)	0.5 ml IM × 1	0.5 ml IM followed by usual schedule	

*ACIP, CDC, 1990.

†body weight

clients and staffs of institutions for the mentally handicapped, hemodialysis patients, sexually active homosexual men, recipients of high-risk blood products, household and sexual contacts of HBV carriers, adoptees from countries with high HBV endemicity, populations with high HBV endemicity (Alaskan natives, Pacific Islanders), prison inmates, sexually active heterosexual persons, and international travelers for 6 months to endemic areas. More recently, the American Academy of Pediatrics and the Advisory Committee on Immunization Practices of the United States Public Health Service have recommended universal immunization of infants. All children should receive three doses of vaccines by the time they are 18 months of age. In our view, even nonimmune adolescents should be considered for HBV vaccination. Hepatitis B vaccine produces protective antibody (anti-HBs) in 90 percent of healthy persons. An adequate antibody response is greater than 10 milliInternational Units (mIU per milliliter) measured after completion of the vaccine series. Available data show that vaccine-induced antibody levels decline steadily over time and that up to 50 percent of vaccinees who respond adequately to vaccine may have low or undetectable levels by 7 years after vaccination. For people with normal immune status, declining antibody levels are still protective against hepatitis B infection, and hence booster doses are not routinely recommended, nor is routine serologic testing necessary within 7 years after vaccination. For immunocompromised and hemodialysis patients for whom vaccine-induced protection is less complete, antibody testing should be done annually, and booster doses be given when antibody levels decline to less than 10 mIU per milliliter.

Postexposure Prophylaxis

Prophylactic treatment to prevent hepatitis B infection after exposure to HBV should be given to newborns of HBsAg-carrier mothers (perinatal exposures), persons exposed to HBsAg-positive blood through accidental percutaneous or permucosal routes, sexual partners of persons with acute HBV infection, and infants less than 12 months of age who have been exposed to primary care givers with acute hepatitis B (Table 3). For accidental percutaneous and permucosal exposure to blood, the decision to provide prophylaxis depends on the HBsAg status of the source of exposure and the vaccination status and vaccine response of the exposed person (Table 4). Although hepatitis B immune globulin (HBIG) has been used with moderate benefit for postexposure prophylaxis, a regimen combining HBIG with hepatitis B vaccine will provide both short- and

Table 4 Recommendations for Prophylaxis Following Percutaneous/Permucosal Exposure to Hepatitis B*

	HBsAg Status of Source		
Exposed Person	Positive	Negative	Unknown
Unvaccinated	HBIG × 1 and initiate HB vaccine	Initiate HB vaccine	Initiate HB vaccine
Previously vaccinated			
Known responder	Test for anti-HBs Adequate – no treatment Inadequate – HB vaccine booster dose	No treatment	No treatment
Known nonresponder	HBIG × 2 or HBIG × 1 plus 1 dose HB vaccine	No treatment	If high-risk source, treat as if source HBsAg positive
Unknown response	Test for anti-HBs Adequate – no treatment Inadequate – HBIG × 1 and HB vaccine booster dose	No treatment	Test for anti-HBs Adequate – no treatment Inadequate – HB vaccine booster dose

*ACIP, CDC, 1990.

long-term protection and is the treatment of choice. For greatest effectiveness, passive prophylaxis with HBIG, when indicated, should be given within 7 days of exposure.

Delta Hepatitis

Since delta hepatitis virus (HDV) is dependent on HBV for replication, prevention of hepatitis B infection, either pre- or postexposure, will suffice to prevent HDV infection for a person susceptible to hepatitis B. At present no products are available that might prevent HDV infection in HBsAg carriers either before or after exposure.

Non-A, Non-B (Predominantly C) Hepatitis

Studies of the efficacy of immunoglobulins in prophylaxis against non-A, non-B hepatitis have provided equivocal data. For persons with percutaneous exposure to blood from a patient with non-A, non-B hepatitis, it may be reasonable to administer a single dose of immune globulin (IG) 0.06 ml per kilogram as soon as possible after exposure. No vaccine for HCV exists at the present.

Hepatitis E

There is no evidence that IG manufactured in the U.S. will prevent this infection. As with other enteric infections, avoidance of potentially contaminated food or water is the best means of preventing hepatitis E.

SUGGESTED READING

Centers for Disease Control. Protection against viral hepatitis. Recommendations of the Immunization Practices Advisory Committee (ACIP). MMWR 1990; 39, S2: 1–26.

Seeff LB. Diagnosis, therapy, and prognosis of viral hepatitis. In: Zakim D, Boyer TB, eds., Hepatology: A textbook of liver disease. Philadelphia: WB Saunders, 1990; 958.

Viral hepatitis management, standards for the future. Proceedings of a Symposium in Cannes, France, May 22–23, 1992. Gut 1993; supplement: S1–S149.

CHRONIC HEPATITIS

EMIL P. MISKOVSKY, M.D.

Chronic hepatitis is a clinicopathologic diagnosis defined as abnormal aminotransferases of 6 months' duration associated with findings of inflammatory liver injury on liver biopsy (Table 1). The diagnosis is confirmed by specific histopathologic features associated with serologic or biochemical determinations. Some clinical entities can imitate chronic hepatitis; chief among them are steatohepatitis and alcoholic liver disease (Table 2). Chronically abnormal liver-related test abnormalities may occur in a variety of disorders that do not fit the classical definition of chronic hepatitis (e.g., systemic lupus erythematosus) and, in general, are not associated with the same long-term hepatic sequelae as classically defined chronic hepatitis. Because many patients with chronic hepatitis may present without symptoms, it is imperative that physicians not neglect the evaluation of asymptomatic, chronically abnormal aminotransferases. The significance of an accurate diagnosis within the rubric of chronic hepatitis can not be overemphasized since the therapeutic options vary dramatically.

When symptoms are present, the most common are fatigue or easy fatiguability, malaise, anorexia, abdominal pain, nausea, arthralgias, myalgias, and occasionally weight loss. Clinical clues, such as related autoimmune phenomena (i.e., hemolytic anemia, ulcerative colitis, Sjögren's syndrome), typical toxicities of hypercupremia (Coombs' negative hemolysis, hypouricemia, Kayser-Fleischer rings, tremor, dystonia, or grand mal seizures), or chronic obstructive pulmonary disease aid in the diagnosis of autoimmune hepatitis, primary biliary cirrhosis, primary sclerosing cholangitis, Wilson's disease, or alpha$_1$-antitrypsin deficiency liver disease, re-

spectively. Recently, important associations have been made between chronic viral hepatitis and vasculitis-glomerulonephritis (chronic hepatitis B or C), type II cryoglobulinemia (chronic hepatitis C), and porphyria cutanea tarda (chronic hepatitis C). In general, symptoms and signs, especially of portal hypertension and/or hyperbilirubinemia, become more evident as the liver disease advances toward end-stage disease, at which point orthotopic liver transplantation may be the only therapeutic option.

This chapter reviews the diagnostic and therapeutic aspects of those causes of chronic hepatitis not covered elsewhere in this book. There is also a chapter on abnormal liver function tests.

EVOLUTION OF THE HISTOLOGIC CLASSIFICATION OF CHRONIC HEPATITIS

The present classification schema of chronic hepatitis was drafted in 1968 (Table 3). Although the lesions of chronic persistent hepatitis (CPH), chronic active hepatitis (CAH), and chronic lobular hepatitis (CLH) were not felt to be immutable, clinical experience (primarily with autoimmune hepatitis) demonstrated that there was a typical clinical prognosis associated with each specific lesion. In particular, CPH and CAH without extensive (i.e., bridging) necrosis were associated with a benign course, and CAH with bridging necrosis was associated with a poor prognosis. These histologic-prognostic associations are still relevant to autoimmune hepatitis. However, the natural history and pathobiology of chronic hepatitis B and the etiologic factor of most non-A, non-B hepatitis, hepatitis C virus (HCV), has led to a reappraisal of the chronic hepatitis histology-prognosis paradigm for viral hepatitis. It is now clear that the characteristic lesions of CPH, CAH, and CLH may occur in the same patient over the course of the viral hepatitis and that there is little clear prognosis to each lesion when taken out of clinical context (which includes serologic and viral replicative status). An

Table 1 Causes of Chronic Hepatitis

Viral	Inherited
Hepatitis B	Wilson's disease
Hepatitis C	
Hepatitis D	Tonic
	Medications
Autoimmune	
Autoimmune hepatitis	Unknown
	Cryptogenic

Table 2 Causes of Chronic Hepatitis-Like Syndromes

Nonalcoholic steatohepatitis
Alcoholic liver disease
Hemochromatosis
Primary biliary cirrhosis
Primary sclerosing cholangitis
Alpha$_1$-antitrypsin deficiency

Table 3 Chronic Hepatitis Histologic Classification

Classification	Characteristic Lesions
Chronic persistent hepatitis (CPH)	Inflammation within the portal triad Small amount of lobular necrosis No fibrosis
Chronic active hepatitis (CAH)	Inflammation crossing the limiting plate, with necrosis extending into the periportal area In severe cases, "bridging necrosis" between portal tracts or portal tracts and central veins Fibrosis in severe cases
Chronic lobular hepatitis (CLH)	Inflammation in the lobule, consistent with acute hepatitis

example is the conversion from HBe antigen (Ag)-positivity to HBe antibody (Ab)-positivity in the course of chronic hepatitis B during which a characteristic flare of hepatitis (with worsening of histology and marked elevation of the serum aminotransferases) occurs, after which the patient may enter into a benign "chronic carrier state" associated with low viral replication. In contrast to this situation, an asymptomatic patient with chronic hepatitis B may develop acute reactivation of the hepatitis B virus (HBV), predictably after a course of corticosteroids, which produces a similar clinicopathologic condition, but is identified by high HBV-DNA levels and the eventual presence of IgM HBc Ab. A similar syndrome is present if the same chronic HBV infection becomes superinfected with either HCV, hepatitis A virus (HAV), or hepatitis delta virus (HDV), which are identified by HCV-RNA, IgM HAV Ab, or IgM HDV Ab, respectively in the serum. Further, some patients with chronic hepatitis C infection display a mild CAH or CPH lesion for many years only to progress inexplicably to cirrhosis and end-stage liver disease, usually after more than 10 to 20 years.

In general, the extent of histologic injury is predicted inconstantly by the level of aminotransferase elevations seen in the various causes of chronic hepatitis. The liver biopsy is of obvious importance in assessing the extent and severity of hepatic injury. Aminotransferases are used, however, to follow the response to therapy in all forms of chronic hepatitis, especially autoimmune hepatitis in which a target response is to decrease aminotransferases to the level of two times normal or less. The amount of "lobular" activity in a liver biopsy of a chronic hepatitis B patient is an accurate means of assessing viral replicative activity, as are serum levels of HBV-DNA or the presence of HBeAg. Similar markers for HCV are not as clearly identified, but quantitative HCV-RNA in serum by polymerase chain reaction (PCR) is roughly correlated with clinical activity of chronic HCV hepatitis.

Recently, characteristic histologic features of HCV infection relative to autoimmune hepatitis and hepatitis B were described. Features suggestive (but not diagnostic) of hepatitis C are lymphoid nodules in the portal tracts, bile duct injury lesions, mild large-drop steatosis, and periportal Mallory bodies. It should be emphasized that although there is a predilection for plasma cells in autoimmune hepatitis, the histologic appearance of chronic viral, drug, or autoimmune hepatitis are not reliably distinguishable by histology alone.

CHRONIC VIRAL HEPATITIS

Diagnosis

Chronic Hepatitis B

Overall, chronic HBV infection accounts for approximately 10 percent of chronic liver disease in the United States. Chronic hepatitis B develops in approximately 5 percent of acute HBV infections in healthy adults. The likelihood of chronic infection is increased if infection occurs in a neonate or child or if the patient has a secondary immunodeficiency state (i.e., dialysis, homosexuality). Although the risk of infection from transfusion is dramatically decreased by routine aminotransferase and HBV screening of all donors, intravenous drug use, tattooing, and sexual promiscuity remain high-risk activities. Vaccination is highly effective, especially in patients younger than 40 years of age, which implies that transmission to health care workers should be completely preventable. The mechanism of hepatocellular damage in chronic HBV hepatitis involves the immune system, particularly cytolytic T cells. Important sequelae of chronic HBV include immune complex disease (vasculitis), liver failure, and hepatocellular carcinoma.

The diagnosis of chronic hepatitis B requires the presence of HBsAg in serum. Clinically, it is useful to divide chronic hepatitis B into two phases: replicative and nonreplicative. Qualitatively, the markers of *replication* (HBV-DNA, HBeAg, and HBV-DNA polymerase) are associated with persistence of viral infection and active liver disease. The severity of the hepatic inflammatory lesion is not predictable using relative levels of any of the markers of replication, however. In general, the *nonreplicative phase* of the infection (marked by loss of HBeAg, HBV-DNA, and HBV-DNA polymerase, and the development of anti-HBeAb) is associated with a marked reduction or frank resolution of hepatic inflammation and incorporation of HBV DNA into the host's genome. The incorporation of HBV-DNA may be critical to the development of eventual hepatocellular carcinoma in patients with chronic hepatitis B. The conversion from replicative to nonreplicative phase is often heralded clinically by an acute exacerbation of hepatitis biochemically and histologically, as previously mentioned. Many patients are already cirrhotic by the time of this conversion. HBeAg may be absent in replicating, chronic HBV infections when the patient is infected with a mutant form of the virus (the so-called precore mutants). If active hepatic inflammation is found in a patient with HBsAg but no HBeAg in the serum, a course of therapy may be indicated, as this precore mutant virus may respond.

Chronic Hepatitis C

Previously called non-A, non-B hepatitis (NANB), HCV is the most common cause of chronic hepatitis in the United States. Acute HCV infection becomes chronic more often than HBV (50 to 75 percent versus 5 to 10 percent). The diagnosis is often made in the setting of minimal symptoms and abnormal aminotransferases associated with anti-HCV antibodies. Antibodies to several presumed structural and nonstructural HCV proteins arise over a period of 4 to 24 weeks after acute infection. These may persist for many years. No evidence is available that these antibodies are protective or that a certain profile of antibodies portends a clearance of actively replicating HCV (as compared to anti-HBe antibody for HBV). When recombinant proteins are used, the sensitivity of these enzyme-linked immunoassays are in the 90 to 100 percent range.

Important false positives still occur in the setting of hyperglobulinemia as a consequence of autoimmune hepatitis, primary biliary cirrhosis, or alcoholic liver disease. The positive predictive value is greatest (approximately 93 percent) for the HCV recombinant immunoblot assay (RIBA) and thus, at this time, the RIBA is the best confirmatory test for HCV infection after the screening, "second generation" antibody tests. The absolute indicator of active HCV infection is HCV-RNA in serum by reverse transcriptase PCR. This marker of replicative activity is not routinely available but is the most accurate indicator of the effect of therapy.

This highly mutable, single stranded RNA virus has been cloned molecularly (and typed into four major strains), but its natural clinico-biologic behavior is less intelligible than that of other hepatotrophic viruses. The epidemiologic factors involved in transmission of HCV are less well characterized than with HBV, although generally, high levels of HCV-RNA in serum, as may occur in concurrent HIV disease, are associated with an increased risk of transmission. As many as 40 percent of HCV patients do not have the usual risk factors of viral hepatitis. Sexual transmission (including homosexual behavior) and vertical transmission, although not absolutely disproved, seem less important routes of transmission than with HBV. It is not clear if the immune system plays a prominent role in the hepatocellular injury in HCV hepatitis even though prominent lymphocyte nodules are seen in many patients' liver biopsies. HCV may express its hepatotoxicity directly without the use of the cytolytic immune system. Much more consistently than with HBV, there is a marked discordance between the clinical and laboratory measures of chronic liver disease and the degree of histologic injury. It is common to find more fibrosis in the liver biopsy of a patient with chronic HCV than was expected on clinical grounds. Jaundice is unusual until late in the course of chronic HCV hepatitis, at which time it portends a poor long-term prognosis.

Hepatocellular carcinoma in the Western world and Japan is associated with HCV and cirrhosis. Most clinical studies in the area of fulminant hepatitis have revealed that HCV is less commonly associated with a fulminant presentation than other viral or toxic hepatitides. Although most cryptogenic cirrhosis (60 to 70 percent) is precipitated by HCV infection, the clinically severe form (aminotransferases in the 500 range, total bilirubin in the 7 range) associated with hyperglobulinemia behaves more like classical type 1 autoimmune hepatitis, including its response to steroids and HLA B8 and A1-B8-DR3 phenotype. Autoimmune phenomena occur in documented HCV hepatitis including Sjögren's syndrome, anti-P450 antibodies (anti-GOR), and anti-liver-kidney-microsomal (LKM) antibodies. The 2b subtype of autoimmune hepatitis, found mainly in older males, is typified by the presence of low titer anti-LKM antibodies, positive anti-HCV, and positive anti-GOR

antibody. This disorder responds to treatment of HCV and not to corticosteroids.

Information about the natural history of chronic transfusion- and non-transfusion-related HCV in the United States suggests that chronic liver disease (either CAH or cirrhosis) is common (approximately 60 percent and 10 to 20 percent, respectively), and that HCV infection can persist without clinical evidence of liver disease, thus providing a potential "reservoir" group. Hepatic failure from chronic hepatitis C occurs after at least 10 years of disease in a minority of cases. Mortality rates due to chronic transfusion-related NANB liver disease are slightly (but statistically significantly) higher than in age-, race-, and sex-matched controls when groups are followed for as long as 18 years. In the same study, overall mortality rates were not statistically different. Further prospective and retrospective data should improve clinicians' insight into the consequences of this chronic infection.

Chronic Hepatitis Delta

HDV is an RNA virus that requires HBV for viability. Chronic HDV hepatitis results more commonly from HDV infection superimposed over a pre-existing HBV infection (*super*infection) than from concurrent HBV and HDV infection (*co*infection). At least two-thirds of patients superinfected with HDV develop chronic HDV infection. The hepatitis is typically more aggressive than isolated chronic HBV hepatitis with consequent severe hepatitis and the rapid development of cirrhosis. The diagnosis is made with a positive HBsAg, high titer IgM HDV antibody (greater than 1:100), or nuclear staining of HDV antigen on liver biopsy. HDV-RNA is detectable in serum and can be followed as a marker of therapeutic response. Most patients are seronegative for HBeAg and have very low levels of HBV-DNA owing to the natural down regulation of HBV replication by HDV. In the United States, HDV infection is rare and shows a propensity for intravenous drug users. The most common areas of the world for HDV infection are the Mediterranean, Middle East, Africa, and South America.

Treatment

Chronic HBV

Therapy for chronic HBV is directed at arresting viral replication. Therapeutic goals include the loss of HBeAg and HBV-DNA from serum which are associated invariably with biochemical, histologic, and clinical remission. Interferon alpha induces clinical and virologic remission in 25 to 40 percent of treated patients. Multiple other therapies, either alone or in conjunction with interferon alpha, have not shown effectiveness (i.e., levamisole, suramin, ribavirin, azathymidine, acyclovir) or have unacceptable toxicities (i.e., adenosine arabinoside, fluoro-iodo-arabinofuransyl uracil). Other therapies have shown promise (i.e., thymosin, 3'-thiacytidine, interferon beta) and are under further evaluation. Outside of carefully designed and monitored clinical trials, corticosteroids should not be used to treat chronic HBV because of the limited utility in certain patient subgroups and increased mortality generally.

Therapeutic interferons replace naturally depressed interferon levels in patients with chronic HBV and cause both decreased HBV replication and increased presentation of intracellular viral proteins to HBV-specific cytolytic T cells. Interferon alpha at a dose of 5 million units (MU) daily or 10 MU three times a week for 4 to 6 months has the best therapeutic efficacy at this time. Patients who relapse after this therapy do not benefit from retreatment. Important contraindications to interferon therapy include decompensated liver disease, pregnancy, autoimmune disease, renal failure, clinical depression, and evidence of advanced hypersplenism or bone marrow insufficiency (i.e., neutropenia, anemia, and thrombocytopenia). Predictors of a favorable response to interferon are HBV-DNA less than 200 pg per milliliter, alanine aminotransferase (ALT) greater than 100 IU per liter, active histology, female sex, acquisition in adulthood, heterosexuality, non-Asian origin, and anti-HDV and HIV negativity. It is useful to check HBV-DNA and HBeAg before instituting therapy and then again at 4 months. If the HBV-DNA level is zero and aminotransferases are normal at 4 months, one should stop therapy and monitor the patient clinically. If the HBV-DNA level and aminotransferases remain unchanged at 4 months, one should abandon interferon therapy alone and/or consider other forms of therapy. For patients who have a partial decrease in HBV-DNA at 4 months, additional therapy could be tried until the aminotransferases are normal and the HBV-DNA is lost. Successful therapy is usually heralded by a flare of biochemical and histological activity, after which the HBeAg and HBV-DNA are lost in serum. The HBsAg may remain for years afterwards, but is lost in approximately 50 percent of responders. It should be mentioned that the effect of interferon alpha treatment in chronic HBV hepatitis on survival or the development of hepatocellular carcinoma is not established.

Orthotopic liver transplantation (OLTx) is not offered to patients with chronic HBV hepatitis because reinfection of the graft occurs uniformly and leads to premature and predictable graft failure in most. Neither alpha interferon nor immune globulin have been able to prevent or treat the graft HBV infection. Hopefully, further advances in the area of HBV therapeutics will enable patients more options (including OLTx) in the future.

Chronic HDV

Long-duration, high-dose interferon alpha therapy for delta hepatitis is successful initially in decreasing aminotransferases and improving histology in 50 percent of cases. Unfortunately, most of the initial responders relapse and thus there is no sustained eradication of delta agent after interferon therapy.

Chronic HCV

Interferon alpha is the only FDA approved therapy for chronic HCV in the United States. Therapeutic trials of interferon alpha for chronic HCV/NANB have selected patients based on abnormal aminotransferases (>1.5 times normal), no significant medical problems including no evidence of liver decompensation, and active histology including cirrhosis in many. Aminotransferases have also been end points of therapy, defining complete and partial responses and relapses. These markers may be much less sensitive than HCV-RNA by PCR. Initial response rates are 40 to 50 percent, with eventual relapse rates of nearly 50 percent for responders, thus making complete response rates around 20 to 30 percent.

Treatment of patients with less active histology is controversial, but evidence indicates that patients with a chronic persistent hepatitis lesion are more likely to respond favorably to therapy with interferon alpha than those with cirrhosis. Other variables that seem to predict response to therapy in chronic HCV are the level of HCV-RNA prior to therapy and its fall during therapy, age less than 40 years, and the HCV genotype(s). Comparison of data from multiple interferon alpha trials suggest that longer duration, higher dose, and possibly tapering the dose of interferon are important in producing complete responses.

Other therapy for HCV includes ribaviron and other forms of interferon (beta, lymphoblastoid, and consensus). Ribaviron is well tolerated and highly effective in reducing aminotransferases and HCV-RNA, but there is a high relapse rate thus far. Further trials are underway with ribaviron. Trials using the other interferons are in progress.

Contraindications to interferon use in chronic HCV are the same as for interferon therapy of chronic HBV. Because interferon therapy for chronic HCV has been associated with symptomatic thyroid disease in some female patients, thyroid function tests should be performed before therapy is begun. If available, HCV-RNA should be measured and quantified before interferon therapy and followed during therapy. Therapy is usually instituted with 3 MU interferon alpha subcutaneously three times a week. If the aminotransferases and HCV-RNA fall to normal or zero by 3 months of treatment, interferon should be continued for 3 more months and a decision can be made to taper the interferon or continue it for up to 1 year. For those that do not respond by 3 months, a 3 month trial of 5 MU three times a week can be tried, but if no normalization of aminotransferases or a decrease in the HCV-RNA occur, there is little hope that further therapy will be effective. There are no controlled data on efficacy of maintenance therapy, although it has been shown that many of the patients that initially respond to interferon and relapse will respond to a second course of interferon. If there is no complete response to the second course of therapy, there is no clear recommendation for further therapy at this time. In contradistinction to the situation with chronic HBV, it is distinctly unusual for a patient with chronic HCV to develop a flare of biochemical and histologic hepatitis during therapy. If this occurs, one should reconsider the possibility that the underlying liver disorder is actually autoimmune hepatitis with a false-positive anti-HCV antibody.

OLTx is an option for patients with decompensated chronic hepatitis C because clinically relevant reinfection occurs at a remarkably lower frequency than with HBV.

AUTOIMMUNE HEPATITIS

Autoimmune hepatitis (AH) is a diagnosis made after the exclusion of toxic, metabolic, and viral causes of chronic liver injury. Although classically defined as lasting greater than 6 months, one should consider this diagnosis before that time point as the early institution of corticosteroids can significantly alter the mortality and morbidity of this liver disease. The major features of the syndrome are a female predominance, a polyclonal hyperglobulinemia (mainly IgG subclass), the presence of autoantibodies (antinuclear and antismooth muscle antibodies), and the prompt response to corticosteroids. Patients may present in three distinct clinical patterns: first, a relatively acute and severe hepatitis often associated with jaundice; second, a relatively asymptomatic presentation of subacute portal hypertension; and third and most frequently, a relatively mild to moderate necroinflammatory liver condition associated commonly with insidious fatigue, malaise, or anorexia but not jaundice until late in the course. Compared to patients with chronic viral hepatitis, patients with AH more often have some symptoms including amenorrhea or delayed menarche, acne, arthralgia, fever, weight loss, and pruritus. Conditions associated with AH include autoimmune thyroiditis, rheumatoid arthritis, Sjögren's syndrome, thrombocytopenic purpura, pernicious anemia, urticaria, Coombs' positive hemolytic anemia, pleuritis, pericarditis, membranoproliferative glomerulonephritis, and ulcerative colitis. Although the presence of ulcerative colitis may adversely effect the outcome of AH (possibly because this subpopulation of patients actually have primary sclerosing cholangitis), the concurrence of AH with any of the above conditions does not effect the overall course of the liver disease. There is a bimodal age distribution with most patients presenting in their second and third decades or their fifth and sixth decades. Of note there is a definite trend toward making this diagnosis in older women and men. The older patients have a less impressive response to corticosteroids and less often have associated autoimmune conditions.

There are now several subtypes of AH and a potential association with HCV (Table 4). Type 1 AH is associated with antinuclear antibody (ANA) approximately 80 percent of the time and antismooth muscle (actin) antibody (SMA) in 60 percent. There are more organ-specific autoantibodies (i.e. antithyroid antibody, antiadrenal antibody) associated with the type 2 group than with type 1. The relative frequency of types 2 and

Table 4 Subtypes of Autoimmune Hepatitis

Subtype	Characteristics
1	Hyperglobulinemia, ANA +, ASMA + *Rx: Corticosteroids ± Azathioprine*
2a	Young women with ANA −, ASMA −, but anti-LKM Ab +, anti-HCV −, and anti-GOR Ab − *Rx: Corticosteroids*
2b	Older men with ANA −, ASMA −, but anti-LKM Ab +, anti-HCV +, and anti-GOR Ab + *Rx: Interferon alpha*
3	ANA −, ASMA −, anti-SLA Ab + *Rx: Corticosteroids*

3 are unknown, but both tend to respond favorably to corticosteroids with the prominent exception of the type 2b subgroup.

Treatment

As mentioned, AH is one of the liver diseases in which therapy is of proven benefit. Corticosteroids have been shown to prolong life, improve symptoms, ameliorate biochemical abnormalities (i.e., serum aminotransferase, bilirubin, and albumin levels), and decrease histologic necroinflammation in symptomatic, hyperglobulinemic patients with relatively severe histopathologic disease (i.e., severe CAH with bridging necrosis/multilobular necrosis or cirrhosis). There is no evidence that corticosteroids reverse cirrhosis or prevent the progression to cirrhosis. Clinical judgement is required in many cases, however, because many patients either have no symptoms or do not display severe histologic features. The histologic lesion of CPH is usually associated with a benign course, and thus an asymptomatic patient with CPH associated with minimally elevated aminotransferases or globulins may not require immunosuppressive therapy, especially if he or she is elderly. A patient with minimal symptoms and CAH with some bridging necrosis probably should be given a trial of therapy the success of which should be judged by aminotransferases and a follow-up liver biopsy. If there is a question of AH versus some other cause of chronic hepatitis (i.e., HCV but not HBV), it is often useful to attempt a course of corticosteroids first as classical AH will respond rapidly and corticosteroids will not dramatically effect hepatitis C. If one treats the presumed hepatitis C with interferon first, however, there is a risk that AH could flare aggressively.

The immediate goals of therapy are to decrease aminotransferases to less than two times normal, normalize the serum bilirubin level, and eradicate symptoms. Initial therapy for severe, symptomatic AH is usually begun with 20 to 60 mg of prednisone per day with or without azathioprine (50 to 100 mg per day). Alternate-day prednisone should not be used as initial therapy because it is not as effective as daily therapy. It is assumed that most patients will require prolonged corticosteroid therapy, so the institution of azathioprine (as a steroid-sparing drug) is especially important in those that may be at increased risk of side effects from corticosteroids (i.e., the elderly, those with recurrent ulcer disease, hypertension, glucose-intolerance, or osteopenia). Azathioprine is ineffective as solo initial therapy for AH and thus should always be used with prednisone initially. Usually, the prednisone dose can be tapered to 20 mg per day relatively rapidly after a therapeutic response is documented and continued at that dose or at an even lower daily dose for a matter of 6 months or so. Duration of therapy is of paramount importance because premature withdrawal of prednisone can lead to aggressive rebound hepatitis and clinical setback. If the patient has had normal aminotransferases and resolved symptoms for 6 months, it is reasonable to attempt to taper the prednisone dose slowly. Many patients, however, require a small dose of prednisone in order to prevent the common relapses of AH. For these patients, remission can be achieved with an even smaller dose of prednisone if azathioprine (at a dose of 50 to 150 mg per day) is added. Alternatively, remission can be maintained using azathioprine alone.

Relapses are more common in patients who have cirrhosis than in those that do not. In order to decrease morbidity, the treatment of recurrence of AH is 20 mg or less of prednisone alone or 10 mg or less of prednisone with 50 mg of azathioprine, followed by clinical observation for a few months. If the clinical activity is controlled, attempt to taper prednisone carefully. Many of these patients require long-term immunosuppression.

In general, patients should be followed carefully during and after therapy for signs of relapse or complications of therapy. Thus, it is reasonable to ask about symptoms and do physical exams (especially blood pressure determinations) and order routine chemistries and blood counts (for those patients on azathioprine) every 1 to 2 weeks for the initial 3 to 6 months. If therapy is progressing smoothly, the same information can then be accumulated every month until disease remission is documented for 6 months or so. After that, it is worthwhile to continue monitoring for biochemical relapse on a regular basis.

OLTx is an effective therapy for decompensated AH liver disease that was either advanced at presentation or unresponsive to therapy. Studies from the Mayo Clinic suggest that patients are less likely to respond to therapy, and therefore more likely to progress to end stage liver disease, if they have a HLA A1, B8 haplotype or do not develop remission within 4 years of onset of therapy. The 5 year survival rate after OLTx is 92 percent and recurrence of AH is rarely, if ever, seen.*

SUGGESTED READING

Alter MJ, et al. The natural history of community-acquired hepatitis C in the United States. N Engl J Med 1992; 327:1899–1905.

Czaja A. Chronic active hepatitis: A challenge for a new nomenclature. Ann Intern Med 1993; 119:510–517.

Davis GL, Balart LA, Schiff ER, Lindsay K, et al. Treatment of chronic hepatitis C with recombinant interferon alfa. N Engl J Med 1989; 321:1501–1506.

DiBisceglie AM, Shindo M, Fong T-L, et al. A pilot study of ribavirin therapy for chronic hepatitis C. Hepatology 1992; 16:649–654.

Johnson PJ, McFarlane IG, Eddleston ALWF. The natural course and heterogeneity if autoimmune-type chronic active hepatitis. Semin Liv Dis 1991; 11:187–196.

Koretz RL, Abbey H, Coleman E, Gitnick G. Non-A, non-B post-transfusion hepatitis: Looking back in the second decade. Ann Intern Med 1993; 119:110–115.

Lefkowitch J, Schiff ER, Davis GL, et al. Pathological diagnosis of chronic hepatitis C: A multicenter comparative study with chronic hepatitis B. Gastroenterology 1993; 104:595–603.

Mutchnick MG, Appelman HD, Chung HT, et al. Thymosin treatment of chronic hepatitis B: A placebo-controlled pilot trial. Hepatology 1991; 14:409–415.

Scheuer P. Classification of chronic viral hepatitis: A need for reassessment. J Hepatol 1991; 13:372–374.

Seeff L, et al. Long term mortality after transfusion-associated non-A, non-B hepatitis. N Engl J Med 1992; 327:1906–1911.

Yoshioka K, Kakumu S, Wakita T, et al. Detection of hepatitis C virus by polymerase chain reaction and response to interferon-alpha therapy: relationship to genotypes of hepatitis C virus. Hepatology 1992; 16:293–299.

*Editor's Note: A recent prospective study from the Mayo Clinic found that patients with HLA class II antigen DR4 had a somewhat better chance of responding to steroid therapy than those with HLA DR3. They also had more evidence of concurrent immunologic disorders (Czaja et al., Gastroenterology 1993; 105:1502–1507).

FULMINANT HEPATIC FAILURE

DAVID H. VAN THIEL, M.D.
STEFANO FAGIUOLI, M.D.
PAOLO CARACENI, M.D.
HARLAN I. WRIGHT, M.D.

Fulminant hepatic failure (FHF) is a clinical syndrome resulting from massive necrosis of liver cells leading to a sudden and severe impairment of hepatic function. FHF was defined initially in 1970 by Trey and Davidson as the development of hepatic failure with encephalopathy occurring within 8 weeks of the onset of the acute hepatic injury in an individual without a history or evidence of pre-existing liver disease. More recently, Bernuau and colleagues in 1986 proposed an alternative definition of FHF as a condition wherein encephalopathy develops within 2 weeks of the onset of symptoms in an individual with acute hepatic injury who has no history or evidence of previous liver disease. Regardless of the specific definition used, it is generally agreed that individuals having a shorter time interval from the onset of symptoms to the point of encephalopathy (Bernuau's definition) have a better prognosis than do those who develop encephalopathy more slowly (Trey and Davidson definition). In contrast, the group defined by Bernuau is more likely to experience cerebral edema than are those with a longer time until the onset of encephalopathy (Trey and Davidson definition). Cerebral edema and brain herniation is the major cause of death in individuals who die with FHF having an early onset of encephalopathy. Conversely, in those with a later onset of encephalopathy, sepsis or renal failure is more likely to be the immediate cause of death. These confounding problems in patients with encephalopathy occurring later than 2 weeks but before 8 weeks from the onset of acute liver disease are typically the precipitating factors for the spiral of multiorgan failure that inevitably leads to the death of most of those who die of FHF. This is discussed in the chapter *Systemic Inflammatory Response Syndrome.*

ETIOLOGY

Viral

Viral liver diseases are the most common causes of FHF. Fulminant type B viral hepatitis (HBV) is the most common type of viral hepatitis that leads to FHF. Most cases of FHF due to HBV occur in young adults 20 to 40 years of age. Hepatitis C is rarely a cause of FHF. In contrast, non-A, non-B, non-C (NANBNC) hepatitis (a putative viral illness) is a common form of FHF that may account for more cases in Western and developed societies than even HBV. Hepatitis A (HAV) leads to FHF when it occurs in individuals older than 40 years of age. Because of the increasing incidence of HAV disease in adults in Western or developed societies, it may account for more cases of FHF in the near future. Hepatitis E virus (HEV) accounts for many FHF cases in central Asia and the Indian subcontinent, as well as in areas in the Western world such as Mexico and Central America. In these areas and during epidemics of HEV infection, pregnant women appear to be particularly susceptible to FHF.

The more unusual forms of viral hepatitis produce FHF primarily, if not exclusively, in individuals who are either endogenously or exogenously immunosuppressed. Examples of endogenous immunosuppression associated with FHF due to unusual causes of viral hepatitis are pregnancy, intrinsic T- and B-cell immunodeficiency states, and lymphoid neoplasms. Examples of exogenous immunosuppression associated with unusual viral forms of FHF include the use of corticosteroids or cytotoxic agents for the treatment of asthma, other autoimmune or inflammatory diseases, and neoplasms.

Drugs

Drug-induced FHF is a less common form of hepatic disease that has been increasing in incidence steadily

Table 1 Causes of Fulminant Hepatic Failure

Infections
  Usual hepatotropic viruses
    Hepatitis A
    Hepatitis B
    Hepatitis C
    Hepatitis B + D
    Hepatitis E
  Unusual forms of viral hepatitis
    Cytomegalovirus
    Epstein-Barr virus
    Herpes simplex
    Varicella
    Adenovirus

Drug-induced hepatic failure
  Halothane
  INH ± pyrazinamide
  Rifampin
  NSAIDs, especially declofenac and acetaminophen
  Antiepileptics
  Disulfiram

Toxin-induced hepatic failure
  Amanita phalloides
  Herbal remedies

Metabolic liver disease
  Fulminant Wilson's disease
  Fatty liver of pregnancy
  Reye's syndrome

Vascular disease
  Hepatic ischemia
  Surgical shock
  Acute Budd-Chiari syndrome

Miscellaneous courses
  Malignant infiltration
  Bacterial sepsis
  Heat stroke

over the past 30 to 40 years with the growth and development of the pharmaceutical industry. Halothane, antituberculous drugs, nonsteroidal anti-inflammatory drugs (NSAIDs), and antiepileptic drugs remain the major causes of drug-induced FHF. Adult women over 40 years of age, and particularly black women, appear to be particularly susceptible to this type of FHF. Acetaminophen is a common cause of self-induced FHF occurring as part of a suicide attempt. Aspirin and valproic acid are common causes of FHF in children. Acetaminophen can occasionally cause FHF in infants and toddlers who are given excessive amounts of the drug in an attempt to control fever. Similarly, alcohol abusers and occasional alcohol-intoxicated revelers experience FHF as a consequence of the use of acetaminophen to treat a hangover that under normal circumstances would not be toxic.

Other Causes

All the other causes of FHF identified in Table 1 occur much less often than do those already described in this text and are not discussed further. The particular circumstances in which these situations occur should suggest the cause of FHF in these unusual cases.

CLINICAL FEATURES (Table 2)

Acute hepatic encephalopathy is a universal feature of FHF, being an intrinsic component of the definition of the condition. Early clinical signs include a change in personality, dizziness, headaches, and nightmares. These can progress to delirium, mania, and other forms of "uncooperative" behavior. Violent acting-out behavior is common in the middle stages of acute hepatic encephalopathy. Fetor hepaticus occurs in the later stages of acute hepatic encephalopathy, whereas asterixis is transient. The clinical grades of hepatic encephalopathy merge almost indistinguishably into

Table 2 Clinical Features of Fulminant Hepatic Failure

Acute hepatic encephalopathy
Cerebral edema
Coagulopathy
Hypoglycemia
Sepsis
Renal dysfunction
Acid-base disturbances
Hypotension
Hypoxia

Table 3 Grades of Acute Hepatic Encephalopathy

Grade 1	Confused or altered mood
Grade 2	Inappropriate behavior or drowsiness
Grade 3	Stuporous but arousable, markedly confused behavior
Grade 4	Coma unresponsive to painful stimuli

each other as the underlying disease progresses, but these should be distinguished whenever possible into four specific grades as shown in Table 3.

Cerebral edema occurs in late stage 3 and stage 4 acute hepatic encephalopathy. It can be recognized by the development of decerebrate rigidity characterized by extension and pronation of the arms and legs, disconjugate eye movements, and a loss of pupillary reflexes. As noted earlier, it occurs in more than 80 percent of patients who die with FHF and meet the criteria of Bernuau and colleagues.

The coagulopathy associated with FHF is the most important prognostic index of the clinical syndrome. A prothrombin time greater than 20 seconds in patients with viral or drug-induced (except acetaminophen-induced) FHF or a prothrombin time greater than 100 seconds in individuals with acetaminophen-induced FHF, and a factor V level less than 20 percent of normal in individuals under 30 years of age and less than 30 percent of normal in those 30 years of age or older with FHF suggest a high likelihood of death. In such cases, bleeding is the usual cause of death and can occur into the lungs, gastrointestinal (GI) tract, or brain.

Hypoglycemia occurs only in patients with an extreme hepatic injury (more than 85 percent of the liver being necrotic) and is more common in children and women than in men.

Sepsis due to gram-negative organisms of enteric bacteria as well as candidiasis and/or an aspergillosis were common causes of infection in cases of FHF before the development of selective enteric decontamination protocols. Since the use of oral antibiotics has become common in patients with FHF, gram-positive organisms, particularly staphylococcus, and multidrug-resistant gram-negative organisms have become more common causes of preterminal sepsis in FHF.

The renal dysfunction seen in FHF is often functional and occurs in response to a progressive shift of renal blood flow from the cortex to the medulla. Endotoxemia occurring as a consequence of the sepsis in FHF also contributes to the high incidence of renal dysfunction. The acid-base and vasomotor consequences of FHF reflect the severity of the underlying hepatic and renal dysfunction in patients with FHF.

PROGNOSIS

The prognosis of FHF with medical therapy alone in cases that progress to stage 3 or 4 encephalopathy is extremely poor and varies between 20 and 40 percent, depending on the specific cause. In general, patients over 40 years of age and those under 10 years are at particular risk of dying. Other clinical signs of a poor prognosis include a rapidly shrinking liver and/or a liver volume of less than 900 ml, necrosis of more than 50 percent of the hepatic lobules assessed by liver biopsy, ascites, decerebrate rigidity, respiratory failure, and a disconjugate gaze.

With the widespread availability of liver transplan-

Table 4 Criteria Used to Identify Individuals Unlikely to Survive Without Liver Transplantation

Group One	Group Two

Prothrombin time >100 sec
or
Any three of the following:
  Age <10 or >40 yr
  Non-A, non-B hepatitis; halothane;
    or other drug reaction etiology
  Duration of jaundice before onset
    of encephalopathy >2 days
  Prothrombin time >50 sec
  Serum bilirubin >20 mg/dl
If acetaminophen induced:
  pH <7.3
    or
  Prothrombin time >100 sec
    and
Creatinine >2 mg/dl in patients with
  grade 3 or 4 encephalopathy
	Factor V < 20%
	  (age <30 yr)
	    or
	Factor V < 30%
	  (age <30 yr)
	Coma or confusion

Data from O'Grady JG, Hamblay H, Williams R. Prothrombin time in fulminant hepatic failure. Gastroenterology 1991; 100:1480; and Bernau J, Samuel D, Durand F, et al. Criteria for emergency liver transplantation in patients with acute viral hepatitis and factor V below 50% of normal: a prospective study. Hepatology 1991; 14:49A.

tation, it has become possible to salvage many patients with FHF who previously would have died. As a result, considerable effort has been made to identify patients with FHF who are unlikely to survive so that they can be listed for transplant before they reach a point of irreversible brain injury or experience an episode of infection that prohibits any attempt at liver transplantation. In addition to the clinical signs mentioned earlier, two groups, who have considerable experience with FHF, have developed criteria for identifying patients unlikely to survive without a liver transplant (Table 4). Although the distribution of specific etiologies of FHF differed markedly at these two centers, the criteria identified at each that characterize patients unlikely to survive are similar if one excludes patients with acetaminophen toxicity from the analysis. These criteria notwithstanding, with the development of intensive care and meticulous attention to details of good supportive care, the survival of individuals with FHF has improved considerably over the last decade and a half.

MANAGEMENT

General Principles

Individuals with FHF require hospitalization in specialized units prepared to manage such patients. Trained nursing personnel are essential. The immediate availability of an established liver transplant program is recommended. Because it takes time to obtain the results of diagnostic serologic testing, all patients except those with a clear-cut history of some other factor that produces FHF should be managed as if they are infectious. All nursing and hospital personnel working in such units should be vaccinated against HBV and more recently with HAV vaccines. Gloves, gowns, and eyewear are essential when patient contact is required. An arterial line can be placed if experienced personnel are available to insert it; if not, it is not essential. A central venous line should be inserted, preferably one with several ports to enable easy infusion of dextrose and other drugs and blood coagulation factors, blood to be drawn as needed, and frequent monitoring of cardiovascular status. In addition, a nasogastric tube and Foley catheter should be inserted to prevent aspiration and to monitor urinary output at regular intervals. If the patient is in grade 3 or 4 coma, endotracheal intubation is recommended to guarantee the airway and prevent aspiration. Patients are best managed in reverse Trendelenburg position to further prevent aspiration and reduce the effects of cerebral edema when advanced stages (III and IV) of acute hepatic encephalopathy are present.

The use of an H_2 blocker or omeprazole combined with a broad-spectrum antibiotic such as norfloxacin is recommended to prevent GI bleeding and translocation of enteric organisms.

Encephalopathy

Acute hepatic encephalopathy is managed by judicious use of protein, 30 to 40 g in a 70 kg individual as an oral or enteral diet, depending upon the patient's level of consciousness, and lactulose administration to produce two to four bowel movements per day. All forms of sedation are to be avoided except when used for intubation or to prevent extubation by the patient.

The use of a short-acting benzodiazepine such as midazolam and an anesthetic such as fentanyl is recommended for this purpose. Both are given intravenously (IV). Their judicious use can prevent central nervous system hemorrhage or oropharyngeal trauma and pulmonary hemorrhage in an uncooperative patient who has both severe coagulopathy and thrombocytopenia. Neomycin should not be used because of the risk of renal injury, particularly in a patient with an edematous leaky bowel due to portal hypertension and low oncotic pressure. Moreover, it is unnecessary if norfloxacin is being used to prevent bacterial translocation.

Cerebral Edema

Cerebral edema, when it occurs, can be treated with mannitol, 1 g per kilogram body weight up to a maximum of 100 g as a 20 percent solution administered as an IV bolus every 4 hours. The use of glucocorticoids to prevent cerebral edema has been shown to be unsuccessful and is associated with an increased risk of GI bleeding and infection in patients with FHF. Mannitol cannot be given in patients with renal failure, but ultrafiltration can and should be used. Thiopental infusions can be used in severe cases no longer responsive to mannitol or ultrafiltration. Extradural intracranial pressure monitoring devices have become popular recently, especially for comatose or anesthetized patients undergoing liver transplantation. Increases in intracranial pressure above 25 to 30 mm Hg that are continuous for 5 or more minutes require treatment. A cerebral perfusion pressure (systolic pressure–intracranial pressure) of 40 mm Hg is considered essential.

Nutrition

Nutrition can be maintained in the initial 3 to 4 days of hospitalization with an IV infusion of 10 percent dextrose up to 3 liters per day. Hypoglycemia often occurs and will not be detected unless frequent blood sugar determinations are made, usually every 2 to 3 hours. Hypoglycemia, when it occurs, should be treated with an emergent 50 percent glucose infusion and an increase in the rate of glucose being infused as 10 percent or, if necessary, 20 percent dextrose. IV infusions should contain sufficient potassium to maintain adequate potassium stores in a patient undergoing diuresis.

Hypotension

Hypotension can be treated early with dopamine, which also guarantees renal blood flow. In patients with a severe reduction in perpheral vascular resistance, norepinephrine (Levophed) in combination with dopamine may be necessary to maintain an adequate blood pressure.

Prostaglandins

Data from uncontrolled studies suggest that prostaglandin infusions (PGE_1) or oral prostaglandin E_2 (100 to 200 μg orally twice a day), either alone or coupled with the oral administration of acetylcysteine or S-adenosylmethionine, can reduce the hepatic injury that occurs regardless of the cause and hastens recovery. The use of these drugs for this purpose, however, is still investigational.

Support Systems

Very recently, the use of an extracorporeal artificial liver consisting of either porcine liver or hepatoblastoma cells contained in a hollow fiber dialysis system wherein plasma is perfused over the cells has been reported to be successful. In all of the cases to date, this therapy has been applied as a bridge to transplantation, maintaining the patient in a state that will enable liver transplantation to occur as soon as an acceptable donor organ can be identified. This usually takes 24 to 72 hours. Even more recently, in 1993 human hepatocytes have been injected successfully into the spleen of patients with FHF for the same purpose.

Transplantation

The decision to transplant a specific patient is best made at the time a donor organ is identified. Such decisions, however, are usually based on the criteria identified in Table 4. Patients with NANB, drug-induced (excluding acetaminophen), and halothane-induced FHF are best served with early liver transplants, which improve the survival of these groups from 12 to 20 percent to 50 to 60 percent. Individuals with other types of FHF are chosen for liver transplantation if they meet the criteria identified in Table 4 when the donor organ is available and if they are still free of sepsis and multiorgan failure.

Editor's Note: The reader is also directed to the three excellent chapters on hepatic transplantation.

SUGGESTED READING*

Bernuau J, Goudeau A, Poynard T, et al. Multivariate analysis of prognostic factors in fulminant hepatitis B. Hepatology 1986; 6:648–651.

Bernuau J, Rueff B, Benhamou JP. Fulminant and subfulminant liver failure: definition and causes. Semin Liver Dis 1986; 6:97–106.

Bernuau J, Samuel D, Durand F, et al. Criteria for emergency liver transplantation in patients with acute viral hepatitis and factor V below 50% of normal: a prospective study. Hepatology 1991; 14:49A.

Blei AT. Cerebral edema and intracranial hypertension in acute liver failure: distinct aspects of the same problem. Hepatology 1991; 13:376–379.

Emond JC, Aran PP, Whitington PF, et al. Liver transplantation in the management of fulminant hepatic failure. Gastroenterology 1989; 96:1583–1586.

Forbes A, Alexander GJM, O'Grady JE, et al. Thiopental infusion in the treatment of intracranial hypertension complicating fulminant hepatic failure. Hepatology 1989; 10:306–310.

Harrison PM, Keays R, Bray GP, et al. Improved outcome of paracetamol-induced fulminant hepatic failure by the administration of acetylcysteine. Lancet 335:1572–1573.

Klein NA, Mabie WC, Shaver DC, et al. Herpes simplex virus hepatitis in pregnancy. Gastroenterology 1991; 100:239–244.

LeRoux PD, Elliott JP, Perkins JD, Winn HR. Intracranial pressure monitoring in fulminant hepatic failure and liver transplantation. Lancet 1990; 335:1291.

Munoz SJ. Prothrombin time in fulminant hepatic failure. Gastroenterology 1991; 100:1480–1481.

O'Grady JG, Alexander GJM, Hayllar KM, et al. Early indicators of prognosis in fulminant hepatic failure. Gastroenterology 1989; 97:439–445.

Rolando N, Harvey F, Brahm J, et al. Prospective study of bacterial infection in acute liver failure: an analysis of fifty patients. Hepatology 1990; 11:49–53.

Schafer DF, Shaw BW Jr. Fulminant hepatic failure and orthotopic liver transplantation. Semin Liver Dis 1989; 9:189–194.

Van Thiel DH. When should a decision to proceed with transplantation actually be made in cases of fulminant or subfulminant hepatic failure: at admission to hospital or when a donor organ is made available? J Hepatol 1993; 17:1–2.

*Editor's Note: A very complete 77-item bibliography is available from the authors or the editor.

LIVER TRANSPLANTATION IN ADULTS: MEDICAL CONSIDERATIONS

SANTIAGO J. MUNOZ, M.D.
SHARON WESTERBERG, B.A.

Three common indications for hepatic transplantation today include alcoholic liver disease and cirrhosis due to hepatitis B and C viruses. It is therefore evident that there is ample room for primary preventive measures to minimize the frequency of these disorders. Alcohol and drug addiction rehabilitation should be implemented before patients develop irreversible liver disease as a consequence of alcohol and drug abuse. Likewise, liberal use of the vaccination against hepatitis B viral infection should be promoted among individuals in high-risk groups. In several states, hepatitis B vaccine, which has a remarkable record of efficacy and safety, is now mandatory as part of the routine immunization schedule for infants.*

INDICATIONS

Almost every liver disorder that becomes life-threatening and has an irreversible and progressive nature is a potential indication for liver transplantation. The most common preoperative diagnoses in adult liver transplant recipients are shown in Table 1. In addition, many uncommon disorders and congenital metabolic deficiencies have been successfully treated by liver transplantation (Table 2). Over the last few years, there has been a remarkable shift in the frequency of liver diseases leading to hepatic transplantation. Primary biliary cirrhosis, primary sclerosing cholangitis, and autoimmune chronic active hepatitis initially constituted the most frequent indications for liver transplantation, but more recently alcoholic cirrhosis, end-stage chronic hepatitis C, and cryptogenic cirrhosis have led the list in many transplant centers. Moreover, it is anticipated that the number of viable candidates with alcoholic liver disease will continue to increase over the next several years because of the high prevalence of alcoholism relative to all other causes of liver disease in the United States.

OPTIMAL TIMING

There are no exact rules to determine the ideal time to perform a liver transplant in a patient with progressive

---

*Editor's Note: This is the first of three chapters on orthotopic liver transplantation.

Table 1 Common Indications for Liver Transplantation in Adults with Chronic Liver Disease

Cirrhosis from previous alcohol abuse
Cirrhosis from chronic hepatitis C
Cryptogenic cirrhosis
Cirrhosis from other viral hepatitides (B, D)
Primary biliary cirrhosis
Primary sclerosing cholangitis
Cirrhosis from autoimmune chronic active hepatitis
Cirrhosis due to alpha$_1$-antitrypsin deficiency
Budd-Chiari syndrome
Hepatocellular carcinoma

From Munoz SJ. Indications for liver transplantation. Int Med March 1994; with permission.

Table 2 Uncommon Disorders Treated with Liver Transplantation

Tyrosinemia	Echinococcosis
Hemophilia A	Organic acidurias
Hemophilia B	Gaucher's disease
Wilson's disease	Familial cholestasis
Protoporphyria	Sanfilippo syndrome
Hemochromatosis*	Wolman's syndrome
Neuroendocrine tumors	Niemann-Pick disease
Glycogen storage disease	Oxalosis, sarcoidosis
Crigler-Najjar syndrome	Galactosemia, amyloidosis
Urea cycle enzyme deficiencies	Hyperlipoproteinemia type II

*Idiopathic hemochromatosis is not an uncommon disorder, but with early diagnosis and appropriate treatment with phlebotomies, it is now uncommon for patients with this condition to require liver transplantation, relative to other etiologies.
Modified from Munoz SJ. Indications for liver transplantation. Int Med March 1994; with permission.

liver disease. Most authorities agree that transplantation should be considered once the estimated life expectancy is less than 1 year. Unfortunately, many life-threatening complications of liver disease develop unpredictably, and with the possible exceptions of primary biliary cirrhosis and primary sclerosing cholangitis, there are no reliable methods to predict the time to death in individual patients. The Child-Pugh-Turcotte classification is useful as a general assessment of the severity of liver disease, but whether this is a reliable tool to determine the best timing for liver transplantation has not been established.

From a practical standpoint, the development of manifestations of liver disease listed in Table 3 should generally signal the need to consider transplantation in the near future. Although there are few prospective studies to support the use of these clinical indicators for liver transplantation, ample experience has demonstrated their ominous prognostic significance.

The waiting time for obtaining a liver donor has become longer over the last several years; currently, most stable candidates wait approximately 2 to 5 months before undergoing liver transplantation. Therefore, it appears reasonable to consider liver transplantation earlier in the course of the natural history of liver disorders. The prolonged waiting time undoubtedly

Table 3 Clinical Indicators for Timing of Liver Transplantation in Adults with Chronic Liver Disease

Ascites resistant to maximal medical therapy
Recurrent spontaneous bacterial peritonitis
Intractable hepatic encephalopathy
Bleeding from esophagogastric varices refractory to sclerotherapy,
  banding, or transjugular intrahepatic portosystemic shunt (TIPS)
Severe progressive malnutrition
Intractable symptomatic coagulopathy
Unrelenting chronic fatigue and weakness
Progressive severe bone disease (hepatic osteopathy)
Recurrent bacterial cholangitis
Symptomatic hepatopulmonary syndrome
Hepatorenal syndrome

From Munoz SJ. Indications for liver transplantation. Int Med March 1994; with permission.

Table 4 Contraindications to Liver Transplantation

Absolute
  Extrahepatic hepatobiliary malignancy
  Severe cardiopulmonary disease
  Acquired immunodeficiency syndrome
  Active alcoholism or drug abuse
  Widespread thrombosis of portal and superior mesenteric veins
  Irreversible severe brain damage

Relative
  Sepsis
  Age > 70 yr
  Previous complex hepatobiliary surgery
  Portal vein thrombosis (with patent SMV)
  Inability to understand magnitude of undertaking

accounts for the increasing death rate of patients with advanced liver disease awaiting a donor organ.

Investigators at the Mayo Clinic have developed and validated prospectively a mathematical model to predict the probability of survival of patients with primary biliary cirrhosis between 1 and 5 years. The model does not require information from a liver biopsy and can be calculated from simple clinical and biochemical parameters, such as serum albumin and bilirubin levels, prothrombin time, age, and the presence of peripheral edema. We have found the Mayo model useful for counseling patients on the timing of transplantation and as a factor in the selection process. The actual survival of patients with primary biliary cirrhosis may be somewhat overestimated by this model, since the equation does not take into account the occurrence of unpredictable life-threatening complications such as variceal bleeding, bacterial peritonitis, or progressive malnutrition. In 1992, a similar prognostic model for patients with primary sclerosing cholangitis was reported from the Mayo Clinic, although its calculation does require information from a liver biopsy.

PREOPERATIVE SCREENING AND SELECTION

The physiologic rigors required to survive liver transplant surgery require thorough evaluation of the major body systems, especially the central nervous system, as well as cardiopulmonary and renal function. The preoperative evaluation can be initiated by the patient's gastroenterologist or primary physician, who can exclude coexisting problems currently considered to be absolute contraindications to orthotopic liver transplantation (Table 4). Patients should also be screened for relative contraindications, which in general are more closely evaluated at the liver transplant center (Table 4).

These general guidelines are suggested to assist in the selection process of liver transplant candidates. The overall goal is to identify individuals who are most likely to benefit from this risky and costly procedure. Flexibility and common sense are essential in the application of these guidelines to individual cases until prospective

studies provide more reliable methods to predict the outcome of liver transplantation for individual patients.

At the transplant center, the evaluation and selection process consist of confirming the diagnosis and establishing the severity of the underlying liver disease, documenting indications and contraindications, and determining the position of the patient in relation to the natural history of the liver disease. On the basis of this information, a multidisciplinary liver transplant team reaches a consensus on the transplant suitability of potential candidates.

LIVER TRANSPLANTATION FOR ALCOHOLIC LIVER DISEASE

Patients with alcoholic cirrhosis represent a huge reservoir of liver transplant candidates. The application of transplantation in this group of patients is controversial because of unresolved ethical and financial issues. So far, small series suggest that highly selected transplanted alcoholic cirrhotics fare as well as nonalcoholic recipients. Additional research is needed to answer key questions regarding predictors of outcome after surgery, medical compliance, frequency of and factors determining recidivism of alcoholism after liver transplantation, and the impact of frequent coexisting problems such as hepatitis C viral infection.

Even with the limited information currently available, many liver transplant programs are actively transplanting patients with alcoholic cirrhosis in response to the pressure of increasing numbers of candidates with alcoholic liver disease. Just as with other liver disorders, the evaluation of candidates with alcoholic liver disease tends to examine certain aspects closer, such as psychosocial status and family support structure, which, coupled with a thorough psychiatric assessment, allows a reasonable prediction of the probability of recidivism. Furthermore, the presence and extent of alcohol-related disease of the brain, pancreas, heart, and other muscles is investigated, since it is thought that significant disease of these organs may decrease the probability of a successful liver transplant operation.

Although the value of requiring a specific period of

abstinence from alcohol before initiation of a liver transplant evaluation has not been established, many programs require 3 to 6 months of abstinence. Furthermore, completion of a formal alcohol rehabilitation program is required for most patients. The referring gastroenterologist is therefore wise to monitor and document alcohol abstinence and to encourage potential candidates with alcoholic liver disease to complete a rehabilitation program as soon as possible, before they reach such a degree of disability that participation in rehabilitation activities becomes nearly impossible. To our knowledge, liver transplantation for acute alcoholic hepatitis has not yet been intentionally performed. Many patients with alcoholic cirrhosis develop pronounced muscle wasting and protein calorie malnutrition. The physician caring for alcoholic patients must keep in mind the possibility of liver transplantation *before* the patient develops profound malnutrition, which may constitute by itself a contraindication to the procedure.

LIVER TRANSPLANTATION FOR ACUTE LIVER FAILURE

Emergency liver transplantation can be a life-saving procedure for patients with fulminant hepatic failure. The combined survival rate in 13 published series is 64 percent at 1 year, which is generally better than that obtained with intensive medical support alone. However, it is unclear in which patients, and at what time during the course of their disease, liver transplantation should be performed. From a practical standpoint, and given the rapidity with which acute liver failure may lead to death, the gastroenterologist should discuss the case and most likely transfer patients to a liver transplant center as soon as they manifest the slightest degree of hepatic encephalopathy (altered personality or sleeping pattern, mild confusion). Cerebral edema is the most common cause of death in these patients and frequently requires highly specialized management, including placement of extradural pressure monitors and barbiturate infusions (Fig. 1). Indications for urgent transplantation in acute liver failure are discussed in the chapter *Fulminant Hepatic Failure*. The factors shown in Table 5 are frequently considered contraindications to transplantation in the setting of acute liver failure. A suggested algorithm for management and transplant decision making in patients with acute liver failure is shown in Figure 2.

MANAGEMENT OF THE PATIENT AWAITING A LIVER DONOR

Candidates with end-stage chronic liver disease awaiting a suitable donor can be relatively stable at home or may be desperately ill in an intensive care unit. All are at risk of developing major complications of liver failure, sometimes in an unpredictable fashion. The prolonged waiting time has made it necessary to monitor ambula-

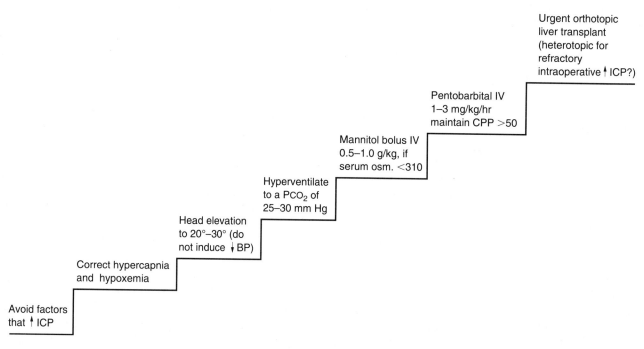

Figure 1 Step-by-step treatment of intracranial hypertension in fulminant hepatic failure. ICP = intracranial pressure; CPP = cerebral perfusion pressure; BP = blood pressure.

tory patients regularly, at least once a month, at the transplant center, and frequently their fragile situation warrants a visit every week or two. Candidates awaiting a liver donor are often managed in a coordinated manner by both the primary gastroenterologist and the liver transplant center. With few exceptions, discussed below, the management of the major complications of chronic liver disease in a patient awaiting liver transplantation does not differ substantially from that of cirrhotic patients who are not transplant candidates. Monthly Doppler ultrasound examinations are performed in many centers to detect intercurrent portal vein throm-

bosis, which may have an impact on the technical feasibility of transplantation. Candidates awaiting a liver donor are often given a combination of nonabsorbable antibiotics, such as neomycin or kanamycin and nystatin, in an effort to sterilize the gut and prevent gram-negative and fungal infections in the immediate postoperative period.

An important aspect of the medical preoperative management is to maintain, and if possible improve, the nutritional status of the candidate. Profound malnutrition and cachexia are not uncommon, and the waiting time for a liver donor is well used in efforts to improve the nutritional status. Implementing a stepwise increase in dietary protein to determine the maximal tolerance in individual patients may be hoped to lead to a nearly ideal dietary intake of 1 to 1.5 g per kilogram per day of protein. Of course, some patients are simply unable to achieve positive nitrogen balance because of intervening hepatic encephalopathy or profound anorexia, and continue to experience progressive muscle wasting and other nutritional deficiencies. A trial of supplemental branched-chain–enriched amino acids may be justified in these admittedly uncommon instances. Occasionally, courses of peripheral parenteral nutrition in patients prone to encephalopathy may be better tolerated than protein administered enterally. Careful monitoring for fat-soluble vitamin deficiencies and appropriate replacement therapy are necessary, especially in candidates with chronic cholestatic disorders such as primary biliary cir-

Table 5 Proposed Contraindications to Urgent Liver Transplantation in Fulminant Hepatic Failure

---

Severe irreversible brain damage
Inability to oxygenate during anesthesia due to severe adult
  respiratory distress syndrome (ARDS)
Active alcohol/drug abuse
Cerebral perfusion pressure <40 mm Hg for >2 hr
Sustained elevation of intracranial pressure to >50 mm Hg
Septic shock
Severe cardiopulmonary disease
Acquired immunodeficiency syndrome
Widespread thrombosis of portal and mesenteric veins
Improving hepatic function
Severe hemorrhagic pancreatitis

From Munoz SJ. Difficult management problems in fulminant hepatocellular failure. Semin Liver Dis 1993;13:395–413; with permission.

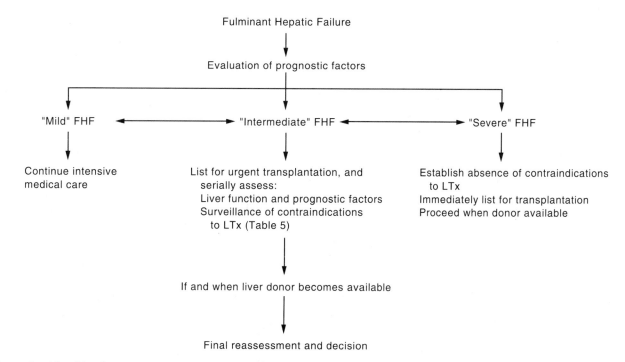

Figure 2 Algorithm for transplant decision making in fulminant hepatic failure. LTx = liver transplant. (From Munoz SJ. Difficult management problems in fulminant hepatocellular failure. Semin Liver Dis 1993;13:395-413; with permission.)

rhosis, primary sclerosing cholangitis, or biliary atresia.

Refractory ascites may require frequent large-volume paracentesis. Replacement with salt-poor albumin is, in our opinion, important in these patients, mainly to prevent the rapid development of protein malnutrition associated with frequent large-volume paracentesis. The use of peritoneovenous shunts is generally discouraged by liver transplant surgeons because of the potential for subsequent intraoperative difficulties, although this is not conclusively proved. Recent preliminary information suggests that selected patients with refractory ascites may experience significant relief by insertion of a transjugular intrahepatic portosystemic shunt (TIPS). There is a separate chapter on this procedure.

Treatment of episodes of spontaneous bacterial peritonitis should be carried out in the standard fashion, and the transplant center should be promptly informed of this or other infectious complications, since many surgeons will not transplant a candidate with an active infection. Evidence is accumulating to suggest that oral antibiotic prophylaxis with neomycin, norfloxacin or ciprofloxacin may confer some protection against recurrent spontaneous bacterial peritonitis. For encephalopathic patients who do not respond to the usual measures, addition of metronidazole to lactulose therapy has been suggested. The recent introduction of TIPS has been used successfully as a bridge to transplantation in patients bleeding from esophagogastric varices who fail sclerotherapy or banding. However, prospective trials of TIPS have just begun and many questions about its indications, timing, and complications remain unanswered. For instance, should a TIPS stent be placed in candidates with primary sclerosing cholangitis awaiting a liver donor? Until controlled studies answer this and other questions, we prefer not to use this device in candidates with primary sclerosing cholangitis because of the frequent presence of multiple intrahepatic abscesses and the inherent risk of septicemia after or during TIPS insertion.

Candidates with renal failure awaiting a liver donor should be supported with hemodialysis in the standard fashion. Similarly, patients with symptomatic hepatopulmonary syndrome awaiting liver transplantation should receive supplemental oxygen as necessary, including home oxygen therapy if indicated.

SURGICAL ASPECTS

Over 100 U.S. centers with liver transplant capability are now active and many surgeons have acquired confidence and expertise in performing this intervention safely. The surgical aspects of liver transplantation are discussed in detail in the next chapter. Some of the recent technical developments include the introduction of the University of Wisconsin preservation solution, which has helped to extend the viability of harvested donor livers by up to 15 to 20 hours. This has probably

led to more efficient organ utilization and allowed improved organ sharing between geographically distant recipients. There is less urgency to perform liver transplantation than in the times when a donor liver was usable for only 6 to 8 hours. However, even with the Wisconsin solution, use of donor livers requiring a prolonged preservation time (over 15 to 20 hours) appears to be associated with an increased frequency of biliary strictures and other complications in the postoperative period.

The introduction of venovenous bypass has also facilitated liver transplantation, in the opinion of many experienced surgeons. The use of reduced-size liver grafts and living liver donors, particularly for pediatric liver transplant recipients, is likely to continue to expand in the near future as one of the responses to the severe donor shortage. There are a few reported cases of successful life-saving heterotopic liver transplantation for patients with fulminant hepatic failure and refractory intraoperative intracranial hypertension. There is a separate chapter on pediatric aspects of liver transplantation.

From a preoperative medical standpoint, it is important to obtain a detailed surgical history in potential liver transplant candidates. Many transplant surgeons feel that a history of multiple intra-abdominal surgeries adds considerable difficulty and risk to a liver transplant operation and may constitute a relative contraindication, depending on the policies and expertise of individual centers. Likewise, confirmation of the patency of the main portal vein is essential in the preoperative evaluation, often requiring a panmesenteric arteriogram and portogram for definitive assessment. While liver transplantation may still be performed with isolated or partial occlusion of the portal vein, most transplant surgeons would consider it impossible to perform such an operation if the occlusion or thrombotic process also extends into the superior mesenteric vein.

POSTOPERATIVE CARE AND COMPLICATIONS

After completion of an orthotopic liver transplant, there are still several potential threats to a successful outcome, and excellent reviews on the postoperative management are included in the Suggested Reading. A multidisciplinary approach is essential to maximize the chances of early diagnosis of and successful therapy for the various possible complications. Thus, a close working relationship must develop among surgeons, hepatologists, intensivists, infectious disease specialists, nephrologists, and other specialists.

The most common problems are caused by bacterial, viral, and fungal infections in the immunocompromised recipient. Acute and chronic forms of liver graft rejection, vascular and biliary tract complications, and so-called primary (idiopathic) graft malfunction are also frequent sources of serious postoperative setbacks. Less common, but not less important, are renal dysfunction, acute respiratory distress syndrome (ARDS), postoperative pancreatitis, seizures, and other neurologic disturbances. Hepatotoxicity and dysfunction of other organs due to toxicity from therapeutic drugs are not uncommon in liver transplant recipients.

Selective bowel decontamination with nonabsorbable aminoglycosides and antifungal agents is currently used in many centers in view of an apparent effect on the frequency of postoperative enterobacterial and fungal infections. Similarly, close monitoring of immunosuppressive therapy has resulted in a reduction of severe rejection episodes. Vascular complications such as hepatic artery thrombosis may occur in the early postoperative period and generally lead to the development of markedly elevated aminotransferase levels and acute hepatic failure. Urgent retransplantation or surgical repair and reanastomosis may be required, depending on the timing of diagnosis, degree of liver graft dysfunction, and extent of the arterial occlusion. Chronic rejection may cause obliteration of the branches of the hepatic artery by an accelerated form of atherosclerosis, the pathogenesis of which is not fully understood. This chronic variety of hepatic artery occlusion may develop in asymptomatic recipients and may be detected only by routine Doppler investigation; alternatively, a dramatic illness characterized by multiple hepatic abscesses and septicemia may ensue. It has been suggested that adult patients given transplants for primary biliary cirrhosis may be at increased risk of developing hepatic artery problems after liver transplantation.

Leaks and strictures of the biliary tract anastomosis are still common complications after liver transplantation. The frequency of biliary tract problems seems to increase as the preservation time for harvested livers extends beyond 15 hours. Strictures can be multiple and involve hilar and intrahepatic biliary radicles, in a pattern suggestive of subclinical ischemic damage or recurrent sclerosing cholangitis in individuals transplanted for this disorder.

Management of biliary anastomotic leaks is generally tailored to the severity of the bile extravasation and impact on the clinical status of the patient. Thus, small or moderate leaks are often managed with observation only or endoscopically placed nasobiliary drains, whereas large leaks or those leading to marked clinical deterioration should be promptly repaired surgically.

It has been reported that as many as 30 to 50 percent of liver transplant recipients experience one or more seizures in the postoperative period. The role of cyclosporine in causing convulsions is unclear. This agent has been associated with the development of white matter cerebral abnormalities, particularly in liver transplant recipients with low serum cholesterol levels. Early reports suggest that the neurotoxicity of FK 506 (see below) may be more limited.

After discharge from the liver transplant center, many recipients choose to see their primary gastroenterologist for common medical problems as well as those related to immunosuppression and liver graft function.

The investigation of abnormal liver graft function tests, anemia, or abdominal pain frequently necessitates gastrointestinal endoscopy and liver biopsy. It is important to establish an expeditious working relationship between the transplant center, generally through a knowledgeable liver transplant coordinator, and the recipient's local physicians.

IMMUNOSUPPRESSION AFTER LIVER TRANSPLANTATION

Cyclosporin A and corticosteroids are the mainstays of immunosuppressive therapy after liver transplantation. Cyclosporine is begun shortly after implantation of the new liver, with careful attention to renal function. This precaution has resulted in a considerable reduction in the early postoperative nephrotoxicity associated with the use of this agent, commonly reported in the 1980s. A modestly elevated serum creatinine level is, however, a frequent observation during the long-term follow-up of liver transplant recipients, and many centers now use a triple regimen by adding azathioprine, which may effectively prevent organ rejection while permitting lower blood levels of cyclosporine. With few exceptions, other adverse effects of cyclosporine are well tolerated by most recipients and easily managed.

A few centers utilize an induction phase of immunosuppression with monoclonal antibodies (OKT3) and high doses of corticosteroids, followed by gradual introduction of cyclosporine and azathioprine. It is claimed that this sequential regimen is associated with a lower incidence of both rejection and renal failure. In most centers, however, cyclosporine and corticosteroids are begun immediately after transplantation, and primary postoperative therapy with monoclonal antibodies is generally reserved for recipients with poor renal function, and for episodes of moderate to severe acute liver graft rejection.

Initial therapy for acute liver graft rejection consists of intravenous boluses of methylprednisolone (0.5 to 1 g daily for 1 to 3 days) followed by a tapered reduction over a week. Liver biopsy is essential before treatment of acute rejection and should be repeated if there are doubts about the response to high doses of corticosteroids. In fact, 20 to 30 percent of episodes of acute liver graft rejection do not respond to corticosteroids, and additional therapy with monoclonal antibodies against the T3-receptor complex of T cells (OKT3) or antilymphocyte globulin may be necessary. These agents are also used by a few centers as primary therapy for episodes of acute rejection of moderate to severe intensity. Less frequently, acute rejection may be resistant to therapy with these agents, and retransplantation of the liver may be required.

Monoclonal antibodies are powerful and selective immunosuppressive agents: reactivation of cytomegalovirus and other opportunistic infections is common during or after a course of therapy with OKT3. Similarly, it has been suggested, but not conclusively proved, that the risk of post-transplant lymphoproliferative disorders may be increased in relation to one or more courses of therapy with monoclonal antibodies. Currently, active research is proceeding on a variety of monoclonal antibodies targeted to various mediators and receptors involved in the pathogenesis of acute graft rejection. Undoubtedly, some of these new agents will reach the level of clinical trials in the future and increase our capability for more selective immunopharmacologic modulation in liver transplant recipients.

Although the macrolide derivative FK 506 has been widely publicized as a breakthrough for transplant immunosuppression, its approval for routine clinical use is not expected for another year or two. On a milligram per milligram comparison, this agent is a considerably more potent immunosuppressant than cyclosporine, but many questions remain unanswered, especially the exact frequency and types of serious adverse effects with its use, such as nephrotoxicity and overimmunosuppression. Its current use is limited to investigational trials and compassionate use when trying to avoid retransplantation in recipients with early chronic rejection or refractory acute liver graft rejection.*

Chronic rejection of a liver graft may pose difficult problems. This process is characterized by progressive loss of intrahepatic small bile ducts, leading to cholestasis, and fibro-obliterative arteriopathy of the medium and large hepatic arterioles. Therapy with FK 506 has been reported to rescue some cases of early chronic rejection, but often the only effective approach has been hepatic retransplantation. The diagnosis of chronic rejection should be carefully documented and frequently requires several liver biopsies and exclusion of chronic viral hepatitis and biliary tract disruption. Chronic liver graft rejection may be preceded by several episodes of acute rejection or may have an insidious course hinted at only by a persistent and isolated elevation of serum alkaline phosphatase levels.

RECURRENCE OF DISEASE

Recurrence of the following entities has been reported after liver transplantation: hepatitis B and C, malignancy (hepatocellular carcinoma, cholangiocarcinoma), Budd-Chiari syndrome, primary biliary cirrhosis, primary sclerosing cholangitis, and autoimmune chronic hepatitis.

The persistence of hepatitis B antigenemia after liver transplantation for chronic hepatitis B is virtually universal. A few recipients may develop a benign form of the disease, in a manner analogous to a healthy hepatitis B carrier, and remain well for many years after trans-

plantation. Most, however, have clinically significant recurrence of liver disease due to reinfection with hepatitis B virus and develop an accelerated progression to chronic hepatitis and cirrhosis. It has been suggested that the preoperative presence of high levels of circulating hepatitis B virus DNA, or HBeAg positivity, may identify candidates likely to have progressive recurrence of hepatitis B after liver transplantation. It should be noted that these putative criteria for selection of HBsAg-positive candidates are not universally recognized.

In contrast, earlier reports indicated that recurrence of hepatitis C in liver grafts was a rare event. Longer follow-up is now available for these recipients, suggesting that the frequency of clinical recurrence of hepatitis C may previously have been underestimated. Most hepatitis C liver recipients remain positive for serum hepatitis C virus RNA by PCR after liver transplantation, and in fact the postoperative levels tend to be markedly higher than the preoperative viremia. The frequency and risk factors determining the development of chronic hepatitis and cirrhosis in these recipients remain to be ascertained.

At the present time, transplants for cholangiocarcinoma and hepatocellular carcinoma are generally performed in two settings: under an experimental protocol including perioperative chemotherapy and/or radiation therapy, and when the tumor is an incidental finding in livers removed from patients with primary sclerosing cholangitis or cirrhosis. Most of the patients receiving transplants solely for the presence of these tumors have developed fatal recurrence shortly after transplantation.

Whereas one group has reported a high rate of recurrence of primary biliary cirrhosis, most centers have not observed this phenomenon to a significant extent. It is generally agreed, however, that antimitochondrial antibodies remain present for at least several years after liver transplantation for primary biliary cirrhosis.

The distinction between recurrence of primary sclerosing cholangitis and multiple intrahepatic biliary strictures due to poor vascular supply can be very difficult. It remains controversial whether primary sclerosing cholangitis recurs after liver transplantation. Recurrence of autoimmune hepatitis is exceedingly rare, if it is ever seen. Patients receiving transplants for Budd-Chiari syndrome should remain on anticoagulant therapy to minimize the postoperative recurrence of hepatic, portal vein, and venal caval thromboses.

RESULTS

The overall results generally reported for liver transplantation in adults with chronic liver disease include a survival of 75 to 85 percent at 1 year and 60 to 70 percent at 5 years. Survival is somewhat lower in candidates with fulminant liver failure (64 percent in 13 published reports). Considering the very short life expectancy of cirrhotic patients with Child C classifica-

---

*__Editor's Note:__ There is a little more information on FK 506 in the next two chapters and in the chapter from the University of Pittsburgh on small bowel transplantation.

tions, these figures clearly illustrate the remarkable results obtained from liver transplantation. Moreover, several centers have reported 1 year survival rates as high as 90 percent, reflecting increasing experience, earlier intervention, and, to some extent, more stringent criteria for selection of candidates. There is little question that the probability of survival in liver transplant patients is closely related to their preoperative status. Thus, critically ill patients in an intensive care unit may have a chance of survival as low as 30 percent after liver transplantation. Conversely, stable outpatients with primary biliary cirrhosis generally have an excellent chance of survival after elective liver transplantation. Equally important is the perception by the recipients themselves of a markedly improved quality of life. This has been documented in several recent prospective studies. Over two-thirds of liver transplant recipients return to gainful employment, often after years of total disability due to chronic liver disease, and report ample satisfaction with their renewed lifestyle.

SUGGESTED READING*

Casavilla A, Gordon R, Wright H, et al. Clinical course after liver transplantation in patients with sarcoidosis. Ann Intern Med 1993; 118:865–866.

de Groen P, Aksamit A, Rakela J, et al. Central nervous system toxicity after liver transplantation. The role of cyclosporine and cholesterol. N Engl J Med 1987; 317:861–866.

---

*Editor's Note: Because of the complexity of issues in the area of liver transplantation, there are three chapters on the subject in this edition. We have also included more references than for most chapters because of the overlap with so many illnesses.

Dickson ER, Grambsch P, Fleming T, et al. Prognosis in primary biliary cirrhosis: model for decision making. Hepatology 1989; 10:1–7.

Dickson ER, Murtaugh P, Wiesner R, et al. Primary sclerosing cholangitis: refinement and validation of survival models. Gastroenterology 1992; 103:1893–1901.

Fagiuoli S, Shah G, Wright H, Van Thiel D. Types, causes and therapies of hepatitis occurring in liver transplant recipients. Dig Dis Sci 1993; 38:449–456.

Gorensek M, Carey W, Washington J, et al. Selective bowel decontamination with quinolones and nystatin reduces gram-negative and fungal infections in orthotopic liver transplant recipients. Cleve Clin J Med 1993; 60:139–144.

Martin P, Munoz S, Friedman L. Liver transplantation for viral hepatitis: current status. Am J Gastroenterol 1992; 87:409–425.

Moritz M, Jarrell B, Munoz S, Maddrey W. Regeneration of the native liver after heterotopic liver transplantation for fulminant hepatic failure. Transplantation 1993; 55:952–954.

Munoz SJ, Maddrey WC. Major complications of acute and chronic liver disease. Gastroenterol Clin North Am 1988; 17:265–287.

Munoz SJ, Friedman LS. Liver transplantation. Med Clin North Am 1989; 73: 1011–1037.

Munoz S, Moritz M, Martin P, et al. Liver transplantation for fulminant hepatocellular failure. Transplant Proc 1993; 25:1773–1775.

Munoz SJ. Difficult management problems in fulminant hepatocellular failure. Semin Liver Dis 1993;13:395–413.

Munoz SJ. Indications for liver transplantation. Intern Med March 1994.

Osorio R, Freise C, Stock P, et al. Non-operative management of biliary leaks after orthotopic liver transplantation. Transplantation 1993; 55:1074–1077.

Schwartz ME, Manzarbeitia C, Miller C. Evaluation, complications and therapy in the immediate postoperative period. In: Fabry T, Klion F, eds. Guide to liver transplantation. New York: Igaku-Shoin, 1992:167–182.

Stampfl D, Munoz S, Moritz M, et al. Heterotopic liver transplantation for fulminant Wilson's disease. Gastroenterology 1990; 99: 1834–1836.

Van Thiel D, Dindzans V, Gavaler J, Tarter R. The postoperative problems and management of the liver transplant recipient. Prog Liver Dis 1990; 9:657–685.

LIVER TRANSPLANTATION: SURGICAL CONSIDERATIONS

ANDREW S. KLEIN, M.D.

Liver transplantation has evolved considerably since the first procedure was performed in humans in 1963. What was once an experimental operation with short-term survival of less than 25 percent is now a well-accepted form of therapy for selected patients with end-stage liver failure. Liver transplant recipients can expect long-term survival in the 70 to 80 percent range, and perhaps more important, in most cases an excellent quality of life.

The factors that have contributed to the growth and development of liver transplantation include improvements in (1) preoperative evaluation and the candidate selection process (described in the preceding chapter); (2) intraoperative management of anesthesia and coagulopathy; (3) organ recovery and preservation; (4) surgical technique, reflected in decreased operating time and blood loss; (5) immunosuppression, including the introduction of new agents such as cyclosporine, FK506, and monoclonal antibodies; and (6) the management of postoperative morbidity, e.g., nonoperative therapy for biliary complications.

PREOPERATIVE EVALUATION

Liver Recipient

The specific liver diseases that in their end stage warrant consideration of a liver transplant are discussed in the preceding and succeeding chapters. Once the indications for liver transplantation have been established, prospective recipients are evaluated to assess both the severity of the liver disease and their capacity to tolerate liver replacement. It is important to identify patients with prohibitive intra- or postoperative risk factors who are unlikely to benefit from a liver transplant (those with inadequate cardiopulmonary reserve, unreconstructable anatomy, extrahepatic malignancy, or psychosocial instability). The risk associated with liver transplantation varies directly with the degree of hepatic decompensation and overall deterioration of the patient. Although 1 year survival rates above 90 percent can be expected for liver recipients followed as outpatients before the transplant, only 50 percent of the recipients requiring intensive care immediately before transplantation will survive 1 year.

Factors that increase postoperative morbidity and/or mortality are cardiopulmonary dysfunction, renal failure, recent infection, malnutrition, ventilator dependency, previous hepatobiliary surgical procedures, and previous portacaval shunt procedures. Pre-existing car-

diopulmonary disorders may compromise the transplant candidate's ability to tolerate the dramatic fluid and electrolyte shifts and stress of liver replacement. All prospective adult patients are screened by cardiology and echocardiography. In those over the age of 45 or with symptoms of heart disease, a stress thallium scan is performed, followed if necessary by cardiac catheterization and coronary angiography. Occult cardiac dysfunction is of particular concern in male cirrhotics and patients of either sex with hemochromatosis or alcoholic liver disease.

Patients with pre-existing renal dysfunction, whether attributable to intrinsic kidney disease or to the hepatorenal syndrome, are often more difficult to manage during and after the transplant procedure. Their postoperative care is further complicated by the fact that two of the commonly used immunosuppressive agents, cyclosporine and FK506, carry a substantial risk of nephrotoxicity. Although pretransplant dependency on dialysis is not a contraindication to liver transplantation, survival rates are lower in this group of patients.

Patients with *active* extrahepatic infections should not undergo liver transplantation. However, septic complications such as spontaneous bacterial peritonitis are common among individuals who have end-stage cirrhosis and who have failing hepatic reticuloendothelial surveillance. Such patients may be reconsidered for liver transplantation if their infection clears with appropriate therapy, but the risk of recurrence or superinfection, particularly fungal, is high in the setting of postoperative immunosuppression.

Previous surgical procedures involving the liver, biliary system, or pancreas may complicate the dissection needed to perform a liver transplant. For this reason, attempts to revise failed biliary reconstructions in patients with sclerosing cholangitis, primary biliary cirrhosis, or biliary atresia should generally be avoided. The presence of a portacaval shunt at the time of liver transplantation is associated with increased (sometimes dramatic!) intraoperative blood product requirements and decreased survival. Before transplantation, patients with portal hypertension and bleeding esophageal varices, who have compensated hepatic function, should be managed preferentially with sclerotherapy, or transjugular intrahepatic portosystemic shunt (TIPS). If surgical decompression of the portal system is required, a mesocaval shunt is the preferred procedure. Unlike portacaval shunts, mesocaval shunts can be performed at a site remote from the porta hepatis, which will not be a reoperative field at the time of subsequent transplantation. It is a simple matter to ligate the mesocaval shunt at the conclusion of the liver transplant.

Anatomic Assessment

Prospective liver recipients undergo an anatomic assessment to aid in planning the surgical approach to the transplant. Abdominal duplex sonography and/or magnetic resonance imaging is used to determine the patency of the portal vein, hepatic artery, and hepatic veins. Portal vein occlusion is no longer thought to be a contraindication to liver transplantation if the superior mesenteric vein (SMV) is patent. In this circumstance, portal blood flow to the donor liver can be re-established via an interposition graft of donor iliac vein sewn end to side to the recipient SMV.

Psychosocial Evaluation

Psychosocial evaluation attempts to ascertain patients' emotional stability, including their understanding of the potential risks and benefits of a transplant, the level of compliance they are likely to exhibit after the transplant, and the support resources among family and friends. For patients with alcohol-related liver disease, it is important to determine whether they have recognized their alcoholism, have been abstinent for a definable time, are committed to remain alcohol free after the transplant, and are willing to contract for participation in a supervised maintenance program such as Alcoholics Anonymous. With such criteria, many programs have found the recidivism rate to be quite low in their alcoholic liver recipients. Equally important is the fact that rehabilitation in this group, as measured by return to employment, is excellent.*

Cadaveric Liver Donor

Most liver transplants performed in the United States use an organ obtained from a brain-dead but heart-beating human. Potential donors are evaluated to assess the likelihood that the various organs removed will tolerate the procurement-preservation process and function adequately in the recipient. Donors are also screened to minimize the risk of transmitting viral agents or other communicable diseases. The common causes of death in potential liver donors include penetrating or blunt head injury, intracerebral hemorrhage, cerebral anoxia (e.g., drowning, hanging, drug overdose, myocardial infarction), and primary brain tumor. Medical contraindications to organ donation are listed in Table 1.

Approximately 10 percent of people who die in the United States could be considered for cadaveric liver donation. However, only a small fraction of this donor pool is actually recovered because of failure on the part of the treating medical team to pursue organ donation, or denial of consent for donation by surviving relatives. As the gap between the number of patients awaiting transplantation and the number of available organs widens, many transplant centers have expanded their criteria for the "minimally acceptable" organ donor. The specific definition of an acceptable organ donor varies not only between centers, but between individuals awaiting transplantation in a single center. One can afford to be more selective for a nonhospitalized

*Editor's Note: The excellent chapter on alcoholism is a useful resource. Obviously, the trauma of transplantation would seem to create a strong motivation for compliance and abstinence.

Table 1 Medical Contraindications to Cadaveric Liver Donation

Cancer, except skin and primary brain tumors
Septicemia
Infectious disease: HIV, HTLV1, HBsAg, RPR
High-risk group for HIV or hepatitis: male homosexuals, intravenous drug abusers, persons recently incarcerated

HIV = human immunodeficiency virus; HTLV = human T-cell leukemia/lymphoma virus; HBsAg = hepatitis B surface antigen; RPR = rapid plasma reagin (test).

Table 2 The "Ideal" Cadaveric Liver Donor

Previously healthy individual with isolated brain injury
Age > 2 yr and < 50 yr
No significant hypotension, hypoxia, or prolonged cardiac arrest
Hemodynamically stable without pressor support
Short hospitalization (< 7 days)
Excellent liver function test results

recipient with chronic liver disease than for a patient with fulminant hepatic failure on life support in the intensive care unit (ICU). The characteristics associated with the "ideal" liver donor are listed in Table 2. However, it should be emphasized that only a small minority of the brain-dead patients who become liver donors satisfy all ideal criteria.

Recipient-Donor Matching

Patients awaiting transplantation are registered with the United Network for Organ Sharing (UNOS), which maintains a national list of all potential recipients. Donated cadaveric livers are matched with recipients on the basis of compatible ABO blood group and weight. The liver is a unique organ from an immunologic perspective, and in fact it is possible to transplant a liver from an ABO-incompatible donor in a patient, albeit with a success rate lower than would be expected for an ABO-compatible transplant. Furthermore, unlike kidney transplantation, human leukocyte antigen (HLA) matching of donor and recipient tissue is not routinely performed for a liver transplant. Before the advances in techniques of organ preservation that expanded the allowable cold ischemia time for liver grafts to 18 to 24 hours, there simply was not enough time to perform tissue typing. Retrospective studies have shown no convincing advantage for well-matched livers compared to those with little or no HLA homology.

A point system based on the severity of disease, the length of time on the waiting list, and the geographic location of the recipient and donor is used to determine which of the matched group will be offered a specific organ.

OPERATIVE PROCEDURE

Orthotopic liver transplantation (OLT), the standard procedure for liver replacement, consists of implantation of a cadaveric liver allograft in the anatomic space previously occupied by the diseased liver, which is removed. OLT should be distinguished from heterotopic liver transplantation ("auxiliary liver transplant"), which involves placing the allograft in a site remote from the native liver, which may or may not be removed. There are three distinct phases of OLT: (1) donor hepatectomy, (2) recipient hepatectomy, and (3) implantation of the donor allograft.

Donor Hepatectomy

To recover as many organs as possible from a single brain-dead donor, a standardized approach to multivisceral organ procurement has been developed. A midline incision is made from sternal notch to pubis to expose the thoracic and abdominal cavities. Although several teams may work in concert during the procedure, the pace of the operation is generally dictated by the liver surgeon, who must recognize the sometimes complicated hepatic vascular anomalies present in nearly 50 percent of all patients. Most anatomic anomalies involve the arterial blood supply to the liver (left hepatic artery originating from the left gastric artery, or right hepatic artery originating from the superior mesenteric artery are most common). Failure to preserve the aberrant arterial blood supply to the liver may result in inadequate infusion of preservation solution to a segment or lobe of the liver, rendering the organ untransplantable.

The basic principles of liver procurement are to make the organ cold and free of blood. After preliminary dissection of the liver, the gallbladder is opened and bile is flushed from it and the transected common bile duct. Vascular cannulas are inserted into the distal abdominal aorta and inferior mesenteric vein. The aorta is cross-clamped above the celiac axis, and cold preservation solution is infused into the cannulas to flush the blood out of the abdominal viscera via the arterial and portal systems. Effluent is drained away through a third cannula inserted into the inferior vena cava at the level of the iliac vein bifurcation. The donor hepatectomy is completed by dividing the hepatic arterial supply, portal vein, and supra- and infrahepatic vena cava followed by the ligamentous, diaphragmatic, and peritoneal attachments of the liver.

A modification of the multivisceral procurement procedure has been dubbed the "scoop" technique. Minimal dissection of the abdominal viscera is performed before infusion of preservation solution, and the liver, pancreas, kidneys, and small intestine are removed en bloc from the donor. The organs are then separated by ex vivo dissection in a basin of cold preservation solution before being distributed for transplantation.

The preservation solution currently in use (Viaspan or "UW [University of Wisconsin] solution") has extended the allowable cold ischemia time for cadaveric livers to 18 to 24 hours. Transcontinental transport of livers is now common, and intercontinental organ sharing is technically feasible.

Recipient Hepatectomy

The recipient operation is performed through a bilateral subcostal incision with a short midline extension. Such an approach provides excellent exposure to the liver, porta hepatis, and suprahepatic vena cava. A thoracic incision is rarely required. The abdominal cavity is explored to identify occult pathology, but exposure may be limited if there are vascularized adhesions and friable venous collaterals. Dissection of the liver begins with division of the falciform, left triangular, and gastrohepatic ligaments. These normally diaphanous structures often contain a rich network of collateral vessels and lymphatics in cirrhotic patients, and thus should be divided and ligated with sutures.

Attention is next turned to the porta hepatis, where the common bile duct, hepatic arteries, and portal vein are dissected free from surrounding tissue, ligated, and divided. At this point, patients may be placed on venovenous bypass (VVB), an external pumping system that accepts blood from cannulas in the portal vein and femoral vein and returns it to the superior vena cava via cannulas percutaneously inserted into the internal jugular vein. During the anhepatic phase of the operation, the inferior vena cava and portal vein are occluded. VVB provides a means of decompressing the venous hypertension that develops in the splanchnic circulation and lower body.

The right lobe of the liver must now be mobilized by dividing the right coronary ligament, exposing the "bare area" of the liver. Hemorrhage from venous collaterals is a particular problem in this region. The Argon Beam Coagulator, a device that rapidly cauterizes large surface areas with less tissue damage than with standard electrocautery, effectively provides hemostasis in this setting. The inferior vena cava is encircled above and below the liver, and all tissue posterior to the vena cava is divided to complete the dissection. Vascular clamps are placed across the supra- and infrahepatic vena cava, which are divided within the hepatic parenchyma to preserve as much caval length as possible for subsequent reconstruction. The liver can then be lifted from the abdominal cavity.

Allograft Implantation

The hepatic allograft is readied for implantation by removing extraneous tissue and preparing the transected vascular structures at the site of proposed reanastomosis. The ex vivo dissection is performed in a basin of iced saline to prevent warming of the organ. The liver is then brought to the operative field and in sequence the suprahepatic vena cava, infrahepatic vena cava, and portal vein are reanastomosed. Before the second caval anastomosis is completed, cold lactated Ringer's solution is perfused through the portal vein to flush preservation solution from the organ. After the portal vein anastomosis is performed, the vascular clamps are removed and blood flow is restored to the liver.

Hepatic reperfusion may be accompanied by transient hypotension and/or cardiac arrhythmias, and not uncommonly the patient's coagulation function temporarily worsens. Once the anastomoses have been inspected for sites of bleeding, hepatic arterial blood flow is re-established. Most vascular thromboses after OLT involve the hepatic artery, and thus the surgeon must take meticulous care in fashioning this anastomosis. Finally, the gallbladder is removed and biliary drainage is re-established either by an end-to-end choledocho-choledochostomy or a Roux-en-Y choledochojejunostomy. The latter procedure is routinely performed for all children, as well as for selected adults with biliary tract disease (e.g., sclerosing cholangitis, injured or scarred distal bile ducts from previous procedures). Patients reconstructed with a choledochocholedochostomy have their anastomosis stented with a T tube inserted into the recipient common bile duct and exited through the abdominal wall. Intraoperative cholangiography is performed to confirm proper placement of the T tube, adequate drainage of the distal bile duct into the duodenum, and absence of anastomotic leak. A postperfusion liver biopsy is obtained before placing several closed suction drains and closing the abdominal incision.

REDUCED VOLUME TRANSPLANTATION

It is possible to transplant an hepatic segment or lobe from an adult donor into a pediatric recipient. The reduced volume transplant, also referred to as the "cut-down" liver transplant, has enlarged the donor pool for pediatric patients awaiting liver replacement. (This subject is also discussed in the next chapter.) Allograft recovery proceeds as for a standard OLT, but the recipient hepatectomy is modified to preserve the entire abdominal vena cava. The diseased liver is dissected free of the cava by carefully ligating and dividing the small veins supplying the caudate and left hepatic lobes.

Depending on the size match of the donor and recipient, the left lateral segment, left lobe, or right lobe of the cadaveric adult liver, along with the blood vessels and bile duct(s) supplying the selected portion of the organ, are carefully dissected from the remainder of the allograft. The dissection is performed ex vivo in a basin of iced saline. For children under the age of 3 years, the left lateral segment is most commonly employed. When dividing the hepatic parenchyma, bridging vessels must be carefully ligated with fine sutures to minimize hemorrhage from the cut surface of the liver after reperfusion.

The reduced-size allograft is implanted by anastomosing the donor hepatic vein(s) to the confluence of the recipient's hepatic veins, followed by the portal vein, hepatic artery, and biliary anastomoses. Iliac artery and vein grafts procured from the cadaveric organ donor may be required to supply additional length for the hepatic artery and portal vein reconstruction, respectively. Although it is possible to obtain more than one transplantable portion of a liver from a single donor, most centers describing such "split liver" transplants also report graft and patient survival rates lower than for full-sized or single-recipient, reduced-volume liver transplants.

LIVING DONOR TRANSPLANTATION

The scarcity of replacement organs from cadaveric sources and the increasing incidence of death among those awaiting liver transplantation, particularly children, has led several institutions to develop a program for living donor hepatic transplantation (LDHT). Countries such as Japan, which lack established brain death criteria, rely almost exclusively on living donation to perform liver transplantation. LDHT is possible owing to the redundant functional capacity and the regenerative potential of a healthy human liver. Simply stated, a portion of the donor's liver (usually the left lateral segment or left lobe) is carefully removed, perfused ex vivo with preservation solution, and then implanted into the recipient. The technique is similar to that used for reduced-volume cadaveric transplants, with the obvious exception that the integrity of the nontransplanted portion of the donor's liver must be preserved. Over a period of months, the donor's liver will regenerate to its normal size and the transplanted segment will grow appropriately with the recipient.

Most living donors have been parents of children with end-stage liver disease, although some centers consider adult siblings or other relatives for donation. The ethical issues must be weighed very carefully before embarking on LDHT. The donor procedure involves a major hepatic resection, and thus the potential for serious morbidity or even mortality of the healthy volunteer cannot be ignored. One reason for limiting the prospective living donor pool to individuals who are both genetically and emotionally related is the perception that the psychological benefit of saving a relative's life is a powerful motivating factor, which enhances the risk-benefit ratio for LDHT. It is very important, however, to consider the psychosocial impact of offering LDHT to a dying child's parent, who may have to provide for a spouse or other children. In this setting it may be difficult for the family to make an informed, uncoerced decision regarding the appropriateness of living donation. The transplant team needs to be sensitive to the emotional as well as the medical issues inherent in LDHT.

Once the decision to proceed with LDHT has been made, the potential donor is evaluated thoroughly by a team of physicians, surgeons, and psychiatrists. The prospective donor should have the same blood type as the recipient, although HLA matching is generally not used in the screening process. The patient must be in excellent general health and should be considered at low risk for a major surgical procedure, which may require 3 to 5 hours of general anesthesia. There should be no history of liver disease, and recent liver function and hepatitis serologic tests should be normal. Volumetric analysis of the liver in conjunction with an abdominal computed tomographic scan is used to determine whether the left lateral segment or entire left lobe of the liver is the appropriate size for the prospective recipient. It is preferable to use the left lateral segment whenever possible, as the morbidity risk is higher when a total left hepatic lobectomy is performed. The final and most invasive component of the evaluation is hepatic artery angiography. Multiple arteries supplying the left lateral segment, or a single artery less than 2 mm in diameter at the proposed site of arterial reconstruction, are considered to be contraindications to living donation, because of the increased risk of hepatic artery thrombosis when such vessels are used.

POSTOPERATIVE CARE

General Measures

Advances in the postoperative care of liver recipients have evolved as a mixture of art and science. The capacity to monitor and manipulate multiple organ systems with increasing precision in the intensive care setting has contributed significantly to our ability to successfully manage patients who have undergone a liver transplant. Nonetheless, the clinical acumen of the experienced transplant surgeon/physician is equally important in developing the appropriate algorithm of care for each individual. The special areas that differentiate the liver transplant recipient from the usual surgical patient are highlighted below.

Evaluation of Graft Function

The assessment of hepatic allograft function begins in the operating room after organ reperfusion with the observation of liver color and texture and bile production, and correction of coagulopathy. If the liver fails to produce bile soon after re-establishment of blood flow, this may be an indication of primary nonfunction of the allograft. Normal bile is usually dark golden to light brown in color. Very dark turbid bile may be a sign of severe hepatic ischemia and/or biliary epithelial necrosis. Bright green bile occurs in the setting of biliary stasis as the stagnant bile within the T tube undergoes conversion of bilirubin to biliverdin.

In the ICU, liver function is evaluated by a battery of clinical parameters and blood tests listed in Table 3. Virtually all patients develop a coagulopathy during the anhepatic phase of the liver transplant, and fibrin split products are usually positive in the early postoperative period. However, adequate synthetic function of the new liver should be reflected by progressive improvement in prothrombin time, activated partial thromboplastin time, and serum fibrinogen levels. Metabolic alkalosis develops largely because of the hepatic metabolism of citrate present in the blood products administered intraoperatively. In general, alkalosis is a good sign. If severe (pH greater than 7.50 or base excess greater than 7), alkalosis may decrease the respiratory drive and delay

Table 3 Postoperative Evaluation of Liver Allograft Function

Hemodynamic stability
Level of consciousness
Quality and quantity of bile produced
Acid-base and electrolyte balance
Ammonia level
Coagulation factors: prothrombin time, activated partial thrombo-
  plastin time, serum fibrinogen
Liver enzymes: AST, ALT, gamma-GTP, alkaline phosphatase
Serum bilirubin
Serum glucose
Renal function: urinary output, serum creatinine, blood urea
  nitrogen

AST = aspartate aminotransferase; ALT = alanine aminotransferase; GTP = glutamyl transpeptidase.

extubation; it should be treated with infusion of 0.1 N hydrochloric acid through a central venous catheter.

Serum transaminase levels may be quite high during the first 24 to 36 hours but may be expected to fall over the ensuing 3 to 4 days. Poor level of consciousness, persistent elevation of serum ammonia or transaminase levels, acidosis, hypoglycemia, hemodynamic dysfunction, and worsening renal function may herald allograft dysfunction due to injury sustained at the time of organ procurement, preservation or reperfusion injury, or hepatic vascular thrombosis. The hepatic artery is most commonly involved if a thrombotic event occurs, and occlusion of the arterial blood supply to the liver should be suspected if there is sudden elevation of liver chemistries along with fever, reduced bile output, or metabolic acidosis. These signs and symptoms are indistinguishable from acute allograft rejection. A Doppler ultrasound examination of the liver should be performed immediately to establish patency of the hepatic vessels. If hepatic arterial flow is undetectable by Doppler, an emergency angiogram should be obtained. Prompt diagnosis and surgical correction of hepatic artery thrombosis will result in the salvage of some allografts, although retransplantation is often necessary.

Immunosuppression

There are almost as many different immunosuppressive protocols as there are liver transplant centers, but almost all employ multiagent regimens. Our choice for routine maintenance is triple drug therapy with steroids, azathioprine (Imuran), and cyclosporine (Sandimmune). Acute rejection is treated with high-dose steroids (500 to 1,000 mg methylprednisolone daily for 3 days) followed by a rapid steroid taper over 5 to 7 days. Steroid-resistant rejection is treated with the monoclonal antibody OKT3, or with FK506, a macrolide antibiotic with potent immunosuppressive properties. Less than 5 percent of the acute rejection episodes are refractory to immunosuppression manipulation and require retransplantation.

The immunosuppressive agents themselves have multiple side effects of varying severity. A consequence of tricking the body's immune system into accepting a foreign organ is interference with normal immune surveillance mechanisms directed against pathogens and neoplasms. Regardless of which immunosuppression protocol is selected, liver transplant recipients are at increased risk for opportunistic infections and malignancies. In addition to receiving drugs that inhibit host defenses, these patients undergo a prolonged surgical procedure during which the biliary and/or intestinal tract may be entered. There is also potential exposure to infectious agents from the donor organ itself, as well as from the blood products administered during the transplant. The pathogenic organisms may be viral, bacterial, or fungal. In the early postoperative period, when graft function is most dependent on high-dose immunosuppression, the risk of infectious complication is highest. Sepsis is the most common cause of early death after liver transplantation. Over the ensuing months, liver engraftment is accompanied by decreased immunosuppression requirements, decreased incidence of acute rejection episodes, and decreased risk of life-threatening infections. It is very unusual to diagnose either acute rejection or opportunistic infection in liver recipients who are otherwise doing well, compliant with their immunotherapy, and maintaining appropriate immunosuppression blood levels more than 1 year after the transplant.

Cyclosporine is a powerful immunosuppressant that has allowed liver transplantation to achieve its present status. Renal toxicity, hepatic toxicity, neurologic toxicity, hypertension, gingival hyperplasia, hirsutism, and hypercholesterolemia are side effects of cyclosporine that are often dose related and controllable to a variable degree by reduction in the amount of drug administered. Adjustments to maintenance cyclosporine dosing are made on the basis of trough serum levels of the parent compound or metabolites. With a whole blood monoclonal radioimmunoassay, desirable trough levels are 250 to 350 ng per milliliter in the immediate postoperative period. By the end of 1 year, target trough levels are reduced to 150 to 250 ng per milliliter.

Corticosteroids interfere with normal immune function at several levels. In addition to inhibiting inflammation and stabilizing capillary membranes, steroids inhibit the production of certain cytokines released during the immune response. The complications of prolonged steroid usage include cushingoid changes, obesity, hyperglycemia, delayed wound healing, osteoporosis, hypertension, peptic ulcer disease, cataracts, hypercholesterolemia, and mood changes. An advantage of multiple drug therapy is the ability to reduce steroid requirements substantially. By the end of their first post-transplant year, most adult patients on a triple-drug regimen receive daily prednisone supplements of 10 mg or less. Carefully supervised trials are under way to totally withdraw exogenous corticosteroids from selected patients with excellent graft function more than 1 year after their transplant.

Azathioprine, a derivative of 6-mercaptopurine, was first used in human renal transplants in 1961. Rapidly dividing cells such as leukocytes are most susceptible to azathioprine, which exerts its immunosuppressive effect by inhibiting DNA and RNA synthesis. Bone marrow suppression as evidenced by leukopenia, erythropenia, or thrombocytopenia occurs commonly with administration of this drug. Some institutions titrate the dosage to changes in the white blood cell count. The use of azathioprine is complicated by the increased incidence of post-transplant leukopenia and thrombocytopenia in patients with chronic active hepatitis. Side effects of azathioprine include hepatotoxicity, pancreatitis, and alopecia.

OKT3 is a monoclonal antibody directed against a membrane-bound glycoprotein (CD3) found on circulating T cells. As opposed to cyclosporine, azathioprine, and corticosteroids, OKT3 is not generally used for maintenance immunosuppression, but rather is given to reverse acute allograft rejection. OKT3 binds to the CD3 complex of molecules that are in close proximity on the cell membrane to the T-cell receptor, and in doing so may produce transient T-cell activation. As a result, the initial one or two doses of OKT3, which is given daily for 10 to 14 days, may be accompanied by fever, chills, arthralgias, a flulike syndrome, meningismus, seizures, respiratory distress, and transient worsening of allograft function. Most of the symptoms resolve spontaneously and can be ameliorated by premedication with steroids, diphenhydramine hydrochloride, and acetaminophen.

The newest addition to liver transplant immunosuppression is FK506 (Prograf). Although U.S. experience with FK506 is limited to those centers investigating the drug under one or more study protocols, it appears to be more potent than cyclosporine; however, it shares some of the same side effects. Excessive FK506 levels are associated with nephrotoxicity, hepatotoxicity, neurotoxicity, and gastrointestinal motility disorders. For some patients, the therapeutic window for FK506 may be quite small.

Biliary Complications

A significant incidence of morbidity and mortality has been attributed to biliary tract complications. Although biliary reconstruction is considered the least technically demanding of the liver transplant anastomoses, bile duct problems account for 7 to 17 percent of post-transplant morbidity. Nonetheless, the following modifications to the transplant operation have diminished the incidence of serious biliary complications: (1) abandonment of the cholecystojejunostomy in favor of the choledochocholedochostomy or Roux-en-Y choledochojejeunostomy, (2) use of absorbable monofilament sutures, (3) recognition of the tenuous hepatic artery–dependent blood supply of the extrahepatic bile ducts, (4) avoidance of excessive dissection of the periductal tissues, and (5) elimination of the electrocautery to control bleeding on or near the bile ducts. Bile duct stricture, obstruction, and leak account for most of the postoperative biliary complications. The traditional approach of reoperative surgery to these problems has been replaced by interventional radiologic or endoscopic techniques. Percutaneous transhepatic cholangiography (PTC) or endoscopic retrograde cholangiography

(ERCP) with drainage, dilatation, and/or stenting is the preferred initial approach to most biliary complications. It is arguable whether the percutaneous or endoscopic technique offers a clear advantage over the other. PTC carries the risks of bleeding, hemobilia, viscus perforation, x-ray exposure, and difficulty in gaining access to a nondilated biliary system. ERCP, on the other hand, is associated with the risk of pancreatitis, bile duct or duodenal perforation, stent migration, the need for repeat endoscopy whenever follow-up imaging is necessary, and a lower probability of technical success. The choice between PTC and ERCP should rest with the local expertise available at the transplant center.

Most biliary complications are avoidable, and those that do develop can usually be managed nonoperatively. Biliary reconstruction should no longer be viewed as the "Achilles heel" of liver transplantation.

FUTURE CONSIDERATIONS

Our ability to rescue individuals with end-stage liver failure remains limited by the shortage of replacement organs. Living donor and split liver transplants offer only a partial solution to the widening gap between organ supply and demand. Exciting developments in xenotransplantation, xenoperfusion, and liver support systems may bring us closer to solving the organ shortage dilemma. Two patients have received liver grafts from nonhuman primate donors, and pig liver perfusion has been used to temporarily support patients awaiting definitive human liver transplantation. Although the immunologic and physiologic consequences of interspecies transplantation are only partially understood, xenotransplantation of the liver is no longer considered science fiction. Ethical as well as medical concerns about this approach must be dealt with thoughtfully.

Bioartificial devices utilizing human or porcine hepatocytes suspended in hemodialysis cartridges have been shown experimentally to reconstitute synthetic and degradative hepatic functions in the setting of fulminant hepatic failure. It is conceivable that patients with fulminant failure (for whom the present treatment of choice is OLT) could be supported long enough for their livers to undergo regeneration and thus obviate the need for liver transplantation. Furthermore, the availability of a liver support system capable of sustaining patients with critical liver dysfunction for an extended period, much as hemodialysis is capable of supporting renal failure patients, would allow us to expand our criteria for the acceptable cadaveric human liver donor and embolden our approach to the "marginal" donor.

SUGGESTED READING*

Brems J, Hiatt J, Millis J, et al. Effect of prior portosystemic shunt on subsequent liver transplantation. Ann Surg 1989; 209:51–56.
Broelsch CE, Whitington PF, Emond JC, et al. Liver transplantation in children from living related donors: Surgical techniques and results. Ann Surg 1991; 214:428–439.
Burdick J, Pitt H, Colombani P, et al. Superior mesenteric vein inflow for liver transplantation when the portal vein is occluded. Surgery 1990; 107:342–345.
Griffith BP, Shaw BW Jr, Hardesty RL, et al. Veno-venous bypass without systemic anticoagulation for human liver transplantation. Surg Gynecol Obstet 1985; 160:270–272.
Gunson BK, Hathaway M, Buckels JAC, et al. HLA matching in liver transplantation: a retrospective analysis. Transplant Proc 1992; 24:2434–2435.
Klein AS, Savader S, Burdick JF, et al. Reduction of morbidity and mortality from biliary complications following liver transplantation. Hepatology 1991; 14:818–823.
Lake JR, Robert JP, Ascher NL. Maintenance immunosuppression after liver transplantation. Semin Liver Dis 1992; 12:73–79.
Lucey MR, Merion RM, Henley KS, et al. Selection for and outcome of liver transplantation in alcoholic liver disease. Gastroenterol 1992; 102:1736–1741.
Makowka L, Stieber A, Sher L, et al. Surgical technique of orthotopic liver transplantation. Gastroenterol Clin North Am 1988; 17:33–52.
Mor E, Klintmalm GB, Gonwa TA, et al. The use of marginal donors for liver transplantation. Transplantation 1992; 53:383–386.
Ring EJ, Lake JR, Roberts JP, et al. Using transjugular intrahepatic portosystemic shunts to control variceal bleeding before liver transplantation. Ann Intern Med 1992; 116:304–309.
Tanaka K, Uemoto S, Tokunaga Y, et al. Surgical techniques and innovations in living related liver transplantation. Ann Surg 1993; 217:82–91.
Todo S, Tzakis AG, Nery J, et al. Extended preservation of human liver grafts with U.W. solution. JAMA 1989; 261:711–714.

*__Editor's Note:__ The preceding and succeeding chapters contain relevant references omitted from this list.

LIVER TRANSPLANTATION IN CHILDREN

PETER F. WHITINGTON, M.D.
ESTELLA M. ALONSO, M.D.

Liver disease requiring orthotopic liver transplantation (OLT) is infrequently encountered in pediatric practice. There are no precise figures for the frequency of life-threatening liver disease in children in the United States. However, using all available data, we estimate an annual U.S. incidence of fewer than 600 children with liver disease that warrants consideration of OLT. From this population come the approximately 300 children who receive transplantation each year. Despite the relative infrequency of OLT in pediatric practice, the subject is not obscure. Practicing gastroenterologists should be prepared to evaluate children with liver disease, to determine whether OLT should be considered in a therapeutic strategy, and to care for children after OLT. The purpose of this chapter is to provide a practical approach to the subject based on our experience at the University of Chicago.

INDICATIONS

The indications for OLT in children can be classified within the following framework: (1) primary liver disease that is expected to progress to hepatic failure; (2) nonprogressive liver disease with morbidity that outweighs the risk of transplantation; (3) primary therapy for liver-based metabolic disease; (4) secondary liver disease, such as occurs in patients with cystic fibrosis; and (5) primary hepatic malignancy. Table 1 gives the frequency of specific disease indications in our experience according to these categories.

Hepatic failure is the major general indication, with biliary atresia alone accounting for over 50 percent of cases. Parenchymal liver diseases, including fulminant hepatic failure, chronic active hepatitis with cirrhosis, and certain metabolic diseases, are also common. Table 2 gives the specific disease indications leading to hepatic failure and OLT in children.

Cirrhosis appears in the literature as a common indication for OLT in children; however, cirrhosis is neither a specific disease entity nor a general indication.

Table 1 Approximate Frequencies of Specific Indications for Pediatric OLT at University of Chicago

Indication	Frequency (%)
Hepatic failure	>95
Biliary atresia	62
alpha$_1$-Antitrypsin deficiency	8
Progressive intrahepatic cholestasis	7
Secondary biliary cirrhosis	4
Fulminant hepatic failure	3
Ductular hypoplasia syndromes	2
Chronic active hepatitis	2
Neonatal hepatitis	2
Postnecrotic cirrhosis	2
Tyrosinemia	2
Wison's disease	<1
Congenital hepatic fibrosis	<1
Nonprogressive liver disease	<1
Arteriohepatic dysplasia	<1
Primary therapy for inborn errors of metabolism	<1
Glycogen storage disease	<1
Urea cycle defects	<1
Crigler-Najjar syndrome	<1
Secondary liver disease	None
Primary hepatic malignancy	<1
Hepatoblastoma	<1
Hepatocellular carcinoma	<1
Sarcoma	<1

Table 2 Classification of Diseases for Which OLT Has Been Performed in Infants and Children for Indication of Hepatic Insufficiency

I. Metabolic diseases
  a. alpha$_1$-Antitrypsin deficiency
  b. Tyrosinemia
  c. Glycogen storage diseases
    1. Type IV
    2. Type III
    3. Type I (?)
  d. Wilson's disease
  e. Perinatal hemochromatosis/iron storage diseases

II. Acute and chronic hepatitis
  a. Fulminant hepatic failure
    1. Viral
    2. Toxin/drug induced
  b. Chronic active hepatitis/cirrhosis
    1. Hepatitis B virus
    2. Hepatitis C virus (non-A, non-B)
    3. Autoimmune
    4. Idiopathic

III. Intrahepatic cholestasis
  a. Idiopathic neonatal hepatitis
  b. Algaille's syndrome (syndromic bile duct paucity)
  c. Nonsyndromic bile duct paucity
  d. Familial intrahepatic cholestasis (Byler's disease)

IV. Obstructive biliary tract disease
  a. Extrahepatic biliary atresia
  b. Sclerosing cholangitis
  c. Traumatic/postsurgical biliary tract diseases

V. Miscellaneous
  a. Cryptogenic cirrhosis
  b. Congenital hepatic fibrosis
  c. Caroli's disease
  d. Cystic fibrosis
  e. Cirrhosis secondary to prolonged total parenteral nutrition

It is an anatomic diagnosis with functional implications, but only when evidence of hepatic decompensation accompanies cirrhosis is there a clear indication for OLT. In our experience, many children with cirrhosis, particularly those with postnecrotic cirrhosis, may be functionally normal, and consideration of liver transplantation should be postponed until hepatic decompensation is evident. Innumerable such children referred to our center are alive and well many years later without transplantation.

OLT has a debatable role in nonprogressive liver diseases such as the chronic intrahepatic cholestasis syndromes, because these are not usually life-threatening. Patients with arteriohepatic dysplasia (Alagille's syndrome), the most common specific disease fitting this criterion, usually do not develop cirrhosis, and the issue arises as to whether OLT should be used to treat only symptoms. Alternative forms of therapy may provide relief from pruritus in some patients, and many complications can be treated by specific administration of vitamins and other nutrients. However, in some instances the cholestasis is refractory to all therapy, and the mortality risks of liver transplantation must be weighed against only the morbidity of the liver disease.

The principal goal of OLT for the primary treatment of inborn errors of metabolism is to correct the metabolic error. To date, most patients with a metabolic error after receiving OLT had hepatic complications, including hepatic insufficiency and hepatocellular carcinoma. However, OLT could be of theoretical benefit to many children with inborn errors that do not injure the liver, e.g., Crigler-Najjar syndrome type I, urea cycle defects, and familial hypercholesterolemia.

Complete replacement of the liver may not be necessary in terms of the treatment of metabolic diseases. The quantity of functioning mass needed to carry critical metabolic functions allows for the use of auxiliary transplants. Recently, we performed orthotopic replacement of the left lobe and completely corrected the metabolic defects in a male infant with ornithine-transcarbamylase deficiency and a female teenager with Crigler-Najjar syndrome. This procedure appears to be safer than orthotopic replacement because it allows for the patient's own liver to support life function in the event of graft failure. Furthermore, should gene therapy become available in the future, the allograft can be safely removed and immunosuppression discontinued.

Some secondary liver diseases are indications for OLT. Over 40 children and young adults with cystic fibrosis and biliary cirrhosis have received liver transplantation. At present, over 60 percent of the recipients are alive and some have actually shown improvement in their other medical condition. Successful OLT has also been performed in several children with biliary cirrhosis secondary to Langerhans' cell histiocytosis. In dealing with secondary liver disease, each patient and set of circumstances must be considered individually to determine whether this approach to therapy is appropriate.

The prognosis is bleak for patients with symptomatic primary hepatic malignancy, and OLT should be avoided. However, some metabolic diseases have a natural history that includes hepatic malignancy. Careful monitoring for the development of carcinoma should be included in the management of these patients. If OLT is performed when cancer is first detectable, or if malignant transformation is found in the hepatic explant, the prognosis is excellent.

CONTRAINDICATIONS

Whenever a child is referred for evaluation for possible OLT, we try to think of reasons why the procedure should not be performed. Obviously, a transplant center wishes to provide OLT for any child needing the therapy, but we judge it to be contraindicated in about one-third of children referred to our center. The reasons for not providing OLT are listed in Table 3 and fall into two broad categories: a reasonable (often better) alternative therapy is available, or the child would not be benefited by OLT, even though it may be indicated.

Many patients referred for OLT are found to be candidates for beneficial alternative therapy. Since liver transplantation carries a significant risk, any potentially effective therapy should be pursued. However, there is also risk involved in another therapy that turns out to be ineffective and thus delays OLT. In many cases, it makes sense to place the patient on the active transplant waiting list while closely observing the effects of other therapeutic interventions.

If the quality of life is expected to be poor after OLT or if the child's general condition makes survival unlikely, OLT should be avoided. Quality of life issues particularly apply to liver diseases that are accompanied by injury to the central nervous system (CNS). Many infants with advanced liver disease have poor psychomotor development, especially of gross motor skills, but these deficits usually recover after OLT. Patients who have developed cerebral edema, either in the setting of fulminant hepatic failure or in hyperammonemic syndromes such as urea cycle defects, can be expected to have poor neurologic function after OLT. Also, we have not considered patients with pre-existing mental retardation to be good candidates for OLT. Frank discussion with the parents of children with CNS impairment is imperative for decision making about proceeding with OLT; when there is undeniable evidence of irreversible injury to the brain, OLT is best avoided. Sometimes it may be impossible to make predictions about the neurologic outcome, such as in a previously healthy child who presents with fulminant hepatic failure in deep hepatic coma. In such cases, OLT should be performed as quickly as possible. Physical or social handicaps are not deemed reasons to deny OLT in our center.

Impairment of other organ systems can significantly reduce the likelihood of survival after OLT. Complex congenital heart disease is observed in association with liver disease in patients with biliary atresia and arteriohepatic dysplasia, and it may be so severe that OLT

Table 3 Contraindications to Orthotopic Liver Transplantation in Children

An acceptable alternative therapy

An expectation of suboptimal quality of life after transplantation

Impairment of other organ systems, either primary or secondary to liver disease, that precludes successful transplantation

A major systemic infection (bacterial, fungal, or viral)

Disease that is expected to recur after liver transplantation, e.g., malignancy or viral infection

cannot be pursued. Renal involvement with severe congenital hepatic fibrosis, alpha$_1$-antitrypsin deficiency, and arteriohepatic dysplasia, and advanced liver disease in children with short bowel syndrome, may require multiorgan transplantation or a decision not to offer OLT. The major intra-abdominal vascular anomalies associated with biliary atresia have been considered as absolute contraindications to OLT, but recent surgical advances have allowed successful transplantation even in children with congenital absence of the portal vein.

Secondary organ failure has a profound negative effect on outcome after OLT, and medical correction of some of the systemic effects of liver disease should be performed before OLT. For example, patients with functional renal insufficiency are managed by establishing an access for renal dialysis before OLT.

Any major acute systemic infection is a contraindication to OLT, but sometimes this cannot be avoided. For example, one of the complications encountered in patients with biliary atresia is ascending cholangitis, which can be refractory to all medical management. Continued antibiotic therapy is unlikely to be effective and liver function can deteriorate rapidly, rendering the patient a less favorable candidate. It seems appropriate under these circumstances to proceed with OLT when a donor becomes available. On the other hand, acute systemic infections, including spontaneous bacterial peritonitis and sepsis, should be treated before proceeding with OLT. Often, a few days of antibiotics are sufficient to render the patient a suitable recipient. Liver transplantation should be deferred in patients with some common childhood viral infections (e.g., upper respiratory infections with respiratory syncytial virus and parainfluenza virus), since the use of immunosuppressive agents will tend to exacerbate these after OLT.

A final reason to avoid OLT is the presence of a disease that is expected to recur after therapy. This principally applies to primary liver cancer, chronic hepatitis B virus infection, and human immunodeficiency virus (HIV) infection.

EVALUATING THE PEDIATRIC OLT CANDIDATE

Our basic pretransplant evaluation is performed in one half-day outpatient visit (Table 4).

Table 4 Key Elements of Pretransplant Evaluation of Children

Confirm diagnosis

Stage patient with regard to urgency of transplantation

Determine intra-abdominal anatomy

Establish status of patient with regard to infectious processes that might present a problem after OLT

Establish relationship with parents and care providers of patient to provide maximal supportive care before and after OLT

Arrange for finances

Arrange mechanism for contacting parents and providing transport when a donor becomes available

The need to confirm a diagnosis is obvious, although sometimes not possible. The course of progression of liver disease cannot be anticipated and proper plans for transplantation cannot be made without a proper diagnosis. However, some children present in end-stage liver failure, and proper diagnosis may require waiting for the availability of explant tissue for proper histologic and biochemical diagnosis.

Careful functional grading of cirrhosis in infants and children has not been performed. We have found that the demonstrated inability of the liver to support a child's growth and development is as good as any measure for the need to proceed with transplantation. Children with chronic liver disease almost invariably develop growth failure and evidence of malnutrition. Every effort should be made to support growth and nutrition, but the nutritional status of children with advanced cirrhosis will decline even if they are provided supranormal quantities of nutrients by intravenous (IV) infusion. This suggests that parenchymal function is critical in order to maintain adequate nutritional status and allow for growth. It is obvious that the child with reduced nutritional reserves will be less able to cope with the rigors of OLT. Thus, when it becomes evident that liver disease is restricting growth, transplantation should be performed as soon as possible, because a child with growth failure cannot improve as a transplant candidate.

A key factor in determining when inevitable hepatic insufficiency will develop is establishment of a primary diagnosis of liver disease with a well-known natural history. Biliary atresia is by far the most common indication for OLT in children, and patients with biliary atresia who have failed the Kasai procedure typically reach end-stage disease between 9 and 18 months of age. Thus, such a patient has a clear indication for liver transplantation and will need the procedure as an infant. Unfortunately, few other pediatric liver diseases have such a clearly defined natural history. alpha$_1$-Antitrypsin deficiency is a common liver disease causing parenchymal failure in children and the most common metabolic disease resulting in the need for pediatric OLT. However, at the time of diagnosis in infancy, the prognosis usually cannot be determined. Less than 20 percent of individuals with the genetic defect have significant liver disease, and only about 15 percent develop macronodular cirrhosis before the age of 20 years. Liver transplantation should be considered for patients with cirrhosis and hepatic insufficiency, whereas those with neonatal cholestasis secondary to alpha$_1$-antitrypsin deficiency should simply be followed closely, since most will not require OLT.

Most children presenting with fulminant hepatic failure require liver transplantation, since most have sporadic non-A, non-B hepatitis, which is associated with over 95 percent mortality. Other etiologies, e.g., acute acetaminophen intoxication, carry a better prognosis for spontaneous recovery. We have developed an aggressive empiric approach to this problem. As soon as the diagnosis of fulminant hepatic failure is established, the child is listed for OLT. If the patient improves while waiting for a donor, the decision can be reversed. If a donor becomes available and the patient has not improved, the decision is made to proceed with OLT.

Considering the intra-abdominal anatomy, the two most important variables are the portal vein and, in patients with biliary atresia, the type of portoenterostomy performed. Some children with biliary atresia have associated congenital absence or thrombosis of the portal vein, hypoplastic portal vein, or other major intra-abdominal vascular anomalies. Knowledge in advance of surgery is essential for proper planning. Some variations on the Kasai portoenterostomy procedure leave the child with long segments of intestine that are essentially defunctionalized and unavailable for cyclosporine absorption after transplant. Advanced knowledge of such anatomy can allow surgeons to reconstruct the intestine to permit improved drug bioavailability.

The candidate must be evaluated with regard to the potential for developing serious infections after OLT. A serologic status for cytomegalovirus determines the risk of infection after OLT, and Epstein-Barr virus is also significant because of its association with lymphoproliferative disorders in transplant recipients. Varicella serologic status should be known so that proper care can be provided in the case of exposure after OLT. Finally, immunization to common childhood viral illnesses, particularly rubeola, should be provided before OLT if possible. We also strongly recommend immunization against hepatitis B, *Streptococcus pneumoniae,* and *Haemophilus influenzae* before OLT.

OBTAINING A DONOR FOR A CHILD

Most children needing OLT are under 2 years of age. This presents a significant problem with obtaining a donor since most cadaver donors are victims of accidents, which have an entirely different epidemiology. Because of the relative paucity of small donors, most large pediatric programs have followed our lead and adopted the routine use of reduced-size transplantation, in which the liver from a larger donor is tailored to fit a small recipient by ex vivo reduction hepatectomy. In our center, over 50 percent of pediatric OLTs are performed with segmental allografts, principally using the left lobe and the left lateral segment. This has resulted in a dramatic reduction in pretransplant mortality of infants, from more than 20 percent to less than 5 percent, while post-transplant survival remains the same or has improved.

Living-related liver transplantation is an important alternative for many families. To date, 50 such transplants have been performed in infants at the University of Chicago. The overall survival has been better than 90 percent, with recent 1 year survival rates exceeding 95 percent. There are two main advantages to this procedure. First, the quality of the graft obtained is uniformly excellent, since it is harvested from a healthy adult with thorough preoperative evaluation. We have not had a single episode of primary nonfunction in living-related recipients, whereas the incidence is approximately 6 percent in recipients of allografts from cadaver donors. The second and more important advantage is the opportunity to schedule the transplant while the patient is an optimal candidate. Because of the shortage of donors, children with end-stage liver disease are often forced to wait until their clinical status worsens, which can be avoided altogether with living-related transplantation. It also appears from our experience that even though the incidence of rejection is not significantly reduced, rejection episodes in recipients of living donor allografts are less severe and more responsive to therapy. No significant morbidity and no mortality have been observed in the donors.

The option of living-related transplantation is presented to the families of all infants evaluated at our center. The donor must be a healthy adult under 50 years of age, preferably a parent of the recipient, and with a compatible blood type. A donor candidate must undergo a complete medical evaluation, including computed tomography of the liver and angiography of the hepatic vasculature, to identify potential contraindications to liver donation. The donor must also be judged emotionally stable and have a reliable support network of family and friends who will be available during the surgical procedure and until the donor is fully recuperated from surgery.

SURGICAL MANAGEMENT*

The surgery involved in pediatric liver transplantation is not too different from that in adults, with some exceptions, listed in Table 5. The use of segmental allografts presents many technical problems that have been overcome in various ways. Positioning of left segmental allografts is an example. In our center, the graft is placed with the cut section to the right, which often requires lengthening of the portal vein and particular care with the hepatic vein anastomosis.

---

*Editor's Note: Although reduced-size transplantation is discussed in the preceding chapter, additional details are given here by members of the group that innovated some of these techniques.

Table 5 Distinctive Features of Intraoperative Management of Children Undergoing Orthotopic Liver Transplantation

Need for segmental allografts
Surgical abdomen: adhesions, etc.
Need for Roux-en-Y choledochoenterostomy
Vascular anomalies and need for vascular reconstruction
No venovenous bypass
Careful flushing of allograft to prevent K$^+$ overload
Difficulty in maintaining body temperature
Difficulty with fluid balance, preventing overload

Arterial anastomosis is effected by an interposition graft extending to the infrarenal aorta. In other centers, the graft is turned upside down, so the cut edge faces to the left, which reportedly results in a more physiologic portal vein anastomosis. Pediatric liver transplant surgeons have been innovative in other ways as well. Complex vascular anomalies have required replacement of the portal vein, which procedure in our center uses cryopreserved saphenous veins. Absence of the inferior vena cava results in the need for direct anastomosis of hepatic veins to the right atrium. Finally, the diameter of the hepatic artery requires microsurgical techniques, particularly for construction of interposition grafts.

Other differences include no venovenous bypass in recipients younger than age 10 years, because this results in temporary interruption of blood flow from the lower half of the body and acute congestion of the portal circulation. Previous surgery, usually hepatoportoenterostomy, results in dense scarring within the abdomen and the need for careful dissection. Small intestinal perforations are common. Virtually all pediatric liver allograft recipients have an inadequate bile duct for direct end-to-end anastomosis, so virtually all need Roux-en-Y choledochoenterostomy. Our studies of cyclosporine absorption have led us to adopt the use of short Roux-en-Ys, with a biliary limb of only 15 cm, entering the intestinal mainstream 10 cm beyond the ligament of Treitz. We use a previously established Roux-en-Y if possible. However, if this is too long or too short, reconstruction may be necessary. Children, particularly small and malnourished infants, have reduced muscle mass and reduced capacity to handle potassium overload. Thus, there is a need to vigorously flush the allograft before unclamping vascular anastomoses, to prevent a rush of potassium into the system and cardiac arrhythmias. Finally, infants and children have increased surface area from which to radiate energy, so careful attention must be paid to maintaining body temperature, including operating in a warm room equipped with radiant heaters.

IMMEDIATE POSTOPERATIVE CARE

A close working relationship between hepatologist and pediatric intensive care personnel has developed around the management of OLT recipients, and their care has become routine. We do not isolate patients, but demand thorough handwashing or gloving before the patient is examined. Routine intensive care monitoring is adequate for these patients, but careful recording of fluid balance and daily weight is essential.

The function of the newly transplanted liver is relatively easily monitored. Important parameters include acid-base balance (persistent metabolic acidosis is indicative of poor graft function), prothrombin time (which should be less than 18 seconds) and aminotransferase levels (values greater than 2,000 IU per liter suggest ischemia-reperfusion injury). We also perform daily duplex ultrasound examinations for the first 3 days after transplant to identify acute vascular thrombosis, which is common in small recipients.

Immunosuppression is provided by a combination of cyclosporine, methylprednisolone, and azathioprine. Cyclosporine is administered IV at 1 mg per kilogram every 12 hours on the first 3 days, increasing to 2 mg per kilogram every 12 hours thereafter. Further changes in dosage are determined by measuring blood cyclosporine levels, which we maintain between 200 and 300 ng per milliliter (whole blood concentration measured by high-performance liquid chromatography). Methylprednisolone is initially given at 1 mg per kilogram every 12 hours, but is tapered to 0.5 mg per kilogram per day by the seventh postoperative day and finally to 0.3 mg per kilogram per day by day 28. Azathioprine is given at a steady dose of 1 mg per kilogram per day.

A carefully constructed regimen of antibiotic prophylaxis can prevent many perioperative and postoperative infections. We use selective bowel decontamination (nystatin, gentamicin, bacitracin) for 2 weeks before surgery in recipients of living donor allografts and whenever possible in recipients of cadaver allografts. This is continued after surgery for 2 weeks. We also administer IV ampicillin and cefotaxime immediately before and during, and for 2 days after, surgery. This antibiotic regimen was tailored to address the specific needs of pediatric recipients, in whom enterococcus and gram-negative enterics are most important. Prophylaxis for cytomegalovirus (CMV) is provided to high-risk patients, which category includes those who are seronegative for CMV and who receive an organ from a seropositive donor, all patients receiving a repeat transplant, and those who have converted from seronegative to seropositive within the previous month. Prophylaxis is provided with ganciclovir, 5 mg per kilogram IV every 12 hours for 14 days, followed by acyclovir, 10 mg per kilogram orally four times a day for the next 3 months.

Pediatric liver transplant recipients can often be transferred from the intensive care unit within 48 hours.

POSTOPERATIVE CONSIDERATIONS

Some considerations of postoperative care with particular importance for pediatric OLT are listed in Table 6.

Several factors have been related to hepatic artery thrombosis, probably the most important being the age of the patient. Arterial thrombosis is two to three times

Table 6 Distinctive Features of Postoperative Management of Children Undergoing Orthotopic Liver Transplantation

High incidence of hepatic artery thrombosis
Prolonged ventilatory insufficiency
Feeding difficulties and problems with restoring nutrition
An unusually high dosing requirement for oral cyclosporine

more common in pediatric liver recipients than in adults, which may relate to two factors: the size of the hepatic artery and the perfusion pressure. Arterial flow is of course related directly to the perfusion pressure and inversely related to the resistance. Diameters of less than 3 mm present a twofold higher risk of thrombosis, and small children's blood pressure are considerably lower. Several medical factors can be related to arterial loss. In our experience, rejection is commonly associated, which is not surprising considering that rejection is often directed against vessels. It causes endothelialitis, with resultant reduced flow and increased risk of thrombosis. The coagulation status may be related to arterial loss, and we routinely use aspirin in low dosage to prevent platelet aggregation. Finally, infection around the hepatic artery can certainly result in thrombosis. Particularly with regard to the reduced-sized grafts in which infection along the resected margin is not rare, this may be an important contributor to arterial thrombosis.

The possible outcomes of hepatic artery thrombosis after liver transplantation are (1) fulminant hepatic failure; (2) subacute hepatic failure, possibly complicated by infection and bile duct disease; (3) focal hepatic infarction with secondary abscess formation, possibly complicated by bile duct problems; and (4) little or no detectable hepatic injury and stable hepatic function. The factors that cause these various outcomes in patients with a singular problem are unknown at present. Arterial collateralization could provide an alternate of oxygenated blood, but collateralization probably develops in most cases long after the outcome has been determined. Conceivably, underlying disease processes such as rejection may make the liver less capable of withstanding arterial loss, but these factors have not been examined.

The manner in which the patient presents with arterial thrombosis is often predictive of the therapy that will be required. Of course, the development of fulminant hepatic failure is a medical-surgical emergency demanding immediate retransplantation. Major changes in transaminase values and evidence of hepatic dysfunction consequent to arterial loss also portend a poor prognosis, and retransplantation should be planned as soon as possible. A patient who develops sepsis with gram-negative enterics, enterococcus, or anaerobes should be investigated for hepatic abscess. If an abscess is found, the arterial supply of the liver should be investigated first, as it has probably been lost. Our experience with hepatic abscess accompanying hepatic arterial loss indicates that this is a hopeless situation, and the patient should be retransplanted as soon as possible. Acutely developing bile duct complications (e.g., bile

drainage from abdominal drains, acute biliary obstruction, and acute biliary distention) or chronic problems (e.g., sludge, strictures, and sclerosing cholangitis) should prompt a thorough evaluation of the arterial vascular supply. If arterial thrombosis is found, retransplantation is almost certainly required. Finally, if arterial loss is discovered serendipitously, but there is no apparent hepatic dysfunction, the patient will probably do well. Our experience and that of others with late-onset asymptomatic hepatic artery thrombosis suggests that collateralization of the arterial supply to these livers is common.

Pediatric patients, particularly very small infants, appear to have an unusually high frequency of pulmonary and ventilatory complications after OLT. We reviewed the records of 80 children transplanted over a 2 year period for specific diagnoses of pulmonary complications, and found that 41 of the patients had one or more in the postoperative period. Five died as a direct result of such complications; 19 had significant right-sided pleural effusions, five requiring placement of a chest tube. Most effusions were associated with a bout of acute rejection; chest fluid contained numerous activated lymphocytes and was thought to be a "sympathetic" effusion from the inflamed liver. No effusion was infected. Ten patients developed pneumonitis, which carried a mortality rate of 30 percent. Influenza B, parainfluenza, and hospital-acquired nosocomial gram-negative bacterial and fungal infections were lethal, while patients with community-acquired bacterial, *Legionella,* respiratory syncytial viral, CMV, and *Pneumocystis* pneumonia recovered. Abdominal abscesses extended into the chest in three patients.

A particular problem in very small children receiving liver transplantation is prolonged dependence on mechanical ventilation, which results from failure of the mechanical aspects of breathing. Small children with chronic liver disease have breathing problems before transplantation. These result from enlarged viscera and/or ascites with elevation of the diaphragm, compression of the pulmonary volume, and flaring of the ribs, all of which reduce the ventilatory efficiency. Added to these mechanical problems is malnutrition, which causes loss of muscle mass and strength. The result is a severely compromised child. Paralysis of the right diaphragm is a moderately common surgical complication that further compromises breathing. As a consequence of these factors, very small and frail recipients often need long-term mechanical ventilatory support. Some patients have been supported for months until malnutrition and poor mechanics have been reversed. Paralyzed diaphragms are plicated to improve breathing efficiency.

Malnutrition and feeding problems are major complications related to medical postoperative care. Parenteral nutrition is usually initiated 2 to 3 days after surgery, and enteral nutrition is begun as soon as tolerated. While complete gut failure is rare in our experience, virtually all small children have some gut-related problem after OLT. Feeding intolerance and vomiting usually indicate delayed gastric emptying, which may be functional (unknown cause) or mechanical (reduced-size left lobe grafts impinging on the stomach). Delayed gastric emptying may respond to medical therapy with metoclopramide, but may necessitate passage of a nasojejunal feeding tube or continued parenteral feeding. Diarrhea and failure to gain weight despite adequate caloric intake indicate malabsorption. It seems obvious that these severely malnourished children should also have secondary digestive insufficiency (exocrine pancreatic insufficiency and hypoplastic villus atrophy), and they often do. Examination of the stool reveals the presence of neutral and split fats. This often improves with pancreatic enzyme replacement therapy, which is continued until nutrition is fully restored. The D-xylose absorption test often indicates mild to moderate malabsorption, which can sometimes be overcome by providing elemental formula in supernormal quantities via continuous drip infusion. Some infants require immense amounts of formula (more than 160 kcal per kilogram per day) to initiate weight gain. Finally, watery diarrhea, often with perianal irritation, commonly indicates carbohydrate malabsorption, which can be corrected by reducing the amount in the formula. More often, it indicates bile acid malabsorption. We have measured fecal bile acid levels in numerous infants with diarrhea after liver transplantation and found high concentrations (more than 1 mmol per liter) in essentially all of them. We now empirically administer a bile acid–binding substance (aluminum hydroxide antacid is usually adequate) in amounts necessary to eliminate diarrhea. A few weeks of treatment are usually all that is required. We assume that time is needed for active ileal transport mechanisms to adapt to the new flux of bile salts after their prolonged absence in the intestine in patients with biliary atresia.

The dosage requirement for cyclosporine varies widely among liver transplant patients, necessitating close pharmacologic monitoring. An observation made in all transplant centers is a requirement for larger dosages of orally administered cyclosporine in children than in adults. We investigated factors, including intestinal length, related to the higher dosage requirement for oral cyclosporine in children after liver transplantation, and found that bowel length was most important. The major determinant of bowel length is age. When viewed as a function of height, which itself demonstrates a pattern of initial rapid increase followed by decelerating change, bowel length increases very rapidly during infancy and the preschool years. Intestinal surface area, in turn, increases by some geometric multiple of its length. From this, we deduced that the intestinal surface available for drug absorption increases very rapidly during early childhood and therefore is an important factor in determining the bioavailability of oral cyclosporine.

Although mostly reflecting this relationship between bowel length and age, the oral dosage requirement can also be affected by surgical bowel removal and exclusion. Standard Roux-en-Y loop construction may exclude 20 to 40 percent of a small infant's intestine from cyclo-

sporine absorption. Superimposed on this is the effect of previous surgery for biliary atresia. As a result of these surgical factors, many young infants lose the use of large portions of what are already short intestines, further restricting cyclosporine absorption. Careful conservation of intestinal length before and during liver transplantation should be a surgical goal when caring for infants with biliary atresia.

Our observations have important implications for the performance of liver transplantation. First, it is difficult to administer enough drug to some infants to achieve a therapeutic level, placing these patients at risk for rejection. Second, the transition from IV to oral dosing can be a problem because of the difficulty in estimating the oral dosage for children. In adults, multiplying the IV dosage by 3 provides a close approximation of the oral dosage. Our results can be used to estimate the oral dosage requirement in infants, which varies from 1.7 to 50 times the IV dosage, if height and excluded bowel length are known. Finally, minimizing the loss of intestine before and during liver transplantation in infants can have an impact on the cost of cyclosporine, which is an important element of the overall cost of liver transplantation.

LONG-TERM CARE AFTER OLT

The median length of hospital stay after transplantation in our center has been reduced to about 20 days, and a child has been discharged after only 9 days. Local follow-up care is provided by a hospice arrangement in the Ronald McDonald House, where patients live for an average of 2 weeks after discharge, during which time they are seen in the outpatient department on a daily basis. As parents gain familiarity with the required care and the patient's condition stabilizes, plans for discharge home are made. Many children are from remote distances, so the local physician must be made familiar with the care regimen. Patients are usually allowed to return home within 4 to 6 weeks of transplant.

The frequency of long-term medical care varies greatly. On average, over the first 3 months, a physician usually sees the patient and biochemistries are measured every 2 weeks. Between 3 and 6 months, monthly visits are usually required. After 6 months, visits are reduced to every 3 months or fewer.

There has been little documentation of the quality of life after liver transplantation, and this issue deserves scrutiny. How adult patients rehabilitate and integrate themselves back into society will certainly be one of the issues considered when policy makers examine liver transplantation from a public perspective. Likewise, pediatric transplantation deserves a closer look with regard to outcome to justify its continued performance.

At present, what has been documented is that patients with growth failure secondary to liver disease will resume growing and that there appears to be a general improvement in lifestyle. Our observations indicate that most resume normal growth within a year after liver transplant, and there appears to be a dramatic increase in general energy and activity. A common request by parents is, "Can you put the old liver back in to slow this kid down?" Liver recipients in our series participate in most age-related activities. All attend school regularly. Most do not participate in interscholastic athletics, but physical education classes are regularly attended. Increased numbers or severity of infectious illnesses do not appear to reduce school attendance. Preschoolers attend day care and participate in other group activities without difficulty. It appears that liver transplantation in children creates a good product, but it is important to study this in greater detail.

SUGGESTED READING

Broelsch CE, Emond JC, Whitington PF, et al. Application of reduced size liver transplants as split grafts, auxiliary orthotopic grafts and living related segmental transplants. Ann Surg 1990; 212:368–377.
Broelsch CE, Whitington PF, Emond JC, et al. Liver transplantine in children from living related donors: surgical techniques and results. Ann Surg 1991; 214:428–439.
Emond JC, Whitington PF, Thistlethwaite JR, et al. Reduced-size liver transplantation: use in the management of children with chronic liver disease. Hepatology 1989; 10:867–872.
Malatack JJ, Schald DJ, Urbach AH, et al. Choosing a pediatric recipient of orthotopic liver transplantation. J Pediatr 1987; 111:479–489.
Shaw BW Jr, Wood RP, Kaufman SS, et al. Liver transplantation therapy for children: part 1. J Pediatr Gastroenterol Nutr 1988; 7:157–166.
Shaw BW Jr, Wood RP, Kaufman SS, et al. Liver transplantation therapy for children: part 2. J Pediatr Gastroenterol Nutr 1988; 7:797–815.
Sokal EM, Veyckemans F, de Ville de Goyet J, et al. Liver transplantation in children less than 1 year of age. J Pediatr 1990; 117:205–210.
Whitington PF. Advances in pediatric liver transplantation. Adv Pediatr 1990; 37:357–389.
Whitington PF, Balistreri WF. Pediatric liver transplantation: indications, contraindications, and pre-transplant management. J Pediatr 1991; 118:169–177.
Whitington PF, Emond JC, Whitington SH, et al. Small-bowel length and the dose of cyclosporine in children after liver transplantation. N Engl J Med 1990; 322:733–738.

ASCITES AND ITS COMPLICATIONS

ANIL K. RUSTGI, M.D.
LAWRENCE S. FRIEDMAN, M.D.

The most common cause of ascites is cirrhosis of the liver. Other etiologies include neoplasms, congestive heart failure, noncirrhotic liver diseases, nephrotic syndrome, and tuberculosis. This chapter deals with the management of ascites in patients with cirrhosis of the liver as well as complications of ascites.

ASCITES IN CIRRHOSIS

Etiology

Several theories have been advanced to explain the development of ascites in patients with cirrhosis. The underfill hypothesis maintains that increased hepatic sinusoidal pressure leads to increased formation of hepatic lymph, which enters the abdominal cavity. Increased portal venous pressure also contributes to the formation of ascites and results in increased splanchnic blood volume. With the expansion of splanchnic extracellular fluid volume, systemic vascular resistance and effective plasma volume decrease, leading in turn to avid renal retention of sodium and water, initially with preservation of the glomerular filtration rate, creatinine clearance, and renal plasma flow. In response to the decrease in effective plasma volume, plasma renin, aldosterone, norepinephrine, and vasopressin activities all increase.

In contrast, according to the overflow hypothesis, renal retention of sodium and water is the primary abnormality leading to the formation of ascites in the absence of central hypovolemia. The triggering event for primary renal sodium and water retention is unclear and is postulated to involve a hepatorenal reflex, perhaps via an intrahepatic baroreceptor mechanism.

The most recent hypothesis, which attempts to reconcile the underfill and overflow hypotheses, is the peripheral arterial vasodilatation hypothesis, in which peripheral vasodilatation is thought to be the initiating event, possibly triggered by endotoxin and cytokines, which reach the portal vein as a result of increased intestinal permeability, and mediated by nitric oxide. (The same factors may account for the formation of arteriovenous shunts seen in the splanchnic, dermal, and pulmonary circulations of patients with cirrhosis.) Peripheral vasodilatation leads to sodium retention as well as a decrease in systemic blood pressure and increase in cardiac output. These physiologic changes may result in an increase in the absolute plasma volume, but not enough to refill the enlarged arterial compartment or to suppress the release of norepinephrine, renin, aldosterone, and vasopressin, all of which contribute to renal sodium and water retention. Paradoxically, plasma levels of atrial natriuretic factor are markedly elevated in patients with severe ascites refractory to diuretics, but not to levels sufficient to overcome the antinatriuretic effects of the renin-angiotensin-aldosterone system.

Ascites indicates decompensated liver disease. The 5-year survival of patients with decompensated cirrhosis is 30 percent, compared with an 80 percent survival for those with compensated cirrhosis. Parameters that correlate with a poor prognosis include small liver size, malnutrition, low urine sodium concentration, high plasma norepinephrine level, low mean arterial pressure, and low glomerular filtration rate. Ascites contributes to the morbidity and mortality associated with cirrhosis by restricting ventilation and leading to umbilical hernias, peripheral venous stasis, and spontaneous bacterial peritonitis.

Management

In any patient with new or worsening ascites, it is important first to perform an abdominal paracentesis with fluid analysis to exclude spontaneous bacterial peritonitis, malignant ascites, chylous ascites, and ascites due to hepatic congestion. Table 1 outlines routine ascitic fluid tests that are helpful. The serum-ascites albumin gradient (SAAG) is a particularly useful marker of the presence or absence of portal hypertension. A SAAG greater than or equal to 1.1 g per deciliter is suggestive of portal hypertension, whereas a SAAG of less than 1.1 g per deciliter suggests that the ascites is not caused by portal hypertension.

Bed Rest and Low-Sodium Diet

Bed rest is advocated as an initial measure. Upright posture in patients with cirrhosis and ascites activates the renin-angiotensin and alpha-adrenergic systems, thereby increasing renal tubular sodium reabsorption. Theoretically, bed rest reduces the plasma renin concentration. Restriction of sodium is prescribed but alone is generally not sufficient therapy, except in outpatients with minimal ascites. Salt restriction to 1 g per day is recommended but is difficult, and many patients are unable to comply. Restriction of water to about 1,000–1,500 ml daily is necessary only if the serum sodium is less than 125 mEq per liter. Impaired water excretion in cirrhosis is due to nonosmotic hypersecretion of vasopressin, decreased delivery of filtrate to the distal tubule in the kidney, and changes in local prostaglandin metabolism in the kidney. Demeclocycline, which antagonizes the renal effects of antidiuretic hormone, may correct the impaired water excretion in these patients but frequently induces renal failure.

Diuretics

Spironolactone is generally the first diuretic agent that is used in the management of ascites. Spironolactone is a mild diuretic that is a specific aldosterone antagonist and spares renal potassium secretion. It induces diuresis in up to 75 to 80 percent of patients, but because of its long half-life and that of its active metabolites, the onset of action of spironolactone is slow. The usual starting dose is 100 to 200 mg per day, initially

Table 1 Ascitic Fluid Tests

Routine	Optional	Selected Cases
Cell count	Total protein for tuberculosis	Smear and culture
Albumin (1st tap)	Glucose	Cytology
Culture (inoculation in blood culture bottles)	Lactic dehydrogenase	Triglycerides
Gram's stain	Amylase	Bilirubin

in divided doses and then in a single daily dose. The dose can be increased by 100 mg every 3 to 5 days as needed up to a maximum of 400 to 600 mg per day, or until the urine sodium to potassium ratio is greater than 1. Potential deleterious side effects of spironolactone include hyperkalemia and painful gynecomastia.

Loop diuretics such as furosemide and bumetanide may be added in patients who respond partially to spironolactone. (Loop diuretics given alone are generally ineffective in the treatment of ascites.) Loop diuretics cause a 20 to 25 percent excretion of filtered sodium and increase the delivery of sodium to the distal tubule, where the ability to reabsorb sodium is exceeded. The usual starting dose of furosemide is 40 mg per day, and can be increased every 1 to 2 days to a maximum of 240 mg per day. Resistance to furosemide may result from impaired furosemide transport into renal tubules. Additionally, furosemide may result in a short-term, rapid decrease in renal perfusion, intravascular volume depletion, electrolyte abnormalities, and encephalopathy.

Thiazides act at the cortical diluting site and proximal tubule to promote natriuresis. In patients with ascites resistant to the aforementioned diuretics, the addition of thiazides may promote a synergistic effect. The usual starting dose of hydrochlorothiazide is 50 to 100 mg per day. Metolazone has the same effect and can be used at a dose of 5 to 10 mg per day.

Diuresis is safer in patients with peripheral edema associated with ascites than in those with ascites alone because of the preferential mobilization of edema. Conventionally, one should aim towards a weight loss of 1 to 2 kg per day in patients with ascites and peripheral edema, whereas a diuresis of 0.5 to 0.75 kg per day should be the goal in those with ascites alone. The urine sodium concentration is a helpful parameter to follow. When the baseline urine sodium is greater than 20 to 25 mEq per liter, treatment with low-dose spironolactone usually suffices. If the urine sodium concentration is in the range of 10 to 20 mEq per liter, high-dose spironolactone with or without low-dose furosemide will likely be required. Finally, when the urine sodium is less than 10 mEq per liter, high-dose spironolactone supplemented with furosemide and possibly thiazides will likely be needed. The dosing schedule requires individualization. A typical starting regimen is spironolactone 100 mg per day with or without furosemide 40 mg per day. The spironolactone can be increased by 100 mg per day and the furosemide by 40 mg per day every 3 to 5 days if no side effects are evident and natriuresis or weight loss have not been achieved. The combination of sodium restriction and diuretic therapy is effective in nearly 90 percent of patients with cirrhotic ascites. If weight loss does not ensue after a trial of maximal doses of diuretics, ascites is considered refractory to diuretic therapy.

Therapeutic Large-Volume Paracentesis

In the 1950s, large-volume paracentesis was the standard therapeutic modality for ascites. It fell out of favor in the 1960s because it was implicated as the cause of orthostatic hypotension, renal insufficiency, symptomatic hyponatremia, and hepatic encephalopathy, especially in cirrhotic patients without peripheral edema. These complications were ascribed to a reduction in intravascular volume due to rapid re-formation of ascites. However, reports of complications were based on limited numbers of patients, and in recent years large-volume paracentesis has re-emerged as a standard therapy for ascites.

In 1985, Kao et al. treated 18 patients with tense ascites and peripheral edema with a 5 L paracentesis, which resulted in relief of symptoms with no changes in plasma volume, electrolytes, or hemodynamics after 24 to 48 hours. Subsequent studies from the Barcelona group concluded that patients with tense ascites treated with large-volume paracentesis had shorter durations of hospitalization without an increase in the complication rate compared to those treated with diuretics. Their observations suggested that supplementation with intravenous albumin was necessary to decrease the frequency of electrolyte and renal disturbances associated with large-volume paracentesis. They and others also demonstrated that large-volume paracentesis could be done safely in patients with ascites but without peripheral edema. In 1987, Ginés et al. randomized 117 cirrhotic patients with tense ascites to large-volume paracentesis supplemented with intravenous albumin versus diuretic therapy alone; those who failed diuretics underwent placement of a peritoneovenous (LeVeen) shunt. There was no difference in survival between the two groups, but the complication rate was lower in the large-volume paracentesis group. Salerno et al., 1987 found that diuretics and large-volume paracentesis plus intravenous albumin were equally effective in mobilizing ascites in 41 patients but that the results were achieved more rapidly with large-volume paracentesis than with diuretics alone. More recently, there have been studies to indicate that tense ascites in cirrhosis can be treated with a single total paracentesis within 1 to 2 hours without adverse renal, hepatic, or hormonal effects, provided intravascular volume is expanded with intravenous albumin. Because of the expense of supplementation with intravenous albumin, alternative synthetic plasma expanders have also been investigated, including dextran-70 and Hemaccel, a polymerized synthetic gelatin, but further study is required before they can be recommended.

One mitigating effect of large-volume paracentesis is the potential to increase the risk of peritonitis. Diuresis has been shown to increase ascitic fluid opsonic activity as well as serum and ascitic fluid complement levels, thereby leading to protection from spontaneous bacterial peritonitis. By contrast, after large-volume paracentesis, ascitic fluid opsonic activity and complement levels remain stable, but serum complement levels decrease, thereby potentially increasing the risk of spontaneous bacterial peritonitis.

In general, repeated large-volume paracentesis of 4 to 6 L per tap supplemented with intravenous albumin (10 gm per liter of ascites removed) is considered the treatment of choice for tense cirrhotic ascites. Compared to diuretic therapy, large-volume paracentesis is hemodynamically safe, shortens the duration of hospitalization, and does not increase the readmission rate to the hospital. Large-volume paracentesis should be considered specifically in patients with respiratory compromise, impending rupture of an umbilical hernia, and severe peripheral venous stasis. It is also appropriate therapy in patients with ascites and peripheral edema and in those with ascites refractory to diuretics. Whether or not large-volume paracentesis is performed, those patients who excrete high amounts of sodium in the urine benefit from salt-restriction and diuretics in the conventional fashion.

The effectiveness of beta blocker therapy in the management of ascites has not been clearly demonstrated, despite the value of beta blockers in decreasing portal venous pressure and preventing variceal bleeding. Certain other medications must be specifically avoided in patients with cirrhotic ascites. These include prostaglandin inhibitors and angiotensin converting enzyme inhibitors. Prostaglandin inhibitors diminish the renal synthesis of vasodilatory prostaglandins (PGE_2 and PGI_2), may adversely affect renal function and natriuresis, and may decrease the natriuretic response to furosemide. Angiotensin converting enzyme inhibitors reduce urinary sodium excretion and lower blood pressure. Other drugs to avoid in patients with cirrhotic ascites include aminoglycosides, which are especially nephrotoxic, and metoclopramide, which may stimulate aldosterone production.

Peritoneovenous Shunt

A variety of therapeutic modalities may be considered in patients with ascites refractory to diuretics (Table 2). Head-out water immersion (HWI) is an effective treatment in some patients with refractory ascites and acts by expanding central blood volume and suppressing renin, aldosterone, vasopressin, and norepinephrine because of reflex vasodilatation. However, use of HWI is cumbersome and is advocated primarily in developing countries where other measures may be too costly.

Peritoneovenous shunts may be considered when large-volume paracentesis and diuretics have failed. The two types of peritoneovenous shunts are the LeVeen and Denver shunts. The LeVeen shunt consists of a perfo-

Table 2 Therapeutic Modalities for Refractory Ascites

Large-volume paracentesis
Head-out water immersion
Peritoneovenous shunt: LeVeen, Denver
Transjugular intrahepatic portosystemic stent shunt (TIPS)
Portosystemic surgical shunt
Liver transplantation

Table 3 Common Complications of Peritoneovenous Shunts

Consumption coagulopathy
Infection
Volume overload
Shunt occlusion

rated intra-abdominal tube connected through a one-way pressure-sensitive valve to a silicone tube that traverses the subcutaneous tissue up to the neck and enters one of the jugular veins. The tip of the intravenous tube is positioned in the superior vena cava near the right atrium or in the right atrium itself. When intraperitoneal pressure exceeds venous pressure by 3 to 5 cm H_2O, the valve opens and ascitic fluid flows into the circulation. Mobilization of ascitic fluid by the LeVeen shunt is associated with continuous expansion of the intravascular compartment. The Denver shunt has a valve which opens at a pressure gradient lower than that of the LeVeen shunt or when the pumping chamber is externally compressed. The Denver shunt was designed to create turbulence within the valve so as to reduce the likelihood of valve obstruction, which is frequently observed with the LeVeen shunt, but the frequency of obstruction of the two shunts is similar. Patients with high protein ascites seem to be particularly prone to shunt obstruction.

Peritoneovenous shunts relieve ascites while simultaneously correcting most of the hemodynamic and renal alterations occurring in these patients. They increase plasma volume and cardiac index; reduce plasma renin activity and plasma levels of aldosterone, norepinephrine, and vasopressin; and lead to a reduction in portal venous pressure, as estimated by the hepatic venous pressure gradient. Immediately after insertion of a peritoneovenous shunt, central volume fluid overload is commonly observed and supplemental furosemide is routinely administered.

The complication rate of the peritoneovenous shunts is high (Table 3). Foremost among the complications are a consumptive coagulopathy caused by delivery of plasmin, plasminogen activator, thromboplastin, and fibrin degradation products to the systemic circulation, and infection, which usually requires removal of the shunt. Recurrent or persistent ascites may result from cardiac and renal failure, decreased shunt flow, or shunt occlusion. Doppler ultrasonography or scintigraphy after the intraperitoneal injection of radioactive technetium will demonstrate the absence of flow through an occluded shunt. Insertion of a 3 cm long titanium tip into the venous limb of the LeVeen shunt is of value in preventing superior vena cava thrombosis. A new heparin-coated Denver shunt has also been advocated for similar purposes.

While peritoneovenous shunts are effective for the initial relief of ascites, long-term efficacy has not been established and ultimate patient survival is not improved. In one large study by Stanley et al., 1989, 299 alcoholic cirrhotic patients with ascites were randomized to medical treatment or LeVeen shunting. LeVeen shunting was associated with more rapid resolution of disabling ascites and a longer time to recurrence of ascites. However, survival was not improved by shunting and correlated instead with the severity of the underlying liver disease. Peritoneovenous shunting has not been compared in a similar fashion with large-volume paracentesis.

Transjugular Intrahepatic Portosystemic Stent Shunts

Recently, a transjugular intrahepatic portosystemic shunt using an expandable metal stent (TIPS) has been introduced as a simple, safe, fast, and inexpensive method of creating a portosystemic shunt without the need for surgery. TIPS is already being used widely in the management of gastroesophageal variceal hemorrhage. Because TIPS functions as a side-to-side portacaval anastomosis, it is of potential value in the management of ascites and the hepatorenal syndrome. Preliminary reports indicate that after placement of a TIPS, ascites disappears or is ameliorated. Clinical improvement is accompanied by an increase in creatinine clearance and improvement in nutritional status. By reducing portal venous pressure and blood flow through esophageal varices, the risk of bleeding from varices is also substantially reduced. TIPS is a particularly attractive procedure for seriously ill patients awaiting liver transplantation. See the separate chapter on TIPS for more information.

Reports of complications of TIPS have begun to appear. The most frequent complication is hepatic encephalopathy, which affects 10 to 20 percent of patients but tends to be mild and easily managed. The second most common complication is stent stenosis, which occurs in 5 to 15 percent of patients and progresses to occlusion in 5 to 10 percent of patients. Other complications include embolization of the stent to the pulmonary artery, puncture of the gallbladder, liver capsule rupture, hemobilia, intraperitoneal hemorrhage, contrast-induced transient oliguric kidney failure, bacteremia, septic shock, and fever. TIPS may be considered in selected patients with ascites, but determining its final place in the treatment of refractory ascites will require studies comparing TIPS with peritoneovenous shunting and other treatment options.*

*****Editor's Note:** Very few of the San Francisco series patients underwent TIPS because of ascites, but several who had ascites did respond.

Other Modalities

Portosystemic surgical shunts are used as a last resort in the management of refractory ascites. A side-to-side portacaval shunt decompresses both the splanchnic and hepatic sinusoidal bed and is therefore advantageous when compared to the end-to-side portacaval shunt, which decompresses the splanchnic bed but not the hepatic sinusoids. In selected patients with refractory ascites, liver transplantation may also be considered.

COMPLICATIONS OF ASCITES AND THEIR MANAGEMENT

Spontaneous Bacterial Peritonitis

Spontaneous bacterial peritonitis (SBP) may be defined as the occurrence of bacterial peritonitis in patients with ascites in the absence of a demonstrable cause of peritonitis, such as bowel perforation or intra-abdominal abscess. Among patients with cirrhotic ascites, the frequency of SBP is 10 to 27 percent. In liver units dedicated to the treatment of ascites, SBP may be diagnosed as many as three times a day and at least once a week. SBP classically occurs in patients with alcoholic cirrhosis, and, initially, it was thought that there was a special relationship between alcoholic cirrhosis and SBP. However, SBP has been reported in patients with a variety of liver disorders, including acute viral hepatitis, chronic active hepatitis, postnecrotic cirrhosis, submassive hepatic necrosis, Wilson's disease, and alpha$_1$ antitrypsin deficiency. The unifying feature of conditions that predispose to SBP is a low protein concentration in the ascitic fluid. Patients who have ascites with a high protein concentration (e.g., ascites due to heart failure or peritoneal carcinomatosis) are unlikely to develop SBP.

Other host factors predisposing to SBP include the severity of the underlying acute or chronic liver disease, which is reflected in reticuloendothelial dysfunction, neutrophil dysfunction, complement deficiency, and impairment in opsonization. Procedures that may predispose to SBP include paracentesis, bladder catheterization, nasogastric intubation, tooth extraction, endoscopic procedures including variceal sclerotherapy, and insertion of LeVeen shunts. Seeding of ascitic fluid generally occurs as a result of hematogenous transmission of organisms from the intestinal lumen or from an extra-intestinal focus of infection. Common causative organisms include *Streptococcus pneumoniae,* group D streptococci, alpha-hemolytic streptococci, and gram-negative enteric organisms, whereas anaerobes rarely cause SBP.

Patients with SBP are usually men with a mean age of 50 years and severe advanced hepatic disease (varices, splenomegaly, and jaundice in greater than 85 to 90 percent of patients). The clinical features of SBP include ascites, fever, new-onset or worsening encephalopathy, abdominal pain, rebound abdominal tenderness, decreased or absent bowel sounds, and hypotension. In 10 percent of cases, fever and abdominal pain are absent, and in 30 percent of patients only subtle findings are observed, including mild hepatic encephalopathy, back pain, hypothermia, refractoriness to diuretics, and deteriorating renal function.

The diagnosis of SBP is supported by the characteristics of the ascitic fluid on paracentesis. The fluid may be cloudy and the protein content is typically low. The most reliable indicator of SBP is an ascitic fluid polymorphonuclear leukocyte (PMN) count of greater than 250 per cubic millimeter in association with characteristic clinical features. Even in the absence of signs and symptoms of SBP, an ascitic fluid PMN count of more than 500 per cubic millimeter strongly suggests SBP. Gram's stain is positive in 30 to 70 percent of centrifuged ascitic fluid specimens. It is important to submit the ascitic fluid for bacterial culture and, if indicated, cultures for tuberculosis. When ascitic fluid from patients with suspected SBP is inoculated into blood culture bottles at the bedside, up to 90 percent of specimens yield a positive diagnosis. Occasionally, blood cultures are positive while ascitic fluid cultures are negative.

Spontaneous bacterial peritonitis must be distinguished from secondary bacterial peritonitis. Features that suggest secondary bacterial peritonitis include an initial ascitic fluid white blood cell count of greater than 10,000 per cubic millimeter, an ascitic fluid protein concentration of greater than 2 per deciliter and multiple bacterial pathogens, including anaerobes.

The treatment of choice for SBP is now cefotaxime 2 g intravenously every 8 hours, pending culture results. Alternatively, amoxicillin-clavulanic acid may be used. Cefotaxime is preferable to regimens that include aminoglycosides, which are potentially nephrotoxic. Treatment is generally continued for up to 10 to 14 days, and paracentesis should be repeated after 48 hours of therapy to confirm a decline in the ascitic fluid PMN count by at least 50 percent.

The mortality of SBP in earlier reports was 80 to 90 percent. In more recent times, mortality rates of 30 to 40 percent have been reported. Adverse prognostic factors include a serum bilirubin level greater than 8 mg per deciliter, serum albumin less than 2.5 g per deciliter, serum creatinine greater than 2.1 mg per deciliter, hepatic encephalopathy, and the development of hepatorenal syndrome. Recurrence of SBP is common in patients surviving one episode, with an approximately 70 percent recurrence rate at 1 year and a high mortality rate. Recent studies suggest that the risk of recurrent SBP can be decreased greatly by the long-term prophylactic use of norfloxacin 400 mg orally once a day. In selected high-risk patients (e.g., those undergoing variceal sclerotherapy), first episodes of SBP may be prevented by initiating therapy with norfloxacin 400 mg once daily.

Hepatorenal Syndrome

The hepatorenal syndrome, the most severe alteration of renal function that occurs in patients with cirrhosis and ascites, is defined as the development of azotemia and oliguria in the absence of any known cause of renal failure. The kidneys are histologically normal or show minimal findings to account for impairment in renal function. Retrospective studies indicate that the hepatorenal syndrome is present in more than 15 percent of patients admitted to the hospital with cirrhosis and ascites. The condition is believed to be a consequence of active renal vasoconstriction leading to impaired renal perfusion and a decrease in the glomerular filtration rate. Contributory pathogenic factors include elevated thromboxane and endothelin levels, impaired renal kallikrein production, and diminished renal synthesis of vasodilating prostaglandins.

The prognosis of hepatorenal syndrome is poor. Attempts to improve renal function in patients with hepatorenal syndrome have included the infusion of renal vasodilators or prostaglandin excretion modifiers and insertion of a peritoneovenous shunt, but in most cases these measures are unsuccessful. In selected cases, patients with the hepatorenal syndrome may be considered for liver transplantation.

SUGGESTED READING

Badalamenti S, Graziani G, Salerno F, Ponticelli C. Hepatorenal syndrome: new perspectives in pathogenesis and treatment. Arch Intern Med 1993; 153:1957–1967.

Ginés P, Arroyo V, Rodés J. Pharmacotherapy of ascites associated with cirrhosis. Drugs 1992; 43:316–332.

Kellerman PS, Linas SL. Large-volume paracentesis in treatment of ascites. Ann Intern Med 1990; 112:889–891.

Moskovitz M. The peritoneovenous shunt: expectations and reality. Am J Gastroenterol 1990; 85:917–929.

Runyon BA. Spontaneous bacterial peritonitis: an explosion of information. Hepatology 1988; 8:171–175.

Schrier RW, Arroyo V, Bernardi M, et al. Peripheral arterial vasodilatation hypothesis: a proposal for the initiation of renal sodium and water retention in cirrhosis. Hepatology 1988; 8:1151–1157.

Warner L, Sorecki K, Blendis L, Epstein M. Atrial natriuretic factor and liver disease. Hepatology 1993; 17:500–513.

ASCITES AND SPONTANEOUS BACTERIAL PERITONITIS

WILLIAM G. RECTOR, Jr., M.D.

ASCITES

Ascites formation in patients with chronic liver disease is one of the most common management problems faced by the hepatologist.

Therapeutic Alternatives

The main methods of treatment are large volume paracentesis, diuretic treatment, and liver transplantation.

Large-Volume Paracentesis

This is the simplest and most direct way to remove ascites. However, it is unsuited to the long-term management of ascites because the diseased liver is often unable to synthesize sufficient protein to replace what has been removed. Thus, paracentesis is principally used for the acute relief of tense ascites.

When large volume paracentesis is performed, as much fluid as possible—ideally all—should be removed. Some employ administration of 50 g of albumin to prevent the minor disturbances of electrolyte and renal

Supported by Public Health Service Grants 1-R29AA07832 and M01-RR00051.

function observed in some patients after large volume paracentesis. However, albumin is expensive, and these biochemical changes have not translated into important complications. Accordingly, I do not use albumin.

Patients with edema will mobilize this extravascular fluid after large volume paracentesis as pressure in the inferior vena cava falls in parallel with intra-abdominal pressure. The resultant expansion in plasma volume causes ascites to re-form rapidly. This overflow of an expanded plasma compartment into ascites does not lead to vascular depletion and renal failure. Patients who re-form ascites from edema simply require further paracentesis or transition to diuretic therapy.

Diuretics

Diuretic therapy is the basis of the long-term management of ascites. The main mechanism by which diuretics mobilize ascites is diminished formation, although increased rates of reabsorption may occur in some patients. The reason diuretics diminish ascites formation is unknown; it is not due to reductions in portal pressure or plasma volume. Increased hepatic lymph flow may contribute.

Diuretic therapy should be instituted with the patient consuming his usual diet. An effective regimen of diuretics when the patient is consuming a minimal amount of sodium in the hospital may become ineffective when intake rises substantially at home. Water restriction is usually unnecessary. Serum sodium concentrations above 125 mEq per liter are well tolerated by patients with cirrhosis. Diuretic requirements will decline in patients with reversible liver disease. For example, alcoholic hepatitis is usually accompanied by sodium retention and ascites formation. However, after months of abstinence, accompanied by improvement in signs of liver disease, sodium excretion often returns to normal; and diuretics should be discontinued. Sodium retention in patients with untreatable forms of liver disease may be expected to remain constant or worsen. Finally, daily weight loss should not exceed 0.5 to 1.0 kg when peripheral edema has resolved and only ascites remains. More rapid weight loss results in plasma volume contraction and renal insufficiency. However, this is reversible when diuretic therapy is discontinued. There is no evidence that nonexcessive diuresis precipitates hepatorenal syndrome.

A variety of diuretics have been used in the treatment of ascites.

Spironolactone, which competitively inhibits the action of aldosterone, produces natriuresis in most patients when given in doses of 100 to 300 mg daily. Up to 1 g or more a day can be given with increasing efficacy to refractory patients. Mild hyperkalemia is commonly observed in patients given high doses of the drug. Significant elevations of the serum potassium concentration may occur in patients with renal insufficiency and in patients who are consuming large amounts of potassium. An often unappreciated source of potassium is artificial salt. Spironolactone is the diuretic of choice in patients with gout, as its use does not elevate serum uric acid levels. Because of its structural resemblance to estrogens, spironolactone may cause painful gynecomastia in some patients. This usually resolves weeks to months after the diuretic is discontinued.

Amiloride and triamterene also are distally-acting, potassium-sparing diuretic agents. They differ from spironolactone in having half-lives of only a few hours; also, they do not competitively inhibit the action of aldosterone. Twenty milligrams of amiloride daily is approximately equivalent in efficacy to approximately 100 mg of spironolactone. As with spironolactone, hyperkalemia may be encountered in patients with renal insufficiency and in patients with a high dietary intake of potassium.

Diuretics that act by inhibiting reabsorption of sodium in the loop of Henle are important in the management of ascites. Furosemide is the principal "loop diuretic" in clinical practice. Furosemide reaches the tubule by both glomerular filtration and tubular secretion and acts from its luminal side. Furosemide normally causes renal blood flow and glomerular filtration rate to increase, perhaps by a prostaglandin-mediated mechanism. Thus, the hemodynamic effects of the drug complement its natriuretic actions. Glomerular filtration rate may not rise or may even fall in response to furosemide in some patients, reducing the filtered load of sodium and its delivery to the loop of Henle. This may be an important mechanism of "diuretic-resistance."

The avidity of the distal tubule and collecting ducts for sodium is increased in patients with ascites. Therefore, sodium not reabsorbed in the loop of Henle is taken up at these avid distal sites, and the natriuretic effect of furosemide is blunted or even lost altogether. Moreover,

as potassium and hydrogen ions are excreted in greater amounts in company with sodium reabsorption, the diminution of diuretic effect is accompanied by a reciprocal worsening of hypokalemia and alkalosis.

Thiazide diuretics and metolazone inhibit sodium reabsorption in the cortical diluting segment of the tubule. Because still more distal sites of sodium reabsorption exist, antinatriuretic efficacy of these agents is blunted when they are used alone, and hypokalemia and alkalosis are frequent complications.

Given in combination, potassium-sparing and potassium-wasting diuretics are highly effective forms of treatment for patients with sodium retention. Side-effects are neutralized, and natriuretic efficacy enhanced. Usually a potassium-sparing agent is given with furosemide. A typical regimen is furosemide (20–160 mg) plus either spironolactone (50–200 mg) or amiloride (10–20 mg). A combination of three diuretics (a loop diuretic, a potassium-sparing agent, and low doses of a thiazide diuretic) will usually produce natriuresis even in patients resistant to two diuretics. Indeed, patients in whom a thiazide is added as a third agent must be observed carefully for excessive weight loss.

Diuretic-Resistant Ascites. A few patients are refractory to diuretic treatment. Causes of "refractoriness" include resistance to natriuresis and accompaniment of even minimal natriuresis by either renal insufficiency or encephalopathy. Some patients are "refractory" as a result of massive salt intake.

Liver transplantation should be considered in all patients with diuretic-resistant ascites. Peritoneovenous shunt may be effective initially, but the morbidity and mortality of the operation and the high incidence of shunt malfunction counterbalance its advantages. Repeated large-volume paracentesis is probably the best and safest method of managing preterminal patients and patients whose liver disease and sodium retention may be expected to improve with time.

The aim of treatment of hepatic hydrothorax is to gain control of sodium retention and ascites formation with diuretics. Diuretic-resistant patients with this additional complication are difficult to manage and may require thoracotomy to close the defect in the diaphragm. Again, liver transplantation should be considered in these difficult patients.

Liver Transplantation

Because ascites usually accompanies advanced liver disease, liver transplantation should be considered in patients in whom it occurs. When ascites is an isolated phenomenon and easily managed, the patient may simply be observed. However, such patients should be monitored closely for deterioration, especially if the waiting time for transplantation exceeds 6 months. There are two chapters on this subject.

Transjugular Intrahepatic Portosystemic Shunt (TIPS)

In TIPS, a stent is inserted by the radiologist between the hepatic and portal veins within the liver, producing a small-diameter, intrahepatic portal-systemic shunt. Portal pressure is thereby reduced, although usually not to normal.

Early reports suggest that TIPS improves sodium handling in many patients with ascites. However, until further data become available, particularly with respect to the nature and duration of the response and the associated complications, this procedure should remain experimental. There is a separate chapter on this subject.

SPONTANEOUS BACTERIAL PERITONITIS

Spontaneous bacterial peritonitis (SBP) is the most serious complication of ascites formation. Earlier recognition and improved therapy have resulted in better survival. Even today, however, over a third of patients with this infection die.

Ascites infection may be divided into several categories based upon the ascites polymorphonuclear (PMN) cell count and the results of culture (Table 1). Culture-negative neutrocytic ascites usually occurs either in patients with SBP in whom antibiotics already have been administered or patients in whom optimal culture methods (bedside inoculation of blood culture bottles) have not been used. Monomicrobial bacterascites represents either early or transient ascites infection. Polymicrobial bacterascites indicates that bowel contents have been inadvertently sampled with the needle. Secondary bacterial peritonitis is ascites infection due to gut perforation.

The usual flora of SBP are facultative gram-negative aerobes and gram-positive streptococci (Table 2). Noteworthy because of their rarity are enterococci, staphylococci, and anaerobes.

Therapeutic Alternatives

SBP is treated with antibiotics. All five categories of ascites infection may be treated. Physicians who wish simply to observe patients with monomicrobial bacterascites or polymicrobial bacterascites are obliged to repeat the paracentesis in 24 to 48 hours to assess the course of the infection.

Preferred Approach

SBP should be treated with cefotaxime 2 g intravenously three times daily for 5 days. Aminoglycosides should be avoided. Calculation of the appropriate dose is difficult owing to distortion of body mass by excess fluid. Also, muscle mass is reduced in patients with cirrhosis. Moreover, renal function may be labile. For these reasons, the serum creatinine concentration may not be an accurate reflection of glomerular filtration rate. Also, patients with cirrhosis may be abnormally sensitive to the nephrotoxic effects of aminoglycosides. Follow-up paracentesis should be done in patients who do not have a rapid clinical response to treatment. The ascites PMN count falls exponentially in adequately treated patients.

Polymicrobial bacterascites and secondary bacterial

Table 1 Usual Flora of Spontaneous Bacterial Peritonitis (SBP)

Organisms	Frequency
Enterobacteriaceae	Common
Non-group D streptococci	Common
Group D streptococci	Uncommon
Staphylococcus aureus	Rare
Anaerobes	Rare

Table 2 Categories of Spontaneous Bacterial Peritonitis (SBP)

Category	Ascites PMN Count	Culture	Organisms
SBP	>250/ml	Positive	One
Culture-negative neutrocytic ascites	>250/ml	Negative	None
Monomicrobial bacterascites	<250/ml	Positive	One
Polymicrobial bacterascites	<250/ml	Positive	Many
Secondary bacterial peritonitis	>250/ml	Positive	Many

PMN = polymorphonuclear neutrophil leukocytes.

peritonitis also require coverage for anaerobes, for example with metronidazole.

Antibiotic therapy is modified appropriately when culture and sensitivity information become available.

Prevention

Prevention has recently been recognized as an important measure. SBP usually arises as a result of seeding of ascites during transient bacteremia. The commonest and most important cause of bactermia in the hospital is catheterization of the bladder. Urinary catheters should be scrupulously avoided in patients with cirrhosis. Infections elsewhere such as cellulitis and pneumonia can also lead to SBP and should be aggressively treated. Severe upper gastrointestinal bleeding is associated with a heightened risk of ascites infection, perhaps as a result of the extensive instrumentation undergone by such patients.

A protein concentration of ascites less than 1 g per deciliter is also associated with enhanced risk of SBP, probably as a result of diminished concentration of opsonins. Diuretic therapy raises the protein concentration of ascites and may help prevent SBP.

The role of continuous oral prophylactic therapy with quinolone antibiotics in patients with recurrent SBP is not fully defined, but early reports suggest it to be safe and effective.

SUGGESTED READING

Cabrera J, Arroyo V, Ballesta AM, et al. Aminoglycoside nephrotoxicity in cirrhosis. Gastroenterology 1982; 82:97–105.

Campra JL, Reynolds TB. Effectiveness of high-dose spirolactone therapy in patients with chronic liver disease and relatively refractory ascites. Dig Dis Sci 1978; 23:1025–1030.

Felisart J, Rimola A, Arroyo V, et al. Randomized comparative study of efficacy and nephrotoxicity of ampicillin plus tobramycin versus cefotaxime in cirrhotics with severe infection. Hepatology 1985; 5:457–462.

Ginés P, Tito LI, Arroyo V, et al. Randomized comparative study of therapeutic paracentesis with and without intravenous albumin in cirrhosis. Gastroenterology 1988; 94:1493–1502.

Gregory PB, Broekelschen PH, Hill MD, et al. Complications of diuresis in the alcoholic patients with ascites. Gastroenterology 1977; 73:534–538.

McHutchinson JG, Pinto PC, Reynolds TB. Hydrochlorothiazide as a third diuretic in cirrhosis with refractory ascites. Hepatology 1989; 10:719.

Perez-Ayuso RM, Arroyo V, Planas R, et al. Randomized comparative study of efficacy of furosemide vs spironolactone in nonazotemic cirrhosis with ascites. Gastroenterology 1983; 84:978–986.

Pinto PC, Amerian J, Reynolds TB. Large-volume paracentesis in nonedematous patients with tense ascites. Hepatology 1988; 8:207–211.

Pockros PJ, Reynolds TB. Rapid diuresis in patients with chronic liver disease: the importance of peripheral edema. Gastroenterology 1986; 90:1827–1833.

Runyon BA, Hoefs JC. Ascitic fluid analysis before, during, and after spontaneous bacterial peritonitis. Hepatology 1985; 5:257–259.

Runyon BA, McHutchison JG, Antillon MR, et al. Short-course vs long-course antibiotic treatment of spontaneous bacterial peritonitis. Gastroenterology 1991; 100:1737–1742.

Runyon BA, Umland ET, Merlin T. Inoculation of blood culture bottles with ascitic fluid: improved detection of spontaneous bacterial peritonitis. Arch Intern Med 1987; 147:73–75.

HEPATIC ENCEPHALOPATHY

ANDRES T. BLEI, M.D.
BARRY FINN, M.D.

A classification of hepatic encephalopathy (Table 1) is not a mere semantic exercise. The management of changes in mental state varies according to the acute or chronic nature of the hepatic disorder. This distinction may require a vigorous diagnostic effort for patients in whom hepatic encephalopathy is the presenting symptom. In fulminant hepatic failure, where a massive necrosis of liver cells is present, severe encephalopathy carries a grave prognosis and the presence of brain edema and intracranial hypertension requires measures seldom used in patients with chronic liver disease. In cirrhosis, liver failure and portal-systemic shunting contribute in a variable degree to the development of encephalopathy, but the appearance of a precipitating factor should always be sought. It is unknown whether chronic hepatic encephalopathy, a fearsome complication of portacaval shunt surgery, will become a clinical problem in patients receiving transjugular intrahepatic portal-systemic stents (TIPS). While the need to treat subclinical encephalopathy is still controversial, consideration may be warranted if subtle coordination abnormalities are detected.

Optimal treatment of hepatic encephalopathy should be based on a thorough knowledge of the

Table 1 Classification of Hepatic Encephalopathy

I. Associated with cirrhosis
  A. Acute portal-systemic encephalopathy
    1. Precipitant induced
      Gastrointestinal bleeding
      Uremia
      Sedatives
      Dietary indiscretion
      Infection
      Constipation
      Hypokalemia
    2. Spontaneous encephalopathy
  B. Chronic hepatic encephalopathy
    1. Chronic recurrent
    2. Hepatocerebral degeneration
  C. Subclinical encephalopathy

II. Associated with fulminant hepatic failure
  A. Stages similar to encephalopathy of chronic disease: lethargy (mania), confusion, stupor, coma
  B. Brain edema evolving to intracranial hypertension

Table 2 Pathogenesis of Hepatic Encephalopathy: Neurotoxins and Postulated Mechanisms

I. Ammonia may act via multiple mechanisms
  A. Direct neurotoxicity
  B. Generation of glutamine (osmotic effect)
  C. Alterations in neurotransmission
    1. Glutamatergic (excitatory)
    2. Serotoninergic (inhibitory)

II. Synergistic neurotoxins potentiate the effects of ammonia
  Mercaptans, short-chain fatty acids, phenols

III. Generation of false neurotransmitters
  A. Entry of aromatic amino acids into the brain is favored by:
    1. Lower levels of plasma branched-chain amino acids
    2. Exchange for brain glutamine, generated from ammonia metabolism
  B. Phenylalanine, tyrosine are precursors of dopamine, catecholamines
    1. Generation of "false" neurotransmitters, e.g. octopamine
    2. Alterations in dopaminergic neurotransmission

IV. GABA-endogenous benzodiazepines
  A. Binding of endogenous benzodiazepines to $GABA_A$ receptor
  B. The nature of the endogenous benzodiazepine is controversial
    1. Diazepam, desmethyldiazepam
    2. Other compounds (endozepines)

pathophysiology of this syndrome. Clinical experience has taught that hepatic encephalopathy arises from gut-derived toxins which gain access to the systemic circulation in the presence of portal-systemic shunts (hence the term portal-systemic encephalopathy, PSE). Precipitating factors that induce coma in fact represent a large load of these putative toxins. However, many views exist as to the nature of these compounds and the mechanisms by which neurotoxicity occurs (Table 2). This has led to the testing of therapeutic agents that specifically antagonize these candidate toxins. Thus, clinical results become the arbiter of the validity of these hypotheses. With all the difficulties in studying brain metabolism in humans, the clinician's experience becomes an invaluable tool to advance research in this area.

ACUTE ENCEPHALOPATHY IN CIRRHOSIS

Search for Precipitating Cause

When cirrhotic patients develop alterations in consciousness, a precipitating factor must be sought (Table 3). Gastrointestinal (GI) hemorrhage, uremia and ingestion of sedatives are the most common factors. In addition, infection and electrolyte disturbances (especially hypokalemia) may be present. In some individuals, excess protein in the diet is enough to cause encephalopathy. Diuretics may result in volume contraction, a rise in blood urea nitrogen and hypokalemia, factors known to usher in changes in mental state.

When the precipitating factor is not clinically obvious, active testing should be pursued. This may include passage of a nasogastric tube to exclude hemorrhage, abdominal paracentesis to rule out an infected ascitic fluid as well as analysis of urinary sediment and renal ultrasonography in cases with abnormal kidney function. Treatment of the precipitating factor should be immediately started. Volume replacement, antibiotic treatment or specific sedative antagonism (in the case of opiates or benzodiazepines) may reverse the encephalopathic state. Although most patients hyperventilate with a primary respiratory alkalosis and have evidence of functional intrapulmonary shunts, oxygen via a nasal cannula is recommended as hypoxemia is common in cirrhosis and may aggravate the effects of the other precipitants. Intravenous fluid should be replaced with

Table 3 Management of Episode of Acute Encephalopathy

1. Removal of precipitating agent (see Table 1)
2. Lactulose
   a) By enema, 300 ml in 700 ml of water
   b) Orally, 30 ml q hour until bowel movement; then 15 to 45 ml q.i.d.
3. If unable to use lactulose, neomycin 2 to 4 g/day or metronidazole (250 mg b.i.d.-t.i.d. in the presence of renal insufficiency)
4. When able to be fed, protein is started at 40 g/day

attention to electrolyte imbalance and volume status. Hypokalemia and/or hypomagnesemia (in the case of diuretic-induced encephalopathy) and intravascular volume depletion with sodium retention (as manifested by ascites and peripheral edema) may be present.

Episodes of encephalopathy, in the absence of a clear precipitating event, have been reported in patients with large spontaneous splenorenal shunts. Patients with acute alcoholic hepatitis and spontaneous encephalopathy are a subgroup whose liver disease, in the appropriate setting, responds to corticosteroids.

General Measures

Catharsis

An increase in stool frequency is a general measure to decrease the neurotoxin load arising from the gut. It acquires special importance in cases with GI bleeding, where blood in the colonic lumen may persist for days. It can be achieved via oral agents (such as lactulose) when the patient is able to swallow; oral mannitol (100 g per liter gastric lavage) has also been administered to patients with GI hemorrhage. In cases with coma, drug administration via a nasogastric tube may be necessary, with appropriate care of the airway. Cleansing enemas with tap water, in the absence of stool acidification, are of limited value.

Dietary Management

When patients are acutely encephalopathic, provision of adequate calories with intravenous dextrose is sufficient. As soon as the patient is able to tolerate oral intake, patients should be fed and protein should not be restricted to values below 0.5 g per kilogram in order to maintain body stores. It is preferable to add another medication rather than curtail protein intake. The provision of branched-chain amino acids in an intravenous formulation (30 to 40 percent of total amino acids) has been tested in cirrhotic patients with acute encephalopathy. The results are equivocal and do not warrant its use in view of their cost.

Nonabsorbable Disaccharides

These compounds benefit patients with hepatic encephalopathy via multiple mechanisms. Fermentation of the sugar by colonic bacteria results in acidification of the colonic lumen, favoring the passage of ammonia from the bloodstream, which is used by bacteria as a nitrogen source. As a consequence of this fermentation, hepatic ureagenesis is decreased. The formation of octanoic acid in the colonic lumen, implicated in the pathogenesis of encephalopathy, is reduced. Colonic acidification promotes catharsis, providing an additional mechanism of action. For patients in coma, lactulose (a synthetic disaccharide composed of fructose-galactose) does not result in immediate beneficial effects. Using a protocol where 30 ml of lactulose is administered hourly until a loose bowel movement is obtained, followed by dosing every 6 hours, 48 to 60 hours elapses before arousal occurs. For patients in whom a more rapid effect is desired, lactulose enemas (300 ml in 700 ml of water) can be administered to be retained over 1 to 2 hours, with the patient in Trendelenburg position to favor passage into the right colon.

Once the patient is awake, oral lactulose is supplied at doses of 15 to 45 ml two to four times daily, aiming for two to three loose bowel movements per day. Abdominal cramping and flatulencè is common. Excessive diarrhea may result in hypertonic dehydration due to the hypotonic nature of colonic fluid. Hypernatremia with associated hyperosmolarity can induce changes in mental state and lead to the erroneous conclusion that further therapy with lactulose is necessary.

Patients who are lactase-deficient which is common in certain parts of the world, can receive lactose as oral therapy. Lactose enemas will be effective regardless of the small bowel enzyme content. Lactitol (a new synthetic disaccharide) appears as effective as lactulose and is associated with better patient tolerance, as the taste is more palatable and appears to result in less abdominal cramping. Lactitol is currently unavailable in the United States.

Antibiotics

Antibiotic therapy is designed to reduce the population of urease-containing bacteria in the colonic lumen. Recent animal studies raise the possibility that the small bowel may be an additional target. In the case of neomycin, the activity of mucosal glutaminase may be reduced by the drug, thus decreasing the generation of ammonia from the small intestine. Neomycin is useful in acute episodes, with doses of 2 to 4 g per day, in divided doses. Although poorly absorbed, 1 to 3 percent of the dose reaches the systemic circulation, and as an aminoglycoside, its use in renal failure is not recommended. Diarrhea, fungal infections and a malabsorption picture are potential complications. Once the precipitating factor is removed, therapy should not be prolonged beyond 1 month.

Metronidazole also appears effective as a measure to reverse PSE. The drug undergoes extensive hepatic metabolism and should be started at a lower dose, 250 mg twice daily, in patients with cirrhosis. Side-effects include an Antabuse-like reaction to alcohol ingestion, peripheral neuropathy, and nausea. Oral vancomycin is an expensive choice and has no role in management. The combination of lactulose and neomycin appears theoretically contradictory in face of the need for colonic bacteria to ferment the nonabsorbed sugar. However, anaerobic species appear to mediate the latter effect and these are not affected by neomycin. Clinical studies have shown effects of combination therapy on nitrogen metabolism that are expected when ammonia moves to the colonic lumen: an increase in fecal nitrogen and a reduction of hepatic ureagenesis. Uncontrolled clinical

testing has also shown efficacy and the combination can be used in face of the failure of either drug alone.

A comment is due on clinical trials in acute hepatic encephalopathy. These are extremely difficult to control, as removal of the precipitating factor is occurring at the same time that therapy is being administered. Different precipitating factors imply a different set of circumstances that require different therapeutic maneuvers. In fact, using rigid criteria, no therapy in acute encephalopathy has been compared to a true placebo.

CHRONIC ENCEPHALOPATHY IN CIRRHOSIS

Patients with chronic encephalopathy seldom exhibit the usual precipitating factors previously discussed and when present, dietary indiscretion or constipation are more frequent. Spontaneous episodes of encephalopathy are common. In some patients, established neurological deficits appear, with prominent extrapyramidal symptoms (acquired hepatolenticular degeneration) or spastic paraparesis. Enthusiasm for portacaval shunt surgery has waned as the ravages of chronic hepatic encephalopathy can be devastating to the individual and family. It is too soon to ascertain whether TIPS, the new noninvasive decompressive procedure, will result in a similar experience causing chronic changes in mental state.

Measures used to treat acute encephalopathy, including protein restriction, nonabsorbable disaccharides and/or poorly absorbable antibiotics, are also used in management of the chronic state. Vegetable protein has the benefit of providing additional fiber and promoting catharsis. Some patients do not tolerate the abdominal cramping associated with this source of protein. Supplements of fiber, such as psyllium, may be very effective. The rationale for the use of oral branched-chain amino acid supplements (0.25 g per kilogram per day) has been questioned. It is based on the theory that normalization of the aromatic/branched chain amino acid ratio will decrease the entry of the former into the brain, thus decreasing the formation of false transmitters. These supplements do not provide a major advantage, are expensive, and should be reserved for patients intolerant of oral protein.

Long-term therapy with lactulose (15 to 45 ml two to three times daily) is difficult to maintain due to subjective complaints with taste and abdominal cramping; lactitol may be more useful in this setting. Long-term use of neomycin (2 to 4 g per day) requires careful attention to potential ototoxicity, and yearly audiograms are necessary. When the first line of therapy is ineffective, metronidazole (500 to 750 mg per day) is considered. Bromocriptine (15 to 30 mg per day) has undergone testing based on its capacity to increase dopamine stores; results have not been encouraging. Initial enthusiasm for L-dopa has waned as clinical studies have not confirmed its efficacy.

Surgical options should be considered for the

chronic patient. Occlusion of the portacaval shunt has been used for cases with intractable chronic encephalopathy. This requires additional measures to ensure that gastroesophageal varices do not recur; this may include angiographic occlusion of the coronary vein or variceal embolization via angiography prior to shunt occlusion. Another drastic surgical approach in non-shunted patients has been colonic exclusion which is seldom used nowadays but the procedure has been effective in selected individuals. Liver transplantation is a real option for suitable candidates and chronic encephalopathy has become a clear indication for this procedure. Even reversal of chronic hepatocerebral degeneration has been recently reported after liver transplantation.

SUBCLINICAL ENCEPHALOPATHY

Subclinical encephalopathy is defined as the presence of abnormal neuropsychological testing in the absence of clinical signs of neurological deficits. It is common with 30 to 70 percent of cirrhotics exhibiting such features. The need to treat these patients is controversial. Lactulose and oral zinc acetate or sulfate (200 mg three times daily) have been shown in controlled studies to improve the performance in neuropsychological testing. Whether this will represent an advantage for patients with cirrhosis is unclear. Cirrhotic patients with subclinical encephalopathy who engage in complex motor activities may be potential beneficiaries.

ENCEPHALOPATHY IN ACUTE LIVER FAILURE

The development of encephalopathy is a serious complication of acute liver failure. Management of encephalopathy is difficult due to the confounding presence of brain edema and intracranial hypertension. During the early stages of encephalopathy, lactulose is administered with special care to avoid electrolyte disturbances associated with catharsis in an already precarious situation. Its efficacy in preventing the progression to deeper stages of encephalopathy has not been formally tested, but does not appear important. Neomycin is not recommended in order to avoid potential deterioration of renal function.

Many patients in stages III to IV encephalopathy (stupor, coma) exhibit a distinct complication of acute liver failure—brain edema and intracranial hypertension. Management of brain edema is symptomatic; the etiology of excessive water accumulation in the brain is still controversial and therapy is thus directed at reducing intracranial pressure. Mannitol, 0.5 to 1 g per kilogram is administered as a bolus; monitoring of intracranial pressure with epidural transducers allows optimization of therapy. Patients are kept at 30°, with avoidance of excessive mobilization. Thiopental coma and hypothermia are used in intractable cases. Liver transplantation is recommended for patients with advanced encephalopathy and poor synthetic function.

NEWER THERAPIES

Zinc is a cofactor for several enzymes in the urea cycle and repletion of depleted stores may improve the efficiency of ammonia conversion to urea. Administered as zinc sulfate or acetate (600 mg per day), it may be useful in patients with associated malnutrition. It has been shown to improve the results of neuropsychological testing in patients with subclinical encephalopathy and is an attractive option if treatment is considered for these individuals.

Sodium benzoate has been used in children with hyperammonemia due to urea cycle enzyme deficiencies. The drug is activated in the liver and combines with glycine (formed from ammonia, bicarbonate, and tetrahydrofolate) to form hippurate, which is now excreted in the urine. In two recent controlled evaluations, the drug was as useful as lactulose in reversing acute encephalopathy in cirrhotics. Benzoate is a ubiquitous food preservative but at this time is not commercially available as a medication. When administered, doses of 5 g twice daily are needed; this represents a sodium load and care should be exercised in patients with ascites.

Flumazenil is a benzodiazepine antagonist available for reversal of excessive sedation due to this group of drugs. Its use to reverse hepatic encephalopathy is based on experimental and clinical evidence that suggests a role for endogenous benzodiazepines in the pathogenesis of hepatic encephalopathy. It is available in an intravenous formulation, and is administered as a 1 mg bolus. Its use as either acute or chronic therapy has not yet been established.

Uncontrolled studies indicate an arousal effect of flumazenil in approximately 70 percent of patients. On most occasions, this effect is transient and does not represent complete normalization of the mental state. More recently, this arousal effect has been noted in a double-blind cross-over study, even when the use of exogenous benzodiazepines had been excluded. These observations are important for the pathogenesis of hepatic encephalopathy. In the meantime, flumazenil is clearly indicated for patients with benzodiazepine-induced precipitation of hepatic encephalopathy. It may be tested in patients in whom other measures have failed but its exact role in the management of encephalopathy of either acute or chronic liver disease has not yet been determined.

SUGGESTED READING

Blei AT. Cerebral edema and intracranial hypertension in acute liver failure. Distinct aspects of the same problem. Hepatology 1991; 13:736–739.

Butterworth RF, Pomier-Layrargues G. Hepatic encephalopathy, pathophysiology and treatment. Clifton: Humana Press, 1989.

Camma C, Fiorello F, Tine F, et al. Lactitol in the treatment of hepatic encephalopathy. A meta-analysis. Dig Dis Sci 1993; 38:916–922.

Conn HO, Bircher J. Hepatic encephalopathy. Management with lactulose and related carbohydrates. East Lansing: Medi-Ed Press, 1988.

Eriksson LS, Conn HO. Branched-chain aminoacids in hepatic encephalopathy. Gastroenterology 1990; 99:604–607.

Mullen KD, Weber FL Jr. Role of nutrition in hepatic encephalopathy. Semin Liver Dis 1991; 11:292–304.

ALCOHOLIC LIVER DISEASE

ANNA MAE DIEHL, M.D.
THOMAS G. TIETJEN, M.D.

The role of alcohol in the genesis of liver disease has been noted for centuries. Early investigators, such as Laennec, identified alcohol's hazardous potential by carefully documenting the prevalence of cirrhosis among heavy drinkers. Modern epidemiologic data from many societies corroborate the correlation between per capita alcohol consumption and deaths from cirrhosis. Although significant progress has been made in our understanding of disease pathogenesis, this has not resulted in effective therapies for most individuals with alcoholic liver disease (ALD). High per capita consumption of alcohol, coupled with the dearth of effective treatments and the failure of most affected individuals to abstain from alcohol, explain why ALD is the most prevalent form of chronic liver disease in the United States.

PATHOGENESIS

For over 30 years, study of the pharmacotoxicology of alcohol has incriminated the compound itself as a potent hepatotoxin. Since alcohol is lipid-soluble, it partitions in lipid bilayers of cell membranes, disordering membrane structure and function. In response, adaptive reorganization of the membrane occurs, resulting in physiologically altered membrane-initiated signaling by mediators such as circulating hormones, growth factors, and cytokines. Once alcohol enters the cell, it is efficiently oxidized by one of several enzyme systems. The intermediates formed in the metabolism of alcohol are responsible for most of the cytotoxic actions of the drug. In the occasional drinker, most alcohol is metabolized by the cytosolic alcohol dehydrogenase-aldehyde dehydrogenase (ADH-ALDH) system. Chronic alcohol consumption, however, induces certain microsomal cytochrome P-450 isozymes (dubbed microsomal enzyme oxidizing system [MEOS]), resulting in a supplemental route for alcohol disposal. The cytosolic and microsomal systems both generate acetaldehyde, an extremely reactive intermediate which forms adducts with critical cellular proteins. Acetaldehyde-protein adduct formation is thought to play a major role in the pathogenesis of ALD. The metabolism of alcohol by the ADH-ALDH system also generates excessive reducing equivalents which, in turn, alter the intracellular redox balance and interfere with the intermediary metabolism of nutrients. Alcohol oxidation by the MEOS requires oxygen, further stressing hepatocytes in the physiologically "oxygen-poor" regions of the liver lobule (zone 3). Since MEOS is involved in the metabolism of numerous drugs and xenobiotics, alcohol induction of MEOS also increases the formation of potentially hepatotoxic metabolites from other drugs. This explains the increased toxicity of acetaminophen in alcoholic individuals. Finally, alcohol may be metabolized by other enzyme systems that contribute relatively little to the overall disposal of alcohol but generate toxic metabolites. One of these systems, fatty acid ethyl ester synthase, is found in tissues (e.g., heart) that have little ADH-ALDH or MEOS activity. The toxic metabolites of alcohol produced by the fatty acid ethyl ester synthase may contribute to the evolution of alcoholic cardiomyopathy.

EPIDEMIOLOGY AND RISK FACTORS

Level of Alcohol Consumption

There is no clear-cut level of alcohol consumption that predictably results in ALD. While evidence suggests that risk increases with habitual intake of 80 g of alcohol per day in men and 20 g per day in women, only a minority of individuals drinking two to three times these amounts will develop significant liver disease. Indeed, only 20 percent of men drinking the equivalent of two six-packs of beer daily for 10 years become cirrhotic. To help reconcile this discrepancy between in vitro and in vivo toxicity of alcohol, a working hypothesis has been formulated. According to this theory, alcohol is viewed as a potential hepatotoxin. In a given individual, the evolution of liver disease depends on the balance between the degree of exposure to the toxin and the presence of other host attributes and/or confounding conditions.

Polymorphisms of Alcohol Metabolizing Enzymes

At least one host factor, genetic polymorphism of ADH-ALDH enzymes, seems to *protect* certain individuals from alcohol toxicity. Asians frequently inherit ADH isozymes that rapidly metabolize ethanol to acetaldehyde but ALDH isoenzymes that sluggishly clear acetaldehyde. Such individuals develop dysphoria and flushing, similar to patients taking disulfiram (Antabuse), after they drink alcohol. Consequently, habitual alcohol use and ALD are rare in this racial group. Emerging evidence suggests that inherited polymorphisms of ethanol-inducible cytochrome P450 isozymes may also influence the tendency to develop alcoholic liver injury.

Female Gender and Gastric ADH

As mentioned, women are more sensitive than men to alcohol-induced liver injury. This increased sensitivity cannot be explained by gender-related differences in tissue composition or alcohol distribution. Recently, unique isoezymes of ADH were identified in gastric mucosa. Gastric ADH activity appears to be lower in women than men, resulting in less gastric detoxification of alcohol and a greater fraction of ingested alcohol reaching the liver. While this discovery may explain gender differences in vulnerability to alcohol toxicity, the physiologic significance of gastric ADH is, at present, hotly contested.

Co-Exposure to Other Hepatotoxins

Chronic consumption of alcohol induces the activity of microsomal enzymes, potentiating the metabolism of drugs and xenobiotics into toxic intermediates which may contribute to liver injury. This is well illustrated by animal experiments in which alcohol-fed rats were treated with subtoxic doses of carbon tetrachloride, a drug metabolized to toxic intermediates by ethanol-inducible isoenzymes of cytochrome P-450. Neither rats fed alcohol alone nor rats treated only with low doses of carbon tetrachloride developed significant liver disease. However, rats treated with both alcohol and carbon tetrachloride developed cirrhosis within weeks. Such findings strongly support the importance of other toxins as potentiators of chronic liver disease in alcoholic patients.

Co-Infection with Hepatotrophic Viruses

Infections with hepatotrophic viruses (especially hepatitis B [HBV] and hepatitis C [HCV]) are prevalent in alcoholic individuals. Indeed, the prevalence of viral infection increases with severity of the underlying chronic liver disease. This has prompted some to postulate that viral infections are intimately involved in the pathogenesis of ALD. However, others argue that the full spectrum of ALD also occurs in the absence of documented viral infection. In any case, the prognosis of both acute and chronic viral hepatitis is worse in alcoholic patients. Furthermore, chronic viral infection appears to increase the risk of hepatocellular carcinoma in alcoholic patients with liver disease.

Immunologic Factors

While impaired immune function has long been recognized in alcoholics and cited as an explanation for the increased prevalence of bacterial and viral infections, recent attention has focused on immune "hyperfunction." Autoimmunity triggered by acetaldehyde-protein adducts has been suggested as a basis for ongoing liver disease in patients who become abstinent. Recently, overproduction of proinflammatory cytokines (e.g., tumor necrosis factor alpha [TNFα] and TNF-inducible cytokines) by macrophages and monocytes has been incriminated in the pathogenesis of both liver injury and multi-organ failure in patients with alcoholic hepatitis because serum levels of these cytokines correlate with mortality in such patients. Active research is directed towards delineating immunologic mechanisms involved in the pathogenesis of ALD.

Nutritional Factors

The role of nutritional status in the pathogenesis of ALD has undergone considerable modification since the 1950s when malnutrition, not alcohol, was considered primarily responsible for the genesis of liver disease in alcoholics. This concept changed radically when Lieber and coworkers demonstrated hepatic fibrosis in alcohol-fed baboons receiving a nutritionally adequate diet. In the years that followed, research focused on understanding why alcohol was hepatotoxic and generally dismissed the etiologic role of malnutrition. Recently, however, the old controversy has been rekindled by evidence that polyunsaturated lecithin prevents hepatic fibrogenesis in alcohol-fed baboons. This has renewed interest in potential nutritional therapies for ALD. Studies are underway to evaluate the efficacy of supplemental choline and cysteine prodrugs (which potentiate the synthesis of metabolically-protective forms of glutathione) in ALD.

HISTOLOGIC STAGING

The clinical features of ALD are, at best, insensitive indicators of the severity (and reversibility) of the underlying liver damage. Hence, hepatic histology remains the most reliable means of defining the stage of ALD.

Alcoholic Fatty Liver (Steatosis)

Alcoholic fatty liver is a reproducible consequence of alcohol oxidation and results when the intracellular redox potential, and redox-sensitive nutrient metabolism, are disturbed. Excessive accumulation of reducing equivalents favors metabolic pathways which lead to the accumulation of intracellular lipid. The excess lipid is stored in large droplets within individual hepatocytes. With abstinence, the normal redox potential is restored, the lipid is mobilized, and the fatty liver completely resolves. While alcoholic fatty liver is generally considered a benign, reversible, condition, a few cases have been reported to have a fatal outcome.

Alcoholic Hepatitis (Steatonecrosis)

The histologic picture of alcoholic hepatitis is characterized by steatosis plus hepatocellular necrosis and acute inflammation. As with alcoholic fatty liver, these findings are most pronounced in zone 3 of the hepatic acinus. Until recently, alcoholic hepatitis was felt to be a necessary prerequisite for alcoholic cirrhosis. However, it is now known that acetaldehyde may initiate fibrogenesis in the absence of demonstrable necroinflammation. Nonetheless, the severity of the clinical syndrome which occurs in some patients with alcoholic steatonecrosis and the lesion's potential to progress to cirrhosis, has made it the target of many therapeutic trials.

Cirrhosis

It is conceptually easy to view cirrhosis as the final, inevitable histologic stage of ALD. While this "progression" is widely accepted, not every patient necessarily follows this course. Indeed, most individuals with alcoholic fatty liver never "progress" to later histologic stages despite prolonged, heavy alcohol abuse. However, in others a fibrogenic response ensues. In some of these individuals, features of all three histologic "stages" coexist. Alcoholic liver damage is typically associated with deposition of collagen around the terminal hepatic vein (i.e., perivenular fibrosis) and along the hepatic sinusoids. This results in a "chicken wire" pattern of scarring which is rarely observed in other causes of cirrhosis. Chronic consumption of alcohol impairs the hepatocellular proliferative response that is normally triggered by liver cell death. Hence, nodules of regenerating parenchyma are typically small (i.e., micronodular) in actively drinking patients with cirrhosis. Abstinence releases the liver from the antiproliferative actions of alcohol and is associated with the evolution of macronodular cirrhosis.

ALCOHOLIC HEPATITIS

Case History. An agitated 36-year-old white female presents with vague, right upper abdominal pain. She has drunk 30 to 40 g of alcohol per day since age 17 and quit 1 week ago. Exam shows a temperature of 39° C, deep jaundice, tender hepatomegaly, and asterixis. Noteable laboratory parameters include: WBC 14.4 K, Hct 55 percent, AST 214, ALT 60, Bili 17.0, PT 19 seconds. Treatment with prednisone results in gradual recovery over 2 weeks but is complicated by hyperglycemia and urinary tract infection.

This patient presents with the "classic" clinical features (fever, jaundice, and tender hepatomegaly) of alcoholic hepatitis. However, other potential etiologies

of fever, jaundice and abdominal pain must be excluded before assuming that the patient's illness results solely from ALD. It is particularly important to exclude impaired hepatic venous outflow, biliary tract obstruction, and intra-abdominal and/or systemic infection, since the treatment of these entities differs drastically from that of alcoholic hepatitis. Hence, ultrasonography of the right upper quadrant and cultures of blood, urine, and ascites fluid are critically important diagnostic tests.

Prognosis

The short-term prognosis of patients with alcoholic hepatitis is best predicted by a combination of clinical and laboratory features which reflect both potentially reversible, alcohol-mediated metabolic toxicity and fixed (irreversible) alcoholic liver damage. Two groups of investigators have independently developed indices which can be used to predict the short-term mortality of patients with alcoholic hepatitis. The Composite Clinical Laboratory Index (CCLI) of Orrego and coworkers is calculated by summing the weighted scores of several clinical and laboratory variables which are known to correlate with mortality in patients with alcoholic liver disease (Table 1). Patients with a low CCLI are likely to survive while those with a high CCLI are at higher risk of in-hospital mortality.

Although the CCLI provides a linear estimate of mortality in patients with alcoholic liver disease, it is not often used in clinical practice because of the large number of variables that must be measured and the complexity of the calculation itself. A more simplified scheme was proposed by Maddrey and coworkers who distilled the risk of acute mortality into a discriminant function (DF), calculated by the formula (4.6 × prothrombin time [sec]) + bilirubin. Patients with a DF of greater than 93 were predicted to have a 50 percent chance of dying during hospitalization. The DF has been validated as a predictor of survival in a subsequent study. However, it provides a relatively crude estimate of prognosis. Recent evidence that serum cytokine levels correlate with acute mortality in patients with acute alcoholic hepatitis suggests that serum cytokine concentrations may be convenient adjunctive tests which could refine the prognostic accuracy of the DF.

Treatment

For all patients with alcoholic hepatitis, optimal treatment centers on the discontinuation of alcohol use and the resumption of a nutritionally adequate diet. Although most patients do not require hospitalization to achieve these goals, they should be urged to enroll in programs to facilitate detoxification and maintain abstinence. The patient described in the case history is predicted to have an acute mortality of greater than 50 percent (DF = (4.6 × 19) + 17 = 94). Hence, she should be admitted to optimize her chance for recovery.

During hospitalization, her withdrawal symptoms, fluid and electrolyte derangements, and malnutrition

Table 1 Composite Clinical and Laboratory Index Scoring

Sign/Symptom	Score
Hepatomegaly	1
Splenomegaly	1
Ascites: 1+	1
2+	2
3+	3
Encephalopathy	
Grade I	1
Grade II	2
Grade III	3
Clinical bleeding	1
Spider nevi	1
Palmar erythema	1
Collateral circulation	1
Peripheral edema	1
Anorexia	1
Weakness	1
SGOT >20 U	1
SGPT >100 U	1
>200 U	2
Alk Phos >80 U	1
Serum albumin <2.59%	1
PT (seconds above control)	
<3	1
3–5	2
>5	3
Bilirubin	
1.2–2 mg/dl	1
2.1–5 mg/dl	2
>5 mg/dl	3

can be treated. Chronic alcohol abuse often causes magnesium, potassium, and phosphate depletion which, in turn, contribute to the metabolic toxicity of alcohol. Hence, these elements should be replenished promptly. If they are administered in a glucose-containing vehicle, it is critical to provide supplemental thiamine to avoid triggering Wernicke's encephalopathy. Gastrointestinal bleeding and occult infections should be sought, and, if identified, efficiently managed. Subsequently, treatment efforts can be directed at improving the risk of mortality from the underlying ALD. Meta-analyses of multiple studies and two prospectively randomized, placebo-controlled trials have demonstrated that patients with clinically severe alcoholic hepatitis benefit from treatment with corticosteroids once serious infections and/or GI bleeding have been controlled. Indeed, a 4-week course of prednisone (32 mg methylprednisolone or the equivalent daily) more than halves the mortality of patients with a DF of greater than 93. It is important to note that these encouraging results were obtained in carefully selected patients who did not have clinically significant diabetes, pancreatitis, hepatocellular carcinoma or hepatitis B. The efficacy of corticosteroids in patients with alcoholic hepatitis and these comorbid conditions has not been established. Although little controlled data is available to guide management decisions in alcoholic hepatitis patients who are infected with hepatitis C or human immunodeficiency virus, we withhold steroid therapy only from otherwise eligible patients who have clinical evidence of AIDS. Although

a significantly higher incidence of infection and diabetes has not been noted in patients randomized to corticosteroid therapy, it is important to monitor with vigilance for potential steroid-induced complications.

Although multiple trials have failed to demonstrate that hyperalimentation alone improves survival in patients with acute alcoholic hepatitis, it is clear that poor nutritional intake is associated with an ominous prognosis. Thus, patients should be encouraged to eat an adequate diet, and, if they cannot, supplemental nutrition should be provided via enteral or parenteral routes. Ideally, the latter is reserved for patients who cannot aliment via their GI tracts. There is no evidence that the intake of nutritionally adequate amounts of dietary protein triggers hepatic encephalopathy in these patients. Similarly, expensive branched chain-enriched amino acid mixtures offer no proven advantage over standard total-parenteral nutrition (TPN) solutions.

Other treatments that have been explored in patients with alcoholic hepatitis include therapies targeted to improve hepatic regeneration (anabolic steroids and insulin/glucagon infusions), decrease oxidative stress (propylthiouracil and cyanidanol), and prevent fibrosis (D-pencillamine and colchicine). None reproducibly improve short-term survival and, hence, these agents cannot be recommended for general clinical use. Despite this, it is premature to conclude that these treatments are devoid of merit since most of the aforementioned trials included relatively small numbers of heterogenous patients and few studies actually determined whether therapy benefited the targeted process.

Once therapy has been initiated in a patient with alcoholic hepatitis, the duration of hospitalization is dictated by the clinical response. Severely ill patients should remain hospitalized until intercurrent conditions have been effectively managed, steady improvement in clinically important indicators of liver dysfunction (e.g., hyperbilirubinemia, prothrombin time prolongation, ascites, hepatic encephalopathy) have been demonstrated, and the patient is able to ingest an adequate diet. There is no need to document histologic resolution of liver injury, since this process typically lags weeks to months behind clinical recovery. Ideally, patients should be discharged to an in-patient alcoholic rehabilitation unit to insure abstinence during the early recovery period. However, in compliant patients, steroid therapy can be continued on an out-patient basis. There is no need to taper the dose of steroids over a prolonged period, since these patients have received a relatively short course of therapy. Rather, the dose can be progressively halved during week 4 of therapy (i.e., 32 mg to 16 mg to 8 mg to 4 mg to 0 mg). Similarly, there is absolutely no evidence that continued treatment with steroids benefit patients with ALD.

Assessing the Risk of Progression to Cirrhosis

Two studies have shown that at least 10 percent of patients with alcoholic hepatitis recover completely normal liver histology and function. While complete recovery requires absolute avoidance of alcohol, many abstinent patients do not achieve resolution of liver disease. Conversely, not all patients who continue to drink alcohol are destined to become cirrhotic. However, nearly half of noncirrhotic patients hospitalized for alcoholic hepatitis ultimately develop cirrhosis. The risk of histologic progression seems related to the severity of the initial bout of alcoholic hepatitis and whether or not the patient becomes abstinent. Female gender also seems to be an independent risk factor for progression of liver disease since abstinent women with initially mild disease often develop cirrhosis.

CIRRHOSIS

Prognosis

As in precirrhotic alcoholic patients, the long-term prognosis of patients with alcoholic cirrhosis is quite variable. By far the most important determinants of prognosis are the degree of irreversible end-organ damage and whether or not the patient continues to drink alcohol. The latter is important because continued alcohol consumption perpetuates the risk of both reversible and irreversible alcohol-induced toxicity. If individuals with clinically-compensated cirrhosis abstain from alcohol, they have a 90 percent 5 year survival rate. If, however, they continue to drink, their survival falls to 60 percent. Abstinent individuals with clinically-decompensated cirrhosis have a 60 percent 5 year survival, while those who continue to drink have a 30 percent chance of surviving for the same period. Hence, abstinence remains the cornerstone of therapy for alcoholic patients, even after cirrhosis has developed.

Treatments to Improve Prognosis*

General Strategies

Some patients deteriorate because of superimposed spontaneous bacterial peritonitis (SBP). Patients with advanced cirrhosis and low (< 1 g per deciliter) ascitic fluid protein concentrations are at high risk of developing "spontaneous" infections of their ascites. The infecting organisms are usually gram-negative enteric flora or gram-positive cocci. Prophylaxis with norfloxacin (400 mg qhs) has proven to decrease the risk of SBP in such patients. Once an infection has developed, intravenous administration of a third generation cephalosporin or amoxicillin-clavulanic acid eradicates the infection in virtually all cases, even if the infecting organism is not very sensitive to these agents in the laboratory. Patients who respond to antibiotic therapy become afebrile and their ascitic fluid WBC counts and cultures normalize within 24 to 48 hours. Studies have shown that treatment

---

*Editor's Note: Some of this information is in other chapters (e.g., Ascites and Spontaneous Bacterial Peritonitis, Ascites and Its Complications, and the liver transplantation chapters).

with 4 days of antibiotics is as efficacious as 10 days of therapy. Hence, there is little justification for prolonged, routine administration of antibiotics in this disease. Once the infection has been cured, norfloxacin prophylaxis should be initiated and attention can be directed to controlling ascites.

Duplex ultrasound evaluation of the portal vein is helpful in excluding portal vein thrombosis as a contributing cause of worsening ascites. Evaluation of renal sodium excretion is useful in gauging the potential efficacy of diuretic therapy. Well-hydrated patients who avidly retain sodium (< 10 mEq sodium per liter) are unlikely to diurese without relatively large doses (200 to 300 mg per day) of spironalactone and typically require adjunctive therapy with furosemide (40 to 120 mg per day) and/or hydrochlorothiazide (50 to 100 mg per day). Patients who fail to diurese despite aggressive diuretic therapy or who develop renal insufficiency or electrolyte abnormalities during therapy should be managed with repeated large volume paracentesis. There is no evidence that intravenous albumin supplements are necessary after paracentesis in ascitic cirrhotic patients with normal renal function. Because one study suggests that large volume paracentesis may trigger renal hypoperfusion in cirrhotic patients with renal insufficiency, some physicians give such patients albumin (6 to 8 g albumin IV per liter of ascites withdrawn) over the 6 hours post-paracentesis. This is discussed in the chapter on ascites and hepatorenal syndrome.

During hospitalization, every effort should be made to optimize nutrition in cirrhotic patients. Since cirrhosis is a state of "accelerated" starvation, prolonged fasts should be discouraged. A recent report suggests that continuous enteral feeding improved morbidity and decreased mortality in one group of cirrhotic patients. There is no need to restrict the protein consumption of cirrhotic patients routinely. Even in patients with encephalopathy, *lactulose* therapy (dose titrated to achieve one to three soft bowel movements per day) should be implemented before protein restriction is considered. Dietary protein can be restricted (40 to 70 g protein per day) if these measures fail to control encephalopathy.

If the patient has not been evaluated for the presence of esophageal varices, diagnostic endoscopy can be considered. If large (grade 3 to 4 +) esophageal varices with stigmata indicative of bleeding risk are identified, prophylactic treatment with beta-blockers (titrated to reduce the heart rate by 25 percent) has been shown to reduce the incidence of bleeding. There is a separate chapter on management of esophageal varices as well as a chapter on portal hypertension.

Colchicine and Propylthiouracil

Few long-term treatment trials of patients with ALD have been conducted. Those that are available have been seriously confounded by noncompliance and large dropout rates. Nonetheless, two prospectively randomized controlled trials have reported treatment-associated improvements in 5 to 10 year survival. In a Mexican trial, a survival advantage was demonstrated in patients with alcoholic cirrhosis who were given daily colchicine therapy. A Canadian group also reported improved long-term survival benefits in patients treated with the antithyroid agent propylthiouracil (PTU). In both studies, treatment-related toxicity was low. However, the small number of patients enrolled in these studies may have been insufficient to detect uncommon adverse reactions. Since the cost and potential toxicity of colchicine are less than PTU, the former may be a better choice for "maintenance" therapy in patients with alcoholic cirrhosis.

Orthotopic Liver Transplantation

It is now clear that orthotopic liver transplantation improves survival in patients with decompensated cirrhosis as compared to historical, medically-treated controls. No "standard" period of abstinence has been found to guarantee survival or to eliminate the risk of recidivism. However, given the value and scarcity of donor organs and the large expenditure of resources involved in orthotopic liver transplantation, most transplant centers require demonstrated commitment to life-long sobriety before transplantation is offered as a therapeutic option. Screening systems currently in place have resulted in recidivism rates of less than 10 percent in transplanted alcoholic patients. Emerging evidence suggests an accelerated form of ALD may develop in patients who resume alcohol abuse after transplantation. This underscores the importance of careful patient selection for this treatment.

FUTURE THERAPIES

The most direct approach to prevent ALD is to eliminate alcohol abuse. Hopefully, active research to define the genetic/biochemical basis of addiction and identify biomarkers of alcohol abuse will improve the ability to limit use of this widely-available hepatotoxin in susceptible individuals. Work is also underway to develop treatments to eradicate coexistent viral infections (e.g., interferon and other antiviral agents); improve cellular tolerance to oxidative stress (e.g., antioxidants and prodrugs of reduced glutathione); block excessive cytokine responses (e.g., pentoxiphylline, soluble cyto-

kine receptors, anticytokine antibodies, and selective gut decontamination); and optimize regenerative responses to liver injury (e.g., supplemental polyamines and growth factors). Refinements in the ability to predict the clinical course of patients with "early", precirrhotic stages of ALD will help target specific treatments to individuals who are most likely to benefit by these therapies.

SUGGESTED READING*

Bird GLA, O'Grady JG, Harvey FAH, et al. Liver transplantation in patients with alcoholic cirrhosis: selection criteria and rates of survival and relapse. BMJ 1990; 301:15–17.

Carithers RL, Herlong HF, Diehl AM, et al. Methylprednisolone therapy in patients with severe alcoholic hepatitis: a randomized multicenter trial. Ann Intern Med 1989; 110:685–690.

Ginés P, Rimola A, Planas R, et al. Norfloxacin prevents spontaneous bacterial peritonitis recurrence in cirrhosis: results of a double-blind placebo-controlled trial. Hepatology 1990; 12:716–724.

Halle P, Pare' P, Kapstein E, et al. Double-blind, controlled trial of propylthiouracil therapy in severe acute alcoholic hepatitis. Gastroenterology 1982; 82:925–931.

Kershenobich D, Vargas F, Garcia-Tsao G, et al. Colchicine in the treatment of cirrhosis of the liver. N Engl J Med 1988; 318:1709–1713.

Kumar S, Stauber RE, Gavaler JS, et al. Orthotopic liver transplantation for alcoholic liver disease. Hepatology 1990; 11:159–164.

Lucey MR, Merion RM, Henley KS, et al. Selection for and outcome of liver transplantation in alcoholic liver disease. Gastroenterology 1992; 102:1736–1741.

Maddrey WC, Boitnott JK, Bedine MS, et al. Corticosteroid therapy of alcoholic hepatitis. Gastroenterology 1978; 75:193–199.

Mezey E, Caballeria J, Mitchell MC, et al. Effect of parenteral amino acid supplementation on short-term and long-term outcomes in severe alcoholic hepatitis: a randomized controlled trial. Hepatology 1991; 14:1090–1096.

Oreggo H, Blake JE, Blendis LM, et al. Long-term treatment of alcoholic liver disease with propylthiouracil. New Engl J Med 1987; 317:1421–1427.

Oreggo H, Kalant H, Israel Y. Effect of short-term therapy with propylthiouracil in patients with alcoholic liver disease. Gastroenterology 1979; 76:105–115.

Ramond M-J, Poynard T, Rueff B, et al. A randomized trial of prednisolone in patients with severe alcoholic hepatitis. N Engl J Med 1992; 326:507–512.

Starzl TE, Van Theil D, Tzakis AG, et al. Orthotopic liver transplantation for alcoholic cirrhosis. JAMA 1988; 260:25–42.

*****Editor's Note:** A 55-item bibliography is available upon request to the authors. I've selected references with obvious therapeutic import.

PORTAL HYPERTENSION

PAUL J. THULUVATH, M.B., B.S., M.D., M.R.C.P. (UK)

The portal vein, about 5 to 8 cm long, is formed by the union of superior mesenteric vein and the splenic vein. In a normal man, the portal blood flow is about 1,200 ml per minute and the portal pressure is less than 8 mm Hg. Although the portal pressure can be measured directly by percutaneous (transhepatic or intrasplenic) or operative catheterization, it is usually measured indirectly as the difference between the wedged and the free pressure of a hepatic venous radicle (hepatic venous pressure gradient) using a balloon catheter. The indirect pressure reading usually reflects the true portal pressure except in presinusoidal portal hypertension where it may underestimate the true pressure. Obstruction to the portal venous blood flow along its course, or rarely from increased portal blood flow as in tropical splenomegaly, results in portal hypertension. Depending on the site of lesion, the portal hypertension may be classified as prehepatic (e.g., portal vein thrombosis, tropical spleno-megaly), hepatic presinusoidal (e.g., schistosomiasis, sarcoidosis, idiopathic), hepatic postsinusoidal (e.g., cirrhosis, acute alcoholic hepatitis), or posthepatic (venocclusive disease). A combination of clinical history, physical findings, duplex-Doppler scans, liver biopsy, wedged hepatic venous pressure readings and angiography will allow the clinician to localize the site of the lesion. A detailed discussion of the various causes of portal hypertension is beyond the scope of this chapter, but it is important to recognize that the major cause in developed countries is cirrhosis whereas schistosomiasis and noncirrhotic portal hypertension (idiopathic portal hypertension or neonatal portal vein thrombosis) account for a significant proportion of portal hypertension in the developing countries.

The pathogenesis of portal hypertension in cirrhosis is a combination of increased portal vascular resistance and a hyperdynamic circulation. The portal vascular resistance is increased in cirrhosis due to the morphological changes and the hemodynamic changes within hepatic vasculature. The hyperdynamic systemic and splanchnic circulation is caused by an increase in vasoactive mediators and a reduced sensitivity to vasoconstrictors. When portal pressure exceeds a certain level (usually 12 mm Hg), due to the unique anatomy of portal venous system, a remarkable collateral circulation develops to decompress the portal system. Despite this collateral circulation, the portal pressure is often sustained due to increased hyperdynamic splanchnic and systemic circulation, and perhaps due to enhanced porto-collateral resistance.

Clinical consequences of portal hypertension include ascites, gastroesophageal varices, hypersplenism, and hepatic encephalopathy. Of all the complications of portal hypertension, variceal bleeding is perhaps the most dangerous. Approximately 30 percent of all patients with documented varices bleed during their lifetime, usually (80 percent) within 24 months after diagnosis. Of those who bleed, 30 to 50 percent die from the first bleed. Fifty to one hundred percent of those who survive the first bleed, will rebleed within 2 years; most bleed within 6 weeks after the first bleed. Thirty percent of all deaths in cirrhotics could be directly attributed to gastroesophageal variceal bleeding.

The prophylaxis against the initial variceal bleeding, the management of acute bleeding and the prevention of recurrent variceal bleeding are all important aspects of the management of portal hypertension and are discussed in this chapter. The management of ascites and hepatic encephalopathy are discussed elsewhere.

MANAGEMENT OF ACUTE VARICEAL BLEEDING

Management may be divided into (1) general resuscitative measures and (2) specific treatment aimed at arresting the variceal bleeding. Aspiration of blood and gastric contents is a major cause of morbidity and mortality in patients with variceal bleeding. Patients may be drowsy and may have reduced pharyngeal reflexes.

Resuscitation

Endotracheal intubation may be necessary in an encephalopathic patient particularly to safeguard the patient during the placement of balloon tamponade or for endoscopic procedures. Pulse oximetry to assess oxygen saturation and thereby to titrate supplemental oxygen through nasal canulae should be mandatory in a patient with active hemorrhage.

Venous access should be safeguarded by using two or three large bore peripheral venous cannulae. Central venous pressure (CVP) and pulmonary capillary wedged pressure (PCWP) measures provide important hemodynamic information which facilitates optimum resuscitation but require expertise for placement and pressure recording. Assessment of blood loss by patients or family members is often inaccurate. Hematemesis is almost always overestimated; conversely significant blood loss may occur without hematemesis. Tachycardia and postural hypotension are useful indicators, but the presence of autonomic neuropathy may influence these measurements. Repeated (over a few hours) hemoglobin and hematocrit provide important serial assessments of blood volume loss and the response to replacement. Measurement of CVP is a sensitive guide to the blood volume status but caution should be exercised in the presence of tense ascites since diaphragmatic compression of the right atrium by the ascites may lead to an overestimation of the readings. PCWP, measured using a pulmonary flotation catheter, is the most accurate guide to control blood volume and may be invaluable in the presence of major ongoing bleeding.

Blood volume restitution should be prompt and as

accurate as possible to protect vital organs, particularly renal function. For practical purposes, one tries to maintain the CVP around 5 to 10 mm Hg. The ideal replacement fluid is blood to maintain the oxygen-carrying capacity of the circulation. Colloid is reserved for immediate infusion until blood becomes available. I prefer gelatin-based colloid solutions since they have less effect on platelet function, partial thromboplastin, and bleeding time, compared with dextran or hydroxy ethyl starch.

Isovolemic replacement should be the aim with care taken to avoid major overexpansion of the circulation which may precipitate further bleeding due to the associated increase in portal pressure. Furthermore, excessive transfusion may worsen thrombocytopenia and cause deficiency of clotting factors either due to disseminated intravascular coagulation or hemodilution. These abnormalities are seen usually after 9 to 15 units of blood are transfused. The role of platelets and fresh frozen plasma is not well established in the management of variceal hemorrhage, but as a general rule it is given when platelet counts are below 50,000 and prothrombin time is prolonged more than 50 percent. The use of fresh frozen plasma every 5 units of blood transfused and platelet transfusion every 8 units is a common practice. Other possible complications of massive transfusion include pulmonary microembolism, citrate toxicity and consequent hypocalcemia and hyperkalemia.

Infection is common after hemorrhage. There is little evidence to support prophylactic antibiotics, however, care should be taken to detect such complications as aspiration pneumonia and spontaneous bacterial peritonitis at the earliest opportunity and to treat aggressively.

Specific Treatment

Since bleeding from a nonvariceal source is not uncommon in chronic liver disease, early endoscopy (after initial resuscitation) is essential to guide specific therapy. There are very few circumstances in which it is justified to initiate specific therapy for variceal bleeding without endoscopic confirmation of the bleeding point.

Endoscopic Therapy

Evidence to support injection sclerotherapy as an important technique for the treatment of active variceal bleeding came from two uncontrolled reports which claimed success rate of over 90 percent. Since then, a number of randomized controlled studies have confirmed its efficacy with control of bleeding in 75 to 90 percent of cases. It is now generally accepted that immediate sclerotherapy is the optimum treatment for active variceal bleeding, but is critically dependent upon available expertise to attain these high success rates and to minimize complications. The chapter *Sclerotherapy and Banding of Gastroesophageal Varices* presents additional information.

An important question that remained unanswered was the optimum timing of injection sclerotherapy with respect to the bleeding episode. The options are immediate treatment with the associated technical difficulties, or delayed treatment after temporary hemostasis is achieved using vasoconstrictive drugs or balloon tamponade. A recent randomized controlled study showed that at 12 hours after presentation, sclerotherapy was superior to vasoconstrictor therapy (88 percent versus 65 percent) for immediate control. The admission mortality was less in the immediate sclerotherapy group than in those managed by vasoconstrictor therapy, but it was not statistically significant (27 percent versus 39 percent).

It is disappointing to note that none of the well-designed trials have shown a consistent reduction in rebleeding (about 30 percent) or in-hospital mortality with sclerotherapy when compared to other modes of treatment. It is possible that the mortality in this group of patients (mainly Child-Pugh Grade C) is determined at an early stage of the bleeding episode, before the institution of treatment and thus masking the benefits of the therapeutic modality applied.

The last 5 years has seen the development and evaluation of two new endoscopic techniques. The tissue adhesive n-butyl-2-cyanoacrylate (Histacryl) solidifies almost instantaneously when brought into contact with blood and by intravariceal injection may produce rapid obliteration of the vessel lumen. The disadvantage is that it has to be handled very carefully, otherwise endoscopic channels may be occluded. Two studies have claimed control of bleeding in approximately 90 percent of cases and of particular note is its use to obliterate fundal varices which respond unreliably to intravarix injection of sclerosant. Reports of cerebral toxicity are a major concern and at present are a restraint on widespread use.

The ability to apply prestressed bands (endoscopic band ligation) to the varices has recently been developed with proven efficacy for both the control of active bleeder and subsequent prevention of rebleeding. No specific benefits have been shown for this technique over the injection of sclerosant during active bleeding and in the light of the extra instrumentation required is probably best reserved for long-term therapy.*

Drug Therapy

The major benefit of pharmacologic therapy is that it can be given immediately without any specialized training. An effective agent offers immediate therapy to hospitals in which the expertise to carry out endoscopic or surgical intervention is lacking and may facilitate transfer of patients to more specialized centers. To date, the low efficacy and complications associated with drugs available have proved a major limitation. The safety margin of the newer preparations appear to be better as discussed in the following section.

---

*Editor's Note: Other views, favoring banding over variceal sclerosis, are presented in the chapters on esophageal varices and upper gastrointestinal bleeding, and in the Suggested Reading list.

Vasopressin and Glypressin. Vasopressin is a peptide hormone which has important splanchnic arterial vasoconstrictor properties, thereby reducing portal blood in flow and portal pressure. Glypressin (triglycl lysine vasopressin) is a prodrug which is converted to lysine vasopressin in vivo. The slow release from the prodrug may explain its prolonged effect (up to 6 hours). This drug has properties similar to those of vasopressin, but can be given as bolus doses (2 mg IV every 4 to 6 hours) through a peripheral line (since it is inactive before conversion) unlike vasopressin which must be given as a continuous infusion (0.4 unit per minute, increased if necessary to 0.8 unit per minute) through a central line. This may be beneficial if patients are being transferred to a specialized center.

The main side effects of vasopressin and glypressin are secondary to non-selective arterial vasoconstriction. These include ischemia of the myocardium, abdominal viscera and lower limbs, left heart failure, hypertension, and arrhythmias. In randomized, controlled studies, up to 25 percent of patients have been withdrawn because of major side effects. Selective infusion of vasopressin into the superior mesenteric artery has not been shown to overcome these adverse effects or improve efficacy.

In a number of studies, a combination of vasopressin and nitroglycerine has been shown to reduce the hemodynamic side effects of vasopressin without attenuating the effect on portal inflow (Table 1). The transdermal route may be preferred because of ease of administration.

There is a wide range (29 to 84 percent) of reported efficacy of vasopressin and glypressin which is difficult to explain (Table 1). There is now little to justify the use of vasopressin as a single agent. Despite vasopressin being the active moiety of glypressin this agent does appear to offer enhanced control of bleeding and fewer side effects. The addition of nitroglycerine to vasopressin is of proven benefit and should be an integral part of such therapy.

Somatostatin and Octreotide. Somatostatin is a 14 amino acid peptide hormone. It has a short half-life (1 to 2 minutes) and has to be given as a continuous intravenous infusion (250 μg bolus dose followed by 250 μg hourly). Octreotide (Sandostatin) is a cyclic octopeptide analog which shares 4 amino acids with somatostatin. It has a longer half-life (1 to 2 hours) and therefore can be administered either subcutaneously or intravenously as bolus doses (50 to 100 μg every 8 hours). Both drugs cause splanchnic vasoconstriction by a direct effect on vascular smooth muscle and possibly by inhibiting the release of vasodilatory peptides such as glucagon. Although both drugs reduce portosystemic collateral blood flow (measured by azygos blood flow), in cirrhotic patients the effect on portal pressure has been variable.

The results of two placebo-based randomized controlled studies of somatostatin have provided conflicting results. Whereas Burroughs et al. showed significant benefit for the somatostatin group (64 versus 41), Valanzuela et al. in a multicenter trial involving 84 patients claimed a completely opposite effect (65 percent versus 83 percent). The very high success rate in the placebo group in this latter study has not previously been observed in any study and may be artifactual reflecting recruitment into the trial of small number of patients from multiple centers. Trials comparing somatostatin with vasopressin have shown the former to be marginally superior for the control of variceal bleeding and to be associated with very few side effects (Table 1).

Two studies have compared somatostatin with tamponade and one study compared octreotide with tamponade. All three studies confirmed similar efficacy for somatostatin or its analog as compared to balloon tamponade (58 to 71 percent versus 50 to 80 percent respectively). In a further study, somatostatin was found to have similar efficacy to injection sclerotherapy.

The major benefit of somatostatin and its analog are their safety margin which permits a longer-term usage over the first few days after presentation with the aim of preventing early rebleeding. In an uncontrolled study, in patients who rebled after initial hemostasis, continuous infusion of octreotide (50 micrograms per hour) stopped bleeding in 30 of 31 with esophageal ulceration and 38 of 42 patients with bleeding varices. It is my usual practice to use octreotide 100 micrograms subcutaneously every 6 hours until the patient had the second endoscopic treatment.

Metoclopramide, Domperidone, and Pentagastrin. These drugs are known to constrict the lower esophageal sphincter and have been shown to reduce varix pressure. A single trial has suggested short-term benefit of these drugs for the control of bleeding, an observation that requires further confirmation.

Balloon Tamponade

Balloon tamponade is a highly effective method of controlling active variceal bleeding. Controlled studies have shown that, in experienced hands, it is superior to pharmacological agents and is equivalent to sclerotherapy for the immediate control of bleeding. However, efficacy extends only to the period of application and in inexperienced hands the morbidity and mortality may be unacceptably high. Balloon tamponade is best reserved for the management of life-threatening bleeding when a risk of exsanguination exists and endoscopic intervention is unlikely to be feasible.

Surgery

While endoscopic therapy at the time of diagnostic endoscopy probably is the optimum approach to an episode of variceal bleeding, surgical intervention has an important and increasing role, particularly in patients who continue to bleed despite early injection sclerotherapy or banding. Most workers would repeat endoscopic therapy on a second occasion before considering it to have failed. However, the decision to progress to surgery should not be further delayed in order to prevent the inevitable escalation of operative risks in a deteriorating

Table 1 Control of Variceal Bleeding: Summary of Controlled Studies Using Vasopressin (VP), Glypressin (GP), VP + Nitroglycerine (NG) and Somatostatin (ST)

Author*	Placebo	VP	GP	VP + NG	ST
Conn 1975 (33)	25%	71%			
Fogel 1982 (33)	37%	29%			
Freeman 1989 (31)	37%		60%		
Soderland 1990 (60)	55%		84%		
Tsai 1986 (39)		47%		55% (SL)	
Gimson 1986 (72)		41%		73% (IV)	
Bosch 1990 (65)		48%		65% (TD)	
Valanzuela 1989 (84)	83%				65%
Burroughs 1990 (12)	41%				64%

*Number of bleeding episodes within parentheses.
SL = Sublingual NG; IV = intravenous NG; TD = transdermal NG.

patient. Bleeding from fundal varices, frequently difficult to diagnose and even more difficult to treat, is a second major indication for surgical therapy. The types of surgery may be divided into shunt and non-shunt procedures. The choice of surgery depends on the local expertise, severity of the liver disease and suitability of the patient for future liver transplantation. There is a subsequent chapter on portal hypertension surgery.

All established shunt procedures have been used to manage active variceal bleeding although the technical difficulties and operating time associated with the selective distal splenorenal shunt makes this generally unsuitable as an emergency procedure. Shunt surgery, especially mesocaval and distal splenorenal shunts, does not preclude subsequent transplantation. The operative mortality of shunting procedures in severe liver disease has been high but in two controlled studies portocaval shunting was shown to be of equivalent benefit to injection sclerotherapy for the management of active bleeding.

Various types of non-shunting procedures are available to control variceal bleeding, but the most common is esophageal transection with varying degrees of devascularization. Three controlled trials have compared sclerotherapy with esophageal transection plus or minus devascularization for control of active variceal hemorrhage. Although there was a trend towards improved control of bleeding with esophageal transection, the survival rates were not different between the groups. However, these studies have confirmed the importance of esophageal transection as a "rescue" procedure for patients who fail endoscopic therapy. The only major concern that arises from the use of devascularization procedures is the adverse effect on liver transplantation. Extensive scar tissue or adhesions, particularly at the hilum, may markedly increase the technical difficulties of transplantation and exacerbate blood loss.

Gastric Varices

The incidence of gastric varices in published reports varies from 6 to 16 percent. Gastric varices are usually seen in association with esophageal varices or rarely in isolation as in splenic vein thrombosis (segmental portal hypertension). The overall mortality from bleeding gastric varices is over 50 percent. Although the management of gastric varices is similar to that of esophageal varices, endoscopic sclerotherapy using sclerosants should be reserved only for lesser curve varices or varices within a hiatus hernia. Tissue adhesives or thrombin may be used to inject fundal varices after the initial bleeding has stopped. It is technically difficult to inject fundal varices when they are actively bleeding. If balloon tamponade is unsuccessful in patients with bleeding fundal varices, one should proceed immediately to transjugular intrahepatic portosystemic shunting (TIPS) or surgery. Splenectomy is curative when varices are seen in association with splenic vein thrombosis.

Ectopic Varices

Bleeding from nongastroesophageal sites varies from 1.6 to 5 percent in the large reported series. The common ectopic sites, usually seen in association with esophageal varices, are duodenum, colon, anorectum and enterostomy. Rarely these varices may be localized, especially in the colon, and result from superior or inferior vein thrombosis, tumor infiltration, adhesions, or congenital malformation.

The management of the bleeding depends on the site of bleeding, the severity of liver disease and the local expertise. Since there are no controlled studies, it is difficult to recommend any special strategy. Shunt surgery may be the best line of management for bleeding varices in the duodenum, jejunum, ileum, and enterostomy. If the expertise for TIPS is available, that should be considered as the first line of management before other forms of shunt surgery. Anecdotal reports suggest that duodenal varices and ileostomy varices can be managed successfully by sclerotherapy or feeding vessel embolization, but one has to consider carefully the postsclerotherapy complications like duodenal perforation and stoma dysfunction and the high recurrence rate after embolization. Colonic varices are usually localized and can be managed by local resection. Again when it is seen in association with esophageal varices, TIPS may be a safer alternative. Anorectal varices can be safely treated with sclerotherapy or by underrunning with an absorbable suture.

Portal Hypertensive Gastropathy

The prevalence of gastrointestinal hemorrhage from gastric mucosal lesions in patients with portal hypertension has been estimated to be between 10 and 60 percent; it is the second most common cause of bleeding in portal hypertension. The risk from mucosal bleeding seems to increase after variceal obliteration by banding or sclerotherapy. The diagnosis of portal hypertensive gastropathy is based on the endoscopic appearance and the histological features. In mild form the mucosa is hyperemic with multiple, small erythematous areas outlined by a white network (mosaic pattern) and in severe form, cherry red spots or diffuse mucosal hemorrhages are seen. These lesions are seen throughout the stomach, but rarely can be localized in the antrum when it may be difficult to distinguish it from watermelon stomach. In doubtful cases characteristic histology (mucosal dilatation of capillaries with edema but without significant inflammation, and submucosal dilatation of veins) may prove useful.

The pathogenesis of these lesions is not completely understood, but portal hypertension and increased gastric blood flow with alteration in microvascular mucosal blood flow are thought to be involved. Although the risk of death from mucosal bleeding is low compared to variceal bleeding, often bleeding is sufficient to require multiple transfusions or hepatic decompensation. Shunt surgery is very effective to arrest the bleeding from portal hypertensive gastropathy, but carries significant mortality.

Two open studies and one randomized controlled study have shown that propranolol may significantly reduce the rebleeding rate. In the 1991 randomized study in 54 cirrhotic patients, 65 percent of those who received propranolol remained free of bleeding at 12 months and 52 percent at 30 months compared to 38 percent and 7 percent in the control group; multivariant analysis showed that the absence of propranolol treatment was the only predictive variable for rebleeding. The mode of action of propranolol in portal hypertensive gastropathy is unclear but may be a combination of reducing portal pressure and altering the blood flow pattern in gastric microcirculation. Although TIPS has not been evaluated in any controlled studies, anecdotal evidence suggests that it is very effective and may become the standard treatment in patients who fail propranolol treatment.

PREVENTION OF RECURRENT VARICEAL BLEEDING (SECONDARY PROPHYLAXIS)

A number of options are available to prevent recurrent bleeding, including endoscopic sclerotherapy, endoscopic banding, propranolol, shunt surgery, esoph-ageal transection, liver transplantation, and more recently TIPS.

Long-Term Injection Sclerotherapy

A number of controlled trials have assessed the efficacy of this form of treatment in reducing the rebleeding rate and mortality. These trials showed an improvement in rebleeding rate, but only three studies showed improved survival. Two meta-analyses have been performed on these controlled trials to clarify the data further. Both showed a significant improvement in survival and reduction in rebleeding rate; however one must interpret these studies with caution since the meta-analysis included heterogeneous studies in which the control arm often received less effective treatment. In spite of these reservations, until recently sclerotherapy was considered the "gold standard" for prevention of recurrent variceal bleeding.

The optimal time interval between the endoscopic sessions is not known. Two studies have compared sclerotherapy at 1 and 3 week intervals and showed that 1 week was probably better than 3 weeks to reduce rebleeding rate as well as for rapid obliteration of varices. On the basis of current evidence I recommend one weekly injection during the first 3 to 4 weeks and thereafter two to three weekly depending on the size of varices and the ulceration. The duration of follow-up after the variceal obliteration is an area of controversy. There is no data to suggest that long-term endoscopic follow-up after variceal obliteration is superior to short-term treatment aimed at obliteration of varices. It may not be necessary to have endoscopic follow-up in patients who are maintained on beta blockers.

Endoscopic Banding

Three controlled studies have compared sclerotherapy with banding. All three reported that banding was marginally more effective and required fewer sessions for variceal obliteration when compared with sclerotherapy. Although one study by Steigman et al. showed improved survival in the group who had banding, the other two studies failed to show any significant survival differences. There was a reduction in the overall complication rate in the banding group in all three studies despite similar ulceration rate. These studies suggest that banding and sclerotherapy are equally effective, but banding may have a slight advantage in terms of the number of sessions required and the treatment-related complication rate. The chapter on esophageal varices provides more details on these techniques.

Beta Blockers

Nonselective beta blockers reduce portal pressure by reducing cardiac output, and by reducing portal inflow via antagonism of the $beta_2$ receptors on the splanchnic vessels. Beta blockers also may increase porto-collateral resistance and hence reduce collateral blood flow.

Results of a meta-analysis by Hayes et al. of secondary prevention studies comparing propranolol with placebo showed that propranolol can reduce the bleeding rate by 39 percent (Confidence Interval [CI] 30,46) and bleeding-related mortality by 40 percent (CI 17,57). The bleeding rate on propranolol in these trials was similar to that of injection sclerotherapy (about 40 percent). More recent trials comparing propranolol with sclerotherapy confirm that both forms of treatment are similar in efficacy. The limited experience with other beta blockers suggests that all noncardioselective beta blockers (e.g., nadolol) may be similar to propranolol in efficacy.

Propranolol With Endoscopic Treatment

Based on the limited data, it appears that addition of propranolol to sclerotherapy may reduce bleeding rate compared to either propranolol or sclerotherapy alone. This may be very useful in patients who are less likely to comply with medical treatment. Unless there are definite contraindications, it is my routine practice to treat patients with propranolol in addition to endoscopic band ligation.

Surgery

Long-term endoscopic sclerotherapy and beta blocker trials suggest that a considerable proportion of patients bleed despite intensive treatment and follow-up. It is therefore important to examine the surgical trials with an open mind.

The only prospective randomized trial of esophageal transection and gastric devascularization was reported by Triger and his colleagues in Sheffield in 1992. They found that this form of surgery conferred no benefit over endoscopic sclerotherapy in terms of long-term survival or cost effectiveness. Decompressive shunt surgery is the most effective way of preventing recurrent variceal bleeding, but it has the significant disadvantage of causing chronic hepatic encephalopathy. Since 1970, 14 randomized trials of various forms of shunt surgery have been performed. None of these trials have shown definite improvement in survival after shunt surgery. Currently shunt surgery (preferably mesocaval shunt or distal splenorenal shunt) is reserved for patients with recurrent bleeding (without advanced liver disease) who fail all other forms of treatment.

TIPS

This is the most exciting recent development in the management of portal hypertension. (There is a separate chapter on this topic.) Preliminary, uncontrolled reports suggest that TIPS is effective and safe in patients who fail endoscopic treatment for acute bleeding. The preliminary data from the only randomized, controlled study confirmed that TIPS is as effective as sclerotherapy for prevention of recurrent variceal bleeding. Unlike shunt surgery, the mortality, even in most advanced cases, appears to be low; the 30 day mortality is between 2 and 16 percent and overall mortality is 6 to 26 percent. This provides the clinician an additional tool in the management of variceal bleeding.

The development of encephalopathy, contrary to expectations, appears to be low although this has not been subjected to intense study. Two large series reported new onset of hepatic encephalopathy as 18 to 20 percent, of which the majority were easily controlled with lactulose. The initial optimism for TIPS as an effective therapy for long-term prevention of variceal bleeding is dampened by reports of very high stent stenosis (7 to 45 percent) and occlusion rate (9 to 14 percent). More randomized trials looking at the long-term outcome of TIPS are necessary before it can be recommended for the routine management of variceal bleeding.

Liver Transplantation

The mortality after variceal bleeding and the long-term survival following the index bleed are directly related to the severity of liver disease. It is difficult to imagine that the various treatment options discussed here are likely to improve liver function and hence survival. Liver transplantation, with survival rate reaching 80 percent, is the treatment of choice for patients with advanced liver disease (Child B & C). There are three chapters on the role of liver transplantation.

PROPHYLAXIS FOR VARICEAL BLEEDING (PRIMARY PROPHYLAXIS)

About a third of all patients with cirrhosis bleed within 2 years of the endoscopic diagnosis of esophageal varices. The chance of bleeding depends on the severity of liver disease (Childs-Pugh grade), the portal pressure (> 12 mm Hg), and the severity of varices (e.g., Beppu score). Mortality depends on the severity of liver disease and varies from 30 to 50 percent. The rationale behind the prophylaxis is based on the high bleeding rate and the very high mortality associated with it. Prophylaxis may be surgical, endoscopic, or pharmacologic.

Surgery

The randomized, controlled, prophylactic shunt trials done before the endoscopic era showed significant reduction in variceal and gastric mucosal bleeding. However, the mortality and the incidence of chronic hepatic encephalopathy were significantly higher in the shunted patients compared to the control group. These poor results and the advent of endoscopy led to the abandonment of shunt surgery for prophylaxis.

A more recent, multi-center study from Japan compared devascularization versus no treatment in a group of patients with high risk of bleeding and claimed lower bleeding rate (7 percent versus 49 percent) and low mortality (22 percent versus 49 percent) in the surgical group compared to the control group. Again the deaths related to bleeding was similar in both groups. It is difficult to draw any conclusions from this study since there was a disproportionate amount of non-bleeding-related mortality in the control group. Unequal randomization due to multi-center trial design (22 centers and 112 patients) may be one explanation for this. Further trials may be necessary to validate these trial results. Moreover, this form of surgery may make future liver transplant technically more difficult as outlined in the chapter *Liver Transplantation: Surgical Considerations.*

On the basis of the current evidence, there is no role for either shunt or non-shunting surgery in the prophylaxis of variceal bleeding.

Sclerotherapy

Prophylactic sclerotherapy has been the subject of many small and large randomized, controlled studies. Earlier reports from Germany showed reduced bleeding rate and improved survival in patients who had sclerotherapy compared to controls, but more recent studies have not confirmed these results. In fact, the multicenter, Veterans Administration trial of prophylactic sclerotherapy involving 282 patients was discontinued prematurely because of the significantly high mortality in the sclerotherapy arm compared to the control group (29 percent versus 17 percent). It has been suggested that these conflicting results may have been due to the differences in patient selection. To examine this, two studies, one from Japan and the other one from Italy, carefully selected patients with high risk of bleeding. While the Japanese study showed reduced bleeding and improved survival, the North Italian study showed identical bleeding rate. However, a meta-analysis done recently on eight controlled studies showed that prophylactic sclerotherapy reduced mortality by 11 percent (95 percent CI 4 to 19 percent); the mortality rate reductions were positively correlated with the bleeding rate reduction and negatively with complication rates. The current evidence suggests that, even in high-risk patients, the benefits from prophylactic sclerotherapy may be marginal and the procedure is not cost effective.

Beta Blockers

Many trials have assessed the efficacy of propranolol for primary prophylaxis and all studies, except one, showed reduction of bleeding. A meta-analysis done on eight of these trials has shown a definite benefit in the treated group with regard to bleeding (47 percent reduction, CI 28 to 61) and mortality (45 percent reduction, CI 10 to 67). There was no evidence for heterogeneity for bleeding events in this analysis, although there was heterogeneity for the total mortality. I recommend propranolol (preferably a long-acting preparation to improve compliance) for primary prophylaxis for all patients with advanced liver disease and large varices.

RECOMMENDATIONS

Active esophageal-gastric variceal bleeding is a medical emergency in which immediate and well-directed resuscitation may improve the early and possibly late outcome. Diagnostic endoscopy, as an essential part of the management, provides the optimum time for intervention by endoscopic methods.

Although sophisticated endoscopic therapy is now widely available, if the expertise for endoscopic intervention is not available, other modes of therapy, primarily pharmacologic and rarely balloon tamponade, should be tried while the patient is transferred to a center where more definitive therapy is available. Pharmacologic treatment is effective in 50 to 70 percent of cases. The choice of therapy lies between vasopressin (or glypressin) with a vasodilator (nitroglycerin) or somatostatin and its analog octreotide. Balloon tamponade is effective in 80 to 90 percent of cases in experienced hands but has major limitations without this expertise. When pharmacologic therapy or balloon tamponade succeeds in controlling the initial bleed, it should be followed immediately by more definitive therapy, usually endoscopic treatment or surgery.

Although banding or sclerotherapy is now frequently the first choice, shunt surgery and esophageal transection are comparable in efficacy to injection sclerotherapy for the management of active bleeding. Surgery should not be delayed when injection sclerotherapy fails on two occasions. Bleeding fundal varices should be managed by early surgery if balloon tamponade fails.

For secondary prophylaxis, endoscopic treatment (banding or sclerotherapy) and propranolol are similar in terms of efficacy. Endoscopic band ligation may be marginally superior to sclerotherapy. A combination of propranolol and endoscopic treatment may be a logical approach for long-term secondary prophylaxis. TIPS may be useful in patients with recurrent bleeding, but further long-term trials are necessary before its routine use. Shunt surgery should be reserved for patients who fail all other forms of treatment. Propranolol should be used for primary prophylaxis in patients with advanced liver disease and large varices. Liver transplantation is the treatment of choice for patients with advanced liver disease.

Editor's Note: I ask authors to review the various options, tell us their choices along with the rationale for those choices, and the results they expect. This author has done that very well. You may not always agree. Fortunately (or unfortunately, if you want pat answers) we've given you several opinions on portal hypertension and esophageal varices. You're the doctor!

SUGGESTED READING

Bosch J. Effect of pharmacological agents on portal hypertension: a hemodynamic appraisal. Clin Gastroenterol 1985; 14:169–183.

Burroughs AK. Somatostatin and octreotide for variceal bleeding. J Hepatol 1991; 13:1–4.

Conn HO. Transjugular intrahepatic portal-systemic shunts: the state of the art. Hepatology 1993; 17:148–158.

Hayes PC, Davis JM, Lewis JA, Bouchier IAD. Meta-analysis of value of propranolol in prevention of variceal hemorrhage. Lancet 1990; 336:153–156.

Laine L, El-Newihi HM, Migikovsky B, et al. Endoscopic ligation compared with sclerotherapy for the treatment of bleeding esophageal varices. Ann Intern Med 1993; 119:1–7.

Lebrec D, Paynard T, Bernuau J, et al. A randomized controlled study of propranolol for prevention of recurrent gastrointestinal bleeding in patients with cirrhosis: a final report. Hepatology 1984; 6:318–331.

North Italian Endoscopic Club for the Study and Treatment of Esophageal Varices: Prediction of the first variceal hemorrhage in patients with cirrhosis of the liver and esophageal varices: a prospective multi-center study. NEJM 1988; 319:983–989.

Smart HL, Triger DR. Clinical features, pathophysiology and relevance of portal hypertensive gastropathy. Endoscopy 1991; 23: 224–228.

Steigman GV, Goff JS, Michaletz-Onody PA, et al. Endoscopic sclerotherapy as compared with endoscopic ligation for bleeding esophageal varices. NEJM 1992; 326:1527–1532.

Westaby D, Williams R. Status of sclerotherapy for variceal bleeding in 1990. Am J Surg 1990; 160:32–36.

BUDD-CHIARI SYNDROME

ANDREW S. KLEIN, M.D.

Budd-Chiari syndrome is a rare form of portal hypertension caused by hepatic venous outflow occlusion. Several distinct pathologic processes can produce hepatic venous obstruction. Discerning the etiology and anatomy of a patient's lesion will determine which therapeutic approach is most appropriate.

Veno-occlusive disease of the liver (VOD) is a proliferative disorder characterized by concentric luminal narrowing at the level of the terminal hepatic venules and sinusoids. VOD is most commonly recognized in allogeneic bone marrow transplant recipients treated with combination chemotherapy and radiotherapy. There is little evidence that surgical intervention has a major role in the management of VOD. It is mentioned primarily to distinguish it from the two major forms of Budd-Chiari syndrome in which thrombosis or occlusion of larger vessels occur: (1) obstruction of the suprahepatic vena cava by a membranous web, and (2) thrombotic occlusion of the hepatic veins and/or suprahepatic vena cava.

Membranous obstruction of the suprahepatic vena cava, the most common cause of Budd-Chiari syndrome worldwide, is unusual in the United States, except in those areas which serve a large population of Asian immigrants. Thrombotic occlusion of the hepatic veins and/or vena cava accounts for most cases in this country. The ensuing approach to managing Budd-Chiari syndrome focuses primarily upon those patients with the thrombotic form of the disease.

CLINICAL PRESENTATION

A variety of predisposing factors have been implicated in the development of hepatic vein occlusion (Table 1) and the incidence of idiopathic Budd-Chiari syndrome is less than 30 percent. Hepatic venous

Table 1 Etiologic Factors in the Development of Budd-Chiari Syndrome

Polycythemia rubra vera
Estrogens/oral contraceptives
Pregnancy
Malignancy
Paroxysmal nocturnal hemoglobinuria
Hepatitis
Trauma
Idiopathic thrombocytopenic purpura
Protein-losing enteropathy
Fungal or parasitic infections

occlusion may present as a fulminant, acute, or chronic illness. The acute form is most common, and is characterized by the sudden onset of ascites, abdominal pain, and tender hepatomegaly. Ascites, which may be massive, is a consistent finding in patients with acute hepatic vein obstruction (>95 percent). Other complications of portal hypertension, such as gastrointestinal hemorrhage, are uncommon (<20 percent) in the early stage of acute Budd-Chiari syndrome. Surprisingly, routine determinations of liver function, including serum transaminases, bilirubin, alkaline phosphatase, and prothrombin time are usually normal or only mildly deranged. Conversely, the serum albumin may be disproportionately low in comparison to other markers of hepatic synthetic function due to the chronic loss of protein in the ascites. Consequently, these tests are not useful in establishing the diagnosis of Budd-Chiari syndrome, nor are they helpful in predicting the patient's clinical course.

In a small fraction of patients, massive destruction of the hepatic parenchyma secondary to acute hepatic venous congestion results in fulminant hepatic failure. If the hepatic venous obstruction is not relieved promptly, these patients develop a rapidly progressive encephalopathy, jaundice, coagulopathy, and acidosis which ultimately results in multiple organ failure and/or lethal cerebral edema. The chronic form of Budd-Chiari syndrome also accounts for a small percentage of patients with this disorder. Patients present with end-stage liver failure, cryptogenic cirrhosis, and portal hypertension. The diagnosis of hepatic vein occlusion may be made during evaluation for a liver transplant or at autopsy.

EVALUATION

The diagnosis of Budd-Chiari syndrome may be suggested by noninvasive procedures including duplex sonography, technetium colloid or gallium-67 hepatic scintiscans, computed tomography, and magnetic resonance imaging. The gold standard, however, for confirming the diagnosis is hepatic venography which will demonstrate either totally occluded hepatic veins or the characteristic spider-web appearance of partially recanalized veins. An important adjunct to hepatic venography is inferior cavography in which imaging of the infrahepatic, retrohepatic, and suprahepatic vena cava is combined with simultaneous measurements of vena caval pressure above and below the liver. Inferior venacavography may reveal (1) patency of the vena cava with no significant caval obstruction or hypertension, (2) patency of the vena cava with caval obstruction (defined as a reduction in luminal diameter by more than 75 percent or a pressure gradient of more than 20 mm Hg from the infra to suprahepatic vena cava), or (3) total occlusion of the vena cava. The caudate lobe drains directly into the vena cava via several short veins which are uninvolved in the thrombotic process producing Budd-Chiari syndrome. In response to the dysfunctional state of the remainder of the liver, the caudate lobe hypertrophies. Compression of the intrahepatic vena cava due to either caudate lobe hypertrophy or pericaval fibrosis, is a common complication of hepatic vein obstruction. In fact, most patients with Budd-Chiari syndrome have either complete occlusion or significant compression of their inferior vena cava at the time of initial presentation.

The percutaneous liver biopsy has been a controversial procedure in the evaluation of patients with Budd-Chiari syndrome. Although the presence of ascites, portal hypertension, and perhaps a mild coagulopathy has dissuaded many physicians from attempting a liver biopsy, recent experience suggests that this technique can be performed safely with a very low incidence of complications. Thirty-two patients with Budd-Chiari syndrome have undergone percutaneous liver biopsy at our institution with no mortality and without significant morbidity. The results of both liver biopsy and inferior cavography have important therapeutic implications which will be discussed.

NONOPERATIVE THERAPY

Although spontaneous resolution of hepatic vein occlusion has been reported, if untreated, this condition generally leads to progressive portal hypertension, end-stage liver failure, and death. Medical management consists of diuresis, anticoagulation, and intensive supportive measures. Unfortunately, the response to such measures is usually limited. In a retrospective study of 12 patients treated by medical means alone at The University of California, Los Angeles, there was but one survivor at 2 years.

Case reports of successful thrombolytic therapy with urokinase or streptokinase have appeared in both the medical and radiological literature. But unless thrombolysis is begun very early in the evolution of hepatic vein thrombosis it is unlikely to succeed. In our experience, most patients present with several months of symptoms. Thrombolytic therapy has only resulted in unnecessary complications and delay in instituting appropriate surgical measures.

OPERATIVE THERAPY

The surgical procedures used to treat Budd-Chiari syndrome can be divided into four categories: peritoneovenous shunts, direct excision of the venous obstruction, portosystemic decompression, and orthotopic liver transplantation.

Peritoneovenous shunts such as the LeVeen or Denver shunt have been used to palliate the tense ascites commonly found in these patients. Unfortunately, shunts of this type fail to address the underlying venous obstruction and portal hypertension, which if uncorrected leads to end-stage hepatic cirrhosis and death. Thus, with the exception of patients who are not acceptable candidates for definitive treatment, peritoneovenous shunts have little role in the surgical management of this disorder.

Successful treatment of Budd-Chiari syndrome by excision of the venous obstruction is generally limited to those patients with vena caval webs. Dorsocranial resection of the liver followed by reconstruction of the vena cava has been attempted when membranous obstruction of the cava has extended into the hepatic veins. Even in the most experienced hands, dorsocranial hepatic resection is a formidable undertaking. Furthermore, patients with the thrombotic form of Budd-Chiari (i.e. most patients treated in the U.S.) can not be managed by direct excision of the offending lesion which often extends into several levels of hepatic venous branches in both hepatic lobes.

Portosystemic Shunt

Alternatively, a number of procedures have evolved which effectively decompress the congested liver by some form of portosystemic or mesenteric systemic shunt. Although a variety of anatomic connections have been proposed (Table 2), all employ the common principle of converting the portal vein from an inflow to an outflow tract. In the absence of cirrhosis or severe synthetic dysfunction, most patients tolerate portosystemic shunting well. Encephalopathy is clinically apparent in only a small fraction of postshunt Budd-Chiari patients, and when it develops it is usually transient and easily controlled with lactulose. The percutaneous liver biopsy is used to establish the presence of pre-existing liver disease which is associated with an increased risk of

Table 2 Portosystemic Shunts for Budd-Chiari Syndrome

Mesocaval
Mesoatrial
Portacaval
Porta-atrial
Portacaval + cavoatrial
Portopulmonary
Splenoazygous
Splenopulmonary
Splenorenal

intractable encephalopathy and liver failure after shunting.

Although portosystemic decompression is felt to be an effective treatment for the acute form of Budd-Chiari syndrome, shunt selection remains controversial. We have chosen the superior mesenteric vein (SMV) for access to the portal circulation since it can be isolated rapidly and safely well away from the congested liver, and the operation can be performed unimpeded by the hypertrophied caudate lobe. Patients with no evidence of vena caval obstruction or significant compression undergo a mesocaval "C" shunt. A 14-mm to 16-mm Dacron graft is sewn end-to-side to the SMV just inferior to the neck of the pancreas. The graft is then navigated in a gentle curve lateral and posterior to the second portion of the duodenum, where it is sewn end-to-side to the inferior vena cava. If the vena cava is totally occluded, a mesoatrial shunt is performed. Although the mesoatrial graft is longer than the mesocaval graft, and the routing is more circuitous (from the SMV, over the pancreas into the lesser sac, over the stomach and left lobe of the liver, and into the right pleural cavity where it is sewn to the right atrium), both effectively divert portal blood flow away from the congested liver into the right atrium. In the setting of a patent vena cava with restricted flow due to compression by surrounding tissues there are two options: (1) mesoatrial shunt or (2) dilatation and stenting of the compressed vena cava with an intravascular metal prosthesis (see below) followed by mesocaval shunt.

As mentioned previously, there is disagreement about which shunt procedure is best for patients with Budd-Chiari syndrome. Orloff et al have strongly advocated the use of side-to-side portacaval shunts and have reported excellent graft patency and patient survival results. Other groups have had less success with the portacaval shunt, due primarily to the caudate lobe hypertrophy which renders this procedure difficult and occasionally impossible. Additionally, should a liver transplant be required in the future, a pre-existing portacaval shunt (but not mesocaval or mesoatrial shunt) has been shown to markedly increase the technical difficulty, average blood loss, operative morbidity, and mortality.

Liver Transplantation

Orthotopic liver transplantation (OLT) was first performed successfully in a patient with Budd-Chiari syndrome in 1974. The enthusiasm for OLT as definitive treatment for end-stage liver disease has led some centers to advocate liver replacement for virtually all patients with Budd-Chiari syndrome. Unfortunately, the demand for donated cadaveric livers in this country has far outstripped the supply, and thus many potential liver recipients die before an appropriate organ can be located for them. We have adopted a somewhat more moderate policy in which OLT is considered for Budd-Chiari patients who have (1) the rare fulminant form of the disease, (2) evidence of severe synthetic dysfunction, (3) a history of pre-existing liver disease documented by liver biopsy, or (4) anatomic abnormalities which would preclude portosystemic shunting (i.e., thrombosed portal vein).

INTERVENTIONAL RADIOLOGY

The skill and expertise of our radiology colleagues has been valuable in the diagnosis and management of Budd-Chiari syndrome. Vena caval webs have been eliminated by transluminal angioplasty or use of the "hot-tip" Nd:YAG laser. However, neither angioplasty nor laser obliteration is likely to be effective in managing those cases caused by hepatic vein thrombosis. We must also consider the risks of caval perforation and pulmonary embolism which accompany these procedures, and would seemingly limit their usefulness to short segment occlusions of the vena cava.

Invasive radiologic maneuvers should be viewed not in competition with, but rather complimentary to surgical treatment of Budd-Chiari syndrome. An emerging technology which has been useful in the management of Budd-Chiari patients is the percutaneous insertion of intravascular stents. Expandable metal prostheses placed across narrowed segments of the vena cava have in some cases eliminated high pressure gradients and functional caval obstruction. Patients who would otherwise require a mesoatrial shunt to decompress their congested liver may be treated with the less complicated mesocaval shunt after caval stenting. Additionally, balloon angioplasty with or without the placement of a vascular stent may be effective in salvaging surgically placed grafts (mesocaval or mesoatrial) which over time become partially occluded as a result of intimal hyperplasia or deposition of laminar clot.

Some patients with the thrombotic form of Budd-Chiari syndrome are found to have patency of a short segment of the main right, left, or middle hepatic vein. There are anecdotal reports of successful transjugular intrahepatic portosystemic stent-shunt (TIPSS) placement in such patients. The TIPSS procedure involves creation of an intrahepatic fistula from the patent hepatic venous segment to a major branch of the portal vein. The fistula is then dilated and supported with a Palmaz or Gianturco-type vascular stent. The advantage of this nonoperative approach is that the entire procedure can be performed under light intravenous sedation via vascular access to the internal jugular vein.

RESULTS AND PROGNOSIS

The 5-year survival rate for patients with Budd-Chiari syndrome treated by mesocaval or mesoatrial shunt is 60 to 80 percent. Despite the fact that Budd-Chiari patients who receive a portosystemic shunt of any type receive warfarin sodium (Coumadin) indefinitely, a major concern is the long-term patency of synthetic grafts in the low pressure venous system. Modifications to the graft to render it less thrombogenic and meticulous attention to the level of anticoagulation (prothrombin times maintained at 1.4 to 1.8 times control) appear to be effective in reducing the graft occlusion rate. Theoretically, the mesoatrial shunts should be most prone to thrombosis, leading some to advocate conversion of an originally-inserted mesoatrial shunt to the shorter mesocaval shunt once the hepatic congestion, caudate lobe hypertrophy, and caval compression have resolved. Recent data, however, suggest that the risk of mesoatrial graft thrombosis resulting in death is quite low, and thus elective conversion of the mesoatrial to the mesocaval shunt exposes the patient to unnecessary risks of reoperative surgery and offers no clear benefit.

Most liver transplant centers are now reporting 1-year survival rates of 75 to 85 percent for adult recipients. Early studies which focused specifically on liver recipients with Budd-Chiari syndrome reported inferior survival (55 to 70 percent) but the series were small, included patients who did not receive postoperative anticoagulation, and were uncontrolled for variable immunosuppressive protocols. As is our practice after portosystemic shunt, patients with hepatic venous occlusion who undergo OLT are anticoagulated indefinitely. Presently, we would expect patients with Budd-Chiari syndrome who receive a liver transplant to have survival rates similar to those of the general adult population transplanted for end-stage liver disease.

The appropriate selection of mesocaval shunt, mesoatrial shunt, or liver transplant should result in the safe and successful treatment of most patients with Budd-Chiari syndrome. Interventional radiologic techniques are an important adjunct to the management of patients with this disorder.

Editor's Note: The past decade has seen a dramatic improvement in survival and quality of life for patients with Budd-Chiari syndrome. The innovative surgical and radiologic techiques described in this chapter, combined with liver transplantation, are a tribute to medical progress. I also cite this as an excellent example of how animal research has benefited specific patients who previously had a dismal outlook.

SUGGESTED READING

Ahn SS, Yellin A, Sheng FC, et al. Selective surgical therapy of the Budd-Chiari syndrome provides superior survivor rates than conservative medical management. J Vasc Surg 1987; 5:28–37.

Bismuth H, Sherlock DJ. Portasystemic shunting versus liver transplantation for the Budd-Chiari syndrome. Ann Surg 1991; 214: 581–589.

Campbell DA Jr, Rolles K, Jamieson N, et al. Hepatic transplantation with perioperative and long term anticoagulation as treatment for Budd-Chiari syndrome. Surg Gynecol Obstet 1988; 166:511–518.

Henderson JM, Warren WD, Millikan WJ Jr, et al. Surgical options, hematologic evaluation, and pathologic changes in Budd-Chiari syndrome. Am J Surg 1990; 159:41–50.

Klein AS, Sitzmann JV, Coleman J, et al. Current management of the Budd-Chiari syndrome. Ann Surg 1990; 212:144–149.

Lopez RR Jr, Benner KG, Hall L, et al. Expandable venous stents for treatment of the Budd-Chiari syndrome. Gastroenterology 1991; 100:1435–1441.

Shaked A, Goldstein RM, Klintmalm GB, et al. Portosystemic shunt versus orthotopic liver transplantation for the Budd-Chiari syndrome. Surgery 1992; 174(6):453–459.

Wang Z, Zhu Y, Wang S, et al. Recognition and management of Budd-Chiari syndrome: Report of one hundred cases. J Vasc Surg 1989; 10:149–156.

TRANSJUGULAR INTRAHEPATIC PORTOSYSTEMIC SHUNTING

ANTHONY C. VENBRUX, M.D.
FLOYD A. OSTERMAN, Jr., M.D.

Patients with portal hypertension due to liver disease may develop portosystemic collateral vessels, the most clinically significant being esophageal varices. Approximately 50 percent of patients with cirrhosis develop esophageal varices. Two-thirds of patients with esophageal varices eventually develop acute bleeding. It is this event that brings the patient to immediate medical attention. Treatment of life-threatening upper gastrointestinal (UGI) hemorrhage in a patient with portal hypertension and bleeding varices requires an aggressive multi-disciplinary approach. Hemodynamically unstable patients are initially managed in an intensive care setting with fluid and blood volume replacement and endoscopic evaluation. Endoscopy is important because it helps localize the source of bleeding; e.g., active esophageal bleeding from other potential sources of UGI hemorrhage such as peptic ulcer disease and gastritis. If bleeding esophageal varices are identified, variceal sclerotherapy and banding are the primary methods of treatment. Approximately 90 percent of acute esophageal variceal hemorrhages can be stopped by this approach. Though highly effective, multiple sessions may be required.

Once stabilized, the radiologist is frequently asked to evaluate a patient with advanced liver disease. The radiologist may be called upon to perform various imaging procedures. Studies include an evaluation of arterial and venous anatomy through catheterization procedures, cross-sectional imaging, i.e., computed tomography, ultrasound, and magnetic resonance imaging. It is frequently necessary to evaluate the arterial and venous anatomy for surgical planning such as a portosystemic shunt or hepatic transplant. Recently a percutaneous technique involving the placement of an intrahepatic portosystemic shunt has been developed. If arteriography is chosen, delayed images obtained during the venous phase of the celiac or superior mesenteric arteriogram will depict the portal venous anatomy in the majority of patients. Wedged and free hepatic vein pressure measurements, an inferior vena cavogram, and a left renal venogram may also be performed from a common femoral or jugular vein approach. This will help the surgeon or radiologist determine which options are available for the patient.

Patients with massive ascites or a coagulopathy due to liver dysfunction in whom a percutaneous transhepatic liver biopsy is risky, may undergo an invasive procedure performed by the radiologist, the transjugular liver biopsy. The biopsy of the hepatic parenchyma is performed with an angulated needle placed through a jugular vein sheath. The angulated needle is used to puncture through the vein wall once the hepatic vein has been engaged. Using the principles of transjugular liver biopsy, combined with a knowledge of hepatic anatomy, the transjugular liver biopsy technique may be applied to create an intrahepatic portosystemic shunt; the so called transjugular intrahepatic portosystemic shunt (TIPS) procedure.

THERAPEUTIC ALTERNATIVES

In general, endoscopic sclerotherapy or banding, balloon tamponade, and systemic pharmacologic therapy are the conventional methods used to treat patients with acute variceal bleeding. Having failed this, patients may be considered for portosystemic shunt surgery. The more common surgically-created portosystemic shunts include the mesocaval shunt, the distal splenorenal shunt (Warren shunt), and the mesoatrial shunt. Patients with severe hepatic dysfunction (e.g., Child C patients) do poorly with shunt surgery. In the past 3 years, a technique has been developed and used clinically which creates an intrahepatic portosystemic shunt between the main right or left portal vein and a hepatic vein. The ability to maintain patency of the hepatic parenchymal tract is dependent on the use of metallic stents. The goal of the TIPS procedure is to decompress the elevated venous pressure into the central (i.e., hepatic) low-pressure venous system. The TIPS procedure shunts blood *away* from esophageal varices and *into* the central venous system similar to surgically-created shunts. The goal is to reduce the elevated pressure in esophageal or other portosystemic collaterals while maintaining some flow into the intrahepatic portal vein radicles. When technically successful, TIPS decom-

presses the portal venous system. With an appropriately-sized shunt, cessation of variceal bleeding, reduction of ascites, and hemodynamic stabilization are a few of the benefits achieved. These results are felt to be related to shunt patency and to the diameter of the shunt. With an appropriately-sized patent shunt, the clinical benefits of decreased variceal bleeding and ascites have been noted.

Long-term studies are currently underway. Because the technique is new, precisely which group of patients will benefit from this procedure is the subject of intensive investigation. The TIPS procedure is a reasonable treatment option in the management of complex patients with portal hypertension and life-threatening UGI hemorrhage who have failed conventional therapy.

The first nonsurgically created decompressive portosystemic shunt was reported by Rosch and colleagues in 1969 in the canine animal model. This "shunt" between a left medial lobe hepatic vein and the portal vein consisted of a percutaneously created hepatic parenchymal tract with a Teflon sleeve, the latter functioning to maintain patency of the hepatic tract. In 1990, Richter et al reported the results of a pilot study in nine humans. Percutaneous creation of a portosystemic shunt was successful in all nine patients with severe portal hypertension. However, the pilot study reported two deaths, one directly related to the procedure, the second 11 days after the procedure from a severe nosocomial infection. Since the earlier reports of several investigators, a fundamental change in the technique has dramatically decreased the morbidity and mortality of this procedure. By avoiding placement of a percutaneous transhepatic catheter in the portal venous system (used as a marker during fluoroscopy), complications such as hemoperitoneum have been significantly reduced in those patients with coagulopathies and ascites.

Of the first eight reported patients undergoing TIPS therapy at the Miami Vascular Institute, there was one episode of stent migration. The stent was nonsurgically retrieved and caused no added morbidity. Of the first 18 patients undergoing TIPS at the Miami Vascular Institute, one patient died 48 hours after the procedure. This patient was septic before the procedure and was actively bleeding from esophageal varices. TIPS therapy was performed as a potential life-saving measure. The cause of sepsis in this patient was felt to be due to an earlier episode of aspiration pneumonia.

TECHNIQUE

After the patient is hemodynamically stabilized, the TIPS procedure is performed electively.

The location of the patent bifurcation of main right and left portal veins is marked on the outside of the patient. Localization is accomplished by ultrasound or based on angiographic landmarks from previous baseline studies. This marker becomes a fluoroscopic landmark during needle passes through the liver.

At our institution, the last eight patients have

undergone pre TIPS placement of a nasobiliary tube. This tube, endoscopically placed in the biliary system with the tip directed into the main right or left bile duct, serves as a radiopaque marker during anterior-posterior and lateral fluoroscopy. The central right or left main portal vein trunks are located posterior to the main right or left biliary ducts. The angled needle is thus directed toward the main right or left portal vein trunk adjacent (posterior) to the course of the previously placed nasobiliary tube. Thus the number of "blind" needle passes through the liver may be reduced using this modified technique.

One percent lidocaine is used to anesthetize the skin and subcutaneous tissues of the right neck. A percutaneous puncture into the right internal jugular vein is made. A vascular sheath is placed into the right internal jugular vein. A guidewire and catheter are advanced caudally and used to catheterize a hepatic vein selectively. Once the hepatic vein is entered, the catheter/guidewire combination is exchanged for a long angulated guiding sheath. With the sheath in the orifice of the hepatic vein, the 16 gauge Colapinto transjugular biopsy needle is directed through the sheath. The needle tip exits the sheath in the hepatic vein and is then directed anteriorly towards the main right or left portal vein. A puncture through the vein wall and hepatic parenchyma is made and the needle is advanced until a portal venous branch is entered. Entry into the main right or left portal vein is desired. The portal vein bifurcation itself is avoided because of possible extrahepatic puncture. Take care to avoid making needle passes peripherally in the liver because of the risk of liver capsule perforation and hemoperitoneum and the technical difficulty of placing the shunt in a peripheral hepatic location. C-arm biplane fluoroscopy is used to confirm proper needle placement. Having punctured the portal vein, a guidewire is directed through the needle into the portal vein. The needle is removed leaving the guidewire in place coursing between hepatic vein, liver parenchyma, and the portal vein. An angiographic catheter is advanced over the guidewire and directed into the portal vein. A pre TIPS direct portal pressure measurement is recorded through the angiographic catheter and the right atrial pressure is recorded through the right internal jugular vein sheath. A portal venogram is obtained. The guidewire is redirected through the catheter and the diagnostic catheter is removed. An angioplasty balloon is next directed over the guidewire into the hepatic parenchyma between the hepatic vein and the portal vein. The tissue tract is dilated with the angioplasty balloon. Because of liver fibrosis, the tract will not remain patent unless a stent is used to hold open the new tract. Stents may be (1) a balloon expandable Palmaz stent, or (2) a self-expanding Wallstent, or (3) Gianturco Z stent. At our institution, the Wallstent is preferred because of its 7 F delivery system and the stent's flexibility.

Once the newly-created tract has been dilated, the balloon is deflated and removed. A nonexpanded Wallstent is directed over the guidewire through the parenchymal tract bridging the distance between the hepatic vein and portal vein. Once the Wallstent is deployed, repeat balloon dilation expands the stent. The stent struts are imbedded in the parenchymal tissue and the stent maintains shunt patency between hepatic vein and portal vein. Care is taken to avoid placing the stents in the inferior vena cava or main portal vein since this may jeopardize possible future hepatic transplantation. Pressure measurements are obtained after the procedure and if necessary the stent may be further expanded to increase the diameter of the intrahepatic shunt. Usually balloon dilation of the stent to 8 to 10 millimeters is usually sufficient to decompress esophageal varices without causing encephalopathy.

If the patient is actively bleeding during the TIPS procedure, the coronary vein (left gastric vein) may be embolized since there is direct access via the TIPS shunt. At our institution, the nasobiliary tube is removed upon completion of the TIPS procedure. Anesthesia support is also used during a TIPS procedure to optimize hemodynamic monitoring of the patients.

After a TIPS procedure, long-term patient management consists of periodic monitoring of hepatic function, directly measuring a shunt pressure gradient by catheterizing the shunt via a femoral or jugular approach, and follow-up esophageal endoscopy. Doppler ultrasound is also used to noninvasively evaluate shunt patency at intervals between the more invasive venous catheterization procedure. Evaluations are done as outpatient procedures. Patients are not kept on long-term anticoagulation. Should a patient rebleed from esophageal varices, it is necessary to evaluate the shunt to check for stenosis or occlusion. If patent but stenotic, the shunt may be redilated. Child A, B, and C patients have all successfully undergone TIPS procedures.

PROS AND CONS OF TIPS

TIPS is an investigational procedure for which Institutional Review Board approval is required. Precisely which patients will benefit from the TIPS procedure is still under investigation. In the largest published series of patients in the United States undergoing the TIPS procedure using the Wallstent endoprosthesis reported by Laberge et al, variceal bleeding was the largest indication for the TIPS procedure (94 of 100 patients). Other indications included: intractable ascites (three patients); hepatorenal syndrome (two patients) and preoperative portal decompression (one patient). Shunts were completed in 96 of 100 patients. Acute variceal bleeding was controlled in 29 of 30 patients. In ten patients, variceal bleeding recurred. Of the group of patients undergoing the TIPS procedure, 15 developed a problem with the shunt—shunt stenosis in six patients, shunt occlusion in nine patients. Patency was reestablished in eight of the nine occluded shunts. Seventeen patients developed new or worsened encephalopathy; i.e., new onset in 14 patients and worsening encephalopathy in three patients, the latter three patients having a history of encephalopathy before the TIPS procedure. Fourteen of 17 patients with new or worsened encephalopathy were controlled with lactulose. An overall frequency of encephalopathy post TIPS procedure in the University of California School of Medicine, San Francisco (UCSF) series was calculated to be 18 percent; however, the frequency of encephalopathy refractory to medical therapy was only 3 percent.

Hepatic decompensation is a recognized complication of surgical portosystemic shunts. In the UCSF series, liver enzyme tests were obtained before and after the TIPS procedure. With regard to the effect of the TIPS procedure on hepatic function, no consistent response was found. Bilirubin levels decreased in approximately 25 percent and remained the same in approximately 50 percent. Nine patients died of liver failure after TIPS, three within 30 days. Based on our experience and that of the UCSF series, deterioration of liver function may be accelerated by the TIPS procedure and therefore, in patients with imminent hepatic failure, TIPS should be undertaken only after careful consideration. In the UCSF series of 96 patients who underwent a successful TIPS procedure, 26 patients have died, 22 have undergone hepatic transplantation, and the remaining 48 patients have survived an average of 7.6 months.

Based on our experience and those of other investigators, the TIPS procedure is an effective and reliable means of lowering portal pressure and controlling variceal bleeding (1) in patients with acute variceal bleeding unresponsive to sclerotherapy and (2) in patients with chronic variceal bleeding awaiting liver transplantation. In general, we feel TIPS should be considered in those patients with significant hepatic reserve who have failed conventional sclerotherapy or banding and who are not yet considered candidates for hepatic transplantation.

As experience with the TIPS technique has accumulated, the following observations are noteworthy:

1. Approximately 10 percent of patients with *acute variceal hemorrhage* will not respond to variceal sclerosis. TIPS is a reasonable alternative for the management of ongoing hemorrhage despite sclerotherapy. The mortality of surgical portacaval shunt procedures in patients with Child C cirrhosis is as high as 50 percent. The 30-day mortality of Child class C cirrhotic patients who underwent TIPS therapy in the UCSF series was 24 percent and therefore substantially less in this high risk group.
2. TIPS appears to be effective in treating patients with chronic recurrent variceal bleeding.
3. Patients with ascites refractory to medical therapy may benefit from the TIPS procedure. A LeVeen shunt is another option but is frequently associated with complications including occlusion.
4. TIPS may play a role in the treatment of patients with Budd-Chiari syndrome. A limited number of patients with Budd-Chiari syndrome have undergone the TIPS procedure to reduce the clinical sequelae of portal hypertension. The procedure is technically difficult in such patients but may be an alternative to other surgical shunt procedures.
5. Patients awaiting liver transplantation may benefit from TIPS in that it does not alter extrahepatic anatomy and may reduce the clinical sequelae of portal hypertension, i.e., esophageal variceal bleeding. There may be a potential added benefit of decreased operative blood loss because of decompression of portal hypertension and retroperitoneal varices. This however is still being investigated.
6. TIPS has been used to treat hepatorenal syndrome in a limited number of patients. TIPS has been performed at UCSF in two patients with hepatorenal syndrome and in eight other azotemic patients treated for bleeding. In five of the eight patients with azotemia and bleeding prior to the procedure, renal function improved post TIPS as evidenced by a sustained decrease in serum creatinine level of at least 1 mg per deciliter (90 μmol per liter) for more than 7 days. In one of the two patients undergoing TIPS for hepatorenal syndrome, renal function also improved. However, results must be interpreted with caution since numbers of patients are small.

Contraindications to TIPS include:

1. Patients with advanced encephalopathy.
2. Patients in whom the hepatic veins or the portal veins are thrombosed have a relative contraindication to the TIPS procedure. TIPS has been performed in limited numbers of patients with documented Budd-Chiari syndrome and in patients with portal vein thrombosis. Recanalization of the occluded (or thrombosed) veins has been technically possible in some patients though this has been difficult and should be attempted only by an experienced interventional radiologist familiar with the procedure. In such patients, the portal vein or hepatic vein is recanalized using guidewires, catheters, and balloon dilation followed by the TIPS procedure; i.e. TIPS with a "nonsurgical reconstruction" of the venous anatomy.
3. Occasionally the anatomy of a patient with advanced cirrhosis may not be favorable for creation of an intrahepatic shunt. In such patients, hepatic or portal vein anatomy may be markedly distorted. With regard to those patients with nonvariceal GI bleeding, there is little information in the literature concerning efficacy of the TIPS procedure in patients with portal hypertensive gastropathy as the primary source of chronic GI bleeding. This is an area of active investigation.

COMMENTS

Although the application of the TIPS procedure in humans is relatively new, the principles of portosystemic decompression for treatment of esophageal hemorrhage are well-established. As with any new procedure, refinements of the technique, shunt patency rates, and precisely which patients will benefit in the long term require further investigation. At present, TIPS is a viable treatment option in a subset of patients with portal hypertension and limited hepatic reserve.

SUGGESTED READING

Haskal ZL, Ring EJ, Laberge JM, et al. Role of parallel transjugular intrahepatic portosystemic shunts in patients with portal hypertension. Radiology 1992; 185:813–817.
Laberge JM, Ring EJ, Gordon RL, et al. Creation of transjugular intrahepatic portosystemic shunts with the Wallstent endoprosthesis: Results in 100 patients. Radiology 1993; 187: 413–420.
Lake JR. A hepatologist's view of TIPS—who needs it and when? Presented at course, Interventional Hepatobiliary Radiology: Percutaneous Portocaval Shunts, Biliary Stents, Tumor Chemoembolization, Lithotripsy. University of California School of Medicine, San Francisco, California. 1992; June 4 to 6, syllabus pp 170–177.
Ostroff JW. Variceal bleeding and non-surgical therapy. Presented at course, Interventional Hepatobiliary Radiology: Percutaneous Portocaval Shunts, Biliary Stents, Tumor Chemoembolization, Lithotripsy. University of California School of Medicine, San Francisco, California. 1992; June 4 to 6, syllabus pp 117–121.
Radosevich PM, Ring EJ, Laberge JM, et al. Transjugular intrahepatic portosystemic shunts in patients with portal vein occlusion. Radiology 1993; 186:523–527.
Richter GM, Noelge G, Palmaz JC, Roessle M. The transjugular intrahepatic portosystemic stent-shunt (TIPPS): Results of a pilot study. Cardiovasc Intervent Radiol 1990; 13:200–207.
Woodle ES, Darcy M, White HM, et al. Intrahepatic portosystemic vascular stents—a bridge to hepatic transplantation. Surgery 1993; 113:344–351.
Zemel G, Katzen B, Becker GJ, et al. Percutaneous transjugular portosystemic shunt: Preliminary communication. JAMA 1991; 266:390–393.
Zemel G, Becker GL, Bancroft JW, et al. Technical advances in transjugular intrahepatic portosystemic shunts. Radiographics 1992; 12:615–622.

PORTAL HYPERTENSION SURGERY

LAYTON F. RIKKERS, M.D.

Until 20 years ago, surgically created portal systemic shunts were the mainstay of treatment for bleeding esophagogastric varices. The first threat to the dominance of shunt surgery for this life-threatening complication of portal hypertension was the discovery in several controlled trials that the portacaval shunt did not result in prolongation of survival of cirrhotic patients who bled from varices when compared to conventional medical management. Soon thereafter, endoscopic sclerotherapy, which was first described more than 50 years ago, was reintroduced and, because it is less invasive than surgery, it became the favored treatment for this problem throughout the world. Recently, development of the transjugular intrahepatic portosystemic shunt (TIPS) has added another treatment option to the nonoperative approach. However, surgeons have remained active participants in the management of these patients by new methods of portal decompression, such as the distal splenorenal shunt, and liver transplantation. The purposes of this chapter are to describe briefly the various surgical alternatives for the treatment of portal hypertension and to present my view of their role in the emergency and elective management of this challenging problem.

OPERATIONS FOR PORTAL HYPERTENSION

The three types of operations used for control of acute variceal bleeding and for prevention of future episodes are (1) portal systemic shunts; (2) devascularization procedures; and (3) liver transplantation.

Portal Systemic Shunts

Surgical portal decompression is the most effective means of controlling acute hemorrhage and of preventing future episodes of bleeding from portal hypertension. However, the price to be paid is diversion of all or a significant fraction of portal venous blood away from the liver. Since portal blood contains important nutrients, hepatotrophic hormones, and cerebral toxins, elimination or diminution of hepatic portal perfusion may have adverse consequences, such as postshunt encephalopathy, liver atrophy, and accelerated hepatic failure. Portal systemic shunts are classified as nonselective, selective, and partial, depending on the degree to which they divert portal flow away from the liver.

Nonselective Shunts

Nonselective shunts reliably decompress the entire portal venous system and eliminate hepatic portal perfusion (Fig. 1). The two hemodynamic types of nonselective shunts are the end-to-side portacaval shunt and several varieties of side-to-side portal systemic shunts. After all of these procedures, the liver is dependent upon hepatic arterial perfusion alone. Because the end-to-side portacaval shunt is relatively easy

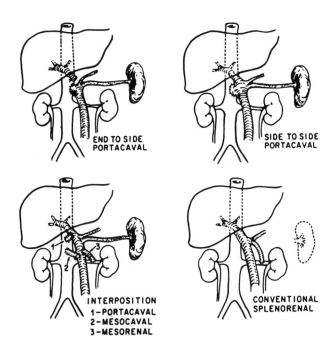

Figure 1 Nonselective shunts. (From Rikkers LF. Portal hypertension. In: Moody FG, ed. Surgical treatment of digestive disease. Chicago: Mosby–Year Book, 1986:416.)

to construct and immediately decompresses the portal venous circulation, it is used by many surgeons in the emergency setting. Side-to-side portal systemic shunts, because they leave the hepatic limb of the portal vein intact, decompress the liver as well as the splanchnic viscera. Since the liver is an important site of ascites formation, these procedures are reliable in relieving medically intractable ascites, as well as controlling variceal bleeding. The end-to-side and side-to-side portacaval shunts create large vein-to-vein anastomoses and, therefore, have excellent long-term patency rates in excess of 95 percent. In addition to complete diversion of portal venous flow, a significant disadvantage of the portacaval shunt is that it makes subsequent liver transplantation a more formidable procedure.

Large diameter interposition synthetic grafts, usually of Dacron or polytetrafluoroethylene material, can be placed in a variety of positions in the portal venous system, but the mesocaval shunt is most commonly used. The hemodynamics of this shunt are identical to those of the side-to-side portacaval shunt. A disadvantage is a high shunt occlusion rate that may approach 35 percent during prolonged follow-up; an advantage is avoidance of the hepatic hilum, which is an important consideration for future transplant candidates.

The conventional splenorenal shunt, which consists of splenectomy and anastomosis of the proximal splenic vein to the left renal vein, is seldom used. The relatively small diameter of the proximal splenic vein makes this shunt prone to thrombosis. Although the conventional splenorenal shunt may initially function as a partial portal systemic shunt, if the anastomosis is large enough to remain patent, it dilates and becomes a total shunt

over time. Splenectomy eliminates hypersplenism, but this is rarely a significant clinical problem in patients with portal hypertension.

Controlled and matched controlled comparisons of the various nonselective shunts to each other have shown no significant clinical differences between these procedures, except for better relief of ascites by side-to-side shunts. Controlled trials of the portacaval shunt versus conventional medical management revealed no significant advantage of this procedure with respect to long-term survival. In addition, encephalopathy rates of 20 to 50 percent are reported in most series of nonselective shunts.

Selective Shunts

The only commonly utilized selective shunt is the distal splenorenal shunt (Fig. 2). The objective of this procedure is to separate the portal venous circulation into two components: a decompressed gastrosplenic division, and a high-pressure superior mesenteric-portal venous circuit which has the potential of continuing to perfuse the liver with portal blood. In addition to constructing a distal splenorenal anastomosis, an important part of the procedure is interruption of all collaterals connecting these newly separated subdivisions of the portal venous circulation. The major contraindications to the distal splenorenal shunt are medically intractable ascites and incompatible anatomy, including prior splenectomy and a small diameter splenic vein (< 7 mm). Although initially considered a technically challenging surgical procedure, the distal splenorenal shunt has been mastered by many surgeons and is presently one of the more commonly performed shunting procedures world-wide with over 3,700 cases being reported in the surgical literature.

Despite the extensive experience with the distal splenorenal shunt, including numerous controlled trials, its superiority over nonselective shunts has not been unequivocally established. Selective variceal decompression clearly preserves hepatic portal perfusion in the short term, but gradual attrition of portal flow occurs over time so that only 40 to 60 percent of patients have evidence of hepatic portal perfusion at 1 to 3 years after the procedure. Portal flow tends to be more effectively preserved in patients with nonalcoholic cirrhosis and noncirrhotic causes of portal hypertension. In alcoholics, portal flow can be better preserved by dissecting the entire length of the splenic vein from the pancreas (splenopancreatic disconnection), but this extension of the procedure makes it considerably more complex. Until clear clinical advantages of splenopancreatic disconnection are proven, it should not be recommended for routine use.

Table 1 presents the combined results of the seven controlled trials of the distal splenorenal shunt versus a variety of nonselective shunts. There was no survival advantage to either operation in any of these investigations; four trials showed a significantly lower frequency of postshunt encephalopathy after the distal

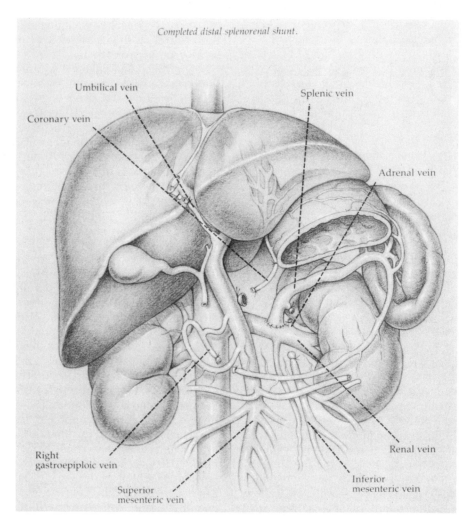

Completed distal splenorenal shunt.

Umbilical vein

Coronary vein

Splenic vein

Adrenal vein

Right
gastroepiploic vein

Superior
mesenteric vein

Renal vein

Inferior
mesenteric vein

Figure 2 Distal splenorenal shunt for portal hypertension. (From Rikkers LF. Distal splenorenal shunt for portal hypertension. In: Surgery Illustrated. New Scotland, NY: Learning Technology Incorporated, 1988.)

Table 1 Seven Controlled Trials of Distal Splenorenal Shunt (DSRS) Versus Nonselective Shunts (NSS)

Procedure	N	Alcoholic Cirrhosis	Operative Mortality	Late Mortality	Encephalopathy	Recurrent Variceal Bleeding
DSRS	181	74%	8%	27%	21%	11%
NSS	190	80%	6%	34%	37%	7%

From Rikkers LF. Portal hypertension: shunting procedures. In: Cameron JL, ed. Current Surgical Therapy. 3rd ed. Toronto: BC Decker, 1989:237; with permission.

splenorenal shunt; and a single investigation revealed better bleeding control following the portacaval shunt than after the distal splenorenal shunt. Based on these observations, as well as data derived from other large series, it can be concluded that selective variceal decompression results in a lower incidence of encephalopathy than nonselective shunts (10 to 15 percent versus 20 to 40 percent). The differences between procedures are most apparent in nonalcoholic causes of portal hypertension, but the alcoholic patient probably also derives a benefit. Shunt failure rates may be slightly higher after the distal splenorenal shunt, but in most series they are below 10 percent. A secondary advantage of the distal splenorenal shunt is that the hepatic hilum is not dissected, thereby making future liver transplantation less challenging.

Partial Shunts

One objective of the partial portal systemic shunt is to leave a significant pressure gradient between portal and systemic venous systems, thereby allowing continuing portal venous flow to the liver. Initial attempts at partial shunting were with small diameter side-to-side portacaval shunts. However, these anastomoses tend to dilate with time, resulting in total portal venous diversion. A newer approach is interposition of a synthetic graft 8 to 10 mm in diameter between the portal vein and the inferior vena cava. Although experience with the small diameter interposition portacaval shunt is limited, initial studies suggest that portal flow may be preserved, and that encephalopathy rates are lower than after total portal decompression. A controlled trial comparing large diameter and small diameter interposition shunts is presently underway, but no results have yet been reported. A potential disadvantage of this approach may be frequent shunt occlusion.

Devascularization Procedures

The objectives of devascularization procedures are to interrupt collateral pathways to varices and/or directly obliterate the varices themselves. They represent the surgical counterpart of endoscopic sclerotherapy. Since devascularization operations generally do not lower portal pressure, the stimulus to formation of varices remains and, therefore, they tend to be less effective than shunts for long-term prevention of recurrent bleeding. The sole exception is splenectomy alone as treatment for bleeding gastric varices secondary to isolated splenic vein thrombosis.

The simplest of devascularization procedures, usually performed in the emergency setting, is distal esophageal transection and reanastomosis using a stapling device, often combined with coronary vein ligation. This technique is generally ineffective for bleeding from gastric varices or portal hypertensive gastropathy, but in some series, it has proved to be an effective method for controlling acutely bleeding esophageal varices. However, the late rebleeding rates after esophageal transection have been considerably higher than after all portal decompressive procedures. Additionally, operative mortality rates after this procedure tend to be similar to those after shunt operations. One controlled trial has demonstrated that esophageal transection is approximately equal in effectiveness to acute endoscopic sclerotherapy.

The Sugiura procedure, which consists of splenectomy, devascularization of the proximal two-thirds of the stomach, devascularization of the distal esophagus, and esophageal transection, is the most extensive of the devascularization operations. Although originally described as a two-stage operation through abdominal and thoracic incisions, most modifications allow the operation to be completed through an abdominal incision alone. In Sugiura's large series of mainly nonalcoholic Japanese cirrhotic patients, the rebleeding rate was less than 5 percent with excellent long-term survival. However, application of the Sugiura procedure to North American alcoholic cirrhotic patients has resulted in rebleeding rates above 25 percent.

The main indications for an elective devascularization procedure are unshuntable patients with diffuse splanchnic venous thrombosis and some individuals with well-preserved hepatic portal perfusion in whom a distal splenorenal shunt is not possible because of prior splenectomy or another anatomic reason. Although less reliable for preventing rebleeding, these procedures are more effective than any shunt in preserving portal blood flow to the liver.

Liver Transplantation

Since liver replacement restores both portal pressure and hepatic functional reserve to normal, it needs to be considered in the therapeutic algorithm of all patients with chronic liver disease who bleed from varices. However, because of a shortage of donor organs, economic factors, and availability of liver transplantation in a limited number of centers, transplantation can be offered to only a small percentage of variceal bleeders. Even when available, many patients are not appropriate candidates because of advanced disease of other organ systems or unresolved alcoholism or other drug abuses. The large number of patients throughout the world with noncirrhotic portal hypertension (e.g., schistosomiasis) are also not transplant candidates. (There are three chapters on orthotopic liver transplantation.)

SURGERY FOR ACUTE VARICEAL HEMORRHAGE

With the availability of more effective nonoperative therapies such as endoscopic variceal sclerosis and variceal banding, emergency surgery plays a lesser, but still important role in the management of acute variceal hemorrhage. Endoscopic sclerotherapy (or esophageal banding) has become the first-line treatment for the patient acutely bleeding from esophageal varices in most centers. Sclerotherapy is successful in controlling acute bleeding in 80 to 90 percent of patients, which allows time for optimization of hepatic function before definitive therapy (chronic sclerotherapy, variceal banding, shunt, or transplantation) is carried out.

The challenge is to recognize those patients who fail sclerotherapy or banding as early as possible so that they can be transported to the operating room or interventional radiology suite for TIPS while they are still salvageable. Failure of sclerotherapy in the acute setting has been defined as persistent bleeding after two sclerotherapy sessions. One series has demonstrated a mortality rate of greater than 50 percent if surgery is not performed after two sclerotherapy sessions have failed to control hemorrhage. Surgical intervention should be considered even earlier in patients who have failed chronic sclerotherapy and in those individuals who bleed from gastric varices or portal hypertensive gastropathy, because nonoperative treatment options are limited for such patients. With sclerotherapy and/or banding now available in many hospitals, one might expect emergency surgery for variceal hemorrhage to be infrequent or even rare. However, in our institution, the percentage of operations done as emergencies (20 percent) has remained the same, because failure of chronic sclerotherapy has become a relatively common indication for emergency surgery.

There is no consensus as to the ideal emergency surgical procedure. An important principle is that a surgeon faced with this situation should perform an operation with which he is familiar and can successfully complete in a relatively short time. For surgeons inexperienced in portal hypertension surgery, the best choice may be esophageal transection with a stapling device. Most experienced surgeons prefer one of the shunt operations because they are more effective in the long-term control of portal hypertensive bleeding from all sites, including gastric varices and portal hypertensive gastropathy. The most frequently used emergency shunt procedures are the portacaval shunt and the interposition mesocaval shunt. The latter is preferable for future transplant candidates. Operative mortality rates after these procedures are clearly higher in the emergency setting than in the elective setting. Operative mortality rates below 20 percent have been reported when only good to moderate risk patients are included (Child's classes A and B). However, Child's class C status is not a contraindication to emergency surgical therapy.

If the expertise is available, very high risk patients may be better served by a TIPS procedure. TIPS is preferable for sclerotherapy failures of all Child's classes if they are candidates for liver transplantation in the near future.

Because of its greater technical complexity and less complete portal decompression in the immediate postoperative interval, the distal splenorenal shunt has generally not been considered an effective emergency surgical alternative. However, we have found the distal splenorenal shunt to be an excellent choice in appropriate patients when the setting is urgent, rather than emergent. Bleeding must be temporarily controlled by intravenous pitressin infusion or balloon tamponade, allowing time for angiographic evaluation. Our operative mortality rate for urgent distal splenorenal shunts (10 percent) compares favorably with that achieved for this operation in the elective setting (6 percent). Additionally, in our experience, control of bleeding has been just as effective after urgent settings as following elective distal splenorenal shunts.

SURGERY AS DEFINITIVE THERAPY FOR VARICEAL HEMORRHAGE

After acute variceal hemorrhage has been controlled, definitive treatment is indicated for most patients because the risk of recurrent bleeding exceeds 70 percent. The algorithm used at our institution is outlined in Figure 3. Patients are first grouped based on their candidacy for liver transplantation. Whether or not they are transplant candidates is based mainly on the cause of portal hypertension, abstinence for alcoholic cirrhotics, and the presence or absence of significant dysfunction of other major organ systems.

Variceal bleeders who fit into the transplant group and who have advanced chronic liver disease (Child's class B or class C) should immediately be referred for transplantation. Additionally, even patients with good hepatic functional reserve (Child's class A and B +), but who have severe symptoms of their liver disease, such as fatigue, persistent ascites, or chronic encephalopathy, should undergo transplantation as soon as a donor organ can be identified. If acute sclerotherapy fails to control bleeding in this category of patients, TIPS should be utilized as a bridge to transplantation.*

Patients who will never be transplant candidates, and those who will probably not require transplantation for several years because of well preserved hepatic function, represent the majority of variceal bleeders. Chronic endoscopic sclerotherapy has become the most commonly used definitive treatment for such patients. However, in trials which have provided long-term follow-up, 45 to 60 percent of patients undergoing chronic sclerotherapy rebled from varices at least once, and up to one-third of patients eventually fail sclerotherapy and either bleed to death or require surgical intervention.

In a recent, controlled trial of the distal splenorenal shunt versus chronic sclerotherapy, we found a survival advantage for those patients undergoing a selective shunt. In contrast, a similar trial completed at Emory University discovered a survival advantage for the sclerotherapy group, one-third of whom required surgical salvage when they failed sclerotherapy. The patient populations of these two trials are quite different. Our patients are derived from a predominantly rural area, and those in the Emory trial were accrued from metropolitan Atlanta. Most of the bleeding deaths in the sclerotherapy group of our trial were in rural patients who were unable to return to our institution for shunt surgery when they failed sclerotherapy. Based on the results of these two trials, we have concluded that chronic sclerotherapy is appropriate, definitive treatment for individuals who bleed from esophageal varices, who are compliant and likely to return for subsequent treatment sessions, and who live in reasonable proximity to the institution responsible for their overall management. However, variceal bleeders living in rural areas, those who bleed from gastric varices and portal hypertensive gastropathy, and those who are incapable of following a treatment schedule are probably better served by initial portal decompression.

Shunt candidates with medically controllable ascites and compatible anatomy should receive a distal splenorenal shunt, because it is associated with a lower

---

*Editor's Note: The astute reader will be picking up more ideas about liver transplantation than "just" those in the chapters on transplantation.

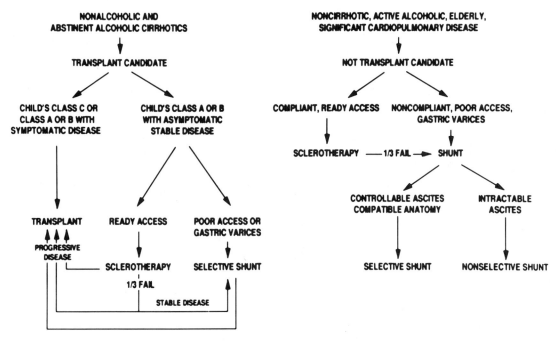

Figure 3 Algorithm for definitive management of variceal hemorrhage used at the University of Nebraska Medical Center. Ready access and poor access refer to availability of portal hypertension surgery based on geographic location or other factors. (From Rikkers LF. Definitive therapy for variceal bleeding: a personal view. Am J Surg 1990; 160:80–85.)

frequency of encephalopathy than nonselective shunts. In contrast, patients with ascites intractable to medical management and portal hypertensive bleeding should undergo a side-to-side nonselective shunt because it is effective in both resolving ascites and preventing recurrent variceal bleeding. A devascularization procedure of the modified Sugiura type should be considered for unshuntable patients with diffuse splanchnic venous thrombosis if they fail endoscopic sclerotherapy. Whether they are undergoing chronic sclerotherapy or have received a portal systemic shunt, future transplant candidates should be carefully monitored so that they can promptly be placed on the transplant list when progressive disease is detected. A key to cost-effective, successful liver transplantation is applying this therapy before the patient has become an extreme operative risk.

TIPS has not been discussed as definitive treatment, other than as a bridge to transplantation. There is a separate chapter on the subject. Most data suggests that TIPS is a total side-to-side shunt with all the advantages and disadvantages of that procedure. Although effective in decompressing varices and in relieving ascites, early series suggest that a disadvantage of TIPS is a relatively high frequency of postshunt encephalopathy. Shunt occlusion or stenosis develops in as many as 50 percent of patients within 6 months, but an effective shunt can often be re-established by interventional methods. The long-term patency rate of TIPS is unknown.

What are the indications for this new approach, other than as a short-term bridge to transplantation? Although the place of TIPS in our treatment algorithm is yet to be determined, it is likely a reasonable option for

nontransplant candidates who fail sclerotherapy and who are high-operative risks for an open shunt procedure because of advanced hepatic dysfunction. Many of these patients are likely to die of liver failure before TIPS occlusion or stenosis develops. On the other hand, patients who may require transplantation in the distant future and nontransplant candidates with adequate hepatic functional reserve are probably better served with a distal splenorenal shunt because both the shunt failure rate and the likelihood of encephalopathy are considerably lower than after TIPS. Although TIPS has been successfully applied to patients with medically-intractable ascites and no history of bleeding, this should be done with caution because of the disadvantages of total portal venous diversion.

SUGGESTED READING

Henderson JM. Liver transplantation for portal hypertension. Gastroenterol Clin North Am 1992; 21:197–213.

Henderson JM, Kutner MH, Millikan WJ, et al. Endoscopic variceal sclerosis compared with distal splenorenal shunt to prevent recurrent variceal bleeding in cirrhosis. Ann Intern Med 1990; 112: 262–269.

Rikkers LF. Definitive therapy for variceal bleeding: a personal view. Am J Surg 1990; 160:80–85.

Rikkers LF, Jin G, Burnett DA, et al. Shunt surgery versus endoscopic sclerotherapy for long-term treatment of variceal bleeding. Am J Surg 1993; 165:27–33.

Rikkers LF, Sorrell WT, Jin G. Which portosystemic shunt is best? Gastroenterol Clin North Am 1992; 21:179–196.

Sugiura M, Futagawa S. Esophageal transection with paraesophagogastric devascularization (the Sugiura Procedure) in the treatment of esophageal varices. World J Surg 1984; 8:673–682.

DRUG-INDUCED LIVER DAMAGE

MACK C. MITCHELL, M.D.

Drug-induced damage is an important cause of liver disease which results most often from idiosyncratic adverse reactions. A wide range of biochemical and histological manifestations of injury may accompany these events. Often the features of drug-induced injury are difficult to distinguish from other causes of liver disease. For this reason, the clinician must maintain a high index of suspicion when evaluating the possibility of drug-related liver damage. Management requires prompt recognition and elimination of exposure to the offending agent. In a few instances, administration of specific agents may be useful in preventing injury or reducing its severity. One example, discussed later in this chapter, is acetaminophen overdose. In most cases, therapy for hepatotoxicity is limited to supportive treatment for the complications of resulting hepatic dysfunction.

CLASSIFICATION

Drug-induced liver damage may be classified according to the histologic features of liver injury (Table 1) or the mechanism of injury (Table 2). Both classifications are useful and are by no means mutually exclusive. Classification based on histopathology is valuable in identifying which of several drugs is the offending agent, since the features of injury are often characteristic for a particular hepatotoxin. For example, chlorpromazine typically causes cholestasis and periportal inflammation, whereas isoniazid most often causes centrilobular necrosis and patchy lobular inflammation. Classification by mechanism of injury is helpful because it provides a rational basis for prevention and treatment of the injury.

As shown in Table 1, both acute and chronic liver diseases may result from drug hepatotoxicity. Furthermore, the time between exposure to the drug and development of clinical manifestations of liver disease varies. Acute injury from exposure to intrinsic hepatotoxins, such as carbon tetrachloride, results in rapid elevation of aminotransferases and clinical signs of

Table 2 Classification of Drug-Induced Liver Damage by Mechanism of Injury

Mechanism	Example
Intrinsic toxins	
Direct	Carbon tetrachloride, arsenic
Metabolite-mediated	Acetaminophen, chlorpromazine, carbon tetrachloride
Idiosyncratic toxins	
Hypersensitivity	Phenytoin, sulfonamides, ticrynafen, p-aminosalicylate, halothane
Host metabolism	Phenytoin (?), valproate, isoniazid (?), halothane?

Table 1 Classification of Drug-Induced Liver Disease by Histopathology

Type of Injury	Biochemical Abnormalities ($\times$ Normal)		Examples
	Aminotransferase	Alkaline Phosphatase	
Hepatocellular			
Acute necrosis	10–500	1–2	Acetaminophen, carbon tetrachloride
Acute hepatitis	10–100	1–2	Isoniazid, aspirin, phenytoin
Chronic hepatitis	5–50	1–2	Isoniazid, alpha-methyldopa, nitrofurantoin
Steatosis/ steatohepatitis	5–10	1–3	Tetracycline, valproate, corticosteroids, nucleoside analogues, ethanol, amiodarone, perhexiline maleate
Cholestasis			
Inflammatory	1–10	3–10	Chlorpromazine, erythromycin, amoxicillin/clavulanate
Noninflammatory	1–5	1–5	Oral contraceptives, rifampicin
Granulomatous inflammation	5–25	2–10	Numerous
Vascular			
Peliosis hepatitis	1–2	1–2	Anabolic steroids, oral contraceptives
Hepatic vein thrombosis	2–5	1–2	Oral contraceptives
Veno-occlusive disease	2–5	2–5	Antineoplastic agents, bone marrow transplants
Tumors			
Hepatic adenomas	Variable	1–3	Oral contraceptives
Hepatocellular carcinoma	Variable	1–3	Anabolic steroids
Angiosarcoma	Variable	1–3	Vinyl chloride

injury when severe. These abnormalities are usually apparent within several days of exposure.

By contrast, idiosyncratic drug hepatotoxicity requires a longer period of exposure before development of damage. Adverse hepatic reaction to medications is more often idiosyncratic since most intrinsic hepatotoxins are eliminated through extensive preclinical testing. With few exceptions, intrinsic hepatotoxins cause liver injury in animals similar to that which might occur in man. Idiosyncratic injury can result from immunologic hypersensitivity or because of metabolic abnormalities that might alter normal drug detoxification within an individual (see Table 2). Hypersensitivity reactions may involve organs other than the liver and frequently produce systemic manifestations such as fever, arthralgias, and rash. Peripheral eosinophilia and granulomatous hepatic inflammation are common. Hypersensitivity usually develops within a few weeks after initiation of therapy, but recurs promptly upon rechallenge after discontinuation.

Reactions due to host metabolic idiosyncrasy require a longer exposure before clinical signs become manifest. In many instances a minor but potentially toxic metabolite of the drug is responsible for the injury. The dose of drug and the rate of formation and elimination of the metabolite(s) will determine the concentration of the metabolite to which the patient is ultimately exposed. For this reason, it is difficult to predict a time for onset of symptoms. Rarely, signs of drug-induced injury emerge weeks after cessation of drug use. Examples include cholestatic injuries from amoxicillin-clavulanic acid and fatty liver with lactic acidosis due to nucleoside analogues.

MONITORING

Since most adverse hepatic drug reactions are idiosyncratic, it is difficult to justify universal monitoring. However, the incidence of hepatic drug reactions is higher in women, in elderly patients, and in those individuals who have a history of drug reactions, including nonhepatic reactions. The incidence of reactions to some agents, although idiosyncratic, may be high enough to justify periodic monitoring of liver enzymes. The anticonvulsants phenytoin and sodium valproate both may cause hepatitis in susceptible individuals. Although hepatitis is rare, it is serious and potentially fatal. Monitoring serum aminotransferase levels may be helpful in predicting which patients will develop serious liver injury. Not all patients with elevated aminotransferase levels develop serious hepatic necrosis, but those who do are at higher risk and thus require closer supervision. Isoniazid causes abnormal aminotransferase levels in 10 percent of those treated, but only 1 percent develop serious toxicity. Nonsteroidal antiinflammatory drugs (NSAIDs), antidepressants, and antiarrhythmics are other categories of drugs for which periodic monitoring of aminotransferases may be indicated. Patients given medications known to cause

hepatotoxicity should be alerted to report immediately symptoms of hepatitis, such as anorexia, nausea, abdominal pain, jaundice, or dark urine.

When confronted with an asymptomatic patient in whom liver enzymes have become abnormal, the physician must decide whether the suspected drug is essential and whether another compound might be equally effective. If the medication is the only effective therapy for a patient's illness, such as life-threatening arrhythmia, the drug could be continued with careful monitoring of enzymes. In these instances liver biopsy may be used to determine the severity of liver damage. If the patient develops jaundice or other symptoms of hepatitis, or hypersensitivity, the drug should be stopped. Continuing therapy in a symptomatic patient with hepatitis is hazardous.

Determining whether abnormal liver enzymes are drug-related or are related to another condition, such as the early stages of viral hepatitis is more difficult. If a drug is responsible for the hepatitis, discontinuation of the presumed offending agent usually results in improvement, although not necessarily complete resolution, in symptoms and liver enzymes within 2 weeks. There are exceptions to this general rule, but failure to improve within a short time suggests an alternative cause for liver disease. Rechallenge is often contemplated as a method of determining whether the presumed agent was responsible for the liver disease. However, rechallenge is inherently risky. The risk is greatest for those drugs that cause allergic hypersensitivity. For example, fatal hepatic necrosis may occur after only the second administration or "rechallenge" with halothane. Rechallenge does not always produce prompt increases in aminotransferases or recurrence of symptoms. In some drug reactions, particularly those that are due to metabolic idiosyncrasy, several weeks or months may be required before recurrence becomes apparent. If rechallenge is carried out, the physician should be prepared for an exaggerated response to readministration of the drug. Hospitalization or close monitoring is advisable in most instances. For these reasons, I do not believe that rechallenge is necessary in most patients with suspected drug-induced liver damage.

TREATMENT

In cases of suspected drug hepatotoxicity, discontinuation of the presumed offending agent is the first and usually the only required step in treatment. Asymptomatic patients do not usually require hospitalization, but should be monitored carefully. Occasionally patients will continue to self-administer medications which they believe to be beneficial for a medical problem other than liver disease. If the patient does not have symptoms of liver disease, he may not recognize the potential danger in continuing therapy. The physician must be alert to such a possibility and instruct the patient carefully. Patients with jaundice or other symptoms of liver injury require more thorough evaluation. Prolongation of the prothrombin time (PT), development of hepatic encephalopathy, hypoglycemia, lactic acidosis, or low albumin are poor prognostic signs. Liver biopsy, when possible, is helpful in determining the severity of injury as well as the histologic pattern of damage.

In patients with fulminant hepatic failure, supportive care and close monitoring in an intensive care unit is indicated. These patients require vasopressor therapy for hypotension, administration of intravenous dextrose solutions to prevent or correct hypoglycemia, fresh frozen plasma for active bleeding, and judicious management of fluid and electrolyte balance. Lactulose may be indicated for encephalopathy and mannitol may be helpful in patients with cerebral edema.

Corticosteroid therapy does not directly alter the cause of fulminant hepatic failure and should not be used routinely. In patients with fever, skin rash, or other signs of allergic hypersensitivity, however, steroids may attenuate the immune response and further reduce hepatic injury. For example, steroids may be beneficial in patients with phenytoin or halothane hepatitis, both of which involve allergic hypersensitivity. Because of the rarity of these reactions, no controlled trial of the efficacy of steroids has been conducted.

Charcoal or resin hemoperfusion has been used successfully in some patients to increase the rate of elimination of highly lipid-soluble drugs with a long half-life. Experience with these techniques is limited and both may cause complications, such as thrombocytopenia. Experimental extracorporeal techniques include hemoperfusion cartridges packed with cultured hepatocytes and use of ex vivo xenografts. Hemodialysis is seldom necessary, except as treatment for associated renal failure, since most drugs that can be easily eliminated with this technique have short half-lives.

These general measures apply primarily to evaluation and management of patients with idiosyncratic drug-induced liver damage. A few drugs and unusual lesions associated with drug injury merit special attention.

Acetaminophen Poisoning

Acetaminophen is becoming the most widely used analgesic in Western countries. In general, the drug has a wide therapeutic index with toxicity occurring at doses more than ten times the usual therapeutic dose of 1 g every 4 hours. In alcoholics and some other individuals, the therapeutic index may be narrower for reasons discussed below. Fulminant hepatic failure and death have occurred in individuals after massive overdoses of this drug. Acetaminophen hepatotoxicity develops because of excessive formation of a highly reactive, electrophilic metabolite which is formed by a minor metabolic pathway of elimination, cytochrome P-450 mediated oxidation. Usually this reactive metabolite is further detoxified by hepatic glutathione; however, after massive overdose, glutathione is depleted, allowing the reactive metabolite to damage cellular macromolecules. Long-term heavy alcohol consumption causes induction of cytochrome P-450 IIe1 and enhances the formation of the toxic metabolite of acetaminophen.

Symptoms of acetaminophen hepatotoxicity usually appear after 24 hours, often resulting in delay in the patient seeking medical attention. The clinical course of hepatotoxicity is outlined in Table 3. Symptoms of liver failure usually begin after 48 to 72 hours. Patients with bilirubin levels over 4 mg per deciliter and prolongation of PT more than two and one-half times that of controls are at highest risk for serious liver damage.

The key to management of acetaminophen overdose is prompt recognition and initiation of treatment. If the patient is seen 24 hours after ingestion, specific treatment with N-acetylcysteine (Mucomyst) can prevent or reduce the severity of liver damage. Treatment may be initiated up to 24 hours after poisoning but is most effective when given early. For oral administration, the recommended dose is 140 mg per kilogram mixed in juice or soft drinks to disguise the unpleasant taste and odor. Repeat doses of 70 mg per kilogram should be given at 4-hour intervals for a total of 72 hours. N-acetylcysteine can be given by gavage. If the patient vomits within 1 hour the dose should be repeated. In Europe intravenous therapy has been used: 150 mg per kilogram in 200 ml of 5 percent dextrose over 15 minutes, followed by 50 mg per kilogram over the next 4 hours, and 100 mg per kilogram over the following 16 hours. Both routes of administration are effective, although at present an intravenous formulation is not available in the United States. If signs of liver failure develop, additional doses should be withheld to prevent worsening of hepatic encephalopathy.

Oral Contraceptives

A variety of liver diseases, including intrahepatic cholestasis, hepatic tumors, Budd-Chiari syndrome, and peliosis hepatis (blood-filled "lakes"), have occurred in patients taking oral contraceptives. *Intrahepatic cholestasis* is usually mild and always responds to discontinuation of the pill. There may be a higher frequency of this lesion in women with a history of jaundice during the third trimester of pregnancy. Hepatic adenomas and hepatocellular carcinoma also occur, although the incidence is low. Hepatocellular carcinoma should be resected, if possible, as medical and radiation therapy are mostly palliative. Although hepatic adenomas may regress after withdrawal of the drug, the propensity of this tumor to bleed massively into the peritoneal cavity suggests that surgical resection is advisable.

Budd-Chiari syndrome and peliosis hepatis are both vascular lesions associated with oral contraceptive use. *Peliosis* may rupture and bleed into the peritoneum. Surgical treatment is recommended only if there is hemoperitoneum. Otherwise, the drug should be withdrawn and the patient followed conservatively. *Budd-Chiari syndrome* is a dramatic illness characterized by abdominal pain, hepatomegaly, and ascites. Although the outlook for these patients is usually poor with only medical management, one report suggests the prognosis

Table 3 Clinical Course of Acetaminophen Hepatotoxicity

Time After Ingestion	Signs and Symptoms	Laboratory Studies
1–8 hr	Nausea, vomiting, anorexia	Normal
24–48 hr	Nausea, vomiting, anorexia, right upper quadrant pain	Elevated AST, ALT, and prothrombin time
48 hr	Jaundice	Elevated AST, ALT, prothrombin time, and bilirubin
72 hr	Jaundice, malaise	Peak of all tests
4–6 days	Encephalopathy, coma, death	Elevated ammonia, decreased glucose

may be better in those women who develop Budd-Chiari syndrome while taking oral contraceptives. In patients in whom there is complete occlusion of both hepatic veins, either side-to-side portocaval, or mesocaval shunting is indicated to relieve the severe outflow obstruction and prevent further loss of hepatocytes. With associated thrombosis of the vena cava, mesoatrial shunting is the preferred operation. When only one vein is obstructed, a trial of medical therapy is permissible although surgery may ultimately be needed. Recently transjugular intrahepatic portal shunts (TIPS) have shown promise as a treatment for the acute hepatic decompensation associated with Budd-Chiari syndrome. There is a separate chapter on Budd-Chiari syndrome.

Anabolic Steroids

Anabolic steroids, particularly methyltestosterone, are widely used by weight lifters and some other athletes. Although the incidence of liver disease in these individuals is low, peliosis hepatis, hepatocellular carcinoma, and angiosarcoma have been reported. Treatment for peliosis is withdrawal of the drug. Hepatocellular carcinoma should be resected, if possible. Angiosarcoma has a dismal prognosis and is not amenable to therapy.

Nonsteroidal Anti-inflammatory Drugs

Many drugs in this class have been reported to cause hepatic damage. Both cholestatic reactions and hepatocellular injury have been observed. In most instances, toxicity is mild. The incidence of serious adverse reactions is low, in the range of 1 case per 10,000 exposed. Abnormal aminotransferase values are seen more frequently. With some drugs, such as diclofenac and oxaprozin, the incidence of enzyme elevations may be as high as 15 percent. More serious liver injury is rare.

Fatal reactions are fortunately rare. A high rate of fatalities occurred with benoxaprofen, although the overall incidence of toxicity was similar to that of other NSAIDs. Benoxaprofen caused unusually severe cholestasis, frequently associated with renal failure. Elderly patients were most severely affected. Of note, this drug has a particularly long half-life, (20 hours) and thus may have accumulated after repeated dosing particularly in those elderly patients with diminished rates of elimination. Interestingly, ibuprofen, another proprionic acid derivative has a much shorter half-life and very little toxicity.

The mechanism of injury from NSAIDs is unclear, but presumably idiosyncratic, mostly the metabolic type. Some of these drugs may be intrinsically toxic as evidenced by a high rate of liver damage following overdoses of phenylbutazone. Because of the potential toxicity of NSAIDs, liver enzymes should be monitored approximately 4 to 6 weeks after the institution of long-term therapy or after substantial increases in the dose. Short-term treatment (<2 weeks) does not require monitoring unless the patient has a history of reactions to other NSAIDs. Those drugs with long half-lives deserve closer attention.

Lipid Lowering Agents

Most drugs which lower serum lipids also produce mild hepatic injury in 10 to 15 percent of recipients. The mechanism of injury has not been established, but the biochemical and histological features suggest hepatocellular damage. Toxicity is dose related which indicates some evidence of intrinsic toxicity. Elevation of aminotransferases less than 3 times the upper limit of normal (ULN) in the absence of clinical symptoms does not require discontinuation of lovastatin, simvistatin, pravastatin or related drugs; however, elevated aminotransferases are a warning that the dose should not be increased. Aminotransferases should be monitored before treatment, at 6 and 12 weeks and then every 2 months for the first year of therapy. Thereafter, monitoring should be done every 6 months or as needed to evaluate symptoms. Approximately 1 to 2 percent of patients treated will have persistent elevations greater than 3 times the ULN. These drugs should be discontinued as soon as symptoms of hepatitis occur or if aminotransferases are persistently greater than 3 times the ULN.

Nicotinic acid (niacin) has been used widely as a lipid lowering agent. Because it is a vitamin, it can be sold over-the-counter without prescription. The lay press has popularized use of this inexpensive, effective drug as part of self-directed health prevention efforts. Elevated aminotransferases are seen in 15 to 20 percent of patients taking niacin. Both the frequency of these abnormalities and the severity are dose related. A number of reports have shown that the slow-release formulations are more likely to produce hepatic injury and at lower doses. In several instances, inadvertent switching from crystalline preparations to a slow-release form led to fulminant hepatic failure. Because the efficacy of regular and slow-release forms is similar, use of the regular form is preferred. To avoid inadvertent toxicity, patients should be cautioned not to switch preparations or to self-prescribe.

Nucleoside Analogues

Nucleoside analogues such as zidovudine, dideoxy-cytidine, and acyclovir have been reported rarely to cause pancreatitis and peripheral neuropathy. Recently, severe microvesicular steatosis complicated by lactic acidosis, hypoglycemia, and other manifestations of fulminant hepatic failure was observed in patients with chronic hepatitis B treated for more than 4 weeks with FIAU (5-fluoro-iodo-arabinofuranosyl-uracil). Little or no toxicity was seen in the early phases of the trial of this antiviral agent, when dosing was limited to 4 weeks. However, a relatively high percentage of patients developed serious liver damage when treated for more than 6 to 8 weeks. A particularly worrisome feature of the toxicity was the relative absence of change in laboratory parameters including AST, ALT, and bilirubin prior to the onset of lactic acidosis which heralded a progressive downhill course. Several patients died or underwent liver transplantation as a result of these adverse events.

There is some evidence that the mechanism of damage was due to inhibition of mitochondrial DNA synthesis. Since other nucleoside analogues may share this potential, careful evaluation of any evidence of liver disease is warranted in patients treated with these antiviral agents.

Occupational Liver Disease

Since discontinuation of the widespread open use of carbon tetrachloride in dry cleaning and other indus-

tries, the incidence of documented hepatotoxicity through occupational exposure has diminished. Nonetheless, there are still many potentially hepatotoxic organic compounds to which workers are exposed which may cause liver damage. Haloalkanes (tetrachlorethane, trichloroethane, and TNT), arsenic, beryllium, and vinyl chloride all cause liver damage or hepatic tumors or both. Pesticides, particularly chlordecone (Kepone), may cause damage to liver and other organs. The herbicides paraquat and diquat have been reported to cause hepatic necrosis, although pulmonary damage is more commonly seen. Prevention of exposure to these potentially hazardous compounds is vital since there is no specific treatment for hepatotoxicity once it has occurred.

SUGGESTED READING

Kaplowitz N. Drug metabolism and hepatotoxicity. In: Kaplowitz N, ed. Liver and biliary diseases. Baltimore: Williams & Wilkins, 1991:82.

Kumar S, Rex DK. Failure of physicians to recognize acetaminophen hepatotoxicity in chronic alcoholics. Arch Intern Med 1991; 151: 1189–1191.

Lee WM. Review article: Drug-induced hepatotoxicity. Aliment Pharmacol Ther 1993; 7:477–485.

Lewis JH, Ranard RC, Carus A, et al. Amiodarone hepato-toxicity: Prevalence and clinicopathologic correlations among 104 patients. Hepatology 1989; 9:679–685.

Newman M, Auerbach R, Feiner H, et al. The role of liver biopsies in psoriatic patients receiving long-term methotrexate treatment. Arch Dermatol 1989; 125:1218–1224.

Pohl LR. Drug-induced allergic hepatitis. Semin Liv Dis 1990; 10:305–315.

Smilkstein MJ, Knapp GL, Kulig KW, Rumack BH. Efficacy of oral N-acetylcysteine in the treatment of acetaminophen overdose. N Engl J Med 1988; 319:1557–1562.

Zimmerman HJ, Maddrey WC. Toxic and drug induced hepatitis. In: Schiff L, Schiff ER, eds. Diseases of the liver. Philadelphia: JB Lippincott, 1993:707.

LIVER DISEASE IN PREGNANCY

SUSAN L. LUCAK, M.D.

Normal pregnancy is associated with physiologic changes which affect the function of many maternal organs including the liver. Liver disease may complicate pregnancy and conversely pregnancy may complicate pre-existing liver disease. Although the association of liver disease and pregnancy is not common (less than 0.1 percent of pregnancies), its occurrence can have serious implications for both the mother and the fetus. In this chapter I discuss the liver changes occurring in normal pregnancy, liver diseases unique to pregnancy, and liver diseases coincident to pregnancy (Table 1). The major emphasis is on treatment and its effects on both the mother and the fetus.

ANATOMIC, PHYSIOLOGIC, AND BIOCHEMICAL CHANGES IN NORMAL PREGNANCY

The size and gross appearance of the liver are not altered during pregnancy. Subtle, nonspecific histologic changes occur. Despite an increase in plasma volume,

Table 1 Liver Diseases in Pregnancy

Liver diseases unique to pregnancy
  Hyperemesis gravidarum
  Intrahepatic cholestasis of pregnancy
  Pre-eclampsia/eclampsia
  Hemolysis, elevated liver enzymes, low platelets (HELLP)
    syndrome
  Acute fatty liver of pregnancy
  Spontaneous hepatic rupture

Intercurrent liver disease
  Acute viral hepatitis
    Hepatitis A, E, B, D, C,
    Other viruses: HSV, EBV, CMV
  Budd-Chiari syndrome

Preexisting liver disease
  Chronic liver disease
    Chronic persistent hepatitis
    Chronic active hepatitis
    Cirrhosis
  Congenital hyperbilirubinemia
    Gilbert's disease
    Rotor's syndrome
    Dubin-Johnson syndrome
  Wilson's disease
  Primary biliary cirrhosis
  Hemochromatosis
  Benign hepatic neoplasms
    Liver cell adenoma
    Focal nodular hyperplasia

HSV = herpes simplex virus; EBV = Epstein-Barr virus; CMV = cytomegalovirus.

the hepatic blood flow is not altered in normal pregnancy. Alterations in liver functions tests (LFT) occur as part of normal pregnancy and are described in Table 2.

LIVER DISEASES UNIQUE TO PREGNANCY

Hyperemesis Gravidarum

Hyperemesis gravidarum (HG) is the condition of severe nausea and vomiting leading to weight loss, ketosis, and dehydration which typically occurs during the first trimester of pregnancy. Liver function abnormalities have been found in up to one-third of affected patients and appear 1 to 3 weeks after the onset of vomiting (Table 3). The cause of HG and HG-related liver abnormalities is unknown. HG generally runs a benign course. In the past, fatal outcomes were the result of starvation and severe dehydration and not of liver failure. Control of vomiting and correction of dehydration and malnutrition leads to reversal of the liver abnormalities. Hospitalization is frequently required to correct fluid, electrolyte, and nutritional abnormalities. Total parenteral nutrition (TPN) has been effective in sustaining fetal growth. Most patients improve symptomatically with IV hydration and TPN. If nausea and vomiting continue, metoclopramide appears safe and very effective (Table 4). Care, however, must be taken in using metoclopramide because neuropsychiatric side effects have been reported in up to 30 percent of nonpregnant subjects.

Intrahepatic Cholestasis of Pregnancy

Intrahepatic cholestasis of pregnancy (IHCP) is the most common liver disease unique to pregnancy occurring in the United States. It is a benign cholestatic disorder that usually begins in the second or third trimester, disappears after delivery, and commonly recurs in subsequent pregnancies. Its etiology is unknown but both genetic and hormonal factors seem to play a role. A strong family predisposition occurs in certain areas of the world, particularly in Chile and Scandinavia. Susceptible women tend to be sensitive to the cholestatic effects of estrogen.

The main clinical manifestations of IHCP are pruritus and jaundice. Steatorrhea has been described but is usually mild and generally does not lead to significant vitamin A, D, E, or K deficiencies. Because of the potential danger of vitamin K deficiency, however, patients with IHCP should be monitored for prolongation of prothrombin time (PT) and treated with vitamin K if necessary. LFT abnormalities and liver pathology are described in Table 3.

In many cases, no specific treatment is necessary. In more symptomatic cases, pharmacologic therapy may be used (see Table 4). Oral cholestyramine relieves pruritus in a large proportion of patients. However, it does not change biochemical markers of cholestasis and may interfere with vitamin K absorption. For this reason PT

Table 2 Liver Tests During Normal Pregnancy

Liver Test (serum)	Change in Pregnancy	Pathophysiology
AP	Progressive increase to 2 times ULN	Released from placenta
GGTP	Low or normal	Impaired release
5'NT	Normal or slight increase	0
LAP	Progressive increase to 3 times ULN	Released from placenta
AST, ALT	No change	0
Bilirubin	Normal or slight increase	Decreased secretion
Bile salts	Progressive increase to 2-3 times ULN	Decreased transport and secretion
Albumin	Decreased by 10-60%	Hemodilution ± decreased synthesis
Globulins (alpha$_1$, alpha$_2$, and beta)	Increased	Increased synthesis
Ceruloplasmin	Decreased	Decreased synthesis
PT	No change	0
Cholesterol	2-Fold increase	Increased synthesis and secretion
Triglycerides	3-Fold increase	Increased synthesis and lipolysis

AP = alkaline phosphatase; GGTP = gamma glutamyl transpeptidase; 5'NT = 5'-nucleotidase; LAP = leucine aminopeptidase; AST = aspartate aminotransferase; ALT = alanine aminotransferase; PT = prothrombin time; ULN = upper limit of normal.

Table 3 Characteristics of Liver Diseases Unique to Pregnancy

	HG	IHCP	PRE/ECL	HELLP Syndrome	AFLP
Trimester	3rd	2nd and 3rd	3rd	3rd	3rd
Symptoms	Severe nausea Vomiting	Pruritus Jaundice	RUQ and epigastric pain Nausea Vomiting	RUQ and epigastric pain Nausea Vomiting	Fatigue RUQ and epigastric pain Nausea Vomiting
Signs	Orthostasis Dehydration	Skin excoriations Jaundice	Hypertension Edema	Hypertension Slight edema	RUQ tenderness Jaundice
Laboratory	Bilirubin 1.3-4.8 AST/ALT 2-3x NL AP slightly increased Ketosis	Bilirubin up to 8.4 AST/ALT 3-4x NL (up to 1,000) AP 2-3x NL Mild steatorrhea	Proteinuria NL or mild hyperbilirubinemia AST/ALT 200-500 U/l (may be >1,000)	Proteinuria Moderate to severe hyperbilirubinemia AST/ALT 200-500 (may be >1,000) Abnormal RBC morphology Low haptoglobin Increased LDH Platelet count 12,000-100,000	Average bilirubin 15.0 AST/ALT 300-500 (may be >1,000) AP moderately increased Evidence of DIC Leukocytosis Increased BUN, creatinine, and uric acid Hypoglycemia Hyperammonemia
Pathology	Normal or slight cholestasis	Centrilobular cholestasis Canalicular bile plugs Bile staining	Sinusoidal fibrin deposition Periportal hemorrhage and necrosis	Sinusoidal fibrin deposit Periportal hemorrhage and necrosis	Microvesicular fatty infiltration
Mortality Maternal	Unaffected	Unaffected	Variable	3%–20%	15% (80% in past)
Fetal	Unaffected	Possible 4-fold increase	Variable	35%	36% (70% in past)
Postpartum recovery of maternal liver disease	Complete	Complete	Complete	Complete	Complete
Recurrence in subsequent pregnancies	Common	Common	Yes	Yes, being reported with increasing frequency	Very rare

HG = hyperemesis gravidarum; IHCP = intrahepatic cholestasis of pregnancy; PRE/ECL = pre-eclampsia/eclampsia; AFLP = acute fatty liver of pregnancy; AST = aspartate aminotransferase; ALT = alanine aminotransferase; RUQ = right upper quadrant; DIC = disseminated intravascular coagulopathy; NL = normal.

Table 4 Treatment of Liver Diseases in Pregnancy

Liver Disease	Treatment or Prophylaxis
Hyperemesis gravidarum	IV hydration
	Total parenteral nutrition
	Metoclopramide 10 mg IV or PO t.i.d.
Intrahepatic cholestasis of pregnancy	Cholestyramine 4 gm PO 4-5x/day
	Vitamin K 10 mg SQ x 3 days if PT prolonged
	Phenobarbital 90 mg PO at bedtime
	Ursodeoxycholic acid 300 mg PO t.i.d.
Pre-eclampsia/eclampsia	Mild: magnesium sulfate
	bed rest
	antihypertensives
	Moderate to severe: delivery
HELLP syndrome	Caesarean section
Acute fatty liver of pregnancy	Mild: careful observation
	Moderate to severe: delivery
Spontaneous hepatic rupture	Hemodynamic support
	Immediate surgery ± prior hepatic artery embolization
Acute viral hepatitis	None or supportive
HSV hepatitis	Acyclovir 30 mg/kg/day for 10 days
CMV and EBV hepatitis	None or supportive
Budd-Chiari syndrome	Orthotopic liver transplantation
Cirrhosis	Mild: none
	Moderate to severe: supportive and sedation during labor
Autoimmune CAH	Prednisone 10-20 mg PO once daily
	Azathioprine up to 50 mg PO once daily
Congenital hyperbilirubinemias	None
Wilson's disease	1st and 2nd trimesters: D-pencillamine 750-1,000 mg PO/day
	3rd trimester: D-penicillamine 250 mg PO/day
	Trientine 500 mg PO t.i.d.
Primary biliary cirrhosis	None
Hemochromatosis	None
Benign hepatic tumors	If large, excise before pregnancy

HSV = herpes simplex virus; CMV = cytomegalovirus, EBV = Epstein-Barr virus; PT = prothrombin time; CAH = chronic active hepatitis.

should be monitored closely. Since cholestyramine is not systemically absorbed, it has no effect on the fetus. The major side effects of cholestyramine are listed in Table 5. Phenobarbital has been effective in the treatment of nocturnal pruritus. Several retrospective studies, however, have shown an association between barbiturates and a higher incidence of fetal abnormalities. For this reason, I would not recommend the use of phenobarbital in pregnancy.

Most recently, ursodeoxycholic acid (UDCA) has been studied in an open pilot study and was found to significantly improve both pruritus and biochemical abnormalities in eight patients with IHCP. The precise mechanism by which UDCA causes its effect is unknown. Its mode of action may rest on the ability of oral UDCA to modify bile acid pool composition replacing endogenous bile acids which are more hydrophobic and cytotoxic to liver cell membranes (Table 6). UDCA was well tolerated with relatively few side effects and caused no fetal abnormalities. Currently, a controlled clinical trial is under way.

The cholestasis of IHCP progresses until delivery or termination of pregnancy. Within hours after delivery, pruritus disappears. Long-term follow-up showed a higher incidence of cholelithiasis but the overall prognosis is excellent. The prognosis for the fetus, however, may not be as benign. Earlier studies reported high rates of premature labor (30 to 60 percent) and neonatal death (fourfold increase). Fetal monitoring has revealed an increased incidence of fetal stress (up to 40 percent) during labor and meconium staining at birth. More recent controlled trials from Scandinavia, however, have failed to demonstrate increased fetal mortality in IHCP. Nevertheless, it is currently recommended that patients with IHCP be monitored closely during the third trimester and to proceed to delivery at the first sign of fetal distress.

Pre-eclampsia and Eclampsia

Among the most serious liver disorders recognized during pregnancy are those associated with pre-eclampsia and eclampsia. Pregnancy-induced or aggravated hypertension is the hallmark of pre-eclampsia. Edema and proteinuria also are common. Renal, hematological, and neurological involvement may be present. When convulsions occur, the condition is termed eclampsia. Pre-eclampsia occurs in 5–10 percent of all pregnancies. It is a disease of unknown etiology. Segmental vasospasm with localized consumptive coagulopathy leading to platelet clumping and fibrin deposition is seen. Impairment of vascular perfusion to a

Table 5 Side Effects of Treatment of Liver Disease in Pregnancy

Treatment	Side Effects
Metoclopramide	No fetal abnormalities reported in HG Extrapyramidal reactions Restlessness Anxiety Insomnia
Cholestyramine	No fetal abnormalities reported in IHCP Prolongation of PT Constipation Nausea Upper abdominal discomfort
Phenobarbital	Fetal abnormalities reported with barbiturates
Ursodeoxycholic acid	No fetal abnormalities reported in a small number of pregnancies Transient abnormalities in transaminases Transient diarrhea
Acyclovir	No fetal abnormalities reported in a small number of studies. Not currently approved for use in pregnancy. Nausea, vomiting, diarrhea Headache Rash
D-penicillamine	No fetal abnormalities reported in Wilson's disease "Allergic-type" reaction on restarting of D-pencillamine Bone marrow suppression Proteinuria, hematuria, nephrotic syndrome, Goodpasture's syndrome Myasthenia gravis Pruritus Dermatitis Arthralgias
Trientine	No fetal abnormalities in a small number of pregnancies Iron deficiency
Prednisone	No fetal abnormalities reported in pregnant women with autoimmune CAH Salt retaining properties Causes varied metabolic effects and modifies immune responses
Azathioprine	No fetal abnormalities in patients with autoimmune CAH where lower doses are used; can cause fetal harm in higher doses Bone marrow suppression Hepatotoxicity Infections
Interferon-alpha	No information available

PT = prothrombin time; CAH = chronic active hepatitis.

Table 6 Mechanism of Action of Medications Used to Treat Liver Disease in Pregnancy

Medication	Mechanism of Action
Metoclopramide	1. Antagonizes central dopamine receptors and blocks stimulation of the medullary vomiting center 2. Sensitizes tissues to the action of acetylcholine and stimulates motility of the upper gastrointestinal tract (intact vagal nerve is necessary)
Cholestyramine	Resin which adsorbs bile acids in the intestine to form a complex which is excreted in the feces and thus interrupts enterohepatic circulation.
Phenobarbital	1. Induces hepatic microsomal enzymes 2. Increases bile salt secretion and bile flow
Ursodeoxycholic acid	1. Replaces endogenous bile acids that are more hydrophobic and cytotoxic to the liver cell membranes 2. Inhibits intestinal absorption of hydrophobic bile acids
Acyclovir	Thymidine kinase encoded by herpes simplex converts acyclovir into acyclovir triphosphate which interferes with HSV DNA polymerase and inhibits viral DNA replication.
Prednisone	Glucocorticoid with potent anti-inflammatory effects
Azathioprine	Immunosuppressive antimetabolite
D-penicillamine	Chelates copper
Trientine	1. Chelates copper 2. Depresses serum iron concentration by an unknown mechanism

number of organs including the liver follows. Liver biopsy findings are as described in Table 3. Liver involvement is seen in at least 10 percent of women with pre-eclampsia and is more common and more severe in eclampsia.

In most cases of pre-eclampsia, liver involvement is mild and largely asymptomatic being detected only by abnormal LFTs. More advanced disease is manifested by right upper quadrant (RUQ) and epigastric pain often accompanied by nausea and vomiting. LFT abnormalities are as in Table 3. When jaundice occurs, it denotes severe liver involvement or pre-existing liver disease. The appearance of severe RUQ pain and hypotension may herald bleeding into the subcapsular liver parenchyma. Rarely, rupture of the liver ensues when bleeding dissects through the liver capsule. Both abdominal sonography and computed tomographic (CT) scanning are useful in the evaluation of women with pre-eclampsia and liver dysfunction. The former is the initial study of choice because of its ready availability and its lack of radiation exposure to the fetus. It is particularly useful in excluding gallbladder disease.

Liver dysfunction in pre-eclampsia requires no special treatment other than that directed at the pre-eclampsia itself (see Table 4). In mild cases that occur early in pregnancy, expectant management with magnesium sulfate, bed rest, and antihypertensives is all that may be required. Because liver disease may be rapidly progressive, the need for careful monitoring cannot be overemphasized. In the latter part of gestation, when the fetus is mature, or in more severe cases, where the risk to the mother is great, prompt delivery is the treatment of choice.

HELLP Syndrome

The association of pre-eclampsia with hemolysis, elevated liver enzymes, and low platelets has been termed the HELLP syndrome. This syndrome probably represents a more severe form of pre-eclampsia rather than a separate clinical entity. Clinical and physical findings are similar to those seen in pre-eclampsia. Characteristic laboratory findings are as in Table 3. Because the HELLP syndrome may worsen suddenly and without warning, delivery by Caesarian section should be accomplished without delay.

Acute Fatty Liver of Pregnancy

Acute fatty liver of pregnancy (AFLP) is another serious and potentially fatal disease unique to pregnancy. Earlier reports commented on its rarity and its extremely high mortality but more recent reports suggest that AFLP is more common and less fatal than previously thought. The most recent figures show an incidence of 1 in 13,000 deliveries. The histological hallmark of AFLP is the infiltration of centrilobular hepatocytes with microvesicular fat. The etiology of AFLP is not known but carnitine deficiency may play a central role. AFLP can present from the 26 to 35th week of gestation and rarely immediately postpartum. The early clinical manifestations may be nonspecific. Signs of liver dysfunction appear 1 to 2 weeks later and may include jaundice, ascites, and liver failure. Laboratory findings are as described in Table 3. Imaging studies of the liver using ultrasound or CT may suggest fatty infiltration. Neither test is reliable enough, however, to either establish or rule out the diagnosis of AFLP. The differential diagnosis may be extensive (Table 7). The diagnosis of AFLP can be confirmed by liver biopsy and appropriate fat stains. Because liver biopsy carries a higher risk in pregnancy, its routine use for diagnosis is controversial. Generally, it should be reserved for those few patients in whom the specific diagnosis is essential and cannot be made otherwise. If the distinction between AFLP and pre-eclamptic liver disease is not possible on clinical grounds, liver biopsy is not indicated as the treatment for both conditions is the same, i.e. delivery. In the case of persistent difficulty with differentiation of AFLP and other diagnoses, liver biopsy is indicated.

There is no specific treatment for AFLP. Most authorities recommend prompt termination of the pregnancy as soon as the diagnosis is made. The only exception may be in very mild cases where careful observation may be attempted. Any deterioration in the condition of the mother or fetus is an indication for immediate delivery. Resolution of the maternal liver disease usually begins within days after delivery. If liver failure does not respond to termination of pregnancy, orthotopic transplantation has been successfully performed.

Table 7 Differential Diagnosis: Acute Fatty Liver of Pregnancy

Acute viral hepatitis
Drug-induced hepatotoxicity
  Acetaminophen
  Tetracycline
  Valproic acid
  Cocaine
Alcoholic hepatitis
Pre-eclampsia associated liver disease
Budd-Chiari syndrome
Acute biliary tract disease

Table 8 Differential Diagnosis: Spontaneous Hepatic Rupture During Pregnancy

Abruptio placentae
Ruptured uterus
Ovarian torsion
Acute cholecystitis
Acute pancreatitis
Perforated viscus
Intestinal infarction

Spontaneous Hepatic Rupture

Hepatic rupture is one of the most catastrophic complications to occur in pregnancy. Ninety percent of cases have pre-eclampsia or eclampsia as a predisposing condition. Hepatic rupture may occur in AFLP and rarely in association with liver cell adenoma, focal nodular hyperplasia, aneurysms, and hemangiomas. Spontaneous rupture occurs late in pregnancy or shortly postpartum. It is heralded by sudden onset of severe abdominal pain followed by shock. The differential diagnosis is outlined in Table 8. Abdominal CT scanning is the most accurate way to detect hepatic hemorrhage and rupture. Treatment requires early diagnosis and vigorous hemodynamic support with volume replacement and correction of any coagulopathy. Immediate surgery or angiographic embolization of the hepatic artery to the involved liver segment followed by delivery is mandatory. Despite such heroic measures mortality is approximately 75 percent for the mother and 60 percent for the fetus.

INTERCURRENT LIVER DISEASE

Acute Viral Hepatitis

Acute viral hepatitis is the most common cause of jaundice during pregnancy accounting for approximately 40 percent of all cases. The incidence in pregnant women is similar to that in nonpregnant women. Other than being associated with a higher incidence of prematurity, uncomplicated viral hepatitis does not significantly alter the course and outcome of pregnancy. In most cases the diagnosis can be made on the basis of serological testing. Management should be conservative and Caesarean section is not indicated. The only major concern is the risk of neonatal transmission. Breastfeeding can be safely recommended as it has not been shown to transmit infection.

Specific clinical features, vertical transmission, and immunoprophylaxis of the different types of acute viral hepatitis are outlined in Table 9. With regard to hepatitis B, the overall risk of transmission of hepatitis B virus (HBV) is 50 percent but the risk approaches 90 percent if the mother is positive for both hepatitis B surface antigen (HBsAg) and e antigen (HBeAg). Most infected fetuses do not get hepatitis but 80 to 90 percent become chronic carriers of HBV and about 35 percent die later because of hepatocellular carcinoma or complications related to portal hypertension. Consequently, if a mother is positive for HBsAg, it is recommended that a newborn be given immunoprophylaxis. Little is known about the natural history of hepatitis C in pregnancy. Recent reports show the risk of neonatal transmission is low. Management guidelines remain to be defined. No information is available on the effect of interferon on human pregnancy.

Other Viruses

Herpes simplex virus (HSV), Epstein-Barr virus, and cytomegalovirus (CMV) rarely cause acute hepatitis during pregnancy. In the case of HSV hepatitis where maternal mortality in untreated patients is as high as 70 percent, prompt diagnosis and treatment can be life saving. Usually there is evidence of HSV infection in other parts of the body (skin, cervix). Liver biopsy shows HSV inclusion bodies. Acyclovir is the treatment of choice. Acute CMV hepatitis in pregnancy is rare and not severe enough to require antiviral therapy.

Budd-Chiari Syndrome

Budd-Chiari syndrome, known to be associated with the use of oral contraceptives, can also occur during pregnancy or shortly after delivery. Of the reported cases, 14 percent are associated with pregnancy. The clinical presentation is dramatic with the sudden onset of RUQ pain, hepatomegaly, and ascites. Orthotopic liver transplantation becomes necessary in most cases. This is the subject of a separate chapter.

PRE-EXISTING LIVER DISEASE

Chronic Liver Disease

Pregnancy rarely occurs in advanced chronic liver disease because advanced liver disease is uncommon in women of childbearing age and when present is associated with markedly diminished fertility. Mild chronic liver disease, however, does not impair fertility and its

Table 9 Acute Viral Hepatitis in Pregnancy

	Hepatitis				
	A	*E (Epidemic NANB)*	*B*	*D*	*C (Classic NANB)*
Transmission	Oral-fecal	Oral-fecal	Parenteral Sexual	Parenteral Sexual	Parenteral Possibly sexual Uncertain
Acute clinical course	Self-limited	Self-limited	Self-limited	Self-limited	Self-limited
Chronicity	No	No	Yes	Yes	Yes
Vertical transmission	Rare	Unknown	Common	Rare	Uncommon
Effect of pregnancy on clinical course	None	Yes Maternal mortality 10-20% (India, Middle East, Mexico)	No	No	Unknown, probably no
Prophylaxis	If mother infected in 3rd trimester, Infant: ISG 0.5 ml IM at birth	None	Infant: HBIG 0.5 ml IM and HBV vaccine IM at 2 sites at birth (HBV vaccine repeated at 1 and 6 months)	Same as for hepatitis B	Infant: ISG 0.06 ml/kg body weight IM
Comment		Not reported in the United States			

NANB = non-A, non-B; ISG = immune serum globulin; HBIG = hepatitis B immune globulin; HBV = hepatitis B virus.

coexistence with pregnancy has not been shown to be harmful to either the mother or the fetus (Table 10).

Chronic persistent hepatitis (CPH) in most instances arises as a sequela of acute viral hepatitis. It is considered to be a benign and nonprogressive disease. Chronic active hepatitis (CAH) which is uncomplicated by cirrhosis generally has little adverse effect on the pregnant patient. Increased fetal wastage, however, is seen. Autoimmune CAH typically occurs in young women. It can be effectively treated with prednisone and/or azathioprine during pregnancy (see Table 4). When pregnancy occurs in the setting of cirrhosis, whether associated with CAH or not, the maternal prognosis is determined by the severity of the underlying liver disease and the presence of portal hypertension. In cirrhosis with portal hypertension, maternal morbidity and mortality are high. Portal hypertension tends to worsen because of the increase in intravascular volume and in intra-abdominal pressure during pregnancy. Most pregnancies in cirrhotic women can be managed conservatively. In general, therapeutic abortion is not justified but should be considered when signs of hepatic decompensation develop or worsen in early pregnancy. Vaginal delivery appears to be safe and Caesarian section is necessary only for standard obstetric indications. Adequate sedation during labor is recommended to avoid excessive straining which may increase the risk of variceal rupture. Because of the high morbidity and mortality seen with pregnancy in cirrhosis, counseling cirrhotic women about the risks of pregnancy is appropriate.

Congenital Hyperbilirubinemias

Gilbert's disease and Rotor's syndrome neither influence nor are influenced by pregnancy. Dubin-Johnson syndrome can cause a marked increase in serum bilirubin leading to deep jaundice. In fact, it may be recognized for the first time during pregnancy. Because of the increased risk of spontaneous abortions and stillbirths in women with Dubin-Johnson syndrome, close fetal monitoring is indicated.

Wilson's Disease

The availability of effective chelation therapy has allowed women with Wilson's disease to expect a normal reproductive life. Pregnancy is tolerated well as long as D-penicillamine therapy is continued throughout the pregnancy. If chelation therapy is stopped, fulminant hepatitis may develop. A lower D-penicillamine dose is used in the third trimester to prevent postpartum wound complications which may be seen with higher doses of the drug. Trientine, a recently introduced copper-chelating agent, has been used successfully in a small number of pregnant patients. There is a separate chapter on Wilson's disease.

Primary Biliary Cirrhosis

Pregnancy is also well tolerated by women with asymptomatic primary biliary cirrhosis (PBC). Increase in serum bilirubin and jaundice near term may bring attention to the presence of PBC. Surprisingly, there appears to be no increase in pruritus in these patients. Pregnancy in symptomatic PBC is rare since the disease usually occurs after the reproductive years.

Hemochromatosis

Little is known about pregnancy in hemochromatosis since women generally present with this condition after menopause or hysterectomy having lost the protective effect of menstrual blood loss. It can be presumed that pregnancy is tolerated well in early hemochromatosis as women diagnosed later in life have had successful pregnancies.

Benign Hepatic Tumors

Focal nodular hyperplasia and liver cell adenoma are estrogen sensitive and may enlarge during pregnancy. Patients typically have RUQ pain. Hepatic rupture has been reported with these tumors. Prophylactic surgical excision should be considered for large lesions in women who wish to become pregnant.

Table 10 Chronic Liver Disease in Pregnancy

	CPH	CAH No Cirrhosis	Cirrhosis +/− CAH
Portal hypertension	No	No	Yes
Fertility	Normal	Normal	Decreased
Effect of liver disease on fetus	None	Increased fetal wastage	Increased fetal wastage (20%) Prematurity
Effect of pregnancy on liver disease	None	None	Jaundice Ascites (20-50%) Variceal bleeding Hepatic encephalopathy
Mortality	Unaffected	Unaffected	~10%

CPH = chronic persistent hepatitis; CAH = chronic active hepatitis.

SUGGESTED READING

Alexander J, Cuellar RE, Van Thiel DH. Toxemia of pregnancy and the liver. Semin Liver Dis 1987; 7:55–58.

Barron WM, Mishra L, Seeff LB, et al. Gastrointestinal and liver problems in pregnancy. Gastroenterol Clin North Am 1992; 21:851–887, 889–903, 905–921, 937–949, 951–960.

Riely CA. Acute fatty liver of pregnancy. Semin Liver Dis 1987; 7:47–54.

Samuels P, Cohen AW. Pregnancies complicated by liver disease and liver dysfunction. Obstet Gynecol Clin North Am 1992; 19:745–763.

Schorr-Lesnick B, Lebovics E, Dworkin B, et al. Liver diseases unique to pregnancy. Am J Gastroenterol 1991; 86:659–670.

Van Dyke RW. The liver in pregnancy. In: Zakim D, Boyer TD, eds. Hepatology: a textbook of liver disease. Philadelphia: WB Saunders, 1990:1438.

Varma RR. Course and prognosis of pregnancy in women with liver disease. Semin Liver Dis 1987; 7:59–66.

Wilkinson ML. Diagnosis and management of liver disease in pregnancy. Adv Intern Med 1990; 35:289–310.

PRIMARY BILIARY CIRRHOSIS

H. FRANKLIN HERLONG, M.D.

Primary biliary cirrhosis (PBC), a disease of unknown etiology that affects predominantly middle-aged women, is characterized by progressive destruction (presumably on an immunologic basis) of septal and intralobular bile ducts. While many patients remain asymptomatic for prolonged periods, eventually symptoms develop and are caused by cholestasis and portal hypertension. The diagnosis of PBC is made by a combination of clinical, biochemical, serologic, and histologic data. The biochemical profile reflects a chronic cholestatic liver disorder. The serum alkaline phosphatase is elevated in virtually all patients, but the height of the elevation does not correlate with the severity of the disease. The aminotransferases are modestly elevated but are not useful in following the course of the disease.

Over 95 percent of patients with this disease have antimitochondrial antibodies in the serum. Antimitochondrial antibodies are nonspecies, nonorgan specific antibodies which can be found in diseases other than PBC. However, a specific antibody directed toward the pyruvate dehydrogenase complex on the inner membrane of the mitochondrion appears specific for PBC (anti-M_2).

The liver biopsy appearance in PBC is graded on a scale of 1 to 4, with the earliest lesion (stage 1) most characteristic of the disease. Intense chronic inflammation, often with granulomata, is seen around septal and intralobular bile ducts. As the disease progresses, bile ducts begin to disappear. With progression to stage IV a true cirrhosis is present and bile ducts are frequently absent. Therapy is directed at controlling the symptoms of PBC and retarding the progression of the liver injury.

COMPLICATIONS OF CHOLESTASIS

Pruritus

Pruritus is the most common symptom of PBC and is worse in the evening and during the summer months. It is most severe on the palms of the hands and soles of the feet and around belt and bra lines. This subject is also discussed in the chapter on cholestasis. Antihistamines are of little value in treating the pruritus of cholestasis, but cholestyramine alleviates pruritus in most patients. Four grams of cholestyramine powder, mixed in a palatable vehicle such as fruit juice or applesauce, is initially given four times a day. In patients with an intact gallbladder, it is important to give the first dose in the morning before breakfast. The other doses are administered 1 hour before each meal. Once pruritus is controlled, the dose can be tapered to the lowest amount that controls the itching. Although the taste and consistency of this agent are unpleasant, it is generally well tolerated. Constipation is the most common side effect, but drinking large quantities of water combined with a stool softening agent such as psyllium will lessen constipation in most patients. Large doses of cholestyramine can lead to malabsorption of fat and fat-soluble vitamins which can be overcome by reducing the dose of cholestyramine or supplementation with water miscible (or parenteral) forms of vitamin A, D, and K. Cholestyramine may affect the absorption of simultaneously administered oral medications such as antibiotics, digoxin, or thyroid hormone. Discontinuation or a sudden reduction in the dose of cholestyramine may change the bioavailability of potentially toxic drugs such as digoxin.

Phenobarbital can be added to the therapeutic regimen for patients who have pruritus refractory to cholestyramine. I use 32 mg as a nighttime dose gradually increasing the dose to a maximum of 100 mg. Phenobarbital is particularly useful at night since pruritus is most severe at this time. Because of its sedative effects I do not use phenobarbital during the day.

Phenobarbital should not be given to patients with hepatic encephalopathy.

Although some patients experience brief amelioration of pruritus with exposure to ultraviolet light, I find that most patients become refractory to this treatment after several weeks.

Oral rifampicin controls pruritus in some patients with PBC, although its mechanism of action remains unclear. It may act by enhancing the urinary excretion of bile salts or by an inhibition of the production of pruritogenic substances by luminal bacteria. Oral rifampicin given at a dose of 150 mg twice a day is generally well tolerated, but potential hepatotoxic and allergic reactions require careful monitoring.

Some preliminary reports suggest that opiate receptor antagonists successfully control the pruritus of PBC, but the parenteral route of the administration of naloxone (Narcan) limits its usefulness. Orally administered nalmefene appears promising. Thalidomide has been used to treat the pruritus of other disorders such as graft-versus-host disease but its efficacy has not been evaluated in PBC.

Malabsorption

Fat malabsorption is common in patients with PBC. If diarrhea develops secondary to steatorrhea, dietary fat should be restricted to 30 grams per day. In patients with weight loss secondary to decreased caloric availability, supplementation with medium chain triglycerides, which do not require bile salts for absorption, may be used. Medium chain triglyceride oil can be used as a salad dressing and Portagen, a powder derived from coconut oil, can also provide a palatable source of additional calories.

Malabsorption of fat-soluble vitamins is common in patients with PBC. Although low serum vitamin A levels are common in patients with PBC, night blindness is rare. Twenty-five thousand units of water-miscible vitamin A (Aquasol A) daily will normalize serum vitamin A levels in most patients. Periodic monitoring of serum vitamin A levels will prevent hypervitaminosis A.

Although malabsorption of vitamin D may contribute to the osteopenia of patients with PBC, osteoporosis is the predominant bone lesion in most patients. Fifty thousand units of ergocalciferol (vitamin D_2), every other day will normalize serum levels of 25-hydroxy-vitamin D in most patients. Hypercalcemia and/or hypercalcuria can result from vitamin D toxicity, so periodic measurement of serum levels of 25-hydroxy-vitamin D should be used to evaluate the efficacy of therapy and monitor for toxicity. Low serum levels of vitamin E have been identified in patients with PBC but symptoms of vitamin E deficiency have not been observed. Because of the possibility of a yet unrecognized benefit of vitamin E supplementation, I recommend 400 IU a day.

Prolongation of the prothrombin time may result from vitamin K deficiency especially in patients on large doses of cholestyramine. Subcutaneous administration of 10 mg of vitamin K (Aquamephyton) will lead to prompt correction of the prothrombin time. Five milligrams daily of oral Synkayvite, a water miscible derivative of menadione (vitamin K_3) may be useful.

Lipid Disorders

Hypercholesterolemia, often with serum cholesterol levels greater than 500 mg per deciliter, is common in patients with PBC. Despite very high levels of serum cholesterol, accelerated atherosclerosis is uncommon. Lipid lowering agents may be considered in patients who develop complications such as painful xanthomata. Plasmapheresis may be required in patients with serum cholesterol levels greater than 1000 mg per deciliter.

MEDICAL THERAPY FOR PBC

Treatment of PBC remains controversial. D-penicillamine was studied in several prospective controlled trials but had no beneficial effect on histologic progression of the disease, relief of symptoms, biochemical tests of hepatic function, or survival. In addition, a third of patients developed serious side effects. The immunosuppressive agents azathioprine and chlorambucil, showed no therapeutic benefit in controlled trials. Colchicine, an agent which decreases collagen synthesis, has been studied for the past 10 years. Modest improvement in biochemical tests of hepatic function was seen when compared to a placebo. A favorable influence on survival was seen in one study, but no beneficial effect on histologic progression or symptoms was seen. Because colchicine has few side effects and a potential, albeit modest, beneficial effect, this agent is still used in many patients. The usual dosage is 0.6 mg twice daily. Preliminary trials of cyclosporine have suggested a favorable effect on serum alkaline phosphatase and aminotransferase levels but potential renal toxicity will likely limit the usefulness of this agent.

Oral low-dose pulse methotrexate therapy at a dose of 15 mg per week resulted in improvement in hepatic biochemical tests and relief of pruritus and fatigue in some selected patients, but secondary thrombocytopenia has limited the use of this agent.

Ursodeoxycholic acid (UDCA, Actigall) improves biochemical tests of liver function and may improve pruritus in some patients with PBC. A beneficial effect on the natural history of the disease is less clear. Three hundred milligrams of oral UDCA three times a day frequently results in reduction in serum alkaline phosphatase, alanine aminotransferase, bilirubin, and IgM concentrations. UDCA therapy is well tolerated with few reported adverse effects. Because of the beneficial effects of UDCA and paucity of side effects, I feel that it is the agent of choice in the medical therapy of PBC.

HEPATIC TRANSPLANTATION

PBC is the second most common indication for liver transplantation in adult patients and accounts for approximately 20 percent of all transplants performed. The results of survival after hepatic transplantation are significantly greater than that expected with conservative management. Most of the transplant recipients for primary biliary cirrhosis are able to return to work. The Mayo Clinic model using five variables (age, total serum bilirubin concentration, total serum bilirubin albumin concentrations, prothrombin time, and edema) has been used to predict the natural history of patients with PBC. Improvement in survival after hepatic transplantation compared with the predicted survival of a simulated control group is significant. Hepatic transplantation should be considered when serum bilirubin levels exceed 10 mg per deciliter, in the presence of incapacitating fatigue or pruritus, ascites, or hepatic encephalopathy refractory to medical therapy, or recurrent esophageal variceal hemorrhage despite sclerotherapy or variceal banding. To date, clinically significant recurrence of PBC in the transplanted liver has not occurred.

SUGGESTED READING

Dickson ER, Grambsch P, Markus BH, et al. Transplantation markedly improves survival in PBC patients: Application of the Mayo model on Pittsburgh transplant patients. Gastroenterology 1988; (abstract) 94:A535.
Gershwin ME, Mackay IR, et al. Primary biliary cirrhosis. Semin Liv Dis 1989; 9:103–157.
Kaplan MM, Knox TA, Arora S. Primary biliary cirrhosis treated with low-dose oral pulse methotrexate: Resolution of symptoms with improvement in biochemical tests of liver function. Ann Intern Med 1988; 109:429–431.
Poupon R, Chretien Y, Poupon RE, et al: Is ursodeoxycholic acid an effective treatment for primary biliary cirrhosis? Lancet 1987; 1:834–836.
Wiesner RH, Grambsch PM, Lindor KD, et al. Clinical and statistical analyses of new and evolving therapies for primary biliary cirrhosis. Hepatology 1988; 8:668–676.

CHRONIC CHOLESTASIS AND ITS SEQUELAE

CARL L. BERG, M.D.
JOHN L. GOLLAN, M.D., Ph.D.

Cholestasis is a clinical syndrome resulting from the interruption of hepatic bile flow. As a consequence of impaired hepatic excretion, selected biliary constituents are depleted in the intestinal lumen and accumulate systemically. For example, intestinal depletion of bile salts may cause impaired absorption of fats and fat-soluble vitamins (A, D, E, K) and lead to steatorrhea and calcium malabsorption. Systemic accumulation of bile salts, bilirubin, and other compounds results in jaundice and pruritus. Conditions which result in chronic intrahepatic cholestasis are listed in Table 1. Any discussion of the medical management of chronic cholestasis assumes that extrahepatic biliary obstruction has been excluded or treated with biliary stenting, dilation, or surgical diversion, as discussed in other chapters. Furthermore, specific medical management for conditions such as primary biliary cirrhosis (PBC) and primary sclerosing cholangitis (PSC) may lead to significant improvement in the associated cholestasis and render

Table 1 Causes of Chronic Intrahepatic Cholestasis

Adults
Primary biliary cirrhosis
Primary sclerosing cholangitis
Chronic total parenteral nutrition
Chronic graft vs host disease
Syndromic and nonsyndromic paucity of intrahepatic bile ducts
Caroli's disease
Cystic fibrosis
Congenital hepatic fibrosis
Drugs
Chronic hepatitis (viral, alcoholic)

Children
Infectious hepatitis
Syndromic and nonsyndromic paucity of intrahepatic bile ducts
Byler's disease
Trihydroxycoprostanic acidemia
Zellweger syndrome
Congenital hepatic fibrosis
Caroli's disease
α_1-antitrypsin deficiency
Cystic fibrosis
Other metabolic disorders
Chronic total parenteral nutrition

the therapies outlined below unnecessary. Thus, the treatment of chronic cholestasis discussed is directed not at the underlying diseases outlined in Table 1, but rather at the management of their associated features and sequelae.

PRURITUS

Conventional therapy for the control of pruritus has centered on the use of cholestyramine, histamine antagonists, androgenic steroids and phenobarbital. More recent therapeutic approaches also have included rifampicin (and other antibiotics), ursodeoxycholic acid and opioid receptor antagonists (Table 2). As with any condition in which a variety of therapies exists, all of the above agents have been employed with only moderate success. The lack of a uniformly effective therapy for pruritus is due largely to our incomplete understanding of the pathogenesis of this debilitating symptom. Various hypotheses have been proposed centering on the role of "toxic" bile salts as the agents responsible for the development of pruritus. One model postulates that retained bile salts, particularly the dihydroxy and unconjugated forms, accumulate in the skin and lead to the excitation of cutaneous nerve endings. Alternatively, other investigators have proposed that high concentrations of bile salts in the liver lead to hepatic membrane disruption, which in turn results in the release of some, as yet unidentified, compound that initiates pruritus. A final theory centers on possible activation of the opioid central nervous system by unidentified pruritogens. With these hypotheses in mind, it is not surprising that most of the therapies outlined below are directed at manipulation of systemic bile salt levels.

Cholestyramine

Cholestyramine is a basic anion exchange resin that is capable of binding bile acids in the intestinal lumen. Often employed in the management of hypercholesterolemia, cholestyramine also is important in the treatment of pruritus associated with cholestatic liver disease.

Cholestyramine sequesters intestinal bile salts which are subsequently eliminated in the feces rather than being recirculated via the enterohepatic circulation. The resin is available as a powder which is mixed with water, juice, or pulpy fruits, such as applesauce or crushed pineapple. Administration before meals (particularly breakfast) is most effective as intestinal bile salts increase with meal-stimulated gallbladder contraction and emptying. The dose of cholestyramine should be titrated to the minimum required to relieve itching; doses of 12 to 16 g of the anhydrous resin per day are commonly necessary. When more than 8 g of anhydrous

Table 2 Therapies with Demonstrated Efficacy in Pruritus

Cholestyramine
Ursodeoxycholic acid
Rifampicin (? and other antibiotics)
Opioid antagonists
Histamine antagonists*
Phenobarbital*
Plasmapheresis†

*Therapy poorly effective and complicated by sedation.
†Effective in a limited experience in refractory cases of pruritus.

resin per day are utilized, cholestyramine should be given before each meal rather than simply before breakfast. Relief of pruritus usually takes several days. As patient acceptance of cholestyramine is often less than enthusiastic, gradual upward titration of the dose is recommended to allow patients to become accustomed to the gritty consistency of the medication.

Adsorption of intestinal contents is not limited to bile salts and thus other oral medications which may be bound by cholestyramine should be administered either 1 hour before or 4 hours after cholestyramine dosing. Some degree of fat and fat-soluble vitamin malabsorption invariably accompanies cholestyramine administration, and thus vitamin supplementation should be considered if long-term therapy is contemplated. Constipation often accompanies cholestyramine therapy particularly when higher doses are employed. Despite the disagreeable taste and consistency of cholestyramine and its side effects, relief from pruritus is often impressive, such that patients gladly accept the inconvenience of therapy in exchange for improvement in their symptoms.

Ursodeoxycholic Acid Therapy

As discussed in the chapters on PBC and PSC, treatment with ursodeoxycholic acid (UDCA) may have beneficial effects on the underlying disease process in these patients. Perhaps as a result of its effects on hepatic histology, or independent of this, UDCA may improve pruritus in patients with cholestasis. The largest number of patients treated have been those with PBC, although patients with Alagille's syndrome (syndromic paucity of intralobular bile ducts), chronic graft versus host disease and TPN-induced cholestasis also have exhibited relief from symptoms. The mechanism of action of UDCA in pruritus is speculative, but may relate to alterations in the composition of the bile salt pool mediated by competition with endogenous bile salts at the level of ileal absorption or by its potential for inducing choleresis.

UDCA is administered orally and is available in 300-mg capsules. Doses of 10 to 15 mg per kilogram per day are typically necessary to relieve pruritus and should be divided in two or three doses. Administration on an empty stomach may lead to improved ileal absorption. If used in conjunction with cholestyramine, UDCA therapy should be staggered in order to minimize binding of the drug to the bile acid binding resin. While this results in a cumbersome medical regimen, the combination of the two therapies may lead to superior symptomatic relief compared to either agent alone. UDCA therapy is associated with few side effects and even in the absence of large clinical trials, its use in the management of pruritus secondary to chronic cholestasis is worthy of consideration.

Rifampicin and Other Antibiotics

Several recent reports have examined the potential efficacy of rifampicin for controlling pruritus in adults with PBC and children with intrahepatic cholestasis. Rifampicin has been reported to increase hepatic microsomal enzyme activities, and thus potential modes of action include (1) enhanced hepatic sulfoxidation of di- and monohydroxy bile acids, resulting in increased bile salt elimination by urinary excretion and (2) enhanced metabolism of non-bile salt pruritogenic substances. Adults are typically treated with an oral dose of 300 mg twice daily while children receive 10 mg per kilogram per day. Relief of pruritus occurs within 7 days of institution of therapy and appears to be maintained long term. Long-term administration, however, has been associated with significant side effects in approximately 10 percent of treated patients. Marked increases in aminotransferases, which resolved with cessation of rifampicin treatment, and the development of an allergic reaction characterized by eosinophilia, cutaneous rash, and facial edema have been observed in patients treated for pruritus. While toxic hepatitis has been reported in approximately 1 percent of all patients treated with rifampicin, the more frequent occurrence of rifampicin-associated deterioration in aminotransferases in cholestatic patients suggests the need for careful monitoring of these patients. Given this side effect profile, rifampicin therapy should be reserved for cholestatic patients in whom cholestyramine and/or bile acid therapy is ineffective.

The beneficial effects of rifampicin on pruritus may not be due solely to enhanced hepatic metabolism of deleterious bile salts, but rather may be a consequence of altered bacterial metabolism of bile salts in the intestinal lumen of cholestatic patients. This hypothesis is based on our observation that both metronidazole and ampicillin are effective in controlling refractory pruritus in some patients with PBC. Intermittent therapy with these antibiotics (metronidazole 250 mg orally three times daily or ampicillin 250 mg orally four times daily for 1 week) has resulted in prompt resolution of pruritus in a small number of individuals. Symptoms typically have returned 4 to 6 weeks after the last dose of the antibiotic (presumably coincident with recolonization of the intestinal lumen with bacteria) and have reproducibly responded to additional short courses of treatment. We have observed no side effects in this small group of patients although allergic reactions and diarrhea are always potential side effects of antibiotic treatment. While limited experience with this therapeutic approach to pruritus precludes its use as a first line therapy, it may be considered as a management option in patients with severe pruritus refractory to conventional therapies.

Antihistamines

While often employed successfully for the management of pruritus in allergic conditions, the use of antihistamines in the treatment of pruritus associated with cholestasis has been disappointing. H_1 receptor antagonists such as diphenhydramine and hydroxyzine have been utilized extensively in the past but with the availability of the other agents outlined above, their use is waning and is not routinely recommended.

Opioid Receptor Antagonists

Recent studies have suggested that the use of opioid receptor antagonists may produce marked improvement in pruritus associated with chronic cholestasis. The two compounds utilized to date are naloxone and nalmefene. Naloxone is available only in parenteral form and thus long-term treatment with this agent is not feasible. Orally administered nalmefene has been studied in a limited number of patients. The mechanism of action by which these compounds are effective remains uncertain but is the subject of intensive ongoing evaluation. The identification of orally active opioid antagonists which are shown to ameliorate the pruritus of cholestasis in controlled trials is still awaited, but the development of such compounds may represent a promising mode of therapy in the future.

HYPERCHOLESTEROLEMIA

Hypercholesterolemia is often apparent in patients with chronic cholestasis. Elevated serum levels of free cholesterol are associated with increased hepatic production of lipoprotein X. Experience suggests that dietary manipulation or the use of cholesterol-binding resins, such as cholestyramine, are generally ineffective in the management of elevated serum cholesterol levels in these patients. Recent reports, however, suggest that in patients with PBC, the serum lipid changes associated with progressive cholestasis are not, in fact, associated with an increased risk of atherosclerotic death. Thus, given the potential hepatotoxic effects associated with many cholesterol lowering agents, and the lack of evidence that hypercholesterolemia due to cholestasis produces significant clinical sequelae, specific treatment of hypercholesterolemia in patients with chronic cholestasis is not routinely recommended.

FAT MALABSORPTION

Severe and prolonged cholestasis may result in significant fat malabsorption with concomitant steatorrhea and weight loss. Steatorrhea results from intestinal bile salt depletion with resultant impaired absorption of monoglycerides and fatty acids. Initial management should center on the institution of a low-fat diet with a goal of 30 to 40 g of fat intake per day. Should this restriction be ineffective, medium-chain triglycerides, which are absorbed even in the absence of bile acid micelles, may be used to supply necessary calories and fat in patients who remain symptomatic on a 30 g fat diet. While medium-chain triglycerides are available as both an oil and in powder form, the unpalatability of the oil causes most patients to prefer the powder. The powder (Portagen) is reconstituted in water or juice and administered two to three times a day. Medium-chain triglyceride use also may improve the absorption of fat-soluble vitamins, although supplementation of these vitamins is often still necessary in cases of severe cholestasis.

FAT-SOLUBLE VITAMIN DEFICIENCY

The magnitude of fat-soluble vitamin deficiency parallels the degree of steatorrhea present in patients with chronic cholestasis. Vitamins A, D, E, and K are normally absorbed with fats. Because most adult patients with chronic cholestasis do not manifest severe steatorrhea, fat-soluble vitamin deficiency is an uncommon problem in this population, but one which should be addressed in the appropriate clinical setting.

Vitamin A

Vitamin A is absorbed from the small intestine as either retinol or β-carotene and is hydrolyzed by esterases prior to absorption. Both compounds are hydrophobic as a consequence of conjugated double bond structure, and thus absorption occurs primarily with mixed micelles. With lumenal bile salt depletion in severe cholestasis, such absorption is impaired. With depletion of liver stores, serum vitamin A levels fall and systemic signs of deficiency may develop. Deficiency is manifest as xerophthalmia, hyperkeratosis, impaired visual adaptation to the dark, and eventual night blindness. Serum levels of vitamin A rather than beta-carotene are most reflective of deficiency, as many Western diets are low in beta-carotene.

Aquasol A is a water-miscible form of vitamin A available in capsules (15 mg per 50,000 IU and 7.5 mg per 25,000 IU). In cases of documented deficiency, oral supplementation should begin with 25,000 IU per day in adults and 10,000 to 15,000 IU per day in children. Alternatively, intramuscular replacement (10,000 IU) may be administered on a monthly basis. Vigilance is required during long-term vitamin A replacement as overdosage may lead to serious clinical sequelae. Periodic monitoring of serum vitamin A levels is therefore mandatory. Signs and symptoms of hypervitaminosis A include fatigue, lethargy, malaise, abdominal discomfort, anorexia, cutaneous desquamation, alopecia, increased intracranial pressure, and hepatic injury.

Vitamin D

Hepatic osteodystrophy is a common consequence of chronic cholestasis and may lead to debilitating vertebral compression fractures and bone pain. The term has been coined to describe a syndrome of bone disease that appears to have characteristics of both osteoporosis and osteomalacia, although features of the former tend to predominate. The etiology of this condition is undoubtedly multifactorial but may be due in part to impaired vitamin D absorption and metabolism as well as decreased intestinal uptake of calcium in the setting of steatorrhea.

Several new modalities of treatment are undergoing investigation including calcitonin therapy, estrogen supplementation, and UDCA treatment. Particular attention is being directed at the effect of these treatments on the relative levels of osteoblast and osteoclast activity in patients with chronic cholestasis. While awaiting data regarding these newer forms of therapy, supplementation with calcium and vitamin D should be considered in patients with chronic cholestasis. Serum levels of vitamin D should be assessed by measurement of 25-OH-vitamin D levels. If documented to be low, vitamin D should be administered. Vitamin D_2 (ergocalciferol, 50,000 USP per tablet) should be administered in doses of 50,000 units three times a week or even daily depending on the severity of deficiency. Alternatively, intramuscular injections of 100,000 units may be administered monthly. If serum levels of 25-OH-vitamin D fail to correct with such therapy, 25-OH-vitamin D (calcifediol, 50 μg tablets) should be administered. Doses of 50 to 100 μg daily to every other day are generally adequate. As is true with vitamin A supplementation, careful monitoring is necessary to prevent overdosage and subsequent clinical sequelae. Signs and symptoms of vitamin D toxicity are related to hypercalcemia and include nausea, vomiting, abdominal pain, and alterations in mental status. Hypercalciuria with coincident renal injury also may result.

In addition to oral or intramuscular supplementation of vitamin D in patients with documented low serum levels, we routinely recommend that all patients with chronic cholestasis engage in activities which preserve bone density: (1) regular exercise, (2) judicious exposure to sunlight including during winter months and (3) consistent dietary intake of calcium-containing foods, or calcium supplements if dietary preferences are low in calcium.

Vitamin E

Deficiency of vitamin E has been documented in both adults and children with chronic cholestasis, although in adults the clinical consequences of vitamin E deficiency remain controversial. Extensive neurologic examination of cholestatic patients with low serum vitamin E levels has documented abnormalities compatible with the neurologic syndrome of vitamin E deficiency in only a minority. Given the disparity between objective findings and measured serum levels, routine replacement of vitamin E in adult cholestatic patients is not routinely recommended. In the adult with neurologic signs or symptoms of uncertain etiology after careful evaluation, supplementation of vitamin E (d-α-tocopherol, 100 to 200 IU orally per day) may be considered.

In contrast, a well-defined neurologic syndrome related to vitamin E deficiency has been documented in cholestatic children. In these individuals, tissue vitamin E levels are diminished as a consequence of impaired intestinal absorption of vitamin E and increased serum binding of vitamin E to elevated levels of lipoproteins. Thus, serum levels of vitamin E must be measured in conjunction with serum lipids. With these determinations, a ratio of vitamin E to lipids may be calculated and a more precise determination of body stores obtained. The clinical syndrome of vitamin E deficiency in cholestatic children includes peripheral neuropathy, cerebellar degeneration, abnormal eye movements, and retinal degeneration. Failure to recognize and promptly treat vitamin E deficiency in such children may result in permanent neurologic damage.

Replacement therapy in children should consist of d-α-tocopherol acetate given orally in a dose of 50 to 200 IU per kilogram per day. This large dose is often necessary as the result of severely impaired intestinal absorption in affected children. If oral supplementation does not produce increased serum levels of vitamin E, parenteral vitamin E (dl-α-tocopherol) should be administered in 50 mg doses at an interval calculated to yield an average daily dose of 1 to 2 mg per kilogram body weight.

Vitamin K

Vitamin K malabsorption may occur in the setting of intestinal bile salt depletion and steatorrhea. The use of cholestyramine and antibiotics to manage pruritus may also further impair normal intestinal production and absorption of vitamin K. Fortunately, deficiency of vitamin K only rarely becomes clinically significant in cholestatic patients. Identification of vitamin K malabsorption may be documented by measurement of the prothrombin time (PT). In patients with an elevated PT due to malabsorption, prompt correction is expected with the administration of subcutaneous vitamin K (phytonadione aqueous colloidal K_1, Aquamephyton) in a dose of 10 mg daily for 3 days. If correction or improvement in PT results, chronic supplementation with vitamin K should be considered. Oral supplementation with a water soluble derivative of vitamin K_3 (menadiol sodium diphosphate, 5-mg tablets, Synkavite) in doses of 5 to 10 mg per day typically is adequate. Monthly subcutaneous injection of 10 mg Aquamephyton represents an alternative to the oral replacement regimen. Doses in children range from 2.5 mg orally twice a week to 5 mg per day. Failure of the prothrombin time to correct with initial subcutaneous replacement of vitamin K suggests the derangement is due to impaired hepatic synthetic function rather than vitamin K deficiency. In such cases, no benefit of regular vitamin K supplementation can be expected.

SUGGESTED READING

Bachs L, Pares A, Elena M, et al. Effects of long-term rifampicin administration in primary biliary cirrhosis. Gastroenterology 1992; 102:2077–2080.

Berg C, Gollan J. Primary biliary cirrhosis: New therapeutic directions. Scand J Gastroenterol 1992; 27S:43–49.

Bergasa N, Talbot T, Alling D, et al. A controlled trial of naloxone infusions for the control of pruritus of chronic cholestasis. Gastroenterology 1992; 102:544–549.

Crippin J, Lindor K, Jorgensen R, et al. Hypercholesterolemia and atherosclerosis in primary biliary cirrhosis: What is the risk? Hepatology 1992; 15:858–862.

Cynamon H, Andres J, and Iafrate R. Rifampicin relieves pruritus in children with cholestatic liver disease. Gastroenterology 1990; 98:1013–1016.

Jeffrey G, Muller D, Burroughs A, et al. Vitamin E deficiency and its clinical significance in adults with primary biliary cirrhosis and other forms of chronic liver disease. J Hepatol 1987; 4:307–317.

Maddrey W. Bone disease in patients with primary biliary cirrhosis. In: Popper H and Schaffner F, eds. Progress in liver diseases. Philadelphia: WB Saunders, 1990:537.

Sokol R. Medical management of the infant or child with chronic liver disease. Semin Liver Dis 1987; 7:155–167.

PRIMARY SCLEROSING CHOLANGITIS

TAMSIN A. KNOX, M.D., M.P.H.
MARSHALL M. KAPLAN, M.D.

Sclerosing cholangitis is a progressive disorder in which inflammation of the intra and extrahepatic bile ducts leads to fibrosis. With time, both large and small bile ducts are oblitered, causing cholestasis, cirrhosis, and liver failure. Most cases are of unknown etiology and termed primary sclerosing cholangitis (PSC). Current data suggest that altered immunity plays a role in pathogenesis. Secondary sclerosing cholangitis may result from damage to the bile ducts due to ischemia, infection, or inflammatory processes. Ischemic injuries occur from radiation, intraarterial floxuridine (FUDR) administration, or from injury to the hepatic artery following liver transplantation. Infectious processes with cytomegalovirus, cryptosporidia, or microsporidia in immunosuppressed patients with AIDS also cause progressive bile duct disease which mimics PSC. Pancreatic inflammation or retroperitoneal fibrosis may involve the extrahepatic bile ducts. Finally, cancer, either cholangiocarcinoma or metastatic disease, may cause focal stricturing similar to PSC. In this chapter, we focus on the treatment of primary sclerosing cholangitis.

The suspicion of PSC should arise in patients with elevations in serum alkaline phosphatase with or without associated symptoms of biliary tract disease. Aminotransferases may be minimally elevated or normal, while bilirubin and albumin levels are typically normal early in the course of the disease. Seventy-five percent of patients with PSC have inflammatory bowel disease which is often quiescent at the time of diagnosis of liver disease. While 90 percent of patients referred to the New England Medical Center have an indolent presentation, the remainder present with an acute form characterized by recurrent episodes of fever, right upper quadrant pain, and jaundice. Defects in immunoregulation are suggested by the presence of antineutrophil cytoplasmic antibodies in about 50 percent of patients with PSC and HLA allele DRw52a in about 60 percent.

DIAGNOSIS

The diagnosis of PSC is made by endoscopic retrograde cholangiopancreatography (ERCP). On ERCP, the normally smooth, tapering bile ducts appear irregular because of areas of stricturing and dilatation involving both large and small bile ducts. Ulcerations may be seen in the extrahepatic ducts. Rare patients have isolated involvement of the intra or extrahepatic ducts.

In addition to ERCP, we perform a liver biopsy to stage the disease, assess the amount of ongoing inflammation, and monitor response to therapy. Stages I and II PSC have inflammation and fibrosis limited to the portal areas with a paucity of normal bile ducts. It is rare to find the onion-skin lesions typical of PSC on liver biopsy. Stage III has evidence of bridging fibrosis and lobular inflammation, where Stage IV implies the presence of cirrhosis. In addition to liver biopsy and ERCP, an assessment of liver synthetic function and evidence of end-stage liver disease should be sought.

THERAPY

The therapeutic approach to PSC can be divided into treatment of the inflammatory process, treatment of the symptoms of PSC (itching, jaundice, and recurrent fevers), and treatment of progressive liver failure (Table 1).

Treatment of the Underlying Disorder

Cholestatic liver diseases such as PSC or primary biliary cirrhosis are unlike diseases affecting the hepatocytes such as hepatitis since hepatocytes successfully regenerate. Bile ducts, when destroyed, do not regenerate. Although liver histology in PSC shows proliferation of atypical bile ductules, these structures do not effectively promote bile drainage. Hence, we believe that treatment for PSC should begin with early disease before there is significant loss of bile duct function. We should stress that at this time no medical treatment has been shown to improve the natural history of PSC. However, our experience suggests that the risk of medical treatment, albeit unproven, is less than the risk of no treatment with the inevitable development of liver failure and the need for liver transplantation.

Table 1 Therapeutic Approach to Primary Sclerosing Cholangitis

Symptom	Treatment
Itching	Cholestyramine Colestipol
Malabsorption	Fat soluble vitamin supplementation Pancreatic enzyme replacement
Recurrent infection	Maintenance antibiotic therapy
Jaundice	Dilation of major strictures Stent placement
Underlying disease	Ursodeoxycholic acid Methotrexate ? Prednisone
Liver failure or intractable symptoms of itching, fevers	Liver transplantation

Table 2 Drugs Tried in the Treatment of Primary Sclerosing Cholangitis

Ineffective and/or Toxic	Promising or Under Investigation
Corticosteroids*	Ursodeoxycholic acid
Azathioprine	Methotrexate
Antibiotics	
Penicillamine	
Colchicine and prednisone	
Cyclosporine	

*May be useful in early, prefibrotic PSC. More data are needed.

Therapeutic Alternatives

A variety of immunosuppressive agents have been tried in PSC, without proven efficacy (Table 2). A double-blind trial of penicillamine compared with placebo showed no improvement with therapy. Other drugs including corticosteroids, azathioprine, and colchicine plus prednisone are either ineffective or associated with unwanted side effects. Colectomy in patients with inflammatory bowel disease and PSC does not favorably affect the course of PSC. In studying the treatment of PSC, disease response is difficult to measure because of the spontaneous fluctuations with occasional dramatic remissions which may account for isolated reports of drug efficacy. Many patients are asymptomatic with indolent disease which progresses only slowly and requires years of surveillance to determine the effect of therapy. Finally, studies of treatment for PSC have been flawed by inclusion of patients with cirrhosis and irreversible loss of bile ducts who cannot be expected to respond to therapy.

Currently, preliminary results with ursodeoxycholic acid (UDCA) and methotrexate are promising in open label trials. O'Brien showed improvement in alkaline phosphatase, aminotransferase, and bilirubin values in 12 patients treated with 10 mg per kilogram per day of

UDCA for 6 and then 18 month periods. There was a trend towards improvement in symptoms of fatigue, pruritus, and diarrhea. Liver biopsies and ERCPs were not performed. Patients relapsed symptomatically and biochemically during the 3 month period of drug withdrawal. Stiehl treated 10 patients with 8 to 12 mg per kilogram per day of UDCA for 12 months. There was a marked improvement in alkaline phosphatase, gamma-glutamyl transpeptidase, and aminotransferases. However, the bilirubin increased slightly from 2.2 to 2.6 mg per deciliter.

UDCA has several potential modes of action in PSC. It does not reduce the concentration of naturally occurring bile acids such as cholate, chenodeoxycholate, or deoxycholate which may be toxic in high concentrations. UDCA appears to stabilize liver cell membranes, thus decreasing serum enzyme levels. In addition, it increases the bile flow and alkalinizes bile which may decrease stone and sludge formation in the bile ducts. This, in turn, may reduce cholestasis and the likelihood of cholangitis.*

We have studied oral pulse methotrexate in the treatment of PSC. In a study of precirrhotic patients with PSC, symptoms and alkaline phosphatase improved after 1 year of treatment. Subsequent liver biopsies showed decreased inflammation. In a small double-blind study of methotrexate in PSC, we found no improvement compared with placebo. However, this included only four precirrhotic patients who were evaluable on methotrexate therapy. In preliminary work, the addition of UDCA to methotrexate gives additional benefit in improving liver function tests.

Preferred Approach

In the absence of ongoing controlled clinical trials of therapy for early PSC, we begin treatment with UDCA in a dose of 10 to 16 mg per kilogram per day in two to three divided doses. Blood tests are repeated at monthly intervals. Biochemical improvements usually occur within several months. If the blood tests become normal, we keep the patient on UDCA and repeat a liver biopsy at 1 year. If the liver biopsy is unchanged or improved, we continue UDCA. More commonly, the blood tests show only mild improvement in 2 to 3 months. At this point, we add methotrexate at a dose of 0.25 mg per kilogram body weight per week (usually 15 mg per week) in three divided doses given 12 hours apart. Patients on methotrexate should have a repeat blood count, platelet count, and liver function tests monthly and a repeat liver biopsy 1 year after starting treatment. We repeat cholangiograms less often, at 2- to 3-year intervals.

Although methotrexate therapy has had a good safety profile at our center, we are concerned with the potential for bone marrow suppression, interstitial pneumonitis (which occurs in 3 to 5 percent of patients

with rheumatoid arthritis treated with methotrexate), potential hepatotoxicity with alcohol, and effects in pregnancy. We counsel patients not to drink alcohol while on methotrexate therapy, to use effective birth control methods, and to report shortness of breath. If there are any signs of toxicity, the methotrexate must be discontinued.

Management of Symptoms Associated with PSC

Cholestasis with PSC may be associated with pruritis, malabsorption, bile duct obstruction, or recurrent episodes of cholangitis. Each requires specific therapy.

Chronic cholestasis can cause intractable itching. Itching is typically worse at bedtime and may be aggravated by dry skin. We don't know the cause of the pruritus. It is not caused by any of the naturally-occurring bile acids or their metabolites. However, itching seems to respond to the nonabsorbed resin cholestyramine. We begin at a dose of 4 g (one packet or scoopful) three times a day. In the absence of complete biliary obstruction (if stool is not clay-colored), itching should improve in 4 to 7 days. Once the pruritus has resolved, a lower maintenance dose is effective at controlling the symptom. If itching does not resolve, the dose of cholestyramine may be increased to 8 g three times a day. Doses above this are rarely effective. Cholestyramine may be constipating and may require additional fluid or laxatives. Some patients find cholestyramine unpalatable. This can be improved by blending with fruit in a food processor or colestipol hydrochloride may be substituted. Mild itching may respond to sedation with antihistamines and treatment of dry skin with emollients. Other potentially effective therapies for itching include activated charcoal capsules, phenobarbital 60 to 90 mg at night which acts as a sedative and may increase bile flow, methyl testosterone, rifampin, naloxone, cimetidine, ultraviolet B light, and large volume plasmapheresis.

Bile obstruction may result in steatorrhea with malabsorption of fat and fat-soluble vitamins, especially in those patients who are chronically jaundiced. Asymptomatic vitamin A deficiency has been found in almost 50 percent of patients. We check serum levels of vitamins A and D (using 25-hydroxyvitamin D). Vitamin K is assessed using the prothrombin time. Oral supplementation is warranted in low or borderline deficiency states. Pancreatic insufficiency has also been associated with PSC. In patients with weight loss or diarrhea, a 72-hour fecal fat collection and trial of pancreatic enzyme supplementation is appropriate.†

Recurrent episodes of cholangitis may occur in bile ducts narrowed by strictures and the development of stones or sludge. Patients present with fevers often associated with right upper quadrant tenderness and jaundice. These may occur frequently as in the acute form of PSC or after manipulation of the biliary system.

---

*Editor's Note: There are also some reports of immunomodulator activity with UDCA. Thus, the effect may be more than just on bile acids.

†Editor's Note: The mechanism for pancreatic insufficiency isn't obvious. Perhaps medium-chain triglycerides might help.

Intravenous antibiotics covering enterococcus and gram-negative organisms should be administered for 7 to 10 days. We find that a prophylactic oral antibiotic regimen using amoxicillin, trimethoprim-sulfamethoxazole, or ciprofloxacin decreases the frequency of attacks in patients with recurrent episodes of sepsis. Changing antibiotics monthly may delay the development of resistant organisms. We administer prophylactic antibiotics before ERCP and for 24 hours after the procedure in any patient with suspected PSC to reduce the risk of bacteremia when injecting dye into a partially obstructed biliary system. We also use prophylactic antibiotics prior to liver biopsy if the bilirubin is elevated.

Biliary obstruction from a dominant stricture should be suspected when patients present with recurrent cholangitis or a rapid worsening in jaundice. We perform ERCP with views 20 to 40 minutes after injection of contrast to look for localized delays in emptying. If balloon dilatation of a dominant stricture is not possible, a plastic stent should be placed across the stricture.* We do not place metal, expandable stents which are not removable because, unlike patients with carcinoma, the life expectancy of PSC patients is longer than the expected patency of expandable stents. We do not perform surgical drainage of obstructed ducts such as roux-en-Y choledochojejunostomy since this seldom relieves intrahepatic cholestasis and makes liver transplantation much more difficult.

Cholangiocarcinoma develops in 7 to 15 percent of patients with long-standing PSC. Unfortunately, it is usually diagnosed postmortem as infiltrating cholangiocarcinoma and is very difficult to differentiate from the progressive scarring of PSC. Malignancy should be suspected in patients with progressive stricturing in the extrahepatic bile ducts or at the bifurcation, with rapid increase in jaundice, weight loss, or abdominal pain.

---

*__Editor's Note:__ Balloon dilatation of most strictures (perhaps with stenting as well) seems anecdotally to allow some patients not yet ready for transplantation to get along without transhepatic stents, which did help dominant bifurcating strictures.

Brushings of the bile ducts at ERCP are low yield. Magnetic resonance imaging or CT scan of the liver may be helpful in distinguishing scar from tumor once the tumor has reached a visible size. However, cholangiocarcinoma remains a difficult diagnosis to make at an early stage and is usually diagnosed at surgery or at the time of liver transplantation.

Liver Transplantation

Liver transplantation has an important role in the management of PSC. Indications for liver transplantation include progressive liver failure with ascites, muscle wasting, jaundice, or portal hypertension. Intractable itching or recurrent infections, unresponsive to prophylactic antibiotics, are also indications for transplantation. This subject is discussed in the chapters on hepatic transplantation in adults.

SUGGESTED READING

Batta AK, Arora R, Salen G, et al. Effect of ursodiol (UDCA) on bile acid metabolism in primary sclerosing cholangitis (PSC). Gastroenterology 1989; 96:A575.

Farrant JM, Hayllar KM, Wilkinson ML, et al. Natural history and prognostic variables in primary sclerosing cholangitis. Gastroenterology 1991; 100:1710–1717.

Kaplan MM. Medical approaches to primary sclerosing cholangitis. Sem Liver Dis 1991; 11:56–63.

Kaplan MM, Knox TA. Primary sclerosing cholangitis (PSC): Response to combination methotrexate and ursodiol. Gastroenterology 1991; 14:194A.

Knox TA, Kaplan MM. Treatment of primary sclerosing cholangitis with oral methotrexate. Am J Gastroenterol 1991; 86:546–552.

O'Brien CB, Senior JR, Arora-Mirchandani R, et al. Ursodeoxycholic acid for the treatment of primary sclerosing cholangitis: A 30-month pilot study. Hepatology 1991; 14:838–847.

Rosen CB, Nagorney DM. Cholangiocarcinoma complicating primary sclerosing cholangitis. Sem Liver Dis 1991; 11:26–30.

Stiehl A, Raedsch R, Theilmann P, Galle P. The effect of ursodeoxycholic acid (UDCA) in primary sclerosing cholangitis (PSC). Gastroenterology 1989; 96:A664.

SCLEROSING CHOLANGITIS: ENDOSCOPIC THERAPY

ANTHONY N. KALLOO, M.D.
PANKAJ J. PASRICHA, M.D.

Primary sclerosing cholangitis (PSC) is a chronic, usually progressive stricturing disease of the biliary tree. The etiology is unknown but current opinion favors an immunologic cause. Medical therapy for this disorder has been generally disappointing although there has been recent enthusiasm for the use of ursodeoxycholic acid. Other forms of therapy have included balloon dilatation (endoscopic and percutaneous) of the biliary tree, reconstructive biliary tract surgery (with or without transhepatic stenting), and liver transplantation.

Despite the immune mechanism for PSC there is a role for endoscopic therapy in these patients. Based on the surgical literature, bypassing dominant extrahepatic strictures even in patients with both intra- and extrahepatic disease appears to improve jaundice and decrease episodes of cholangitis. This suggests that the extrahepatic obstructive disease plays a role, at least in part, in the pathogenesis of the syndrome. Therefore it stands to reason that endoscopically alleviating the extrahepatic

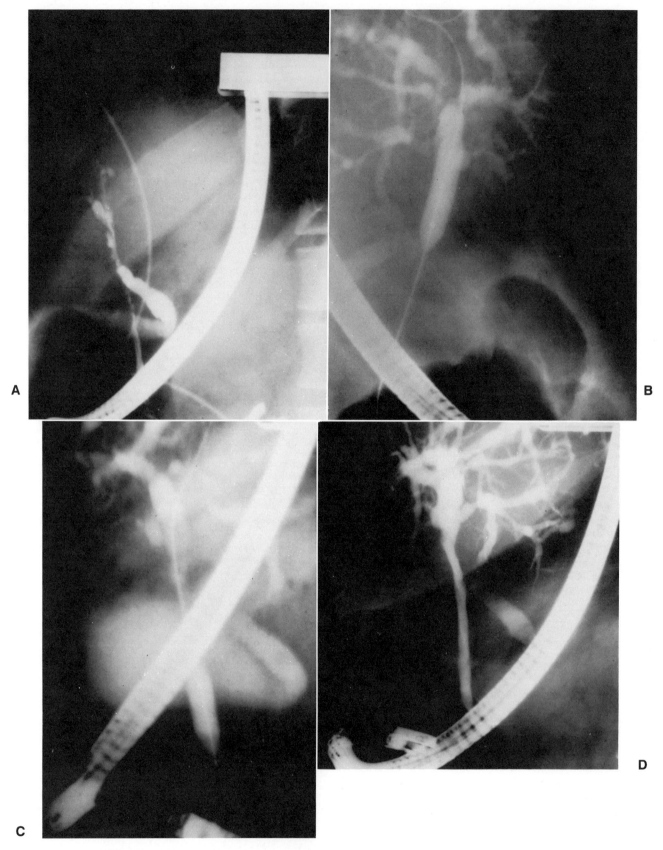

Figure 1 *A,* Cholangiogram of a patient with significant intra and extrahepatic disease. In this patient the diameter of the cystic duct is greater than that of the common bile duct. *B,* The endoscopic wire deeply inserted into the biliary tree with the balloon inflated at the common hepatic duct. *C,* The endoscopic wire deeply inserted into the biliary tree with the balloon inflated at the distal common bile duct. *D,* The appearance of the biliary tree after aggressive endoscopic therapy.

obstruction may accomplish the same goal as nontransplant surgical intervention but in a far less invasive way.

The goal of endoscopic therapy is *dilatation of strictures* to a point that bile flow is improved, thereby decreasing episodes of cholangitis and alternating jaundice. The first description of the use of endoscopic therapy in patients with PSC was by Siegel and Guelrud. They treated two patients with PSC using balloon catheters inflated at the site of the strictures to 75 psi for 2 to 3 minutes with good success in one patient. Since Siegel's initial description, there have been several published uncontrolled trials in which endoscopic therapy has been used to treat PSC. In these trials endoscopic therapy has been directed to patients with dominant strictures of the biliary tree.

In addition to balloon dilatation of bile duct strictures, several other endoscopic forms of therapy have been tried with varying degrees of success. These include endoscopic sphincterotomy, placement of biliary stents, and placement of nasobiliary catheters with subsequent lavage with saline or infusion of steroids.

The largest published series of endoscopic therapy in PSC is by Johnson and others who reviewed the results of an uncontrolled trial of 35 patients with dominant strictures. This was a follow-up report to their earlier published results on 10 patients. They used endoscopic balloon dilatation in patients with dominant strictures. In some patients, nasobiliary lavage was performed if the stricture could not be dilated. Eleven patients in this group had stents placed. The indications for stent placement was not specified. They found an improvement in the clinical parameters of liver function tests and hospitalization rates after a mean long-term follow-up of 24 months. Six patients (five with endoscopic stents) had cholangitis following endoscopic therapy. The five patients with stents had resolution of the cholangitis on stent removal.

Cotton reported on 20 patients with PSC who had endoscopic therapy consisting of balloon dilatation of extrahepatic and bifurcation strictures using an 8 mm balloon. If the dilatation was felt to be unsuccessful (by lack of a ductal diameter increase), endoscopic stenting of the strictures was performed. Most patients improved biochemically and clinically with a minimum follow-up of 6 months.

Several other smaller series have shown substantial improvement in clinical and biochemical parameters with the use of endoscopic balloon dilatation with or without endoscopic stenting. The disadvantages of endoscopic stenting include the need for repeat endoscopy for stent change or removal and possible increased risk of cholangitis if the stents become occluded.

The use of nasobiliary lavage was felt to be helpful in patients with PSC because of the observation that these patients frequently had thickened bile and sludge and that endoscopic irrigation may improve biliary flow. However a randomized trial of steroids versus normal saline endoscopic irrigation showed no benefit to either approach but an increased rate of infectious complications.

We used endoscopic therapy to aggressively treat patients with PSC. Instead of only dilating dominant strictures we dilated the total extrahepatic tree up to and including the hepatic bifurcation. Endoscopic sphincterotomy was performed in all patients because, in our experience, the Oddi sphincter is inevitably thickened, probably as a result of involvement by the sclerosing process. After endoscopic sphincterotomy, hydrophilic coated wires are used to access the strictures. These new wires have made it possible to cannulate strictures hitherto impossible to dilate. High pressure inflation balloons were used to dilate the bifurcation and common duct. This was performed by first inserting the balloon catheter to the hepatic bifurcation and then sequentially dilating by withdrawing the catheter in stations until the total extrahepatic tree was treated (Fig. 1). Inflation pressures of 150 psi were used at each station for a duration of 1 minute. Patients required one to three procedures to successfully dilate the extrahepatic tree. If more than one procedure was required, additional procedures were performed on an outpatient basis. Our initial results after a 6 month follow-up of five patients, all of whom had hyperbilirubinemia, demonstrated normalization of the bilirubin and an improved Mayo risk score for survival analysis.

Endoscopic therapy is a useful adjunct in the therapy of PSC. Ultimately many of these patients will require liver transplantation. The main advantages of endoscopic therapy are that it is relatively noninvasive and can be repeated serially if necessary. Endoscopic therapy may improve the quality of life of patients who may potentially be transplant candidates and may delay the need for transplantation.

SUGGESTED READING

Cotton PB, Nickl N. Endoscopic and radiologic approaches to therapy in primary sclerosing cholangitis. Semin Liver Dis 1991; 11:40–48.

Hutson D, Russell E, Jeffers L, et al. Balloon dilatation of biliary strictures in primary sclerosing cholangitis through choledochojejuno-cutaneous fistula: A new therapeutic approach. Gastroenterology 1986; 90:1470.

Johnson GK, Geenen JE, Venu RP, et al. Endoscopic treatment of biliary tract strictures in sclerosing cholangitis: A larger series and recommendations for treatment. Gastrointest Endosc 1991; 37: 38–43.

Kalloo AN, Miskovsky EP, Harris ML, et al. Aggressive endoscopic therapy in patients with sclerosing cholangitis. Gastroenterology 1991; 100:758A.

Kozarek RA. Hydrostatic balloon dilatation of gastrointestinal stenoses: A national survey. Gastrointest Endosc 1986; 32:15–19.

Lillemoe KD, Pitt HA, Cameron JL. Sclerosing cholangitis. Adv Surg 1987; 21:65–92.

Lombard M, Farrant M, Karani J, et al. Improving biliary-enteric drainage in primary sclerosing cholangitis: Experience with endoscopic methods. Gut 1991; 32:1364–1368.

Martin M. Primary sclerosing cholangitis. Annu Rev Med 1993; 44:221–227.

Siegel JH, Guelrud M. Gastrointest Endosc 1983; 29:99–103.

WILSON'S DISEASE

IRMIN STERNLIEB, M.D.
I. HERBERT SCHEINBERG, M.D.

Wilson's disease is an inherited metabolic defect as a result of which copper in small amounts — essential to life — accumulates to toxic levels. The pathologic effects of the excess copper on the liver and central nervous system (CNS) are progressive and fatal unless specific treatment is given.

CLINICAL COURSE AND DIAGNOSIS

Clinical onset of the disease may occur at any age between 5 and 50 years. In childhood, the initial symptoms are usually hepatic, manifested by jaundice, portal hypertension, hepatic insufficiency with ascites or bleeding varices, sometimes accompanied by hemolytic anemia. Later in life, the first clinical manifestation is more likely to be of a tremulous, dystonic, dysarthric or other motor neurologic or psychiatric disorder. Such a CNS disorder — which is what Wilson described — always eventually appears if the hepatic disease has not first proved fatal.

A confirmed diagnosis of Wilson's disease is essential before life-saving specific treatment is instituted. The demonstration of any two of the following suffices to confirm the diagnosis: corneal Kayser-Fleischer rings, deficiency of serum ceruloplasmin (<20 mg per deciliter), elevation of hepatic copper concentration (>250 µg per gram dry tissue), and hypercupriuria (>100 µg per 24 hours without penicillamine administration). Rarely, a radiocopper loading test may be required to confirm or rule out the diagnosis. In the latter case, penicillamine or any other treatment specific for Wilson's disease is useless.

TREATMENT

Penicillamine

Regardless of the presence or absence of clinical manifestations of Wilson's disease, its confirmed diagnosis mandates treatment with D-penicillamine. One gram of penicillamine daily, administered in four divided doses, at least half an hour before meals, constitutes the basic therapeutic regimen. Children weighing less than 40 kg should receive 0.02 g per kilogram body weight daily rounded to the nearest quarter of a gram. A daily dose of 25 mg of pyridoxine is recommended to counteract the weak antipyridoxine effect of penicillamine. We have not found it necessary to supplement penicillamine treatment with minerals, except for the occasional need for iron in adolescent girls or women with excessive menstrual losses of blood. A stringent low copper diet is not necessary, but shellfish, liver, mushrooms, nuts, broccoli, and chocolate should be avoided.

Early Sensitivity Reactions

Early sensitivity reactions to penicillamine occur in about 20 percent of patients. For the first month of treatment, such a reaction must be watched for by taking the temperature at night; having a physician examine the patient for a morbilliform rash or adenopathy; ascertain that leukopenia or thrombocytopenia does not occur by determining white blood cell, differential, and platelet counts; and check urine for proteinuria at weekly visits. If all has gone well, the frequency of subsequent visits can be progressively decreased.

If fever, rash, lymphadenopathy, leukopenia, thrombocytopenia, or some combination of these occurs, the drug should be stopped immediately until the reaction has completely subsided. Then it is reinstituted gradually in increasing dosage from an initial 125 mg daily to 1 g a day over several weeks, accompanied by the administration of 30 mg of prednisone daily. The latter is started 2 or 3 days before and continued after the reinstitution of full penicillamine dosage for about 5 days. If no reaction recurs, the dosage of prednisone is tapered slowly over 2 or 3 weeks. Recurrent sensitivity is treated by more gradual desensitization.

Neurologic Symptom Response

In about 10 percent of patients, neurologic symptoms may first appear or worsen during the first weeks or months of penicillamine therapy. The patient should be warned of this possibility before the regimen is begun. However, in most neurologically-affected patients, there is generally significant — sometimes dramatic — improvement within a few months of starting therapy; in a minority, significant improvement may not be noticeable for 6 to 12 months; and in a very few, there may be no improvement or continued progression of neurologic symptoms.

Liver Disease Response

Overt liver disease responds more slowly with improvement of jaundice, ascites, edema, and bruisability after several months of penicillamine treatment supplemented with appropriate dietary salt restriction and diuretics. In patients with severe, irreversible pathologic changes and in those with the clinical picture of relentlessly progressive or fulminant hepatitis, pharmacologic therapy may be ineffective, and only a liver transplant may be lifesaving.

Late Adverse Reactions

Late reactions to penicillamine* include:

---

*Except possibly for lupus, any of these reactions require substitution of triethylene tetramine (trientine) for penicillamine.

1. Nephropathy, manifested as proteinuria, which usually resolves with substitution of trientine for penicillamine
2. Lupus erythematosus, often accompanied by arthralgias, and usually controlled by slight reduction of penicillamine dosage and the addition of 5 to 10 mg prednisone daily
3. Thrombocytopenia, unrelated to hypersplenism, and of concern only when the platelet count drops to less than 50,000 per cubic millimeter
4. Pemphigus or pemphigoid lesions
5. Myasthenia
6. Macromastia
7. Penicillamine dermatopathy—discoloration and thinning of the skin, and the appearance of milia-like white papules—occurring in patients receiving 2 g or more of penicillamine daily for many months.
8. Elastosis perforans serpiginosa—raised, arcuate lesions on the neck and axillae of some patients receiving penicillamine for 6 to 8 years

Long-term Course

Most patients improve often to the point of normality. Indeed, in patients in whom therapy is started before the appearance of symptoms, good health and normal longevity can virtually be assured provided the prescribed regimen is adhered to indefinitely and monitored periodically.

Penicillamine treatment may require simultaneous psychotherapy or the judicious use of psychotropic drugs when the emotional or psychiatric disturbances are severe.

Almost invariably, girls who have never menstruated or who have irregular or abnormal periods, as a consequence of Wilson's disease, establish normal cycles with effective penicillamine treatment. Puberty, occasionally delayed in the untreated boy or girl, generally progresses normally with specific therapy. Repeated miscarriages, although not uncommon in untreated patients with Wilson's disease, are rare in treated patients, whose ability to conceive and deliver healthy babies is generally unaffected. This topic is also discussed in the chapter *Liver Disease in Pregnancy*.

Periodic monitoring is required to assure the continued effectiveness of treatment with penicillamine and absence of adverse reactions. Monitoring should include relevant physical, neurologic, and slit-lamp examination of the corneas; measurements of the non-ceruloplasmin copper fraction of serum; complete blood counts; tests of liver chemistries; and routine urinalysis at least twice yearly, and more often if feasible. Patients must remain under a physician's care for life.

British Antilewisite (Dimercaprol) Therapy

Treatment with British Antilewisite, 2,3-dimercaprol (BAL) may be helpful if a patient with severe neurologic manifestations—mutism, drooling, rigidity, involuntary movements, uncontrollable tremors—does not show significant improvement after 3 to 4 months of treatment with 1 to 3 g of D-penicillamine daily. Five intramuscular injections of 3.0 ml of BAL weekly should be administered while penicillamine is continued. Several months of this regimen may be required before significant improvement takes place.

Trientine Hydrochloride

Trientine hydrochloride is a chelating agent that appears to be as clinically effective as penicillamine. It is the drug of choice for patients intolerant to penicillamine. Although this drug is not as cupriuretic as is penicillamine, its continued use in divided doses of 1 to 1.5 g daily is generally therapeutically effective. Side effects are rare and to date seem limited to sideroblastic anemia and possibly lupus erythematosus.

Zinc

Daily doses of 75 to 300 mg of elemental zinc administered as the sulfate, acetate, or gluconate, have been used by several investigators for symptomatic and asymptomatic patients with Wilson's disease. However, published data on the effectiveness of zinc as therapy in patients with severe neurologic symptoms or hepatic decompensation are scanty, though zinc appears able to prevent progression of stabilized hepatic disease. Headaches, abdominal cramps, gastric irritation and loss of appetite occur in some patients receiving large amounts of zinc. Zinc can cause sideroblastic anemia, alter immune responses, and affect the serum lipoprotein profile. Zinc should not be given to a patient who is also receiving simultaneous treatment with penicillamine or trientine.

Tetrathiomolybdate

Tetrathiomolybdate is an investigational agent that appears to block the absorption of copper holding the absorbed metal in a tight, metabolically inert bond. It has been used in a few patients intolerant to both penicillamine and trientine.

Liver Transplantation

Orthotopic liver transplantation is indicated in patients suffering from severe hepatic insufficiency not responding to medical therapy and in those presenting with a clinical picture of fulminant hepatitis.

Adjunctive Therapy

Psychotherapy, physiotherapy, speech therapy, and surgery for lengthening of tendons in patients with contractures of joints may be indicated in individual patients. Splenectomy for hypersplenism is hardly ever indicated.

Editor's Note: Astute users of this series of books will remember that Drs. Sternlieb and Scheinberg wrote a chapter for the first edition 10 years ago. We appreciate their sharing their updated experience with us (the readers).

SUGGESTED READING

Scheinberg IH, Sternlieb I. Wilson's disease. Philadelphia: WB Saunders, 1984.

Walshe JM, Yeolland M. The management of neurological Wilson's disease. Experience with one hundred and thirty-seven patients. QJ Med, 1993 86:197–204.

HEMOCHROMATOSIS

HERBERT L. BONKOVSKY, M.D.

Hemochromatosis is the term used to describe states of iron overload. Since humans lack an efficient pathway for the excretion of iron (only small amounts are excreted in the bile or urine in the absence of hemobilia or hematuria), iron overload occurs whenever there is excessive net absorption of iron from the gut or excess parenteral iron administration. The usual schemes for classifying causes of iron overload are based on this dichotomy (Table 1), although, of course, the two may coexist. Excess gut absorption may occur due to chronic ingestion of excessive quantities of iron, usually in the form of medicinal iron, or due to an inherited or acquired defect in normal function of gut mucosa that leads to increased net iron absorption. Parenteral iron overload nearly always is due to repeated transfusions of blood, given for therapy of chronic anemias. For example, patients with aplastic anemias may require hundreds of blood transfusions, each pint of which contains 200 to 250 mg of iron. Patients with ineffective or dyserythropoiesis who may have had far fewer blood transfusions, may nevertheless also develop heavy iron overload due to the additional contribution of increased net gut absorption of iron. Due to the anemia, such patients continue to absorb inappropriately large amounts of iron from the gut despite a surfeit of total body iron.

HEREDITARY HEMOCHROMATOSIS

Among Caucasians, the most frequent cause of iron overload is hereditary hemochromatosis, which is among the most common autosomal recessive disorders. Although, as of this writing, the precise molecular cause of hereditary hemochromatosis has not been identified, studies have shown that the genetic locus is on the short arm of chromosome 6, closely linked to the HLA A and B loci. Furthermore, due to a founder effect, most patients with hereditary hemochromatosis have HLA types A3, B7, or A3, B14. A single dose of the abnormal hemochromatosis gene occurs in 8 to 10 percent of Caucasians and produces a mild degree of gradually progressive iron overload, with levels of serum ferritin, transferrin saturation, and hepatic iron concentrations that are at the upper end of the normal range or mildly increased. However, in the absence of other factors that cause or promote excess iron accumulation, heterozygotes for hereditary hemochromatosis do not develop heavy, pathological iron overload.

In contrast, heavy iron overload does occur in the homozygous recessive state which occurs in 0.3 to 0.45 percent of Caucasians. The major defect in such patients resides in an inappropriately high degree of absorption of iron from the gastrointestinal (GI) tract for the degree of total body iron present. Since the fraction of ingested iron absorbed by the gut is controlled in part by body iron stores, and since this control mechanism is not entirely missing in homozygous hemochromatosis, such patients when heavily iron-loaded, may absorb iron only to a

Table 1 Cause of Iron Overload in Humans

Due to excess enteral absorption of iron
  Hereditary hemochromatosis (genetic, primary, idiopathic)
  Congenital atransferrinemia
  Anemia due to ineffective erythropoiesis*
    Hereditary spherocytosis
    Sideroblastic anemias
    Thalassemias
    Other forms with dyserythropoiesis
  Increased oral intake of iron
  African dietary iron overload (Bantu siderosis)†
  Excess medicinal intake of iron
  Iron overload complicating chronic liver disease
    Alcoholic liver disease
    Porphyria cutanea tarda
    Portosystemic shunting of blood

Due to excess parenteral absorption of iron
  Multiple blood transfusions*
  Excessive parenteral iron injections
  Associated with chronic hemodialysis with transfusions
  Neonatal hemochromatosis

*Iron overload complicating chronic anemia may be due both to enteral and parenteral iron overload.
†A genetic contribution to the iron overload observed in Black Africans has been suggested (Gordeuk et al).

normal extent. Nevertheless, it is abnormally increased in the setting of total body iron overload.

IRON OVERLOAD IN NONHEMOCHROMATOTIC LIVER DISEASE

Although patients with chronic liver disease not primarily due to iron overload may develop heavy hepatic iron loading, this is a rare event. When such patients are encountered, the possibility of the coexistence of hereditary hemochromatosis and alcoholic or other liver disease should be considered.

The degree of hepatic iron overload associated *per se* with alcoholic liver disease, chronic viral hepatitis, porphyria cutanea tarda, and other chronic liver diseases is relatively mild (less than four times the upper limit of normal). Only in porphyria cutanea tarda is such iron clearly pathogenic, in that it plays a major role in the hepatic overproduction of uroporphyrin and heptacarboxyporphyrin, which produces the clinical and biochemical hallmarks of this form of porphyria.

Neonatal hemochromatosis is a rare, poorly understood disorder that occurs at or shortly after birth. It is characterized by failure to thrive, severe hepatic dysfunction, and early death unless liver transplant is carried out. Although familial occurrence of neonatal hemochromatosis has been described, it is not associated with hereditary hemochromatosis. It probably represents a form of neonatal hepatitis, perhaps of diverse etiology.

CLINICOPATHOLOGIC FEATURES OF HEMOCHROMATOSIS

Regardless of the underlying causes of iron overload, it is toxic whenever sufficient concentrations are present for sufficient time. The toxicity of chronic iron overload is thought to relate chiefly to oxidant damage to key macromolecules, causing organelle and cell damage and death with subsequent fibrosis and hepatic cancer.

The organs chiefly involved are the liver, pancreas, heart, pituitary gland, and joints. A full account of the variegated clinical manifestations of advanced hemochromatosis is beyond the scope of this chapter. However, it is important to stress that hemochromatosis can and should be detected and treated in the early, pre-symptomatic stage, before the development of "bronze diabetes," arthropathy, gonadal failure, or cardiac dysfunction.

Early detection and vigorous treatment of hereditary hemochromatosis can totally prevent the eventual development of end-organ damage and liver cancer. The same is true of other forms of hemochromatosis in which therapy by venesection is feasible. Unfortunately, in those forms of hemochromatosis in which venesection cannot be performed due to the presence of anemia, the chelation therapy currently available is not as effective, such that the toxic effects of chronic iron excess are not entirely preventable. Even in these diseases, however, where iron overload can be anticipated, early, vigorous, and continuing therapy has been shown to decrease morbidity and mortality.

The most important step in making the diagnosis of hemochromatosis is to think of it in the first place. This should not be difficult in patients with chronic ineffective erythropoiesis who have required multiple transfusions. In such patients, the minimum total body iron burden in grams is approximately equal to the number of units of blood transfused divided by four. In addition, such patients have a hyperabsorption of iron from the GI tract which further increases the total body burden.

Because of the high gene frequency of hereditary hemochromatosis among Caucasians, and the high sensitivity and low cost of screening tests, a cogent argument can be made that all Caucasian adults should be screened for this condition. Screening should include serum iron, serum transferrin or total iron-binding capacity (TIBC), and serum ferritin (Table 2). In the absence of other causes of liver disease or inflammation, the level of the serum ferritin is a reasonably accurate, minimally invasive reflection of total body iron stores. However, it is often increased in alcoholic liver disease, viral hepatitis, or other causes of liver injury, as well as by numerous other inflammatory diseases. Thus, as shown in Table 3, serum ferritin is sensitive, but not specific, for diagnosis of hemochromatosis.

The serum iron while of some use in screening, is often within the normal range (50 to 150 μg per deciliter) in hemochromatosis. More useful is the serum transferrin iron saturation, which is usually increased due to the combined effects of a high normal or high serum iron and low serum transferrin and TIBC. Often in homozygous hereditary hemochromatosis, the serum transferrin iron saturation is high even when patients are not iron-overloaded (e.g., following therapy), because of their genetic propensity for abnormally increased iron absorption from the gut. Thus, although useful for initial diagnosis, the transferrin iron saturation is not very useful as a guide to therapy of such patients.

Analysis of HLA A and B types is not routinely required for diagnosis of hemochromatosis. The chief usefulness of HLA typing is in evaluation of siblings of patients with definite homozygous hereditary hemochromatosis since siblings with HLA types identical to the patients' are virtually certain also to have inherited hemochromatosis. Although HLA types A3, B7 or A3, B14 occur with increased frequency in hereditary hemochromatosis, they also occur in about 30 percent of all Caucasians. Thus, the presence of these haplotypes is not diagnostic of hemochromatosis, even when the serum ferritin is elevated, unless a sibling with documented homozygous disease has the identical HLA type.

Although excess iron in the liver increases hepatic CT attenuation and shortens proton relaxation times in hepatic MRI scans, these expensive imaging modalities cannot be recommended at present for hemochromatosis screening (Table 3). Although abdominal MRI

Table 2 Tests for Iron Overload

Test	Typical Reference Range*	Category of Patient	
		Symptomatic	Asymptomatic
Indirect, screening tests			
Serum transferrin iron saturation	20%–50%	Marked increase	Usually increased
Serum ferritin	F 21-99, M 30-270 ng/ml	Marked increase	Normal or increased
Direct, definitive tests			
Quantitative liver iron	300-1,200 μg/g dry wt (5.35-21.4 μmoles/g dry wt)	Marked increase	Mild-moderate increase
Venesection assay	< 12 units to achieve iron depletion	Marked increase	Mild-moderate increase

*Normal values vary somewhat depending upon laboratory and methods used.

Table 3 Diagnostic Efficacy of Screening Tests for Heavy Iron Overload*

Variable Studied	Reference Range‡	Sensitivity	Specificity	Predictive Value	
				Of Positive	Of Negative
Serum ferritin	F 21-99, M, 30-270 ng/ml	1.00	0.21	0.32	1.00
Serum iron	30-210 μg/dl	0.27	0.94	0.60	0.80
Serum transferrin iron saturation	20-50%	0.91	0.42	0.34	0.93
Urinary iron excretion†	<2 mg/24 hours	0.75	0.50	0.36	0.84
Hepatic CT attenuation	<70 HU	1.00	0.64	0.48	1.00
Hepatic MRI scan					
T2, uncorrected	>37ms	0.90	0.61	0.43	0.95
SI2, (L/M)§	>0.5	1.00	0.92	0.83	1.00

*Heavy iron overload was defined as hepatic iron concentration > 107 μmole/g dry liver (>5 × upper limit of normal).
†Urinary iron measured after administration of deferoxamine, 10 mg/kg IM.
‡Normal values vary somewhat, depending upon laboratory and methods used.
§SI2 (L/M) is the ratio of the intensity of the second echo from the liver to that of paraspinous muscle, measured in the same scan slice.
Adapted from Bonkovsky HL, Slaker DP, Bills EB, Wolf DC. Usefulness and limitations of laboratory and hepatic imaging studies in iron-storage disease. Gastroenterology 1990; 99:1079-1091; with permission.

scanning as routinely done is very sensitive, only mild increases in hepatic iron concentrations are sufficient to produce an abnormal "black hole" appearance of the liver on T2-weighted images. Thus, in addition to high cost, we have shown that routine MRI scanning lacks the ability to predict the degree of iron overload with acceptable accuracy and cannot be recommended for routine evaluation of hemochromatosis. In the future, specialized algorithms for abdominal MRI scans may provide results that are both sensitive and specific enough to be useful; however, they will require special expertise and scan sequences and likely will be available in only a few specialized centers.

The diagnosis of hemochromatosis is established definitively either by liver biopsy with quantitative iron measurement and/or by therapeutic venesection (see Table 2). Since in hereditary hemochromatosis iron accumulation is progressive with age, the hepatic iron concentration is best interpreted in light of the patient's age. The ratio of the liver iron concentration to the age of the patient has been termed the "hepatic iron index," and several studies have shown that the value of this index can distinguish untreated homozygous from heterozygous hereditary hemochromatosis or other forms of liver disease (Table 4). The index may be increased in secondary hemochromatosis as well as in homozygous primary disease, and it will, of course, be decreased in patients who have lost appreciable amounts of blood either due to natural or iatrogenic (therapeutic) causes. Thus the hepatic iron index must be interpreted thoughtfully in the light of the patient's history. Five to ten milligrams of liver (i.e., a core of 0.5 to 1.0 cm in length obtained with a 16 gauge needle) is sufficient for quantitative iron measurement as done in our or other reference laboratories. An extra "pass" of the biopsy needle ordinarily is not necessary.

EVALUATION OF RELATIVES AT RISK

After a diagnosis of hereditary hemochromatosis has been established, we urge that all first-degree relatives be screened for iron overload. This should include all children over the age of 10 years since severe

Table 4 Hepatic Iron Index (HII)* in Differential Diagnosis of Iron Overload

Study	Normal	ALD	Diagnosis Hereditary Hemochromatosis Heterozygous	Homozygous
Bassett et al, 1986, *Hepatology*	< 1.0	< 1.4	< 1.8	> 2.0
Bonkovsky et al, 1990, *Gastroenterology*	< 0.7	< 1.1	< 1.8	> 2.0 (17/19)
				1.2-2.0 (2/19)†
Kowdley et al, 1991, *Hepatology*	< 1.0	< 1.0	–	> 2.0 (14/18)
				1.25-2.0 (4/18)
Olynyk et al, 1990, *Hepatology*	< 1.1	< 1.6	–	> 2.1
Sallie et al, 1991, *Gut*	–	< 1.6	–	> 2.0
Summers et al, 1990, *Hepatology*	–	–	< 1.5	> 1.9

*HII is concentration of liver iron (μmoles Fe/g dry wt) divided by age of patient in years.
†The two patients with HII < 2.0 were both women with histories of heavy menstrual blood loss and multiple births.
ALD = Alcoholic liver disease.
—indicates results not reported.

disease has rarely been described in persons of this age. If initial results of routine serum studies are normal, first-degree relatives should be retested every 2 to 3 years, since an abnormal phenotype may not become detectable until later in life. Men over 35 or women over 50 who have not shown elevations in serum ferritin or transferrin iron saturation do not require further testing, unless they have a history of abnormal blood loss. HLA typing is indicated only in siblings as already described. In view of the high gene frequency of hereditary hemochromatosis in Caucasians, the screening of spouses of patients is rational both for their information and for their descendants. It is likely that, within 3 years, the gene for hereditary hemochromatosis will be identified and a definitive test for the disease developed. Such a test should facilitate early, definitive diagnosis and obviate the need for repeated testing of relatives-at-risk.

MANAGEMENT

Hereditary or Primary Hemochromatosis

Initial Therapy

Repeated venesection is the most effective, least expensive method for iron removal (Table 5). The usual prescription for adults is for weekly phlebotomy of 1 pint of blood. Children and some small women may benefit from IV replacement of the blood volume lost with normal saline or tolerate removal of only 300 ml of blood per session. Many men tolerate removal of 2 pints per week. The most common therapeutic mistake is not recommending or assuring a sufficiently vigorous regimen of iron removal. The initial target is to make the patient mildly iron-deficient with a fall in prevenesection hematocrit to a slightly low value (men < 38 percent, woman < 34 percent). When these values have been reached, no blood should be removed but patients should return the following week for repeat testing and

Table 5 Management of Hemochromatosis

Primary (Homozygous hereditary) hemochromatosis
Initial Therapy
　Weekly phlebotomy of 1 unit until patient mildly anemic
　Confirm iron depletion with serum ferritin
Maintenance Therapy
　One unit phlebotomy every 2–3 months
　Patient to keep record of phlebotomies
　Check serum ferritin yearly; adjust frequency of phlebotomy to keep serum ferritin 20–100 ng/ml

Secondary hemochromatosis (Due to Anemias or Transfusions)
Chelation therapy with parenteral deferoxamine (Desferal)
　Begin therapy early in course of disease prior to heavy iron accumulation
　Administer nightly by slow SC infusion
　Maximal daily dose 70 mg/kg
　Add vitamin C, 1 g/day orally after first 3 months of therapy
　(Possible future therapies: oral chelators; iron-binding resin perfusion)

Diet for both Primary and Secondary Hemochromatosis
　No liver; minimal red meat
　Drink tea with meals

phlebotomy if the hematocrit has risen, as will often be the case. When patients have remained mildly anemic for 2 or more weeks in succession, in all likelihood, they are iron depleted. This can be confirmed by measurement of the serum ferritin which should be less than 30 ng per milliliter. (The serum iron or transferrin iron saturation may still be elevated at such times depending upon the amount and recency of iron intake; thus repeated measurements of these are not recommended.) Repeat liver biopsy, although the most definitive test to confirm iron depletion is not usually necessary unless other disease is a concern (e.g., hepatoma or hepatitis).

Removal of the last bits of excess body iron is more difficult than the first. Some authorities recommend the addition of vitamin C (500 to 1,000 mg per day), after the first 4 to 6 months of phlebotomy therapy since vitamin

C is known to enhance iron mobilization. However, it also enhances iron absorption from the gut, making its use something of a two-edged sword. We have not found its routine use necessary.

To decrease the accretion of new iron, we recommend that patients moderate their intakes of foods high in readily absorbed iron, especially liver and red meat (see Table 5). It is impractical to recommend avoidance of grains and vegetables high in iron since iron fortification regrettably is so ubiquitous. Fortunately, absorption of iron from such sources is lower than from animal sources. We also recommend that patients drink tea with one or more meals per day, especially those containing meat, since tea decreases gut iron absorption presumably by chelating the iron to poorly-absorbed tannins. Avoidance of meat altogether can further decrease iron absorption but most patients prefer to donate a few extra pints of blood rather than to alter radically their dietary habits. Because of the likely synergy between iron and alcohol in producing iron injury, abstinence from alcohol should be encouraged for all patients and strongly advised in those with hepatic fibrosis or cirrhosis.

The symptoms of heavily iron-loaded patients typically improve noticeably after a few months of phlebotomy with decreased abdominal discomfort and fatigue. Typically, liver, cardiac, and pancreatic dysfunction improve but arthritis and hypogonadism do not. Although the plasma removed by phlebotomy could be harvested and returned to the patient, this is rarely necessary since the synthesis of plasma proteins can keep pace with the amounts removed even in patients with cirrhosis. Chelator therapy with deferoxamine is rarely indicated in hereditary hemochromatosis, its use being reserved to those few, usually young patients with severe myocardial dysfunction.

Maintenance Therapy

After initial iron depletion has been achieved, the object of therapy is to prevent reaccumulation of iron. This usually requires 1 unit venesections every 2 to 3 months. Patients should not be kept chronically anemic. The adequacy of therapy is best monitored by insisting that the patient keep a record of phlebotomies to be brought to each follow-up visit and reviewed by the physician, and by yearly serum ferritin measurements which should remain between 20 to 100 ng per milliliter. Regular follow-up (at least annually), with reminders that hereditary hemochromatosis requires life-long therapy is essential lest patients slip into iron reaccumulation and toxicity due to inattention.

The life expectancy of noncirrhotic patients with hereditary hemochromatosis who undergo chronic, adequate therapy is normal. Those with cirrhosis have an improved prognosis but remain at increased risk of eventual development of hepatoma, emphasizing the importance of early diagnosis and therapy. Although it is intuitive to screen cirrhotic patients for the presence of early, asymptomatic hepatomas, the meager available evidence does *not* indicate that such screening prolongs

life. These studies used semiannual hepatic ultrasound alternating with serum alpha-fetoprotein measurements. Perhaps use of CT or MRI scanning would detect hepatomas earlier although costs would be higher. Rarely, hemochromatotic patients without cirrhosis develop hepatomas; routine periodic screening of such patients is even more difficult to justify.

Secondary Hemochromatosis

Some patients with secondary hemochromatosis, e.g., those with relatively mild degrees of anemia who perhaps have taken medicinal iron in the erroneous belief that the anemia was due to iron deficiency, can also tolerate regular therapeutic venesection albeit less frequently than just described. This possibility, coupled with therapy with large doses of vitamin B_6, B_{12}, folate, and/or erythropoietin should be considered carefully. If such therapy proves impossible or ineffective, chronic chelation therapy with deferoxamine (Desferal) is the only available alternative.

Although deferoxamine can be given intramuscularly or intravenously (e.g., at the times of transfusions), it is most effective when given by slow, continuous infusion. For nearly all patients this means nightly for 10 to 12 hours by use of a constant infusion pump. The amount given should generally be 25 to 50 mg per kg per day and should not exceed 70 mg per kg per day because of a high risk of toxicity at higher doses. Toxic effects include local reactions at sites of infusion, rare anaphylactic reactions, coma, seizures, growth retardation, cataracts, retinal damage with decreased visual acuity, ototoxicity with sensorineural hearing loss and tinnitus, renal toxicity, thrombocytopenia, musculoskeletal pain, and increased risk of infection with unusual organisms (*Rhizopus, Yersinia, V. vulnificus*). Risks of toxicity are higher in patients with minimal body burdens of iron who are treated with standard doses of deferoxamine. In practice, the lowest necessary daily dose of deferoxamine is best. This can be estimated from periodic measures of 24 hour urinary excretions of iron during therapy, assuming that two-thirds of the iron is excreted in the urine and one-third in the stool during deferoxamine therapy. Total amounts excreted must be compared to amounts gained through transfusions (250 mg iron per unit), which are minimal estimates since patients also absorb iron from the gut. Another method for estimating the daily dose of deferoxamine required is to measure the serum iron and TIBC during deferoxamine infusions. A proposed target dose rate is that which produces 50 to 150 µg per deciliter unbound iron-binding capacity during infusions (UIBC = TIBC − serum iron).

After deferoxamine therapy has been instituted for several months, vitamin C (ascorbic acid) should be added to the regimen to enhance iron mobilization. The best route and dose of the vitamin are somewhat controversial. Low doses (50 to 100 mg per day, given strictly in conjunction with deferoxamine) and larger doses (1,000 mg per day) have both been shown effective in increasing iron excretion.

The greatest impediments to effective, long-term deferoxamine therapy are high cost and noncompliance particularly among adolescents and young adults. A cheap, effective, nontoxic orally-effective iron chelator would represent a major therapeutic advance.

SUGGESTED READING

Bonkovsky HL, Slaker DP, Bills EB, Wolf DC. Usefulness and limitations of laboratory and hepatic imaging studies in iron-storage disease. Gastroenterology 1990; 99:1079–1091.

Edwards CQ, Cartwright GE, Skolnick MH, Amos DB. Homozygosity for hemochromatosis: Clinical manifestations. Ann Intern Med 1980; 93:519–525.

Fosburg MT, Nathan DG. Treatment of Cooley's anemia. Blood 1990; 76:435–444.

Milder MS, Cook JD, Stray S, Finch CA. Idiopathic hemochromatosis, an interim report. Medicine (Baltimore) 1980; 59:34–49.

Neiderau C, Fischer R, Sonnenberg A, et al. Survival and causes of death in cirrhotic and non-cirrhotic patients with primary hemochromatosis. N Engl J Med 1985; 313:1256–1262.

Slaker DP, Bonkovsky HL. Hemochromatosis—the forgotten disease. Emory J Medicine 1988; 2:177–191.

PRIMARY HEPATIC NEOPLASM

SEYMOUR I. SCHWARTZ, M.D.

Benign and malignant neoplasms develop within the hepatic parenchyma. Benign lesions are relatively common, and both benign and malignant lesions are diagnosed with increasing frequency because of the liberal use of imaging procedures.

BENIGN TUMORS

Hamartoma

Mesenchymal hamartoma of the liver is a rare benign tumor that usually presents in children before the age of 2 as an abdominal mass. The lesion is characterized by a mixture of ductal structures in a copious, loose, connective tissue stroma and has a tendency to undergo cystic degeneration. Many of the lesions are pedunculated or superficial and encapsulated; these are easily removed. Asymptomatic lesions located deep within the parenchyma should be left alone because they do not grow rapidly or undergo malignant transformation. If the tumor is adherent to the inferior vena cava it can be treated by partial excision and marsupialization. Radiotherapy often reduces the size of large lesions by hyalinization of the mesenchymal components. Reduction in size should be followed by resection.

Hemangioma

Hemangioma is the most common benign tumor of the liver and the liver is the visceral organ most frequently affected by this lesion. In the adult age group, most patients are women and most lesions are smaller than 5 cm and are asymptomatic. The diagnosis can be established by computed tomography (CT), preferably with intravenous contrast material, technetium 99m sulfur colloid scan, ultrasonography (US), or T2 phase of magnetic resonance imaging. Percutaneous needle biopsy is hazardous because of the danger of hemorrhage.

Infants with hemangioma frequently present with an abdominal mass and high output congestive heart failure. In these infants, a variety of treatments has been successful. Some children have been managed expectantly and spontaneous regression of symptoms has been documented. Steroids have resulted in resolution of extensive nonresectable tumors. A regimen of digitalis and 350 Gy has resulted in dramatic reduction of size and rapid reversal of cardiac failure. Hepatic artery ligation and also hepatic resection have been effective.

Most hemangiomas in adults should not be removed. Lesions smaller than 5 cm in diameter rarely grow significantly. Pregnant women with small tumors should be followed with serial US, and although an occasional significant increase in size has been noted, this is uncommon. In adults, the indications for surgical excision are a palpable mass in an area potentially subject to trauma, rapid growth of the hemangioma, platelet trapping causing thrombocytopenia, and rupture. Intraperitoneal bleeding is extremely rare and the potential for rupture does not constitute an indication for surgery. The relation of the tumor to female sex hormones has not been resolved. It is generally believed that the presence of a small hemangioma does not preclude pregnancy and that estrogen replacement therapy can be used. An alternative to estrogen or progesterone should be advised for contraception.

Surgical excision is the treatment for clinically-significant hemangiomas. Resection of the tumor with minimal hepatic parenchyma is the treatment of choice; often even large lesions can be enucleated. Very extensive tumors require anatomic resection. The operative mortality is negligible and postoperative compromise of hepatic function is not anticipated. In the adult, radiation therapy, hepatic arterial ligation, and embolization are rarely effective.

Adenoma

Hepatic adenoma is a benign tumor that was rarely reported before the introduction of oral contraceptives.

More than 60 percent of patients were exposed to mestranol only and 80 percent were exposed to a mestranol product. More than half the patients used the pill continuously for more than 5 years, but lesions have become manifest even years after discontinuation of the drug. The lesions also develop during pregnancy, in patients with diabetes mellitus, glycogen storage disease, and rarely as adenomatosis, which is defined as more than ten adenomas in an otherwise normal liver.

Hepatic adenomas in patients who were contraceptive users tend to be larger and have higher rates of intratumoral and intraperitoneal hemorrhage. Bleeding has also been noted during pregnancy. Transformation into hepatocellular carcinoma has been documented; this occurs more frequently in patients with adenomatosis.

The diagnosis is typically made in women of childbearing age. Eighty percent are symptomatic with pain or mass effect generally related to intratumoral or intraperitoneal bleeding. The latter can cause shock. The hepatic lesion is usually identified by US or CT. At times a small lesion is not detected but the diagnosis is suggested by a subglissonian hematoma. Percutaneous biopsy is contraindicated because it is associated with a high risk of bleeding.

Although regression and disappearance of hepatic adenomas have been reported after the discontinuation of contraceptives, the potential for bleeding and malignant transformation coupled with the current safety of removing the lesions, favors routine resection. Deaths associated with elective resection are rare while an 8 percent mortality is reported for emergency resection. The lesions are readily identified by their pale yellow, homogenous appearance. They often can be removed by enucleation with a narrow rim of normal hepatic parenchyma. Because of the diffuse nature and potential for malignancy, transplantation has been advised for patients with adenomatosis.

Focal Nodular Hyperplasia

Focal nodular hyperplasia (FNH) is generally included among the benign tumors of the liver. FNH might not be a neoplasm or a hamartoma but rather a reaction to injury or to a noxious agent. It has been suggested that FNH is a hyperplastic response to a pre-existing spider-like malformation. There is no consistent relation to oral contraceptives. US and CT frequently fail to define the lesion because it is isodense. The angiogram demonstrates a typical sunburst hypervascular pattern. Most lesions are not suspected until they become apparent at celiotomy.

In order to establish the diagnosis histologically, it is essential to take a deep wedge biopsy to incorporate the characteristic central fibrosis. The remaining lesion is made up of normal hepatocytes with a normal architecture. Resection of large lesions and those in critical locations is rarely indicated because of the risk-benefit ratio. Smaller lesions should be removed because there

is a suggestion that FNH might be a precursor to follicular hepatocellular carcinoma and there is minimal risk from resection.

MALIGNANT TUMORS

Malignant neoplasms include sarcomas, hepatoblastomas, and hepatocellular carcinomas.

Sarcoma

The sarcomas are vascular lesions classified as angiosarcomas; they are extremely rare with an incidence of 0.014 per 100,000 population. Etiologically they have been related to exposure to vinyl chloride, and patients who had angiograms performed with thorium dioxide are at risk, usually manifesting the tumor decades after the procedure was performed. Thrombocytopenia is present in over half the cases and hypercalcemia, due the production of an ectopic parahormone-like substance, is noted in 7 percent of the patients; a situation that also pertains to hepatocellular carcinomas. The angiogram demonstrates a characteristic diffuse increased vascular pattern. Needle biopsy readily establishes the diagnosis and there is no treatment available. Transplantation has been performed with no long-term success; immunosuppression resulted in widespread dissemination of what is usually a localized malignancy. Chemotherapy and radiation therapy have failed to alter the rapid progression to death, usually within months.

Hepatoblastoma

Hepatoblastoma occurs principally in children under age 3 but it has been reported in older children and adults. Unlike hepatocellular carcinoma, there is no association with cirrhosis or chronic hepatitis. There are two types of tumors. The first occurs in infants and children up to the age of 3 years and is characterized by a combination of embryonal liver parenchyma and mesenchyme. The second type occurs in older children and is characterized by increased mitochondria and irregular endoplasmic reticulum.*

In over half the cases, the first clinical evidence is an abdominal mass. Hemihypertrophy is noted in 2 percent of cases and sexual precocity secondary to ectopic gonadotropin production can be present. The alpha-fetoprotein is usually elevated. The treatment is surgical excision followed by chemotherapy using doxorubicin and cisplatin. In one series, 21 of 27 children under 2 years, were alive and well with no evidence of disease for a mean of 53 months. In some children with tumors that were deemed unresectable at celiotomy, chemotherapy and radiation therapy effected reduction in tumor size

---

*Editor's Note: The increased risk for this tumor in patients genetically destined to develop familial adenomatous polyposis was described in an earlier chapter.

allowing resection during a second procedure and at times resulted in permanent cure.

Hepatocellular Carcinoma

The incidence of primary hepatocellular carcinoma varies from less than 1 case per 100,000 in parts of the western world to over 60 per 100,000 in areas of Africa. In the South African Bantus, the tumor is responsible for over 80 percent of all carcinomas. In southeast Asia, autopsy series have reported rates of 2.4 percent. Two to six men are affected for every woman, but the fibrolamellar variant that occurs mainly in young adults has an equal sex distribution.

Almost three quarters of adult cases have an associated cirrhosis or chronic hepatitis. The frequency of cirrhosis in the liver cell group is reported at 89 percent, contrasted with 24 percent for the bile duct group. The question remains unanswered whether hepatitis B and C viruses are direct etiologic factors or whether they act through their ability to produce cirrhosis. Another factor associated with hepatocellular carcinoma is aberrant alpha 1-antitrypsin-pi Z. In areas in which the incidence reaches endemic proportions, screening with US has detected lesions 2 cm and smaller in diameter which were removed; cures resulted.

Among the major problems in diagnosis is the differentiation between clinical manifestations attributable to cirrhosis and those related to the development of superimposed hepatic carcinoma. A rapid increase in symptoms and signs associated with cirrhosis is suggestive of tumor. The sudden onset of acute abdominal pain is often related to intraperitoneal rupture or intraparenchymal bleeding. It should be remembered that the sudden amelioration of diabetes and hypoglycemic episodes also is suggestive of neoplastic change. CT defines the space-occupying lesions and angiography demonstrates the characteristic hypervascularity.

The only potentially curative treatment for primary hepatocellular carcinoma or intrahepatic cholangiocarcinoma is surgical excision. Certain criteria must be met before resection is performed. The carcinoma should be localized to a resectable portion of the liver so that an adequate amount of functional hepatic parenchyma remains. The minimum is 20 percent of hepatic mass. There must be no evident lymph node, blood vessel, or extrahepatic bile duct involvement and the presence of distal metastases should be ruled out.

In order to make these assessments preoperatively and thereby obviate a nonproductive celiotomy, selective arterial infusion CT and angiography have been used. The catheter is initially positioned in the hepatic artery or arteries and during infusion of dye, the CT is carried out, lighting up the tumor. The catheter is then positioned in the superior mesenteric artery, and during the venous phase of infusion, CT is repeated. This demonstrates the tumor as a radiolucency. Intraoperative US is particularly helpful in defining resectability by determining the relation of the tumor to the major hepatic veins and the inferior vena cava.

Resection of liver tumors superimposed on cirrhosis is compromised by the increased vascularity of the liver and attendant increased operative morbidity and inability of the remaining liver to regenerate. It is my contention that resection of a lobe or trisegmentectomy is not feasible in a cirrhotic patient with significant ascites, hypoalbuminemia, or coagulation abnormalities. With the exception of fibrolamellar carcinomas, orthotopic liver transplantation results have been discouraging in patients with hepatic malignancies. Almost all patients have demonstrated recurrence or metastases within a year.

Several Asian studies have reported 5 year survivals of 35 percent after subsegmental resection or segmentectomy of tumors smaller than 5 cm in diameter in cirrhotic livers. Primary hepatic tumors of that size are rarely encountered in the western experience and cures following resections are extremely rare. In the Mayo Clinic experience, the 5 year survival after curative resection of a primary hepatic malignancy was 27 percent. Cholangiocarcinoma, nodal metastases, cirrhosis, hypocalcemia, and increased alkaline phosphatase and prolonged prothrombin time were associated with decreased survival. In some cases, patients with fibrolamellar carcinoma had significantly better survival. In the Pittsburgh series, the 5 year survival was 32 percent; similar survival rates were achieved with partial hepatic resection and total hepatectomy with orthotopic transplantation. In children with hepatocellular carcinoma, the alpha fetoprotein is almost always elevated. The prognosis following resection and/or chemotherapy and radiation therapy is extremely poor.

HEPATIC RESECTION

The management of benign and malignant neoplasms of the liver is based on hepatic resection. Removal of up to 80 percent of the liver is compatible with life, but current appreciation of the functional division into eight segments has resulted in the use of segmentectomy and bisegmentectomy rather than lobectomy on many occasions. In patients undergoing lobectomy for tumors, postoperative hepatic function is largely dependent on the extent of compensation that has occurred preoperatively. Patients generally maintain normal prothrombin times, fibrinogen production, and ammonia levels. With major resection, transient elevation of the serum bilirubin is often noted. Clinical jaundice is a transient phenomenon. The most profound change after lobectomy or trisegmentectomy is hypoalbuminemia that usually corrects by the third week.

After extensive resections, infusion of 10 percent glucose postoperatively is indicated to obviate severe hypoglycemia. Albumin 25 to 50 g should be administered daily to maintain the serum level above 3 g per liter. Usually a second generation cephalosporin is administered intraoperatively and continued for 3 days. Analgesics and hypnotics that are detoxified by the liver should be used sparingly.

ADJUVANT THERAPY

In general, primary hepatic malignancies have not responded to radiation therapy or intravenous chemotherapy. Dramatic temporary reduction in tumor size has been achieved in some patients treated with intra-arterial infusion of chemotherapeutic agents. A catheter is positioned in the hepatic artery; infusion uses a pump implanted in the subcutaneous tissue of the abdominal wall. This allows daily infusion of the drugs at a rate of 0.3 mg per kilogram in 2 week cycles alternating with saline and percutaneous refilling of the pump. The response has been variable and the toxicity has been equivalent to intravenous therapy. In addition, the complication of chemically-induced sclerosing cholangitis has been reported.

SUGGESTED READING

Brady MS, Coit DG. Focal nodular hyperplasia of the liver. Surg Gynecol Obstet 1990; 171:377–381.
DeMaioribus CA, Lally KP, et al. Mesenchymal hamartoma of the liver: A 35-year review. Arch Surg 1990; 125:598–600.
Gutierrez O, Schwartz SI. Diagnostic atlas of hepatic lesions. New York: McGraw-Hill, 1984.
Huguet C, Bona S, et al. Repeat hepatic resection for primary and metastatic carcinoma of the liver. Surg Gynecol Obstet 1990; 171:398–402.
Iwatsuki S, Starzl TE, et al. Hepatic resection versus transplantation for hepatocellular carcinoma. Ann Surg 1991; 214:221–229.
Kanematsu T, Takendaka K, et al. Limited hepatic resection effective for selected cirrhotic patients with primary liver cancer. Ann Surg 1984; 199:51–56.
King DR, Ortega J, et al. The surgical management of children with incompletely resected hepatic cancer is facilitated by intensive chemotherapy. J Pediatr Surg 1991; 26:1074–1081.
Leese T, Farges O, Bismuth H. Liver cell adenomas: A 12-year surgical experience from a specialist hepato-biliary unit. Ann Surg 1988; 208:558–564.
Moazam F, Rodgers BM, et al. Hepatic artery ligation for hepatic hemangiomatosis of infancy. J Pediatr Surg 1983; 18:120–123.
Nagasue N, Yukaya H, et al. Clinical experiences with 118 hepatic resections for hepatocellular carcinoma. Surgery 1986; 99:694–702.
Nagorney DM, Adson MA, et al. Fibrolamellar hepatoma. Am J Surg 1985; 149:113–119.
Nagorney DM, van Heerden JA, et al. Primary hepatic malignancy: Surgical management and determinants of survival. Surgery 1989; 106:740–749.
Ni YH, Chang MH, et al. Hepatocellular carcinoma in childhood: Clinical manifestations and prognosis. Cancer 1991; 68:1737–1741.
Paquet KJ, Koussouris P, et al. Limited hepatic resection for selected cirrhotic patients with hepatocellular or cholangiocellular carcinoma: a prospective study. Br J Surg 1991; 78:459–462.
Shortell CK, Schwartz SI: Hepatic adenoma and focal nodular hyperplasia. Surg Gynecol Obstet 1991; 173:426–431.
Schwartz SI, Husser WC. Cavernous hemangioma of the liver. Ann Surg 1987; 205:456–465.
Stanley P, Geer GD, et al. Infantile hepatic hemangiomas: clinical features, radiologic investigations, and treatment of 20 patients. Cancer 1989; 64:936–949.

METASTATIC CANCER OF THE LIVER

PAUL H. SUGARBAKER, M.D.

Most gastrointestinal cancers present in an advanced stage. To improve survival, one may attempt to prevent the disease or to bring about its early detection. Although these strategies should be more widely used, for various political and economic reasons, they have not been effective. Another strategy by which to improve the survival with intra-abdominal cancer is to successfully treat metastatic disease. For primary colorectal cancer, early disease is curable in most patients with a simple surgical procedure. Metastatic disease to the liver presents a major challenge to achieve a long-term survival.

NATURAL HISTORY OF COLORECTAL METASTASES TO THE LIVER

The concept of step-wise dissemination of colorectal cancer provides the biologic rationale for the surgical removal of hepatic metastases. There are vascular and lymphatic networks that temporarily interrupt cancer dissemination as a systemic process. The filtration systems that develop metastatic cancer and yet can be made surgically disease-free with curative intent are the adjacent lymphatics, liver parenchyma, and lung parenchyma. Also, a curative approach to peritoneal implantation has been described. In patients who are treated relatively early in the natural history of large bowel cancer, recurrent cancer is more likely to show first recurrence at a single anatomic site. Therefore, reoperative surgery is more likely to be successful. Hughes and co-workers reported a 35 percent 5 year survival rate in liver resection for Dukes stage B cancer and a 28 percent survival rate for Dukes stage C cancer. This phenomenon of isolated sites of local-regional disease progression can occur only if all malignant tissues are removed with negative margins of excision (surgical complete response). This concept of cancer dissemination necessitates a redefinition of the reasonable surgical limit of resection for advanced primary and recurrent large bowel cancer.

An important feature of cancer surgery for metastatic disease involves the surgeon's ability to definitively locally control the primary cancer. The ability to gain control of the primary cancer distinguishes large bowel cancer from other gastrointestinal malignancies such as gastric cancer, pancreatic cancer, and visceral sarcoma. Only with local control can the surgical benefits of the removal of metastatic disease result in long-term survival.

Also, successful liver surgery for metastatic disease demands selection of patients who have no other sites of metastatic disease. Lung metastases, retroperitoneal lymph node metastases, hepatic lymph node metastases and peritoneal seeding must be meticulously ruled out before liver resection is initiated.

Third, successful liver resection for metastatic disease requires complete extirpation of cancer from the liver. Survival of patients with nonradical liver resections will be the same as if no cancer removal occurred.

Although the metastatic process from primary colorectal cancer to liver occurs by way of the portal vein, the blood supply to hepatic tumors is arterial. The transition from portal venous to hepatic arterial supply occurs early in the progression of the metastases. Even tumors 1 cm or less in diameter are nourished by hepatic arterial blood. For this reason, if one wants to infuse cytotoxic agents into liver tumors, the hepatic artery has been the most frequently used route of drug delivery and may prolong life in carefully selected patients.

NONCOLORECTAL LIVER METASTASES

From a tumor biology perspective, the only cancers that can be resected for cure are those whose primary site is anatomically located within the hepatic portal system. These cancers invade host tissues, gain access to venules (venous invasion), and then implant and grow within the hepatic portal system. Metastases that gain access to the hepatic parenchyma through the portal system are theoretically treatable for cure, if they can be detected and eradicated completely. Rarely should one attempt the resection of liver metastases that result from primary tumors outside the portal system.

SURGICAL ANATOMY OF THE LIVER

The liver is a large parenchymal structure secured by the evolutionary process beneath the right rib cage so that it is not injured by vigorous exercise or extensive abdominal or chest trauma. This makes it surgically difficult to approach. However through large abdominal incisions and the use of self-retaining retractors, the surfaces of the liver can be inspected in their totality and the parenchyma bimanually palpated. The external markings on the liver are helpful in attempting to define its internal anatomy and the position of tumors. The falciform ligament defines the left hepatic plane. An imaginary line between the inferior vena cava and the gallbladder (Cantlie's line) defines the middle plane. A deep fissure on the posterior surface of the liver defines the caudate body on the left; the caudate process on the right is less clearly defined.

Lymphatics

The liver is richly supplied by lymphatics. Most of the lymph flow is retrograde along the portahepatis toward the hepatic and then the celiac lymph nodes (Fig. 1). Metastases from the liver typically are seen within the hepatic lymph nodes. Lymph flow does occur along the right triangular ligament, left triangular ligament, and falciform ligaments up into the mediastinum. Isolated tumor deposits within the mediastinal lymph nodes from liver metastases have been observed. A final lymphatic channel from the liver is along the hepatogastric ligament to periesophageal lymph nodes. Before a hepatic tumor is removed, it is important to examine the lymph nodes that receive drainage from the liver. Patients with lymphatic metastases from hepatic metastases do not show long-term survival after hepatic resection.

Within the liver itself there is a rich lymphatic plexus; nearly 25 percent of lymph flow in the thoracic duct is from the liver. The lymph plexus contains no

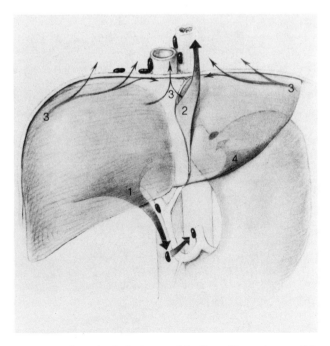

Figure 1 Lymphatic drainage of the liver (From August CA, et al. Lymphatic dissemination of hepatic metastases. Cancer 1985; 55:1490–1494; with permission.)

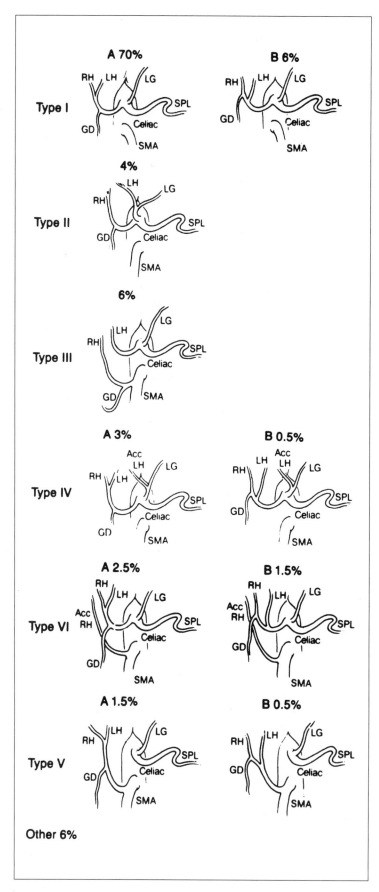

Figure 2 Variations of the extrahepatic arterial anatomy of the liver. (From Daly JM, et al: Longterm hepatic arterial infusion chemotherapy. Arch Surg 1984; 119:936–941; with permission.)

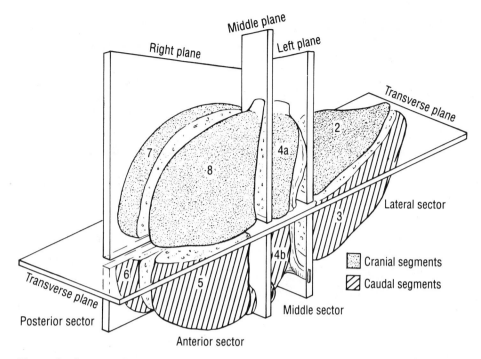

Figure 3 Segmental anatomy of the liver defined by the portal system and major hepatic veins. (From Sugarbaker PH. Surgical management of primary and metastatic cancer of the liver. In: Schiff L, Schiff ER, 7th ed. Diseases of the liver. Philadelphia: JB Lippincott, 1993:1303; with permission.)

valves. Tumor emboli may move within the liver parenchyma along lymphatic channels. With metastatic liver tumors, this results in satellitosis. Satellitosis seldom, if ever, is seen with small liver tumors. It indicates a relative metastatic efficiency of liver tumors and is associated with a poor prognosis.

Vascular Anatomy

The variations in the extrahepatic arterial anatomy are shown in Figure 2. Type I anatomy occurs in about 70 percent of people. It presents the ideal situation for hepatic arterial infusion through side-branch cannulation. This allows continuous infusion of the common hepatic artery by way of a catheter inserted through the gastroduodenal artery. There is a profuse and rapid hepatic arterial collateralization if all or some of the hepatic artery is ligated. Therefore, if an accessory right or accessory left artery exists and one wants to perform hepatic arterial infusion, the accessory branch is ligated.

In the normal adult, about two-thirds of the liver's blood supply comes from the portal vein. The hepatic artery of a normal liver can be ligated with only transient liver function abnormalities. The major portal pedicles bifurcate to the right and left as they enter the base of the liver. They define the transverse plane. This important anatomic landmark cuts the liver in a skewed manner transversely and equally divides the liver into cranial and caudal segments (Fig. 3). The transverse plane is perpendicular to the portal vein on a tangent through the right and left portal pedicles.

The right and middle hepatic veins define their respective vertical planes. The left plane is defined by the origin of the left hepatic vein cranially and by the left paramedian branch of the portal vein caudally. Externally, it is approximated by the falciform ligament. These vertical planes define the posterior, anterior, medial, and lateral sectors. Each sector is cut by the transverse plane to define eight of the nine liver segments.

The caudate segment (perhaps more accurately referred to as the caudate sector or sector 1) is located above the transverse plane within the cranial half of the liver. It occupies the space between the middle hepatic vein superiorly and the bifurcation of the right and left portal pedicles inferiorly. A prominent fissure to the left of the portal vein distinguishes the caudate sector from its direct relation to liver segment 4. The hepatogastric ligament arises from this fissure and the fissure may be referred to as the hepatogastric fissure. A less prominent fissure to the right of the portal vein distinguishes the caudate process from liver segment 7 (1 to 7 fissure).

RADIOLOGIC LIVER IMAGES

New radiologic techniques have allowed precise anatomic descriptions of the liver in vivo. In the United States, the computed tomographic portogram (CTP) has been the most useful test in this regard. Figure 4 shows a CTP through the midportion of the cranial liver segments. The smooth walls of the left, middle, and right

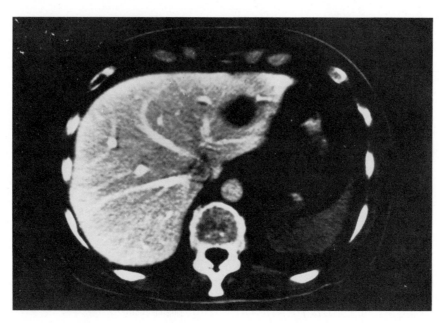

Figure 4 Computed tomographic portography of the liver. (From Sugarbaker PH. Surgical management of primary and metastatic cancer of the liver. In: Schiff L, Schiff ER, 7th ed. Diseases of the liver. Philadelphia: JB Lippincott, 1993:1303; with permission.)

hepatic veins are prominent. They enter into the superior vena cava as the liver is cut by the plane of the computed tomogram (CT). The spiculated appearance of the portal segmental branches to segment 8 are well defined. The segment 8 portal blood supply is almost always composed to twin vessels oriented anteroposterior to each other. Small portal segmental veins to liver segments 7 and 4 are also imaged. By clearly defining the vascular anatomy of the liver, the CTP enables the surgeon to precisely relate liver tumors to the portal and hepatic venous vasculature and has become the standard radiologic study by which to define hepatic tumors preoperatively.

Intraoperative ultrasound has been reported to be of benefit in the evaluation of liver tumors at the time of a surgical procedure. This new technology can identify liver tumors located deep within the liver parenchyma. Also, it can define the anatomic relation of liver tumors to portal structures and to major branches of the hepatic veins. Along with the external anatomy of the liver, intraoperative ultrasonography allows the surgeon to define the segmental anatomy of the liver. This may facilitate the planning of a resection, especially if the adequacy of the surgical margins are in question.

The CT portogram is the most accurate test to define the total number and anatomic position of liver tumors. Yet, magnetic resonance imaging and intraoperative ultrasonography provide some additional information. All three of these modern radiologic techniques need to be available on request to the surgeon if any optimal surgical event is desired because each provides useful information in selected patients.

PATIENT SELECTION

Patients with isolated hepatic metastases represent a subset of primary colorectal cancer patients. Patients with resectable metastases may constitute only 10 percent to 20 percent of the entire population with large bowel cancer. The major determinant of prognosis is the complete resection of the cancer. To separate patients with curative surgical options from those who will receive palliative or no treatment, the groups usually are divided into those with one to four liver metastases and those with five or more metastases. In unresectable patients who have chemotherapy as an option, the duration of survival depends, in large part, on the volume of intrahepatic tumor, the performance status of the patient, and the response to intra-arterial chemotherapy.

For patients with resectable disease, the clinical features with prognostic importance include the following:

1. Number of metastases (1 to 3 versus 4 or more)
2. Margin of resection (negative vs positive)
3. Lymph node status of the primary tumor (Dukes B versus Dukes C)
4. Preresection carcinoembryonic antigen (<5 versus ≥5)
5. Time interval from primary resection until diagnosis of the hepatic metastases (>1 year versus ≤1 year)

These clinical features constitute independent prognostic information, yet they provide data that only relatively contraindicate surgery and seldom, if ever, rule out liver resection. A useful approach to patient selection is to identify patients who have absolute contraindications to resection. These include patients with uncontrolled disease at another site, patients with hepatic lymph nodes positive for cancer, and patients with more than four metastases.

Excluding Extrahepatic Disease

In operating on a patient with liver tumors, even before one contemplates the liver resection, one must rule out disease at other sites. Exclusion of patients with extrahepatic disease from resection constitutes the most powerful means whereby one can improve the results of surgery. Patient selection is accomplished preoperatively through a meticulous radiologic evaluation. A CT scan of chest, abdomen, and pelvis is mandatory. Also, a second primary cancer or recurrent disease within the colorectum must be ruled out. This requires a complete colonoscopy or barium enema.

At the time of surgery, a complete intra-abdominal exploration is necessary before liver dissection begins. Despite a negative preoperative physical and radiologic evaluation, nearly 30 percent of patients at laparotomy have extrahepatic disease. The most common site is hepatic and celiac lymph nodes. The second most common site to find disease intraoperatively is peritoneal surfaces or the omentum. Patients who have liver resections with disease left behind within the liver or at other anatomic sites within the abdominal cavity do not profit from the liver resection.

TECHNICAL ASPECTS OF LIVER RESECTION

Parenchymal Transection Techniques

Numerous techniques have been used to minimize blood loss while transecting liver parenchyma. Early on, the finger fracture technique was used. This technique is still used for major resections with acceptable results at many institutions. It does not lend itself, however, to parenchyma-sparing procedures, such as metastasectomy or segmental resections. In these instances, a narrow margin of resection is necessary and the liver fracture may extend into the tumor itself, causing the dissemination of tumor cells within the liver or within the abdominal cavity. Tumor spill results in high incidence of local recurrence and must be avoided.

A second widely used technique is the suction dissection method. This was first described by Foster and has been refined by Sugarbaker. Ultrasonic dissectors have recently been shown to be of value in that they allow precise anatomic dissections of liver segments. Also, they minimize blood loss. Using these techniques, branches of the hepatic veins crossing the liver planes can be isolated, ligated, and then divided, thereby preventing the hemorrhage formerly thought to be an inevitable part of liver surgery. Other parenchymal transection techniques that have been described include electrocautery, microwave coagulation, yttrium aluminum garnet (YAG) laser, and water-pick.

The major resections performed in liver surgery are shown in Figure 5. They include the right lobe resection, right trisectorectomy, left lobe resection, left trisectorectomy, left lateral sectorectomy (polysegmentectomy 2 and 3), transverse hepatectomies (polysegmentectomy 4a, 7, and 8 or 4b, 5, and 6), and mesohepatectomy (polysegmentectomy 4a, 4b, 5, and 8).

In planning a major liver resection, one must determine the relation of the tumor mass to the caudate segment (segment 1). This should be done by CTP obtained preoperatively. Involvement of the caudate segment may be difficult to determine from intraoperative inspection of the liver tumor. Figure 6 shows the importance of caudate lobe anatomy in liver resections. The position of the caudate lobe with respect to the portal vein is variable. The caudate lobe may be spared in many right and left lobe resections. This facilitates the dissection and conserves liver parenchyma. An extended right hepatectomy usually is well tolerated if liver segments 1, 2, and 3 remain intact after liver resection. If only segments 2 and 3 remain (true right trisectorectomy), the vascularity of the left hepatic duct may be compromised and the remaining parenchyma may be inadequate to sustain life in the postoperative period.

If the caudate segment is to be removed in a right or left lobe resection, then its venous drainage must be secured before beginning parenchymal transection. As shown in Figure 7, the caudate veins are isolated, ligated in continuity, and then divided along the vena cava. This allows the caudate lobe to be elevated off of the surface of the inferior vena cava. This avoids excessive blood loss that may occur if one attempts to secure these veins from within the liver parenchyma.

An important maneuver often used if hemorrhage occurs at any time during liver transection is the Pringle maneuver. This involves inflow occlusion of the hepatic artery and portal vein. In performing a right or left lobectomy, we prefer to use selective occlusion of the appropriate hepatic artery and portal vein before initiating parenchymal transection. A Romel tourniquet is placed around the appropriate vessel. The division of major vessels outside the liver is an unnecessary and time-consuming part of the procedure. It is unnecessary to secure the right or left hepatic duct before parenchymal transection.

To minimize tumor embolization into the lungs that may occur with liver trauma during resection, preliminary division of the relevant hepatic veins is performed before initiating parenchymal transection. Small, stiff vascular clamps are placed across the hepatic veins outside the liver. The vessels are secured proximally and distally with a running suture. If the hepatic veins are approached from beneath the liver after division of the caudate lobe veins, one can safely skeletonize about 1 cm of hepatic vein in nearly all patients. In addition to preventing intravascular tumor dissemination with manipulation of the cancer during resection, preliminary

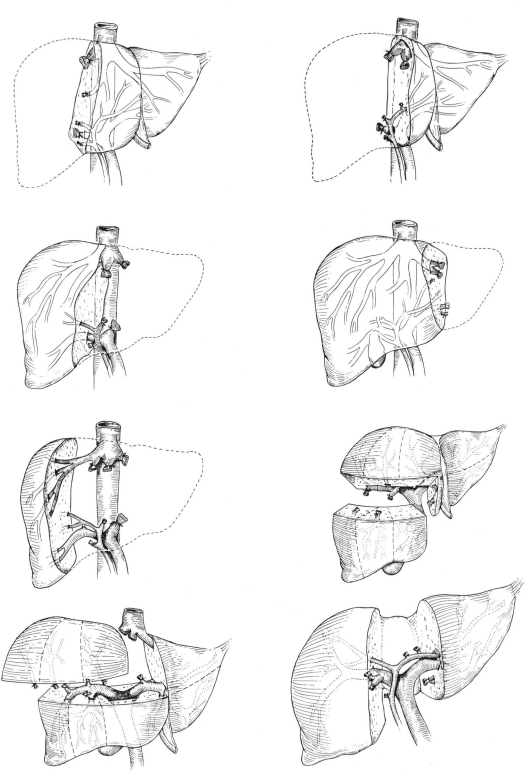

Figure 5 Major liver resections utilize planes between the liver segments defined by the portal vein. Major hepatic veins that cross these boundaries are isolated, ligated, and then divided as parenchymal transection proceeds. *A,* Right lobe resection. *B,* Right trisectorectomy. *C,* Left lobe resection. *D,* Lateral sectorectomy. *E,* Left trisectorectomy. *F,* Transverse hepatectomy—polysegmentectomy 4b, 5, 6. *G,* Transverse hepatectomy—polysegmentectomy 4a, 7, 8. *H,* Mesohepatectomy. (From Sugarbaker PH. Surgical management of primary and metastatic cancer of the liver. In: Schiff L, Schiff ER, 7th ed. Diseases of the liver. Philadelphia: JB Lippincott, 1993:1309–1310; with permission.)

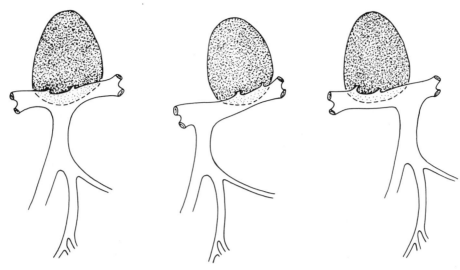

Figure 6 Variable position of the caudate lobe in relation to the portal vein. (From Couinaud C. Principes directeurs des hepatectomies reglees. Chirurgie 1980; 106:8–10; with permission.)

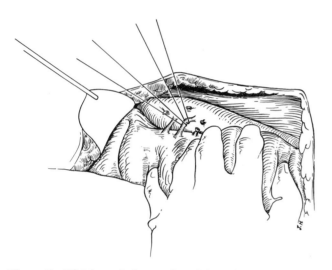

Figure 7 Division of the caudate lobe veins prior to the initiating parenchymal transection is necessary in procedures that require removal of the right or left portion of the caudate sector. (From Sugarbaker PH. Left hepatectomy. In: Daly JM, Cady B, eds. Atlas of Surgical Oncology. St. Louis: Mosby–Year Book, 1993:361–368; with permission.)

division of the hepatic veins adds greatly to the mobility of the portion of the liver to be resected. If one places the tissue being transected on strong traction, identification of vascular structures within the liver is greatly facilitated and the time required for parenchymal transection is greatly reduced.

Segmental Resections

Rarely, if ever, are deep transections of liver parenchyma performed that cross intersegmental planes. Although small tumors near the liver surface are

removed by metastastectomy procedures (wedge resections), a tumor more than 3 cm in diameter is removed as a segmentectomy procedure. As many different segmentectomies have been performed as there are conceivable combinations. Segmental resections on the caudal liver segments (4b, 5, or 6) are easily performed and associated with minimal blood loss. Resections of cranial liver segments (4a, 7, or 8) are considerably more difficult and require amputation of the relevant hepatic vein close to the vena cava. In performing these segmental resections, one does not transect any portal structures until most of the parenchymal transection has been completed. This surgery can be conceptualized as hepatic vein surgery. As one appreciates by direct vision the relevant portal segmental structures as they arise from the major right or left portal pedicles, the segmental vein, artery, and bile duct are ligated, sutured, ligated, and then transected.

Cytoreductive Approach to Liver Tumors

Combining intra-arterial chemotherapy with surgical or radiotherapeutic cytoreductions of intrahepatic tumor deposits is a new approach to regional dose intensity for colorectal metastases to the liver. New strategies for control of liver tumors have recently been described whereby numerous tumor nodules with the liver are resected or in some other way devitalized. Cytoreduction implies complete devitalization of all visible tumor within the liver. To achieve complete liver cytoreduction, one often may use several cytoreductive techniques in the same liver. Surgical, radiotherapy or cryosurgical techniques are not competitive but complementary, in that together they may devitalize all tumor nodules with the liver.

Either before or after complete cytoreduction of liver tumor, intra-arterial chemotherapy is initiated. This treatment is an attempt to prevent the outgrowth of undetected foci that usually are present in the liver in patients with multiple liver metastases. Also, systemic chemotherapy is given because it may be of some benefit in suppressing the progression of disseminated disease.

Intra-Arterial Chemotherapy

Because the liver has a solitary arterial blood supply and the hepatocyte has such marked resistance to chemotherapy toxicities, direct intra-arterial administration of chemotherapy frequently has been used. The high response rates seen with regional drug delivery come about because of two pharmacologic principles. First, there is a first-pass effect that results from increased concentration which is inversely proportional to the fraction of total blood flow through the artery that has been cannulated. Second, many drugs have a first-pass effect because of drug metabolism. These chemotherapeutic agents are metabolized at least in part by a single pass through the liver (such as floxuridine [FUDR] or fluorouracil [5-FU]). Systemic toxicities are greatly reduced, so that a markedly increased total dose of regional drug instillation is possible. If adverse effects occur, the toxicities may be first expressed within the liver itself and usually by the biliary tree. The ductal structures do not have the capability to metabolize drug or to replicate as do hepatocytes. Therefore, without special monitoring, the biliary tree may be severely damaged by the intra-arterial administration of drugs such as FUDR.

The goal in intra-arterial infusion chemotherapy is to change the natural history of colorectal hepatic metastases by helping to control intrahepatic disease. There have been four major problems with intra-arterial chemotherapy treatments in the past. First, agents such as FUDR that were metabolized by a single pass through the liver were used. These agents manifested little or no systemic toxicities. This approach resulted in extensive complications within the biliary tree. Second, the absence of effective systemic treatment resulted in a higher likelihood for development of disseminated disease. Third, clinicians often failed to meticulously rule out extrahepatic disease, especially with anatomic sites difficult to image by radiologic tests. Hepatic lymph nodes and peritoneal surfaces are involved in a significant proportion of patients. Only surgical exploration with careful inspection of the entire abdominal cavity and biopsy of suspicious lesions can rule out the presence of extrahepatic disease. Fourth, substantial regressions of intrahepatic tumors were not consolidated through the use of other multidisciplinary treatments that could be added onto the chemotherapy. Dose-intensive treatments used to augment intra-arterial chemotherapy include cytoreduction by surgery or by radiation therapy. If consolidation treatments are not used, drug resistance occurs within several months. Because of the Gompertzian nature of tumor growth, little benefit, in terms of prolonged survival, resulted.

ENTIRE HEPATIC FROM CELIAC

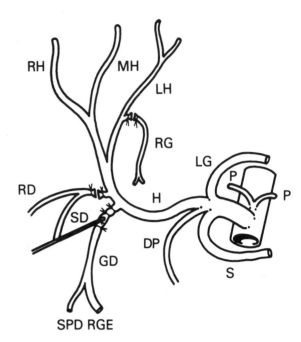

Figure 8 Hepatic artery cannulation through the gastroduodenal artery. RH = right hepatic; MH = middle hepatic; LH = left hepatic; RG = right gastric; LG = left gastric; H = hepatic; RD = right duoden; SD = superior duodenal; GD = gastroduodenal; SPD = superior pancreatic duodenal; RGE = right gastroepiploic; P = phrenic; S = splenic; CE = celiac; ReLH = replaced left hepatic; CE = cardioesophageal; AcLH = accessory left hepatic; AcLG = accessory left gastric. (Modified from Sugarbaker PH, Schneider PD. Technique of hepatic infusion chemotherapy. In: Velde C van de, Sugarbaker PH (eds). Liver Metastases. Boston: Martinus Nijhoff, 1984:339–345; with permission.)

Technical Aspects of Hepatic Artery Catheterization

Figure 8 shows the technical aspects of hepatic artery cannulation. If only three to four monthly cycles of intra-arterial chemotherapy are contemplated, a port catheter system is adequate. If multiple cycles over many months are planned, a continuous infusion pump may be preferable. The Infusaid pump maintains patency of the hepatic artery in many patients for years. The continuous administration of heparin at the tip of the catheter prevents platelet thrombi and the eventual arterial thrombosis observed with other catheter systems.

TREATMENT RESULTS

Surgical Resection

The results of surgery for colorectal metastases isolated to the liver are shown in Figure 9. Overall survival at 5 years approaches 30 percent. These results

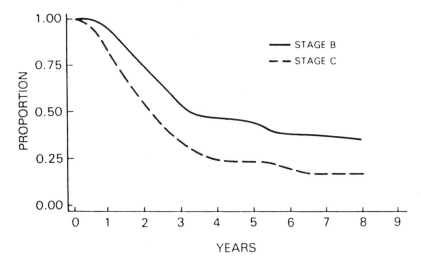

Figure 9 Survival after resection of isolated colorectal liver metastases. (Modified from Hughes KS, et al. Surgery for metastatic colorectal cancer to the liver: optimizing the results of treatment. Surg Clin North Am 1989; 69:339–359; with permission.)

continue to improve with time as clinicians gain expertise in eliminating occult distant metastases in this group of patients. Although liver transplantation has been attempted in liver metastases patients, no favorable long-term results have been reported.

Long-term survival after surgical treatment is limited to patients whose primary tumors occur within the hepatic portal system.

Intra-Arterial Chemotherapy

In the protocols using intra-arterial FUDR in which survival was an endpoint, significant prolongation in survival was documented in the patients with no extrahepatic disease. As the cytoreductive approach is tested in clinical trials, it is possible that the median survival of these patients will show additional improvement.

Failure Analysis for Patients Treated by Surgery

The hepatic resection effectively controls disease within the liver in about two-thirds of patients. Both liver and lungs together were the most common sites at which recurrent disease was detected. Recently subgroups of patients who had recurrences in liver only have been reported. These patients probably have progression of occult disease in the liver that was metastatic from the primary tumor. These patients do not represent the cascade phenomenon. If the isolated repeat recurrence is detected in the liver, these patients represent a favorable group for long-term control. It is clear that metastatic disease is not a uniformly fatal process with large bowel cancer. Furthermore, recurrence of liver metastases after hepatic resection is not necessarily a lethal process. Careful follow-up may select patients for curative repeat resection in the liver or curative resection of metastases from the lungs.

FOLLOW-UP AFTER LIVER RESECTION

Recommendations for follow-up of these patients includes radiologic assessments of the patients for metastatic disease in addition to liver imaging. Carcinoembryonic antigen assay is the most useful follow-up test and should be performed every 3 months. Follow-up continues for five years.

Editor's Note: This is certainly not the area for therapeutic nihilists. The author has pursued the "holy grail" of curative resection through a variety of scientific and technical advances. We thank him for sharing his views and experience.

SUGGESTED READING

August DA, Ottow RT, Sugarbaker PH. Clinical perspective of human colorectal cancer metastasis. Cancer Metastasis Rev 1984; 3:303–324.

August DA, Sugarbaker PH, Schneider PD. Lymphatic dissemination of hepatic metastases. Cancer 1985; 55:1490–1494.

Couinaud C. Principes directeur des hepatectomies reglees. Chirurgie 1980; 106:8–10.

Daly JM, Kemeny N, Oderman P, Botet J. Long-term hepatic arterial infusion chemotherapy. Arch Surg 1984; 119:936–941.

Foster JH, Berman MM. Solid liver tumors. Philadelphia: WB Saunders, 1977.

Hughes KS, Scheele J, Sugarbaker PH. Surgery for metastatic colorectal cancer to the liver: Optimizing the results of treatment. Surg Clin North Am 1989; 69:339–359.

Sugarbaker PH. Surgical decision-making for large bowel cancer metastatic to the liver. Radiology 1990; 174:621–626.

Sugarbaker PH, Nelson RC, Murray DR, et al. Liver computerized tomography for hepatic resection: A segmental approach. Surg Gynecol Obstet 1990; 171:189–195.

BILIARY TRACT

LAPAROSCOPIC CHOLECYSTECTOMY

KEITH D. LILLEMOE, M.D.

Laparoscopic cholecystectomy has likely influenced abdominal surgery more than any previous surgical procedure. This technique has within a few short years become not only the primary operation for gallbladder disease, but has also led to the development of a new generation of minimally invasive surgical procedures. This development has occurred at an extraordinary pace driven by both unprecedented patient acceptance and industrial technological advances. Yet, this tremendous progress has also led to controversies with respect to management of subgroups of patients with gallstones and concerns with respect to complications, often associated with inadequate training of surgeons anxious to perform laparoscopic procedures.

Approximately 10 to 15 percent of the adult population or more than 20 million people in the United States have gallstones. It is estimated that there are about 1 million newly diagnosed patients annually. In 1991, approximately 600,000 patients underwent cholecystectomy. Gallbladder stones may present in one of three clinical stages: (1) asymptomatic, (2) symptomatic, and (3) with complications. This chapter will focus on the role of laparoscopic cholecystectomy in the treatment of gallstone disease and its complications. Furthermore, the limitations and complications of this technique will be reviewed.

ASYMPTOMATIC GALLSTONES

Most patients with gallstones are asymptomatic. Existing data suggest that 1 percent to 4 percent of asymptomatic patients will develop symptoms per year with most becoming symptomatic in the first 5 years after diagnosis. Almost all patients will experience symptoms before developing a complication of gallstones. The role of cholecystectomy for silent gallstones has been debated for years. The introduction of the "minimally invasive"

laparoscopic cholecystectomy has led some to advocate cholecystectomy for asymptomatic patients. Despite patient acceptance of laparoscopic cholecystectomy, there appears to be no indication for extending the procedure to asymptomatic patients. This includes diabetic patients in whom morbidity and mortality is increased after emergency cholecystectomy for complications. The risk of gallbladder cancer in patients with asymptomatic gallstones is so low that concern for malignancy is not a reasonable justification for cholecystectomy.

SYMPTOMATIC GALLSTONES

In contrast to silent gallstones, patients with symptoms are likely to experience recurrent complaints and are at risk (25 percent within 10 years) to develop complications. Therefore, with few exceptions, patients with symptomatic gallstones should be treated. The alternatives for treatment of gallstones include nonoperative methods such as oral bile salt dissolution, contact dissolution therapy, and extracorporeal shock wave lithotripsy. It is not the focus of this chapter to discuss these therapies, but with exception of significant comorbid conditions precluding general anesthesia, there appears to be no reason to consider these techniques over laparoscopic cholecystectomy. (There is a separate chapter on non-surgical approaches.)

The indications for choosing laparoscopic cholecystectomy over open or traditional cholecystectomy has evolved significantly since its introduction. During the initial "learning curve" for laparoscopic cholecystectomy, increased technical difficulty and concern for a greater risk of complications led many surgeons to develop contraindications, which included patient-related factors such as pregnancy, cirrhosis with or without portal hypertension, coagulopathy, previous abdominal surgery, morbid obesity, and significant operative risks. Disease-related factors considered contraindications for laparoscopic cholecystectomy included acute cholecystitis, jaundice, gallstone pancreatitis, cholangitis, suspected common bile duct stones, known gallbladder cancer, or cholecystoenteric fistula.

As experience has developed, most of these contraindications have been overcome. Laparoscopic cholecystectomy has been reported during pregnancy but it is recommended that operations be limited to the second trimester. Cholecystectomy performed in a patient with cirrhosis with or without portal hypertension is a technical challenge. Increased morbidity, mortality, and operative blood loss can be expected regardless of whether the open or laparoscopic technique is used. In the elective setting an attempt at laparoscopic cholecystectomy is appropriate with the realization that conversion to the open technique may be necessary. Specific limitations which may be encountered include difficulty in retraction of the gallbladder with the hard cirrhotic liver, extensive vascular adhesions to the gallbladder, and oozing from the gallbladder bed. The use of the laparoscopic argon beam coagulator may be useful for the latter problem and also in patients with pre-existing, uncorrectable coagulopathies.

Adhesions from previous upper abdominal operations were originally felt to preclude laparoscopic cholecystectomy. Now with the use of the open approach for placement of the Hasson cannula, a pneumoperitoneum can be safely obtained in virtually all cases. At that point, the skilled laparoscopic surgeon can usually place the remaining trocars and gain access to the right upper quadrant to complete the cholecystectomy. Laparoscopic cholecystectomy in the morbidly obese patient can also be technically difficult; however, the availability of longer cannulas has eliminated this as a contraindication. This group of patients would appear to have significant benefits with the laparoscopic approach. Finally, patients with comorbid medical conditions, representing greater operative risks, were originally considered poor candidates for laparoscopic cholecystectomy due to the initial prolonged operative times and concern for intraoperative or postoperative complications. Certainly for most experienced laparoscopic surgeons, these concerns no longer exist and the laparoscopic approach is viewed as a favorable alternative for such patients. Carbon dioxide used for insufflation of the abdominal cavity may be absorbed resulting in hypercarbia and acidosis, and therefore, close monitoring is necessary in patients with significant chronic obstructive pulmonary disease.

The management of patients with disease-related factors or complications of gallstone disease is discussed later in this chapter. It can be concluded, however, that with appropriate preoperative evaluation and therapy, and a skilled laparoscopic surgeon, there are very few existing contraindications to laparoscopic cholecystectomy. A known gallbladder carcinoma or cholecystoenteric fistula likely are the only current exceptions. An aggressive "all-comer" approach to laparoscopic cholecystectomy is therefore appropriate with two caveats. First, the surgeon must be aware of the limitations of his personal experience and laparoscopic skills. Secondly, any surgeon regardless of his or her experience should not consider conversion to an open cholecystectomy a complication or failure, but rather in most cases, a demonstration of good judgement.

ELECTIVE LAPAROSCOPIC CHOLECYSTECTOMY

Interpretation of the published results for laparoscopic cholecystectomy can be difficult on several counts. First, the early published reports in most cases include the initial learning curve with morbidity and conversion rates higher than what might be expected as individual series grew larger. Many of these "second generation" series are just beginning to appear in the literature and as expected the results have improved. Secondly, most published series have come from the leaders or pioneers in this field and therefore, may not be applicable to the average surgeon performing laparoscopic cholecystectomy. The large number of series of bile duct injuries managed at major medical centers would suggest that these injuries are appearing at an increased rate following laparoscopic cholecystectomy. Finally, and most importantly, it is generally accepted that the rates of conversion to open cholecystectomy and the incidence of complications, specifically bile duct injury, can be directly correlated to the experience of the surgeon. It is the obligation, therefore, of every surgeon performing this procedure to obtain appropriate training and supervision during this "learning curve" period and to maintain an appropriately low threshold to convert a patient to an open cholecystectomy rather than risk complication.

The reported conversion rate for elective laparoscopic cholecystectomy by an experienced surgeon is currently less than 2 percent. Operative findings of inflammation or unclear anatomy remain the leading reasons for conversion. Perioperative mortality is extremely uncommon in reported series, however, this may not reflect the overall status of the procedure outside of reporting centers. The overall complication rates reported are generally less than 5 percent. The incidence of bile duct injury is 0 percent in a number of large series with total number exceeding several thousand. Yet, if one analyzes confidential audit series giving a more accurate view of the practice outside reporting centers, the incidence would appear to be between 0.2 and 0.5 percent. This incidence is better than the initial reports of laparoscopic cholecystectomy but still exceeds the expected incidence following open cholecystectomy. There is also no evidence that routine operative cholangiography will decrease the incidence of bile duct injury.

Postoperative hospital stay is less than 2 days in almost all series, with a number of centers advocating outpatient procedures in selected patients. A return to normal activities, including strenuous labor, in less than 2 weeks can be anticipated for most patients. Postoperative pain and patient satisfaction clearly favor laparoscopic cholecystectomy over traditional cholecystectomy. Although hospital stay and postoperative disability has been shortened by laparoscopic cholecystectomy, there has been no translation of this benefit to reduced hospital costs. This fact can be directly attributed to additional costs of disposable laparoscopic trochars and instruments.

LAPAROSCOPIC CHOLECYSTECTOMY FOR ACUTE CHOLECYSTITIS

Approximately 20 percent of patients requiring cholecystectomy present with acute cholecystitis. Initially these patients were not considered candidates for laparoscopic cholecystectomy, recognizing that the acute inflammation and edema would distort the biliary ductal and vascular anatomy resulting in a higher incidence of major complications. Yet, as experience has been gained, most surgeons no longer consider an acute presentation a contraindication to attempting the laparoscopic approach. It must be emphasized, however, that initiating an attempt at laparoscopic cholecystectomy does not mandate that the operation be completed by the same technique.

The preoperative discussions with the patient should clearly state that acute cholecystitis increases the technical difficulty of laparoscopic cholecystectomy and therefore, the conversion rate. It should be emphasized that conversion does not represent a complication, but rather, in the judgement of the surgeon, a step to minimize operative complications. With this attitude by both the surgeon and the patient, laparoscopic cholecystectomy can be successfully completed in most patients with acute cholecystitis without a significantly increased rate of major complications.

The patient presenting with typical symptoms and signs of acute cholecystitis (right upper quadrant pain and tenderness, fever, and leukocytosis) should be maintained NPO, receive intravenous rehydration, and be started on broad-spectrum intravenous antibiotics. It has been recognized for decades that a "golden period" of approximately 7 days exists for performing open cholecystectomy in the face of acute cholecystitis. Although no objective data exists, most laparoscopic surgeons favor early intervention, within 48 hours, to maximize the chances of successful laparoscopic cholecystectomy for acute cholecystitis. (See also the subsequent chapter on acute cholecystitis.)

The operative technique in cases of acute cholecystitis varies little from standard laparoscopic cholecystectomy. It is not uncommon that an additional trochar is necessary to aid in retraction of the gallbladder. A common intraoperative occurrence is a tear in the gallbladder wall allowing the spillage of purulent bile and/or stones. Efforts should be made to control spillage, retrieve dropped stones, and irrigate the abdomen copiously with antibiotic solution to minimize the effect of peritoneal contamination. Bile and stone spillage, however, should not be the sole reason to convert to an open cholecystectomy. Although late abscesses have been reported, in general, such spillage is seldom of consequence. A closed suction drain can be placed through a lateral 5 mm trochar site if necessary.

The postoperative recovery in many patients undergoing laparoscopic cholecystectomy for acute cholecystitis is often not dissimilar from an elective procedure. In most patients, postoperative abdominal pain is minimal and the patient can resume liquid diet shortly after surgery. Intravenous antibiotics should be continued postoperatively for a minimum of 48 hours or until the patient is afebrile and the white blood cell count returns to normal. Oral antibiotics are usually continued for 5 to 7 days after hospital discharge.

In published series, the success rate of laparoscopic cholecystectomy for acute cholecystitis has been 75 to 85 percent, the incidence of complications ranging from 1 to 17 percent. There have been no reported deaths or major bile duct injuries in these series. The mean postoperative hospital stay is between 2 and 4 days after successful laparoscopic cholecystectomy versus approximately 7 days in those patients converted to an open procedure.

Laparoscopic cholecystectomy appears to be the procedure of choice for patients with acute cholecystitis provided the surgeon has significant experience (>50 cases). Therefore, the benefits of laparoscopic surgery can be extended to 75 percent or more of these patients without increasing the likelihood of major ductal or vascular injuries. An appropriately low threshold for conversion to an open laparotomy, if extreme difficulty in dissection is encountered, remains key to obtaining good results.

LAPAROSCOPIC CHOLECYSTECTOMY AND SUSPECTED COMMON BILE DUCT STONES

The management of suspected common bile duct stones in the era of laparoscopic cholecystectomy has been one of the most controversial points since the introduction of this procedure. The presence of jaundice, cholangitis, and/or suspected common bile duct stones were originally considered relative contraindications to laparoscopic cholecystectomy. Early in the development, some authors advocated routine preoperative endoscopic retrograde cholangiography for all patients to define biliary anatomy and to detect unsuspected choledocholithiasis. Since that time intraoperative cholangiography has become universally available and has eliminated the need for preoperative cholangiography in all but selected cases. Using fluoroscopic techniques, intraoperative cholangiography can be performed successfully in over 90 percent of patients, usually adding less than 10 minutes to operative time. Currently, the management of choledocholithiasis is undergoing further evolution as reports of successful laparoscopic management of common bile duct stones are appearing.

The current management of patients with suspected common bile duct stones depends on both the degree of suspicion that stones exist and the local expertise in biliary endoscopy, interventional radiology, and laparoscopic surgery. In patients with symptomatic gallstones felt to have a high likelihood of harboring common bile duct stones, such as patients presenting with jaundice and/or cholangitis, preoperative evaluation of the biliary tree should be performed. Endoscopic retrograde cholangiography can successfully visualize the biliary tree in virtually all patients with minimal morbidity. If common bile duct stones are identified, successful stone clearance can be achieved by an accomplished endoscopist in over 90 percent of patients. It is recommended that all these patients undergo preoperative clearance of the biliary tree to eliminate the risk of postoperative complications and the small chance that reoperation may be necessary if postoperative choledocholithiasis develops that cannot be managed endoscopically. (There is a separate chapter on biliary therapeutic endoscopy techniques.)

The other extreme of the spectrum are those patients with no clinical history or laboratory findings suggesting choledocholithiasis. In the presence of normal liver function tests and a nondilated biliary tree on ultrasound, preoperative cholangiography appears illogical. Debate does exist concerning the role of routine versus selective intraoperative cholangiography for these patients. This argument existed for years before the introduction of laparoscopic cholecystectomy. It would appear that the selective use of intraoperative cholangiography will result in postoperative symptoms suggesting retained common bile stones and necessitating the need for postoperative endoscopic retrograde cholangiography in less than 3 percent of patients with sphincterotomy for documented and retained stones in less than 1 percent of patients.

The final group of patients fall in the middle of the spectrum where there is some suspicion of common bile duct stones based on preoperative evaluation. The management of these patients depends primarily on the local expertise. If an accomplished biliary endoscopist is available, preoperative cholangiography can be successfully completed with few if any complications. Laparoscopic cholecystectomy should follow within 24 to 48 hours to eliminate the possibility of passage of other gallstones out of the gallbladder. If endoscopy skills are limited, intraoperative cholangiography should be performed to assess the biliary tree for the presence of stones. If the study is normal, laparoscopic cholecystectomy is completed without further concerns.

There are multiple options for the management of common bile duct stones detected intraoperatively at the time of laparoscopic cholecystectomy. The newest most attractive option is laparoscopic management. In most cases this involves transcystic bile duct exploration employing a number of techniques including passage of stone baskets, flexible laparoscopic choledochoscopes, or simply flushing or irrigating stones through the sphincter often after pharmacologic dilatation using glucagon or nitroglycerin. Fluoroscopic imaging, a variety of new laparoscopic instrumentation, and significant technical expertise are necessary to attempt this procedure. However, the results from the initial published series are encouraging with 75 to 95 percent of patients successfully managed. The most common complication of transcystic duct exploration has been hyperamylasemia. Few major complications have occurred. A more aggressive approach involves laparoscopic choledochotomy. Although success with this procedure has been reported, it would appear that very few surgeons

have the operating room equipment or laparoscopic expertise to attempt this approach.

If common duct stones are detected by laparoscopic cholangiography and either access to the common bile duct via a tortuous cystic duct cannot be achieved or instrumentation or laparoscopic skills are lacking, the surgeon is faced with two options: (1) convert to open choledochotomy; or (2) complete the laparoscopic cholecystectomy and plan postoperative management for the retained stone. Both procedures can be associated with morbidity and mortality particularly in older patients. Furthermore, if the choice is postoperative management, the surgeon risks the small chance (less than 10 percent) that endoscopic sphincterotomy will not be successful. On the other hand, for a number of patients in whom the delayed option is chosen, no intervention is necessary suggesting either asymptomatic passage of the stone or the possibility of a false-positive cholangiogram. In some cases, the surgeon can hedge his or her bet by maintaining access to the biliary tree with a catheter to allow postoperative cholangiography and a route to assist in postoperative stone extraction.

In conclusion, there is no right or universally accepted answer to this question. The decision must be individualized based on the nature of the common bile duct stone or stones, the size of the common bile duct, the available expertise in performing endoscopic sphincterotomy, the age and medical condition of the patient, and importantly, the wishes of the patient. An older patient with multiple or large common bile duct stones and a dilated biliary tree may be best managed by an immediate open procedure, whereas the younger patient with small stones and a nondilated system may be best suited for postoperative management.

LAPAROSCOPIC CHOLECYSTECTOMY IN PATIENTS WITH GALLSTONE PANCREATITIS

Gallstone pancreatitis complicates the course of approximately 5 percent of patients with cholelithiasis. Fortunately, the majority of cases are self-limited and abdominal pain and systemic manifestations pass quickly. On the other end of the spectrum, a full-blown attack with cardiovascular collapse, respiratory and renal insufficiency, and pancreatic necrosis with secondary infection can occur with associated significant mortality. As with the management of other complications of gallstones, the role of laparoscopic cholecystectomy in patients with acute gallstone pancreatitis has expanded. This role has been aided by two realizations. First, the recognition that open cholecystectomy can be safely performed during the same hospitalization after resolution of signs and symptoms of acute pancreatitis; and secondly, the safety and favorable results of early endoscopic retrograde cholangiopancreatography (ERCP) and endoscopic sphincterotomy in patients with gallstone pancreatitis. Two prospective randomized studies have shown an advantage for endoscopic stone clearance when performed within 24 to 72 hours of hospital admission. Furthermore, early endoscopic treatment was not associated with worsening complications of pancreatitis or biliary or pancreatic sepsis.

The current recommendations, therefore, for patients with acute gallstone pancreatitis include initial fluid resuscitation and intravenous antibiotics. If biochemical evidence of biliary obstruction exists, early ERCP should be performed with the addition of endoscopic sphincterotomy if indicated. Laparoscopic cholecystectomy can follow during the same admission after signs and symptoms of pancreatitis have resolved. If, as is the case with many patients, the acute pancreatitis resolves early after hospital admission, many surgeons forego preoperative ERCP and perform laparoscopic cholecystectomy with operative cholangiography after complete resolution of symptoms. The risk of finding a common bile duct stone is relatively high (15 to 20 percent). Therefore, the surgeon must be prepared to manage the common bile duct stone by techniques discussed previously in this chapter.

COMMENTS

In September of 1992, the National Institutes of Health convened a consensus development conference and subsequently published a consensus statement entitled "Gallstones and Laparoscopic Cholecystectomy." This statement and the papers presented to the panel are included in the selected reading list. A complete list of the conclusions of this panel cannot be included in this chapter, but the key point concerning laparoscopic cholecystectomy is as follows: "Laparoscopic cholecystectomy provides a safe and effective treatment for most patients with symptomatic gallstones. Indeed, it appears to have become the treatment of choice for many of these patients." The ability to extend this procedure to almost all patients and their complications depends on the skill and experience of the laparoscopic surgeon. It remains the obligation of every surgeon to obtain adequate training and initial proctoring in this technique to minimize the risk of significant complications during the initial "learning curve" of laparoscopic cholecystectomy. Finally, surgeons, patients, and referring physicians must remember that conversion to open cholecystectomy is not a complication, but usually represents a demonstration of sound surgical judgement.

SUGGESTED READING

Cushieri A, Dubois F, Mouiel J, et al. The European experience with laparoscopic cholecystectomy. Am J Surg 1991; 161:358–387.
Deziel DJ, Millikan KW, Economou SG, et al. Complications of laparoscopic cholecystectomy—results of a national survey of 4292 hospitals and analysis of 77,604 cases. Am J Surg 1993; 165:9–14.
Lillemoe KD, Yeo CJ, Talamini MA, et al. Selective cholangiography: Current role in laparoscopic cholecystectomy. Ann Surg 1992; 215:669–676.
MacFadyen BV, Ponsky JL (eds): Laparoscopy for the General Surgeon. Surg Clin North Am 1992; 72:997–1107.
Macintyre IMC, Wilson RG. Laparoscopic cholecystectomy. Br J Surg 1993; 80:552–559.
Proceedings of the NIH Consensus Development Conference on Gallstones and Laparoscopic Cholecystectomy. Am J Surg 1983; 165:387–548.
Soper NHJ, Stockman PT, Dunnegan DL, Ashley SW. Laparoscopic cholecystectomy—the new gold standard. Arch Surg 1992; 127: 917–923.

ACUTE CHOLECYSTITIS

ROGER G. KEITH, M.D., F.R.C.S.C., F.R.C.S., F.A.C.S.

Biliary calculus disease is a very common problem facing practitioners worldwide. Gallbladder pathology is the most frequent sequela of cholelithiasis, although many patients remain asymptomatic through life. Since the advent of laparoscopic cholecystectomy, the incidence of complicated gallbladder disease has been reduced due to the increasing operative rates related to accelerated patient acceptance of surgical treatment for minimally symptomatic cholelithiasis. Nonetheless, the significant morbidity and mortality associated with acute cholecystitis remain unchanged. Understanding the spectrum of gallbladder disease and utilizing the most effective investigations and treatment while avoiding life-risking complications become a significant responsibility for the health care provider of the current decade.

SPECTRUM OF DISEASE

Calculus Related

Biliary colic is a pain syndrome related to cholelithiasis. This is the most benign form of obstructive gallbladder disease, wherein a calculus temporarily obturates the outflow lumen of the gallbladder. This results in a short-lived episode of pain of variable severity which by spontaneous dislodgement of the gallstone terminates the clinical problem. Recurrence is the rule at unpredictable frequency related to stimulation of gallbladder contraction by food ingestion, primarily. Most patients present for cholecystectomy because of unacceptable recurrences of biliary colic.

Acute cholecystitis occurs with progressive obstruction of the gallbladder neck or duct by a gallstone, which through failure to dislodge initiates a cascade of circulatory compromise affecting the end arterial flow of the cystic artery. The complexity of inflammation and ischemia of the gallbladder wall results in local and systemic clinical findings which distinguish this process from biliary colic. Untreated ischemia leads to focal gangrenous necrosis, usually involving the fundus and Hartmann's pouch.

Perforation of the gallbladder wall by increasing secretory pressure exerted at necrotic sites may cause local or generalized spillage of contents. A pericholecystic abscess will result from localization of the leak by the regional viscera and omentum. Failure to contain the leak will lead to biliary peritonitis with risk of septic shock and 40 to 45 percent mortality if not recognized early.

Severity of inflammation of acute cholecystitis is characterized by a palpably tender, enlarged gallbladder associated with fever and leukocytosis greater than 14,000 per milliliter. Hemodynamic instability heralds bacteremia and risk of septic shock. Jaundice of mild degree is not uncommon and is usually due to extending periportal inflammation and not common duct stone. The impacted stone precipitating acute cholecystitis precludes subsequent passage of gallstones to the bile duct, unless this was a pre-existing condition.

Risk factors which lead to acceleration of the gallbladder inflammation and ischemia are related to local impairment to arterial flow such as atherosclerosis with or without diabetes mellitus and systemic factors which compromise host immune responsiveness. Advanced liver disease and portal hypertension not only blunt the response to inflammation but increase the morbidity of surgery by the derangement of local anatomy and abnormal bleeding risk.

Noncalculus Related

Acalculous cholecystitis is an acute complication of critical systemic illness. It most frequently occurs in hospitalized patients undergoing intensive care management or having immune compromising systemic therapy for unrelated diseases. Prolonged fasting and deranged gastrointestinal function are common factors in most patients who predispose to gallbladder stasis. Imaging studies delineate the pathogenetic "biliary sludge" implicated in acute acalculous cholecystitis. The other factor required to initiate the progressive necrotizing inflammation is hypoperfusion of the gallbladder relevant to critical illness caused by trauma, sepsis, or cardiopulmonary failure.

This form of cholecystitis has a more formidable course because of the blunted systemic response and the more rapid progression of gallbladder ischemia to gangrenous necrosis and perforation. Lack of awareness and compromise of signs by the pre-existing illness contribute to the delay in treatment which leads to the increased morbidity and mortality associated with the acalculus form of acute cholecystitis.

DIFFERENTIAL DIAGNOSIS

Distinction between acute cholecystitis and other causes of right upper quadrant inflammation must be based on clinical evaluation and cost effective laboratory examinations. Prior existence of gallstones lends credibility to the diagnosis of cholecystitis but does not eliminate the possibility of common bile duct stones and acute cholangitis, which may be anicteric in up to one-third of cases. Rigors and sepsis are more likely to indicate cholangitis and with high probability the gallbladder will not be palpable or tender. Immediately evident jaundice, indicating at least a threefold increase in serum bilirubin, is predictive of common duct stone not cholecystitis. Painless cholestasis with or without fever may indicate periampullary neoplasm.

Generalized peritonitis with associated cholelithiasis should be considered acute biliary pancreatitis until proved otherwise. Elevations of serum amylase greater than 1,000 IU per liter are diagnostic. Whereas normal or intermediate elevations can be found with pancreatitis, other causes of peritonitis should be ruled out. Perforation of a duodenal ulcer may mimic pancreatitis or cholecystitis. In such patients, a history of ulcer may be absent; however, most cases are confirmed by radiographic evidence of free intraperitoneal air.

Acute hepatitis of viral or toxic etiology may be difficult to differentiate from acute cholecystitis as the enlarged liver with distended Glisson's capsule may be mistaken for the gallbladder. However, the entire liver is tender to percussion over the lower chest cage on both right and left sides with acute hepatitis. Acute alcoholic hepatitis is more readily confused with extrahepatic cholestasis from stone disease as the liver tenderness is severe and the biochemical liver function tests are similar with significantly disproportionate elevation of alkaline phosphatase compared to transaminase.

Diagnostic Imaging Studies

The laboratory examination which will yield the maximal diagnostic information at least cost with greatest accessibility, is ultrasound scanning of the abdomen with reference to the gallbladder, liver, biliary tract, and pancreas. Although operator-dependent, current technology will confirm pathology of the biliary tract including gallbladder in 95 percent of cases. Cholelithiasis will be substantiated in more than 95 percent and false negative studies should be under 5 percent.

Criteria to support the clinical diagnosis of acute cholecystitis include gallbladder distention with a thickened, edematous wall. The impacted calculus may be observed in the cystic duct or neck of the gallbladder. Pericholecystic fluid indicates transmural inflammation and gas in the gallbladder wall is an ominous finding.

Empyema of the gallbladder is confirmed by finding gas in the lumen. Portal edema and lymphadenopathy indicate severity and duration of the inflammatory process. Transducer tenderness over the imaged gallbladder fundus corresponds to the findings on initial abdominal examination, but is not organ specific.

Dilatation of the intrahepatic bile ducts is most easily recognized by the ultrasonographer and suggests extrahepatic biliary obstruction. However, this is not diagnostic of common duct stones unless visualized. Distal common duct dilatation is highly suspicious for the presence of stones in the duct or the less frequent periampullary tumor, confirmed by the additional finding of a mass in the pancreas or region of the ampulla.

Acute liver disease is suggested by liver enlargement and heterogeneity of texture. Splenomegaly and a contracted liver are pathognomonic of cirrhosis.

Radionucleotide biliary scanning using technetium 99–labelled HIDA derivatives is especially valuable in acute acalculous cholecystitis or clinically apparent cholecystitis in which stones cannot be visualized on ultrasound scan. Although less readily accessible, time consuming, and more expensive, this study may confirm cystic duct obstruction and delayed bile duct emptying in selected cases. I would not recommend biliary scintigraphy as the first study for acute cholecystitis and would reserve this examination for patients in whom ultrasound proved equivocal in the face of high probability clinical findings.

Patients with minimal leukocytosis, low-grade fever, and ultrasound evidence of extrahepatic bile duct dilatation without severe cholecystitis on scanning should have preoperative endoscopic retrograde cholangiopancreatography (ERCP) for confirmation of common duct stones, followed by endoscopic sphincterotomy and stone extraction. Subsequent cholecystectomy without operative bile duct exploration will have reduced morbidity compared to cholecystectomy with operative exploration of the duct. This is particularly important in the current era of laparoscopic biliary surgery.

Percutaneous transhepatic cholecystography is only indicated when interventional radiographic techniques will be considered for emergency therapy. Transhepatic cholangiography and biliary drainage should be considered in management of cholangitis as discussed in the chapter *Choledocholithiasis*.

The ultimate imaging study is diagnostic laparoscopy. This study should only be considered as part of definitive therapy for cholecystitis and should be conducted by a qualified abdominal surgical specialist with experience in open and laparoscopic biliary surgery.

INITIAL MANAGEMENT

Self-limited biliary colic rarely requires hospitalization and subsequent management is efficiently conducted on an ambulatory care basis. However, the clinical diagnosis of acute cholecystitis should initiate hospital admission. Baseline hemoglobin, white blood cell

Table 1 Indications for Systemic Antibiotic Therapy (One or More Criteria)

Clinical parameters on admission or within 8 hours:
 Temperature > 38°C
 Clinical jaundice
 Generalized peritonitis

Laboratory parameters:
 Leukocytosis > 14,000/ml
 Elevated bilirubin
 Amylase > 500 IU/L
 Elevated blood glucose

Ultrasound scan parameters:
 Pericholecystic fluid
 Gas in gallbladder wall or lumen
 Dilated intra or extrahepatic bile ducts

Table 2 Criteria Indicating Urgent Operative Intervention

Clinical and laboratory (any two at least):
 Temperature 39°C or greater
 BP < 90 mm systolic
 Jaundice and rigors
 Local or generalized peritonitis
 Leukocytosis 20,000/ml or greater

Ultrasound findings (at least one):
 Pericholecystic fluid
 Gas in gallbladder wall
 Gas in gallbladder lumen
 Edematous gallbladder wall and free abdominal fluid

count, amylase, blood sugar, and liver profile biochemistry are obtained at presentation. Blood cultures should be obtained in the febrile patient after initiation of intravenous crystalloid infusions. The abdominal ultrasound scan should be obtained. Triple antibiotic therapy (aminoglycoside, metronidazole, and ampicillin) should be added when indicated (Table 1). Repeated clinical assessment including temperature and vital signs, combined with ultrasound findings, will determine the subsequent decision for or against urgent operative intervention. The criteria to guide the physician to consider urgent operation are presented in Table 2.

Clinical improvement or absence of surgical indications during the first 48 hours support the continuation of nonoperative treatment, with or without antibiotic therapy. Deterioration or presentation of surgical indications should deter the physician from further conservative management.

Nonoperative treatment during initial management is proposed in order to promote resolution of acute inflammation and present an increased opportunity for minimal access surgery. This proves successful in less than one-third of cases initially diagnosed as acute cholecystitis. In this group of patients, the theoretic interval to complete resolution by 6 weeks is rarely achieved because of residual subacute inflammation or recurrent acute attacks. Therefore, I advise same admission surgery for any patient with residual pain or tenderness after the first week of otherwise effective conservative treatment. Only those with complete freedom of symptoms at 1 week will be planned for an interval cholecystectomy at 6 weeks.

NONOPERATIVE INTERVENTIONAL MANAGEMENT

Interventional Radiologic Treatment

A small percentage of patients with acute cholecystitis and surgical indications have compromising medical conditions which contraindicate general anesthesia. Although mini-laparotomy for open cholecystostomy could be performed under local anaesthesia, a preferable approach is ultrasound-guided percutaneous transhepatic gallbladder drainage. An 18-Fr catheter is placed for emergency decompression and left in place for continued drainage. Unaltered disease progression indicates established gallbladder necrosis and probable bacteremia. Intensive care may be successful in reversing sepsis in these critically ill patients. Failure to respond will mitigate open cholecystectomy under general anesthesia despite high risk in this selected population. Most patients respond favorably to gallbladder drainage. Subsequent management of residual cholelithiasis may utilize the established tract for graduated dilation and percutaneous extraction of stones or consideration may be given to contact lithotripsy or instillation of dissolution agents.

Interventional Endoscopic Management

Patients with acute cholecystitis associated with cholestasis and ultrasound documented dilatation of the extrahepatic biliary tract should have urgent preoperative ERCP and possible sphincterotomy with stone extraction if identified. This is particularly so if the patient is septic and the focus is not defined as gallbladder or bile duct. If stones cannot be extracted at ERCP, a nasobiliary catheter should be placed for proximal biliary decompression. Subsequent to control of sepsis, an urgent cholecystectomy and required biliary exploration should be undertaken by the appropriate open or laparoscopic route. Successful endoscopic sphincterotomy and stone extraction will quickly reverse sepsis if the cause was cholangitis. This leaves an interval opportunity before cholecystectomy, recognizing a small number of cases wherein the gallbladder stones have entirely cleared from the gallbladder without clinical incident. If the sepsis was due to cholecystitis and ERCP failed to identify common duct stones or incidental common duct stones were cleared without alteration of the septic process, urgent cholecystectomy must follow.

OPERATIVE MANAGEMENT

The developments in laparoscopic surgery have changed the approach to calculus disease of the biliary tract significantly. The recognized advantages of reduced hospital stay and earlier return to work attributed to

Table 3 Indications for Conversion to Open Cholecystectomy

At laparoscopy:
    Fixed fundic adhesions
    Free fundus; fixed Calot's triangle
    Perforated necrotic cholecystitis

On attempted cholecystectomy:
    Perforation of necrotic gallbladder on adhesolysis
    Disruption of artery or duct on dissection of obliterated porta
    Nonvisualization of cystic duct–common duct junction
    Inadvertent injury to common bile duct

laparoscopic cholecystectomy have driven surgeons toward minimal access surgery whenever feasible.

The documented increase in frequency of bile duct injury since the advent of laparoscopic cholecystectomy must be considered with any proposal for operative treatment of acute cholecystitis. The maximal derangement of biliary anatomy occurs with severe inflammation of the gallbladder. Technical aspects of open cholecystectomy are most significantly challenged during operation for acute cholecystitis. This has not changed with the improved visual technology of laparoscopic surgery. Thus, the initial guidelines for laparoscopic cholecystectomy contraindicated this technique for acute cholecystitis. This is no longer an absolute contraindication; however, the abdominal surgeon must be prepared to convert to open surgery at the least difficulty (Table 3).

Early Operation

Patients with indications for urgent intervention and those with unremitting pain in the hospital should proceed to cholecystectomy as soon as stabilized. Parenteral antibiotic therapy should continue after the operation for at least 20 hours. Perioperative fluid and electrolyte therapy is delivered based on maintenance requirements per body mass and measured losses. Colloid and blood products are not required unless unusual bleeding occurs during surgery.

The initial approach in most urgent cases is laparoscopic cholecystectomy. The first procedure should be to decompress the gallbladder by laparoscopic-directed percutaneous needle aspiration. Thereafter, exposure and dissection will be easier. A prograde cholecystectomy should begin at the neck of the gallbladder. The impacted stone will be readily identified and the cystic duct will be exposed by blunt dissection of the edematous tissues in Calot's triangle. Identification of the cystic artery should precede division of either structure. Then the decision for laparoscopic cholangiography must be made. I prefer selective cholangiography and perform the study through the cystic duct. Indications for selective cholangiography are outlined in Table 4. The surgeon must recognize that the impaction of a gallstone in the gallbladder neck or cystic duct causes this disease and commonly prevents migration of gallstones to the common duct.

If completion cholangiography precludes exploration of the duct, the gallbladder should be removed

Table 4 Indications for Selective Cholangiography in Acute Cholecystitis

Preoperative:
  Ultrasound demonstration of extrahepatic duct dilatation
  Ultrasound demonstration of common duct stones
  Ultrasound evidence of pancreatitis or pancreatic mass
  Acalculus cholecystitis

Intraoperative:
  Dilated common bile duct
  Palpable common duct stones
  Nonimpacted gallbladder stone at neck
  Empty gallbladder
  Pancreatic mass or inflammation

prograde after stepwise clipping and division of the cystic duct and artery. I prefer coagulation, not laser, for dissection and hemostasis. Removal of the severely-diseased gallbladder may require extension of the umbilical incision. If the gallbladder fossa is dry and bleeding is controlled, no drainage is required.

If cholangiography reveals small common duct stones, I prefer to perform a postoperative ERCP with endoscopic sphincterotomy and stone removal. Laparoscopic duct exploration is only considered for larger stones with a wide diameter cystic duct which will allow transcystic duct introduction of a flexible choledochoscope for stone extraction or lithotripsy. If there are multiple large stones or the surgeon is not experienced with laparoscopic duct exploration, then open cholecystectomy and choledochotomy should be the procedure of choice.

Conversion to open operation should be followed by prograde or retrograde dissection according to the surgeon's preference and experience. Cholangiography should be selected by the same criteria. As open surgery will be performed in more severe cases, meticulous care should be taken during dissection around the porta. If pathology is extenuating, the decision should be taken early to perform a cholecystostomy and remove gallstones, leaving a tube exteriorized at the fundus.

Elective Operation

A small percentage of patients with acute cholecystitis settle and can return electively for definitive treatment. The same operative approach is recommended. The fibrosis of healed cholecystitis may make the adhesolysis so difficult that the surgeon will be forced to convert to open cholecystectomy.

The advantage of preoperative ERCP must be recognized. I favor this method of study for any patient with preoperative indications for cholangiography based on ultrasound examination.

The presence of edematous inflammation should not be the reason to select early treatment if a patient is clinically improved. Most elective operations are technically satisfactory and the risks of duct injury in face of acute inflammation are reduced by the delay for resolution.

POSTOPERATIVE MANAGEMENT

Following laparoscopic cholecystectomy, the recovery phase is shorter than open, even with severe acute cholecystitis.

After early resolution of ileus, oral feedings are initiated without restriction of fats. Normal activity is encouraged soon after surgery, and with small laparoscopic wounds, no restriction in exertion is necessary. Return to full employment is expected after 1 week.

Laparoscopic surgery for necrotizing or perforated cholecystitis may be complicated by umbilical wound infection by the extracted gallbladder. Acute inflammation is evident about the 5th day and local drainage is effective treatment.

Intra-abdominal abscess may occur in the subhepatic or subphrenic spaces or even in the pelvis. More significant sepsis occurs without wound signs. Ultrasound scanning is the preferred first imaging technique. It is diagnostic in over 80 percent of cases. Failed localization requires CT and nuclear medical scanning.

Residual stones may be quiescent and present years after operation, or early evidence of fluctuating cholestasis may be seen within weeks. Ultrasound scans should be followed by diagnostic and therapeutic ERCP and stone extraction. Cholangitis is uncommon in the early postoperative phase, but urgent biliary decompression must be initiated under triple antibiotic coverage.

Bile duct injury presents with rapid onset of progressive cholestasis if complete occlusion of the common duct resulted from inadvertent clipping or ligation. Bile duct leaks may present as biliary fistula if open surgery was performed; or bile peritonitis or ascites may present after a delay of several weeks. Cholangiography will be required by the endoscopic or transhepatic route; in some cases both techniques may be utilized to define the exact nature and extent of the complication. Biliary intestinal continuity should be restored by reconstruction techniques using a roux-en-Y limb of jejunum. Primary end-to-end repair should only be considered when recognition of injury is apparent at the primary operation.

Open cholecystectomy prolongs hospital stay and return to full activity. Wound infection may be more frequent and cause greater morbidity. Otherwise, postoperative complications are not significantly different than for the laparoscopic procedure, except for the recognized increase of bile duct injury attributed to laparoscopic cholecystectomy.

SUGGESTED READING

Flowers JA, Bailey RW, Zucker KA. Laparoscopic management of acute cholecystitis. Am J Surg 1991; 161:388–392.
Hermann RE. The spectrum of biliary stone disease. Am J Surg 1989; 158:171–173.
Jacobs M, Verdeja JC, Goldstein HS. Laparoscopic cholecystectomy in acute cholecystitis. Surg Endosc 1991; 1:174–175.
McSherry CK. Cholecystectomy: the gold standard. Am J Surg 1989; 158:174–178.
Unger SW, Edelman DS, Scott JS, et al. Laparoscopic treatment of acute cholecystitis. Surg Endosc 1991; 1:14–16.

CHOLELITHIASIS

ELDON A. SHAFFER, M.D., F.R.C.P.C., F.A.C.P.

Gallstone disease is a major health care problem, afflicting 20 to 30 million people and resulting in over 500,000 cholecystectomies each year in the United States. It is now the most common operation after Caesarean section. The resultant burden costs the U.S. economy $4 to 5 billion each year, representing 2.5 percent of all health care dollars. The variance in the performance of cholecystectomy is significant: it is six to sevenfold higher in the U.S. and Canada than in Europe. The frequency of gallstone disease, though high, is not different. Such variance suggests overuse of the health care system, particularly as few patients ever become symptomatic.

The management of cholelithiasis has changed significantly with better understanding of its natural history, the introduction of new medical therapies and advances in surgical technologies. A balanced perspective is in order.

NATURAL HISTORY

Cholesterol gallstones (composed of >50 percent cholesterol) are the most common type, representing over 85 percent of all stones in the Western world. They are more frequent in women especially with early menarche and parity; the obese and those undergoing rapid weight loss; older age groups and certain ethnic groups, such as American Indians. The remainder are pigment stones containing bilirubin polymers plus several insoluble calcium salts.

Cholesterol gallstones form in three stages (1) chemical stage in which the liver secretes bile supersaturated with cholesterol; (2) physical stage in which the excess cholesterol precipitates from solution as microcrystals; and (3) gallstone growth in which these crystals aggregate and grow into macroscopic stones.

Gallstones grow at about 1 to 2 mm per year over 5 to 20 years before symptoms develop. They frequently are clinically "silent," some being incidentally detected on a routine ultrasound examination performed for another purpose. Indeed, over 80 percent of people with gallstones never develop symptoms. Problems, if they do arise, usually do so in the form of biliary pain during the first 5 to 10 years. Most will experience some symptoms for a period of time before developing a complication. No gallstone-related deaths have been reported from patients followed for asymptomatic gallstone disease. Because of this, prophylactic treatment of asymptomatic patients is no longer justified. The same applies to diabetic patients; they are not at greater risk of complications but have a high mortality if acute cholecystitis supervenes. In general, the risk of gallbladder cancer in patients with gallstones is so very low as to not justify prophylactic cholecystectomy. Prophylactic cholecystectomy is only warranted when the risk of coexistent carcinoma of the gallbladder is high, such as in the presence of a calcified gallbladder ("porcelain gallbladder"), gallstones > 3 cm in diameter and possibly solitary gallbladder polyps > 1 cm in diameter.

Symptomatic gallstones are best defined by the development of true biliary pain. Although termed "biliary colic," the upper abdominal pain typically is steady, not spasmodic. It begins suddenly, becomes severe and persists for 1 to 5 hours, and then gradually disappears over 30 to 60 minutes, leaving a dull ache. Its duration may be somewhat less than 1 hour but is not as brief as 30 minutes. "Fatty food intolerance," a vague discomfort which follows a heavy or spicy meal, is not specific for biliary tract disease. Rather, biliary pain is significant enough to awaken the individual from sleep or require narcotics for relief. Episodes of pain occur irregularly, separated by pain-free intervals lasting from days to years. Symptomatic patients are likely to have recurrent episodes of biliary pain; obviously some go on to complications, such as cholecystitis or biliary obstruction. Those with symptoms warrant therapeutic intervention.

AVAILABLE THERAPIES

Expectant Management

No therapy other than watching is necessary for most individuals with gallstones who are not experiencing symptoms.

Medical Therapy

Oral Dissolution with Bile Acids

Chenodeoxycholic acid and ursodeoxycholic acid when taken orally can effectively dissolve cholesterol gallstones; neither works for pigment stones. The only structural difference between these two molecules is the orientation of the hydroxyl group in the seven position. This epimeric difference confers unique physical-chemical properties to each bile acid, accounting for their differences in mechanisms of action, dosage, and side effects. The 7α-hydroxyl group of chenodeoxycholic acid provides it with an axial orientation. It is therefore more soluble in water and has a greater detergent action. For ursodeoxycholic acid, the equatorial position of its 7β-hydroxyl lessens its water solubility and detergent action. Ursodeoxycholic acid is thus less injurious to biological membranes, does not cause secretory diarrhea and is not hepatotoxic.

Both bile acids reduce the hepatic secretion of cholesterol into bile, lowering cholesterol saturation of bile. Chenodeoxycholic acid decreases hepatic cholesterol synthesis. Ursodeoxycholic acid facilitates conversion of hepatic cholesterol to bile acids and reduces cholesterol absorption in the intestine. Ursodeoxycholic acid, being less of a detergent, does not carry as much cholesterol into bile. Further, ursodeoxycholic acid may have a different mechanism by which it solubilizes cholesterol molecules from gallstones—incorporating the cholesterol into phospholipid vesicles rather than just micelles.

Pharmacologic properties also differ. Ursodeoxycholic acid is less well absorbed because of reduced water solubility, but its 7-β-OH group is removed more slowly by intestinal bacteria. This resistance to bacterial hydrolysis permits a lower therapeutic dose. Chenodeoxycholic acid should be administered at 13 to 15 mg per day, ursodeoxycholic acid at 8 to 10 mg per kilogram per day. Obese individuals may require dosages up to 50 percent higher.

Trials of clinical efficacy are controversial. Complete dissolution in patients with cholesterol gallstones varies from 0 to 64 percent for chenodeoxycholic acid and 9 to 83 percent for ursodeoxycholic acid. Methodological differences in patient selection, sample size, and reporting bias likely account for most of these discrepancies.

The initial enthusiasm for chenodeoxycholic acid became tempered by a major National Institutes of Health study which revealed that only 14 percent of patients could expect complete dissolution of radiolucent gallstones after 2 years of therapy. Many experienced diarrhea and a few developed reversible hepatic toxicity. Although many have written off chenodeoxycholic acid based on this work, most patients in the study actually were on a sub-therapeutic dose. As a result, ursodeoxycholic acid, which does not induce diarrhea or elevate serum transaminase or cholesterol levels, is now the drug of choice. Consolidating all ursodeoxycholic acid trials in a meta-analysis indicates that complete dissolution occurred in 37.3 percent of patients. Combination therapy with 7.5 mg chenodeoxycholic acid plus 6.5 mg of ursodeoxycholic acid per kilogram per day might even be faster and better, succeeding in 63 percent, although only limited studies are available.

Factors for success are patient dependent, related to gallbladder function and stone size and composition. Gallbladder visualization on an oral cholecystogram or ultrasound evidence of a decrease in gallbladder size after a fatty meal or cholescintigraphy demonstrates adequate gallbladder function and patency of the cystic duct. Gallstones should be radiolucent, indicating that they are likely composed of cholesterol. Unfortunately pigment stones are not necessarily radiopaque. Small stones with a high surface-to-volume ratio are more likely to dissolve. Ideal candidates are tiny (<5 mm), radiolucent stones which float on oral cholecystography, indicating a higher likelihood of cholesterol rather than calcium. Ninety percent of such cases will undergo total dissolution when treated for 6 to 12 months. Unfortunately only about 3 percent of all patients fall into this category. Radiolucent gallstones with diameters of 10 mm or less, representing 15 percent of all gallstones,

yield a near 60 percent success rate. Dissolution rates are lower with broader selection criteria and for obese individuals.

Side effects with ursodeoxycholic acid are minimal; any symptoms likely relate to the gallstone disease per se. Biliary pain may even be less frequent while on bile acid therapy. The leading management problem is the need for prolonged therapy (up to 2 years), plus the risk of recurrence once therapy is discontinued. Fifty percent will redevelop stones over a 5-year period; most are not symptomatic and a second dissolution is quite feasible.

Oral dissolution therapy is most appropriate in those with symptomatic gallstones which are small, the informed patient who wishes to avoid surgery, or when a comorbid condition precludes a safe operation. Use of a low cholesterol diet and ingestion of the bile acid dose at bedtime improve the success rate with chenodeoxycholic acid but are unproven for ursodeoxycholic acid where no guidelines exist. While on bile acid therapy, ultrasonographic follow-up at 6 to 9 months can determine if dissolution is proceeding. Once dissolution is complete, bile acid therapy should be continued for another 3 months to eliminate any stone remnants that might be too small for ultrasonographic detection. Then annual ultrasonography may be useful for a few years. Detection of stone recurrence indicates consideration for another course of bile acid therapy. There is no established therapy to prevent recurrent stone formation, but common sense suggests eliminating obvious risk factors such as obesity.

Bile acid therapy compared to cholecystectomy is not cost effective in younger patients. In those over 65 years, bile acids become more cost effective.

Extracorporeal Shock Wave Lithotripsy

Shock waves are an ultrashort, high pressure form of sound wave. Their multiple frequencies provide higher energy and greater tissue penetration. Generated outside the body and transmitted via water, shock-wave energy travels through human tissue with little attenuation or damage. Acoustic impedance abruptly changes at the interface between body tissues and the surface of the stone, causing wave deflection. Shock wave energy is released, yielding tear-and-shear forces. The formation and violent collapse of macroscopic gas bubbles in the liquid bile adjacent to the stone's surface produces a cavitation effect. Fissures develop, and fragmentation leads to progressive stone disintegration.

The three techniques to generate shock waves use a spark gap, piezoelectric, or electromagnetic source. They differ in terms of the energy delivered to the stone. Higher energy produces better stone fragmentation but causes more discomfort for the patient. Current systems use a small focal volume, lessening the requirement for anaesthesia or analgesia and making biliary lithotripsy an outpatient procedure.

Disintegration of gallstones into fragments permits the spontaneous passage of small particles (<2 to 3 mm) from the biliary tract into the intestine. If gallbladder contraction is impaired, mechanical ejection is less effective. Shock-wave lithotripsy therefore requires adjuvant bile acid therapy to dissolve residual fragments. The standard is a combination of 7 to 8 mg of chenodeoxycholic acid plus 6 to 7 mg ursodeoxycholic acid per kilogram per day. Several months may be necessary before clearance of stone fragments is complete.

Inclusion criteria embrace symptomatic patients with biliary pain, a functioning gallbladder, and radiolucent stones. The patient may have up to three stones, but none should be larger than 20 mm and their total diameter should be less than the equivalent of a 30 mm stone. Excluded are gallstones associated with complications (acute cholecystitis or pancreatitis), concomitant bile duct stones, coagulopathy, pregnancy, or local pathology which would either obscure targeting of the stones or present a structural risk (e.g., vascular aneurysm). Treatment times average about 1 hour; usually one to two sessions are required. The aim is to produce fragments less than 3 to 5 mm which will clear spontaneously. The ideal is a solitary, non-calcified gallstone less than 20 mm in diameter; success can be 95 percent in experienced hands. Broadening the standards to patients with 20 to 30 mm gallstones and those with up to three stones in a functioning gallbladder yields a lesser clearance rate of 60 percent. About 7 to 16 percent of all patients with symptomatic stones fall into these two categories.

Complications of shock wave lithotripsy are minor: biliary pain (25 percent), presumably from passage of stone fragments; pancreatitis (1 to 2 percent), which usually is uncomplicated; and hematuria (3 to 5 percent). The recurrence rate is less than after bile acid dissolution, perhaps reflecting the natural history of solitary stones. Twenty percent develop stones at 4 years; most remain asymptomatic.

The procedure is not widely approved in North America. For older patients, shock-wave lithotripsy is cost effective compared to cholecystectomy but not in younger persons. It is especially useful in patients with a high surgical risk. Shock-wave lithotripsy of bile duct stones is also reasonable in selected cases in which large ductal stones cannot be crushed or extricated by ERCP or the percutaneous transhepatic route. This is discussed in the chapter *Choledocholithiasis*.

Direct Contact Dissolution

Instillation of solvents into the common bile duct to dissolve retained stones has evolved from using ether (which becomes volatile at body temperature producing pain) to a medium-chain triglyceride derivative, monooctanoin (glyceryl-1-monooctanoate), approved and marketed as Capmul 8210. Monooctanoin perfusion of the biliary tract via T-tube, nasobiliary tube, percutaneous transhepatic catheter, or cholecystectomy drain clears the common duct in 26 to 50 percent. Significant side effects including pulmonary edema, peptic ulceration, and systemic acidosis, plus the advent of sophisticated

endoscopic and percutaneous methods to extract ductal stones, has obviated the need for monooctanoin infusion.

Methyl tert-butyl ether (MTBE), a liquid at body temperature, is a powerful solvent but also is potentially explosive and toxic. Its use in dissolving gallstones is invasive, requiring direct instillation via a percutaneous transhepatic catheter placed in the gallbladder. Small volumes (about 4 ml to prevent outflow from the gallbladder) are continuously infused and aspirated, facilitated by an automated pump. Dissolution occurs in 95 percent after repeated cycles lasting 6 to 7 hours. Adverse effects such as hemolysis and somnolence have been surprisingly mild. Use is limited to very highly specialized centers and then only for those who are high surgical risks.*

Other percutaneous techniques are mechanical, technically demanding, and experimental. Cholecystolithotomy removes the stone from the gallbladder. Rotary contact lithotripsy crushes the stone in a metal basket containing rotary blades.

SURGERY

Open Cholecystectomy

Cholecystectomy via an "open" abdominal incision has been standard treatment for symptomatic gallstone disease. It is curative, removing gallstone and the gallbladder. The mortality is <0.5 percent when electively performed for biliary colic, but reaches 3 percent for emergency surgery in acute cholecystitis or for common duct procedures. It is even higher in the elderly. Hospitalization averages about 1 week. There are few contraindications to classical cholecystectomy. Variations including a mini-incision somewhat reduce the postoperative pain and shorten the convalescent time slightly. This procedure is discussed in the chapter on cholecystitis.

Laparoscopic Cholecystectomy

This new operation employs laparoscopic visualization of the gallbladder and surrounding vital tissues while the peritoneal cavity is insufflated with carbon dioxide gas. This procedure is discussed in detail in a separate chapter. The procedure is a variant of the standard cholecystectomy. Operative cholangiogram can be performed through a small incision in the cystic duct; in common practice this is only done in about 5 percent of cases. Postoperative recovery is phenomenal. Many are discharged within 24 hours and return to normal physical activity within 1 week. Patient comfort and the cosmetic effects highlight this procedure.

Contraindications are sepsis, peritonitis, and dis-

---

*Editor's Note: The gallbladder can be examined 1 week later via a fiberscope passed through the perfusing catheter. Remaining small fragments, which may not be detectable on sonography, can be retreated before the catheter is withdrawn.

tended bowel. Conversion to an open cholecystectomy is necessary in about 5 to 10 percent of cases. The most ominous complication is bile duct injury, usually the result of mistaking the common bile duct for the cystic duct or an inaccurately placed clip. Retained common duct stones are a further problem necessitating an increased use of ERCP for their removal.

The popularity of laparoscopic cholecystectomy has spread throughout North America. About 80 percent of cholecystectomies are now performed in this manner. Critical assessment of safety, training standards, cost-effectiveness, and outcome are necessary as the potential for overuse is great.

SUGGESTED READING

Bachrach WH, Hofmann AF. Ursodeoxycholic acid in the treatment of cholesterol cholelithiasis: Part I, II. Dig Dis Sci 1982; 27:737–761, 833–856.
May GR, Sutherland LR, Shaffer EA. Efficacy of bile acid therapy for gallstone dissolution: A meta-analysis of randomized trials. Aliment Pharmacol Ther 1993; 7:139–148.
Ransohoff DF, Gracie WA, Wolfenson LD, Neuhauser B. Prophylactic cholecystectomy or expectant management of silent gallstones: A decision analysis to assess survival. Ann Intern Med 1983; 99: 199–204.
Sachmann M, Pauletzki J, Sauerbruch T, et al. The Munich gallbladder lithotripsy study: Results of the first 711 patients. Ann Intern Med 1991; 114:290–296.
Schoenfield LJ, Lachmin JM and the National Cooperative Gallstone Study Group. Chenodiol, (chenodeoxycholic acid) for dissolution of gallstones: A controlled study of efficacy and safety. Ann Intern Med 1981; 95:257–282.
Strasberg SM, Clavien P-A. Cholecystolithiasis: Lithotherapy for the 1990s. Hepatology 1992; 16:820–839.
Thistle JL, May GR, Bender CE, et al. Dissolution of cholesterol gallbladder stones by methyl-tert-butyl ether administered by percutaneous transhepatic catheter. N Engl J Med 1989; 320: 633–639.

CHOLEDOCHOLITHIASIS

ROBERT E. HERMANN, M.D.

Choledocholithiasis, stones in the bile ducts, may be identified in several settings. They may be found at the time of either laparoscopic or open cholecystectomy, they may be identified after the gallbladder has been removed as retained or recurrent stones, or they may present as an acute septic cholangitis or as a cause of acute pancreatitis.

Most stones in the bile ducts are secondary, arising in the gallbladder and passing from there into the bile ducts. Primary bile duct stones also occur in some patients without stones in the gallbladder or in patients in whom the gallbladder has previously been removed. In Asian countries, primary intrahepatic bile duct stones are found in association with a chronic stenosing cholangitis, a condition termed oriental cholangiohepatitis. Primary bile duct stones are probably the result of stasis of bile flow with the secondary element of infection as a contributing factor.

Choledocholithiasis is a relatively common problem in the United States and in most Western societies with a frequency which ranges from 10 percent to 20 percent of all adult patients with gallstones. The incidence of cholelithiasis and choledocholithiasis appears to increase with increasing age of the patients studied.

Stones in the bile duct may be initially asymptomatic and unsuspected, but as they grow they may cause bile duct obstruction with the development of pain symptoms or secondary infection. The most common symptom is colicky right upper abdominal pain (biliary colic) from partial or intermittent bile duct obstruction. The next most common symptom is jaundice from obstruction of bile flow. The third most common symptom is fever caused by the infection which so frequently develops in patients with bile stasis and large stones. The incidence of bacteria cultured from the biliary system in patients with choledocholithiasis is approximately 90 percent. A mixed flora of gram-negative bacilli, some gram-positive aerobes, and anaerobes can be frequently cultured from bile.

If a bile duct stone becomes impacted in the distal bile duct or ampulla of Vater, acute gallstone pancreatitis may result from the obstruction of the distal pancreatic duct or from the common channel which may develop between the obstructed biliary and pancreatic duct systems. Pancreatitis is potentially the most severe complication of choledocholithiasis.

In patients suspected of having bile duct stones, basic laboratory studies should include a complete blood count, liver function studies to include bilirubin levels, alkaline phosphatase, and serum transaminase levels, as well as serum amylase and lipase determinations. Other useful studies include a serum creatinine and blood urea nitrogen level to assess renal function, serum electrolyte levels, and a serum glucose.

Important radiologic studies include ultrasonography (US) of the liver and biliary system which is the most rapid and inexpensive technique to assess the biliary system for gallstones or for evidence of dilatation in patients with low-grade jaundice. Computed tomography (CT) scans provide more precise definition of the dilated biliary system and also help to provide more detail in the radiographic examination of the liver, porta hepatis, and head of the pancreas.

For further definition of the cause of biliary dilatation, endoscopic retrograde cholangiopancreatography (ERCP) and percutaneous transhepatic cholangiography (PTC) provide direct visualization of the biliary and pancreatic ducts. For patients with suspected choledocholithiasis as the cause of pain, jaundice, or fever, antibiotics should be started prior to the study. ERCP is our study of choice since the entire biliary system can be visualized from the ampullary orifice to the intrahepatic radicles. Additionally, if the patient has bile duct stones, endoscopic sphincterotomy can be performed and the stones can be removed during the procedure.

THERAPEUTIC ALTERNATIVES

In the past 20 years, the treatment of bile duct stones has changed dramatically. Years ago, surgical exploration and removal of the stones was the only method of treatment. Bile duct stones can now also be removed by endoscopic sphincterotomy and extracted during endoscopy, they can be fragmented by shock wave lithotripsy and dissolved by chemical dissolution agents, and can be removed after percutaneous transhepatic intubation of the biliary system through the matured catheter tract. Each of these techniques has merit and may be utilized in selected situations.

Since choledocholithiasis presents in a variety of ways, the pros and cons of various methods of treatment are discussed in relation to these various clinical syndromes.

Choledocholithiasis in Patients with Cholecystitis

Bile duct stones are found in 10 to 20 percent of patients having symptoms of acute or chronic cholecystitis. In many of these patients, the bile duct stones may be unsuspected, but in a number of patients symptoms of biliary colic, elevated bilirubin or alkaline phosphatase levels, jaundice, or a dilated common bile duct on US alert the surgeon to the presence of choledocholithiasis.

If laparoscopic cholecystectomy is planned and choledocholithiasis is suspected preoperatively, we schedule ERCP prior to the operation. If bile duct stones are found, they can be removed by endoscopic sphincterotomy and extraction during this procedure. If all the stones can be removed, the surgeon can then schedule laparoscopic cholecystectomy as soon as possible. If all the bile duct stones cannot be removed by endoscopic techniques, open operative cholecystectomy and common bile duct exploration are scheduled. (There is a chapter on biliary tract manipulation by endoscopy.)

If choledocholithiasis is unsuspected preoperatively, but is identified by intraoperative cholangiography during laparoscopic cholecystectomy, we attempt to remove these stones during the laparoscopic procedure. The cystic duct can be gently dilated and small wire baskets or balloon catheters passed down into the

common bile duct to attempt extraction of the bile duct stones. Some skilled laparoscopic surgeons are now performing bile duct exploration, opening the bile duct, removing stones, and closing it over a T-tube catheter, all during the laparoscopic procedure. Most of us have not, as yet, achieved the skills to do a complete bile duct exploration as just described. If the stones cannot be easily removed by the wire basket or balloon catheter techniques, a decision must be made as to whether to leave the stones in place, leave a small catheter in the cystic-common bile duct, complete the laparoscopic cholecystectomy, and plan ERCP removal of the stones at a future time; or to convert the laparoscopic procedure to an open common bile duct exploration and remove the stones at this time.

This decision will be guided, to some extent, by the size and number of the bile duct stones; if the stones are large or if more than two or three stones are present, we convert to an open common bile duct exploration. If the stones are small and only one or two stones are present, we complete the laparoscopic procedure and plan to remove the stones later by ERCP.

If the patient is scheduled for open cholecystectomy and choledocholithiasis is identified by intraoperative cholangiography, operative common bile duct exploration and stone removal should be performed during this operative procedure. Having removed the bile duct stones, the only final decision is whether the bile duct should be closed over a T-tube or whether a biliary drainage operation (choledochoduodenostomy, choledochojejunostomy, or sphincteroplasty) should be added. If all stones could not be removed, if a stone is impacted in the ampulla of Vater, or if the common bile duct is significantly dilated, (larger than 15 mm) with evidence of distal stenosis, the chance of recurrent stone formation is high and a biliary drainage operation should be added to the common bile duct exploration.

Retained Bile Duct Stones

In patients who have had either laparoscopic cholecystectomy or open cholecystectomy with common bile duct exploration, one or more stones may occasionally be left in the bile ducts as retained stones. If a T-tube has been left in the bile duct, these stones may be removed through the T-tube tract 6 weeks to 2 months postoperatively, a period necessary for the T-tube tract to become matured or walled off from the peritoneal cavity.

The matured T-tube tract can be utilized by the radiologist in the outpatient Radiology Department, to gently dilate the tract and pass wire baskets under fluoroscopic guidance into the bile ducts, manipulate the basket around the stone and extract it through the tract. This technique of stone extraction, the Burhenne technique, has been used successfully for the past 15 years. (This procedure is discussed in a separate chapter.) If, at laparoscopic cholecystectomy, the surgeon could only pass a small drainage catheter into the bile duct through the cystic duct, it is unlikely that the radiologist will be able to work through such a small tract. However, chemical solvents which dissolve cholesterol, such as monooctanoin, can be used to irrigate the bile duct and attempt to dissolve the stones.

For most patients who have retained stones after laparoscopic cholecystectomy, ERCP and endoscopic sphincterotomy with subsequent removal of the stones should be performed.

Recurrent Bile Duct Stones

In patients who develop biliary colic or jaundice 2 or more years after a previous cholecystectomy, with or without bile duct exploration, recurrent bile duct stones should be suspected. ERCP and endoscopic sphincterotomy (all patients should be started on antibiotics prior to this procedure) with extraction of the stones by nonoperative means is our treatment of choice. If the bile duct has become greatly dilated or if there is significant distal bile duct stenosis, or if there are multiple large earthy (primary) bile duct stones in the duct, we favor an open operative exploration to remove these stones and to perform a biliary drainage procedure (choledochoduodenostomy or choledochojejunostomy).

If endoscopic sphincterotomy and extraction of several of the bile duct stones can be accomplished, but one or more large stones cannot be removed, endoscopic direct contact lithotripsy or extracorporeal shock wave lithotripsy directed at these stones may be successful in fragmenting them, so that the fragments can be removed. If the stones are rich in cholesterol, a nasobiliary catheter can be placed up into the bile duct endoscopically and the duct infused with monooctanoin solution over a period of several weeks to attempt to dissolve the stones or reduce their size. Chemical dissolution has about a 60 percent success rate.

Acute Suppurative Cholangitis

Occasionally, in elderly patients or in patients with diabetes or immune-compromised states, choledocholithiasis with bile duct obstruction and jaundice will present as an acute, septic, or suppurative cholangitis. Such patients are acutely and critically ill. They may have symptoms of biliary colic, high fever, and jaundice (Charcot's triad), with hypotension, and coma (Reynold's pentad). They should be rapidly started on intravenous antibiotics designed to combat a broad spectrum of mixed gram-negative bacteria and anaerobes, given supportive intravenous fluids, and scheduled for drainage of the obstructed biliary system as rapidly as possible. Nonoperative endoscopic drainage of the obstructed biliary system by ERCP, endoscopic sphincterotomy, and extraction of the bile duct stones, or by passing a catheter or stent retrograde into the biliary system to drain it into the duodenum is our first choice for treating this acute problem.

If endoscopic drainage of the biliary system cannot be immediately and successfully accomplished, percutaneous transhepatic catheter drainage of the obstructed biliary system is a second choice which also avoids open operative exploration. In some patients, however, neither of these nonoperative drainage procedures may be effective or successful. In this situation, there should be no hesitancy to move as quickly as possible to the operating room where, under general anesthesia, an open operative exploration of the common bile duct with removal of all stones and T-tube drainage should be performed.

Acute Gallstone Pancreatitis

Choledocholithiasis may be a cause of acute pancreatitis. As mentioned previously, the offending bile duct stone may pass through the distal bile duct into the ampulla of Vater and temporarily cause obstruction of both the biliary and pancreatic duct systems or may block the ampullary orifice so that there is a common channel created behind the stone. In either regard, it is the obstruction of the biliary and pancreatic duct systems with resultant infection behind the obstruction which is thought to cause acute pancreatitis.

Although in the past, gastroenterologists and surgeons were reluctant to obtain ERCP studies in patients with acute pancreatitis for fear that the pancreatitis might be made worse, we now know from the experience of several endoscopists that a careful endoscopic retrograde cholangiogram, using just enough contrast medium to outline the ampulla of Vater and avoiding injection of the pancreatic duct system, followed by endoscopic sphincterotomy and extraction of the stones, is a safe and effective procedure for acute gallstone pancreatitis. This procedure when skillfully performed, carries less morbidity and mortality than does open operative exploration of the abdomen, palpation of the pancreas, common bile duct exploration and operative exploration to remove bile duct stones. (The chapter on endoscopic management of gallstone pancreatitis provides details and results.)

Intrahepatic Stones

It is relatively uncommon to find intrahepatic bile duct stones in patients in the United States or other Western countries. This problem, however, occurs frequently in the Orient, and, when associated with chronic stenosing cholangitis of the intrahepatic ducts, is termed oriental cholangiohepatitis. It is thought to be due to chronic parasitic infections in the biliary system or liver and seems to be related to the traditional oriental diet and the oriental preference for raw or uncooked fish and vegetables in these traditional diets.

Patients with this problem frequently have recurring episodes of fever, chills, and jaundice. US or CT scans of the liver will show intrahepatic cystic dilatation of the bile ducts with multiple small stones and debris in these obstructed segments of the biliary system. Both ERCP and PTC have been used to further delineate the intra and extrahepatic bile ducts and the extent of the disease.

Open operative drainage of the obstructed bile ducts or resection of these bile ducts and their liver segments is the most effective treatment. Usually, only one or several segments of the intrahepatic biliary system are involved, most commonly in the left lobe of the liver. If multiple segments throughout the liver, both right and left lobes, are involved, biliary cirrhosis is the end result and liver transplantation may eventually be necessary.

SUGGESTED READING

Bernhoft RA, Pellegrini CA, Motson RW, Way LW. Composition and morphologic and clinical features of common duct stones. Am J Surg 1984; 148:77–85.

Chetlin SH, Elliott DW. Biliary bacteremia. Arch Surg 1971; 102:303.
Choi TK, Wong J. Current management of intrahepatic stones. World J Surg 1990; 14:487–491.
Cotton PB, Lehman G, Vennes J, et al. Endoscopic sphincterotomy complications and their management: An attempt at consensus. Gastrointest Endosc 1991; 37:383–394.
Hermann RE: Bile duct stones. In: Moody FG, Carey LC, Jones RS, et al., ed. Surgical Treatment of Digestive Disease. 2nd ed. Chicago: Year Book 1990: 285.
Miller JS, Ferguson CM. Current management of choledocholithiasis. Am Surg 1990; 58:66–70.
Patti MG, Pellegrini CA. Gallstone pancreatitis. Surg Clin North Am 1990; 70:1277–1295.
Reynolds B. Daugen E: Acute Obstructive Cholangitis. Annals of Surgery, 1959; 150:299.

BILIARY STRICTURES AND NEOPLASMS

JOEL J. ROSLYN, M.D.
FRANCIS D. FERDINAND, M.D.

OVERVIEW

Extrahepatic biliary obstruction can occur secondary to a benign or malignant stricture of the bile duct, as well as occurring as a consequence of gallstones. Benign biliary strictures may be a manifestation of chronic pancreatitis, diffuse processes such as sclerosing cholangitis, or result from an operative misadventure and injury. Unfortunately, this latter setting is the most common scenario for a benign bile duct stricture. Most strictures of the bile duct occur postoperatively and over 90 percent of these postoperative strictures occur after cholecystectomy. Therefore, it seems intuitively clear, that most bile duct strictures are potentially preventable. The increased risk of bile duct injury which has been reported with laparoscopic cholecystectomy underscores the importance of developing a rational approach to the management of patients with benign bile duct strictures.

Bile duct tumors tend to be small, focal lesions which are difficult to manage because of their location and intimate relationship to major vascular structures. Although therapeutic goals for these lesions includes surgical resection for cure, this is often not possible and palliation becomes the priority. During the last 15 years, the management of patients with extrahepatic biliary obstruction whether secondary to a benign or a malignant process, has been greatly influenced by innovative advances and developments in interventional radiology and endoscopy as well as in surgical techniques including transplantation. These advances when coupled with our increasing understanding of the effects of hyperbiliru-binemia on renal, hemodynamic, and immune function have greatly facilitated our care of these challenging and often frustrating patients. This chapter focuses on clinical strategies for the management of patients with benign or malignant biliary strictures. Decision making should be based on a number of factors including etiology, location, and clinical setting.

PRINCIPLES OF MANAGEMENT

Therapeutic Goals

The vast majority of patients with either benign or malignant strictures present with jaundice and hyperbilirubinemia. Management priorities include definition of the pathologic process, relief of jaundice, assessment for resection if appropriate, and internal biliary drainage if possible.

Hyperbilirubinemia can result from primary hepatocellular pathology or as a consequence of extrahepatic biliary obstruction. This distinction can often be made based on clinical history, examination, and simple serum studies. In patients with a presumptive diagnosis of biliary obstruction, noninvasive imaging with either ultrasonography or computed tomography (CT scan) should be employed initially to define the presence and level of biliary dilatation and also to exclude any masses. In patients with an intact gallbladder, the identification of a collapsed gallbladder indicates a lesion proximal to the cystic duct—common bile duct junction, whereas a distended gallbladder suggests the blockage is distal to this site. The presence of fluid or a mass may be of particular help in defining the problem in patients with an unrecognized bile duct injury or a tumor.

The next step in the diagnostic schema is often the definition of biliary anatomy. This can be most readily accomplished by either a percutaneous transhepatic cholangiogram (PTHC) or an endoscopic retrograde cholangiopancreatogram (ERCP). The decision to proceed with one or the other of these modalities is dependent on presumed location and etiology of the suspected lesion. Precise definition of the anatomic defect allows for appropriate therapeutic intervention, which may be accomplished either radiologically, endoscopically, surgically, or by a combination of one or more of these methods.

Percutaneous Biliary Drainage

A number of early studies have correlated the degree of hyperbilirubinemia with outcome following surgery. These observations prompted the investigation of the role of preoperative transhepatic biliary drainage (PTBD) as an adjunctive therapy in patients with obstructive jaundice. Although early anecdotal reports suggested some benefit, prospective, randomized, controlled studies failed to support this observation. While PTBD should not be routinely employed in all patients with benign or malignant biliary strictures, it may be of enormous benefit in selected patients.

POSTOPERATIVE BILIARY STRICTURES

Most series indicate that the incidence of bile duct injury and/or stricture associated with open cholecystectomy is 0.1 to 0.2 percent. Recent experience with laparoscopic cholecystectomy suggests that the incidence of this complication is probably fivefold as frequent in this setting. Therapeutic options and strategies for the management of these patients should be based on the nature of the injury, timing of recognition, and local expertise.

Timing of Recognition

Intraoperative

Unfortunately, most bile duct injuries are not recognized acutely and are discovered later when they are manifested as strictures. If injury to the bile duct is recognized during cholecystectomy, the surgeon should assess the situation in terms of his own ability to deal with the problem. In general, bile duct injuries that are discovered during surgery should be dealt with immediately. The nature and extent of injury, as well as its anatomic location, should be carefully determined. Goals of repair are to maintain proximal duct length and viability with minimal sacrifice of tissue and to minimize the chance of a postoperative anastomotic leak or fistula. There is growing evidence that a well-done reconstruction at the time of initial injury may have a greater chance of success than operations performed subsequently. Surgeons who are not experienced in complicated biliary reconstructions may opt to provide external biliary drainage by means of proximal intubation and then refer the patient for definitive management to a center with experience in the complexities of these problems.

Early Postoperative

Most iatrogenic injuries to the bile duct are recognized within days or weeks after the index operation and are manifest by bile peritonitis, biliary fistula, or jaundice. The goals for managing patients with bile peritonitis and/or fistula are similar and focus on the need to establish good drainage and control of the biliary leak. This can often be accomplished by the judicious placement of tubes, either percutaneously or endoscopically, without resorting to surgical intervention. Anecdotal experience points to the efficacy of endoscopic stent placement with and without biliary sphincterotomy in patients with blown cystic duct stumps or lateral ductal injuries. In one series, 40 of 52 patients with biliary fistulae (77 percent) were successfully managed in this fashion without need for surgery. As with other clinical settings the duration that a stent should be left in place for these patients remains controversial and has not been well defined. Transhepatic tubes are of particular benefit in controlling biliary leaks in patients with transection of the bile duct. Early definitive repair may not be feasible in these patients due to the associated inflammation, and the goal should be long-term external drainage. The status of the leak and resolution of the inflammatory process can be monitored by clinical course and periodic fistulography or transhepatic cholangiography. In patients with jaundice following cholecystectomy, it is important to define the etiology—retained stones, biliary fistula, transected or ligated bile duct. Complete transection of the bile duct (Fig. 1) will require early operation, although often the situation may be temporized if necessary, by transhepatic tube placement. In this situation, biliary reconstruction with Roux-en-Y hepaticojejunostomy is the preferred treatment.

Delayed Presentation

Occasionally, bile duct strictures do not become manifest until months or even years after an injury to the

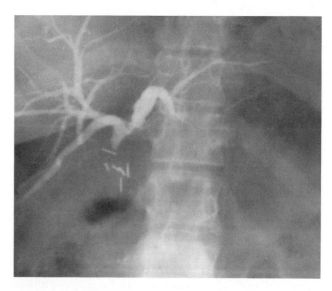

Figure 1 Complete transection of common bile duct.

duct during cholecystectomy or some other abdominal procedure. In virtually all of these delayed situations, the presenting symptom is jaundice. The diagnosis and location of the stricture is most readily confirmed by transhepatic cholangiography or ERCP (Fig. 2). The potential role of PTBD for these patients has been discussed previously. The goal of any intervention should be to re-establish bile flow into the proximal gastrointestinal tract. Depending on the site of the stricture, this may be theoretically accomplished by surgery, nonoperative balloon dilatation, or endoprostheses. Distal lesions are most amenable to direct surgical repair and bypass. More proximal lesions, particularly Grade IV strictures as defined by Blumgart are especially challenging, and may be best treated by stent placement (Fig. 3, *A* and *B*).

Surgical Procedures

The goal of reoperative surgery for biliary strictures should be to re-establish bile flow into the proximal gastrointestinal tract with a tension-free anastomosis. Optimal surgical management is facilitated by the preoperative placement of at least one and sometimes bilateral percutaneous transhepatic tubes. These tubes help the surgeon identify the bile duct and separate it

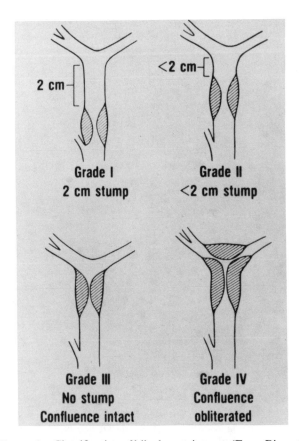

Figure 2 Classification of bile duct strictures. (From Bismuth H. In: Blumgart LH, ed. The biliary tract. Vol 5. New York: Churchill Livingstone, 1982; with permission.)

from other structures in the hepatoduodenal ligament. Specific principles include (1) adequate exposure of the ductal system, (2) satisfactory drainage of all segments of the liver, (3) excision of scar tissue from the duct so as to insure adequate blood supply, and (4) performance of mucosa to mucosa anastomosis between defunctionalized limb of bowel and bile duct in tension-free setting. Over the years, a number of surgical options have been proposed. These have included end-to-end choledochojejunostomy, loop choledochojejunostomy, choledochoduodenostomy, and intrahepatic cholangiojejunostomy. Most experienced biliary surgeons now recommend that a Roux-en-Y hepaticojejunostomy be performed. This procedure avoids a large amount of reflux of enteric contents into the biliary system. Occasionally, this procedure will not be feasible and a mucosal graft biliary reconstruction, as described by Lord Smith, can be performed. Recent reports indicate that the success rate with conventional surgical reconstruction ranges from 75 to 88 percent. In a review of 185 consecutive patients with bile duct strictures managed by surgery at UCLA between 1955 and 1980, a good to excellent outcome was achieved in 80 percent.

The issue of whether to stent all biliary reconstructions performed for benign strictures continues to be controversial. Although some authors state that the size of the duct dictates the need for a stent, we routinely stent all cases. Placement of a transanastomotic tube not only helps to maintain patency, but also decompresses the biliary tree in the event of a leak, and provides access to the biliary tract for postoperative cholangiography. The length of time that stents should be left in place has also been the subject of some debate. Data from the recent UCLA study indicates that stent placement for less than 1 month was associated with approximately a twofold increase in restricturing and need for further therapy. Although these data are not conclusive, we continue to believe that placement and maintenance of long-term stents for 6 to 9 months enhances the likelihood of long-term therapeutic success.

Balloon Dilatation

During the last several years, a number of reports have advocated the use of radiologic or endoscopic balloon dilatation of postoperative benign strictures. Early proponents suggested these modalities had significant theoretical advantages over conventional surgical intervention; obviating the need for reoperation and its associated risks and resulting in better long-term patency. Although initial reports indicated an acceptable success rate of 85 percent with balloon dilatation, further analysis revealed an increasing incidence of recurrent stricture formation that became apparent with longer follow-up. The high rate of recurrent stricture after single balloon dilatation mandates repeated balloon dilatation in most patients being managed in this manner. Many people now believe that transhepatic or retrograde balloon dilatation should be reserved for

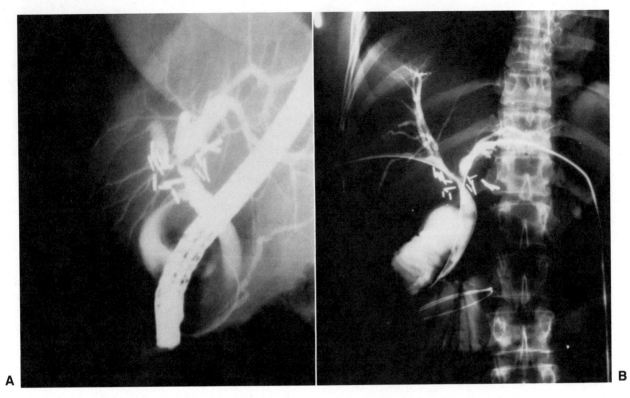

Figure 3 *A,* Proximal bile duct stricture. *B,* After stent placements across stricture.

those patients with stricture of a biliary-enteric anastomosis.

ANASTOMOTIC STRICTURES

Anastomotic strictures after biliary reconstruction present a different problem than primary lesions. Endoscopic access to these lesions is often difficult and a satisfactory resolution of the problem typically requires surgery or radiologic balloon dilatation. In a recent review from Johns Hopkins, long-term success was achieved in only 51 percent of patients undergoing balloon dilatation as compared to 86 percent of patients treated surgically, with a follow-up period of 72 months. In a separate study, balloon dilatation was successful in 13 of 14 patients with anastomotic strictures but in only 50 percent of patients with primary bile duct strictures. These data suggest that balloon dilatation should be reserved for patients with anastomotic strictures or with hilar, right or left hepatic ductal strictures that are not readily amenable to a surgical solution (Fig. 4). The reason for the apparent improved results in patients with anastomotic versus primary strictures is unclear, but is likely due to inherent differences in the nature of these lesions. Anastomotic strictures tend to be short and discrete, and maybe even weblike. In contrast, primary strictures tend to be long and the area of scarring frequently extends far beyond the area where the original stricture is located.

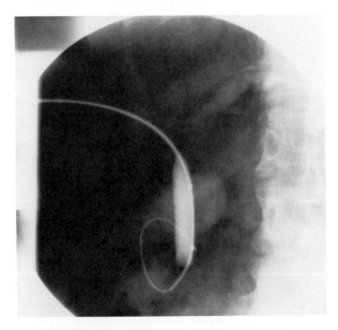

Figure 4 Balloon dilatation of biliary duct stricture.

PRIMARY SCLEROSING CHOLANGITIS

Primary sclerosing cholangitis (PSC) is an unusual idiopathic, inflammatory process, which tends to progress to diffuse intra- and extrahepatic scarring of the biliary ductular system. (There is a separate chapter on this subject.) Although the precise cause of this disorder is unknown, considerable evidence suggests that its pathogenesis is immunologic in nature. Most patients with PSC present with episodic jaundice or cholangitis. While many of these patients have an indolent course, some experience a more fulminant and rapidly progressive disease with death ultimately resulting from complications of biliary sepsis and/or hepatic failure. A myriad of treatments have been proposed including drug therapy, balloon dilatation, aggressive surgical management with resection, and most recently, liver transplantation. The advent and documented role of organ transplantation has revolutionized the approach to this very challenging group of patients. While aggressive surgical management in some patients with primarily extrahepatic PSC may provide good long-term treatment without the risks inherent with hepatic transplantation, it is now being used in only selected cases as it may compromise the ability to subsequently perform a transplant. Aggressive endoscopic treatment with balloon dilatation and stenting may offer a better solution in selected patients, without affecting subsequent transplantation. Whether or not endoscopic management influences the natural history of this disease remains unclear. There is a chapter on endoscopic procedures in patients with PSC.

MALIGNANT STRICTURES

Bile duct tumors account for about 15 to 20 percent of the approximately 15,000 new cases of liver and biliary tract cancer diagnosed each year in the United States. Thus, an estimated 2,250 to 3,750 new cases of bile duct tumors are diagnosed each year. The infrequency with which these tumors are seen and our inability to prospectively evaluate different treatment options, has impaired our ability to precisely define ideal strategies for management. The location of tumors within the extrahepatic biliary tract have been classified according to specific anatomic boundaries. In most large series of patients, over 50 percent of lesions are considered to be upper third: located between the egress of the right and left hepatic ducts from the hepatic parenchyma into the common hepatic duct to the insertion at the level of the cystic duct. Middle third lesions (15 to 20 percent) are those in the area bounded by the cystic–common bile duct junction to the superior border of the pancreas. A similar number of patients have lower third lesions with tumors being identified in the intrapancreatic portion of the common bile duct. Less than 10 percent of these tumors are diffuse in nature.

Management Principles

Definition of the site of obstruction and extent of disease, and delineation of the intra- and extrahepatic ductal system need to be accomplished in order to proceed with the development of a rational therapeutic plan. The goals of management should include relief of

jaundice, tumor resection if possible, and restoration of internal biliary drainage if possible. Alleviating the obstruction and accomplishing these goals can be facilitated by a multidisciplinary approach and appropriate utilization of expertise in surgery, interventional radiology, or endoscopy. The role of adjuvant therapy in the management of patients with malignant strictures remains unclear due to the lack of suitable prospective, randomized, controlled clinical trials. Nonetheless, most experienced clinicians recommend a course of external radiation therapy for patients with bile duct cancer regardless of whether or not a curative resection has been performed.

Upper Third Malignant Strictures

Management of these lesions can be particularly challenging due in large measure to anatomic considerations. The role of aggressive resectional therapy and or transplantation for these patients continues to be ill defined and is controversial. Recent data suggest an improvement in survival for patients undergoing resection of proximal lesions with reconstruction by hepaticojejunostomy. These complicated operations are best carried out at centers with specific expertise in this area. Unfortunately, most patients with hilar lesions are not candidates for resection. Considerable experience indicates that radiologic placement of a single or bilateral transhepatic tube will provide reasonably good palliation. With lesions at this level, endoscopic stent placement is more difficult. Several studies have attempted to address the efficacy of surgical intervention versus radiologic or endoscopic tube placement in providing palliation. Although patient groups may not be completely comparable, data suggests that patients will have less days in the hospital, fewer episodes of cholangitis, and in general a better quality of life when managed surgically. Clearly, the ideal means to palliate a patient with a malignant stricture which is unresectable, must be selected based on the individual circumstances.

Middle and Lower Third Lesions

Curative resection is more likely to be possible for middle and lower third lesions (66 percent) as compared to more proximal lesions (18 percent). In addition, the prognosis and 5 year survival rate is more favorable in the distal lesions. Typically, curative resection requires a pancreaticoduodenectomy, although occasionally, small mid-duct lesions can be locally resected and proximal reconstruction achieved. In patients who are not suitable candidates for resectional therapy, good palliation can often be achieved with either radiologic or endoscopically-placed stents (Fig. 5).

New innovations in biliary endoprostheses have allowed for satisfactory internal drainage of bile without the need for external catheters. Early experience focused on plastic catheters. In more recent years, their use has been limited by problems with recurrent occlusion and episodic cholangitis. Larger diameter

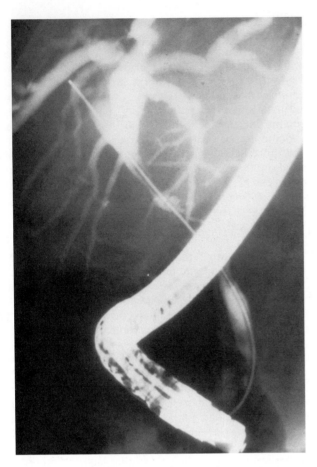

Figure 5 Bile duct stenting.

expandable metallic stents have been developed. These include the Gianturco Z stent, Strecker stent, and most recently the self-expanding Wallstent. This latter stent is delivered on an *8-Fr gauge system and expands to 30-Fr gauge in its fully expanded form. The primary theoretical advantage of this stent over more conventional stents is the avoidance of stent exchanges. Preliminary studies suggest that this type of device may prolong the time of stent occlusion and may therefore, be a suitable alternative for the management of patients with unresectable bile duct cancers.

SUGGESTED READING

Adam A, Chetty N, Roddie M, et al. Self-expandable stainless steel endoprostheses for treatment of malignant bile duct obstruction. AJR Am J Roentgenol 1991; 156:321–325.

Huibregtse K, Carr-Locke DL, Cremer M, et al. Biliary stent occlusion – a problem solved with self-expanding metal stents? Endoscopy 1992; 24:391–394.

Lillemoe KD, Pitt HA, Cameron JL. Primary sclerosing cholangitis. Surg Clin North Am 1990; 70:1381–1402.

Millis JM, Tompkins RK, Zinner MJ, et al. Management of bile duct strictures: An evolving strategy. Arch Surg 1992; 127:1077–1084.

Morrison MC, Lee MJ, Saini A, et al. Percutaneous balloon dilatation of benign biliary strictures. Radiol Clin North Am 1990; 28: 1191–1201.

Pitt HA, Kaufman SL, Coleman J, et al. Benign postoperative biliary strictures: Operate or dilate? Ann Surg 1989; 210:417–427.

Tompkins RK, Saunders K, Roslyn JJ, Longmire WP Jr. Changing patterns in diagnosis and management of bile duct cancer. Ann Surg 1990; 211:614–621.

PERCUTANEOUS MANAGEMENT OF BILIARY TRACT DISORDERS

SCOTT J. SAVADER, M.D.

INDICATIONS

The primary role of percutaneous biliary drainage (PBD) is to relieve biliary tract obstruction in patients with benign or malignant disease of the intra or extrahepatic biliary system. While PBD is used most commonly to relieve obstructive jaundice in patients with malignant disease, its indications have expanded greatly over the years and many benign biliary tract disorders can now effectively be treated without surgery, using only percutaneous interventional techniques. In patients without parenchymal disease, the serum bilirubin level can be expected to decrease by 50 percent in 7 to 15 days after PBD, depending on the type of drainage system and the French (Fr) size of the drain. Other liver function tests such as alanine aminotransferase, aspartate aminotransferase, and alkaline phosphatase can be expected to improve concurrently.

PBD is used in patients with benign disease to relieve obstruction secondary to strictures, to provide improved drainage in cases of iatrogenic or traumatic bile duct injury which result in bile leakage, and to provide access to the biliary tract for adjunctive therapy such as percutaneous stone removal and stricture dilatation.

In patients with malignant disease, PBD is used to relieve obstruction of the intrahepatic and extrahepatic biliary tree secondary to tumor. When jaundice is a result of extrahepatic cholestasis, death most commonly occurs from progressive liver failure rather than from tumor involvement of the liver or metastatic disease. Thus, re-establishment of bile flow with biliary decompression is absolutely necessary. In addition to a marked improvement in liver function tests, pruritus is relieved and patient comfort and overall health are improved. PBD may be utilized as the primary palliative procedure in patients with one or more of the following findings: (1) a prohibitively high surgical risk; (2) tumor shown to be unresectable based on computed tomography (CT), magnetic resonance imaging (MRI), and angiographic criteria; (3) metastatic disease; (4) metastatic obstruction of the extrahepatic biliary tree; (5) primary biliary duct tumor with extension into both the right and left lobes of the liver; and (6) patients who refuse surgical management. PBD may also be used as part of a two-stage therapeutic procedure when surgical resection for cure or palliation is planned.

CONTRAINDICATIONS

PBD is absolutely contraindicated in patients with coagulopathies resulting in a significant elevation of the prothrombin time (PT) or partial thromboplastin time (PTT) or a significant decrease in platelet count. We do not perform PBD in patients with either a PT or PTT greater than 1.3 times control or with a platelet count less than 50,000 per microliter. Correction of the coagulopathy with fresh frozen plasma, whole blood, or platelets is required prior to initiation of the procedure. Colonic interposition between the liver and chest or abdominal wall is another absolute contraindication to PBD. This is relatively uncommon and in almost all cases, effective drainage can usually be established through the opposite hepatic lobe. The presence of ascites is a relative contraindication to PBD. Ascites displaces the liver away from the lateral chest and abdominal wall. This results in a greater risk of injury during the initial percutaneous transhepatic cholangiogram (PTC) and catheter placement and greatly increases the incidence of inadvertent catheter dislodgment from the biliary tract. In addition, we have also found it very difficult to prevent constant pericatheter drainage of ascitic fluid regardless of the catheter size. In patients with ascites who require PBD, drainage of the fluid prior to PBD is mandatory.

PATIENT PREPARATION

Patients receive clear liquids only for at least 8 to 12 hours prior to the procedure. Intravenous antibiotics are administered 30 to 60 minutes prior to the procedure. We usually recommend a broad spectrum cephalosporin such as cefoxitin (1 gram) or a combination regimen of ampicillin (0.5 to 1.0 gram) and gentamicin (1 to 1.5 mg per kilogram). In patients with biliary sepsis, triple antibiotic therapy consisting of ampicillin, gentamicin, and metronidazole (15 mg per kilogram loading dose) is

utilized. Vancomycin (500 mg) can be substituted for ampicillin in patients allergic to penicillin and its derivatives. A narcotic such as Demerol or morphine and an anxiolytic such as Valium or Versed are administered about 30 minutes before the procedure. We then use Fentanyl (50 μg aliquots) and Versed (1 mg aliquots) liberally during the procedure to maximize patient comfort. After PBD, antibiotic therapy is continued for 24 hours or until sepsis resolves and the patient remains afebrile for 24 hours. If patients are scheduled to undergo multiple contrast-enhanced procedures (CT, intravenous urography), the total contrast load must be considered as patients can receive a considerable dose of intravenous contrast medium during PBD. This is especially true in patients with nondilated or minimally dilated biliary ductal systems. To avoid the risk of contrast-induced renal failure, multiple procedures involving intravenous contrast should not be scheduled for the same day when possible.

In addition, patients with known allergies to iodinated contrast and those with significant risk factors (e.g., asthma, allergies, cardiac disease, previous documented contrast reaction) require a complete antianaphylactic protocol with steroids and antihistamines. We use methylprednisolone (32 mg by mouth) or Solu-Medrol (100 mg IV) administered 12 and 2 hours prior to the procedure. In addition, an H_2 blocker such as cimetidine (400 mg IV) or famotidine (20 mg IV) is given 2 hours prior to the procedure. Although there are questions as to the actual benefit, nonionic contrast rather than ionic contrast is also used.

TECHNIQUE

The patient is placed in a supine position with the right arm elevated and hand behind the head. Under fluoroscopic control, the patient is instructed to take a deep inspiration so that the most inferior position of the lung can be noted. In most patients, the typical entry site for the catheter is between the tenth and eleventh or eleventh and twelfth intercostal space along the midaxillary line. Once the maximum inspiratory level of the lung is noted, the intercostal space below this is infiltrated with 1 percent lidocaine. A 22 gauge Chiba needle is then passed through the liver towards the midline and parallel to the posterior ribs under fluoroscopic control. The needle is then connected to a syringe of contrast by a short tube and as the needle is slowly withdrawn, contrast is gently injected through the needle. When the needle crosses a bile duct, the distinctive pattern of contrast spreading through the biliary tree is appreciated. About 5 to 10 ml of bile is then drained from the liver and specimens are sent for gram stain and culture and sensitivity. Contrast is used to opacify the biliary tract and delineate the point of obstruction. A second needle is then placed into another duct which is chosen for its relative course and position in relationship to the obstruction. A guidewire is passed through this needle into the biliary tract to "secure access". The needle is removed and a dilator sheath assembly is passed over the guidewire and into the intrahepatic biliary tract. The guidewire and dilator are then removed, leaving the sheath in place. Through the sheath, a 5 Fr hockey stick catheter and angled guidewire are passed into the intrahepatic biliary tree and manipulations of the two in tandem are performed in order to bypass the obstruction. Once the guidewire bypasses the obstruction, the catheter is passed over the guidewire and positioned within the duodenum. The initial guidewire is then removed and a stiff guidewire is passed through the catheter and into the duodenum for final catheter placement. The 5 Fr catheter is removed from the guidewire and an 8.3 Fr Ring biliary catheter is passed over the stiff guidewire and positioned with the distal tip in the duodenum. The Ring biliary catheter is a multi-sidehole catheter and it is positioned so that the most proximal sideholes are at the point where the catheter enters the biliary tree and the distal sideholes are within the duodenum. In 24 to 48 hours, the Ring biliary catheter can be exchanged over a guidewire for a softer, better-tolerated catheter such as a Cope biliary catheter or Percuflex biliary drain. If during the initial procedure we are unable to cross the obstruction, an external biliary drain is left in place and the patient is returned on a subsequent day for a second attempt. In most cases, the obstructing lesion can usually be bypassed at this time. If not, then the patient is left to external drainage.

POST-PBD CARE

After PBD, patients are maintained on external biliary drainage for 24 to 48 hours or until sepsis resolves. A repeat cholangiogram is obtained to fully evaluate the site of obstruction. If the obstruction was not initially crossed, a second attempt is made to cross the obstruction and to establish duodenal drainage. If intervention is planned, the size and type of catheter is appropriately chosen (although up-sizing more than one tube may be required) and the Ring biliary catheter is exchanged. If the patient is to be discharged with a PBD catheter and further therapy is not planned (i.e., unresectable malignancies), the patient returns every 2 to 3 months for a routine biliary tube change. As an alternative, the PBD catheter can be exchanged for an internal polymer endoprosthesis (10 to 12 Fr) or a self-expanding metallic biliary stent (up to 30 Fr).

COMPLICATIONS

Because PBD is an invasive procedure, complications are inevitable, although most patients do relatively well. The most common complication is post-PBD cholangitis which can occur in 13 to 47 percent. This complication can usually be resolved with intravenous antibiotics and change of the patient's biliary drain. Biliary tube migration, blockage, and dislodgment can

occur in up to 23 percent of patients. This can also be handled relatively easily by a simple tube repositioning or change. In addition, fever (11 percent), hemobilia (3.5 to 9.6 percent), pancreatitis (1 to 10 percent), sepsis (3.9 to 8.0 percent), bile hypersecretion with electrolyte imbalance and hypertension (5 percent), leaking ascites (3 percent), bile peritonitis (1 percent), and pleural effusions (1 percent) can occur. Death after PBD in patients with benign disease is exceedingly rare, however, the 30-day mortality rate in patients with malignant disease may range from 3 to 5.6 percent.

TREATMENT OF BENIGN BILIARY TRACT DISEASE

Strictures

Up to 80 percent of benign bile duct strictures are secondary to surgical trauma which occur during operations performed on the ducts (e.g., common duct exploration) or in the vicinity (e.g., laparoscopic cholecystectomy). Other causes of benign bile duct strictures are shown in Table 1. Traditionally, these patients have been managed with surgery, either by primary repair with an end-to-end anastomosis or by creation of a biliary-enteric anastomosis (choledochojejunostomy or hepaticojejunostomy with Roux-en-Y loop). Success rates for surgical repair range from 65 to 90 percent, however, this constitutes a major operation and without long-term biliary stenting, a significant number of patients may experience restenosis. Percutaneous management, though not a benign procedure, offers a reasonable alternative to surgical repair and can be performed through either a surgically created T-tube tract or percutaneous transhepatic or transjejunal tract. Success rates for percutaneous management of biliary strictures ranges from 70 to 78 percent. Although this technique is not as successful as surgical repair, the morbidity and mortality is significantly lower and percutaneous techniques can be repeated multiple times without precluding eventual surgical repair. In addition, percutaneous stricture dilatation may be preferred in patients at high risk for surgical repair, for strictures not amenable to surgical means, and in cases of failed surgical repair.

Regardless of the route chosen for percutaneous therapy, the first step is to gain access to the biliary tract. This is often accomplished transhepatically using standard PBD techniques. Accessing the biliary system retrograde via a tacked Roux-en-Y loop is also possible if the appropriate planning has been taken at the time of surgery. A surgically-created T-tube tract will also serve as an acceptable route, with intervention possible either proximal or distal to the communication with the duct. Once access is gained, the stricture must be crossed. I prefer using a 0.035 inch angled hydrophilic coated guidewire in conjunction with a short 5 Fr hockey stick (JB1) catheter. This combination of catheter and guidewire allows for maximum versatility when trying to cannulate a small orifice which may not be centered

Table 1 Causes of Benign Bile Duct Strictures

Postoperative strictures
Injury at cholecystectomy and common bile duct exploration
Injury at other operative procedures
    Gastrectomy
    Hepatic resection
    Portacaval shunt
    Pancreatic surgery
Biliary-enteric anastomosis

Inflammatory strictures
Chronic pancreatitis
Cholelithiasis and choledocholithiasis
Primary sclerosing cholangitis
Sphincter of Oddi spasm
Duodenal ulcer
Crohn's disease
Bacterial infections
Viral infections (CMV)
Protozoal infection (cryptosporidium)
Parasitic infection (clonorchis, ascaris)
Toxic drugs (chemotherapeutic agents)
Radiation therapy
Graft versus host disease

Miscellaneous
Blunt or penetrating trauma
Congenital
    Isolated stricture
    Choledochal cyst associated stricture(s)

within the duct. The shape of the catheter may have to be altered depending on the anatomy as determined by the cholangiogram. If the stricture cannot be crossed with the hydrophilic guidewire, a small gauge (0.014 inch to 0.016 inch) platinum-tipped coronary guidewire or graduated hydrophilic guidewire (0.020 inch tip, 0.035 inch shaft) can be used. Once the stricture is crossed, a JB1 catheter is passed over the guidewire and into the bowel (or intrahepatic biliary tract in cases utilizing a retrograde approach). The guidewire used to cross the stricture is then exchanged for a stiff guidewire over which serial tract dilatations can be performed. Strictures can be dilated either using serial dilators or a standard balloon angioplasty catheter. I prefer the latter method as it is less traumatic to the stricture itself and requires a smaller access tract. Eventual dilatation of the access tract is usually required prior to final stenting, but this can then be accomplished without repeated trauma to the stricture. Our goal is to eventually place a 16 Fr biliary stent across the stricture, thus we typically dilate ductal strictures with at least a 6 mm balloon. Biliary-enteric anastomoses can be dilated with balloons up to 8 to 10 mm in size. Balloon inflation times vary, but unlike vascular angioplasty, the balloon may be left inflated across the stricture for 5 minutes or more at a time. Dilatations are repeated if necessary based on the postprocedure cholangiogram. Reaching the desired endpoint may require two or three procedures in some patients. A 16 Fr multi-sidehole catheter is positioned across the stricture with sideholes both proximal and distal to allow for internal-external drainage. Patients with hilar, biliary-enteric, or multiple intrahepatic strictures may require multiple catheters simultaneously to achieve adequate drainage and stricture dilatation. The catheter(s) can be internalized within 6 to 8 hours if the patient remains afebrile. Antibiotic therapy is continued for at least 24 hours in all patients.

Patients at our institution are typically stented for at least 1 year as continuous fibrotic healing of the biliary tract can occur for extended periods after therapeutic dilatation. During this period, patients are maintained on internal biliary drainage and routine changing of the biliary stent(s) is performed every 2 to 3 months or should patients become febrile, develop pericatheter bile leakage, or encounter difficulty flushing their stents.

After adequate stenting, the patient's biliary stent(s) are exchanged for modified biliary stent(s) which enter the biliary ducts but do not cross the stricture. A cholangiogram with emphasis on the treated region is obtained. Patients are then discharged for a 2 to 3 week "clinical trial". Patients who become symptomatic, (e.g., right upper quadrant pain, nausea, vomiting, fever, chills) are admitted for replacement of their biliary tube(s) and antibiotic therapy if necessary. Stenting in these patients is extended an additional 6 to 12 months, and often the stent is increased in size to 18 or 20 Fr. Patients who remain asymptomatic during the clinical trial are admitted for a biliary pressure-flow study analogous to the renal Whitaker test.

To perform this test, the patient's biliary stents (which are proximal to the treated region) are connected to an automatic injector and 50 percent contrast material is injected at a rate of 1.9, 3.8, 7.6, 15, and 20 ml per minute for 5, 5, 5, 3, and 2 minutes respectively. Intrahepatic pressure is continuously monitored in patients with more than one tube and at the end of each injection period in patients with only one tube. Normal intrahepatic pressure should remain less than 20 cm water throughout the test. Based on this exam and the cholangiographic appearance of the treated stricture, the patient's tubes may be removed or additional stenting may be necessary. Patients who fail this test two times are probably best treated surgically if possible. The use of this test as a predictor of long-term patency in these patients is still new and we continue to collect data in order to better assess its value.

Cumulative results from multiple studies indicate that at a 3 year follow-up, percutaneously-treated biliary duct strictures have a primary patency rate of 67 to 87.5 percent for anastomotic primary biliary duct strictures and 72.5 to 76 percent for iatrogenic primary bile duct strictures, yielding an overall success rate of 70 to 78 percent.

Biliary Stone Disease

About 600,000 cholecystectomies are performed each year in the United States. Of these patients, 30,000 (5 percent) experience retained or recurrent common duct stones. Nonoperative management is the treatment of choice. Methods of nonoperative stone extraction include (1) percutaneous stone extraction (through T-tube tract if available); (2) percutaneous electrohydraulic lithotripsy; (3) chemodissolution with stone solvents; (4) extracorporeal shock wave lithotripsy; (5) endoscopic sphincterotomy with stone extraction; and (6) combined therapy utilizing more than one of the above-mentioned procedures. All of these methods except endoscopic sphincterotomy are available to the interventional radiologist, however this section focuses on percutaneous extraction utilizing stone retrieval baskets.

Retained bile duct stones are usually detected on the postoperative cholangiogram. Four to 6 weeks are typically allowed for T-tube tract maturation prior to percutaneous techniques, however, we have performed T-tube tract dilatation in preparation for peripheral stone removal as early as 3 weeks. If a transhepatic tract is to be used, PBD is performed on day 1 with placement of an 8.3 Fr Ring biliary catheter, followed by tract dilatation (up to 16 Fr) on day 2, and stone extraction on day 3. Using standard interventional techniques, a safety wire and working wire are passed into the duodenum using a sheath carefully sized to allow for stone removal. If it is desired to push the stones into the bowel, the tract does not need to be as large (10 to 12 Fr), but a sphincterotomy should be performed prior to attempting stone removal. If this has not been done, the ampulla can be dilated with a 10 mm angioplasty balloon passed over the safety wire. After the calculi are located on an air-free preprocedure cholangiogram, a 5 Fr JB1 catheter and guidewire are steered to the calculus via the PBD or T-tube tract. Initial attempts at flushing the stone fragments from the ducts can be made by attaching the catheter to a power flush of 20 to 30 percent contrast at 10 to 15 ml per second and directing the catheter either at or just beyond the stones. Once stones are flushed into the common bile duct distal to the catheter tip, the 5 Fr catheter is removed and a balloon catheter is passed over the working guidewire, inflated gently, and used to push the stones beyond the ampulla. If flushing does not result in passage of stone fragments into the distal common bile duct, a torque-control catheter is manipulated adjacent to the calculi and a stone basket (e.g., Burhenne, Dormia, Segura, etc.) is passed through the guiding catheter and used to entrap the calculus. Basket size and shape are matched to the size of the calculus and anatomy of the biliary system. The guiding catheter with the snared stone is then passed beyond the ampulla where the stone is released or it can be removed through the transhepatic or T-tube tract if size allows. Three-prong graspers or alligator forceps passed through a guiding catheter may also be utilized in a similar fashion. After completion of the stone removal, a multi-sidehole drainage catheter is placed across the ampulla and left to external drainage for 12 to 24 hours. Antibiotic therapy should also be continued during this period. A repeat cholangiogram is obtained in 2 to 4 days. If stones are still present, the procedure is repeated electively; if stones are not present and the intrahepatic biliary tree is also clear of residual stones, the catheter is removed.

The morbidity associated with percutaneous stone removal is about 4 to 5 percent. In two large series totaling 1,231 patients, no deaths were reported. Potential complications include tract perforation, which in most cases can be avoided by using sheaths to remove the stones. Vasovagal reactions may occur following advancement of large stones through the ampulla or when pulling stones through small tracts that are not sheathed. This can be avoided by breaking up large stones into multiple fragments and, again, using sheaths to remove the stones. Fever and sepsis are avoided with proper antibiotic therapy before and after the procedure. Pancreatitis has been documented to occur after manipulations near or trauma to the pancreatic duct. Judicious use of proper stone removal techniques combined with stone fragmentation and minimal, unnecessary stone basket manipulation can help minimize the incidence of this complication. Subhepatic bile collections can occur following an extremely traumatic procedure resulting in extrahepatic bile duct laceration. Again, this is avoided by fragmenting larger stones and using reasonable care when trying to push stones through the common duct and ampulla.

Bile Leaks

Leakage of bile into the peritoneum may occur after blunt or penetrating trauma, iatrogenic bile duct injury, surgery to create a biliary-enteric anastomosis, or liver transplantation. The function of PBD is the same, in principle, in each of these cases: (1) stent the injured area until healing occurs, (2) divert bile away from the injured site, and (3) provide a method for detailed anatomic monitoring of the healing process. These leaks may be significant and in some patients take weeks to resolve. In addition, some patients may require a second drainage catheter within the biloma itself in order to provide the degree of biliary diversion required to facilitate healing of the injury.

Bile duct injuries may occur in 0.1 to 0.2 percent and 0.5 percent of patients who undergo conventional and laparoscopic cholecystectomy, respectively. Trerotola, et al reported on a series of 13 patients who had undergone laparoscopic cholecystectomy and experienced a ductal injury. Six patients (46 percent) presented with postoperative bilomas or bile leaks. Of these, two (33 percent) were managed effectively by percutaneous means alone, thus avoiding a second operation. In almost all such cases, patients can undergo a trial of PBD before repeat surgery.

After liver transplantation, bile duct complications can occur in up to 26 percent of patients. Postoperative leaks from the common bile duct anastomosis are not common, but if severe, can result in significant morbidity. PBD is the preferred method of handling this complication, and in most cases, will successfully decompress the biliary system adequately enough to promote healing.

Sclerosing Cholangitis

Primary sclerosing cholangitis is an idiopathic inflammatory disease characterized by fibrous strictures of the extrahepatic and intrahepatic bile ducts. Approximately 50 percent of cases are associated with inflammatory bowel disease, suggesting an immune etiology, although multiple mechanisms of injury most likely play a role in its manifestations. The clinical presentation is variable. Most frequently, patients experience right upper quadrant pain, intermittent jaundice, pruritus, and fatigue. Patients may experience mild or severe symptoms with repeated exacerbations, extended periods of quiescence, or even remission. Cholangiographic evaluation performed by either endoscopic retrograde cholangiopancreatography (ERCP) or PTC offers the most sensitive method for evaluating the progress of the disease. Diffuse involvement of both the extrahepatic and intrahepatic biliary tract is by far the most common pattern.

PBD is used to decompress the obstructed biliary tree in cases of symptomatic cholestasis and biliary sepsis. Since the common hepatic duct bifurcation is very commonly involved, bilateral PBD catheters are often required. However, since the disease tends to be diffuse, segmental areas of ductal obstruction may occur regardless of how many drainage catheters are placed. Balloon dilatation of the strictured ductal segments has been tried with limited success. Multiple dilatations are usually required, restricturing commonly occurs, and the most severely affected areas may simply be inaccessible due to anatomic location and the severity of the disease.

Aggressive surgical therapy consists of resection of the involved extrahepatic biliary tree usually at the bifurcation with long-term transhepatic intubation with 16 Fr or larger Silastic stents. The biliary stents are maintained indefinitely with routine changes every 2 to 3 months or more frequently, if needed. Treatment with this protocol has yielded an actuarial survival rate of 77 percent at 5 years. Patients with primary sclerosing cholangitis and documented biliary cirrhosis require liver transplantation. In this group of patients, the 1 and 3 year survival rates are 71 percent and 57 percent, respectively.

Pancreatitis

Pancreatitis in both the acute and chronic forms is a relatively uncommon cause of biliary obstruction. In a review of multiple series in which 132 patients with benign biliary obstruction were evaluated, only one (0.8 percent) had pancreatitis as the etiology of their stricture. In patients with only a single episode of pancreatitis, biliary tract obstruction is exceedingly uncommon. Strictures of the common bile duct occur more frequently in patients with chronic pancreatitis. These patients may present with typical signs and symptoms of biliary tract obstruction in addition to those of pancreatitis. In these patients, ERCP is more commonly performed than PTC for evaluation of the extrahepatic biliary tree and pancreatic duct. In those

uncommon cases in which obstruction of the extrahepatic biliary tree is demonstrated, a polymer stent would most likely be placed from an endoscopic approach. This also applies to those cases in which a pancreatic duct obstruction is noted (unless surgery is the desired method of treatment). However, PBD is an option in patients with both acute and chronic pancreatitis. In patients with acute disease, PBD is used to maintain biliary-enteric continuity and prevent critical ductal stricturing during the healing phase of the disease. PBD would most likely be maintained for 6 to 12 weeks after resolution of the inflammatory process. In patients with chronic disease, PBD may be used in conjunction with balloon dilatation. Long-term stenting in the 6- to 12-month range would most likely be necessary to salvage the extrahepatic biliary tree.

Patients with pancreatitis far more commonly develop pancreatic duct obstruction. Although this is usually treated endoscopically and surgically, percutaneous techniques are an option. In patients with chronic pancreatic duct strictures and moderate to significant pancreatic duct dilatation, the pancreatic duct can be cannulated percutaneously from an anterior approach, using either ultrasound or CT as the guiding modality. After cannulation of the pancreatic duct, typical catheter and guidewire manipulations are used to cross the stricture and obtain duodenal access. Balloon dilatation of the stricture can then be performed followed by stenting using either a biliary drainage type catheter or a balloon expanded or self-expanding metallic stent. The advantage of this technique over the more commonly pursued surgical approach is that it is far less invasive and has a lower morbidity and mortality rate. The disadvantage is that eventual blockage of the stents can occur secondary to sludging or endothelial overgrowth, and even though recannulization can be performed, this technique at the present time is best reserved for those patients unsuitable for more conventional intervention.

TREATMENT OF MALIGNANT BILIARY TRACT DISEASE

The most common causes of malignant biliary tract obstruction are shown in Table 2. Regardless of the etiology of the obstruction, the goal of PBD in patients with malignant disease is to relieve obstructive jaundice, thus decreasing the risk of biliary sepsis and liver failure. PBD can provide dramatic relief with marked improvement (50 percent decrease) in serum bilirubin and liver function tests within 7 to 15 days. One PBD catheter is usually sufficient for patients with infrahilar disease, however, patients with hilar obstruction will most likely require both a right and left biliary stent for adequate decompression. Because the size of the left lobe is so variable, I always obtain a CT scan of the liver prior to left lobe drainage in order to avoid inadvertent transgastric or transcolonic catheter placement. Patients with intrahepatic metastatic disease are not candidates for PBD as poor liver function in this group is more likely

Table 2 Causes of Malignant Bile Duct Strictures

Primary tumors
Pancreatic carcinoma
Cholangiocarcinoma
Gallbladder carcinoma
Ampullary and duodenal carcinoma
Hepatoma

Metastatic disease
Pancreatic carcinoma
Colon carcinoma
Breast carcinoma
Melanoma
Lung carcinoma
Ovarian carcinoma

secondary to parenchymal disease rather than obstructive jaundice. In addition, the number of lesions present usually renders PBD impractical.

Preoperative PBD has been demonstrated by some authors to significantly decrease operative morbidity and mortality; however, other studies have not shown this to be the case. Surgeons at our institution use percutaneously placed biliary stents in patients with malignant disease as an aid in surgical reconstruction. PBD catheters are used to provide anatomic landmarks for the extrahepatic biliary system. This can be extremely helpful in patients with large bulky tumors. In addition, the presence of the PBD catheters allow surgical dissection deep into the liver hilum by simply following the course of the stents. After surgical resection of the tumor has been performed, a Roux-en-Y loop is formed over the stents prior to closure of the biliary-enteric anastomosis. During the early postoperative period (less than 30 days), the stents provide access to the surgical site for evaluation of any complications (e.g., minor leaks, anastomotic dehiscence) and prevent biliary-enteric anastomotic stricturing from edema or early scarring. In the late postoperative period (greater than 30 days) the stents prevent stricture formation at the biliary-enteric anastomosis caused by the extensive fibrotic scarring common to this area. In addition, biliary-enteric continuity is maintained in those patients who prove to have disease unresectable for cure and allows for close monitoring of tumor recurrence at the surgical site in patients resected for "cure". In this last group, stenting is typically maintained for 1 to 2 years during which time routine tube changes are performed every 2 to 3 months on an outpatient basis, concurrent with noninvasive imaging.

In patients who are not surgical candidates because of the extent of their disease, percutaneous biliary decompression performed for palliation has several advantages over surgical decompression, including a shorter hospital stay, decreased costs, the ability to use local and intravenous analgesia versus general anesthesia, and a markedly decreased mortality rate of 3 percent versus 20 to 30 percent for surgical decompression. Percutaneous biliary decompression is not without risks, however. This group of patients can experience the same types of complications as those previously mentioned for patients with benign disease, and in addition, a 30-day mortality rate of up to 5.6 percent. Debilitated patients may find having an external drainage tube inconvenient or psychologically wearing, because they are continuously reminded of the presence of their disease. Patients in whom duodenal access is not obtained will also have to wear an external drainage bag indefinitely, which can be very demanding in terms of tube care, drainage bag care, and oral bile salt and fluid replacement, in addition to the psychological stress involved. Despite the benefits of internal-external biliary drainage catheters, including the ease with which these catheters can be replaced should they become obstructed, patients with a relatively short life expectancy who are treated for palliation only, may benefit greater from internal biliary drainage with either a polymer or metallic endoprosthesis.

More specifically, internal biliary prostheses are indicated for the following group of patients: (1) those with tumor involving the biliary tract which is unresectable for cure, with an associated short predicted life span; (2) those with terminal stage disease metastatic to the porta hepatis with biliary obstruction, and (3) those with obstructive jaundice secondary to tumor involvement of the extrahepatic biliary tree who are incapable of providing for themselves routine tube and bile-collecting bag care, or those in a setting such as a nursing home where this care cannot be provided for them. In patients meeting these criteria, conversion from an internal-external type drainage catheter to an internal biliary prosthesis can be very desirable. Improvement in the overall quality of life can occur as the daily maintenance requirements of external biliary drainage catheters are eliminated. In addition, patients are no longer at risk for local skin infections (where biliary catheters exit the liver), pericatheter bile leakage, or rib erosion.

The endoprosthesis may be placed from either a transhepatic approach as an extension of PBD, or an endoscopic technique may be used. PBD-directed placement of an endoprosthesis is most desirable in patients with intrahepatic, hilar, or common hepatic duct obstruction, whereas ERCP-directed placement is most applicable with low-lying unresectable tumors. In these patients, ERCP, sphincterotomy, and retrograde stent placement can usually be accomplished in one procedure.

The polymer endoprostheses typically range in size from 10 to 12 Fr. Smaller prostheses tend to encrust and occlude at too great a rate (3 to 6 months) to be useful for long-term drainage. Larger polymer endoprostheses ranging in size from 14 to 24 Fr have not demonstrated patency rates that are significantly improved over those achieved with the smaller 10 to 12 Fr endoprostheses. In addition, when placed transhepatically, larger endoprostheses are associated with increased complication rates. Recently, metallic self-expanding biliary stents have been developed for patient use. These stents typically consist of a woven or soldered wire device formed into a tubular structure. Each stent has a predetermined radial expansile force and maximum diameter which is dependent on the wire gauge, the length of the legs, and the number of legs on the stent (or density of wire weave). These stents are low profile (7 to 10 Fr) for improved ease and decreased trauma during placement. Because of their low profile, these stents can usually be placed at the same time the initial PBD is performed. Upon release from the guiding catheter, these stents self-expand from 30 to 36 Fr (depending on design and manufacture) in the fully-open position. Even though these stents are obviously of a much greater caliber than the typical polymer designed endoprosthesis, the long-term patency rates have been disappointingly low as a result of multiple factors including mucosal hyperplasia from stent irritation of the biliary endothelium and tumor ingrowth through the walls of the stent. Additional modifications of these metallic stents will most likely be necessary in order to improve their long-term patency rates and justify their increased cost. Metallic self-expanding stents are also discussed in the chapters on Budd-Chiari syndrome and on palliation of esophageal carcinoma.

The most significant complications which occur during percutaneous placement of biliary endoprostheses include hepatic vascular injuries, bilomas, hematomas, and abscess formation. These complications occur at a collective incidence of approximately 10 percent. These complications tend to be more a direct result of the PBD rather than actual placement of the endoprosthesis itself. A 30 day mortality rate has been reported, ranging from 26 to 32 percent in patients with terminal disease. Patency rates for biliary endoprostheses are difficult to determine because many patients die after a short time, often before occlusion of the stent has occurred. Various studies have noted occlusion rates ranging from 18.5 percent at 24 weeks up to 30 percent at 1 year. When polymer endoprostheses become obstructed, most can be exchanged relatively easily using endoscopic techniques.

SUGGESTED READING

Castaneda-Zuniga WR, Irving JD, Herrera MA, et al. Interventional techniques in the hepatobiliary system. In: Castaneda-Zuniga WR, Tadavarthy SM, eds. Interventional radiology. 2nd ed. Baltimore: Williams and Wilkins, 1992:1053.

Gordon RL, Shapiro HA. Nonoperative management of bile duct stones. Surg Clin North Am 1990; 70:1313–1328.

Irving JD, Adams A, Dick R, et al. Gianturco expandable metallic biliary stents: Results of a European clinical trial. Radiology 1989; 172:321–326.

Klein AS, Savader SJ, Burdick JF, et al. Reduction of morbidity and mortality from biliary complications after liver transplantation. Hepatology 1991; 14:818–823.

Lillemoe KD, Pitt HA, Cameron JL. Primary sclerosing cholangitis. Surg Clin North Am 1990; 70:1381–1402.

Lillemoe KD, Pitt HA, Cameron JL. Current management of benign bile duct strictures. Adv Surg 1992; 25:119–174.

Mathieson JR, Cooperberg PL, Murray DJ, et al. Pancreatic duct obstruction treated with percutaneous antegrade insertion of a metal stent: Report of two cases. Radiology 1992; 185:465–467.

McLean GK, Burke DR. Role of endoprostheses in the management of malignant biliary obstruction. Radiology 1989; 170:961–967.

Trerotola SO, Savader SJ, Lund GB, et al. Biliary duct complications following laparoscopic cholecystectomy: Imaging and intervention. Radiology 1992; 184:195–200.

Yee ACN, Ho CS. Complications of percutaneous biliary drainage: Benign vs malignant disease. AJR 1987; 148:1207–1209.

ENDOSCOPIC MANAGEMENT OF BILE DUCT OBSTRUCTION AND SPHINCTER OF ODDI DYSFUNCTION

QAZI E. KHUSRO, M.B., Ch.B.
GLEN A. LEHMAN, M.D.

Endoscopic retrograde cholangiopancreatography (ERCP) has undergone major transformation since its inception. The ability to perform therapy with a lower morbidity than the alternatives such as surgery has led to improved patient care and shorter hospital stays. Techniques such as lithotripsy can help with the management of difficult choledocholithiasis, and sphincter of Oddi manometry may detect an additional cause for biliary-type pain.

INDICATIONS

The American Society for Gastrointestinal Endoscopy guidelines for performing diagnostic ERCP are as follows:

1. Evaluation of the jaundiced patient suspected of having biliary obstruction.
2. Evaluation of the highly symptomatic patient without jaundice whose clinical presentation suggests pancreatic or biliary tract disease.
3. Evaluation of signs and symptoms suggesting pancreatic malignancy when results of indirect imaging, for example, ultrasonography (US), computed tomography (CT), and magnetic resonance imaging (MRI), are equivocal or normal.
4. Evaluation of recurrent or persistent pancreatitis of unknown etiology.
5. Preoperative evaluation of the patient with chronic pancreatitis.

6. Evaluation of possible pancreatic pseudocyst undetected by CT or US and for known pseudocyst prior to planned surgical therapy.
7. Evaluation of the sphincter of Oddi and bile duct by biliary and pancreatic manometry.
8. For endoscopic therapy such as endoscopic sphincterotomy (ES), stent placement, balloon dilation of biliary strictures, and nasobiliary drain placement.

CONTRAINDICATIONS

Contraindications to ERCP include patient refusal, unstable hemodynamic status, and the lack of personnel trained to manage identified disease, especially biliary obstruction. Relative contraindications include poor patient cooperation during the procedure (which can be circumvented by general anesthesia as in the case of children and some adults), coagulopathy, and the lack of appropriate radiologic or surgical backup.

ERCP is generally not indicated in the following circumstances:

1. Evaluation of vague abdominal pain of obscure origin in the absence of objective findings that suggest biliary or pancreatic disease.
2. Evaluation of suspected gallbladder disease without evidence of bile duct disease.
3. As further evaluation of pancreatic malignancy that has been demonstrated by US or CT, unless management will be altered.

COMPLICATIONS

ERCP shares some of the complications that can occur with any upper endoscopic procedure, including reaction to medications, respiratory depression, and perforation. Complications more specific to ERCP and ES include acute pancreatitis, bleeding, and infection and occur in approximately 2 percent and 6 percent of diagnostic and therapeutic studies, respectively. Bleeding can usually be managed endoscopically and small retroperitoneal perforations after ES and pancreatitis can be managed conservatively. The instillation of dye into a closed space (obstructed biliary tree or large pseudocyst) without achieving endoscopic drainage may precipitate serious infection and usually requires help from radiology and, less often, from surgery.

PATIENT PREPARATION

We administer preprocedure antibiotics to all patients, usually a third generation cephalosporin. Penicillin-allergic patients are given ciprofloxacin intravenously. Patients with prosthetic heart valves, history of rheumatic valvular heart disease, or bacterial endocardi-

tis receive the preprocedure antibiotics recommended by the American Heart Association. Recent hemoglobin, platelet count, plasma thromboplastin, partial thromboplastin time, electrolytes, blood urea nitrogen, liver chemistries and amylase are checked. All patients are advised to stop nonsteroidal anti-inflammatory drugs for at least 1 week prior to the procedure, if circumstances allow. During the procedure, patients are monitored for pulse, oxygen saturation, and blood pressure. Sedation is titrated and given according to the type of procedure being performed, with a benzodiazepine alone being used initially if sphincter of Oddi manometry is to be performed.

In jaundiced patients, consent for percutaneous biliary decompression is obtained beforehand in case there is failure to cannulate. A standard video endoscope with a 2.8 mm biopsy channel is used in most cases, including manometry, and the 4.2 mm biopsy channel endoscope is used for biliary stenting.

Endoscopic views of the esophagus, stomach, and duodenum are obtained with the side-viewing instrument. The papilla and adjacent duodenal wall are carefully examined for signs of extrinsic pressure, tumors, or ulceration. The size and patency of the papillary orifice is noted. If indicated, manometry is performed first before any drugs expected to alter sphincter pressure or duodenal motility are administered. The intraductal position of the catheter is generally confirmed by aspirating bile or clear pancreatic juice or by contrast injection, and full ductography is performed with the manometry catheter. Pancreatograms are obtained with 60 percent meglumine diatrizoate. If the main interest is the pancreatic duct, filling of secondary branches is obtained, with the aim of minimizing the chances of acinarization, by slow injection and fluoroscopic monitoring. Cholangiograms are obtained with half-strength contrast to allow for better visualization of stones. Early films with minimal ductal filling are recommended. Dye will often flow into an intact gallbladder preferentially. In this case the catheter may be moved proximally into the common hepatic duct, the contrast is injected more rapidly, and the patient tilted head-down 10 to 20 degrees. Although ERCP does not provide optimal images of the gallbladder, if it is to be studied radiographs should be taken at early stages of filling, because a large amount of contrast may obscure intraluminal lesions. Delayed films of the gallbladder (4 to 8 hours) may detect small stones. In patients with an intact gallbladder, nonfilling indicates obstruction of the cystic duct due to stone or tumor.

TECHNIQUES OF CANNULATION

The papilla is initially viewed in the upper half of the field when cannulation of the bile duct is attempted. Occasionally, the papilla is hidden behind a fold or is located on the rim of a diverticulum. The cannulating catheter may be used to manipulate the folds or pull the papilla out of the diverticulum. Engaging the catheter into the papilla from below will help select for the bile duct. The endoscope is then shortened, tipping the catheter somewhat downwards and aiming it perpendicular to the duodenal wall. At this point, if cannulation of the bile duct has been obtained, contrast will be seen to fill the duct. The catheter can then be inserted deeper using information from both the fluoroscopic and endoscopic views. The catheter will readily slide in when it is aligned with the axis of the bile duct. Pushing on the papilla without satisfactory alignment is usually counterproductive as it leads to further distortion of the anatomy.

Alternative approaches that we use to obtain selective deep cannulation include the use of a papillotome and the use of a guide wire. An initial cholangiogram, perhaps obtained by cannula impaction only, may be helpful in determining the precise cannulating angle. A partly bowed papillotome may be used to give additional upwards curvature to the catheter. The endoscope is then pulled back into a shorter position while simultaneously relaxing the amount of bow on the catheter and withdrawing it. This decreases the cephalad angle on the tip, generally allowing it to advance into the bile duct. A 0.035-inch guide wire with 3 to 4 mm protruding from the tip of a catheter or sphincterotome can also be used to cannulate selectively. The wire is gently advanced under fluoroscopy until it is deeply seated.

With the use of these techniques, precutting papillotomy is needed infrequently. We use it when deep cannulation of the bile duct is considered necessary, for example, in order to enter a definitely obstructed biliary tree. We generally use a needleknife and initiate cutting at the papillary orifice, extending cutting for 6 to 8 mm in a 12 o'clock direction. The depth of the cut is determined by the length of the wire protruding from the sheath and should be limited to 3 to 5 mm. An alternative approach is to use a precutting papillotome with the cutting wire starting at or very close to the tip. This allows cutting to be performed with a minimal amount of catheter engaged into the orifice. The problems with either approach are reduced control over the direction and depth of the cut.

Cannulation of the common bile duct may also be difficult because of unusual anatomy. The endoscope may not be able to reach the papilla as in the case of Roux-en-Y surgery. However, successful ERCP can be performed in patients with a previous Billroth II operation, although sphincterotomy is less successful. We initially intubate with the side-viewing duodenoscope; if the first limb entered is not the afferent limb, it is marked with a pinch biopsy. When the afferent limb cannot be intubated, rolling the patient into a supine position and advancing the guidewire and catheter ahead into the lumen may facilitate entry. An alternative is to use a forward-viewing instrument to place a guidewire into the afferent limb, and follow it down with the duodenoscope. The smooth wall of the duodenal bulb is an easy landmark to recognize. The papilla can then be identified by careful examination, bearing in mind that the direction

of the ducts is an upside-down image of the normal orientation, with the bile duct taking off at 6 o'clock and the pancreatic at 1 o'clock. The bile duct is best cannulated with the papilla seen at some distance.

GALLSTONE DISEASE

The gallbladder is usually evaluated by transcutaneous ultrasonography or oral cholecystography. Occasionally (2 to 5 percent), ERCP will find gallbladder stones that were missed by these techniques. Bile can also be aspirated from the duodenum or biliary tree for crystal (microlithiasis) analysis.

Cholelithiasis

Cholecystectomy, especially via laparoscopy, is the main treatment for acute cholecystitis and symptomatic cholelithiasis. Alternatives such as extracorporeal shockwave lithotripsy are less attractive and still leave the gallbladder behind with its risk of reformation of stones and a small risk of gallbladder cancer. Management of ductal stones in the laparoscopic cholecystectomy (LC) era is evolving. Routine use of ERCP before LC is *not* justified as the prevalence of ductal stones is only 5 to 10 percent. We recommend ERCP *before* laparoscopic cholecystectomy for patients with a serum bilirubin, ALT and/or alkaline phosphatase persistently elevated to at least 1.5 times normal. ERCP is also recommended for those patients with common bile duct diameter greater than 8 mm by ultrasonography. The frequency of finding ductal stones correlates with the magnitude of biochemical abnormality, the degree of ductal dilation, and the presence of cholangitis. Acute suppurative cholangitis associated with ductal stones is a serious infection that usually requires urgent drainage of the biliary tree. Such cholangitis can generally not be treated adequately by antibiotics. Surgery, too, has unacceptable mortality rates in the 5 to 20 percent range if performed in the acute, toxic setting. Percutaneous biliary catheter drainage will relieve obstruction and help resolve infection. However, endoscopic sphincterotomy has a high success rate in achieving bile duct clearance (90 percent) and lower mortality. It is considered the procedure of choice for obtaining duct clearance in such patients. If this is not possible, perhaps owing to the presence of stones above a stricture, a biliary stent or nasobiliary catheter should be placed. If cholangitis was the major pathology, the patient should defervesce rapidly and the cholecystectomy may be performed electively. In the absence of rapid improvement, urgent cholecystectomy may be needed for unresolved cholecystitis.

Patients with obvious evidence of cholestasis, but failed ERCP, present a special problem. Such patients may be managed by open cholecystectomy and common duct exploration, percutaneous cholangiography, percutaneous stone extraction techniques, or combined procedure with passage of a percutaneous guidewire into the duodenum and repeat ERCP. Alternatively, the patient may be referred to an ERCP center with more experience. Patients with only minimal evidence of cholestasis, however, can generally be managed by proceeding on to laparoscopy. Intraoperative cholangiography is then performed. Only a small number, perhaps 25 percent, of such patients will have common duct stones in the final analysis. A decision must then again be made as to whether to handle these by duct exploration or passage of a guidewire into the common duct and on into the duodenum for subsequent ERCP extraction.

Once successful duct clearance has been achieved via ES, patients usually undergo elective cholecystectomy, especially after an episode of acute cholecystitis. However, the risk of surgery needs to be viewed in the context of the chances of becoming symptomatic over time. In younger patients (less than 60 years of age) the mortality rate from elective cholecystectomy is less than 0.5 percent, and surgery is generally recommended. Older patients, or patients with multiple medical conditions, will be at a higher risk. Because clinically significant biliary symptoms recur at 3 to 5 percent per year, it appears to be reasonable to defer surgery in patients with multiple medical conditions until such time that they become highly symptomatic again.

Choledocholithiasis (After Cholecystectomy)

The incidence of retained bile duct stones after laparoscopic cholecystectomy is approximately 5 percent. This obviously depends on the aggressiveness with which attempts to clear the duct are made before laparoscopic cholecystectomy. After gallbladder surgery, ERCP is recommended if obvious biliary colic recurs or laboratory evidence suggests cholestasis. Additionally, if intraoperative cholangiography shows residual ductal stones, ERCP and sphincterotomy are recommended.

Postoperative patients with a T-tube or catheter in the bile duct may be managed by percutaneous techniques, once the tract matures over a 4- to 6-week interval. Simple distal bile duct stones can generally be removed by standard percutaneous basketing techniques; however, larger impacted stones may require passage of a small-caliber bronchoscope into the T-tube's tract and laser or electrohydraulic lithotripsy of the stone. (See the preceding chapter for a discussion of percutaneous techniques.) Proceeding with sphincterotomy and stone extraction in such patients is warranted if patients are highly symptomatic during the 4- to 6-week tract maturation interval, bile loss via the T-tube causes electrolyte abnormalities, or the T-tube dislodges.

Biliary colic and cholelithiasis occurring several years after cholecystectomy are handled in a similar manner to that identified earlier. ERCP and sphincterotomy can remove 85 to 95 percent of such stones. The routine addition of mechanical lithotripsy has improved stone fragmentation and retrieval by approximately 10 percent. Especially difficult stones include those occurring in the setting of coagulopathy, ductal strictures, duodenal diverticula, or unusually large stones. Once

ductal access is obtained, stones that can be basketed can almost always be crushed by mechanical lithotripsy. Stones that cannot be basketed must generally be managed by some fragmentation technique such as mother-baby scope with retrograde use of a pulsed-dye laser or electrohydraulic lithotripsy. Occasionally, percutaneous access needs to be obtained and such fragmentation techniques need to be applied again by percutaneous miniscope approach.

Patients with failed stone removal must be temporized with nasobiliary catheter drainage or stenting. Preliminary evidence indicates that treatment of such patients for an interval of 1 year with ursodeoxycholic acid will result in stone softening and permit stone removal in many such cases at follow-up. Overall, current evidence indicates that nearly all stones can be removed by percutaneous or endoscopic techniques if the patients are willing to travel to a specialized center. Alternatively, management of such stones by common duct exploration remains an acceptable alternative.

ACUTE PANCREATITIS

The most common cause of pancreatitis in females worldwide is gallstones. Alcohol ingestion is the most common cause in males. Patients presenting with pancreatitis and bilirubin greater than 2.5 mg/dl will generally have bile duct stones. Surgical studies have shown that common-duct exploration in patients with acute gallstone pancreatitis results in unacceptable morbidity and mortality. Two randomized controlled trials of early endoscopic sphincterotomy (within 1 to 3 days) have shown decreased complication rates and a trend toward lower mortality rates in patients treated by endoscopic sphincterotomy and stone extraction. Overall, our current recommendation is to treat patients with presumed gallstone pancreatitis with intravenous fluids, analgesics, and antibiotics. If toxicity and pain resolution are evident in those first 24 hours, the ductal stone has probably passed or disimpacted, and management becomes elective. If pain or toxicity persists, urgent ERCP is seemingly warranted. Attempts to clear ductal stones, or at least decompress the biliary tree with a stent or nasobiliary tube, is warranted. Pancreatography should generally be restricted to partial duct filling or avoided altogether.

NONCALCULOUS BILIARY OBSTRUCTION

Benign Strictures

Narrowing of the bile duct can result after penetrating trauma; a surgical procedure (cholecystectomy, choledochoenterostomy); inflammation (primary sclerosing cholangitis); extrinsic compression (such as by pancreatic disease), or a variety of other rare causes.

Postsurgical strictures can be managed surgically, radiologically, or endoscopically. Surgery has a high initial success rate but is difficult in the postoperative abdomen and has a 25 to 35 percent recurrence rate. Percutaneous approaches allow easy access for repeated dilation and stenting, but involve the discomfort and inconvenience of percutaneous catheters. ERCP allows further diagnostic studies, such as brushings or biopsies, as well as therapy of the stricture. Depending on the diameter of the stricture, initial dilation is carried out with a 6 mm to 8 mm balloon inflated to a pressure of 8 atmospheres. The long-term goal is to place two or three 10 Fr stents across the stricture and maintain these for approximately 12 months. The patient is then followed clinically and biochemically. Further ERCPs are carried out only if indicated by the development of symptoms or obstructive chemistries. The most frequent complication is cholangitis due to inadequate dilation or stent occlusion. Duct rupture rarely occurs. Initial intermediate duration results (3 years) indicate a 25 percent stricture/cholestasis recurrence rate after endoscopic therapy.

Primary Sclerosing Cholangitis

This disease is characterized by multiple intrahepatic and extrahepatic biliary strictures. Approximately one fourth of the patients have one or two dominant main-duct strictures that can be treated percutaneously or endoscopically with the aim of providing relief from pruritus and cholestasis. Balloon dilation of the stricture is generally followed by the placement of one or two plastic stents for 3 to 4 months. We generally avoid placing expandable metal stents because these are not removable. Brushings and biopsies can also be performed as indicated. The advantage of ERCP is that symptomatic relief is provided without altering the surgical anatomy. (An earlier chapter discusses endoscopic management of strictures in patients with sclerosing cholangitis.)

Malignant Obstruction

Pancreatic cancer and primary bile duct cancers account for most cases of malignant biliary obstruction, with metastases accounting for only a small proportion. Less than 20 percent of patients with pancreatic cancer and 30 percent of patients with cholangiocarcinoma are eligible for a resection for attempted cure at the time of presentation. However, although ampullary carcinoma accounts for only 10 percent of biliary tract malignancies, resection is recommended in suitable operative candidates. Because Whipple's procedure carries mortality rates of 2 to 10 percent, adequate preoperative assessment for disease spread is essential. This optimally includes the use of endoscopic ultrasound, which can image for local spread and vascular invasion.

Palliative treatment for biliary obstruction is indicated in most patients. Surgery and endoscopy provide similar survival rates but endoscopic stenting of the malignant stricture entails shorter hospital stay. This is of considerable importance in patients whose mean survival is 6 to 8 months. Endoscopic stenting is obtained either with a large diameter plastic stent or an expandable metal stent. Either will provide adequate drainage for 3 to 4 months on average, although the latter may have longer patency.

Hilar or high bile duct strictures are more difficult to traverse with an endoscopic stent and are amenable to a combined approach if endoscopy alone fails. A guidewire is passed through a percutaneous stent into the duodenum, where it is pulled out via the endoscope. An internal stent is then placed over the wire. It is preferable to convert an external stent into an internal stent, because the former is associated with pain and a more frequent cholangitis.

Gastric bypass surgery is needed in patients with duodenal obstruction, and a biliary bypass can also be carried out. In some cases, patients operated on with the aim of a curative resection will be found to have widely spread disease and will undergo palliative biliary surgery only.*

SPHINCTER OF ODDI DYSFUNCTION

Sphincter of Oddi dysfunction refers to benign noncalculous obstruction occurring at the pancreatobiliary duodenal junction that results in cholestasis, pancreatitis, or pancreatobiliary-type pain. The latter pain is typically right upper quadrant or epigastric in location with radiation to the back occurring in the absence of acid peptic disease or response to acid peptic disease therapy. Histologically, such patients commonly have edema, fibrosis, or inflammation of the papilla, although one-third of such patients have no identifiable histopathology and may represent motor disorders. In patients with recurrent pancreatitis, cholestasis, or recurrent pancreatobiliary-type pain in whom no stones, tumor, or other mechanical lesions can be found to cause the pathology, sphincter dysfunction will be found in a significant percent (pending additional factors such as chronic alcohol ingestion, hyperlipidemia, psychological factors, and so on).

Sphincter of Oddi manometry has evolved as probably the best tool to identify sphincter of Oddi dysfunction. Such manometry is generally performed by ERCP but also can be performed intraoperatively or percutaneously. Manometry is technically more demanding than standard ERCP and is generally performed with only the use of a benzodiazepine sedative (no narcotics, anticholinergics, or glucagon). Manometry has generally been found to be reproducible with a low intraobserver variability when performed in large centers. Patients with suspected sphincter of Oddi dysfunction are commonly grouped according to the constellation of symptoms. Those with pain, obstructive liver chemistries, dilated common bile duct, and slow drainage of contrast

---

*Editor's Note: Optimal patient care seems to be best served by a team of experienced and cooperating endoscopists, surgeons, and radiologists.

from the bile duct, in the absence of ductal stones and tumors, have a high probability of sphincter dysfunction and are commonly classified as type I. Patients with pain and one or two of the findings mentioned earlier are listed as type II, and patients with suggestive pain but *no* other objective evidence are classified as type III. Sphincter manometry is found to be abnormal in approximately 80 percent of type I patients, 50 percent of type II patients, and 25 percent of type III patients. Some of the type I patients with normal manometry probably really have common bile duct microlithiasis masquerading as sphincter dysfunction.

Noninvasive testing to evaluate the sphincter includes the Nardi test (morphine-neostigmine provocative test), secretin-stimulated ultrasonography of the pancreas, fatty meal, or cholecystokinin-stimulated ultrasonography of the common bile duct, or nuclear scintigraphy of the bile duct. Each of these studies has been demonstrated to have high sensitivity in selected patients (usually type I patients) but generally low sensitivity in type III patients (i.e., the very group of patients in which clinical judgement alone is least helpful). Overall, we have found these studies of limited clinical value.

Therapy

Type I patients should generally be treated with sphincterotomy without further diagnostic testing. Type II and type III patients should generally receive trials of medical therapy before possibly proceeding with invasive therapy. Limited studies indicate that trials of low-fat diet, anticholinergics, calcium channel blockers, nitrates, and antidepressants all have some benefit in relieving or controlling pain. We find these agents to be of some value, but they usually do not leave the patient asymptomatic. We generally recommend that patients with continued or refractory pain then be studied with manometry. Patients with abnormal manometry are then recommended for sphincterotomy. Therapeutic outcome after sphincterotomy again varies according to clinical presentation. Nearly all type I patients will have symptom relief after sphincterotomy. Approximately 80 percent of type II patients will respond to sphincterotomy, whereas only 50 to 60 percent of type III patients will respond to sphincterotomy. Two randomized controlled trials have shown that endoscopic sphincterotomy is two to three times more effective than sham therapy in controlling the pain associated with sphincter dysfunction. One study demonstrated that this beneficial effect remained over a 4-year follow-up interval.

The risks and benefits of performing sphincterotomy in sphincter of Oddi dysfunction patients must be carefully assessed before proceeding with sphincterotomy. The complication rate, predominately pancreatitis but also perforation, is approximately twofold that of common duct stone patients. Because most sphincter of Oddi patients are middle-aged females, the devastation to the patient and family are obvious when a major complication occurs. Risks and benefits should, therefore, be thoroughly discussed before proceeding with therapy.

Patients with documented sphincter abnormalities who fail to respond to sphincterotomy generally may have one of several residual conditions. Residual biliary sphincter stenosis may be present, but this is uncommon. More commonly, residual pancreatic sphincter narrowing is present. The frequency with which such patients respond to pancreatic sphincterotomy or septotomy, however, is not well defined. Residual evidence of chronic pancreatitis is a common finding. Such patients may or may not have had abnormal pancreatography but commonly have abnormal pancreatic parenchyma by endoscopic ultrasound evaluation or analysis of pure pancreatic juice. Alternatively, some patients appear to have a very sensitive bile duct, in that biliary distension or dye injection continues to provoke typical pain, despite obviously patent biliary sphincter. The cause of this is unknown. Occasionally, patients respond to celiac ganglionectomy, although much more work is needed, in these cases, with bile duct hyperesthesia.

Overall, our understanding of sphincter of Oddi dysfunction is increasing, but the area remains open for extensive additional research on diagnosis and therapy.

SUGGESTED READING

Cotton PB, Baillie J, Pappas TN, Meyers WS. Laparoscopic cholecystectomy and the biliary endoscopist (editorial). Gastrointest Endosc 1991; 37:94–97.

Davids PHP, Groen AK, Rauws EAJ, et al. Randomised trial of self-expanding metal stents versus polyethylene stents for distal malignant biliary obstruction. Lancet 1992; 340:No 8834:1488–1492.

Fan ST, et al. Early treatment of acute biliary pancreatitis by endoscopic papillotomy. N Engl J Med 1993; 328:228–232.

Geenen JE, Hogan WJ, Dodds WJ, et al. The efficacy of endoscopic sphincterotomy after cholecystectomy in patients with sphincter-of-Oddi dysfunction. N Engl J Med 1989; 320:82–87.

Hawes R, Jamidar P. Endoscopic diagnosis and treatment of ampullary tumors. Gastroenterol Clin North Am 1992; 2:529–542.

Johnson GK, Geenen JE, Venu RP, et al. Endoscopic treatment of biliary tract strictures in sclerosing cholangitis: A larger series and recommendations for treatment. Gastrointest Endosc 1991; 37: 38–43.

Kozarek R. Endoscopic management of bile duct injury. Gastroenterol Clin North Am 1993; 3:261–270.

Sherman S, Hawes RH, Lehman GA. Management of bile duct stones. Semin Liver Dis 1990; 10:205–221.

THE PANCREAS

ACUTE PANCREATITIS

JOHN H.C. RANSON, B.M., B.Ch., M.A.

The term "acute pancreatitis" is used to describe a broad spectrum of etiologic, pathologic, and clinical entities. Etiologic associations include factors as varied as gallstones and the bite of the black scorpion of Trinidad. Pathologic findings range from edema through hemorrhagic necrosis, and the clinical course ranges from mild, self-limiting symptoms through a fulminant, rapidly lethal illness. It is clear, therefore, that management of patients with acute pancreatitis must be individualized.

ETIOLOGY

Our knowledge of the actual pathogenesis of acute pancreatitis is fragmentary and incomplete. In most instances, etiologic factors have been identified primarily on the basis of epidemiologic associations. Sixty to 80 percent of patients have either *biliary lithiasis* or a history of long-standing *alcohol abuse*. Clinical pancreatitis is recognized in 0.9 percent to 9.5 percent of alcoholic patients and pathologic evidence of pancreatitis is found in 17 percent to 45 percent of this group. Cholelithiasis is present in 60 percent of nonalcoholic patients with pancreatitis and pancreatitis has occurred in 4 percent to 5 percent of patients treated surgically for biliary stones. Some of the other etiologic associations of pancreatitis are listed in Table 1.

CLINICAL MANIFESTATIONS AND DIAGNOSIS

An accurate diagnosis of acute pancreatitis depends primarily on a careful evaluation of the patient's history and physical examination. The clinical presentation may be variable with symptoms closely mimicking those of acute biliary disease, peptic ulcer, and intestinal obstruction or infarction. The predominant symptom is usually pain that is characteristically located in the epigastrum

Table 1 Etiologic Factors in Acute Pancreatitis

Metabolic:	*Vascular*:
Alcohol	Postoperative
Hyperlipoproteinemia	Atherosclerosis
Hypercalcemia	Vasculitis
Drugs	Periarteritis nodosa
Genetic	
Scorpion venom	*Infection*:
	Mumps
Mechanical:	Coxsackie B
Cholelithiasis	Cytomegalovirus
Postoperative	Cryptococcus
Pancreas divisum	
Post-traumatic	
Retrograde pancreatography	
Pancreatic duct obstruction	
Pancreatic ductal bleeding	
Duodenal obstruction	

and may radiate to the back and to both flanks. The pain is constant in character and may be extremely severe.

Nausea and vomiting are almost invariably present and often a prominent early feature. The findings on physical examination also vary widely. Patients may be restless with a rapid pulse and respiratory rate. The blood pressure may be mildly elevated, normal, or decreased. The temperature is usually 99° F to 100° F. The abdomen is usually mildly distended and may exhibit a characteristic epigastric fullness. Tenderness is usually most marked over the epigastrum and upper abdomen. It may be diffuse, especially in more severe cases.

Laboratory Findings

Determination of serum and urine amylase levels are the most widely used tests for the diagnosis of pancreatic disease. Elevated serum levels are observed at hospital admission in 95 percent of patients with acute pancreatitis compared to only 5 percent of patients with other acute intra-abdominal conditions. Among patients with pancreatitis who have normal serum amylase levels, approximately 40 percent have hyperlipidemia with lactescent serum. In large groups of patients with acute abdominal conditions, approximately 20 percent have elevated serum amylase levels. Of these, approximately 75 percent have pancreatitis, and among the 25 percent with extrapancreatic disease, only about 50 percent have conditions that might be confused with acute pancreatitis.

Radiographic Findings

Plain radiographs of the abdomen and chest demonstrate findings that may support a diagnosis of acute pancreatitis in approximately 80 percent of patients. The most common is segmental dilation or ileus of a loop of small bowel in the left upper quadrant, the so-called "sentinal loop." Dilation of the transverse colon and loss of the psoas margins are other relatively common findings.

Computed tomography (CT) provides the most accurate available noninvasive imaging of the retroperitoneum. The most frequent findings in patients with acute pancreatitis are diffuse pancreatic enlargement, obliteration of the peripancreatic fat planes, and inflammation of the left anterior pararenal space. Peripancreatic fluid collections may also be visualized. It must be recognized that early CT findings may be interpreted as normal in a significant portion of patients judged to have acute pancreatitis. In most such instances the pancreatitis is mild.

Diagnostic Celiotomy

In most patients, the diagnosis of acute pancreatitis can be made with reasonable certainty on the basis of clinical, radiographic, and laboratory findings. In some cases, however, other diseases may closely mimic acute pancreatitis, and diagnostic celiotomy may be required to exclude or treat acute life-threatening extrapancreatic disease in up to 5 percent of patients. In this regard, it should be stressed that strong positive evidence of acute pancreatitis does not exclude the possibility of concomitant extrapancreatic disease in an occasional patient.

PROGNOSTIC ASSESSMENT

Because the spectrum of severity of acute pancreatitis ranges so widely, the early identification of the risk of life-threatening complications is helpful in permitting the appropriate application of monitoring and therapeutic interventions. For the evaluation of proposed treatments, objective means to stratify the diverse population of patients with pancreatitis are essential.

In 1974, we reported the eleven early objective prognostic criteria listed in Table 2. These signs were developed from a statistical analysis of the relationship between early measurements and overall morbidity and mortality of acute pancreatitis. The relationship between the number of signs present and morbidity in a group of 450 patients is shown in Figure 1. The acute physiology and chronic health evaluation (APACHE II) illness grading system has been applied to prognostic assessment of pancreatitis. The accuracy of this system appears to be comparable to that of the specific multiple

Table 2 The 11 Early Objective Signs Used to Classify the Severity of Pancreatitis

At admission or diagnosis
Age > 55 yr
White blood-cell count > 16,000/cu mm
Blood glucose > 200 mg/dl
Serum lactic dehydrogenase > 350 IU/l
Serum glutamic oxaloacetic transaminase > 250 Sigma-Frankel units %

During initial 48 hr
Hematocrit fall > 10 percentage points
Blood urea nitrogen rise > 5 mg/dl
Serum calcium level < 8 mg/dl
Arterial PO_2 < 60 mm Hg
Base deficit > 4 mEq/L
Estimated fluid sequestration > 6000 ml

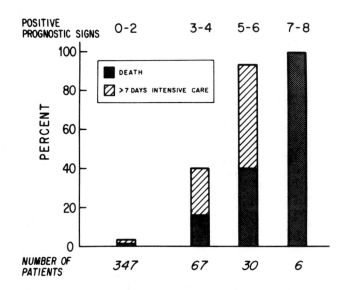

Figure 1 Correlation of positive prognostic signs and morbidity in acute pancreatitis.

prognostic criteria. APACHE II is more complex but has the advantage that it may be applied at times other than at diagnosis. A relationship between prognosis and the volume and color of fluid obtained by paracentesis, early hemodynamic measurements, coagulation factors, complement levels, antiproteases, and C-reactive protein have also been described.

In recent years, there has been renewed interest in the relationship between pancreatic necrosis and the pathogenesis of the complications of pancreatitis. Correlations have been reported to be between alpha-1 protease inhibitor, alpha-2 macro proteins, complement factors C3 and C4, and C-reactive protein and trypsinogen activation peptides and necrotizing pancreatitis. Most intriguing has been the use of contrast-enhanced CT. Radiographic enhancement of the pancreas following contrast injection has been interpreted as evidence of tissue viability. Failure of enhancement has been interpreted as evidence of tissue necrosis. The finding of nonenhancement of pancreatic tissue is, in our experi-

Table 3 Measures Proposed for the Treatment
of Acute Pancreatitis

A. To limit severity of pancreatic inflammation
  1. Inhibition of pancreatic secretion
     a) Nasogastric suction
     b) Pharmacologic: anticholinergics, glucagon, 5-fluorouracil, acetazolamide, cimetidine, propylthiouracil, calcitonin, somatostatin
     c) Hypothermia
     d) Pancreatic irradiation
  2. Inhibition of pancreatic enzymes
     a) Aprotinin, epsilon-aminocaproic acid, soybean trypsin inhibitor, insulin, snake antivenom gabexate mesilate, camostate, fresh frozen plasma, chlorophyll, xylocaine
  3. Corticosteroids
  4. Prostaglandins
  5. Operative biliary procedures
  6. Endoscopic biliary intervention

B. To interrupt the pathogenesis of complications
  1. Antibiotics
  2. Antacids, cimetidine
  3. Heparin, fibrinolysin
  4. Low-molecular-weight dextran
  5. Vasopressin
  6. Peritoneal lavage
  7. Thoracic duct drainage
  8. Operative pancreatic drainage
  9. Pancreatic resection
  10. Debridement of necrotic tissue

C. To support the patient and treat complications
  1. Restoration and maintenance of intravascular volume
  2. Electrolyte replacement
  3. Respiratory support
  4. Nutritional support
  5. Analgesia
  6. Heparin
  7. Debridement and drainage of pancreatic infection
  8. Drainage of pseudocysts

ence, associated with an approximately 70 percent risk of late pancreatic sepsis.

TREATMENT

Multiple measures have been proposed for the treatment of patients with acute pancreatitis. It is convenient to categorize these various proposals by their therapeutic objectives. These are (1) to limit the severity of pancreatic inflammation itself; (2) to ameliorate complications by interrupting their pathogenesis; and (3) to support the patient and treat complications as they arise. Measures that have been proposed for the treatment of acute pancreatitis are listed in Table 3 under these three headings.

To Limit Severity of Inflammation

Nasogastric Suctioning and the Timing of Oral Feeding

Nasogastric suction has traditionally been instituted in patients with acute pancreatitis to reduce vomiting and abdominal distension. It has also been suggested that the aspiration of gastric acid may decrease pancreatic exocrine secretion by reducing secretin release. The therapeutic efficacy of nasogastric suction has been evaluated recently in controlled clinical trials. Although none of these trials demonstrated any significant benefit from nasogastric suction, it should be noted that the great majority of patients studied had mild, alcoholic pancreatitis. In addition, the number of patients in individual studies was small. Hence, the present data indicate that nasogastric suction is not essential for recovery from mild pancreatitis, especially that associated with alcohol abuse. I believe that further studies are needed to evaluate the role of this measure in more severe pancreatitis and in other etiologic subgroups. I continue to recommend nasogastric suction for most patients with acute pancreatitis of moderate or severe degree because of the symptomatic relief that is often reported. Inhibition of gastric acid production by the administration of H_2 blockers, and attempts to inhibit pancreatic exocrine secretion by administration of anticholinergics, calcitonin, somatostatin and glucagon, have not been of benefit in controlled clinical trials.

The concept that the severity of acute pancreatitis and of its complications may be reduced by inhibitors of pancreatic enzymes has received much attention over the past 30 years. The most extensively studied agent has been aprotinin. Controlled studies of this and other enzyme inhibitors have provided no convincing evidence that any of these agents would have significant clinical benefit.

Adrenocorticosteroids have been administered to patients with acute pancreatitis because of their anti-inflammatory effects. No adequate clinical studies have been reported.

Studies have recently been reported evaluating the influence of prostaglandins and drugs that influence their metabolism on the course of acute pancreatitis. A randomized double-blind clinical trial evaluated indomethacin administered by suppository (50 mg twice daily). Only 30 patients were studied, but a significant reduction in pain was reported.

Biliary Procedures

Evaluation of the treatment of patients with gallstone-associated pancreatitis has been clouded by difficulty in determining the presence or absence of actual pancreatic inflammation. Of patients who have abdominal pain, elevated serum, or urinary amylase levels and gallstones, 39 to 75 percent (60 percent average) have no significant pancreatitis demonstrable at early operation or autopsy. Such patients respond well to management of their biliary disease and behave clinically as if they had no pancreatitis. Furthermore, approximately 80 percent of patients with true pancreatitis have mild disease and will recover uneventfully. A controlled clinical trial has shown that early operative intervention to correct associated gallstones is associated with increased morbidity, especially in those who have severe pancreatitis.

Recently, endoscopic sphincterotomy and removal of stones impacted in the ampulla of Vater have been advocated for patients with gallstone-associated pancreatitis. A recent controlled clinical trial indicated that emergency endoscopic retrograde cholangiopancreatography and endoscopic papillotomy, if common bile duct stones were present, were associated with a reduction in biliary sepsis, compared to noninterventional treatment. Unfortunately, however, there was no significant difference in the incidence of either systemic or local complications of pancreatitis following early endoscopic intervention.

To Interrupt the Pathogenesis of Complications

Pharmacologic Therapy

Antibiotics have traditionally been recommended in the treatment of acute pancreatitis. Prospective controlled clinical trials of ampicillin in patients with mild acute pancreatitis have failed to effect any reduction in septic complications with this particular antibiotic. I continue to recommend broad-spectrum antibiotics in patients who have gallstone-associated pancreatitis, because of the frequency of biliary infection in this group. In addition, antibiotics may be beneficial in those patients judged to have severe pancreatitis.

Antacids should be administered to patients with pancreatitis in order to reduce the frequency of acute gastroduodenal ulceration or bleeding.

Anticoagulants have been recommended on the basis of experimental studies. It has, however, been my experience that administration of heparin in the first few days of acute pancreatitis is associated with a very high risk of significant retroperitoneal hemorrhage and should be avoided, if possible. Attempts to improve pancreatic blood flow by the administration of low-molecular-weight dextran and vasopressin have been recommended on the basis of experimental studies, but not evaluated clinically.

Peritoneal Lavage

Controlled clinical studies of the efficacy of peritoneal lavage in the treatment of acute pancreatitis have produced conflicting results. Our initial experience suggested that peritoneal lavage was a significant adjunct to the management of early cardiovascular, respiratory complications.

We have considered any patients who were experiencing their first or second episode of acute pancreatitis and who had "severe" pancreatitis on the basis of prognostic signs (Table 1) to be candidates for peritoneal lavage. We have attempted to minimize the risk of visceral injury by introducing lavage catheters through an open incision about 4 to 5 cm in length with direct visualization of the peritoneum. Local infiltration anesthesia is used. The lavage fluid is an approximately isotonic electrolyte solution containing 15 g per liter of dextrose (Dianeal). Potassium, 4 mEq per liter; heparin, 500 USP; and ampicillin, 125 mg are usually added to each liter of lavage fluid. In general, 2 L of the fluid are allowed to run into the peritoneal cavity over about 15 minutes to remain intraperitoneally for about 30 minutes and then drained out by gravity over 15 minutes. The cycle is usually repeated hourly using 48 liters of lavage fluid during each 24-hour period. Lavage has been instituted within 48 hours of diagnosis in all patients. It has been discontinued after 48 hours to seven days, depending upon the patient's course.

Initially we had limited the period of lavage to 4 days because of fear of introducing infection into the peritoneal cavity, if the catheters were allowed to remain longer. However, a chance observation in 1979 led to a study of the duration of peritoneal lavage that was reported in 1990. This study suggests that a longer period of lavage is associated with a reduced risk of late pancreatic infection and of death from this complication. Although this observation requires confirmation by others, the morbidity of long-term peritoneal lavage is small compared to its benefits. I would recommend peritoneal lavage for patients who have severe pancreatitis, on the basis of prognostic criteria and CT findings.

Because pancreatic enzymes can enter the blood stream by way of lymphatic channels, it has been proposed that drainage of the thoracic duct may ameliorate the course of acute pancreatitis. Reports of the efficacy of this approach have been too limited to allow evaluation.

Early Operative Drainage

Early operative drainage of the pancreas may be associated with a dramatic reduction in early cardiovascular instability. It is, however, followed by dramatically increased respiratory and pancreatic septic complications.

The concept that formal pancreatic resection may ameliorate the course of very severe pancreatitis has received extensive evaluation, especially in Europe. Recent critical evaluation of this measure has shown no convincing benefit, and this measure has, at present, few, if any advocates.

Surgical debridement of necrotic tissue without formal pancreatic resection and with postoperative lavage of the peritoneal bed has recently been advocated. A low overall mortality has been reported. Many patients subjected to this intervention have, however, had uninfected necrosis, and it is difficult to be certain how many of these patients might have recovered without any form of surgical therapy.

To Support the Patient and Treat Complications

Until better measures are available that will limit the severity of acute pancreatitis and prevent its complications, the most important aspects of treatment are supportive and symptomatic.

Intravascular Volume Management

Evaluation and monitoring of intravascular volume and cardiovascular function require regular measurements of pulse rate and blood pressure. In most patients, a central venous catheter should be placed and an indwelling urethral catheter introduced for regular measurement of central venous pressure, venous blood gases, and hourly urine output. In those with associated cardiovascular disease, large fluid requirements or severe respiratory complications, monitoring of pulmonary arterial pressures and cardiac output using a Swan Ganz catheter may be essential for appropriate management. In most patients, intravascular volume can be satisfactorily restored and maintained using crystalloid solutions. Serial measurements of hematocrit may indicate the need for blood transfusion. If colloid administration is required, fresh frozen plasma may theoretically be superior to albumin because of the presence of trypsin inhibitors. Hypokalemia is frequent and potassium replacement usually is required. Intravenous replacement of calcium and magnesium has also been recommended. Symptoms and complications referable to hypocalcemia, however, are uncommon and because hypercalcemia has been implicated in the genesis of pancreatitis, calcium administration should be done cautiously.

Respiratory Monitoring and Support

Clinically occult respiratory failure is a frequent feature of acute pancreatitis and may occur in patients who do not have severe disease, by the usual clinical criteria. Changes in oxyhemoglobin affinity during acute pancreatitis may increase the physiologic consequences of respiratory failure, and hypoxemia certainly may be lethal if diagnosed or untreated. It is essential, therefore, that arterial blood gas values be determined at the time of diagnosis and at intervals of not less than 12 hours for the initial 48 to 72 hours of treatment. Subsequent measurements depend on the patient's course.

In most patients, early hypoxemia resolves as the underlying pancreatitis subsides, and the only management necessary is close observation and administration of oxygen. Progressive pulmonary insufficiency, pulmonary infiltrates, and effusions tend to occur in those patients who have severe acute pancreatitis and following early operative intervention. They should be anticipated in these groups. The most appropriate management is early endotracheal intubation and institution of mechanical respiratory support with positive end expiratory pressure.

Nutritional Support

The occurrence of marked nutritional depletion in patients with acute pancreatitis is well known. In those with mild pancreatitis, oral feedings can usually be resumed within a few days. In patients with severe pancreatitis, oral feedings usually are not tolerated for prolonged periods of time and alternative nutritional support must be instituted as early as possible. Initially, the only possible route is intravenous alimentation. After intestinal peristalsis returns, enteral feedings are a possible alternative route.

For most patients, standard total parenteral nutrition, initiated as soon as early cardiovascular instability has subsided, is the most practical form of nutritional support. Glucose levels should be carefully monitored and insulin given as needed. The safety of intravenous lipid as a caloric source has been controversial. Although it is probably safe, we limit administration of lipids to that required to provide essential fatty acids. It should be emphasized that total parenteral nutrition is only appropriate for patients in whom oral feedings are not possible for a substantial period of time.

Analgesia

The pain associated with acute pancreatitis may be very severe and it is traditional to administer meperidine or pentazocine rather than morphine because of the spasm of the ampulla of Vater that is associated with the latter drug.

Heparin

Although early administration of heparin may be hazardous, patients with severe pancreatitis may develop a hypercoagulable state late in their course. If this occurs, heparin may be indicated during the second or third weeks of severe pancreatitis, to reduce thrombotic complications.

Diagnosis and Treatment of Infected Pancreatic Necrosis

Pancreatic infection is usually recognized after the first 14 days of treatment in patients with acute pancreatitis who have not undergone early laparotomy. The diagnosis should be suspected in all patients who have persisting fever or leukocytosis after the early phase of disease. CT scan is also helpful in identifying patients at high risk for infection. Specifically, patients who have fluid identified on their initial CT scan have an approximately 50 percent risk of late infection. Furthermore, those who have more than 50 percent of their gland failing to enhance on early contrast CT scan have an approximately 70 percent risk of developing infection. The clinical and laboratory findings at the time sepsis was diagnosed in patients who developed sepsis after early nonoperative treatment of acute pancreatitis is shown in Table 4. The most prominent findings are fever, abdominal distension, and leukocytosis, with a palpable abdominal mass. Laboratory findings are nonspecific. Clearly, the occurrence of positive blood cultures that cannot be attributed to nonpancreatic sources indicate probable pancreatic sepsis. The presence of gas outside the gastrointestinal tract, either on plain abdominal film or on CT scan, usually indicates sepsis and is present in approximately 14 percent of patients with sepsis. If the presence of infection is uncertain on the basis of clinical and laboratory findings, needle aspiration of the pancreas under CT guidance with bacteriologic examination of the aspirate may be helpful in determining the presence or absence of infection.

Pancreatic infection secondary to acute pancreatitis is almost always associated with extensive necrosis of pancreatic or peripancreatic tissues. The infected material is semisolid, and attempts at percutaneous catheter drainage are usually futile. Operative treatment is, therefore, required in virtually all patients. The approach that we have favored is illustrated in Figure 2. It consists of wide exploration of the whole peripancreatic retroperitoneum and institution of sump drainage. A feeding jejunostomy is constructed, and if gallstones are identified, appropriate surgical treatment is carried out.

An alternative surgical approach has been to debride and pack infected pancreatic necrosis. Essential features of this approach are to debride necrotic tissue and cover the viscera with nonadherent porous gauze

followed by packing of the wound with moist laparotomy pads. The dressings are changed under general anesthesia every 2 or 3 days, until sufficient granulation has formed to permit changes on the ward. Although adequate debridement and drainage is essential for these patients, they are usually critically ill as a result of their underlying pancreatitis and superimposed sepsis. Vigorous supportive care is, therefore, essential and includes meticulous care to respiratory management, fluid and electrolyte balance, prevention of gastroduodenal bleeding, and nutritional support. Current morbidity remains high from this complication and mortality with either closed drainage or with packing followed by an overall mortality of approximately 15 percent.

Pancreatic Pseudocysts

Pseudocysts are defined as persistent localized collections of enzyme-rich fluid with a clearly defined wall made up of fibrous tissue and adjacent viscera. They occur most commonly in patients with chronic pancreatitis. Only 1 to 2 percent of patients with acute pancreatitis develop pseudocysts. The overwhelming majority of fluid collections in acute pancreatitis resolve, if they do not become infected. Such acute collections may take weeks or months to resolve but do not require intervention.

When a symptomatic pseudocyst or enlarging pseudocyst is present following acute pancreatitis, drainage is required. External drainage, either by surgery or by percutaneous catheter placement under radiographic guidance, is the simplest approach. They are, however, associated with a significant risk of pancreatic fistula. Internal drainage of a pseudocyst into the stomach, duodenum, or jejunum is applicable to the majority of mature pseudocysts. Resection may be required for

Table 4 Incidence of Clinical and Laboratory Features in Patients with Infected Pancreatic Necrosis

Fever >101° F	100%
Abdominal distension	94%
Palpable mass	71%
Hypotension (BP <90 mm Hg)	39%
Respirator support	39%
Renal failure	39%
Coma	28%
Elevated serum amylase	28%
White cell count >10,000/mm³	78%
Platelet count <175,000/cm	55%
Bilirubin >1.5 mg/dl	67%
Serum albumin <3.5 g/l	75%

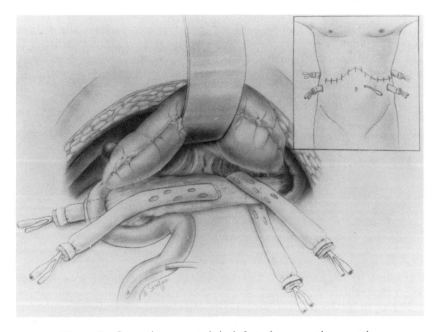

Figure 2 Operative approach in infected pancreatic necrosis.

anatomical reasons or in those cysts that are accompanied by major vascular communication.

PREVENTION OF RECURRENCE

Biliary Lithiasis

In patients with associated cholelithiasis, the risk of recurrent pancreatitis may be reduced from 36 to 63 percent down to 2 to 8 percent by correction of the underlying biliary disease. This can usually be accomplished safely during the same hospital admission.

Pancreas Divisum

Pancreas divisum is a congenital anomaly in which there is no communication between the dorsal and pancreatic ducts. It has been suggested that in patients with this anomaly, there may be relative obstruction to drainage to the major portion of the pancreas served by Santorini's duct with resultant pancreatitis. There are a few well-documented cases in which the anomaly of pancreas divisum has been associated with histologically demonstrated pancreatitis with the dorsal pancreas drained by the duct of Santorini while the ventral pancreas drained by Wirsung's duct is normal. However, the frequency with which this anomaly is the primary etiology of pancreatitis and, indeed, the mechanism by which it may initiate pancreatitis, are unknown. It has been reported that transduodenal sphincteroplasty may yield good results in 50 to 68 percent of patients with pancreas divisum and recurrent acute pancreatitis. However, this therapeutic intervention can be hazardous, and further studies are required to develop criteria to identify those patients who may benefit from treatment.

RECOMMENDATIONS

Our current approach to the management of patients with acute pancreatitis includes close observation and re-evaluation of the diagnosis. Laparotomy is reserved for those in whom there is significant concern about life-threatening extrapancreatic disease. Patients require monitoring, restoration, and maintenance of intravascular volume. Respiratory status should be closely monitored by serial measurements of arterial blood gases for at least 48 to 72 hours with the institution of respiratory support when needed. Broad spectrum antibiotics are administered to patients who have gallstone-associated or severe acute pancreatitis. Nasogastric suction is recommended for most patients who have pancreatitis of moderate or severe degree. Oral feedings should be withheld until evidence of pancreatitis has subsided. In patients with marked cardiovascular instability or renal failure, early institution of peritoneal lavage may result in dramatic clinical improvement.

We continue to use the prognostic criteria listed in Table 2 to identify patients at a high risk of developing life-threatening complications. In patients with suspected severe disease, CT scans with contrast enhancement are helpful in delineating the anatomy of the retroperitoneum. In patients who have high risk of late complications, peritoneal lavage for seven days may reduce this risk.

In patients who develop evidence of pancreatic infection, wide debridement, and either sump drainage or packing is required. With this approach, overall mortality from acute pancreatitis is approximately 5 percent.

SUGGESTED READING

Beger HG, Buchler M, Bittner R. Necrosectomy and postoperative local lavage in patients with necrotizing pancreatitis: results of a prospective clinical trial. World J Surg 1988; 12:255–262.

Fan S-T, Lai ECS, Mok FPT, et al. Early treatment of acute biliary pancreatitis by endoscopic papillotomy. N Eng J Med 1993; 328:228–232.

Kelly TR. Gallstone pancreatitis: a prospective randomized trial of the timing of surgery. Surgery 1988; 104:600–604.

Ranson JHC. Necrosis and abscess. In: Bradley EL ed. Complications of pancreatitis. Philadelphia: WB Saunders, 1982;72–95.

Ranson JHC, Berman RS. Long peritoneal lavage decreases pancreatic sepsis in acute pancreatitis. Ann Surg 1990; 211:708–716.

Ranson JHC, Spencer FC. The role of peritoneal lavage in severe acute pancreatitis. Ann Surg 1978; 187:565–575.

PANCREATITIS: SURGICAL CONSIDERATIONS

DAVID W. RATTNER, M.D., F.A.C.S.

ACUTE PANCREATITIS

There is no single operative treatment and probably no operation that cures pancreatitis. Surgery in acute pancreatitis is reactive to the local complications created by inflammation and necrosis.

The diagnosis of acute pancreatitis rests on synthesis of clinical and laboratory information. In cases with severe peritoneal irritation, laparotomy can be the safest means to establish a diagnosis and avoid missing a surgically correctable disease. When acute pancreatitis is found unexpectedly at laparotomy, it should not be a source of embarrassment and may even provide an opportunity to correct the underlying cause (such as gallstones or ampullary stenosis).

It is the development of necrosis which differentiates mild from severe pancreatitis. Clinical scoring systems are widely employed to obtain an early estimate of the severity of an attack of pancreatitis. The most widely utilized system is the Ranson criteria, consisting of 11 easily obtainable clinical parameters at admission and 48 hours later. The presence of three signs or less suggests a favorable outcome whereas patients with four or more positive signs are likely to have a complicated course. (See the preceding chapter by Ranson.) Recently the APACHE II score has been used to stratify patients with acute pancreatitis. Although initially designed for use in critical care, it can also provide useful discrimination between mild and severe cases of pancreatitis upon admission to the hospital (without the 48 hour delay required to collect the Ranson criteria). Furthermore, it can be recalculated daily to reflect continuing disease activity with rising scores suggesting ongoing and untreated complications. Dynamic contrast enhanced computed tomography (CT) scanning has been shown to accurately identify areas of the pancreas that are not perfused and are likely to subsequently undergo necrosis. Since the extent of necrosis correlates with severity of illness, early CT scans can predict the likelihood of subsequent complications.

Gallstone Pancreatitis

Early Biliary Surgery

The demonstration that gallstones can be recovered from the stools of most patients with gallstone pancreatitis emphasized the importance of gallstones passing into the common bile duct and then obstructing or traumatizing the pancreatic duct orifice. Proving that early stone removal is beneficial has been problematic. First, many of the patients studied have undoubtedly had only chemical hyperamylasemia induced by the obstructing stone, not true pancreatic inflammation. Second, the differentiation of gallstone induced from other forms of pancreatitis is often difficult. Third, even when cholangiography demonstrates the presence of common duct stones, less than 5 percent are impacted at the ampulla. Nonetheless, 60 percent of patients who die from gallstone-induced pancreatitis are found at autopsy to have choledocholithiasis. This has led some to propose that nonimpacted stones may intermittently obstruct the pancreatic duct, thus playing a key role in either preventing resolution of mild pancreatitis or promoting progression from mild to severe pancreatitis.

Biliary surgery in the face of ongoing acute pancreatitis is associated with a high rate of complications. Because 95 percent of cases of gallstone pancreatitis "quiet down" with medical management and without progression to a fulminant form, and 95 percent of stones pass spontaneously in the first week, surgical intervention to remove the stone within the first 48 hours does not seem justifiable at present. Laparoscopic cholecystectomy with intraoperative cholangiography (and if still necessary, common duct exploration) may be safely and effectively performed after pancreatitis subsides, generally during the same hospital admission.

Early Endoscopic Retrograde Cholangiopancreatography

An alternative to early surgery is endoscopic retrograde cholangiopancreatography (ERCP) which may be carried out safely by experienced endoscopists in up to 90 percent of cases of gallstone pancreatitis. Prophylactic antibiotics should be employed and injections into the pancreatic duct avoided. The earlier ERCP is performed, the more frequently common duct stones are found. When an impacted stone is found and endoscopic sphincterotomy with stone removal successfully performed, most authors report a rapid improvement in the clinical course. In patients with an impacted stone with complicating cholangitis, a situation that is rare, urgent decompression is clearly beneficial.

Two prospective randomized clinical trials of early ERCP and endoscopic sphincterotomy (ES) have been published. In the first trial by Neoptelemos et al, overall complications appeared to be less in the patients undergoing early ERCP and ES (17 percent versus 34 percent) and the mortality rate to be diminished (2 percent versus 8 percent) though the numbers were too small to achieve statistical significance. Endoscopic sphincterotomy was of no benefit in patients with mild pancreatitis. When the data were analyzed only for those patients with severe pancreatitis, there was a significant decrease in both morbidity (24 percent versus 61 percent) and mortality (4 percent versus 18 percent). This study has been criticized because the control group was significantly older than the ERCP and ES group and because only 12 patients who underwent urgent ERCP and ES actually had common duct stones. Therefore the rather important conclusion was based on a small number of patients. Nonetheless, the implication of this study is that early removal of common duct stones in patients with severe pancreatitis may be beneficial. Recently, Fan et al published a larger trial and failed to confirm that local and systemic complications of pancreatitis were reduced by early ERCP and ES. Hospital mortality was reduced in those patients undergoing early ERCP and ES but the difference was not statistically significant. However Fan et al conclusively demonstrated that early ERCP and ES resulted in a reduction in biliary sepsis in both mild and severe pancreatitis. In all patients who had unrelenting biliary sepsis, persistent ampullary or common duct stones were identified. From these studies one can conclude that patients with evidence of cholangitis clearly benefit from early ES. Patients who present with indices of severe nonalcoholic pancreatitis (either by clinical scoring system, CT scan, or serum markers) should be considered for early ERCP and ES if a highly skilled endoscopist is available. If early ES is to have an impact it should be performed within 48 hours of the onset of the illness.

Early Pancreatic Resection

Major distal pancreatic resection can be accomplished in the face of acute pancreatitis with a mortality of approximately 40 percent, while pancreaticoduodenectomy or total pancreatectomy raises mortality to 60 percent or more. A key question is how to select those patients likely to benefit. The surgeon must decide which part of the pancreas to resect and how much to resect. This decision can be very difficult, because surface changes may not represent the degree of central pancreatic injury and because several days are required for the changes of pancreatic devitalization to become visible. In the first few days there is only massive swelling with or without hemorrhagic staining. Early dynamic contrast enhanced CT pancreatography can identify areas of necrosis which could be targeted for early debridement. Nonetheless there are patients with substantial areas of necrosis who remain well clinically and there have been no reports demonstrating improved survival in patients with pre-emptive early resection compared with those treated by later debridement of clearly demarcated necrotic tissue. In a recent trial comparing early pancreatic resection versus peritoneal lavage, resection was not found to be superior to intensive conservative management (including peritoneal lavage) and led to a longer intensive care unit (ICU) and hospital stay. Since the operative mortality of early pancreatic resection is high, it seems preferable to delay surgery until areas of necrosis are clearly demarcated or there is proven bacterial infection.

Peritoneal Lavage

The precise role of peritoneal lavage is controversial. Peritoneal lavage is not a treatment of pancreatitis itself, but only reverses some of the early phase systemic effects which are mediated by circulatory toxins. It is therefore of no benefit in mild to moderate pancreatitis and it does not alter the progression of pancreatic injury or prevent the intermediate or late phase developments of pancreatic necrosis and abscess. No study has yet been performed which addresses the use of peritoneal lavage in the treatment of early phase shock or even identifies a subset of patients in early phase shock. These are precisely the patients in whom striking immediate improvement is commonly seen. Therefore, many still feel that peritoneal lavage is beneficial when there is early evidence of major plasma volume loss, hypotension, pulse greater than 140 beats per minute, or continued clinical deterioration. Lavage should be instituted within 24 hours of the onset of illness. Ranson recently reported a small but intriguing series in which prolonged peritoneal lavage for 7 days reduced the incidence of late pancreatic sepsis and death. Although the number of patients in this study was small, the results are exciting and await confirmation from other centers.

Pancreatic Necrosis

It is only after several days of acute pancreatitis that irreversible tissue destruction becomes recognized. Liquefaction may occur in small well-defined geographic patches or even in large segments such as the distal two-thirds of the gland, with extension of the necrotizing process into the retroperitoneum, pararenal spaces, and mesentery. This process is really regional necrosis, rather than just pancreatic necrosis.

The real benefit of dynamic contrast enhanced CT scans may be in patients who are in the middle or late phase of acute pancreatitis. In these patients, with smoldering symptoms and inflammation, routine CT scans often demonstrate solid appearing inflammatory masses which do not appear amenable to debridement or drainage. However, dynamic contrast enhanced CT scans often delineate substantial areas of necrosis. This can direct subsequent intervention to hasten resolution of the process.

When necrosis develops, several factors that determine the ultimate outcome are the amount and extent of necrosis, bacterial contamination of necrosis, and perhaps most importantly the overall status of the patient as reflected in the APACHE II score. Since the factors affecting outcome are multiple, no single parameter, except the presence of infection, is an absolute indication for debridement. There is virtually universal agreement that infected necrosis must be surgically debrided. Percutaneous radiologic guided drainage is not capable of removing infected solid material. Therefore, while percutaneous radiologic intervention plays a major role in the management of collections which are primarily fluid, it should not be utilized as an initial therapy for patients with necrosis.

The management of patients with sterile necrosis is extremely controversial. Several authors have reported high mortality rates in patients with sterile necrosis, casting doubt on the primacy of infection as the major determinant of outcome. Operative mortality is rare in patients with sterile necrosis operated upon after the first week. However, postoperative complications (fistula, abscess) are frequent (13 to 24 percent) leading some to question whether or not sterile necrosis should be operated on at all. If necrotic areas are small, sterile collections may resolve. When signs of inflammation are present, percutaneous aspiration should be undertaken to determine if infection is present. When bacteria are found in the aspirate, debridement and drainage are indicated. Larger necrotic areas are problematic because of concern that they will become infected before there is sufficient time to reabsorb and heal. If large collections are truly asymptomatic, they can be managed nonoperatively with the expectation that a small percentage will become infected and require debridement and drainage. However, the decision to operate on large collections is often made because of clinical signs of inflammation, and thus the actual bacteriologic status of the necrotic tissue does not necessarily alter the clinical decision. Many sterile collections produce symptoms by mass effect or local inflammation. Patients who are symptomatic (systemically ill, can't eat, anoretic, febrile, or in pain) should not be denied a laparotomy simply because a necrotic collection is sterile. Symptoms due to mass effect and local inflammation can only be relieved by debridement and drainage.

There are three main surgical approaches for debridement of necrosis. I have performed aggressive initial debridement of the lesser sac and retroperitoneum, often via a transmesocolic approach. In this technique it is imperative that the initial operation be thorough and therefore the results are best in the hands of experienced pancreatic surgeons. At the time of laparotomy, the entire pancreas from head to tail must be explored. Reference to the preoperative CT scan provides a road map to direct the operation. Often the capsule of the pancreas must be incised to find a necrotic sequestrum. All necrotic tissue must be removed. Simply placing drains adjacent to dead tissue is not adequate therapy.

Because the necrotizing process may not stop after the initial operation, two alternative approaches have been developed. Both aim to provide continuing debridement in the lesser sac as more tissue is sloughed. One technique popularized by Beger and colleagues involves necrosectomy and continuous postoperative lavage of the lesser sac. In this technique necrotic tissue is debrided and irrigation catheters are placed in the lesser sac. Two days after surgery, lavage with isotonic solution begins at a rate of 7 to 48 L per day. The median duration of lavage is 25 days and the median hospital stay in Beger's series was 60 days. Lavage may be discontinued when the effluent no longer contains particulate debris and the amylase content of the effluent is similar to serum levels. In spite of lavage, however, reoperation was required in 31 percent of patients with infected necrosis and 21 percent of patients with sterile necrosis. The technique requires substantial nursing care to manage the lavage system. In spite of these drawbacks, the mortality rate in Beger's series was impressively low (8.1 percent).

Another popular technique is open packing. After blunt debridement, the lesser sac is packed with moist gauze and the abdominal wound partially closed. The patient is returned to the operating room every 48 hours for further debridement and packing change until all necrotic debris is removed and healthy granulation tissue appears. After the first four or five debridements, these reoperations can be performed in the ICU. When healing occurs the abdomen can be closed over drains, with or without delayed lavage of the cavity. Good results have been reported with this technique despite the relatively high rate of enteric fistulae (15 to 40 percent), with mortality rates as low as with the previously described methods. This technique, however, requires repeated use of general anesthesia and requires the surgeon to return with the patient to the operating room every other day.

It is very difficult to compare the results of these three techniques because published series contain patients with differing severity of illness, differing indications for surgery, and differing levels of paramedical and ancillary support. Circumstances in which greater than 100 grams of necrotic tissue are removed, in which there is poor delineation of viable from nonviable tissue, or in which there is extensive peripancreatic necrosis with extension into the root of the mesentery, pararenal spaces, and lateral gutters are most likely to require more than one debridement. If there is concern that the initial debridement is likely to be incomplete, greater consideration should be given to open packing or continuous postoperative lavage.

Hemorrhage, a highly lethal complication, is caused by erosion of major blood vessels by elastase and other proteases. The initial lesion is a pseudoaneurysm. Infection is almost always present. If rupture occurs, life-threatening hemorrhage into a pseudocyst or retroperitoneum occurs. Angiography should be the initial step in management for this problem. Surgery is inevitably required at some point for debridement of the associated regional necrosis and to control sepsis. If the affected area is inadequately drained or debrided, progression of sepsis and/or recurrence of bleeding will surely follow and kill the patient.

Pancreatic Pseudocysts

Pseudocysts occur in 10 to 20 percent of cases of acute pancreatitis. Pseudocysts occurring as part of the ongoing necrotizing process are different and more dangerous than the pseudocysts which are common in chronic pancreatitis. Symptomatic pseudocysts which fail to resolve should be decompressed to relieve symptoms and prevent complications. The management of asymptomatic cysts is controversial. Ideally, surgical drainage of pancreatic pseudocysts should be performed when the cyst wall is fibrotic enough to allow placement of sutures (so-called mature cyst wall). A rule of thumb is that most cyst walls are mature within 6 weeks of the onset of symptoms.

Percutaneous drainage has gained acceptance in the treatment of pancreatic pseudocysts. Simple aspiration of acute pancreatic pseudocysts is associated with a recurrence rate of 75 percent or more. Drainage of pseudocysts with indwelling catheters is more successful and may be akin to external drainage without debridement of associated necrotic debris. The ideal patients for percutaneous drainage are those who are relatively well with a discrete fluid collection. Patients with multiple pseudocysts and ongoing inflammation are probably best managed with surgical techniques.

Endoscopic techniques have been used to drain pseudocysts in patients with chronic pancreatitis, but the complication rate in acute pancreatitis appears to be much higher. One must resist the temptation to utilize endoscopic and percutaneous drainage procedures inappropriately just because they seem easy to perform. All forms of intervention carry defined risks of complications and thus the indications and timing of intervention should be the same regardless of whether one employs surgical, percutaneous, or endoscopic techniques. Endoscopic pseudocyst drainage is discussed in a separate chapter, as well.

Persisting Pancreatitis

Some patients have lingering symptoms such as inability to eat, abdominal pain, or even intermittent fever long after a bout of acute pancreatitis. Most of these patients require intravenous nutritional support either at home or in the hospital. At some point (usually 2 to 3 months after the onset of illness) one must look for a reversible problem which will alter the course of the illness.

Surgically correctable causes of persisting pancreatitis include undrained collections, irreversible injury to the pancreatic duct, or inflammatory masses pressing on the stomach or duodenum. If a focal collection is seen on a CT scan, debridement or drainage is the obvious intervention which is required. Persisting collections generally require surgical therapy. By the time these patients are referred to a surgeon, it is not uncommon for several attempts at percutaneous drainage to have been made and failed. If no obvious collection is identified by CT scan, ERCP may identify irreversible injury to the pancreatic duct causing persistent obstructive pancreatitis distal to the ductal injury. Distal pancreatectomy is indicated in symptomatic patients when the pancreatic duct becomes obstructed by the necrotizing process and its healing by scar.

A few patients continue to have low-grade signs of pancreatic inflammation for many weeks or even several months, without focal collections or areas of necrosis demonstrable by CT scan which might be suitable for debridement or drainage. In those patients who have persistent swelling or phlegmon, particularly in the head of the pancreas, pancreatic duodenectomy, however radical that may seem, may be the only option left.

Usually the resected specimen demonstrates microabscesses or unrecognized duodenal wall injury. Pancreatic duodenectomy in this setting is technically demanding and should only be performed by experienced pancreatic surgeons.

CHRONIC PANCREATITIS

Presently there is no therapy which alters the natural history of chronic pancreatitis. Therefore surgery is indicated for relief of pain, relief of obstruction of the bile duct and duodenum, and to exclude the presence of malignancy. Most cases of chronic pancreatitis are due to alcohol abuse and therefore surgery is only part of the treatment for these patients. Patients who continue to drink following surgical procedures to relieve pain in chronic pancreatitis are likely to have recurrent symptoms.

In evaluating patients with chronic pancreatitis for surgery, pancreatic duct morphology plays a pivotal role in selecting the surgical procedure. Patients with chronic pancreatitis may be divided into two groups based on the diameter of the pancreatic duct. Those whose pancreatic ducts are less than 7 mm in diameter are best treated by partial pancreatic resection. Pain relief for those whose ducts are larger than 7 mm can be achieved by ductal decompression which preserves the remaining endocrine parenchyma.

Ductal Decompression

Patients with dilated pancreatic ducts are best served by longitudinal pancreaticojejunostomy. It is critical that the entire pancreatic duct from the head to the tail be opened and drained into a Roux-en-Y loop of jejunum. Failure to achieve pain relief following this procedure is usually due to inadequate drainage of the pancreatic duct. Therefore, the surgeon must unroof the duct in the head of the gland, to the right of the gastroduodenal artery. At times resection of the anterior portion of the head of the pancreas is necessary to expose the proximal pancreatic duct. When a bile duct stricture is present, a choledochojejunostomy may be performed into the same loop of bowel which drains the pancreas. Patients with multiple pseudocysts and a dilated pancreatic duct can undergo combined pseudocyst and ductal drainage with this procedure. Longitudinal pancreaticojejunostomy has an extremely low morbidity and mortality rate. Immediate pain relief is achieved in over 80 percent of patients and 60 percent of patients are pain free 5 years following surgery.

Pancreatic Resection

Pancreatic resection provides effective relief of pain and excludes the presence of malignancy in carefully-selected patients. Pancreatic resection is most successful in patients with a dominant mass (i.e., focal pancreatitis). Distal pancreatic resection should be considered when the bulk of the disease appears to be in the tail of the gland and the pancreatic duct is obstructed in its midportion by scar. Although it seems logical that such patients are likely to achieve pain relief when the obstructed segment of pancreas is removed, the historical results of this operation are poor. Furthermore the tail is rich in islets and precious endocrine reserve may be sacrificed. Therefore, I do not recommend distal or distal subtotal pancreatectomy for pain relief unless the head of the pancreas appears normal at the time of laparotomy and disease is truly confined to the left side of the gland.

In many patients, the most severe inflammation is found in the head of the gland. Such patients get excellent pain relief from a pylorus preserving pancreaticoduodenectomy. The long-term results are superior to pancreatic drainage procedures. Preservation of the pylorus during Whipple procedure avoids postgastrectomy and nutritional problems associated with the traditional Whipple operation. Although new operations such as duodenum-sparing resections of the head of the pancreas have been proposed, they do not appear to offer any advantage over pylorus-preserving pancreaticoduodenectomy. Pancreaticoduodenectomy also prevents or corrects biliary and duodenal obstruction from the cicatrizing process of chronic pancreatitis.

Total pancreatectomy should be reserved for those patients who have failed either Whipple procedures or distal pancreatectomies. Often these patients will have dense retroperitoneal fibrosis and continue to have pancreatic type pain following a total pancreatectomy. The development of diabetes is a certainty following this procedure and thus it is useful only in highly selected patients. Celiac ganglion blocks are an alternative to completion (total) pancreatectomy. Some centers have reported excellent results using a combination of steroids and long-acting local anesthetics but this experience has not been widely duplicated. Neurotoxic solutions may be used as well with relief of pain for 6 months to 1 year, but most patients will develop recurrent pain and repeated blocks are ineffective. The utility of nerve blocks may be to allow a period of time to wean the patient from narcotics or to check on abstinence from alcohol prior to proceeding with a major resective procedure.

SUGGESTED READING

Beger HG, Bittner R, Block S, Buchler M. Bacterial contamination of pancreatic necrosis: A prospective clinical study. Gastroenterology 1986; 91:433–438.

Beger HG, Krautzberger W, Bittner R, et al. Results of surgical treatment of necrotizing pancreatitis. World J Surg 1985; 59: 972–978.

Fan ST, Lai ECS, Mok FPT, et al. Early treatment of acute biliary pancreatitis by endoscopic papillotomy. N Engl J Med 1993; 328:228–232.

Neoptolemos JP, London N, Slater ND, et al. A prospective study of ERCP and endoscopic sphincterotomy in the diagnosis and treatment of gallstone acute pancreatitis. Arch Surg 1986; 121:697–702.

Ranson JHC. The timing of biliary surgery in acute pancreatitis. Ann Surg 1979; 189:654–661.

Rattner DW, Legermate DA, Lee MJ, et al. Early surgical debridement of symptomatic pancreatic necrosis is beneficial irrespective of infection. Am J Surg 1992; 163:105–110.

Schroder T, Sainio V, Kivisaari L, et al. Pancreatic resection versus peritoneal lavage in acute necrotizing pancreatitis. A prospective randomized trial. Ann Surg 1991; 214:663–666.

PANCREATITIS: ENDOSCOPIC THERAPY

RICHARD A. KOZAREK, M.D.

The endoscopic approach to pancreatitis can be subdivided into therapy for acute or chronic pancreatitis. Treatment of the former has usually consisted of biliary sphincterotomy for choledocholithiasis or microlithiasis in conjunction with sphincter dysfunction. Treatment of the latter, on the other hand, has included a variety of interventional techniques traditionally applied to the biliary tree. These include pancreatic duct sphincterotomy, stent or drain placements, stone extraction, and treatment of pancreatic ductal disruption with concomitant pseudocyst, pleural effusion, or pancreatic ascites.

ACUTE PANCREATITIS

Endoscopic retrograde cholangiopancreatography (ERCP) can be utilized both to diagnose and treat causes (Table 1) of severe acute or relapsing pancreatitis (choledocholithiasis, choledochocele, pancreas divisum, sphincter dysfunction).

Sphincterotomy—Major Papilla

From the standpoint of presumed acute biliary pancreatitis, prospective surgical and endoscopic studies suggest that cholangiograms undertaken within 1 to 3 days will show a high likelihood of stones. Moreover, patients with severe pancreatitis as defined by the Ranson or Glasgow criteria will be less likely to have spontaneously-passed calculi. In contrast, cholangiography done several weeks later at time of elective cholecystectomy is much less likely to demonstrate a retained bile duct stone. Prospective studies have

Table 1 Endoscopic Therapy for Acute Pancreatitis

Gallstone pancreatitis	ES, stone extraction
Sphincter dysfunction	ES, septotomy
Choledochocele	ES
Pancreas divisum	Minor sphincterotomy, DPD stent

ES = endoscopic sphincterotomy (biliary); DPD = dorsal pancreatic duct.

demonstrated that urgent ERCP and sphincterotomy for documented choledocholithiasis in conjunction with severe acute pancreatitis significantly ameliorates the disease process. For instance, one British group noted statistically significant reduction in mortality (1.7 percent versus 17.9 percent), hospitalization length (9.5 versus 17 days), and complications (24 percent versus 61 percent) when compared to patients treated conservatively or with acute cholecystectomy and common bile duct exploration.

In addition to treatment of choledocholithiasis associated with severe pancreatitis, endoscopic sphincterotomy has been utilized to treat sphincter dysfunction associated with relapsing pancreatitis. Previous pancreaticobiliary manometry data by the Geenen group suggest that up to one-sixth of patients with acute relapsing pancreatitis have a hypertensive pancreaticobiliary sphincter. Most of these patients responded to biliary sphincterotomy although a few required surgical septoplasty to prevent recurrent attacks of pancreatic inflammation. Although data such as the above can be construed to suggest that some patients with relapsing pancreatitis have primary sphincter dysfunction, an alternative explanation may be that a subset of these individuals have microlithiasis that is etiologic for both the pancreatitis and the sphincter dysfunction, the latter as a consequence of gravel-induced papillitis and papillary stenosis. Recent articles seem to confirm this.

Sphincterotomy—Minor Papilla

Finally, endoscopic therapy has been utilized in patients with relapsing pancreatitis thought to be a consequence of pancreas divisum. The latter, occurring in 5 to 10 percent of autopsy and ERCP series, has been felt by some authors to offer a relative obstruction to dorsal pancreatic ductal (DPD) flow and to eventuate in a form of obstructive pancreatitis in a subset of such patients. Unfortunately, most of the reports utilizing endoscopic therapy for pancreas divisum admix patients with chronic pain, recurrent attacks of acute pancreatitis, and those with ductal changes of chronic pancreatitis. Three major approaches have been used in patients with divisum and relapsing pancreatitis. Our group has previously shown that up to 25 percent of such patients have hypertension of the sphincter of Oddi and that biliary sphincterotomy has precluded recurrent pancreatitis in two-thirds of these patients for up to 4 years. It is possible that some or all of these patients had been passing biliary gravel; abnormal liver function tests during attacks was a helpful, but not invariable, finding.

Some authors believe that patients with relapsing pancreatitis are best treated with 5 to 7 Fr pancreatic ductal stents which are changed at 3 to 4 month intervals over a period of 1 to 2 years. The Racine group has excellent open label and patient-blind data to suggest this technique is useful in many relapsing pancreatitis patients who have divisum but no other discernible etiology for their pancreatitis. Because I have previously published data on the induction of chronic pancreatitis-like lesions in patients who have endoprostheses inserted into normal pancreatic ducts, I would discourage such a practice. Such lesions, potentially initiated by stent or sidebranch occlusion, or a direct consequence of tip pressure on the pancreatic duct epithelium, are occasionally irreversible.

The approach I prefer in patients with divisum, particularly in individuals who appear to manifest ductal obstruction by a secretin ultrasound test, was popularized by Lehman and his colleagues. The latter includes placement of a short (1 to 3 cm) DPD endoprosthesis and, using the stent as a strut, effecting a minor duct sphincterotomy with the needle-knife. The Indianapolis group has reported a reduction in acute pancreatitis attacks in 15 of 20 such patients after a 6 to 54 month follow-up. Only 38 percent of patients with chronic pain, in turn, experienced clinical improvement after sphincterotomy of the minor ampulla, a figure that may approximate the placebo response.

CHRONIC PANCREATITIS

The endoscopic approach to chronic pancreatitis has been directed at obstructing calculi or stenoses or various forms of ductal disruption (Table 2). Such treatment assumes that ductal leakage or obstruction play a role in the pain patterns or relapsing attacks of pancreatitis in chronic pancreatitic patients. That pseudocysts or pancreatic ascites can be symptomatic or be associated with subsequent complications needs little emphasis. Supporting the concept that ductular obstruction can be symptomatic is the ductal dilation that develops distal to a stone or local stenosis, an elevation of main pancreatic duct pressure in chronic pancreatitis patients when compared to controls, and the relief of symptoms many patients experience after a longitudinal pancreaticojejunostomy.

Sphincterotomy

There is very little evidence that pancreatic duct sphincter dysfunction causes either chronic pain or relapsing pancreatitis in individuals with documented chronic pancreatitis. Papillary stenosis does occur in a subset of such individuals, however, and endoscopic section of the pancreatic duct sphincter mechanism is associated with decrease in duct size. Moreover, pancreatic sphincterotomy can be utilized to facilitate other therapeutic maneuvers such as stone extraction or endoprosthesis placement.

Historically, endoscopic pancreatic duct (PD) sphincterotomy had been felt to be contraindicated, both because of uncertainty regarding its application as well as fear of inducing fulminant pancreatitis. More recently, a number of groups including our own, have reported their experience with the technique. Most individuals have adopted conventional sphincterotomes to the pancreatic duct although ductal septotomies can also be performed utilizing a needle-knife sphincterotome over a transpapillary endoprosthesis. Over the past 4 years, we have undertaken 56 endoscopic PD sphincterotomies at our institution, all but two in the setting of chronic pancreatitis. Indications included obstructing calculi (26), ductal disruption (12), papillary stenosis (10), and dominant ductal stenosis (8). All but four patients had short endoprostheses placed across the sphincterotomy site. Acute complications were noted in 8 percent cholangitis (2), pancreatitis exacerbation (4) and an additional 15 percent developed self-limited ductal changes related to stent placement. Sphincterotomy stenosis, perhaps related to small incisions early in our experience, was ultimately noted in eight patients (16 percent). All of the latter patients required repeat endoscopic sphincterotomy of the pancreatic duct. Data such as the foregoing, while not defining efficacy, suggest at least that the procedure is relatively safe in this group of patients.

Table 2 Endoscopic Therapy for Chronic Pancreatitis

Sphincter stenosis	PD sphincterotomy (major, minor)
Obstructing calculi	PD sphincterotomy, stone extraction
Dominant stenosis	Endoprosthesis
Pseudocyst	Transgastric, transduodenal drainage, transpapillary drainage
Pancreatic ascites/effusion	Endoprosthesis
Biliary stricture	Biliary endoprosthesis

Stone Extraction (Fig. 1)

Conventional wisdom suggests that pancreatic duct calculi are the consequence as opposed to the cause of chronic pancreatitis. Stones can become obstructive, however, particularly when situated distal to a local ductal stricture or in the setting of papillary stenosis. In our series, we have been able to retrieve calculi in 23 of 26 patients (88 percent) with resolution of relapsing attacks of chronic pancreatitis in 90 percent and decrease in chronic pain in an additional 50 percent. The largest series of such patients have been reported by the Cremer group following sphincterotomy, extracorporeal shock wave lithotripsy (ESWL), endoscopic stone fragment extraction, and endoprosthesis placement. In their series, stone fragmentation was effected in 99 percent of 104 patients and complete stone clearance was possible in one-half. All patients were purported to experience initial pain relief although 41 percent developed subsequent recurrence related to stone migration, relapsing stricture or stent placement. Given the foregoing, I currently utilize PD sphincterotomy and stone extraction in patients with amenable anatomy, absence of tight stenoses, and one to four proximal calculi.

Endoprosthesis Placement (Fig. 2)

Pancreatic duct stents can be placed with or without a pancreatic sphincterotomy. When they are used to protect a fresh sphincterotomy, I tend to utilize short stents for 1 to 4 weeks, taking care not to utilize a diameter that will eventuate in side branch occlusion.

Although endoprostheses can also be placed beyond obstructing stenoses or calculi without sphincterotomy, they are not a long-term solution to an obstructive problem. Not only do endoprostheses occlude secondary to bacterial biofilm development plus clogging with mucus and calcium-rich secretions, their mere presence

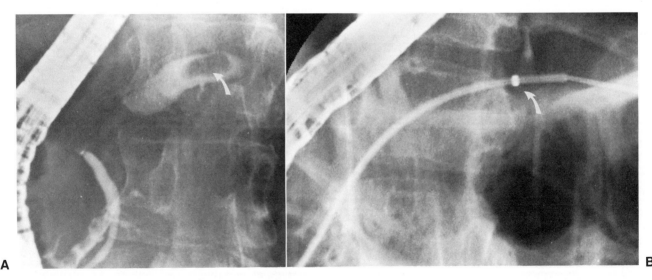

A   **B**

Figure 1 Pancreatogram demonstrating chronic pancreatitis, large stone *(arrow)*, mid-body *(A)*. Balloon catheter *(arrow)* placed over guidewire and used to extract calculus following PD sphincterotomy *(B)*.

is associated with development of significant ductal stenoses and side branch ectasias. Rather, stents should be used in the latter settings as a diagnostic tool with resultant pain relief postendoprosthesis to be used as a clinical guide to direct subsequent medical, endoscopic, or surgical intervention. The Brussels group has published one of the largest series utilizing endoprostheses in this way, successfully inserting stents in 75 of 76 chronic pancreatitis patients.

Endoprostheses are quite useful in the setting of pancreatic ductal disruption. Pseudocysts are discussed in the next section. Pancreatic ascites, in turn, has traditionally been treated with large volume paracenteses, hyperalimentation, and more recently, somatostatin analog. Nevertheless, ultimate surgical intervention is required in more than one-half of these patients. I currently have treated four patients with pancreatic ductal disruptions and refractory pancreatic ascites, inserting 6 to 7 Fr stents through the papilla and beyond the ductal disruption. Two of these patients had concurrent pseudocysts. All underwent a subsequent single large volume paracentesis and did not develop recurrent ascites with refeeding. Stents were retrieved at 4 weeks and mean patient follow-up is now 1 year. No patient has developed recurrent problems. This limited experience suggests that endoprosthesis insertion should be considered in selected patients with pancreatic ascites before surgical intervention.

Pseudocyst Drainage (Fig. 3)

Pancreatic pseudocysts can either be drained through the gastric or duodenal wall or via a transampullary approach. Our group has published the largest series utilizing the latter technique. In this series, 17 patients with pancreatic duct disruption and associated fluid collections underwent transpapillary drain or stent placement. Nine patients had acute and eight had chronic pancreatitis. Fourteen patients had successful

resolution of their fluid collection and closure of their ductal disruption. Mild pancreatitis occurred in two patients and an additional two developed stent occlusion with recurrent pseudocyst (one) or infection in a pseudocyst (one). Both of the latter complications resolved with stent exchange. The purpose was to avoid acute but not necessarily elective surgical intervention; surgery was ultimately required in one-third of the patients.

Transgastric or transduodenal drainage of a pseudocyst requires a cyst contiguous with an amenable segment of bowel, less than 1 cm of intervening soft tissue, and absence of varices at the puncture site. This anatomy usually requires a baseline computed tomography (CT) examination and may be better defined with endoscopic ultrasonography. I currently utilize a fistulotome with two additional channels for aspiration, contrast injection, or guidewire placement. After antibiotic coverage and having undertaken a baseline ERCP to define the anatomy to include presence or absence of active ductal disruption, I fistulize through the contiguous gut wall, obtain an aspirate for gram stain, culture and sensitivity and amylase; and place two guidewires into the cyst cavity. I utilize a 10-Fr, 3-cm double pigtail stent for initial drainage then usually insert a 7-Fr nasocyst drain for 24 to 48 hours. The latter can be simply removed or exchanged for a second stent in several days. Stents can be retrieved in 4 to 6 weeks after ascertaining cyst resolution with follow-up CT or ultrasound examinations. Although I initially described this technique, the largest experience with it has been in Europe and there are currently three series describing in excess of 30 patients so treated. Combined technical success rates approximate 95 percent and complications, usually bleeding or infection, 10 percent. Ultimate cyst resolution without recurrence has been noted in 80 to 90 percent.

The previous data need to be put into the perspective of more traditional surgical or percutaneous ap-

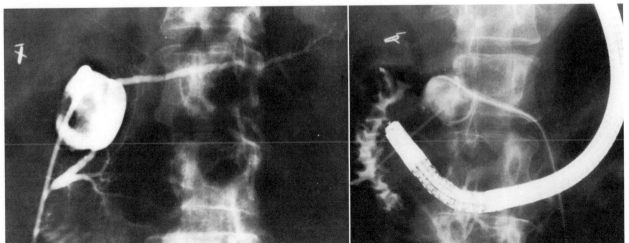

Figure 2 Percutaneous drainage of pancreatic pseudocyst in head of gland *(A)*. Transpapillary pancreatic stent *(B)* in patient depicted in *(A)*. Percutaneous drainage stopped within 24 hours, pseudocyst resolved in 1 week.

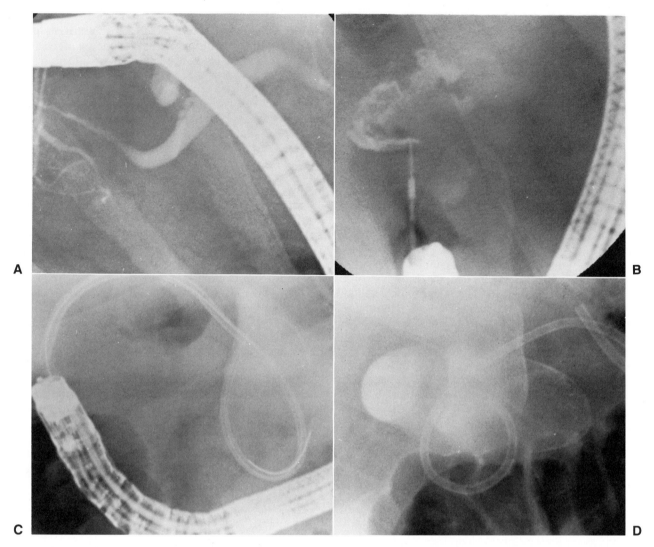

Figure 3 ERCP demonstrating distal CBD stenosis, obstruction of PD in head *(A)*. Transduodenal contrast injection into retroduodenal pseudocyst in patient depicted in A *(B)*. 10 Fr double pigtail stent inserted into retroduodenal pseudocyst *(C)*. 10 Fr double pigtail inserted through duodenal bulb to drain pseudocyst *(D)*. Note gallbladder contrast from previous ERCP.

proaches to pseudocyst drainage. They must also be placed into the perspective of amenable anatomy and local subspecialty expertise. Even in our own institution, less than one-third of pancreatic pseudocysts undergo endoscopic decompression as I do not think it is wise to drain huge, compartmentalized cysts through a single puncture. Nor does it seem reasonable to expect small diameter internal stents to drain pseudocysts with copious debris and persistent phlegmonous changes.*

Biliary Stricture

Acute edema or cicatrization of the distal bile duct within the head of the pancreas may be associated with cholestasis and even bouts of cholangitis. Moreover,

prolonged stenosis has been associated with the development of secondary biliary cirrhosis in a small subset of such patients.

It seems reasonable to place a 10- or 11.5-Fr biliary stent in patients with the acute onset of cholestasis or cholangitis associated with pancreatitis. Data do not support resolution of long-term biliary strictures following endoprosthesis placement in patients with chronic pancreatitis. Rather, large series from Amsterdam and Brussels suggest a prohibitively high rate of stent occlusion with subsequent cholangitis, liver abscess, and even death.

PERSPECTIVE

The endoscopic approach to pancreatic disease remains in its infancy. Most of the techniques described

---

*Editor's Note: Unless you're good, "don't try this at home."

above are adaptations of procedures previously utilized within the biliary tree and are likely to undergo an evolutionary process contingent upon patient and endoscopist needs and the results of controlled clinical trials. Moreover, the ability to apply a technology does not mean that application of that technology is right in all situations. I am particularly concerned about long-term, indwelling pancreatic endoprostheses in patients with ostensibly normal ductal systems. I am also concerned about proliferation of PD sphincterotomy as an attempt to treat all patients with chronic pancreatitis or the generalization that because sphincterotomy is safe in patients with fibrotic pancreases, it is also safe in those with normal pancreatic ducts. There are no data to support the latter assumption. Finally, I am concerned about the European experience regarding metal stent placement to treat pancreatic ductal stenoses. As such prostheses imbed in the epithelial wall, they cannot be removed endoscopically and would seem to make surgery, if needed, considerably more difficult.

Nevertheless, I look forward to an evolving endotherapy directed against acute and chronic pancreatic pathology in the years to come.

SUGGESTED READING

Amman RW. A critical appraisal of interventional therapy in chronic pancreatitis. Endoscopy 1991; 23:191–193.

Cremer M, Deviere J, Delhaye M, et al. Non-surgical management of severe chronic pancreatitis. Scand J Gastroenterol 1990; 25:77–84.

Geenen JE, Rolny P. Endoscopic therapy of acute and chronic pancreatitis. Gastrointest Endosc 1991; 37:377–382.

Kozarek RA. Endoscopy and the pancreas. In: Cotton PB, Tytgat CNJ, Williams CB, eds. Annual of gastrointestinal endoscopy. London: Current Science, 1992:81.

Lang JI, Geenen JE, Johanson JF, Hogan WJ. Endoscopic therapy in patients with pancreas divisum and acute pancreatitis: A prospective, randomized, controlled trial. Gastrointest Endosc 1992; 38: 430–434.

Lee SP, Nicholls JF, Park MZ. Biliary sludge as a cause of acute pancreatitis. N Engl J Med 1992; 326:589–593.

Lehman GA, Sherman S, Nisi R, Hawes RM. Pancreas divisum: Results of minor papilla sphincterotomy. Gastrointest Endosc 1993; 39:1–8.

Neoptolemos JP, London NJ, Carr-Locke D, et al. Controlled trial of urgent endoscopic retrograde cholangiopancreatography and endoscopic sphincterotomy versus conservative treatment for acute pancreatitis due to gallstones. Lancet 1988; 2:979–983.

Venu RP, Geenen JE, Hogan WJ, et al. Idiopathic recurrent pancreatitis—An approach to diagnosis and treatment. Dig Dis Sci 1989; 34:56.

CHRONIC PANCREATITIS: EXOCRINE AND ENDOCRINE INSUFFICIENCY

SUDHIR K. DUTTA, M.D.

DIAGNOSIS

The diagnosis of chronic pancreatitis is generally considered in patients who present with upper abdominal pain, chronic diarrhea, or significant weight loss. In a given case, any combination of these symptoms may be present. Furthermore, in many cases, recurrent attacks of acute pancreatitis may precede the onset of chronic pancreatitis. However, 10 to 15 percent of patients with chronic pancreatitis present initially with only diarrhea or weight loss or both. The development of malabsorption in a patient with chronic pancreatitis indicates more than 90 percent loss of exocrine pancreatic function.

The abdominal pain associated with chronic pancreatitis is characterized by a mid-epigastric location, a dull and continuous nature, and radiation to the back that is relieved by forward bending. Diarrhea in these patients is chronic, with a frequency ranging from only one bowel movement per day to as many as six or more per day. Weight loss is often significant (10 lb or more) and frequently associated with clinical manifestations of uncontrolled diabetes mellitus. As a result of weight loss, protein energy malnutrition of the marasmus type is initially present in 30 to 50 percent of cases of chronic pancreatitis. It is important to assess the extent of malnutrition carefully in order to determine the response to pancreatic enzyme or nutritional therapy. It is equally important to record the symptoms in detail, because the response to medical therapy is generally evaluated in relation to the presenting symptoms.

Irreversible Structural Damage

The diagnosis of chronic pancreatitis is often difficult to establish in clinical situations, particularly in patients with early disease associated with only mild to moderate pancreatic dysfunction. Evidence of irreversible structural damage or permanent functional impairment of the pancreatic gland should be obtained by various clinical tests available. Clinical evidence of irreversible structural damage generally includes (1) pancreatic calcification, (2) pancreatic duct strictures, and (3) chronic inflammation on histologic views of the pancreatic gland. Pancreatic calcification is noted on plain radiographs of the abdomen or on computed tomographic (CT) scans. Pancreatic duct abnormality is delineated by pancreatography, which can be obtained endoscopically and occasionally at the time of surgery. Pancreatic histologic findings are available in a few patients who undergo pancreatic biopsy or resection. In clinical practice, chronic pancreatitis is frequently diagnosed on the basis of pancreatic calcification and/or abnormal pancreatographic appearance.

Permanent Functional Impairment

The presence of permanent functional impairment of the pancreatic gland can be determined by traditional tests such as the secretin stimulation test or one of the newer tests of pancreatic function, such as the bentiromide nitroblue tetrazolium-para-aminobenzoic acid (NBT-PABA) test. It should be emphasized that although the secretin stimulation test is tedious and inconvenient because of the need for duodenal intubation, it is still the most sensitive test for diagnosing early pancreatic disease in patients who have not yet developed malabsorption. Among a large number of "tubeless" pancreatic function tests, the bentiromide test appears to be the most convenient, inexpensive, and easily available for diagnosing advanced chronic pancreatitis. Because of these features, sequential bentiromide tests are being used to evaluate the response to pancreatic enzyme therapy in patients with exocrine pancreatic insufficiency. However, the bentiromide test and similar "tubeless" pancreatic function tests have low sensitivity for diagnosing early or mild pancreatic gland dysfunction. Furthermore, it is essentially a urine test, which requires normal renal function, sufficient diuresis, and proper intestinal absorption. Bentiromide is a synthetic tripeptide that is specifically cleaved by pancreatic chymotrypsin. The cleavage of this molecule by chymotrypsin in the duodenum releases para-aminobenzoic acid (PABA), which is rapidly absorbed, conjugated in the liver, and excreted in the urine. Patients with chronic pancreatitis consistently excrete less PABA in the urine than healthy controls, because of impaired chymotrypsin secretion.

TREATMENT

Treatment of patients with chronic pancreatitis is generally directed toward (1) relief of upper abdominal pain and (2) correction of diarrhea, weight loss, and malnutrition.

Treatment of Abdominal Pain

Abdominal pain is the most difficult problem to treat for several reasons. First, pain is a subjective sensation, with no objective parameter to document or monitor its occurrence. Second, alcoholism is an underlying problem in many of these patients, and alcoholics have a drug-dependent personality. Not infrequently, alcoholic patients feign abdominal pain in order to obtain analgesics, sedatives, and narcotics. Consequently, it is often difficult to determine whether the abdominal pain is truly due to an underlying organic disease. Abstinence from alcohol is obviously desirable and should be strongly recommended. In the management of abdominal pain from chronic pancreatitis, I have found a five-step strategy exceedingly helpful (Table 1). The first step is documentation of pancreatic inflammation. Biochemical or radiologic evidence of pancreatic inflammation tends to suggest a pancreatic origin for such pain. Elevated serum amylase or lipase activity or evidence of an abnormal pancreatic gland on imaging suggests active pancreatic inflammation. However, patients with chronic pancreatitis sometimes have normal serum amylase and lipase levels and a fibrotic calcified pancreatic gland without any evidence of edema. The second step in management of pancreatic pain involves careful evaluation of complications such as pseudocyst or phlegmon. Again, pancreatic gland imaging by ultrasonography or CT helps to confirm or rule out these complications. The third step is to rule out other gastrointestinal (GI) lesions that can present clinically with upper abdominal pain, including peptic ulcer disease, penetrating ulcer, gastritis, and cholelithiasis. Upper endoscopy, ultrasonography, and a profile of liver function tests can help the differential diagnosis. The fourth step includes careful re-evaluation of the diagnosis of chronic pancreatitis in terms of irreversible structural damage or permanent impairment of pancreatic gland function; this often involves repeat pancreatography or CT scan. The fifth and final step is a close follow-up, monitoring the severity of pain, and the analgesic needs of the patient for 4 to 6 months. Again, abstinence from alcohol is essential. Alcoholism is the subject of a separate chapter.

After a thorough evaluation of pancreatic pain, a number of treatment measures can be instituted (Table 2).

Patient Education

The first step is educating patients about the natural history of this chronic ailment, its associated complications, and its likely long-term outcome. Each patient with chronic pancreatitis should understand that after 5 to 10 years the episodes of pancreatic pain generally diminish in frequency and often disappear altogether. However, at about the time that abdominal pain diminishes, most patients with chronic pancreatitis also develop hyperglycemia and malabsorption.

Analgesics

The second step involves generous use of non-narcotic analgesics (e.g., acetaminophen, ibuprofen, and nonsteroidal analgesics) to control abdominal pain. In my experience, a large percentage of patients with

Table 1 Evaluation of Patients With Abdominal Pain Associated With Chronic Pancreatitis

Step 1 Seek evidence of active pancreatic inflammation during painful periods (elevation of serum amylase, lipase, or urinary amylase activity).

Step 2 Seek evidence of complications of pancreatitis (pancreatic pseudocyst or phlegmon).

Step 3 Rule out other upper gastrointestinal diseases (peptic ulcer disease, gastritis, and gallstone disease).

Step 4 Re-evaluate evidence of irreversible structural abnormality or permanent functional impairment of exocrine pancreatic gland.

Step 5 Closely follow-up patient's abdominal pain for 4 to 6 months.

Table 2 Management of Abdominal Pain From Chronic Pancreatitis

Patient education (about natural history of chronic pancreatitis, risk of prolonged analgesic abuse, and need for alcohol abstinence)
Administration of non-narcotic analgesics (acetaminophen, ibuprofen, and nonsteroidal analgesics)
Exogenous pancreatic enzyme therapy
Periodic administration of narcotic analgesics
Somatostatin therapy
Endoscopic intervention
Celiac ganglionectomy
Surgical intervention
  Pancreaticojejunostomy
  Pancreatectomy

chronic pancreatic pain can be managed for a long time with these two measures. Limited prescription of narcotic analgesics such as acetaminophen with codeine is also reasonable during episodes of severe abdominal pain. Patients should always be reminded that long-term use of narcotic analgesics can result in drug dependence. If a patient's requirements for narcotic analgesic appear to be gradually increasing, strong consideration should be given to possible enrollment in a pain relief program and the use of pain control by other means. Pain due to chronic pancreatitis is frequently intermittent and postprandial, but when abdominal pain becomes more frequent, persistent, and affects the lifestyle of the patient, relief of pain becomes the most crucial part of the overall management. In these situations, celiac ganglionectomy and surgical intervention should be considered.

Pancreatic Enzyme Therapy

There has been significant interest in the use of oral pancreatic enzymes to ameliorate pancreatic pain because these preparations are relatively innocuous and inexpensive. The rationale for their use is based on presence of protease-sensitive feedback regulation of exocrine pancreatic secretion in normal human subjects. It has been postulated that reduced pancreatic enzyme

secretion in chronic pancreatitis causes increased and sustained stimulation of pancreatic gland, resulting in development of pancreatic pain.

The goal of pancreatic enzyme therapy in the treatment of chronic pancreatic pain is suppression of pancreatic stimulation, reduction in exocrine pancreatic secretion, decrease in pancreatic ductal and tissue pressure, and amelioration of pancreatic pain. Four clinical trials testing this hypothesis, involving a total of 69 patients with chronic pancreatitis, have been reported in the literature. Three studies (two controlled and one uncontrolled) have shown some benefit with pancreatic enzyme replacement therapy in pancreatic pain relief. Most of the benefit has been observed in patients with idiopathic chronic pancreatitis. In my experience, the use of oral pancreatic enzyme has not been effective in reducing chronic abdominal pain in patients with alcoholic pancreatitis. To examine this issue more definitively, a controlled, double blind clinical trial is needed in carefully selected patients with well-documented alcoholic and nonalcoholic chronic pancreatitis. Based on available information, a 4 week trial of oral pancreatic enzymes seems reasonable in patients with chronic abdominal pain from idiopathic pancreatitis. If abdominal pain is ameliorated or relieved, pancreatic enzyme therapy should be continued on a long-term basis. The precise dose of pancreatic enzymes necessary to restore normal feedback regulation of exocrine pancreatic secretion in patients with chronic pancreatitis has not been defined. I have used the same dose of pancreatic enzymes which is employed in the treatment of pancreatic steatorrhea (i.e., approximately 32,000 lipase units per meal).

Somatostatin Therapy

Somatostatin is a potent inhibitor of exocrine pancreatic enzyme secretion directly and indirectly via inhibition of cholecystokinin secretion. It has been proposed that a long-acting analog of somatostatin octreotide (Sandostatin) may ameliorate pancreatic pain by reducing exocrine pancreatic secretion, diminishing pancreatic ductal pressure, and minimizing exposure of pancreatic nerves to pancreatic enzyme. However, to date there is no published controlled clinical trial evaluating the effectiveness of octreotide therapy in this group of patients. Anecdotal case reports and data from octreotide compassionate need program have provided encouraging results about amelioration of abdominal pain in patients with chronic pancreatitis. A multicenter-controlled clinical trial designed to assess the short-term efficacy of octreotide therapy in the treatment of abdominal pain associated with chronic pancreatitis, has recently been completed in the U.S.A. In this trial, octreotide therapy was administered subcutaneously at a dose of 50 μg three times per day to a maximum of 200 μg three times per day to obtain adequate pain relief. Results of this and other similar clinical trials are eagerly awaited. Based on limited available information, it seems reasonable to consider octreotide therapy in a given case with persistent pseudocyst, pancreatic fistulae, pancreatic ascites, and chronic pancreatic pain. Limitation of octreotide therapy include lack of availability of oral preparation and development of side effects such as nausea, pain at the infection site, hyperglycemia, steatorrhea, and cholelithiasis.

Endoscopic Intervention

In the last 5 years, several published reports have documented the technical feasibility of pancreatic stent placement and pancreatic stone removal to overcome intraductal obstruction. These interventional modalities are designed to ameliorate pancreatic pain by establishing better drainage of main pancreatic duct and by reducing intrapancreatic pressure. These reports are preliminary and require further confirmation by larger controlled clinical studies. Significant concerns about the application of endoscopic techniques in this group of patients include (1) frequent occlusion of pancreatic stents, (2) distal migrations of the stent, (3) development of progressive histological changes of chronic pancreatitis, (4) development of acute pancreatitis, and (5) onset of pancreatic infection. The precise role of these endoscopic therapeutic modalities in the treatment of chronic pancreatic pain will be better defined in the next few years. The chapter on therapeutic endoscopy of the pancreas provides additional information.

Celiac Ganglionectomy

If medical treatment fails to control abdominal pain and the patient continues to consume narcotic analgesics frequently, more invasive measures should be considered. Local anesthetic agents such as lidocaine have been injected in the celiac ganglion under fluoroscopic guidance to reduce abdominal pain in patients with chronic pancreatitis. If pain relief is significant, the celiac ganglion can be destroyed by injecting alcohol at the same site (celiac ganglionectomy). Alternatively, complete destruction of celiac ganglion can be achieved surgically. The duration of pain relief after celiac ganglion destruction is approximately 6 months in the 50 percent of patients who respond to this treatment. In view of the limited long-term benefit and controlled clinical experience with this procedure, it should be used with caution in the management of chronic pancreatitis-related abdominal pain. The use of this technique for pancreatic cancer is discussed in the chapter on pancreatic and peripancreatic cancer.

Surgery

The final measure used to control pancreatic pain is surgical intervention. However, a decision for surgery is often difficult because the clinical course of this disease is unpredictable and pain frequently disappears spontaneously after a few years in a subgroup of patients. Patients should be advised of this possible outcome and encouraged to avoid surgery whenever possible.

Patients with chronic pancreatitis who have a dilated main pancreatic duct due to fibrotic strictures are generally treated by surgical drainage of the duct. Although a dilated, abnormal pancreatic duct and pancreatic pain are not well correlated, pain relief for a significant time has been well documented in some patients after a pancreatic drainage procedure. The choice of operation for abdominal pain from chronic pancreatitis includes (1) caudal pancreaticojejunostomy (DuVal procedure), (2) longitudinal pancreaticojejunostomy (Puestow procedure), and (3) subtotal pancreatectomy. The Puestow is the most popularly used drainage procedure in patients with chronic pancreatitis associated with a dilated main pancreatic duct. The entire main duct is opened in a longitudinal manner and all the pancreatic stones are extracted. A loop of jejunum is then opened longitudinally and sewn over the open duct so that the pancreatic juice can empty into the lumen of the jejunum. The results of surgery are generally better in patients who are neither alcoholic nor drug dependent. The surgical mortality rate from longitudinal pancreaticojejunostomy is less than 4 percent. As many as 50 percent of patients with chronic pancreatitis have been reported to derive relief from pain for 5 years. In those who do not respond favorably, an endoscopic pancreatogram should be obtained to verify the patency of pancreaticojejunal anastomosis. Anastomotic revision or pancreatic resection may provide pain relief in a subgroup of these patients. Marked pancreatic pain relief is achieved with distal pancreatectomy in patients with chronic pancreatic inflammation confined to the tail of the pancreas. Total and subtotal resections of the pancreatic gland have been largely abandoned by most tertiary care centers due to major metabolic and nutritional sequelae and unpredictable pain relief. There is a chapter *Pancreatitis: Surgical Considerations.*

Treatment of Diarrhea and Weight Loss

Pancreatic enzyme therapy is the cornerstone of management of pancreatic malabsorption. Symptomatic diarrhea is significantly improved with oral pancreatic enzyme therapy, but complete correction of steatorrhea is exceedingly difficult even with large amounts of pancreatic enzyme supplementation. Before pancreatic enzyme therapy is prescribed a number of points should be considered (Table 3).

Type of Enzyme Preparation

Many pancreatic enzyme preparations are commercially available; only those with a significant amount of lipase should be used. Well-known preparations include Ilozyme, Cotazym, Viokase, and Ku-Zyme HP. The pH-sensitive, enteric-coated preparations include Pancrease and Cotazym-S. There should be at least 8,000 units of lipase per capsule or tablet. More recently available pancreatic enzyme preparations contain as much as 10 to 25,000 units of lipase per capsule (Pancrease MT10, MT16, MT25; Creon 10 or 25). In general, capsules are preferable to tablets because there

Table 3 Selection of Exogenous Pancreatic Enzyme Therapy

Type of preparation: Any potent preparation that contains 8,000 units of lipase activity per capsule or more (e.g., Cotazym, Vikase, Ilozyme) can be used

Amount of preparation: Approximately 30,000 units of lipase per meal (2 to 8 capsules or tablets per meal)

Form of preparation: Capsules are preferable to tablets; powder form is of dubious value

Time of administration: With meal; total dose distributed evenly during ingestion of meal (two capsules in beginning, two in middle, and two at end)

Adjuvant therapy: H$_2$-receptor antagonists; antacids

pH-sensitive, enteric-coated pancreatic enzyme preparations (Pancrease, Cotazym-S)

New more potent enzyme preparations: Creon, Pancrease M25

is no unpalatable flavor and smell in the encapsulated preparation. Smaller capsules are preferred because of the ease with which they can be swallowed. The powder form of pancreatic enzyme preparation should not be used because of extensive inactivation by the acidity in the food articles and the stomach. Low-potency enzyme preparations do not provide adequate concentrations of pancreatic enzymes in the upper small intestine. In my experience, prescription of a few potent capsules of pancreatic enzyme preparation results in better patient compliance.

Amount of Pancreatic Enzyme

The dosage of the pancreatic enzyme preparation should be adequate to reduce steatorrhea significantly and improve symptoms satisfactorily. Large amounts of these enzyme preparations are inactivated in the stomach and only 5 to 10 percent of the orally ingested enzymes reach the upper small intestine. It has been estimated that about 30,000 units of lipase are necessary with a standard meal to provide a significant reduction in steatorrhea. Once ingested, lipase activity is inactivated below a pH of 4.0 and trypsin is inactivated below a pH of 3.0. These pH values are frequently reached in the stomach and in the upper small intestine during the postprandial period in this group of patients. Clinical studies have shown that as many as six to eight tablets or capsules (24,000 to 32,000 units of lipase) of potent pancreatic enzyme preparations per meal can provide a significant concentration of pancreatic enzymes in the upper gastrointestinal tract. Adequate amount of pancreatic enzymes can be provided by 2 to 3 capsules of high potency preparations such as Creon and Pancrease M25. These amounts of pancreatic enzymes are generally able to reduce steatorrhea by 60 percent and fecal nitrogen loss by 75 percent.

In order to improve the efficacy of pancreatic enzyme preparations, antacids and sodium bicarbonate have also been used. It has been reported that antacids such as aluminum hydroxide and sodium bicarbonate are effective as adjuvant therapy. However, magnesium and calcium-containing antacids should not be used, because they precipitate fatty acids and bile acids. Histamine$_2$ (H$_2$) receptor antagonists (H$_2$ blockers) as adjuncts to pancreatic enzyme supplementation have been shown by clinical studies to reduce steatorrhea significantly. H$_2$ blockers are likely to be more helpful in patients with hyperchlorhydria than in patients with low gastric acid secretion. H$_2$-blocker therapy should be added only in patients with an inadequate response to conventional pancreatic enzyme therapy alone.

Enteric-Coated Products

In order to protect pancreatic enzymes from the hostile acidic environment of the gastric acid, pH-sensitive, enteric-coated pancreatic enzyme preparations have become available. These preparations have pancreatic enzymes rolled into microspheres 1.5 to 2.5 mm in diameter, packed in a capsular form. The pH-sensitive enzyme coatings dissolve only at pH of 5.5 to 6.0 and release pancreatic enzymes into the environment. The enteric-coated preparations have been shown to be effective in reducing steatorrhea, but have not proved more effective than potent conventional enzyme preparations in alcoholic patients with pancreatic insufficiency. However, patients with cystic fibrosis seem to do better with enteric-coated preparations than with conventional preparations. The different responses of cystic fibrosis and alcoholic pancreatitis patients to enteric-coated preparations may be related to higher gastric acid secretion and gastric emptying in young patients with cystic fibrosis. The enteric-coated preparations are generally more expensive than conventional ones.

Hyperuricemia

There are no significant side effects from pancreatic enzyme therapy. Pancreatic extracts contain large amounts of nucleic acid and large doses have been reported to lead to hyperuricemia in some patients.

Poor Compliance

Compliance with pancreatic supplements is generally poor because of the large number of tablets or capsules that a patient with exocrine pancreatic insufficiency has to take with each meal. The preparations also have an unpleasant taste, so that capsules are much better tolerated by patients than the tablets. Cost can also be a factor.

Therapeutic Goals

The goal of pancreatic enzyme therapy is generally to help patients control diarrhea and gain body weight. A number of objective parameters can be used to evaluate the efficacy of pancreatic enzyme therapy in patients with exocrine pancreatic insufficiency (Table 4). With adequate pancreatic enzyme therapy, patients

Table 4 Parameters for Evaluation of Clinical Response to Pancreatic Enzyme Therapy in Exocrine Pancreatic Insufficiency

Weight gain and growth (in children)
Reduction in frequency and volume of bowel movements
Improvement in intestinal absorption
    Decrease in fecal fat excretion
    Increase in bentiromide excretion
Nutritional improvement
    Height-weight relationship
    Midarm muscle circumference
    Serum albumin
    Creatinine height index

Table 5 Management of Patients With Poor Response to Pancreatic Enzyme Therapy

Increase pancreatic enzyme therapy
Add adjuvant therapy
    H_2-blocker therapy
    Antacid therapy
    Sodium bicarbonate
Switch to pH-sensitive, enteric-coated pancreatic enzyme therapy
Check for noncompliance
Search for other associated disorders
    Celiac sprue
    Altered gastric emptying (status gastric surgery)
    Uncontrolled diabetes mellitus
    Bacterial overgrowth
    Ileal disease or resection
    Pancreatic cancer

should gain 1 or 2 lb each week and stabilize at about 10 percent below ideal body weight. In addition, anthropometric and biochemical parameters of nutritional assessment should also show improvement. Patients who do not respond well to pancreatic enzyme therapy should be carefully evaluated for noncompliance or for the presence of other associated disorders such as celiac sprue, altered gastric emptying, or bacterial overgrowth (Table 5). Specific steps to diagnose and treat each of these disorders are necessary in such individuals.

Treatment of Protein Energy Malnutrition

Nutritional support is also of paramount importance in patients with exocrine pancreatic insufficiency. As many as 40 percent of patients with chronic pancreatitis have clinically significant protein energy malnutrition.

These patients generally have diminished muscle mass as demonstrated by anthropometric and biochemical parameters of nutrition evaluation. Factors responsible for the development of protein energy malnutrition include diminished caloric intake and malabsorption due to impaired pancreatic enzyme secretion by the pancreatic gland. Not infrequently, uncontrolled diabetes mellitus and protein loss from a fistula also contribute significantly to protein energy malnutrition.

Besides generalized protein energy malnutrition due to maldigestion and malabsorption of fat, proteins, and carbohydrates, specific nutrient depletion can occur in these patients. Depletion of fat-soluble vitamins (particularly vitamins A and E) has been described in children with exocrine pancreatic insufficiency due to cystic fibrosis, and in adult patients with chronic alcoholic pancreatitis. Zinc deficiency manifesting as perioral and perianal eczematous rash has also been reported in patients with alcoholic pancreatitis. Vitamin B_{12} malabsorption can be documented in 40 to 50 percent of patients with untreated exocrine pancreatic insufficiency, but severe vitamin B_{12} deficiency and related anemia are rare in this group of patients. The physician should be aware of potential nutritional problems and should treat them appropriately when indicated. I do not routinely screen or treat patients with chronic pancreatitis for these specific nutrient deficiencies. However, patients with poor response to pancreatic enzyme therapy or with recurrent attacks of pancreatitis

are carefully evaluated for deficiencies of fat-soluble vitamins and minerals.

Management of protein energy malnutrition due to exocrine pancreatic insufficiency requires not only correction of malabsorption but also administration of a high-protein high-calorie diet. Poor caloric intake is a significant problem in some of these patients and is generally related to postprandial pain, dietary restrictions due to a recurrent flare-up of pancreatitis, and anorexia. Nutritional supplementation entails (1) assessment of the most appropriate nutritional support (e.g., total parenteral nutrition [TPN] or an elemental diet), (2) assessment of the duration of anticipated nutritional support, and (3) identification of the underlying problem contributing to the severe malnutrition.

If patient with chronic pancreatitis is severely malnourished, early TPN may be the treatment of choice. The pancreatic gland is very nutrition sensitive, and severe malnutrition has been reported to lead to atrophy and fibrosis. Nutritional repletion in these patients is associated with an improvement in pancreatic gland function.

In patients with mild-to-moderate severe malnutrition, elemental diets, protein hydrolysate preparations, or other supplemental diet therapies should be carefully considered. Medium chain triglyceride (MCT) preparations are attractive sources of lipid calories in this group of patients. Most MCT preparations contain primary fatty acids with 8 to 10 carbon chains as an energy source, and do not require lipase activity for absorption; they are derived mainly from coconut oil. However, poor taste and the development of nausea frequently limit the use of MCT in the treatment of severe malnutrition due to pancreatic insufficiency. MCT is available in a formula diet (Portagen) and also as a pure oil preparation for food. A specific nutrition supplemental therapy plan should be developed for each patient in consultation with the dietitian and nutrition support team.

Management of Diabetes Mellitus

The principal steps in the management of diabetes mellitus associated with chronic pancreatitis consist of correction of irregular food intake, malabsorption, and malnutrition and elimination of alcohol intake. Most patients require low doses of insulin, 5 to 15 units per day, to correct the hyperglycemia. The insulin requirement fluctuates between 10 and 40 units daily. Because of erratic and partial absorption of carbohydrates, these patients have a propensity to develop hypoglycemia; this may also be related to impaired glucagon secretion in chronic pancreatitis. Episodes of hypoglycemia have been reported in as many as one-third of patients being treated with insulin. The most prudent course to avoid hypoglycemia in this group of patients is to achieve higher-than-normal blood glucose levels, using the minimal doses of insulin necessary to avoid significant glucosuria. This approach appears to be reasonable, since the development of ketoacidosis and microvascular complications is relatively uncommon in these patients, and hypoglycemic episodes are frequent. Once the malabsorption is corrected with an appropriate diet plus pancreatic enzyme supplements, and after the body weight is stabilized, finer adjustment of blood glucose should be made. The importance of patient education about insulin administration and the management of its potential complications, cannot be overemphasized.

SUGGESTED READING

Adsor MA, McIlrath DC. Surgical treatment of chronic pancreatitis. In: Go VLW, et al, eds. The exocrine pancrease: biology, pathobiology and diseases. New York: Raven Press, 1986:587–599.

Cremer M, Deviere J, DeMaye M, et al. Non-surgical management of severe chronic pancreatitis. Scand J Gastroenterol 1990; 25:77–84.
DiMagno EP, Go VLW, Summerskill WHJ. Relations between pancreatic enzyme outputs and malabsorption in severe pancreatic insufficiency. N Engl J Med 1973; 288:813–815.
DiMagno EP, Malajelada JR, Go VLW, Moertel CG. Fate of orally infested enzymes in pancreatic insufficiency. N Engl J Med 1977; 296:1318–1322.
Dutta SK, Hubbard VS, Appler M. Critical examination of therapeutic efficacy of a pH-sensitive enteric-coated pancreatic enzyme preparation in the treatment of exocrine pancreatic insufficiency secondary to cystic fibrosis. Dig Dis Sci 1988; 33:1237–1244.
Dutta SK, Rubin J, Harvey J. Comparative evaluation of the therapeutic efficacy of a pH-sensitive coated pancreatic enzyme preparation with conventional pancreatic enzyme therapy in the treatment of exocrine pancreatic insufficiency. Gastroenterology 1983; 84:476–482.
Graham DY. Enzyme replacement therapy of exocrine pancreatic insufficiency in man. N Eng J Med 1977; 297:1314–1317.
Owyang C, Louie D, Tatum D. Feedback regulation of pancreatic enzyme secretion. J Clin Invest 1986; 77:2042–2047.
Regan PT, Malagelada JR, DiMagno EP, et al. Comparative effects of antacids, cimetidine, and enteric coating on the therapeutic response to oral enzymes in severe pancreatic insufficiency. N Engl J Med 1977; 297:854–858.

CYSTIC FIBROSIS

J.N. ROSENSWEIG, M.D.
A.J. KOVAR, M.S., R.D.

Cystic fibrosis (CF) is a genetic syndrome with autosomal recessive inheritance characterized by ductular obstruction of many organ systems as a result of thickened mucus secretions. Median life expectancy has improved from 10 years in 1960 to 29 years at present. With new medical therapies, it is anticipated that the median lifespan in patients with CF will reach 40 years. Carrier frequency in the Caucasian population is one in 25, and one in 2,500 neonates are affected; CF remains the most commonly inherited disorder in Caucasians of Northern European extraction. Other ethnic groups including African Americans, Askenazi Jews, and Southern Europeans are affected to a lesser extent.

There is a defect in the ability of epithelial cells throughout the body to transport chloride anions. Now it is clear that defects in many steps in transcription and translation and intracellular transport may be involved. In CF epithelium, one or more of these types of defects occurs, resulting in thickened secretions obstructing the respiratory tree, reproductive tract and pancreatic, intestinal, and hepatobiliary systems.

The CF gene was localized to chromosome seven in 1985 by Dr. Lap-Chee Tsui. Collaboration with several investigators using restriction fragment length polymorphisms, known DNA sequences, and gene jumping and gene walking (positional cloning), resulted in identification of the cystic fibrosis transmembrane conductance regulator (CFTR) gene 4 years later. The gene is composed of 230 kilobases and includes 27 exons. A three-base pair deletion in exon 10 resulting in the loss of phenylalanine at the 508 position of the 1,480 amino acid long transmembrane protein (ΔF508 defect), and accounts for 67 percent of those affected with CF. More than 300 other mutations account for the remainder of CFTR gene defects, although 20 non-ΔF508 defects comprise the majority of this group. The CFTR protein contains two hydrophobic transmembrane domains, two nucleotide-binding domains, and a regulatory region where phosphorylation occurs. In 1991 to 1992, the chloride channel defect in epithelial cells was corrected by transfection of wild-type CFTR. In 1993, the first

Table 1 Gastrointestinal and Nutritional Complications of Cystic Fibrosis

Area Affected	Type of Complication	Frequency
Pancreas	Pancreatic insufficiency	85%
	Pancreatic sufficiency (pancreatitis may develop)	15%
Biliary tract	Cholelithiasis	<10%
	Microgallbladder, nonfunctioning gallbladder	up to 50%
	Distal common bile duct stricture	30%
Liver	Focal biliary cirrhosis	40%
	Multilobular biliary cirrhosis	<10%
	Portal hypertension	<5%
GI tract	Gastroesophageal reflux with esophagitis	?
	Meconium ileus	10-15%
	Distal intestinal obstruction syndrome	<10%
	Rectal prolapse	<5%
Nutrition	Growth failure	Variable
	Fat-soluble vitamin deficiencies	Variable
	Salt depletion	Variable

From Gaskin KJ. Cystic fibrosis. In: Bayless TM, ed. Current therapy in gastroenterology and liver disease. 3rd ed. Philadelphia: BC Decker, 1990:559.

clinical trials of CFTR gene transfer in nasal epithelium using an adenovirus vector were initiated.

The clinical presentation of CF can take many forms: meconium ileus in the newborn period (15 percent), abnormal stools or steatorrhea secondary to pancreatic insufficiency (25 percent), failure to thrive (34 percent), and respiratory symptoms (40 percent). Progressive pulmonary disease and its complications, including recurrent infections, pneumothorax, hemoptysis and respiratory failure, account for 95 percent of the morbidity and mortality. Gastrointestinal (GI) complications are seen in 85 to 90 percent of patients, involve the pancreatic, hepatobiliary, and the intestinal tracts and will serve as the focus of this discussion. Table 1 lists the GI complications seen in CF.

DIAGNOSIS

Prenatal diagnosis of CF is possible by chorionic villus sampling or amniocentesis for high-risk families. The findings of meconium ileus, failure to thrive, abnormal stooling, respiratory symptoms, electrolyte imbalance, and rectal prolapse account for most of the clinical signs leading to a CF diagnosis. Once CF is suspected, the pilocarpine iontophoresis sweat test is performed at an experienced center. This remains the standard diagnostic method, requiring two samples with sweat chloride greater than 60 mEq per liter. In borderline cases, CFTR mutational analysis, measurement of nasal transepithelial potential difference, and analysis of pancreatic secretion after pancreozymin-secretin stimulation may be useful. Several statewide neonatal screening programs using the immunoreactive trypsinogen (IRT) assay, confirmed with sweat testing,

have shown no improvement in pulmonary outcomes as a result of early diagnosis and intervention. However, these screening tests have identified nutritional deficiencies of fat-soluble vitamins, abnormal growth, and chest x-ray abnormalities in most infants with CF. The nationwide acceptance of newborn screening for CF awaits clearcut proof of its benefit as well as resolution of ethical considerations. As a result of heightened physician awareness more children are diagnosed before their first birthday; 48 percent of patients were diagnosed within the first year of life in 1974 compared to 68 percent in 1991.

GASTROINTESTINAL COMPLICATIONS

Meconium Ileus

This complication of CF occurs in 15 percent of patients and presents in the first few days of life. CF is the underlying cause of meconium ileus in most cases, yet 1 to 2 percent of infants with meconium ileus have a pancreatic abnormality other than CF. Pancreatic insufficiency (PI) occurs in most patients with meconium ileus, but not all. A history of polyhydramnios is common in these infants who typically present with signs of intestinal obstruction: bilious vomiting, abdominal distension, and delayed passage of meconium. Firm, distended intestinal loops may be palpable. The rectum is usually empty, although a mucus plug or thick meconium may be present.

The pathogenesis is unclear although it is suspected that abnormal intestinal mucoprotein secretions and pancreatic exocrine deficiency are contributory. The meconium is abnormally viscid, containing serum proteins, calcium, and lysosomal enzymes in higher concentrations compared to normal meconium. Complications of perforation, meconium peritonitis, or pseudocyst and associated volvulus, atresia, or stenosis may be present.

Although x-ray findings are not specific for meconium ileus, abdominal films may show a distended proximal small bowel, with right lower quadrant "soap bubble" or ground glass appearance, as air is trapped within the thickened meconium. Contrast enema may show microcolon, commonly outlining meconium collections in the proximal colon. In uncomplicated cases, Gastrograffin enemas (diluted with normal saline 3:1, to reduce the hypertonicity) may be therapeutic in clearing the obstruction. Those who fail to clear the obstruction with enemas (30 percent of patients in some series) require surgery, usually involving an enterostomy. A diagnosis of CF is suspected in the setting of meconium ileus, yet a definitive diagnosis requires a sweat test. In addition, it is generally suggested that all infants diagnosed with volvulus, microcolon, jejunal or ileal atresia, and meconium plug syndrome should undergo a sweat test.

Meconium Plug Syndrome

Patients with CF may also present with meconium plug syndrome, a transient distal colonic obstruction associated with the passage of a meconium plug. A small series reported an incidence of 5 to 10 percent, yet the incidence of meconium plug syndrome has not been examined systematically. This condition may represent a mild form of meconium ileus, differing from meconium ileus primarily in the location and severity of the obstruction. Infants may present with abdominal distention and/or vomiting or merely with passage of a meconium plug. Bowel loops may be prominent; a leading edge of a meconium plug may be palpated on rectal exam.

Clinical examination may not differentiate meconium plug syndrome from meconium ileus, Hirschsprung's disease, or ileal atresia. Abdominal radiographs may show a gas-filled proximal bowel. Filling defects may be evident on contrast enemas, as meconium is mixed with contrast, yet the caliber of the colon is normal in contrast to meconium ileus and ileal atresia. Management, if needed, may include mild digital manipulation, enemas, rectal suppositories, or nasogastric infusions to clear the colon.

Pancreatic Insufficiency

PI, the most common GI manifestation of CF, affects only 85 percent of patients, although pancreatic secretions from all patients are abnormal. Elevated serum concentrations of trypsinogen are present at birth, probably due to obstruction of ductular flow, and serve as the basis for the IRT newborn screening test.

Unlike other clinical aspects of CF, PI strongly correlates with the ΔF508 defect, as essentially all homozygotes for this most common mutation develop PI.

When a ΔF508 mutation combines with a mutant CFTR gene associated with pancreatic sufficiency (PS), pancreatic function is preserved. PS is associated with fewer pulmonary symptoms, lower sweat chloride values, and a longer life expectancy. Yet nearly 10 percent of patients with PS develop pancreatitis, as residual enzymatic activity initiates autodigestion.

The clinical result of PI is intraluminal deficiency of pancreatic lipase, colipase, and trypsin, and fat malabsorption. Steatorrhea is defined in infants as greater than 15 percent fat malabsorption, and greater than 7 percent malabsorption in children and adults, as measured during a 72 hour fecal fat collection with a simultaneous record of dietary fat intake. Steatorrhea and creatorrhea do not occur until lipase and trypsin activities are less than 2 to 10 percent of normal, reflecting the large pancreatic reserve capacity. Stool chymotrypsin quantitation and pancreatic stimulation tests can define the degree of PI, yet are rarely used in our patients.

Pathological findings include collections of secretory material within the pancreatic ducts obstructing the lumen. Over time, acini atrophy and are replaced by fibrotic tissue and fat. Calcification and cystic changes may develop in the childhood years in those with PI. Typically, endocrine function is spared relative to exocrine function, as approximately 5 percent of patients develop insulin-dependent diabetes mellitus, although glucose intolerance is more common.

Management

CF-associated fat malabsorption can be managed with pancreatic enzyme supplementation, enteric-coated acid-resistant microspheres which dissolve at the duodenal pH of 5.5 to 6.0. The dose of pancreatic enzymes can be empirically adjusted so that steatorrhea is controlled and stools are reduced to an acceptable frequency and consistency. Others suggest that changes in dosing be based on results of quantitative fecal fat studies. In the presence of large amounts of enzyme supplements, refractory steatorrhea may respond to increasing duodenal pH to the range in which lipase is most active. Gastric acid production can be reduced with H_2-receptor antagonists and synthetic prostaglandins (misoprostol).

The older nonenteric-coated pancreatic enzyme replacement products are largely degraded by gastric acid before reaching the duodenum. While still in use with infants due to their ability to be mixed with formula, large doses are required to compensate for the degree of inactivation. Exposure of these preparations to skin surfaces can result in perioral and perianal irritation, as well as allergic reactions.

Children too young to swallow the capsules whole are advised to take the microspheres mixed in a nonbasic medium. Often strained fruits (such as applesauce), jam, or ketchup are used. These foods must be swallowed without chewing the microspheres, so that enzymes will not be released then degraded before reaching the duodenum. Infant formulas are an inappropriate liquid in which to dissolve enzyme capsules due to their alkaline pH.

Technological improvements have allowed for the enzyme preparations to contain more units of lipase, protease, and amylase than in the past. At present, capsules containing up to 32,000 units of lipase are available. It is hoped that compliance will improve as fewer capsules are required per meal. These also allow us to prescribe higher enzyme doses, which some recent studies propose may better normalize absorption. Yet, with these newer preparations there is less flexibility in delivering an intermediate dose with the same prescription, necessitating multiple prescriptions for different concentrations of enzyme. Additionally, these high lipase–containing enzymes can be confusing for patients in dosing meal versus snack regimens. Snack dosages are approximately one half the meal dosage. This may require the family to obtain two enzyme formulations rather than one.

Approximately 10 percent of patients on pancreatic enzyme supplementation fail to respond adequately. Noncompliance, inadequate dosing, inappropriate technique (mixing microspheres with high pH foods or chewing microspheres), or an acidic intestinal pH may explain the lack of response. Objective methods to tease these situations apart include 3 day fecal-fat study and nasogastric intubation test to assess gastric pH.

Gastroesophageal Reflux and Esophagitis

There appears to be an association between respiratory symptoms in CF and gastroesophageal reflux (GER) and esophagitis. Durie reports that more than half of those with significant respiratory symptoms have been diagnosed with esophagitis. The etiology is probably multifactorial, involving increased intra-abdominal pressure during coughing and wheezing, inverted position during physiotherapy, and medications which reduce lower esophageal sphincter pressure.

Patients with GER may report regurgitation, vomiting, or abdominal pain, while those with erosive esophagitis may also develop hematemesis, heme positive stools, anemia, failure to thrive, decreased appetite, irritability, or changes in behavior.

Evaluation for these conditions should include an upper GI contrast study to ascertain the patency of the upper GI tract, excluding malrotations, strictures, atresias, webs, and fistulas. In persistent GER and when esophagitis is suspected, endoscopic evaluation is performed and biopsies obtained. Endoscopic examination can be used to identify the presence of esophageal varices, candidiasis, Barrett's esophagus, Crohn's disease, and to assess the extent of mucosal injury. The typical findings of chronic GER may reveal esophagitis: basal cell hyperplasia of the esophageal mucosal epithelium, increased length of the stromal papillae, acute and chronic inflammation. Gastric and duodenal biopsies may exclude Helicobacter pylori and giardiasis.

When anatomic causes have been excluded, GER is managed in infants with small, more frequent feedings,

thickened feedings, and/or continuous nasogastric feedings. Positioning prone with the head elevated 30 degrees may be effective. Prokinetic agents such as bethanecol (0.6 mg per kilogram per day divided three times a day) or cisapride (0.2 mg per kilogram per dose four times a day), can be used in GER. Symptoms and endoscopic findings of esophagitis typically normalize with antacids and H_2-receptor antagonists (ranitidine 2 to 4 mg per kilogram per day divided two times a day for 8 to 12 weeks). In refractory cases, omeprazole, a proton pump inhibitor, (1.0 mg per kilogram per day, up to 3.3 mg per kilogram per day) is used. Recent reports of safety of omeprazole in children after long-term use validate use of this treatment long-term if other methods fail, titrating the dose to gastric pH. Surgery is reserved for those with refractory symptoms on omeprazole, esophageal stricture, or evidence of Barrett's esophagus.

Radiographic Abnormalities

Radiographic studies in patients with CF, before the use of endoscopy, suggested an increased frequency of peptic ulcer disease. At present, it is felt that peptic ulcer disease does not occur more frequently in CF, but that filling defects, perhaps due to mucus collections, were misinterpreted as ulcers. Small intestinal radiographic abnormalities have been reported in 80 percent of patients with CF: thickened folds, nodular filling defects, and variable dilatation. Yet these findings do not correlate with endoscopic findings, nor are they specific for CF. The etiology and significance of these changes is unclear.

Rectal Prolapse

Rectal prolapse is the presenting sign in approximately 2 percent of those with CF, yet nearly 20 percent of CF patients develop this complication before age 3, usually recurrently. Prolapse may involve the mucosa alone or the entire rectal thickness. Factors thought to be responsible for this complication include poor muscle tone, frequent bowel movements, malnutrition, and increased intra-abdominal pressure with coughing. Rectal prolapse resolves in conjunction with routine nutritional and pancreatic enzyme replacement therapies. However, if prolapse develops while patients are receiving enzyme supplements, spontaneous resolution is less likely, and intervention with pararectal saline injections has been reported.

Clostridium Difficile Infections

Reports of intestinal colonization with *Clostridium difficile* range from 17 percent to 50 percent, yet the incidence of *C. difficile* infections in CF appears to be quite low, considering that chronic use of antibiotics is a known risk factor. Asymptomatic carriage, diarrhea, pseudomembranous colitis, and marked bowel wall edema have been reported in this group. It is speculated that the relative protection against *C. difficile* may be due to the absence of an intestinal toxin A receptor or differences in intestinal flora.

Diagnosis is confirmed with stool cytotoxin B production, and supportive evidence may be obtained from stool culture and stool exam for leukocytes. Radiographic findings are variable; bowel wall edema, thumbprinting, and dilatation with air-fluid levels may be seen. Contrast radiographs are relatively contraindicated since toxic megacolon and perforation may develop. A pseudomembranous exudate consisting of fibrin, mucus, and leukocytes as well as an erythematous, friable, mucosa and scattered epithelial necrosis can be identified endoscopically.

Perhaps the most important treatment in *C. difficile* infection is to remove any pre-existing antibiotics which may have contributed to the illness. This may be all that is needed until symptoms resolve. However, oral vancomycin (20 to 60 mg per kilogram per day divided four times a day for 10 days) or oral metronidazole (15 to 20 mg per kilogram per day divided three times a day) may be used. If ileus is present, an intravenous route is used. Enteric precautions are implemented to minimize crossinfection. Relapses are not uncommon and usually respond to repeated courses of antibiotics. Persistence of cytotoxin positivity in the absence of clinical symptoms is not an indication to renew or prolong treatment. Prophylaxis with vancomycin prior to initiation of antibiotics for pulmonary infections in patients who have had *C. difficile* infection is not recommended but its use has been reported.

Distal Intestinal Obstruction Syndrome (DIOS)

DIOS, previously called meconium ileus equivalent, generally affects 10 percent of patients over 10 years of age, causing partial or complete intestinal obstruction due to impaction of tenacious mucuscontaining fecal masses in the ileum and proximal colon. Patients report recurrent crampy abdominal pain yet little difficulty passing stools. The examination may reveal a right-sided palpable fecal mass. Diagnostic studies may be needed to differentiate DIOS from intussusception, appendicitis or appendiceal abcess, volvulus, constipation, Crohn's disease, peptic ulcer disease, cholelithiasis, and pancreatitis. Abdominal radiographs suggest fecal material in the ileum, cecum, and proximal colon.

Medical management of DIOS is effective in most cases by increasing the dose of pancreatic enzymes and adding mineral oil. In addition, oral or rectal N-acetylcysteine or lactulose may help loosen the impaction. In patients with significant DIOS that does not respond to mineral oil and enemas, intragastric polyethylene glycol is the treatment of choice.

Constipation

Constipation occurs commonly in CF and may accompany DIOS. Typically, constipation presents with abdominal cramping and delayed and painful passage of stools. Abdominal radiographs typically suggest fecal matter throughout a dilated colon. Nasogastric infusion of polyethylene glycol (10 to 20 ml per kilogram per hour, for 24 to 72 hrs, until stools are clear) is used for disimpaction if initial attempts with enemas are unsuccessful. After the cleanout, oral laxatives (mineral oil and lactulose) are used daily for several months as the colonic caliber and function presumably return to normal.

Appendicitis and Intussusception

Appendicitis occurs in 1 to 2 percent of patients with CF, less frequently than in the general population (7 percent), and its diagnosis may be delayed as more common causes of abdominal pain in these patients are pursued. Differentiating appendicitis or appendiceal abcess from DIOS remains a diagnostic challenge. Imaging studies with CT or sonography may be helpful. It is speculated that chronic antibiotic use may explain the decreased incidence of appendicitis in CF.

Similarly, a high index of suspicion of intussusception, which occurs in 1 percent of patients with CF, is needed in the evaluation of patients with CF who present with abdominal pain. In contrast to most cases of intussusception in the general population in which there is usually no obvious lead point, in patients with CF, the predisposing lesion may be a luminal collection of intestinal secretions mixed with fecal matter. When treatment for other causes of abdominal pain are not helpful, a contrast enema can be diagnostic.

Hepatobiliary Disease

CF-associated liver disease (CFLD) has developed into an important clinical problem, with a prevalence of 10 percent in those under 10 years old to over 30 percent in those older than 20 years. It is expected to become more common as therapies for pulmonary complications prolong life. Liver disease and its complications remain the second most common specific cause of mortality in patients with CF.

The clinical presentation of CFLD may take many forms. Neonatal cholestasis may be the first manifestation. CFLD may come to medical attention when a nodular liver and splenomegaly are noted, raising the likelihood of cirrhosis and portal hypertension. A soft enlarged liver in an otherwise well patient suggests steatosis. More dramatically, an acute hemorrhage from an esophageal varix may be the first sign of liver disease. Yet more commonly, CFLD presents as a mild elevation in serum aminotransferase concentrations. Rare, but of great import, is the patient with end-stage cirrhosis who may present with coagulopathy, jaundice, and encephalopathy, with a shrunken liver or one that appears multinodular.

Focal biliary cirrhosis (FBC), the hallmark of CFLD, is characterized by inspissated granular eosinophilic material within biliary ductules. Chronic inflammation, variable degrees of fibrosis, and FBC are present on postmortem liver biopsy in 11 percent of infants and 27 percent of children over age 1 year. Seventy percent of adults with CF have findings of FBC postmortem. More commonly, CFLD reduces quality of life because of ascites (which may compromise pulmonary function) and inanition (which contributes to fatigue, depression, and impaired immune function). The significance of steatosis, which is seen in up to 30 percent of CF patients, is unclear. Portal hypertension and its complications of esophageal varices, hypersplenism, and thrombocytopenia are reported, but their incidence is unknown in CF.

The most common biliary tract complication of CF is gallstones, reported in up to 10 percent of patients. Microgallbladder, sclerosing cholangitis, and intrahepatic and extrahepatic obstruction are reported, although the incidence of these conditions is unknown.

Diagnosis of CFLD remains problematic, as serum chemistries, sonography, CT imaging, and percutaneous liver biopsy are not consistently reliable, yet each of these studies has a role. Hepatobiliary scintigraphy with technetium-labeled compounds is becoming more widely used in the evaluation of CFLD.

Isolated portal hypertension requires no specific treatment. Management of the complications of CFLD is the same as the treatment of these conditions from other causes. Sclerotherapy for variceal hemorrhage, general supportive care for those with decompensated liver disease with attention to fluid and electrolyte balance, and correcting hyperammonemia and coagulopathy are the primary management issues. Orthotopic liver transplantation can be lifesaving in patients with end-stage liver disease.

Preliminary clinical trials with ursodeoxycholic acid (UDCA, 10 to 25 mg per kilogram per day) improve biochemical markers of CFLD. UDCA is a safe and effective therapy used initially for dissolution of gallstones and for treatment of primary biliary cirrhosis. UDCA is thought to exert its effect in two ways: a cytoprotective effect due to replacement of hydrophobic bile acids with UDCA which is comparatively hydrophilic, and stimulation of a bicarbonate rich choleresis within the biliary system. Studies of duodenal bile acids in patients with CF have shown that the bile acid pool is enriched up to 32 percent after UDCA administration from a baseline of 12 percent. UDCA may also have immunomodulating effects, and further studies are underway to define the role of UDCA in treating and ultimately preventing CFLD.

Associated Disorders

Celiac disease, Crohn's disease, and alpha$_1$ antitrypsin deficiency have been reported in patients with CF. Hernia, hydrocele, and undescended testes are reported to occur more commonly in CF patients than the general population. There is no evidence that GI cancers are increased in CF and CF is not a risk factor for lactase deficiency.

NUTRITIONAL SUPPORT

With appropriate nutritional support, individuals with CF can grow normally in terms of height, weight, and anthropometric analysis. Over the last 10 to 15 years since nutritional recommendations in CF have been revised to allow liberal fat intake, we have corrected much of the malnutrition in this group. Our efforts to correct all nutritional deficiencies in these patients is supported by evidence that improved nutritional status slows the decline in lung function and improves lung function in some patients. A key component in nutritional management is the enzyme therapy explained above. However, this must be coupled with dietary manipulations to supply additional nutrients needed as a result of malabsorption, pulmonary involvement, and specific micronutrient repletion if additional complications exist.

Much of the growth failure seen in the past was largely due to the lack of caloric intake while patients were prescribed a low-fat diet. The enzyme therapy available today controls malabsorption well enough that dietary control of steatorrhea is no longer necessary. Instead, individuals with CF should consume a liberal fat diet, containing approximately 40 percent fat. While essential fatty acid needs can be met with the provision of 5 percent total energy intake from fat, additional dietary fat serves as a concentrated source of calories.

Caloric intake should amount to 30 to 50 percent above recommended dietary allowances initially. This varies according to presence of lung infections and GI complications. Nutritional needs are assessed in the clinic setting by a dedicated nutritionist with whom patients can develop a consistent relationship. Growth charts are kept up to date, as frequent monitoring of growth parameters is needed. Protein needs are usually set at 50 percent above expectations of non-CF peers. Carbohydrate is generally not restricted, and even with the complication of insulin dependent diabetes mellitus, dietary management with regard to carbohydrate is liberal.

Individuals with PI are also at risk for fat-soluble vitamin deficiency and supplementation is advised (Table 2). Fat-soluble vitamins, when prescribed, should be given in a water-miscible form. While some CF centers follow serum vitamin levels, others provide routine prophylactic vitamin supplementation. Subgroups of patients, such as those with liver disease complicating their CF, are particularly likely to need supplemental fat-soluble vitamins. We prescribe vitamin E to all PI patients (5 to 10 IU per kilogram per day, to a maximum of 400 IU per day). Tocopheryl polyethylene glycol 1000 succinate (TPGS), which contains tocopherol esterified to an emulsifying agent, forms micelles at low concentrations and thus can be absorbed in the absence of bile salts. This water-miscible form of vitamin E serves as a low cost alternative to the commonly used Aquasol E preparation. TPGS is commercially available as Liqui-E, only

Table 2 Vitamin and Mineral Supplementation

Vitamins:

A*	500–1,000 IU/day
D*	400-800 IU/day
E	5-10 IU/kilogram (water-miscible form) maximum dose–400 IU/day
K†	5 mg/week
Multivitamin	1-2 times RDA/day

Minerals:

Salt	Add ¼ tsp salt/day to infant formula Liberal use of salt shaker and salty foods (older children and adults)

*Can be provided in multivitamins.
†Supplementation not needed unless deemed low by laboratory analysis.

in liquid form (26.7 IU per ml). A daily multivitamin supplement is also recommended.

CF patients are also at risk for sodium depletion, as a result of increased losses via sweat. While salt tablets have been prescribed in the past, the current recommendation is to add table salt liberally at meals and to include high-salt foods within the diet. Patients must also be cautioned regarding exercise and hot weather when their sodium replacement needs are likely to increase. Keeping salty snacks available at these times often is sufficient. For young infants not yet consuming solid foods, families are advised to add salt to the formula being consumed (1/4 teaspoon salt per day).

Despite the nutritional interventions described above, some patients remain malnourished. When oral supplementation with high-calorie foods has been exhausted, intragastric supplemental feedings can be considered. Sinusitis and nasal polyps are relative contraindications to nasogastric feedings; in these situations we have found that many patients and their families accept the gastrostomy approach. Supplemental enteral feedings have proven to enhance growth and reverse malnutrition in CF patients. Further, this improvement in nutritional status often improves the prognosis with regard to respiratory status.

The choice of formulas to use via enteral feedings is controversial. Our center uses the polymeric varieties, which are less costly, and supplement these with pancreatic enzymes. This approach also has a lower osmolarity, and thus advancement to higher caloric density may be more achievable. We use formulas which contain medium chain triglycerides, as they are directly absorbed into the enterocyte without the need for bile salts. Alternatively, elemental formulas are favored by other CF centers. When using these products, pancreatic enzyme supplements are not needed.

Enzyme therapy in conjunction with the enteral feedings may be managed in several ways. Patients may take their enzymes at the beginning, midpoint, and/or the end of their continuous (typically overnight) infusion. The benefit of any single enzyme dose lasts approximately 90 minutes. In our clinic, we use a single enzyme dose at the beginning of the cycle. We only suggest a morning dose when a patient's growth is not progressing as desired and do not interrupt their normal sleeping patterns to take medications. The alternative method is to mix the enzyme directly into the formula. The older, nonenterically coated enzymes serve this purpose, as they are compatible to mix with most products. We usually add one-half teaspoon of Viokase powder per 120 ml formula.

Although TPN is more expensive and risks more complications than enteral nutrition, it remains an option when enteral feedings are not tolerated or are contraindicated. We aim to provide 100 to 120 percent of the patient's RDA for energy via the parenteral route. Because TPN bypasses the intestinal tract, malabsorptive issues are nonexistent. Since vitamins and minerals are supplied parenterally, additional supplementation is not necessary for those receiving TPN.

COMMENTS

Patients with CF now commonly live into adulthood and are increasingly cared for by adult clinicians. Dramatic progress at the genetic and molecular levels promises to produce more effective therapies in the not too distant future. Replacement of pancreatic enzymes in those with PI and attention to total calorie, macro- and micronutrient status to prevent deficiencies and growth failure, and consideration of the many approaches to provide enteral nutrition will hopefully provide these patients with a better outlook. These efforts are essential in conjunction with aggressive treatment of pulmonary infections and management of complications, and constitute the mainstay of therapy for CF at present.

SUGGESTED READING

Bowser EK. Evaluating enteral nutrition support in cystic fibrosis. Top Clin Nutr 1990; 5:55–61.

Collins FS. Cystic fibrosis: Molecular biology and therapeutic implications. Science 1992; 256:774–779.

Durie PR. Cystic fibrosis: Gastrointestinal and hepatic complications and their management. Int Sem Pediatr Gastroenterol Nutr 1993; 2:3–9.

Gaskin KJ. Cystic fibrosis: Nutritional problems and their management. Int Sem Pediatr Gastroenterol Nutr 1993; 2:9–15.

Luder E. Nutritional care of patients with cystic fibrosis. Top Clin Nutr 1991; 6:39–50.

Park RW, Grand RJ. Gastrointestinal manifestations of cystic fibrosis: A review. Gastroenterology 1981; 81:1143–1161.

Ramsey BW, Farrell PM, Pencharz P, and Consensus Committee: Nutritional assessment and management in cystic fibrosis. Am J Clin Nutr 1992; 55:108–16.

Schidlow DV, Taussig LM, Knowles MR. Cystic fibrosis foundation concensus conference report on pulmonary complications of cystic fibrosis. Pediatr Pulmonol 1993; 15:187–198.

PANCREATIC AND PERIPANCREATIC NEOPLASIA

STEVEN A. AHRENDT, M.D.
HENRY A. PITT, M.D.

Periampullary neoplasms include adenocarcinomas of the head of the pancreas, ampulla of Vater, duodenum, and distal common bile duct. These lesions present with jaundice, weight loss, and abdominal or back pain. Less commonly they can present with new onset diabetes mellitus, pancreatitis, or exocrine pancreatic insufficiency. Recent improvements in operative morbidity and mortality have led to a predominantly operative approach for patients with potentially resectable periampullary cancer. Pancreatoduodenectomy is now being performed with low operative mortality (0 to 3 percent) and reasonable 5-year survival for those resected for cure (15 to 25 percent). Results of surgical palliation have also improved for patients with periampullary malignancies. In contrast, most patients with cancer involving the body or tail of the pancreas are unresectable at presentation and have limited survival.

DIAGNOSIS AND STAGING

The therapeutic approach to pancreatic and other periampullary malignancies is determined by the clinical stage at presentation. Patients with a suspected pancreatic neoplasm undergo a diagnostic evaluation which usually includes computed tomography (CT) and cholangiography. Angiography may also provide useful information in staging, but its routine use is more controversial. Operative exploration provides an opportunity to determine resectability, establish a tissue diagnosis, and, if the tumor is not resectable, to offer palliation with biliary and/or duodenal bypass as well as chemical splanchnicectomy. Some patients who are at very high operative risk, have advanced metastatic disease, or have clearly unresectable tumors may be better palliated nonoperatively. Thus, the goal of preoperative staging of pancreatic and periampullary tumors should be to determine the optimal treatment for each patient.

CT is the initial imaging study of choice for the patient with a suspected pancreatic or periampullary tumor. CT scanning can detect pancreatic and peripancreatic masses as small as 2 cm, dilatation of the main pancreatic and/or bile ducts, and hepatic or other extrapancreatic metastases. Dynamic CT scanning with a continuous bolus of intravenous contrast as well as the new spiral techniques have improved the ability of CT to detect small liver metastases and vascular invasion. In addition, local tumor extension and invasion of contiguous organs is more clearly defined with these techniques

than with older CT methodology. CT is less dependent on the observer and the patient's body habitus than ultrasound and, as a result, has a slightly higher sensitivity (80 to 85 percent) and specificity (90 to 95 percent) in establishing the diagnosis of pancreatic cancer. The additional staging information provided by spiral CT gives it clear advantages over ultrasound in the evaluation of a patient with a suspected pancreatic tumor. Comparative studies of CT scanning and magnetic resonance imaging have demonstrated no obvious advantage for the latter.

Percutaneous transhepatic cholangiography (PTC) is very accurate in establishing the level and cause of bile duct obstruction. However, for pancreatic and periampullary neoplasms, endoscopic retrograde cholangiopancreatography (ERCP) has the advantages of visualizing the duodenum and ampulla and providing a pancreatogram as well as a cholangiogram. As a result, most diagnostic algorithms recommend ERCP for patients with distal bile duct obstruction and reserve PTC for more proximal lesions (Fig. 1). ERCP has a higher sensitivity and specificity than CT in diagnosing pancreatic cancers. The presence of a "double duct sign" may be diagnostic of a pancreatic cancer even when the CT scan does not demonstrate a mass, and the patient is not jaundiced.

Angiography is no longer used to establish a diagnosis of pancreatic or periampullary carcinoma. However, it provides additional valuable staging information in patients who appear resectable by CT scan. A recent study at the Johns Hopkins Hospital evaluated 90 patients with periampullary tumors with visceral angiography. Among 62 patients with normal angiograms, 48 (77 percent) were resectable. In 17 patients with angiograms suggesting vessel encasement, the resectability rate was 35 percent. None of the 11 remaining patients with vessel occlusion were resectable. This study concluded that major vessel occlusion rules out resection and that major vessel encasement makes resection unlikely. In addition to providing useful information about tumor stage, angiography also delineates vascular anatomy. A replaced right hepatic artery originating from the superior mesenteric artery occurs in up to 20 percent of patients and is prone to injury during pancreatic resection if not recognized. In patients with significant celiac axis stenosis, hepatic arterial supply may be via the pancreaticoduodenal arteries. Angiography may alert the surgeon to the potential need for hepatic artery revascularization after pancreatic resection.

Numerous serologic tumor markers have been proposed for the early diagnosis of pancreatic cancer. However, none are sufficiently sensitive or specific to reliably differentiate pancreatic cancer from other diseases. CA 19-9 and CA 50 are the best available markers; however, serum levels are often normal in patients with small, resectable tumors. After resection, CA 19-9 levels fall and become secondarily elevated with tumor recurrence. Thus, CA 19-9 is more useful in patient follow-up than for early diagnosis.

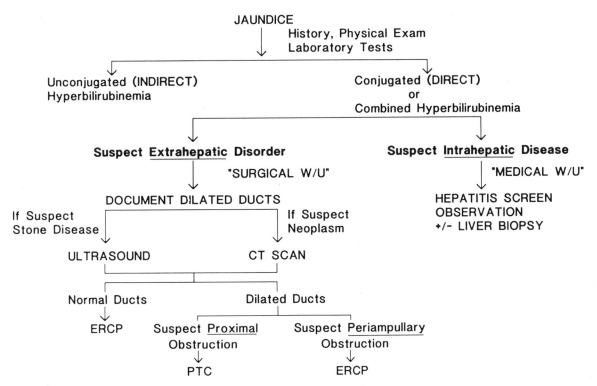

Figure 1 An algorithm for the evaluation of jaundice. CT = computed tomography; ERCP = endoscopic retrograde cholangiopancreatography; PTC = percutaneous transhepatic cholangiography. (From Lipsett P, Pitt H. Jaundice: mechanisms and differential diagnosis. In: Toouli J ed. Surgery of the biliary tract. London: Churchill Livingstone, 1993:49, with permission.)

Diagnostic laparoscopy has been used by several investigators as an additional staging modality in the evaluation of patients with pancreatic and periampullary malignancies. Peritoneal, omental, and hepatic metastases less than 1 cm in size are often not visualized by CT but may be identified laparoscopically. Nevertheless, preoperative staging including laparoscopy has not improved the resectability rate over that at our institution where laparoscopy is not routinely used. In addition, we believe that surgical palliation offers advantages over nonoperative methods with respect to recurrent jaundice and gastric outlet obstruction. The finding of distant metastases at laparoscopy would not alter our palliative approach; therefore, we believe that laparoscopy should not be routinely performed as a staging procedure.

Endoscopic ultrasonography (EUS) is the newest imaging technique being used for both the diagnosis and staging of patients with pancreatic and peripancreatic cancer. EUS may be better than CT at detecting lesions less than 2 cm. These two techniques are similar in their assessment of portal vein involvement, but CT is more accurate in detecting superior mesenteric artery involvement. In addition, EUS appears to be more accurate than CT or conventional ultrasound in detecting lymph node metastases. However, the ultimate role of EUS in detecting and staging pancreatic and periampullary tumors awaits further analysis.

A preoperative tissue diagnosis of pancreatic or other periampullary malignancy can be obtained by several methods. Duodenal and ampullary lesions can be biopsied at the time of ERCP. Bile or pancreatic juice aspirated at ERCP or via transhepatic catheters can be sent for cytology. The low sensitivity of these techniques may be improved by brushing biliary or pancreatic strictures. Nevertheless, an indeterminate or negative biopsy does not rule out a cancer in patients with a suggestive history and radiologic findings. Moreover, some recent data suggest that preoperative needle biopsy may adversely affect long-term survival in patients with resectable tumors. Therefore, patients who appear resectable on the basis of CT and angiography should undergo exploration without attempts at establishing a preoperative tissue diagnosis. Percutaneous fine-needle aspiration cytology should be reserved for those patients with a pancreatic mass that is clearly unresectable on CT and/or angiography, with metastatic liver lesions, or who are prohibitive operative risks.

PREOPERATIVE PREPARATION

Accurate assessment of a patient's operative risk is key in deciding whether and when to operate. Little has defined a mortality index which employs serum albumin, serum creatinine, and a cholangitis score to determine operative risk in patients with obstructive jaundice. With the use of such a predictive model, a small percentage of patients can be identified in whom the risk of major pancreatic surgery is high. In these patients preoperative biliary drainage and nutritional support may decrease operative morbidity and mortality.

Several prospective, randomized studies in the mid-1980s failed to demonstrate a benefit for preoperative percutaneous biliary drainage. However, in these studies the length of preoperative drainage was only 10 to 18 days, bile was often drained externally, and nutritional status was not assessed. Recent studies suggest that the internal drainage of bile salts into the gut lumen may decrease the incidence of gut-derived endotoxemia and thereby, prevent its role in the development of postoperative renal failure. Furthermore, one Italian study suggests that a combination of preoperative alimentation and biliary drainage is better than biliary drainage alone in decreasing operative risk. We, therefore, favor a 2 to 3 week period of internal biliary drainage and enteral and/or parenteral alimentation in patients judged to be at greatest risk by Little's mortality index. On the other hand, most patients will not need either preoperative biliary drainage or nutritional support.

All patients receive perioperative prophylactic antibiotics. Nonjaundiced patients and patients without indwelling stents receive a first generation cephalosporin started immediately prior to surgery and continued for 24 hours. Patients with indwelling stents or previous episodes of cholangitis receive a broad-spectrum penicillin or antibiotic(s) specifically directed against known biliary tract organisms. Coagulation defects are common among jaundiced patients and should be corrected preoperatively. A prolonged prothrombin time is corrected with vitamin K. If the partial thromboplastin time is prolonged, fresh frozen plasma may be required before invasive procedures.

THERAPEUTIC ALTERNATIVES

The initial approach to the patient with a periampullary cancer is determined after completion of the staging evaluation. Patients with potentially resectable lesions, good risk patients with a low chance for resection, and those with gastric outlet obstruction all undergo operative exploration. Patients with biliary obstruction, an open duodenum, and who are felt to be poor operative candidates as well as patients with large unresectable body and tail lesions are palliated nonoperatively.

Surgical Resection

Exploratory laparotomy is performed via an upper midline or extended subcostal incision. A careful search is made for any hepatic or peritoneal metastases which would preclude resection. Lymph nodes outside the limits of a pancreatoduodenal resection including those along the celiac axis are examined. Any suspicious areas are biopsied and sent for frozen section. In the absence of any distal spread, the duodenum is mobilized, and the superior mesenteric vein, superior mesenteric artery, and portal vein are assessed for any involvement in the tumor.

Periampullary cancers are resected with either a classic Whipple procedure or using a pylorus-preserving pancreaticoduodenectomy. The Whipple operation includes en bloc resection of the antrum, duodenum, pancreatic head, distal common bile duct, and gallbladder. The pylorus-preserving pancreatoduodenectomy (PPPD) was described in 1978 and preserves the antrum, pylorus, and proximal 2 cm of duodenum. PPPD has the late advantage of avoiding most postgastrectomy sequelae and providing a better long-term nutritional status. Moreover, PPPD has not demonstrated any survival disadvantage when compared with the classic Whipple operation. Therefore, we currently use the pylorus-preserving modification in approximately 80 percent of our pancreatoduodenal resections. Rarely, a lesion in the body or tail of the pancreas will be resectable for cure. In these instances a distal pancreatectomy is performed.

Surgical Palliation

Some patients explored with an intent to resect are unresectable due to locally advanced or metastatic disease. An additional group of patients will be explored to palliate symptoms of gastric outlet or biliary obstruction. Establishing a tissue diagnosis is important so that these patients know where they stand and can be treated with radiation and chemotherapy. If liver or lymph node metastases are present they can be biopsied. Fine-needle aspiration cytology or transduodenal needle biopsy of the pancreatic mass should be performed if metastatic disease is present.

Surgical palliation should include relief of jaundice, treatment or prevention of gastric outlet obstruction, and relief of pain. For relief of jaundice choledochojejunostomy is preferred to cholecystojejunostomy as the latter procedure is associated with a higher incidence of ascending cholangitis and recurrent obstruction from cephalad tumor growth. Cholecystojejunostomy may be preferred in the patient with portal hypertension secondary to portal or superior mesenteric venous occlusion by the tumor. A gastrojejunostomy is routinely performed at Johns Hopkins for palliation as approximately 20 percent of patients require reoperation or die with gastric outlet obstruction if this procedure is not performed at the initial laparotomy. Chemical splanchnicectomy with 50 percent alcohol is also performed in all patients for the palliation of pain. This procedure has recently been shown in a prospective, randomized trial to reduce pain when present and to delay its onset in patients without significant pain at the time of surgery.

Nonoperative Palliation

Patients who are poor operative risks or have very advanced disease at presentation can be palliated nonoperatively. Nonoperative palliation is directed at relieving obstructive jaundice and controlling pain. Jaundice can be relieved either endoscopically or percutaneously. The endoscopic placement of an endoprosthesis has been associated with fewer complications than transhepatic stents and is successful in 85 to 90 percent of patients. In randomized trials nonoperative palliation has had a lower initial mortality, but late problems with recurrent jaundice and gastric outlet obstruction have favored surgery. Symptoms of gastric outlet obstruction are poorly palliated nonoperatively. In patients with advanced disease a percutaneous endoscopic gastrostomy can prevent recurrent vomiting.

Pain is the most disabling symptom in patients with unresectable pancreatic cancer. A percutaneous celiac plexus block should be considered in patients with advanced disease at presentation, lesions of the body and tail of the pancreas not associated with jaundice or duodenal obstruction, or in whom operative splanchnicectomy has produced inadequate pain relief.

THERAPEUTIC OUTCOME

Since 1980, the operative morbidity and mortality for major pancreatic resection has improved considerably. Between 1980 and 1992 the operative mortality for pancreatoduodenectomy at the Johns Hopkins Hospital has been 2.5 percent. Improvements in operative technique including a decrease in operative time and blood loss as well as improved pre- and postoperative care have led to this decrease in operative mortality. Similar results have been achieved in several other centers with an interest in pancreatic surgery.

Postoperative complications still occur in approximately 50 percent of patients. Delayed gastric emptying requiring prolonged nasogastric decompression is the most common complication increasing hospital stay. Delayed gastric emptying is often associated with postoperative pancreatitis or a pancreatic fistula and usually resolves as these problems improve. Pancreatic fistulas occur in 15 to 20 percent of patients after pancreatoduodenectomy. Most fistulas close spontaneously with parenteral hyperalimentation, adequate drainage of pancreatic secretions, and perhaps the addition of octreotide.

Similar to the results for pancreatic resection, the operative morbidity and mortality have improved for palliative operations for pancreatic cancer. In a recent series of 118 patients undergoing laparotomy for unresectable periampullary cancer at the Johns Hopkins Hospital, the operative mortality was 2.5 percent (Table 1). Seventy-five percent of these patients had undergone biliary bypass and gastrojejunostomy. Operative complications were seldom life threatening and included wound infection, cholangitis, and delayed gastric emptying.

The prognosis for patients undergoing pancreatoduodenectomy for pancreatic or periampullary cancer varies with the site of tumor origin. Recent 5-year survival for patients with pancreatic and peripancreatic

Table 1 Results of Resection and Operative Palliation of Pancreatic and Peripancreatic Cancer at the Johns Hopkins Hospital

	Resection	Operative Palliation
Operative results		
Number of patients	145	118
Hospital mortality	0%	2.5%
Postoperative morbidity	52%	37%
Postoperative hospital stay	19 days	14 days
Survival		
Number of patients	89	118
Actuarial survival		
1 yr	50%	30%
2 yr	28%	4%
5 yr	19%	0%
Mean survival	11.9 months	7.7 months

Data from Cameron JL, et al. Am J Surg 1991; 161:120; Cameron JL, et al. Ann Surg 1993;217:430; and Lillemoe KD, et al. Surg Gynecol Obstet 1993;176:1.

cancer resected for cure at the Johns Hopkins Hospital has been 15 to 25 percent. Moreover, patients without tumor spread to regional lymph nodes have a 5-year survival of 50 percent. Also, patients receiving two or fewer units of blood at the time of operation have a significantly prolonged median survival of 24 months versus 10 months in those receiving more than two units. Patients with nonpancreatic periampullary malignancies involving the bile duct, ampulla, or duodenum resected for cure have an actuarial 5-year survival of 40 to 50 percent.

The survival results for patients with unresectable periampullary malignancies are understandably less encouraging. Mean survival for patients undergoing surgical palliation of periampullary carcinoma at the Johns Hopkins Hospital was 7.7 months. In those undergoing both biliary bypass and gastrojejunostomy, only 4 percent of patients developed late gastric outlet obstruction and 2 percent developed recurrent jaundice. In addition, a recent study has also demonstrated that in the subset of patients with severe pain at the time of surgery, chemical splanchnicectomy with alcohol significantly prolongs survival compared to patients receiving saline placebo. Patients with cancer involving the body or tail of the pancreas continue to do poorly with a median survival of 4 months.

RADIOTHERAPY AND CHEMOTHERAPY

Despite recent improvements in operative morbidity and mortality for patients with both resectable and unresectable pancreatic cancers, survival is limited for most patients with this disease. Postoperative radiation therapy and chemotherapy have been shown in a randomized trial to improve survival after curative resection of pancreatic cancer and to palliate symptoms and improve survival in patients with unresectable lesions.

Combination chemotherapy and radiation therapy have yielded better results in the postoperative adjuvant setting than either modality alone. The Gastrointestinal Tumor Study Group compared surgery alone versus surgery followed by radiotherapy (40 Gy) plus 5-fluorouracil (5-FU). Median survival in the combined therapy group (20 months) was significantly longer than in the control patients (11 months). Five year survival was also improved in the combined modality group (18 percent versus 7 percent). Thus, adjuvant radiation and chemotherapy should be offered to patients after curative resection of a pancreatic malignancy.

Radiation therapy has also been administered intraoperatively to increase the radiation dose to the tumor bed. In the only prospective, randomized trial of intraoperative radiation therapy (IORT), operative morbidity and mortality were high. Once operative deaths were excluded, IORT provided some improvement in median survival. Whether IORT offers any advantages over standard postoperative external beam radiation remains unclear. Phase II trials of preoperative radiation and chemotherapy are also being performed. Whether this strategy will improve resectability rates and survival with an acceptable morbidity and mortality have yet to be determined.

Results of chemotherapy for advanced pancreatic cancer remain dismal with median survivals of only 3 to 6 months. Only 5-FU has provided a greater than 20 percent response rate, although whether chemotherapy improves survival remains questionable. Several prospective randomized trials of combination chemotherapy and radiotherapy in patients with locally advanced pancreatic cancer have demonstrated a benefit over either modality alone. Median survivals of 10 months have been achieved in these patients with some treatment-related toxicities.

SUGGESTED READING

Cameron JL, Crist DW, Sitzmann JV, et al. Factors influencing survival following pancreaticoduodenectomy for pancreatic cancer. Am J Surg 1991; 161:120–125.
Cameron JL, Pitt HA, Yeo CJ, et al. One hundred forty-five consecutive pancreaticoduodenectomies without mortality. Ann Surg 1993; 217:430–438.
Lillemoe KD, Cameron JL, Kaufman HS, et al. Chemical splanchnicectomy in patients with unresectable pancreatic cancer: A prospective randomized trial. Ann Surg 1993; 217:447–457.
Lillemoe KD, Sauter PK, Pitt HA, et al. Current status of surgical palliation of periampullary cancer. Surg Gynecol Obstet 1993; 176:1–10.
Little JM. A prospective evaluation of computerized estimates of risk in the management of obstructive jaundice. Surgery 1987; 102:473–476.

ENDOCRINE TUMORS OF THE PANCREAS

CHARLES J. YEO, M.D.

Endocrine tumors of the pancreas are seen rarely in clinical practice, with a recognized annual incidence of five cases per 1 million population. These tumors are best divided into functional and nonfunctional varieties. Most pancreatic endocrine tumors discovered clinically are functional, indicating that they elaborate one or more hormonal products into the blood, leading to a recognizable clinical syndrome. By convention, functional tumors are named according to the predominant clinical syndrome and hormonal product (Table 1). Patients with endocrine tumors of the pancreas with no recognizable clinical syndrome and normal serum hormone levels (excluding pancreatic polypeptide) are considered to have nonfunctional pancreatic endocrine tumors.

Editor's Note: There is some overlap of this chapter with the chapter *Zollinger-Ellison Syndrome*, but I believe diagnosis is a major part of management of these syndromes. Please refer to the other chapter for some details.

Patients with suspected functional endocrine tumors of the pancreas are managed using a three step approach. First, the characteristic syndrome and associated pathophysiology must be recognized. Characteristic clinical syndromes are well described for insulinoma, gastrinoma, vasoactive intestinal peptide-secreting tumors (VIPoma), and glucagonoma. The somatostatinoma syndrome is nonspecific, much more difficult to recognize, and exceedingly rare. The second step in patient management involves the detection of hormone elevation in serum by radioimmunoassay (RIA). RIAs are widely available for the measurement of insulin, gastrin, VIP, and glucagon. Assays for somatostatin, pancreatic polypeptide, prostaglandins, and other hormonal markers are not widely commercially available, but may be obtained from selected laboratories or investigators. The third step in patient management involves localization and staging of the tumor in preparation for possible operative therapy.

LOCALIZATION AND STAGING OF THE TUMOR

The standard preoperative techniques currently in use for pancreatic endocrine tumor localization include computed tomography (CT) with intravenous and oral contrast, visceral angiography, and transhepatic portal

Table 1 Classification of Functional Pancreatic Endocrine Tumors

Tumor (Syndrome)	Clinical Features	Extrapancreatic Location	Malignancy Rate
Insulinoma	Hypoglycemia	Rare	10%
Gastrinoma (Zollinger-Ellison)	Peptic ulcer Diarrhea	Frequent	50%
VIPoma (Verner-Morrison)	Watery diarrhea Hypokalemia Achlorhydria	10%	Majority
Glucagonoma	Hyperglycemia Dermatitis	Rare	Majority
Somatostatinoma	Hyperglycemia Steatorrhea Gallstones	Rare	Majority

venous hormone sampling. The accuracy of CT in detecting the primary pancreatic tumor varies widely in the literature, ranging from 35 to 85 percent, with larger lesions being more easily detectable. The CT scan is also used to assess for lymph node and hepatic metastases. Using the combination of CT, angiography, and portal venous hormone sampling, more than 90 percent of functional pancreatic islet cell tumors can be localized preoperatively.

A new technique that is gaining acceptance and shows promise for improving preoperative localization of pancreatic endocrine tumors is endoscopic ultrasonography. In recently published data, Rosch and colleagues were able to correctly localize 32 of 39 tumors (82 percent) using endoscopic ultrasound after prior negative CT scans. In their experience endoscopic ultrasonography was more sensitive than both CT and visceral angiography. As further experience with this technique is gained, it may play a more prominent role in the localization of endocrine tumors of the pancreas. There is a separate chapter on use of endoscopic ultrasound in gastrointestinal malignancies.

Another technique that holds promise for pancreatic endocrine tumor localization is somatostatin-receptor imaging. Early studies utilizing nuclear medicine techniques scanning with ^{123}I-labeled Tyr^3-octreotide have been reported, identifying primary tumors as well as metastases in patients with pancreatic endocrine tumors. This somatostatin-receptor imaging technique may prove helpful in identifying extrahepatic metastases from pancreatic endocrine tumors, entities that are not well localized by other radiographic modalities.

SURGICAL EXPLORATION

At the time of surgical exploration, a thorough evaluation of the pancreas and peripancreatic regions is undertaken. The body and tail of the pancreas are exposed by dividing the gastrocolic ligament; this portion of the pancreas can be partially mobilized by dividing the retroperitoneal attachments inferior to the gland. The pancreatic head and uncinate process are palpated bimanually after elevating the second portion of the

duodenum out of the retroperitoneum using the Kocher maneuver. The liver is carefully assessed for evidence of metastatic disease. Potential extrapancreatic sites of tumor are evaluated with particular attention to the duodenum, splenic hilum, small bowel and its mesentery, and peripancreatic lymph nodes. One technique that may provide additional information in the intraoperative setting is real-time ultrasonography, which may assist in tumor identification. The goals of surgical therapy for pancreatic endocrine tumors include control of symptoms from hormone excess, safe resection of maximal tumor mass, and preservation of maximal pancreatic parenchyma. Management strategies, both preoperative and intraoperative, differ for the various types of pancreatic endocrine tumors.

INSULINOMA

Insulinoma is the most common pancreatic endocrine tumor (Table 2). The insulinoma syndrome is associated with Whipple's triad (1) symptoms of hypoglycemia during fasting, (2) documentation of hypoglycemia with blood glucose less than 50 mg per deciliter, and (3) relief of hypoglycemic symptoms following administration of exogenous glucose. Autonomous insulin secretion from insulinomas leads to spontaneous hypoglycemia with symptoms that can be characterized into neuroglycopenic symptoms (confusion, personality change, obtundation, seizure, and coma) and hypoglycemia-induced catecholamine-surge symptoms (tremulousness, diaphoresis, and tachycardia). Typically, the prevention or relief of these symptoms is achieved via the consumption of carbohydrate-rich foods.

Whipple's triad is not specific for insulinoma. Apart from insulinoma, the differential diagnosis of adult hypoglycemia is extensive and includes reactive hypoglycemia, functional hypoglycemia associated with gastrectomy or gastroenterostomy, hypopituitarism, nonpancreatic tumors (such as pleural mesothelioma, sarcoma, adrenal carcinoma, hepatocellular carcinoma, and carcinoid), extensive hepatic insufficiency, chronic adrenal insufficiency, and surreptitious administration of insulin or ingestion of oral hypoglycemic agents. Of these

Table 2 Insulinoma

Characteristic			
Symptoms	Whipple's triad		
	Neuroglycopenia	→	Confusion, personality change, coma
	Catecholamine surge	→	Tremulousness, diaphoresis, tachycardia
Diagnosis	Monitored fast		
	Insulin/glucose ratio		
	C peptide and proinsulin levels		
Anatomic localization	Evenly distributed throughout pancreas		

entities, reactive hypoglycemia is most commonly seen, causing symptoms of hypoglycemia 3 to 5 hours following meals. Reactive hypoglycemia is typically not associated with fasting hypoglycemia.

The most common mistake made in the evaluation of a patient with suspected insulinoma is to commence the evaluation with an oral glucose tolerance test. Rather, the diagnosis of insulinoma is most reliably made using the technique of a monitored fast. Blood for glucose and insulin determinations is sampled every 4 to 6 hours during the fast, and at the time of symptom occurrence. Hypoglycemic symptoms typically occur when glucose levels are less than 50 mg per deciliter, with concurrent serum insulin levels often being greater than 25 μU per milliliter. Additional support for the diagnosis of insulinoma comes from the calculation of the insulin to glucose ratio (I:G ratio) at different time points during the monitored fast. Normal individuals have ratios less than 0.3, while patients with insulinoma typically demonstrate I:G ratios greater than 0.4 after a prolonged fast. Other measurable beta cell products synthesized in excess in patients with insulinoma include C-peptide and proinsulin. The possibility of surreptitious insulin or oral hypoglycemic agent administration should be considered in all cases of suspected insulinoma. C-peptide and proinsulin levels will not be elevated in patients self-administering insulin, while the presence of oral hypoglycemics such as sulfonylureas can be assessed using standard toxicologic screening.

After confirming the diagnosis of insulinoma by biochemical analyses and performing the appropriate localization and staging studies, the treatment of insulinoma is surgical in nearly all cases. Insulinomas are found evenly distributed within the pancreas with one-third located in the head and uncinate process, one-third in the body, and one-third in the tail of the gland. Up to 90 percent of patients have benign solitary adenomas amenable to surgical cure. Less than 10 percent of patients with insulinoma have some form of the multiple endocrine neoplasia-1 (MEN-1) syndrome, with the possibility of multiple insulinomas being present. Insulinoma metastatic to peripancreatic lymph nodes or to the liver will be present in 10 to 15 percent of cases. Small benign insulinomas not in close proximity to the main pancreatic duct may be resected by enucleation, independent of their location within the gland. In the body and tail of the pancreas, insulinomas

greater than 2 cm in diameter or those in close proximity to the pancreatic duct are best excised by distal pancreatectomy. Large insulinomas deep in the head or uncinate process of the pancreas may not be amenable to local excision, and may require pancreaticoduodenectomy.

If after careful exploration no insulinoma is identified by visualization, palpation, and intraoperative real-time ultrasonography, a management dilemma exists. Some authors have in the past recommended a "blind" distal pancreatic resection to the level of the superior mesenteric vein (70 percent pancreatectomy), in the hopes of excising a previously unidentified insulinoma or of reducing the islet cell mass in patients with islet cell adenomatosis. Others have suggested that a "blind" pancreaticoduodenectomy would be more appropriate, as the thickness of the head and uncinate process render this region of the pancreas most likely to harbor an unidentified insulinoma. However, the most rational approach to this situation may be to avoid any form of a "blind" resection, and to defer resection in favor of postoperative selective transhepatic portal venous insulin sampling, to allow for specific tumor localization and directed surgical excision.

In cases of malignant insulinoma (less than 10 percent of insulinomas), cautious and safe resection of the primary tumor and accessible metastases should be performed. Tumor debulking can be quite helpful in reducing problematic hypoglycemic symptoms. Patients with limited numbers of hepatic metastases are candidates for local resection of these metastases.

In those patients with unresectable insulinoma, dietary manipulations including judicious spacing of carbohydrate-rich meals and nighttime snacks can minimize dangerous hypoglycemia. Drugs that may be used to inhibit insulin release include diazoxide and octreotide. Chemotherapeutic agents with some efficacy against malignant insulinoma include streptozocin, dacarbazine (DTIC), and doxorubicin.

GASTRINOMA (ZOLLINGER-ELLISON SYNDROME)

In 1955, Zollinger and Ellison described two patients with severe peptic ulcer disease and pancreatic endocrine tumors, postulating that an ulcerogenic agent originated from the pancreatic tumor. Today, approximately one in 1,000 patients with primary duodenal ulcer disease and two in 100 patients with recurrent ulcer following ulcer surgery are found to have gastrinoma. Seventy-five percent of gastrinomas occur sporadically, whereas 25 percent are associated with the MEN-1 syndrome. In the past most gastrinomas were found to be malignant based on the findings of metastatic disease at the time of exploration. More recently, with increased awareness and earlier screening for hypergastrinemia (Tables 3 and 4), the diagnosis of gastrinoma is being made earlier, leading to the discovery of a higher percentage of benign curable neoplasms. See the chapter *Zollinger-Ellison Syndrome* for details of biochemical diagnosis.

After biochemical confirmation of the diagnosis of gastrinoma, patient management follows two routes. First, gastric acid hypersecretion is pharmacologically controlled. Omeprazole in doses of 20 to 200 mg per day is now considered the drug of choice for antisecretory therapy in patients with gastrinoma. The dose is adjusted to achieve a nonacidic gastric pH during the hour immediately prior to the next dose of the drug. (Acid suppression is discussed in detail in the chapter on Zollinger-Ellison syndrome.) Second, after the initiation of omeprazole therapy, all gastrinoma patients should undergo radiographic studies in an effort to localize the primary tumor and to assess for metastatic disease. The modalities appropriate for localization and staging of gastrinoma patients include dynamic CT scan with intravenous and oral contrast, selective visceral angiography, endoscopic ultrasonography, and percutaneous portal venous sampling for gastrin.

A relatively new localization test for gastrinoma was first proposed by Imamura in 1987. This selective arterial secretin stimulation test is doubly invasive, involving the placement of vascular catheters at the level of the hepatic vein and in the abdominal aorta and its branches. Thirty units of secretin are then serially injected via the arterial catheter into the splenic, gastroduodenal, and inferior pancreaticoduodenal arteries. Venous blood samples are then drawn from the hepatic vein at time intervals after the arterial secretin injections. The artery which feeds the gastrinoma can be determined based on which selective secretin injection causes a large increment in hepatic vein gastrin concentration.

Gastrinoma patients whose localization and staging studies are suspicious for unresectable hepatic metastases should undergo percutaneous or laparoscopic-directed liver biopsy for histologic verification. If unresectable gastrinoma is confirmed, surgical exploration is not performed, and the patient is maintained on long-term omeprazole therapy. In the absence of documented unresectable disease, all patients with gastrinoma should undergo surgical exploration with curative intent. The entire abdomen should be carefully examined for areas of extrapancreatic and extraduodenal gastrinoma. As the vast majority of gastrinomas have been identified to the right of the superior mesenteric vessels within the pancreas or the duodenum ("gastri-

Table 3 Indications for Serum Gastrin Measurement

Peptic Ulcer Disease:
  Initial diagnosis
  Recurrent ulcer
  Failure of medical therapy
  Postoperative ulcer
  Postbulbar ulcer
  Family history
  Ulcer with diarrhea
Prolonged undiagnosed diarrhea
MEN-I kindred
Nongastrinoma pancreatic endocrine tumor
Prominent gastric rugal folds on upper gastrointestinal series

Table 4 Disease States Associated with Hypergastrinemia

Nonulcerogenic (Normal to decreased acid secretion)	Ulcerogenic (Excess acid secretion)
Atrophic gastritis	Antral G cell hyperplasia or hyperfunction
Pernicious anemia	
Post vagotomy	Gastric outlet obstruction
Renal failure	Retained excluded antrum
Short-gut syndrome	Zollinger-Ellison syndrome

noma triangle"), particular attention is focused on these areas. Intraoperative ultrasonography may assist in tumor localization. Additionally, intraoperative endoscopy may be helpful in allowing transillumination of the duodenal wall for identification of small duodenal gastrinomas. At surgery, any suspicious peripancreatic lymph nodes are excised and submitted for frozen section. Tumors within the substance of the pancreas that are small (less than 2 cm) and well encapsulated may be carefully enucleated. Pancreatic tumors without defined capsules or situated deep in the parenchyma often require partial pancreatic resection. In the absence of an identifiable pancreatic tumor, a longitudinal duodenotomy may be performed at the level of the second portion of the duodenum, and the duodenum can be bimanually palpated and everted in a further search for duodenal gastrinomas. Tumors identified within the duodenal wall are resected locally, with closure of the duodenal defect. Uncommonly, gastrinomas may be located deep within the substance of the pancreatic head or uncinate process, and pancreaticoduodenectomy may be required for tumor excision.

Despite thorough preoperative and intraoperative localization efforts, in some patients (5 to 20 percent) no tumor may be demonstrable at laparotomy. In the face of such a negative exploration, two surgical options are available. First, parietal cell vagotomy has been proposed as a means of reducing antisecretory drug dose requirements in patients on high dose antisecretory drug therapy, but without previous life-threatening complications. However, the usefulness of parietal cell vagotomy to decrease dose requirements was established in patients taking histamine H_2-receptor antagonists, and not in patients being treated with omeprazole. The second surgical option for patients with a negative exploration is total gastrectomy. While in the past total gastrectomy provided the most reliable means of controlling the ulcer diathesis, the availability of omeprazole has drastically reduced the need for total gastrectomy. However, there is still a role for total gastrectomy in patients whose tumors cannot be localized or whose tumors are unresectable, if those patients cannot or will not take adequate doses of antisecretory medications.

There has been a notable improvement in the outlook of patients with gastrinoma in recent years. In the 1950s and 60s gastrinoma patients were often diagnosed late in the course of their disease without the benefit of gastrin radioimmunoassay. At that time effective medical therapy for hyperchlorhydria was not available, and sophisticated localization and staging techniques did not exist. These patients often suffered multiple ulcer complications, required total gastrectomy to control the ulcer diathesis, and typically succumbed to continued tumor growth following gastrectomy. In contrast, recent series of gastrinoma patients treated surgically provide room for optimism. For example, of 130 patients who have undergone exploration in recent years, 81 percent had the gastrinoma located at the time of surgery, while only 19 percent had a negative exploration. Primary tumors were identified in 64 percent of the patients explored, with 29 percent of patients having pancreatic primaries, 14 percent having duodenal primaries, and 21 percent having primaries located in other regions. Thirty-five percent of the patients explored were considered to be surgically cured, as defined by postoperative fasting eugastrinemia, negative secretin stimulation tests, and negative imaging studies. Considering only those patients explored and thought to be successfully resected, the cure rate was 60 percent. These recent results represent a major improvement in the management of gastrinoma patients over the past decades, and support the practice of initial pharmacologic control of gastric hypersecretion, followed by aggressive tumor localization and staging in hopes of curative resection. The earlier chapter on Zollinger-Ellison syndrome provides information on postoperation gastrin and acid levels.

The cause of death in most patients with incurable gastrinoma is tumor growth and dissemination. Multiple treatment modalities have been utilized in an effort to treat patients with metastatic gastrinoma. The overall objective response rate to chemotherapy appears to be less than 50 percent. A recent prospective study of monthly cycles of streptozocin, 5-fluorouracil, and doxorubicin in ten patients with metastatic gastrinoma showed a partial response rate of 40 percent and a 60 percent no response rate. Survival has not been improved by chemotherapy. Hormonal therapy with octreotide has been reported to improve symptoms, reduce hypergastrinemia, and diminish hyperchlorhydria in patients with metastatic gastrinoma. Anecdotal reports suggest that octreotide may occasionally reduce tumor volume. However, the role of octreotide, which must be parenterally administered, remains limited because adequate doses of omeprazole can control hyperchlorhydria and peptic symptoms in nearly all patients. Hepatic transplantation, hepatic artery embolization, and interferon therapy have all been used in small numbers of patients with gastrinoma metastatic to the liver. The efficacy of these therapies remains to be proven.

VIPOMA (VERNER-MORRISON SYNDROME)

Endocrine tumors of the pancreas associated with *w*atery *d*iarrhea, *h*ypokalemia, and either *a*chlorhydria or hypochlorhydria comprise the rare clinical entity known as the Verner-Morrison syndrome (WDHA syndrome). Verner and Morrison are credited with the definition of this secretory-type diarrhea syndrome, following their report of two cases in 1958. Additional information is provided in the chapter *Secretory Diarrhea*. The characteristic clinical finding is that of intermittent severe diarrhea, often of a watery nature, averaging 5 liters per day. Malabsorption and steatorrhea are not common. Hypokalemia results from the fecal loss of large amounts of potassium (up to 400 mEq per day) and may be associated with muscular weakness, lethargy, and nausea. Half of the patients have hyperglycemia and hypercalcemia while cutaneous flushing occurs in 20 percent of patients. The diagnosis of VIPoma is typically made after excluding other more common causes of diarrhea (Table 5). The circulating hormones felt to be the active agents in this syndrome include vasoactive intestinal polypeptide (VIP), peptide histidine-isoleucine (PHI), or prostaglandins. Fasting VIP levels should be measured in all patients with suspected VIPomas. Because VIP secretion may be episodic, a single low VIP level does not rule out the syndrome.

Tumor localization and staging begins with dynamic abdominal CT scan with intravenous and oral contrast, and is followed by visceral angiography if the CT is negative. In addition, because 10 percent of VIPoma patients have extrapancreatic tumors located in the retroperitoneum or thorax, thoracic CT scan is also indicated.

Preparation for surgery must include correction of fluid and electrolyte losses via intravenous fluid administration and electrolyte replacement. Therapy with octreotide has been proven effective in the preoperative setting, leading to a reduction in circulating VIP levels and control of the diarrhea. Prior to the availability of octreotide, corticosteroids and indomethacin were used preoperatively to control diarrhea and associated fluid and electrolyte losses. Surgical excision of the tumor is recommended in all patients with the Verner-Morrison syndrome. The majority of pancreatic primaries are located in the distal pancreas and are amenable to resection via distal pancreatectomy. If no tumor is found in the pancreas, a careful exploration of the retroperitoneum, including both adrenals, should be performed. Metastases have been present in half of the reported cases. In these cases, safe palliative debulking of the

Table 5 Verner-Morrison Syndrome:
Differential Diagnosis

Entity	Work-up
Villous adenoma	Lower GI endoscopy
Laxative abuse	Stool exam for phenolphthalein
Celiac disease	Fecal fat measurement
	D-xylose tolerance test
	Small bowel biopsy
Parasitic and infectious diseases	Stool culture
	Ova and parasites
Inflammatory bowel disease	Lower GI endoscopy
	Upper GI and small bowel series
Carcinoid syndrome	Urinary 5'-HIAA
	Upper GI and small bowel series
	Abdominal CT scan
Gastrinoma	Serum gastrin
	Gastric acid analysis
	Secretin stimulation test

metastatic tumor is indicated. The chapter *Secretory Diarrhea* provides additional therapeutic details.

In patients with recurrent or unresectable VIPoma, therapy with octreotide is used to reduce circulating VIP levels and control diarrhea. Chemotherapy in VIPoma patients has not been studied prospectively. Streptozocin or interferon appear to be the drugs of choice based on limited data.

GLUCAGONOMA

The glucagonoma syndrome is characterized by severe dermatitis, mild diabetes, stomatitis, and anemia. The characteristic skin rash is termed necrolytic migratory erythema. The rash exhibits cyclic migrations with erythematous patches that spread serpiginously with central healing points of resolution. It is thought that the hypoaminoacidemia seen in patients with glucagonoma is responsible for the dermatitis. Glucagonoma patients may also demonstrate malnutrition, weight loss, hypertrophic intestinal villi, hypoproteinemia, and venous thrombosis.

The diagnosis of glucagonoma may be suggested by biopsies of the skin lesions and is secured by the documentation of elevated levels of fasting serum glucagon (normal levels up to 150 pg per millimeter). Demonstration of hypoaminoacidemia may help to confirm the diagnosis, but is extremely expensive and rarely necessary.*

In patients with biochemical documentation of hyperglucagonemia, radiographic localization and staging should commence with an abdominal CT scan with both intravenous and oral contrast. Because these tumors are usually large and solitary, the CT scan localizes the tumor in the majority of patients. Angiography is the next step in tumor localization should the CT

---

*Editor's Note: Occasionally, recognizing enlarged small intestinal villi by their "smudgy" appearance on contrast radiograph arouses suspicion of this syndrome.

scan be nondiagnostic. Prior to exploration, attention should be given to the management of malnutrition. Total parenteral nutrition has been used to improve the catabolic state created by hyperglucagonemia. Octreotide can be used to reduce the circulating glucagon levels and allow improved response to total parenteral nutrition.

Most glucagonomas are located in the body and tail of the pancreas. Surgical resection typically involves distal pancreatectomy. Metastases have been found in up to 80 percent of patients and safe debulking of these metastatic lesions should be considered.

Glucagonoma patients with incurable or recurrent disease have had low response rates to chemotherapeutic agents such as streptozocin, dacarbazine, and doxorubicin. Octreotide has been successful in reducing the elevated glucagon levels and in controlling the hyperglycemia and dermatitis associated with incurable glucagonoma.

SOMATOSTATINOMA

The somatostatinoma syndrome is the least common pancreatic endocrine syndrome with an estimated annual incidence of one in forty million people. The clinical features of the somatostatinoma syndrome are nonspecific and include steatorrhea, diabetes, hypochlorhydria, and cholelithiasis. The test used to confirm the diagnosis of a somatostatinoma is a fasting somatostatin level. While the normal plasma level is below 100 pg per millimeter, patients with somatostatinomas have high levels of circulating somatostatin, often measured in the nanogram per millimeter range.

Most somatostatinomas have been located in the head of the pancreas, with less common sites being the body and tail of the pancreas and the periampullary region. The most useful test for localization and staging has been the abdominal CT scan, which has been used to document and stage these typically large tumors. Preoperative management of patients with somatostatinoma involves treatment of hyperglycemia and malnutrition. At surgery, resection for cure has been uncommon, because of the presence of metastatic disease in most cases. Safe resection of the primary tumor and careful debulking of hepatic metastases appear indicated. At the time of exploration, cholecystectomy is indicated, even in the absence of documented gallstones, because of the known increased incidence of cholelithiasis with persistently elevated somatostatin levels.

NONFUNCTIONAL ISLET CELL TUMORS

Up to one-third of endocrine tumors of the pancreas are found to be nonfunctional, based on the absence of a defined clinical syndrome and a lack of elevated serum insulin, gastrin, VIP, glucagon, and somatostatin levels. The one hormone that may be elevated in the serum in these nonfunctional tumors is pancreatic polypeptide

(PP), which appears to be a marker for pancreatic endocrine tumors without being the mediator of any specific PP-related clinical syndrome. Nonfunctional endocrine tumors of the pancreas usually present with clinical manifestations such as abdominal pain, weight loss, and jaundice. These clinical manifestations are similar to those found in patients with ductal adenocarcinoma arising from the head of the pancreas. Nonfunctional tumors are most commonly located in the head of the pancreas or in the periampullary region. The malignancy rate for nonfunctional tumors ranges from 50 to 90 percent. However, in contrast to the poor prognosis associated with ductal adenocarcinoma of the pancreas, these nonfunctional tumors tend to be slower growing and are associated with a longer survival.

Localization and staging studies are performed in similar fashion to patients with the more common diagnosis of ductal adenocarcinoma of the exocrine pancreas. The abdominal CT scan is used for evaluation of the primary tumor and to assess for hepatic metastases. Visceral angiography can be used to locate the primary tumor and assess for arterial anomalies. The venous phase of the angiogram provides information regarding encasement or occlusion of the main portal venous structures by tumor. At surgery, most of these nonfunctional tumors are larger than 2 cm in size and it is rarely safe to excise them by local techniques. Tumors in the head or uncinate process of the pancreas may require pancreaticoduodenectomy for safe resection while tumors arising in the body or tail of the pancreas are treated by distal pancreatectomy. Patients with unresectable tumors in the head of the pancreas are candidates for surgical palliation of obstructive jaundice and gastric outlet obstruction by biliary-enteric and gastroenteric bypass, respectively. The overall 5-year survival rate in all patients with nonfunctional tumors approaches 50 percent, greatly in excess of the 10 to 20 percent 5-year survival rate reported for resected ductal adenocarcinoma of the exocrine pancreas.

In patients with unresectable nonfunctional islet cell tumors, partial responses to combination chemotherapy have been reported. In a recent multicenter trial reported by Moertel and associates, 105 patients with advanced islet cell carcinoma were randomly assigned to one of three treatment regimens. The combination of streptozocin plus 5-fluorouracil was associated with a 45 percent response rate, the combination of streptozocin plus doxorubicin was associated with a 69 percent response rate, while chlorozotocin alone was associated with a 30 percent response rate. Streptozocin plus doxorubicin therapy was associated with a significant survival advantage when compared to the other two treatment arms. The most common toxic reactions to the chemotherapy included nausea and vomiting, leukopenia, and mild renal insufficiency.

SUGGESTED READING*

Delcore R Jr, Cheung LY, Friesen SR. Characteristics of duodenal wall gastrinomas. Am J Surg 1990; 160:621–624.

Frucht H, Norton JA, London JF, et al. Detection of duodenal gastrinomas by operative endoscopic transillumination. A prospective study. Gastroenterology 1990; 99:1622–1627.

Imamura M, Takahashi K, Adachi H, et al. Usefulness of selective arterial secretin test for localization of gastrinoma in the Zollinger-Ellison syndrome. Ann Surg 1987; 205:230–239.

Lamberts SWJ, Bakker WH, Reubi J-C, Krenning EP. Somatostatin-receptor imaging in the localization of endocrine tumors. N Engl J Med 1990; 323:1246–1249.

Moertel CG, Lefkopoulo M, Lipsitz S, et al. Streptozocin-doxorubicin, streptozocin-fluorouracil, or chlorozotocin in the treatment of advanced islet-cell carcinoma. N Engl J Med 1992; 326:519–523.

Norton JA, Shawker TH, Doppman JL, et al. Localization and surgical treatment of occult insulinomas. Ann Surg 1990; 212:615–620.

Rosch T, Lightdale CJ, Botet JF, et al. Localization of pancreatic endocrine tumors by endoscopic ultrasonography. N Engl J Med 1992; 326:1721–1726.

Udelsman R, Yeo CJ, Hruban RH, et al. Pancreaticoduodenectomy for selected pancreatic endocrine tumors. Surg Gynecol Obstet 1993; 177:269-278.

Von Schrenck T, Howard JM, Doppman JL, et al. Prospective study of chemotherapy in patients with metastatic gastrinoma. Gastroenterology 1988; 94:1326–1334.

Yeo CJ. ZES: Current approaches. Contemporary Gastroenterol 1990; 3:17–29.

*Editor's Note: There are other pertinent references in the chapter on Zollinger-Ellison syndrome in an earlier section of the book.

PANCREATIC AND ISLET CELL TRANSPLANTATION

HANS W. SOLLINGER, M.D., Ph.D.

This chapter reviews the current status of vascularized pancreas transplantation as well as clinical islet transplantation. Because of the significant increase in the number of vascularized pancreas transplants over the past 5 years and the high success rate of this procedure, most of the chapter deals with this treatment modality. Islet transplantation, still considered experimental, has not yet achieved long-term clinical success and therefore is briefly discussed at the end of the chapter.

VASCULARIZED PANCREAS TRANSPLANTATION

In 1980, the International Pancreas Transplant Registry reported a 1-year survival rate for pancreas transplantation of 21 percent and patient survival of 67 percent. Thirteen years later, at the Fourth International Congress on Pancreatic and Islet Transplantation held in Amsterdam, tremendous progress has been reported in the area of pancreas transplantation by a number of groups, predominantly from the United States and Europe. The areas in which giant strides were made and that are responsible for the current success of vascularized pancreas transplantation include organ procurement and preservation, surgical technique, immunosuppressive therapy, and the treatment and diagnosis of rejection. Furthermore, information regarding the influence of the pancreatic transplantation on secondary diabetic complications is now accumulating that suggests a beneficial influence of the pancreatic transplant on diabetic neuropathy, recurrence of diabetic nephropathy in the transplanted kidney, and most recently, diabetic retinopathy.

Types of Pancreas Transplantation

Pancreas transplantation has been performed in three settings. In the uremic diabetic patient, simultaneous pancreas-kidney transplantation (SPK) with both organs from the same donor is currently the most frequently performed surgical procedure. Pancreas transplantation after successful kidney transplantation and pancreas transplantation alone in nonuremic diabetic patients are less frequently performed. The advantages of SPK are that the recipient requires only one surgical procedure and identical immunosuppressive therapy as compared to kidney transplantation alone. In contrast, in the nonuremic diabetic patient, the side effects and complications of immunosuppressive therapy must be balanced against the possible secondary diabetic complications that may or may not occur in the future. In my own view, in most patients the complications of immunosuppressive therapy are predictably worse than the expected diabetic complications, and therefore I do not perform pancreas transplantation in nonuremic diabetic patients. Furthermore, it is important to note that the success rate for pancreas transplantation and pancreas transplantation after a kidney transplantation are significantly worse than the results achieved in SPK transplantation. In our own series of approximately 340 kidney transplantations, the vast majority are SPK transplantations. For these reasons, my comments in this chapter primarily address SPK transplantation.

Technical Aspects of SPK Transplantation

One of the key events in successful SPK transplantation is organ procurement and preservation. With the increasing number of pancreas transplants performed, surgeons worldwide have become familiar with a rapid and efficient surgical technique for safe removal of the pancreas. Most transplantation centers in the United States are now performing combined liver-pancreas procurement so that the liver as well as the pancreas from the same donor can be used for transplantation. In our own experience, more than 95 percent of multi-organ donors serve both as liver and pancreas donors. The liver and pancreas are procured en bloc, with the blood supply between the pancreas and liver not dissected during the procedure. En bloc removal minimizes the chance of injuring the hepatic blood supply, especially if an aberrant hepatic artery exists. After combined liver-pancreas retrieval, the pancreatic arterial blood supply must be reconstructed with donor iliac Y-graft. This modification has not only allowed the use of both liver and pancreas from the same donor, but has also facilitated the transplantation procedure for the pancreas.

One of the most significant advances in pancreas transplantation has been the introduction of the University of Wisconsin organ preservation solution. For optimal preservation of the pancreas, an aortic flush consisting only of University of Wisconsin solution is utilized. The International Pancreas Transplant Registry has compiled data from nearly 2,000 pancreatic grafts with varying preservation times. It now seems clear that preservation times for up to 30 hours can be considered safe if University of Wisconsin solution is used. In our own center we have reviewed 253 patients receiving SPK transplantation. There was *immediate insulin independence in 99.6 percent of patients.* There was only one primary nonfunction, and the rate of vascular thrombosis was 0.8 percent. Postoperative hemodialysis for the simultaneously transplanted kidney occurred in 2.4 percent. Once procured, all kidneys and pancreata were utilized for transplantation, resulting in a 0 percent nonutilization rate.

Patient Selection

With the increasing success of SPK transplantation, an increasing number of patients is seeking this treatment modality, especially in centers with a large experience. At the University of Wisconsin-Madison, approximately 100 to 120 patients per year are being evaluated for SPK transplantation. Our selection criteria are based on the fact that we believe that a successful pancreas transplantation will exhibit its beneficial effects in the long term, possibly 5, 10, 15 or 20 years after transplantation. Therefore, we select patients who, as judged by general medical criteria, have a life expectancy for this period of time. We feel that it is unreasonable to select a patient for SPK transplantation who has severe vascular disease that might significantly limit life expectancy. Specifically, we expect the patient to have a normal thallium stress test. If the thallium stress test is suggestive of coronary artery disease, we request coronary angiography. If coronary angiography suggests that an intervention such as balloon angioplasty or coronary artery bypass is necessary, we recommend kidney transplantation alone. We also feel that it is inappropriate to accept patients who have already undergone major amputations secondary to atherosclerotic vascular disease. In addition, the patient must be able to understand the complex nature of the procedure and be able to comply with the demanding follow-up regimen. Funding for SPK transplantation has been a problem in the past, but an increasing number of insurance companies has agreed to cover SPK transplantation. Medicare is investigating the possibility of extending coverage for SPK transplantation.

Surgical Procedure

The first series of pancreas transplantation was performed at the University of Minnesota by Kelly and colleagues in 1966. The first operation was a segmental pancreas transplantation with duct ligation, and the second was a whole pancreas transplantation with duodenostomy. For the past 25 years, the best surgical procedure for pancreas transplantation has been a matter of great controversy among transplant surgeons. In principle, three types of surgical procedures have been most frequently advocated. These include enteric drainage, either using a segmental graft anastomosed to a Roux-en-Y loop, duct injection using fast-hardening polymeric substances injected into the pancreatic duct, and bladder drainage, first described at the University of Wisconsin.

The major problem with enteric drainage was leakage of the pancreatico-enteric anastomosis, which had a high potential to develop into significant septic complications. In their initial series, the Stockholm group reported a 58 percent complication rate requiring reoperation. More recently, they have changed their technique to whole pancreas transplantation with side-to-side anastomosis of the duodenal segment to the jejunum. This technique is safer and associated with a lower complication rate and better 1-year graft survival.

In an attempt to avoid anastomosis between the pancreas and the draining organ, the Lyon group suggested, in 1978, to inject the pancreatic duct with prolamin, a fast-hardening amino acid solution. Although this technique initially seems to be safe, graft pancreatitis and graft fibrosis lead to a high incidence of early vascular thrombosis and later, pancreaticocutaneous fistulas. Even in the world's best series, 2-year graft survival does not exceed 55 percent. The high incidence of chronic wound complications, as well as the high incidence of vascular thrombosis, has led the majority of surgeons to abandon this technique.

Laboratory work at the University of Wisconsin performed by Dr. Katie Cook and myself in the early 1980s demonstrated the feasibility of *draining the pancreatic duct into the urinary bladder*. After a successful series of transplantation in a dog model, we proceeded in 1982 to perform the first bladder drained pancreatic transplantation in man. Initially, a segmental pancreas transplantation was anastomosed to the bladder (in the later stages modified to use the whole pancreas with the anastomosis of a duodenal button to the bladder), and further modified by Corry and Nghiem from the Iowa group, who suggested the use of a *side-to-side anastomosis of the duodenal segment to the bladder*. This technique has now become the preferred technique in more than 95 percent of pancreas transplantation centers worldwide.

For the operation to be performed, the patient is placed in supine position and the pelvis is slightly extended. A midline incision starting at the symphysis pubis and extending superiorly to about 5 to 10 cm below the xiphoid is needed for exposure. The right colon, small bowel, and sigmoid colon are reflected medially and superiorly, allowing access to the iliac vessels. The pancreas is placed on the right and the kidney on the left. The right common and external iliac veins are freed of all posterior branches from the inguinal ligament to the inferior vena cava bifurcation. The common, external, and iliac arteries are exposed. After excision of a narrow ellipse of the iliac vein, the portal vein is anastomosed lateral to the iliac arteries. Freeing of the iliac vein of posterior branching and completing the anastomosis laterally ensures a tension-free anastomosis. When the pancreas swells postoperatively, the portal vein may be tented. Freeing the iliac vein obviates the need for an interposition vein graft. The arterial anastomosis is performed between the common iliac artery of the reconstructed Y-graft and the common iliac artery of the recipient. Heparin is not used during the venous or arterial anastomosis or postoperatively. This has not been associated with an increased incidence of clots or thrombosis, which has been less than 1 percent in our entire series of more than 250 SPK transplantation. After completion of the vascular anastomosis, the clamps are released in a manner calculated to minimize pressure within the graft vascular system. Undue pressure causes graft edema and may lead to pancreatitis. First, the proximal venous clamp is released and the graft vessels are examined for bleeding. Next, the clamp on the iliac artery is released. With each clamp release, the graft is in turn inspected for bleeding. Next, the distal iliac arterial clamp is removed, followed by the proximal arterial clamp. The distal venous clamp is removed last. Pancreaticoduodenocystostomy is performed between the midpoint of the duodenal segment in the most accessible portion of the bladder using a two-layer anastomosis of absorbable suture material. Prior to the anastomosis, the duodenal contents are aspirated and submitted for culture. The kidney is placed in the left iliac fossa using standard renal transplantation technique. The Liche technique is used for ureteroneocystostomy.

It is important to emphasize that no drains are used, but attention to absolutely secure hemostasis is essential. No anticoagulation is administered, with the exception of one aspirin daily.

Surgical Complications

Hematuria

Hematuria is a common finding following surgery, but in most instances the urine clears within a few days. Of greater concern is blood loss, especially with clot formation. This usually indicates bleeding from the duodenocystostomy anastomotic site. If the bleeding and clots do not clear, cystoscopy is done to evacuate the bladder and fulgurate the bleeding point if clearly identified. Persistent or recurrent hematuria occuring any time after transplantation is due to granulation tissue at the anastomotic site or ulcers in the duodenal segment. If hematuria persists despite appropriate therapy, conversion to enteric drainage is indicated.

Urinary Leak

Urinary leak may occur from three sources: the ureteral implantation site, the duodenocystostomy anastomosis, and the duodenal segment itself. Ureteral leaks are rare and may be corrected either by operative intervention or percutaneous stent placement. Leaks at the site of the duodenocystostomy usually occur within the first few weeks after transplantation and can be managed in the following ways. Small leaks are initially treated with prolonged Foley catheter drainage. Usually these leaks close spontaneously. Larger leaks either need surgical closure or enteric conversion. Late leaks most frequently are caused by ulcers in the duodenal segment. In approximately 50 percent of these ulcers, cytomegalovirus is cultured. In all of these instances, enteric conversion with prior excision of the ulcerated segment is necessary.

Graft Pancreatitis and Hyperamylasemia

Early postoperative hyperamylasemia occurs in about one-third of SPK recipients. The rise in the serum amylase levels usually declines rapidly and is asymptomatic. Persistent or marked elevation of the amylase levels indicates possible technical errors such as ligation or injury to the primary or accessory pancreatic duct. Preservation injury is another cause of post-transplant hyperamylasemia. Sudden lower abdominal pain with hyperamylasemia and perigraft tenderness usually indicates reflux pancreatitis. These patients are best treated with Foley catheter drainage. Serum amylase levels may also be elevated during rejection, infected ascites, and duodenocystostomy leak.

Bicarbonate Loss

Bicarbonate replacement is necessary in about 80 percent of patients to maintain an HCO_3 level of 20 mg/dl or above. The bicarbonate loss is accompanied by loss of fluid so that low serum bicarbonate levels are frequently accompanied by dehydration. Fortunately, this problem usually stabilizes with time and is an infrequent indication for conversion from bladder to enteric drainage.

Urethritis

Patients with chronic urethritis complain of persistent dysuria. Perforation of the urethra usually involves the membranous segment and patients may present with perineal and testicular swelling. The treatment is prompt conversion from bladder to enteric drainage. The incidence of urethritis, which usually occurs only in males, is about 5 percent, and the cause remains unclear.

Immunosuppression

In SPK transplantation, rejection occurs earlier and with greater frequency than when the kidney is transplanted alone. We estimate that more than 85 percent of our patients have at least one rejection episode, which is usually manifested as a renal rejection episode.

Quadruple drug immunosuppression has been the backbone of SPK immunosuppressive therapy at our center. Currently, *OKT3* (5 mg) is given intra-operatively and for 12 to 14 days postoperatively. Although it is not clear that OKT3 offers significant advantages in terms of graft survival or reduction in infectious complications in comparison with Minnesota antilymphocyte globulin, it is our impression that the incidence of serious rejection episodes is lower. The other three drugs used are *prednisone, azathioprine,* and *cyclosporine.* Prednisone is rapidly tapered to 30 mg per day on day 4 and to 20 mg per day 4 weeks after transplantation. Cyclosporine dose is adjusted to maintain a whole blood level between 350 and 500.

Graft rejection is initially treated with high-dose *steroid* therapy for 3 to 4 days, and if there is no response, a second course of OKT3 is initiated. Patients unresponsive to OKT3 receive a 10- to 14-day course of *antilymphocyte globulin.* Patients retreated for rejection with antibody therapy receive prophylactic *ganciclovir.* With early and aggressive therapy, more than 90 percent of rejection episodes are reversed.

Effect of Pancreas Transplantation on Secondary Diabetic Complications

As expected, it took many years before the effect of pancreas transplantation on secondary diabetic complications could be assessed. The first observation was that patients with a successful pancreas transplantation demonstrated normalization or near normalization of glycosylated hemoglobin A_1C. This is an observation that was uniformly made throughout all transplantation centers worldwide. There is also an accumulation of reports that show that lipid levels in recipients of SPK transplantation are better than in well-matched diabetic recipients of a kidney transplantation alone. In our own series, cholesterol levels in SPK recipients were significantly lower than in a well-matched group of diabetic living-related-donor recipients, despite the fact that the weight gain in the SPK group was twice as high.

Recurrent nephropathy in the transplanted kidney has been a concern of transplantation surgeons for many years. Fortunately, it usually takes more than 10 years before the recurrence becomes clinically significant. The Stockholm group reported that a simultaneously transplanted pancreas will prevent recurrent diabetic nephropathy in the co-transplanted kidney. The University of Wisconsin and University of Minnesota are currently collaborating on a trial (sponsored by the National Institutes of Health) to document the influence of simultaneously transplanted pancreas on the kidney transplantation in a systematic long-term, prospective trial.

Most clinicians performing pancreas transplantation have noted significant improvement in peripheral and autonomic neuropathy. However, to distinguish the improvements caused by normalization of creatinine versus the contribution of the pancreatic graft is only possible in well-matched series comparing the progression of neuropathy in recipients of a kidney transplantation alone versus SPK recipients. There are now numerous reports available demonstrating the long-term effect of a successful pancreatic graft. Solders and colleagues from the Stockholm group were the first to demonstrate that objective parameters such as nerve conduction will take several years before significant improvement can be measured, which was in contrast to their earlier report. Autonomic neuropathy was studied by Gaber and colleagues comparing 13 patients receiving a kidney transplantation alone versus 16 patients receiving SPK. In almost all parameters studied, including gastric emptying, recipients with SPK fared better.

The first report on the influence of SPK transplantation on diabetic microangiopathy came from Abendroth and Land's group in Munich. Transcutaneous oxygen determination demonstrated significant improvement in peripheral muscle after SPK, but no change after kidney transplantation alone. The same was true for reoxygenation time, which was significantly shortened in patients who had undergone SPK, but was not changed in isolated kidney transplant recipients. At this time, however, we have no clear-cut information as to whether the changes in microangiopathy will translate into a reduced amputation rate. Nevertheless, the experience in our own center suggests that recipients of SPK have fewer amputations, as well as diabetic ulcers in their lower extremities, but it is difficult to find a comparable control group to study this issue.

One of the more recent and most exciting observations regarding diabetic microvascular disease has come from the laboratory of Dr. Anthony Cheung in Sacramento. Dr. Cheung, in collaboration with Dr. Bill Bry from San Francisco, is measuring the time from the injection of fluorescein to the time when capillary leakage occurs. Using a sophisticated camera, as well as computer equipment, he could show that recipients of SPK have leakage 2 years post-transplant, which compares to normal control, while the pretransplant value compared to a group of diabetic patients.

For the patient, one of the most significant incentives to undergo SPK transplantation is the hope of stabilization or improvement of diabetic retinopathy. Unfortunately, an earlier report by Ramsay and his colleagues from Minneapolis demonstrated progression of diabetic retinopathy after pancreas transplantation. This study included a group of patients who had received pancreas transplantation alone. In contrast, a recent study by Klein and coworkers from our group, comparing several parameters of diabetic retinopathy in recipients of SPK transplantation versus well-matched diabetic recipients of kidney transplantation alone, demonstrated significant improvement in overall changes. In 43 percent of SPK recipients, regression was noted, as compared to 23 percent of recipients of a kidney alone. In about 50 percent of patients in both groups, no change was noted; however, only 7 percent of the SPK recipients have progression of disease, although progression was noted in 27 percent of the isolated kidney transplantation recipients.

Finally, the issue of quality of life has been addressed by several groups. Following the first report by Nakache and colleagues from Stockholm, several other groups, most notably from Iowa, Minnesota, and Wisconsin, have investigated the quality of life of SPK recipients versus recipients of kidney transplantation alone. All of these studies are in agreement that SPK recipients enjoy a higher quality of life as determined by multiple parameters.

The success rate in terms of patient and graft survival as reported by the International Pancreas Transplant Registry has significantly improved over the past decade. Between October 1987 and November 1992, 1,604 patients underwent SPK transplantation in the United States. Patient survival at 1 year is 91 percent, kidney survival 84 percent, and pancreas survival 75 percent. In our own center, 5-year actuarial survival in 236 consecutive patients with SPK transplantation and bladder drainage is 90 percent for patients, 82 percent for kidneys, and 80 percent for the pancreatic graft. These results are as good or better than kidney transplantation alone from haplotype-matched living related donors or diabetic recipients of cadaver kidneys.

For the reasons discussed earlier, as well as the

patient and graft survival achieved, we now consider SPK transplantation the procedure of choice for selected uremic diabetic patients.

ISLET CELL TRANSPLANTATION

There is little doubt that if pancreatic islet transplantation were to become a clinical reality, it would be the treatment of choice for juvenile onset diabetic patients, as the procedure itself would consist of little more than an injection, with virtually no discomfort or risk to the patient. In addition, pretreatment of the islets with organ culture or monoclonal antibodies could decrease the immunogenicity of these grafts, and therefore, transplantation might be possible with little or no immunosuppressive therapy. In the 1970s, early results with islet transplantation in rodents suggested that this treatment modality might become a clinical reality in the very near future. Successful islet transplantation requires automated separation of pancreatic islets and successful preparation for injection either into the spleen, omentum, or portal vein. Many of these more technical aspects, such as fully automated islet separation as well as high-quality cryopreservation, have already been accomplished. Nevertheless, the successful transplantation of pancreatic islets, even under immunosuppressive coverage, has been restricted to a few patients. The longest successful pancreatic islet graft was performed in Edmonton, Canada. This patient received islets separated from several adult donors in conjunction with a renal allograft. To our knowledge, this graft was fully functional for approximately 2.5 years. Other longer-term functioning islet transplantations were performed at the University of Minnesota with graft survival of 6 and 12 months, respectively. The most disturbing aspect of these initially successful transplantations was their *abrupt cessation of function.* Previous studies in large animals using autologous tissue predicted such an occurrence. It is not clear if the islets failed from recurrent autoimmune diabetes or if it is necessary for the long-term function of islets that they be imbedded in the exocrine pancreatic tissue mass to receive the necessary nutrients and growth factors.

Another approach already clinically attempted is the transplantation of *immunoisolated islets.* Unfortunately, the first series of this transplantation was performed very recently and it is too early to make conclusions about the long-term success. Even more worrisome is the fact that several investigators have now demonstrated that islets, but not whole pancreas, are susceptible to autoimmune recurrence of the disease. An additional question will be the effect of successful islet transplantation on secondary diabetic complications. There are contradictory reports in the literature indicating that islets do not exert the same beneficial effect on secondary diabetic complications as pancreatic grafts will do.

In my opinion, the limited mass of adult islets currently available in the United States (under optimal circumstances, transplantation would only be possible for 400 to 600 patients) limits this technology significantly. Much more promise is therefore in the area of fetal pancreas transplantation, where significantly more material is available.

Holding even more promise for the future may be early experiments of genetic engineering. Several groups around the world have cloned the insulin gene and are now inserting appropriate control and regulatory elements. It must be expected that within a short time a fully functional insulin gene will be available. Once the problem of in vivo transfection of genetic material has been overcome, it is quite likely that gene therapy will become the preferred and ultimate method for the treatment of type I diabetes.

SUGGESTED READING

Bohman SO, Tyden G, Wilczek H, et al. Prevention of kidney graft diabetic nephropathy by pancreas transplantation in man. Diabetes 1985; 34:306–308.

Cheung ATW, Cox KL, Ahlfors CE, Bry WI. Reversal of microangiopathy in long-term diabetic patients after successful simultaneous pancreas-kidney transplants. J Microvasc Surg (in press).

Martin X, Lefrancois N, Dawhara M, et al. Pancreas transplantation in the uremic patient: a random trial of total pancreas with bladder drainage versus duct obstruction of segmental grafts. Transplant Proc 1993; 25:1182–1183.

Nghiem DD, Corry RJ. Transplantation with urinary drainage of pancreatic secretions. Am J Surg 1987; 153:405–406.

Pirsch JD, Groshek M, Reed A, et al. Effect of simultaneous pancreas-kidney transplantation on serum cholesterol. Proceedings of the Third International Congress on Pancreatic and Islet Transplantation 1991; Abstract 105.

Ploeg RJ, Eckhoff DE, D'Alessandro AM, et al. Urological complications and enteric conversion after pancreas transplantation with bladder drainage. Transplant Proc (in press).

Sollinger HW, Messing EM, Eckhoff DE, et al. Urological complications in 210 consecutive simultaneous pancreas-kidney transplants (SPK) with bladder drainage. Ann Surg (in press).

Sollinger HW, Vernon WB, D'Alessandro AM, et al. Combined liver and pancreas procurement with Belzer-UW solution. Surgery 1989; 106:685–691.

INDEX

677

Gastric epithelial dysplasia, 171
Gastric hypersecretion, in short bowel syndrome, 312
Gastric lymphomas, 170
Gastric pH, for diagnosis of Zollinger-Ellison syndrome, 127
Gastric polyps
  hyperplastic, 171
  mucosal, 171
Gastric remnant, premalignant conditions, 172, 174(t)
Gastric surgery, nausea and vomiting after, 179
Gastric ulcers
  Helicobacter pylori and, 106
  from nonsteroidal anti-inflammatory drug use, treatment, 120
Gastric varices, management, 537
Gastrin, serum, measurement, indications, 667(t)
Gastrinomas, 666-668, 667(t)
  with hepatic metastases, 130-131
  metastatic, 130-131
  surgical therapy, 125-126
  in Zollinger-Ellison syndrome, control of, 129-131
Gastrin output, for diagnosis of Zollinger-Ellison syndrome, 127
Gastritis
  antral, diffuse, 145
  atrophic
    corporal, with pernicious anemia, 172-173
    multifocal, 171, 174(t)
  autoimmune, 172-173, 174(t)
  chronic
    classification, 144-147, 145(t)
    Sydney system for, 147
    management, 147-151, 149(f)
    with dyspepsia, 148
    pathophysiology, 145
  cytomegalovirus, from human immunodeficiency virus infection, 218
  eosinophilic, 146
  follicular, 174
  granulomatous, 146, 146(t)
  Helicobacter pylori and, 106
    with nonulcer dyspepsia, 148
  lymphocytic, 146-147
  metaplastic
    autoimmune, 145
    environmental, 146
  postgastrectomy, 150
Gastrocolic fistula, after percutaneous endoscopic gastrostomy, 159
Gastroduodenal cancer, Nd:YAG laser therapy for, 91
Gastroduodenal Crohn's disease, surgical management, 338
Gastroduodenal disease, *Helicobacter pylori*, 105-109. *See also Helicobacter pylori* gastroduodenal disease
Gastroduodenocutaneous fistulas, 342
Gastroenterologists, allegations against, 9
Gastroenterostomy, with truncal vagotomy, for peptic ulcer disease, 122
Gastroesophageal reflux
  from cystic fibrosis, 656
  gastrostomy tubes and, 48
  in infants and children, 46-48
Gastroesophageal reflux disease (GERD)
  diagnosis, 29, 30, 34-35
  extraesophageal manifestations, 30-33
    management, 31(f), 31-32.32(t)
    surgical therapy, 33
  medical therapy, 24-29, 35, 35(f)
    drugs for, 25-28, 26(t), 32, 32(t)
    lifestyle changes for, 24-25, 25(t)
  surgical therapy, 29, 34-39
    choice of procedure for, 37-38
    esophagectomy for, 39
    failed, reoperation for, 39
    patients benefiting from, 36-37
  vs. peptic ulcer disease, 110(t)
Gastroesophageal varices, 73-76
  combination therapy, 75, 75(f)
  therapeutic alternatives, 73, 74(f)

Gastrointestinal bleeding
  after bone marrow transplantation, 231
  lower, 465-468
    causes, 465-466, 466(t)
    definition, 465
    diagnostic approach, 466(f), 466-467, 467(t)
    treatment, 467-468, 468(t)
  upper, 132-139
    causes, 132(t), 132-133
    clinical presentation, 133-135
    endoscopy for, 135-137, 136(t)
    hemodynamic status in, 134
    investigation, 135
    management, 133-135
    of continued hemorrhage, 137-139
    transjugular intrahepatic portosystemic shunt for, 544-548
Gastrointestinal cancer. *See also* Gastric cancer
  BICAP tumor probe, 93-94
  injection therapy, 94
  Nd:YAG laser therapy, 89-92, 91(t), 96
  photodynamic therapy, 92-93, 93(t), 95
  radiation therapy, 95
  stents, 94-95
  therapeutic options, 89, 89(f), 95-96
Gastrointestinal-cutaneous fistulas, as indication for perioperative nutritional support, 274
Gastrointestinal diseases, oral manifestations, 22-23
Gastrointestinal hemorrhage, after percutaneous endoscopic gastrostomy, 159
Gastrointestinal infections, after bone marrow transplantation, 233-234
Gastrointestinal polyposis syndromes, oral manifestations, 23
Gastrointestinal tract, upper
  functional disorders, 176-181
  laparascopic surgical procedures, 103
  lesions, staging, 76-80. *See also* Upper gastrointestinal tract lesions, staging
Gastrojejunostomy, for peptic ulcer disease, 122
Gastroparesis, 151-154
  clinical presentation, 151
  diagnosis, 151-152
  etiology, 151
  treatment, 152-154
Gastropathy
  hypertrophic, Ménétrier's, 172, 174(t)
  with portal hypertension, 538
  reflux, 146
Gastroplasty, Collis, 38
Gastroscopy, for diagnosis of gastric cancer, 162
Gastrostomy tubes. *See* Percutaneous endoscopic gastrostomy
  and reflux, 48
Gaviscon, for gastroesophageal reflux disease, 25-26, 26(t)
Gemfibrozil, for hyperlipidemia, 322
GERD (gastroesophageal reflux disease). *See* Gastroesophageal reflux disease (GERD)
GGTP (gamma-glutamyltranspeptidase), for investigation of elevated alkaline phosphatase, 475-476, 476(t)
Giardia lamblia, and traveler's diarrhea, 242
Giardia lamblia infections, 251, 252(t), 253
  antimicrobial therapy, 238(t), 241, 429(t)
Gingivostomatitis, herpetic, primary, 17
Globus pharyngeus, 179
Glossitis, migratory, benign, 18, 18(f)
Glucagonoma, 326
Glucagonomas, 669
Glucocorticoids, for ulcerative colitis, 384-385
Glucose galactose malabsorption, 307
Glutamine
  infusion, for short bowel syndrome, 315
  for prevention of systemic inflammatory response syndrome, 223
Gluten-sensitive enteropathy, 298-302
Glypressin, for variceal bleeding, 536
Graft versus host disease
  after bone marrow transplantation, 230(t)-231(t), 230-231, 233
  after small bowel transplantation, 318

Granulomatous gastritis, 146, 146(t)
Groin, hernias, 380-381
Group health maintenance organizations, 1
Growth, delayed, in Crohn's disease, in children and adolescents, 335
Guidewires, for dilation of esophageal strictures, 53(t), 55
Gut-associated lymphoid tissue (GALT), 170
Gut-body barrier, and systemic inflammatory response syndrome, 220

H

Habit training, for constipation, in children, 370
Hairy leukoplakia
  with acquired immunodeficiency syndrome, 21-22, 22(f)
  oral, 217
Halitosis, 20-21
Hamartoma, hepatic, 585
Hamartomatous polyposis syndromes, 449-451
Health foods, 288
Health maintenance organizations (HMOs), practice in, 1-4
Height-weight tables, 182(t)-183(t)
Heineke-Mikulicz pyloroplasty, for peptic ulcer disease, 122
Helicobacter pylori gastroduodenal disease, 105-109
  detection, 106
  epidemiology, 105-106
  treatment, 106-108, 107(t), 112
Helicobacter pylori infections
  and chronic gastritis, 145
    with nonulcer dyspepsia, 148
  and nonulcer dyspepsia, 176
  with peptic ulcer disease, treatment, 111-112
Heller myotomy, for achalasia, 68
HELLP syndrome, 560(t)-561(t), 563
Helminth infections, treatment, 255(t)-256(t), 255-257
Hemangiomas, hepatic, 585
Hematochezia, 465-468. *See also* Gastrointestinal bleeding, lower
Hematuria, after pancreas-kidney transplantation, 673
Hemochromatosis, 580-585
  causes, 585(t)
  clinical features, 581-582
  differential diagnosis, 582, 583(t)
  evaluation of at-risk relatives, 582-583
  hereditary, 580, 583-584
  management, 583(t), 583-585
  neonatal, 581
  in pregnancy, 565
  screening, 581, 582(t)
Hemodialysis, nutritional support, 269, 269(t)
Hemodynamic status, in upper gastrointestinal bleeding, 134
Hemophilus ducreyi infections, treatment, 429(t)
Hemorrhage
  diverticular, 472
  gastrointestinal, after percutaneous endoscopic gastrostomy, 159
  upper gastrointestinal. *See also* Gastrointestinal bleeding, upper
  variceal, surgical therapy, 551-552, 553(f)
Hemorrhoids, 431-433
Heparin, for acute pancreatitis, 635
Hepatectomy
  donor, 504
  recipient, 504
Hepatic. *See also* Liver entries
Hepatic adenomas, 585-586
Hepatic artery
  catheterization, for intra-arterial chemotherapy, 596, 596(f)
  thrombosis, after liver transplantation, in children, 513-514
Hepatic biopsy, transjugular, for diagnosis of veno-occlusive disease, after bone marrow transplantation, 228
Hepatic cancer, chemotherapy, intra-arterial, 595-596, 596(f)